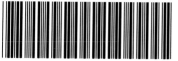

ABDOMINAL-PELVIC MRI

Volume 1

ABDOMINAL-PELVIC MRI

Third Edition

Volume 1

Richard C. Semelka, M.D.

Director, Magnetic Resonance Services
Professor, Vice Chairman of Clinical Research and
Vice Chairman of Quality and Safety
Department of Radiology
University of North Carolina at Chapel Hill

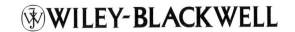

A JOHN WILEY & SONS, INC., PUBLICATION

Wiley-Blackwell is an imprint of John Wiley & Sons, formed by the merger of Wiley's global Scientific, Technical, and Medical business with Blackwell Publishing.

Published by John Wiley & Sons, Inc., Hoboken, New Jersey
Published simultaneously in Canada

For general information on our other products and services or for technical support, please contact our Customer Care Department within the United States at (800) 762-2974, outside the United States at (317) 572-3993 or fax (317) 572-4002.

Wiley also publishes its books in a variety of electronic formats. Some content that appears in print may not be available in electronic formats. For more information about Wiley products, visit our web site at www.wiley.com.

ISBN   978-0-470-48775-4

Library of Congress Cataloging-in-Publication Data is available

Cover Art by Diane Armao, M.D., copyright 2010
Cover Design by Lauren Keswick, M.S., medicalarts

Printed in the United States of America

10 9 8 7 6 5 4 3 2

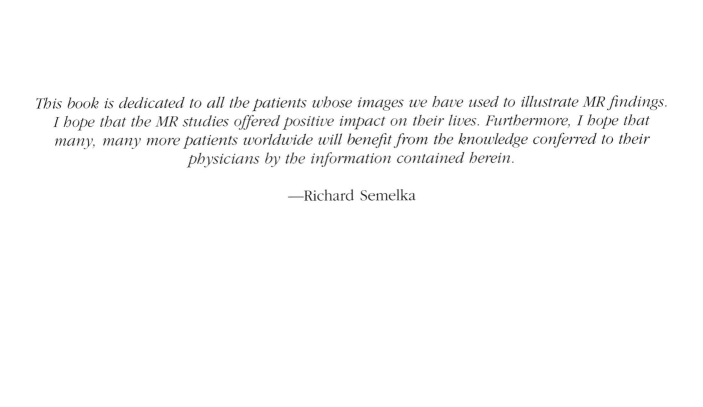

This book is dedicated to all the patients whose images we have used to illustrate MR findings. I hope that the MR studies offered positive impact on their lives. Furthermore, I hope that many, many more patients worldwide will benefit from the knowledge conferred to their physicians by the information contained herein.

—Richard Semelka

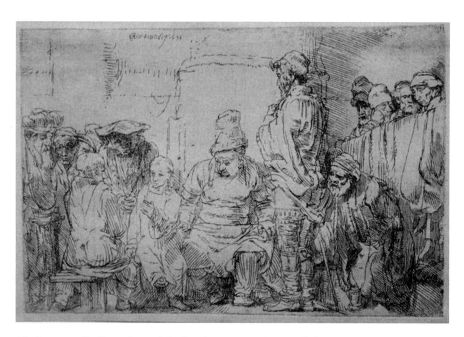

Christ seated, disputing with the doctors. Etching, 1654. Rembrandt. This etching describes evolution in human thought. New individuals challenge prevailing wisdom, and the end result is the improvement of the human condition.

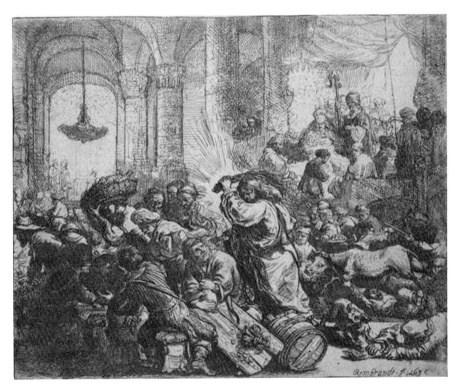

Christ driving the money-changers from the temple. Etching, 1635. Rembrandt. This etching describes the necessity of being ever vigilant against the excesses of greed. We must constantly challenge ourselves and others that this is not a prime motivation for conduct.

CONTENTS

PREFACE

uch change has occurred in imaging since the writing of the previous edition of this work. The entity of nephrogenic systemic fibrosis (NSF) has been identified and its association with gadolinium-based contrast agents (GBCAs), especially the linear nonionic agents, has been recognized. Further recognition by the main-stream radiological community of the detrimental nature of excessive medical radiation, that may result in malignancy, and contrast-induced-nephropathy related to the use of iodine-based contrast agents (IBCAs) have simultaneously occurred. These lapses in attention on the subject of safety by the radiology community serve to remind ourselves of our duty to patients of Primum Non Nocere, emphasizing the age-old wisdom of "everything in moderation" and the importance of being ever vigilant when it comes to patient welfare. Positive steps have been taken by individual radiologists and radiological societies and equipment manufacturers to lessen the potential harmful effects of what we have previously assumed to be innocuous imaging studies. Almost all centers have adopted a restrictive GBCA policy that has largely vanquished NSF, and will progressively make the elimination of this condition complete. Policies and programs related to medical radiation, currently foremost amongst them being the Image Gently campaign, a program designed to minimize the amount of radiation sustained by pediatric patients in imaging studies, and operated as a joint venture between many of the large radiology societies, have been developed and instituted.

At the same time, positive advances in MRI have occurred. These include the more widespread adoption and development of 3 T MRI to study diseases of the chest, abdomen and pelvis. 3T possesses higher signal-to-noise, greater image quality especially with 3D-gradient echo imaging, greater sensitivity to GBCA enhancement, and thinner section acquisition. This has allowed further expansion of MRI into more applications in torso imaging.

In recognition of these changes in the imaging terrain, this current edition addresses many of these above mentioned issues and advances. A new chapter on Contrast Agents is included to address the use of MR contrast agents, but also describes GBCA and IBCA issues and safe practice. New chapters on Fetus and Pediatric imaging draw attention to the capacity of MRI to accurately investigate young subjects, to ameliorate the problems with excess medical radiation in this group, who are the most sensitive to radiation damage. Breast imaging has also come of age and is included as a new chapter in this work. Additionally, many of the new images throughout the book are 3T images, emphasizing the high image quality provided at ultrahigh field strength, and illustrating its growing importance.

Despite all these changes, the principles of this book remain unchanged. The emphasis remains on short duration imaging studies that combine comprehensive information and consistent image quality. The major step to widespread implementation of MRI in replacement of other modalities, remains reproducibility and generalizability of information acquired. MRI has to replicate CT images and studies need to be generated with comparable and not excessively longer duration, and image quality must be reliable and consistent, but with the addition of greater and more comprehensive information, and greater safety. Although we touch on new applications in Chapter 1, such as diffusion-weighted imaging and MR elastography, at present I do not consider their roles established in main-stream MRI practice, paying attention to the above mentioned principles, and I recommend that at present their use be restricted to research centers. This text again emphasizes multiple examples of disease processes both rare and common, so that the reader has guidance on the appearances of virtually all diseases processes in the abdomen, pelvis, chest and breast, to compare their own cases against. With all the advances in MRI, and perhaps despite the advances in CT, coupled with the recognition of the hazards intrinsic to CT, especially CT performed with multiple passes of the torso, this work aims to show that much of imaging of these areas can be performed with MRI, by virtue of the depth and breadth of disease processes that can be evaluated well. In many organ systems, as this book reveals, MRI performs extremely well at diagnosing most disease entities, and outperforms CT in many areas, notably the liver. MRI may be the best tool to evaluate cancers in most of the organs described in this text, and much of the inflammatory diseases. CT remains dominant for major trauma, diffuse lung parenchymal diseases, and renal stone diseases. What remains exciting is that despite the comprehensiveness of this work, it is not the omega work of MRI. We anticipate further exciting advances that may further alter imaging management, perhaps especially, making inroads into more indica-

tions in trauma. Those developments may need to wait for the future next edition. With further exciting advances we have to remain vigilant on the subject of safety, MRI is not an innocuous tool, and as we move to even higher field strengths, safety must be cautiously assessed.

RICHARD SEMELKA, M.D.

CONTRIBUTORS

ERSAN ALTUN, M.D., Department of Radiology, University of North Carolina, Chapel Hill, Chapel Hill, North Carolina

DIANE ARMAO, M.D., Department of Radiology, University of North Carolina, Chapel Hill, Chapel Hill, North Carolina

SUSAN M. ASCHER, M.D., Department of Radiology, Georgetown University, Washington, DC

TILL BADER, M.D., Associate Professor of Radiology, Medical University of Vienna, Austria

N. CEM BALCI, M.D., Department of Radiology, St. Louis University, St. Louis, Missouri

KATHERINE R. BIRCHARD, M.D., Department of Radiology, University of North Carolina, Chapel Hill, North Carolina

LARISSA BRAGA, M.D. Ph.D, M.P.H., Department of Radiology, University of Nebraska Medical Center, Omaha, Nebraska

MICHÈLE A. BROWN, M.D., Associate Professor of Radiology, University of California, San Diego, California

REENA CHOPRA, M.D., Clinical Fellow, Department of Radiology, University of California, San Diego, California

BRIAN M. DALE, Ph.D., Siemens Medical Solutions, Inc., Morrisville, North Carolina

RAFAEL DE CAMPOS, M.D., Clinical Research Scholar, MR Section, Department of Radiology, University of North Carolina, Chapel Hill, North Carolina

CORINNE DEURDULIAN, M.D., Imaging Department, VA Medical Center, Salisbury, North Carolina

DRAGANA DJILAS-IVANOVIĆ, M.D., Ph.D., Associate Professor of Radiology, University of Novi Sad, Oncology Institute of Vojvodina, Sremska Kamenica, Serbia

LARA B. EISENBERG, M.D., Chairman of Radiology, Suburban Hospital, Bethesda, Maryland

MOHAMED ELAZZAZI, M.D., Ph.D., Clinical Research Scholar, MR Section, Department of Radiology, University of North Carolina, Chapel Hill, North Carolina; Professor of Radiology, Al-Azhar University, Cairo, Egypt

JORGE ELIAS, JR., M.D., Ph.D., Professor of Radiology, Faculty of Medicine of Ribeirao Preto, University of Sao Paulo, Brazil

CARLOS GONZALEZ, M.D., Clinical Research Scholar, MR Section, Department of Radiology, University of North Carolina, Chapel Hill, North Carolina

VASCO HEREDIA, M.D., Clinical Research Scholar, MR Section, Department of Radiology, University of North Carolina, Chapel Hill, Chapel Hill, North Carolina

NIKOLAOS L. KELEKIS, M.D., Associate Professor of Radiology, National and Kapodistrian University of Athens, General University Hospital "ATTIKON," Athens, Greece

YOUNG HOON KIM, M.D., Clinical Research Scholar, MR Section, Department of Radiology, University of North Carolina, Chapel Hill, North Carolina; Seoul National University College of Medicine and Seoul National University Bundang Hospital, Seongnam-si, Gyeonggi-do, Korea

KATARINA KOPRIVSEK, M.D., Ph.D., Associate Professor of Radiology, University of Novi Sad, Diagnostic Imaging Center, Oncology Institute of Vojvodina, Sremska Kamenica, Serbia

YOUNG MI KU, M.D., Clinical Research Scholar, MR Section, Department of Radiology, University of North Carolina, Chapel Hill, North Carolina; Assistant Professor, Department of Radiology, Uijongbu St. Mary's Hospital, Catholic University of Korea, Uijongu, Korea

RAHEL A. KUBIK, M.D., M.P.H., Department of Medical Services, Cantonal Hospital, Baden, Switzerland

CHANG-HEE LEE, M.D., Ph.D., Clinical Research Scholar, MR Section, Department of Radiology, University of North Carolina, Chapel Hill, North Carolina; Associate

Professor, Department of Radiology, Korea University Guro Hospital, Korea University College of Medicine, Seoul, Korea

DIEGO R. MARTIN, M.D., Professor and Director of MR, Department of Radiology, Emory University, Atlanta, Georgia

TARA NOONE, M.D., President, SEA Imaging, LLC, Mt. Pleasant, South Carolina; Clinical Associate Professor, Medical University of South Carolina, Charleston, South Carolina

SAMEER A. PATEL, M.D., Clinical Fellow, Department of Radiology, University of California, San Diego, California

DAG PAVIC, M.D., Assistant Professor of Radiology, University of North Carolina, Chapel Hill, North Carolina

MIHAELA I. POP, M.D., Clinical Fellow, Department of Radiology, University of California, San Diego, California

WAQAS QURESHI, M.D., Clinical Research Scholar, MR Section, Department of Radiology, University of North Carolina, Chapel Hill, North Carolina

MIGUEL RAMALHO, M.D., Clinical Research Scholar, MR Section, Department of Radiology, University of North Carolina, Chapel Hill, North Carolina

CAROLINE REINHOLD M.D., M.Sc., Professor of Radiology, Gynecology, and Internal Medicine; Director, MR Imaging, McGill University Health Center, Montréal, Québec, Canada

LORENE ROMINE, M.D., Assistant Professor of Radiology, University of California, San Diego, California

HELMUTH SCHULTZE-HAACK, Siemens Medical Solutions USA, Inc., Santa Ana, California

RICHARD C. SEMELKA, M.D., Professor of Radiology, University of North Carolina, Chapel Hill, North Carolina

FAIQ SHAIKH, M.D., Clinical Research Scholar, MR Section, Department of Radiology, University of North Carolina, Chapel Hill, North Carolina

PUNEET SHARMA, Ph.D., Clinical MR Physicist, Department of Radiology, Emory Healthcare, Inc., Atlanta, Georgia

SANG SOO SHIN, M.D., Clinical Research Scholar, MR Section, Department of Radiology, University of North Carolina, Chapel Hill, North Carolina; Assistant Professor, Department of Radiology, Chonnam National University Medical School, Gwanju, Korea

MILENA SPIROVSKI, M.D., Diagnostic Imaging Center, Oncology Institute of Vojvodina, Sremska Kamenica, Serbia

PENAMPAI TANNAPHAI, M.D., Clinical Research Scholar, MR Section, Department of Radiology, University of North Carolina, Chapel Hill, North Carolina

NACIYE TURAN, M.D., Resident, Department of Radiology, University of North Carolina, Chapel Hill, North Carolina

BUSAKORN VACHIRANUBHAP, M.D., Clinical Research Scholar, MR Section, Department of Radiology, University of North Carolina, Chapel Hill, North Carolina

THUY VU, M.D., Resident, Department of Radiology, University of North Carolina, Chapel Hill, Chapel Hill, North Carolina

DIAGNOSTIC APPROACH TO PROTOCOLING AND INTERPRETING MR STUDIES OF THE ABDOMEN AND PELVIS

PUNEET SHARMA, DIEGO R. MARTIN, BRIAN M. DALE, BUSAKORN VACHIRANUBHAP, AND RICHARD C. SEMELKA

High image quality, reproducibility of image quality, and good conspicuity of disease require the use of sequences that are robust and reliable and avoid artifacts [1–5]. Maximizing these principles to achieve high-quality diagnostic MR images usually requires the use of fast scanning techniques, with the overall intention of generating images with consistent image quality that demonstrate consistent display of disease processes. The important goal of shorter examination time may also be achieved with the same principles that maximize diagnostic quality. With the decrease of imaging times for individual sequences, a variety of sequences may be employed to take advantage of the major strength of MRI, which is comprehensive information on disease processes.

Respiration and bowel peristalsis are the major artifacts that have lessened the reproducibility of MRI. Breathing-independent sequences and breath-hold sequences form the foundation of high-quality MRI studies of the abdomen. Breathing artifact is less problematic in the pelvis and high-spatial and contrast-resolution imaging have been the mainstay for maximizing image quality for pelvis studies.

Disease conspicuity depends on the principle of maximizing the difference in signal intensities between diseased tissues and the background tissue. For disease processes situated within or adjacent to fat, this is readily performed by manipulating the signal intensity of fat, which can range from low to high in signal intensity on both T1-weighted and T2-weighted images. For example, diseases that are low in signal intensity on T1-weighted images, such as peritoneal fluid or retroperitoneal fibrosis, are most conspicuous on T1-weighted sequences in which fat is high in signal intensity (i.e., sequences without fat suppression). Conversely, diseases that are high in signal intensity on T1-weighted images, such as subacute blood or proteinaceous fluid, are more conspicuous if fat is rendered low in signal intensity with the use of fat suppression techniques. On T2-weighted images, diseases that are low in signal intensity, such as fibrous tissue, are most conspicuous on sequences in which background fat is high in signal intensity, such as single-shot echo-train spin-echo sequences (fig. 1.1). Diseases that are moderate to high in signal intensity, such as lymphadenopathy or ascites, are most conspicuous on sequences in

Abdominal-Pelvic MRI, Third Edition, edited by Richard C. Semelka. Copyright © 2010 John Wiley & Sons, Inc.

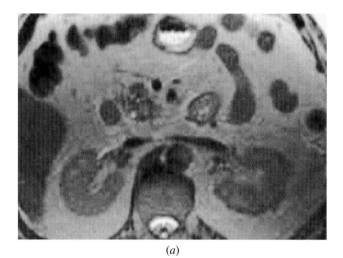

(a)

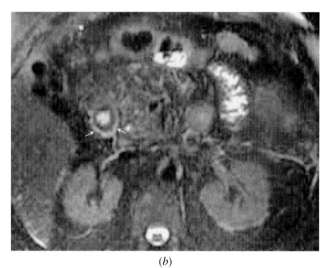

(b)

FIG. 1.1 Maximizing contrast between abnormal and background tissue. T2-weighted single-shot echo-train spin-echo, standard (a) and fat-suppressed (b) in a patient with mild pancreatitis. On the non-fat-suppressed image (a), the small-volume peripancreatic fluid is most clearly seen because background fat is high signal and of comparable signal intensity. With application of fat suppression (b), fat is rendered dark and the small-volume fluid surrounding the pancreatic head and duodenum (arrows, b) is readily appreciated.

which fat signal intensity is low, such as fat-suppressed sequences.

Gadolinium chelate enhancement may be routinely useful since it provides at least two further imaging properties that facilitate detection and characterization of disease, specifically the pattern of blood delivery (i.e., capillary enhancement) and the size and/or rapidity of drainage of the interstitial space (i.e., interstitial enhancement) [6]. Capillary phase image acquisition is achieved by using a short-duration sequence initiated immediately after gadolinium injection. Two- or three-dimensional (2D or 3D) gradient echo sequences, performed as multisection acquisition, are an ideal sequence

to use for capillary phase imaging. The majority of focal mass lesions are best evaluated in the capillary phase of enhancement, particularly lesions that do not distort the margins of the organs in which they are located (e.g., focal liver, spleen, or pancreatic lesions). Images acquired 1.5–10 min after contrast administration are in the interstitial phase of enhancement, with the optimal window being 2–5 min after contrast administration. Diseases that are superficially spreading or inflammatory in nature are generally well shown on interstitial phase images. The concomitant use of fat suppression serves to increase the conspicuity of disease processes characterized by increased enhancement on interstitial phase images including peritoneal metastases, cholangiocarcinoma, ascending cholangitis, inflammatory bowel disease, and abscesses [7, 8].

The great majority of diseases can be characterized by defining their appearance on T1, T2, and early and late postgadolinium images. Throughout this text the combination of these four parameters for the evaluation of abdomino-pelvic disease will be stressed.

T1-WEIGHTED SEQUENCES

T1-weighted sequences are routinely useful for investigating diseases of the abdomen, and they supplement T2-weighted images for investigating disease of the pelvis. The primary information that precontrast T1-weighted images provide includes 1) information on abnormally increased fluid content or fibrous tissue content that appears low in signal intensity on T1-weighted images and 2) information on the presence of subacute blood or concentrated protein, which are both high in signal intensity. T1-weighted sequences obtained without fat suppression also demonstrate the presence of fat as high-signal-intensity tissue. The routine use of an additional fat attenuating technique permits reliable characterization of fatty lesions.

In the abdomen and pelvis, gradient echo (GE) sequences including spoiled gradient echo (SGE) or three-dimensional gradient echo (3D-GE) sequences are preferred to spin-echo sequences. Gradient-echo sequences have a number of advantages:

1. With GE sequences, T1 tissue contrast can be generated similar to that of spin-echo sequences with much shorter scan times. The scan time reduction can be achieved either by exciting all required slices within one TR (multislice) or exciting one slice per very short TR (single slice). The spoiling in the SGE minimizes the influence of T2 weighting.
2. The shorter scan time of GE sequences allows breath-hold imaging to minimize motion artifacts. Breath holding obviates other, often time-consuming,

methods of artifact reduction such as signal averaging and phase reordering.

3. GE sequences allow chemical shift imaging for the detection of relatively small amounts of fat in organs (e.g., fatty infiltration of the liver) and lesions (e.g., adrenal adenomas, liver cell adenomas). In contrast, frequency-selective fat-suppression methods suppress the signal in tissues or lesions with larger amounts of fat like intraperitoneal fat or dermoid cysts.

4. SGE, which is a two-dimensional (2D) technique, allows multislice imaging that acquires central k-space lines, which determine tissue contrast, of 20–24 slices within 4–5 s. 3D-GE can also acquire central k-space lines volumetrically, in a segmented fashion within the early portion of data acquisition. These properties are useful to perform contrast-enhanced dynamic exams of the upper abdomen with distinct arterial, portal, and venous phases in breath hold times.

5. Currently, 3D-GE sequences, in combination with robust segmented fat suppression techniques, overlapping reconstruction, and in-plane as well as through-plane interpolation of the MR data, allow high-quality imaging with larger volume coverage in breath hold times. 3D-GE sequences can be obtained with sufficient anatomic coverage, very thin sections, and high spatial resolution matrices in scan times of only 15–20 s. 3D-GE is particularly suitable for dynamic contrast-enhanced MR imaging because of its excellent inherent fat suppression and sensitivity to enhanced tissues and abnormalities. The spatial resolution depends on matrix size, section thickness, and field of view (FOV). In 3D-SGE, the actual spatial resolution depends on the chosen FOV and is often different in three orthogonal dimensions: spatial resolution$_x$ = FOV$_x$/N$_x$; spatial resolution$_y$ = FOV$_y$/N$_y$; spatial resolution$_z$ = section thickness. Currently, most of the 3D-GE sequences used for dynamic gadolinium-enhanced MR exams employ sequential k-space filling as opposed to the sequences with centric or elliptic-centric k-space filling used in MR angiography in most centers. The 3D-GE sequences with sequential k-space filling can be combined with segmented fat suppression techniques that result in very reliable and homogenous fat suppression without significant increase in scan time. These beneficial features, in combination with clinically viable acquisition breath hold times, makes 3D-GE the primary technique over 2D-SGE for dynamic contrast-enhanced imaging of the abdomen and pelvis.

Gradient Echo (GE) Sequences

The most commonly used gradient echo sequences for routine abdominal imaging are SGE and 3D-GE sequences.

SGE sequences are one of the most important and versatile sequences for studying abdominal disease. SGE sequences are two-dimensional sequences and can also be used as a single (breathing independent) or multiacquisition (breath hold) technique. They provide true T1-weighted imaging and, with the use of phased-array multicoil imaging, may be used to replace longer-duration sequences such as T1-weighted spin-echo (SE) sequence. Image parameters for breath-hold SGE sequences involve: 1) relatively long repetition time (TR) (approximately 150 ms) and 2) the shortest in-phase echo time (TE) (approximately 6.0 ms at 1.0 T, 4.4 ms at 1.5 T, 2.2 ms at 3.0 T), both to maximize signal-to-noise ratio and the number of sections that can be acquired in one multisection acquisition [2]. For routine T1-weighted images, in-phase TE are preferable to the shorter out-of-phase echo times (4.0 ms at 1.0 T and 2.2 ms at 1.5 T, 1.1 ms at 3.0 T), to avoid both phase-cancellation artifact around the borders of organs and fat-water phase cancellation in tissues containing both fat and water protons. Flip angle should be approximately 70–90° to maximize T1-weighted information. With the body coil, the signal-to-noise ratio of 2D-SGE sequences is usually suboptimal, with section thickness less than 8 mm, whereas with the phased-array multicoil, section thickness of 5 mm results in diagnostically adequate images. On new MRI machines, more than 22 sections may be acquired in a 20-second breath hold.

An important feature of multisection acquisition of SGE is that the central phase encoding steps (which determine the bulk signal in the image) are acquired over 6 s for both the entire data set and each individual section. The data acquisition, therefore, is sufficiently short to isolate a distinct phase of enhancement (e.g., hepatic arterial dominant phase), while at the same time the data acquisition of each individual section is sufficiently long to compensate for slight variations in patient cardiac output, peak lesion enhancement, and injection technique.

In addition to its use as precontrast T1-weighted images, SGE may be routinely used for capillary-phase image acquisition after gadolinium administration for investigation of the liver, spleen, pancreas, and kidneys.

In single-shot techniques, all of the k-space lines for one slice are acquired before acquiring the lines for another slice, that is, in sequential rather than interleaved fashion. SGE may be modified to a single-shot technique, by minimizing TR, to achieve breathing-independent images for noncooperative patients.

GE sequences can be performed as a 3D acquisition, which can be used both for volumetric imaging of organs such as the liver and for pre- and postgadolinium administration.

A 3D-GE sequence is typically performed with minimum TR and TE and a flip angle between 10° and

15°. The flip angle is related to the TR to maximize T1 signal. With a minimum TR, flip angle can also be relatively low and still achieve good T1 contrast. As TR and TE of these sequences have minimum values (TR < 5 ms and TE < 2.5 ms), the flip angle will mainly determine the contrast in the images. In 3D-GE, a volume of data is obtained rather than individual slices. There are several advantages of 3D versus 2D gradient echo sequences:

1. Higher inherent signal-to-noise ratio (SNR) than 2D gradient echo sequences
2. Higher in-plane resolution with larger matrices (>192 × >256)
3. Contiguous, thinner sections for higher through-plane resolution, which facilitates reformats in other planes; thin sections are often possible because of interpolation of the MR data in the z-direction.
4. Homogenous fat-suppression (most vendors apply segmented fat suppression, i.e., fat suppression pulse is applied after every nth k-space lines [n can typically be up to 60–70]; this allows scan times that are still short enough to perform breath-hold imaging with fat suppression.
5. The enhancement of vessels and tissues with gadolinium is more obvious because of the fat suppressed nature of the sequence.

Gadolinium-enhanced 3D-GE sequences also are the most clinically effective techniques for MR angiography (MRA) of the body (see Chapter 10, *Retroperitoneum and Body Wall*).

Fat-Suppressed Gradient Echo Sequences

Fat-suppressed (FS) SGE sequences are routinely used as precontrast images for evaluating the pancreas and for the detection of subacute blood. Image parameters are similar to those for standard SGE; however, it is advantageous to employ a lower out-of-phase echo time (2.2–2.5 ms at 1.5 T), which benefits from additional fat-attenuating effects and also increases signal-to-noise ratio and the number of sections per acquisition. On state-of-the-art MRI machines, FS-SGE may acquire 22 sections in a 20-s breath hold with reproducible uniform fat suppression.

Fat-suppressed-SGE images are often used to acquire interstitial-phase gadolinium-enhanced images. The complementary roles of gadolinium enhancement, which generally increases the signal intensity of disease tissue, and fat suppression, which diminishes the competing high signal intensity of background fat, are particularly effective at maximizing conspicuity of diseased tissue. The principle of maximizing signal difference between diseased tissue and background tissue is achieved in the majority of MRI examinations with this approach. Fat-suppressed 3D-GE sequences can also be routinely used for the acquisition of fat-suppressed pre-contrast T1-weighted images. Although the contrast resolution of fat-suppressed 3D-GE is mildly lower compared to fat-suppressed SGE, the acquisition of thin sections with higher matrices is advantageous.

If fat-suppressed-GE sequences cannot be performed on an MRI system, then fat-suppressed spin-echo sequences can be substituted, with little loss of diagnostic information.

Out-of-Phase Gradient Echo Sequences

Out-of-phase (opposed-phase) SGE images are useful for demonstrating diseased tissue in which fat and water protons are present within the same voxel. A TE of 2.2 ms is advisable at 1.5 T, 4 ms at 1.0 T, and 1.1 ms at 3T. A TE of 6.6 ms is also out of phase at 1.5 T, but the shorter TE of 2.2 ms is preferable as more sections can be acquired per sequence acquisition, signal is higher, the sequence is more T1-weighted, and in combination with a T2-weighted sequence, it is easier to distinguish fat and iron in the liver. At TE = 6.6 ms both fat and iron in the liver result in signal loss relative to the TE = 4.4 ms in-phase sequence, while on TE = 2.2 ms out-of-phase sequences fat is darker and iron is brighter relative to TE = 4.4 ms, facilitating their distinction (fig. 1.2). At 3.0 T, the shortest in-phase and out-of-phase values are 2.2 ms and 1.1 ms, respectively. It is challenging to acquire the first echoes at these optimal in-phase and out-of-phase TE times due to gradient capabilities unless imaging bandwidth is increased, or highly asymmetric echoes are utilized in a single scan. With these adjustments, asymmetric TE values can achieve low in-phase (2.5 ms) and out-of-phase (1.58 ms) echoes. These values vary depending on the vendor. When acquiring in-phase/out-of-phase GE sequences, it is essential to use an opposed-phase TE that is less than the in-phase TE. Additionally, it is also possible to acquire in-phase and out-of-phase 3D-GE sequences, although this technique is still developing.

The most common indications for an out-of-phase sequence are to detect the presence of fat within the liver and lipid within adrenal masses to characterize them as adenomas. Another useful feature is that the generation of a phase-cancellation artifact around high-signal-intensity masses, located in water-based tissues, confirms that these lesions are fatty. Examples of this include angiomyolipomas of the kidney and ovarian dermoids. In addition to out-of-phase effects, the different TE, for the out-of-phase sequence compared to the in-phase sequence, provides information on magnetic susceptibility effects that increase with increase in TE. This can be used to distinguish iron-containing structures (e.g., surgical clips, Gamna–Gandy bodies in the

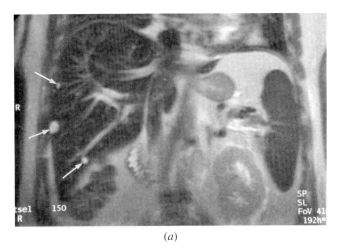

(a)

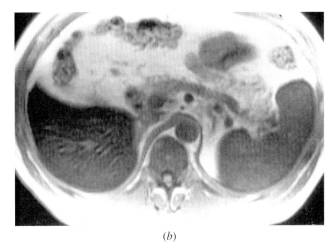

(b)

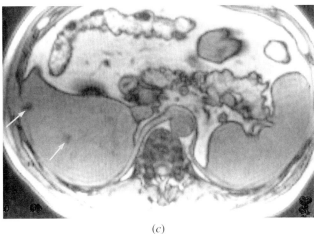

(c)

F I G . 1.2 Iron effects. Coronal T2-weighted single-shot echo-train spin-echo (*a*), TE = 4 ms in-phase (*b*), and TE = 2 ms out-of-phase (*c*) sequences. Iron in the reticuloendothelial system from transfusional siderosis results in low signal of the liver and spleen on T2-weighted images (*a*). The liver and spleen are low signal on the longer-TE in-phase sequence (*b*) and increase in signal on the shorter-TE out-of-phase (*c*) sequence, because of decreasing susceptibility effects on the shorter-TE sequence. Note the excellent conspicuity of small liver cysts on the T2-weighted image (arrows, *a*). The high fluid content of cysts in a background of iron-deposited liver renders them very high in signal. On T1-weighted images, the low signal of cysts results in no signal difference from liver on the TE = 4 ms in-phase sequence because of the concurrent low signal of liver. On the TE = 2 ms sequence, liver becomes higher in signal and the cysts are visible (arrows, *c*).

spleen) from nonmagnetic signal-void structures (e.g., calcium). To illustrate this point, the signal void susceptibility artifact from surgical clips increases in size, from a shorter TE (e.g., 2.2 ms) out-of-phase sequence to a longer TE (e.g., 4.4 ms) in-phase sequence, whereas the signal void from calcium remains unchanged.

Magnetization-Prepared Rapid-Acquisition Gradient Echo (MP-RAGE) Sequences

MP-RAGE sequences include turbo fast low-angle shot (turboFLASH). In 2D, multisection varieties, these techniques are generally performed as a single shot, with image acquisition duration of 1–2 s, which renders them relatively breathing independent. Magnetization preparation is currently performed with a 180° inversion pulse to impart greater T1-weighted information. The inversion pulse may be either slice or non-slice selective. Slice-selective means that only the tissue section that is being imaged experiences the inverting pulse, while non-slice-selective means that all the tissue in the bore of the magnet experiences the inverting pulse. The

advantage of a non-slice-selective inversion pulse is that no time delay is required between acquisition of single sections in multiple single-section acquisition. A stack of single-section images can be acquired in a rapid fashion. This is important for dynamic gadolinium-enhanced studies. A non-slice-selective inversion pulse results in slightly better image quality, particularly because flowing blood is signal void (fig. 1.3). Approximately 3 s of tissue relaxation is required between acquisition of individual sections, which limits the usefulness of this sequence for dynamic gadolinium-enhanced acquisitions. Current versions of MP-RAGE are limited because of low signal-to-noise ratio, varying signal intensity and contrast between sections, unpredictable bounce-point boundary artifacts due to signal-nulling effects caused by the inverting 180° pulse, and unpredictable nulling of tissue enhanced with gadolinium. Research is ongoing to alleviate these problems with MP-RAGE so that it may assume a more important clinical role. Routine use of a high-quality MP-RAGE sequence would further increase the reproducibility of MR image quality by obviating the need for breath holding, particularly in patients unable to suspend

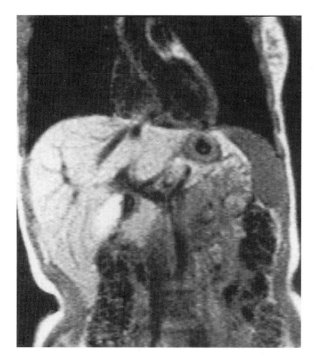

FIG. 1.3 Non-slice-selective 180° magnetization prepared gradient echo. A coronal image through the liver demonstrates good T1 weighting, evidenced by a moderately high-signal-intensity liver and moderately low-signal-intensity spleen. The infracardiac portion of the left lobe is artifact free. Blood vessels in the liver and the cardiac chambers are seen as signal void.

respiration. 3.0 T MR imaging particularly improves the image quality of MP-RAGE sequences due to higher signal-to-noise ratio and greater spectral separation [9].

T2-WEIGHTED SEQUENCES

The predominant information provided by T2-weighted sequences are 1) the presence of increased fluid in diseased tissue, which results in high signal intensity, 2) the presence of chronic fibrotic tissue, which results in low signal intensity, and 3) the presence of iron deposition, which results in very low signal intensity.

Echo-Train Spin-Echo Sequences

Echo-train spin-echo (ETSE) sequences are termed fast spin-echo, turbo spin-echo, or rapid acquisition with relaxation enhancement (RARE) sequences. The principle of ETSE sequences is to summate multiple echoes within the same repetition time interval to decrease examination time, increase spatial resolution, or both. ETSE has achieved widespread use because of these advantages. Conventional T2 spin-echo sequences are lengthy and suffer from patient motion and increased

examination time, factors that are lessened with ETSE. In addition, ETSE sequences allow higher matrices within relatively shorter acquisition times. One of the disadvantages of echo-train sequences is that T2 differences between tissues are reduced, in part because of averaging of T2 echoes, which has the greatest effect of diminishing contrast between background organs and focal lesions with minimal T2 differences. This generally is not problematic in the pelvis because of the substantial differences in the T2 values between diseased and normal tissue. In the liver, however, the T2 difference between diseased (solid tissue) and background liver may be small and the T2-averaging effects of summated multiple echoes blur this T2 difference. These effects are most commonly observed with hepatocellular carcinoma. Fortunately, diseases with T2 values similar to those of liver generally have longer T1 values than liver, so that lesions poorly visualized on ETSE are generally apparent on precontrast GE as low-signal lesions or on postgadolinium GE images as low- or high-signal lesions depending on enhancement features.

ETSE, and T2-weighted sequences in general, are important for evaluating the liver and pelvis. T2-weighted sequences are often useful for the pancreas, in demonstrating the pancreatic and common bile ducts, evaluating cystic masses and pseudocysts, and detecting islet cell tumors. Breathing-independent single-shot T2-weighted sequences are useful for the investigation of bowel and peritoneum. Use of the single-shot technique for many applications of a T2 sequence is recommended, because the image quality is consistent, in large part because of the breathing-independent nature of these sequences. Although the detection of lesions with subtle T2 difference from background organ/tissue is compromised (e.g., hepatocellular carcinoma), the major role for T2-weighted sequences is to provide information on fluid content of disease processes for disease characterization. This information is reliably provided by single-shot echo-train spin-echo.

Fat is high in signal intensity on ETSE sequences, in comparison to conventional spin-echo sequences in which fat is intermediate in signal intensity. The MR imaging determination of recurrent malignant disease versus fibrosis for pelvic malignancies illustrates this difference. Recurrent malignant disease in the pelvis (e.g., cervical, endometrial, bladder, or rectal cancer) generally appears high in signal intensity on conventional spin-echo sequences because of the higher signal intensity of the diseased tissue relative to the moderately low-signal-intensity fat. In contrast, fat is high in signal intensity on ETSE images, and recurrent disease will commonly appear relatively lower in signal intensity. The fact that abnormal tissue is not high signal on T2-weighted images relative to fat cannot be relied upon to exclude recurrence. Caution must therefore be exercised not to misinterpret recurrent disease as fibrotic tissue, by making the assumption that recurrence is higher in signal intensity than background fat. Fat may also be problematic in the liver because fatty liver will be high in signal intensity on ETSE sequences, thereby diminishing contrast with the majority of liver lesions, which are generally high in signal intensity on T2-weighted images. It may be essential to use fat suppression on T2-weighted ETSE sequences for liver imaging. Alternative fat-suppressed T2-weighted sequences for the liver such as echo-planar imaging have also been employed at some centers (further description is provided in the 3T section of this chapter).

ETSE sequences, acquired as contiguous thin 2D sections, as 3D thin sections, or as a thick 3D volume slab, form the basis for MR cholangiography (see Chapter 3, *Gallbladder and Biliary System*) and MR urography (see Chapter 9, *Kidneys*). The greatest concern with high-resolution 3D ETSE sequences is the significant increase in specific absorption rate (SAR). This is particularly relevant since most 3D implementations must increase the echo-train length compared to 2D varieties because of the added data that need to be acquired. Recently, newer MR systems, in combination with advances in gradient and software design, have allowed the development of efficient long echo-train 3D ETSE using variable flip angle refocusing pulses. Concerns of SAR are offset by using smaller (constant or variable) flip angles during data acquisition. With this strategy, T2 information can be maintained throughout the echo train, or used more effectively, for high-SNR imaging. Efficiency is further aided by implementing an additional "restore" pulse at the end of data collection to expedite magnetization recovery, allowing shorter TRs (~1200 ms) to be used for T2 imaging. These recent modifications to conventional 3D-ETSE imaging have made high-resolution isotropic ($1 \, mm^3$) T2 imaging of the pelvis and biliary system feasible in a relatively short acquisition time (~5 min).

Single-Shot Echo-Train Spin-Echo Sequence

Single-shot echo-train spin-echo sequence [e.g.,: half-Fourier acquisition single shot turbo spin-echo (HASTE), single-shot fast or turbo spin echo (SSFSE or SSTSE), or single-shot echo-train spin echo (SS-ETSE)] is a breathing-independent T2-weighted sequence that has had a substantial impact on abdominal imaging [3]. Typical imaging involves a 400-ms image acquisition time, in which k-space is completely filled using half-Fourier reconstruction. Shorter effective echo time (e.g., 60 ms) is recommended for bowel-peritoneal disease, and longer effective echo time (e.g., 100 ms and greater) is

recommended for liver-biliary disease. Since the technique is single shot, the echo train length is typically greater than 100 echoes, while the effective TR for one slice is infinite. A stack of sections should be acquired in single-section mode in one breath hold to avoid slice misregistration; however, the method lends itself to free-breathing application under uncooperative imaging circumstances. Recently, 3D versions of this technique have been implemented. Motion artifacts from respiration and bowel peristalsis are obviated; chemical-shift artifact is negligible; and susceptibility artifact from air in bowel, lungs, and other locations is minimized, such that bowel wall is clearly demonstrated. Similarly, susceptibility artifact from metallic devices such as surgical clips or hip prostheses is minimal (fig. 1.4). All of these effects render SS-ETSE an attractive sequence for evaluating abdomino-pelvic disease. In patients with implanted metallic devices and extensive surgical clips, SS-ETSE is the sequence least affected by metal susceptibility artifact.

Fat-Suppressed (FS) Echo-Train Spin-Echo Sequences

Fat suppression in spin-echo sequences may be useful for investigating focal liver disease to attenuate the high signal intensity of fatty infiltration, if present. Fatty liver is high in signal intensity on ETSE, in particular single-shot versions, which lessens the conspicuity of high-signal-intensity liver lesions. Diminishing fat signal intensity with fat suppression accentuates the high signal intensity of focal liver lesions (fig. 1.5). FS SS-ETSE is also useful for evaluating the biliary tree. Fat suppression appears to diminish the image quality of bowel because of susceptibility artifact from air-bowel wall interface and is not recommended for bowel studies, although bowel-related extraluminal disease (such as appendical abscess) may be well shown with this technique.

Fat suppression in ETSE is achieved through either spectral-selective or non-spectral-selective preparation pulses. Non-spectral-selective fat suppression, which is termed short-tau inversion recovery (STIR), is performed with a slice-selective inversion pulse timed to suppress the T1 of fat (TI = 150 ms at 1.5 T). Since the pulse is broadband, both water and fat are magnetization prepared, resulting in suppression of fat signal, alteration of contrast from water signal, and depression of water signal from equilibrium. While fat signal is uniformly suppressed (given ideal inversion pulses and consistent T1 over the imaging FOV), the remaining soft tissue (water signal) has lower signal as a direct consequence of the inversion pulse. Since soft tissue in the abdomen has long T1 relative to fat, adequate SNR is still maintained. Although STIR is sensitive to nonuniform

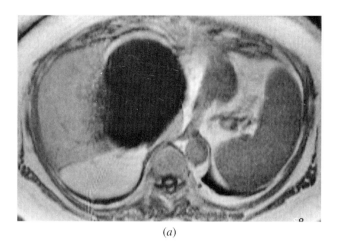

(a)

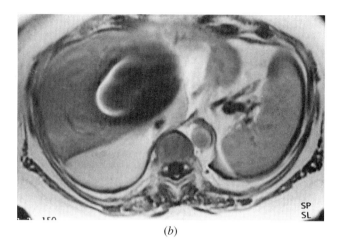

(b)

FIG. 1.4 Metallic susceptibility artifact. SGE (*a*), T1 spin-echo (T1-SE) (*b*), and HASTE (*c*) images. Severe susceptibility artifact is present on the SGE image (*a*), with the result that the images of the liver are not interpretable. T1-SE (*b*) is relatively resistant to image degradation by susceptibility artifact; however, substantial artifact still renders much of the liver uninterpretable. The HASTE image (*c*) is the least sensitive MR sequence, and less sensitive than CT imaging for artifacts generated by metallic devices. Only a small portion of the liver is not interpretable with HASTE (*c*).

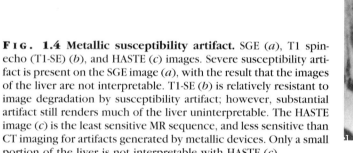

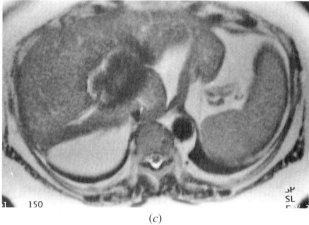

(c)

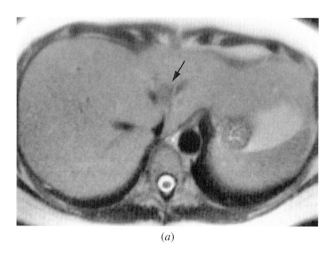

(a)

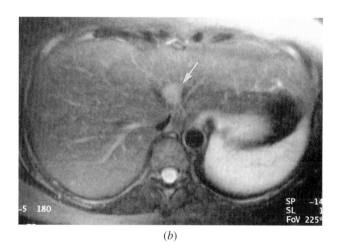

(b)

FIG. 1.5 Focal liver lesion in a fatty liver. Single-shot echo-train spin-echo (SS-ETSE) (*a*) and fat-suppressed (FS)-SS-ETSE (*b*) images. The liver appears high in signal intensity on the SS-ETSE image (*a*) because of the presence of fatty liver. A focal liver lesion (focal nodular hyperplasia, arrow, *a*) is identified that is mildly lower in signal intensity than liver parenchyma. On the FS-SS-ETSE image (*b*), the liver has decreased in signal intensity, and the liver lesion (arrow, *b*) now appears moderately high in signal intensity relative to liver. Good liver-spleen contrast is also apparent on the fat-suppressed image (*b*), with no liver-spleen contrast on the nonsuppressed sequence (*a*).

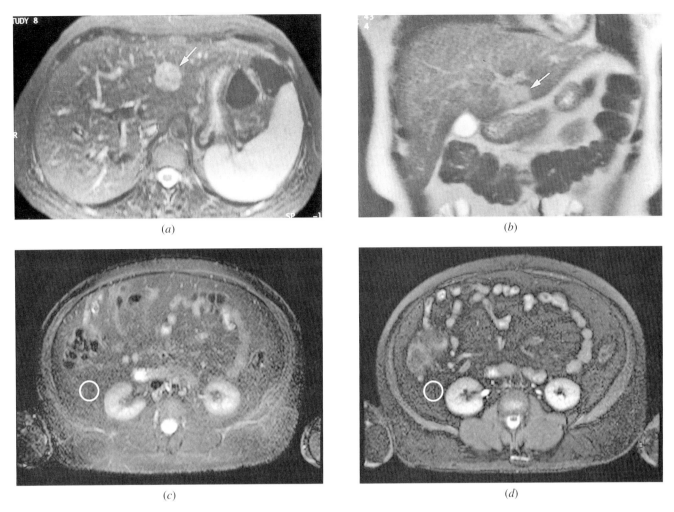

(a)

(b)

(c)

(d)

F I G . 1.6 Echo-train STIR and SS-ETSE. Transverse echo-train STIR (*a*) and coronal SS-ETSE (*b*) images in a patient with colon cancer liver metastases. A moderately high-signal-intensity metastasis is present in the left lobe of the liver on the echo-train STIR (arrow, *a*). Background fat is nulled. The liver metastasis is also shown on the coronal SS-ETSE image (arrow, *b*). Background fat is high in signal intensity. Variations in the signal intensity of the background fat provide differing contrast relationships. Comparison of axial STIR (*c*) and SPAIR (*d*) fat suppression on SS-ETSE. The bowel and kidneys are more defined on SPAIR because of the preservation of water signal. Region-of-interest measures (white circle, *c*, *d*) reveal a significant difference in soft tissue SNR and CNR ($P < 0.01$).

inversion (due to B1 field effects), the method is well-accepted as a robust technique for fat suppression in the abdomen using spin echo-based sequences. As the sequence is fundamentally different from SS-ETSE, it may be useful to combine both short-duration sequences for the liver in place of longer, breathing-averaged ETSE (fig. 1.6).

An alternate method of fat suppression involves spectral selection of fat resonances exclusively. Preparation pulses (inversion or saturation) can be spectrally tuned to fat signal, while avoiding undue suppression or alteration of water signal, as seen with STIR techniques. Conceptually, the technique is similar to STIR, in which magnetization (in this case, only fat) is prepared with an inversion pulse timed to suppress fat. Ideally, other soft tissue will remain unaffected,

preserving high contrast-to-noise ratio. Since spectral fat suppression is frequency-specific, it is sensitive to spatial susceptibility, which creates an inhomogeneous magnetic field. The water and fat resonances are not clearly delineated in this circumstance, causing fat-water frequency "overlap," and potentially a significant number of fat spins to be unsuppressed. This effect is also prevalent at the edges of the FOV, or any regions away from the magnet isocenter.

Further improvement in uniform fat suppression can be achieved by incorporating adiabatic pulses, which are a specially designed class of RF pulses that provide B1-insensitive spin nutation. Recently, spectral (fat)-selective adiabatic inversion pulses, termed "SPAIR," have been used in T2-weighted imaging of the abdomen [10]. The uniformity of fat suppression is more robust than traditional spectral-selective techniques, making it the method of choice for liver and bowel imaging. Moreover, its inherent high CNR provides important diagnostic advantages over STIR, since soft tissue signal is preserved. The effects of inhomogeneous main magnetic field still pose challenges for SPAIR, due to spectral overlap. But the improved inversion profile and frequency cutoff of SPAIR alleviates the degree of poor fat suppression (fig. 1.6). Implementation of SPAIR fat suppression takes longer than its other counterparts, because of the longer pulse length required for the adiabatic condition. This may increase scan times for segmented T2 and T1 acquisitions.

GADOLINIUM-ENHANCED T1-WEIGHTED SEQUENCES

Gadolinium contrast agent is most effective when it is administered as a rapid bolus, with imaging performed with T1-weighted SGE or 3D-GE sequences obtained in a dynamic serial fashion. After the intravenous injection of gadolinium, a minimum of two postcontrast sequences are needed, one acquired in the hepatic arterial dominant phase, within 30 s of contrast administration, and the second in the hepatic venous or interstitial phase at approximately 2–5 min. For liver imaging, an intermediate-timed third pass, termed portal venous or early hepatic venous, at 1 min postcontrast, is useful as well [6]. Little additional information is provided if more than four sequences are acquired. Features of these phases of enhancement are as follows.

Hepatic Arterial Dominant (Capillary) Phase

The hepatic arterial dominant (capillary) phase is the single most important data set when using a nonspecific extracellular gadolinium chelate contrast agent [6]. This technique is essential for imaging the liver, spleen, and pancreas, and it provides useful information on the kidneys, adrenals, vessels, bladder, and uterus. The timing for this phase of enhancement is the only timing for postcontrast sequences that is crucial. It is essential to capture the "first pass" or capillary bed enhancement of tissues during this phase. Demonstration of gadolinium in hepatic arteries and portal veins and absence of gadolinium in hepatic veins are reliable landmarks (fig. 1.7). At this phase of enhancement, although contrast is present in portal veins, the majority of the gadolinium present in the liver has been delivered by hepatic arteries. The absolute volume of hepatic artery-delivered gadolinium is greater in this phase of enhancement than acquiring the data when gadolinium is only present in hepatic arteries; therefore, more hepatic arte-

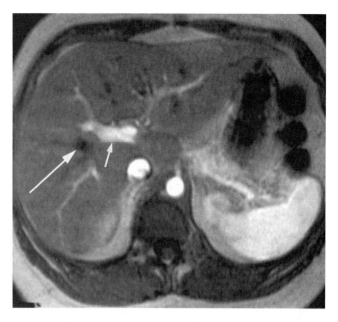

F I G . 1.7 Hepatic arterial dominant phase. Image demonstrates gadolinium in portals veins (short arrow) and lack of contrast in hepatic veins (long arrow).

rial enhancement information is available. This is important since most focal liver lesions, especially metastases and hepatocellular carcinoma, are fed primarily by hepatic arteries. Imaging slightly earlier than this, when only hepatic arteries are opacified (hepatic arteries-only phase) may approach the diagnostic utility of the hepatic arterial dominant phase if the injection rate of contrast is very fast (e.g., 5 ml/s) and data are acquired late in the hepatic arteries-only phase (within 1 or 2 s of gadolinium appearing in the portal veins). It is very difficult to achieve these objectives in the hepatic arteries-only phase, and it is also difficult to judge whether image acquisition is too early in this phase, when the liver is essentially unenhanced. Appropriate timing, as judged by vessel enhancement, also is important for the evaluation of surrounding organs. Too little pancreatic enhancement is consistent with pancreatic fibrosis or chronic pancreatitis, and too little enhancement of renal cortex may imply ischemic nephropathy or acute cortical necrosis. This can be reliably judged on hepatic arterial dominant phase images, because of the fixed landmarks of contrast in portal veins and absence in hepatic veins. In the hepatic arteries-only phase, minimal enhancement of pancreas or renal cortex may reflect too early image acquisition rather than disease process. Since this immediate postgadolinium phase of enhancement is also used to diagnose adequate perfusion of these organs, it is oxymoronic to use enhancement of these organs as the determination of the appropriateness of the phase of image acquisition timing. Although enhancement of pancreas or renal cortex is used as ancillary information for assessment of timing, it is not the major determinant, since the extent of enhancement of these organs is also evaluated at this phase. In the liver, imaging too early in the hepatic arteries-only phase diminishes the ability to recognize the distinctive patterns of lesion enhancement for different lesion types, because the absolute volume of hepatic artery-delivered contrast may be too small and may cause lesions to be mischaracterized (fig. 1.8).

On hepatic arterial dominant phase T1-weighted SGE or 3D-GE images, various types of liver lesions have distinctive enhancement patterns: Cysts show lack of enhancement, hemangiomas show peripheral nodules of enhancement in a discontinuous ring, nonhemorrhagic adenomas and focal nodular hyperplasia show intense uniform enhancement, metastases show ring enhancement, and hepatocellular carcinomas show diffuse heterogeneous enhancement. The ability to use this information to characterize lesions as small as 1 cm may be unique to MRI. Appearances of less common liver lesions on immediate postgadolinium images have also been reported, many of which show overlap with the above-described patterns of common liver lesions. To a somewhat lesser extent, appreciation of the capillary phase enhancement of lesions in the pancreas, spleen, and kidneys provides information on lesion characterization that will be described in the respective chapters of these organ systems. Clinical history is often important, despite the high diagnostic accuracy of current MRI imaging protocols. In addition, many different histologic types of liver lesions when they measure less than 1 cm, demonstrate virtually identical uniform enhancement, for example, hemangiomas, adenomas, focal nodular hyperplasia, metastases, and hepatocellular carcinoma. Ancillary information to assist in characterization of lesions is crucial, which includes T2-weighted images that demonstrate lesion fluid content (e.g., high for hemangioma and often high for hypervascular metastases, and relatively low for adenoma, focal nodular hyperplasia, and hepatocellular carcinoma), appearance of other concomitant large lesions, and clinical history (e.g., history of known primary tumor that can result in hypervascular metastases, such as gastrointestinal leiomyosarcoma).

Various enhancement patterns of liver and other organ parenchyma are also demonstrated on hepatic arterial dominant phase images. One of the most common perfusion abnormalities observed in the liver is transient increased segmental enhancement in liver segments with compromised portal venous flow due to compression or thrombosis. Other hepatic diseases that demonstrate perfusion abnormalities on immediate postgadolinium images include Budd–Chiari syndrome, with different enhancement patterns for acute, sub-acute, and chronic disease, and severe acute hepatitis with hepatocellular injury. Perfusion abnormalities of the kidneys are also relatively common and are clearly shown on early- and late-phase gadolinium-enhanced images.

Examination for liver metastases may be the most common indication for liver MR examination. Liver metastases have been classified as hypovascular (typical examples are colon cancer and transitional cell carcinoma) or hypervascular (typical examples are islet cell tumors, renal cell carcinoma, and breast cancer). A third category of vascularity has not been described well in the past and this is near-isovascular with liver. Near-isovascular refers to lesion enhancement that is very comparable to that of liver on early and late postgadolinium images. Near isovascularity is most readily appreciated when lesions are poorly seen on postgadolinium images but well seen on precontrast images (fig. 1.9). Liver metastases from primaries of colon, thyroid, and endometrium may show this type of enhancement pattern. The most common setting is postchemotherapy, although this may also be observed in untreated patients. Fortunately, many of these tumors are moderately low signal intensity on T1-weighted images, rendering them readily apparent, and on occasion they may also be moderately high signal intensity on T2-weighted images. Rarely they may also be near isointense on T1-weighted and T2-weighted images, and therefore can escape detection. The rarity of this occurrence illustrates one of the great strengths of MRI over sonography and computed tomography: The greater the number of distinctly different data sets that are acquired, the less likely it is for disease to escape detection. MRI has more acquisitions of different types of data than ultrasound or CT.

Chemotherapy-treated liver metastases deserve special mention in that chemotherapy is routinely given to the majority of patients with liver metastases and chemotherapy alters the imaging features of metastases. Chemotherapy induces change in the signal intensity and imaging features of metastases such that they may resemble cysts, hemangiomas, or scar tissue [6]. As mentioned above, they may also become near isovascular on postgadolinium images.

Portal Venous Phase or Early Hepatic Venous Phase

This phase is acquired at 45–60 s after initiation of gadolinium injection. In this phase hepatic parenchyma is maximally enhanced so hypovascular lesions (cysts, hypovascular metastases, and scar tissue) are best shown as regions of lesser enhancement. Patency or thrombosis of hepatic vessels are also best shown in this phase.

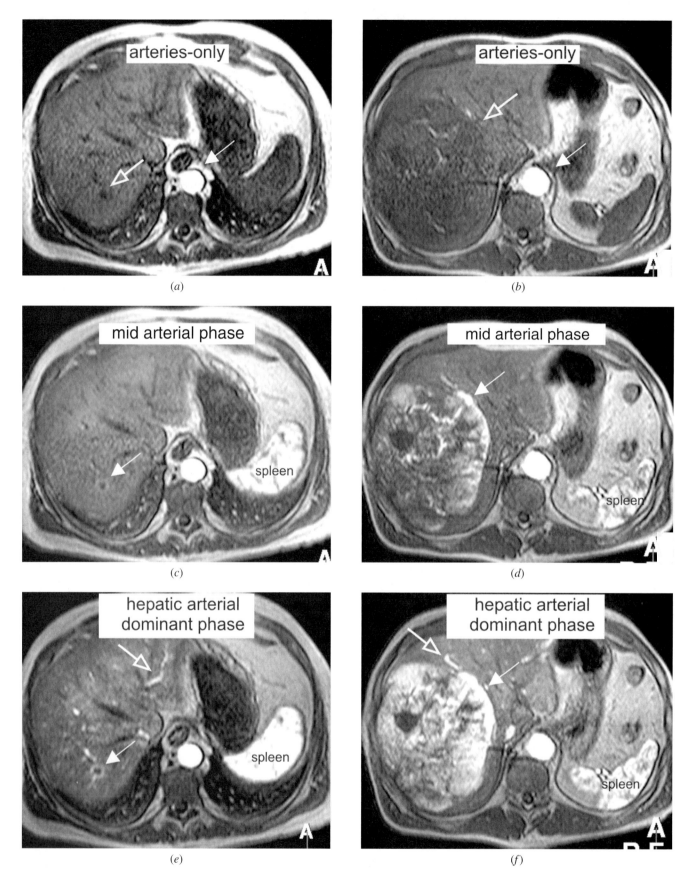

F I G . 1.8 Hepatic arteries-only, hepatic early arterial phase and hepatic arterial dominant phase. Images from a series of time-resolved 2D dynamic gadolinium-enhanced spoiled gradient echo with parallel imaging (parallel MRI acceleration factor 2; scan time of 7 s per image) in two different patients with a neuroendocrine metastasis (*a, c, e*) and with a pathology-proved hepatocellular carcinoma (HCC) in a noncirrhotic liver (*b, d, f*), respectively. Very early after the injection of gadolinium, only the arteries are visible (arrows in *a* and *b*). In the following phase, little enhancement of the lesions is present (arrows in *c* and *d*). In the hepatic arterial dominant phase, optimal enhancement difference is visible between the liver and the lesions because of more enhancement of the lesions (solid arrows in *e* and *f*). Note also the enhancement of the portal vessels in this phase (open arrows in *e* and *f*). Data acquisition in the arterial phase provided better diagnostic information on the enhancement features of the two hepatic lesions.

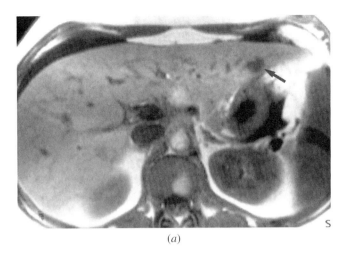

(a)

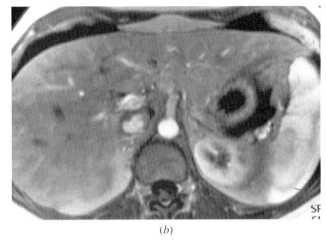

(b)

F I G . 1.9 Near-isovascular liver metastases. SGE (*a*) and hepatic arterial phase gadolinium-enhanced SGE (*b*) images. In this patient with liver metastases who is at 9 months after initiation of chemotherapy, liver metastases are clearly shown on noncontrast T1-weighted images (arrow, *a*) but poorly seen after gadolinium administration. This enhancement pattern, termed near-isovascular, is most commonly observed in liver metastases in a subacute phase of response to chemotherapy.

Hepatic Venous (Interstitial) Phase

Hepatic venous phase or interstitial phase is acquired 90 s to 5 min after initiation of contrast injection. Late enhancement features of focal liver lesions are shown that aid in lesion characterization, such as persistent lack of enhancement of cysts, coalescence and centripetal progression of enhancing nodules in hemangiomas, homogeneous fading of enhancement of adenomas and focal nodular hyperplasia to near isointensity with liver, late enhancement of central scar in some focal nodular hyperplasias, peripheral or heterogeneous washout of contrast in liver metastases, washout to hypointensity with liver in small liver metastases and hepatocellular carcinoma, heterogeneous washout of hepatocellular carcinoma, and delayed capsule enhancement in hepatocellular carcinoma (less commonly adenoma). Enhancement of peritoneal metastases, inflammatory disease, bone metastases (fig. 1.10) and circumferential, superficial spreading cholangiocarcinoma are also well shown at this time frame. Concomitant use of fat suppression is essential for optimized demonstration of these findings. Additional documentation of vascular thrombosis is also provided on these images.

MULTIPLE IMAGING VARIABLES

On MR images, it is common that multiple imaging properties are concurrently present. The contributions of these various properties must be separately determined so that appropriate diagnosis is made. Common potentially competing imaging characteristics include T2 and fat suppression effects; T1 out-of-phase and magnetic susceptibility effects; and gadolinium washout and

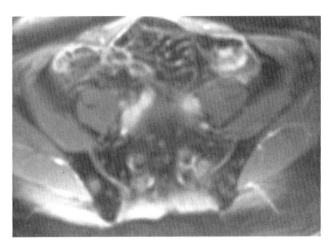

F I G . 1.10 Bone metastases. Two-minute gadolinium-enhanced T1-weighted fat-suppressed SGE image demonstrates multiple rounded enhancing bone metastases that are clearly defined in a background of suppressed fatty marrow.

fat suppression effects. T2 and fat suppression effects can usually be separated by employing both nonsuppressed and fat-suppressed T2-weighted sequences. Low signal due to fat suppression effects can be correctly ascertained by the demonstration of higher signal intensity of the structure on non-fat-suppressed T2 sequences relative to the T2 fat-suppressed sequences. Out-of-phase and magnetic susceptibility signal loss can be separated by observing that susceptibility effects increase with increasing TE on SGE sequences and are generally also observed as low signal on T2-weighted sequences, whereas out-of-phase lipid signal effects cycle with in- and out-of-phase echo times. Distinction between gadolinium washout and fat suppression effects on the 2-min postgadolinium T1-weighted fat-suppressed GE sequence must also be established. In problem cases, there is the observation of low signal of a structure on later postgadolinium fat-suppressed sequences, that appeared high signal on early postgadolinium nonsuppressed sequences. The question arises whether this reflects a fat suppression effect rather than a gadolinium washout effect. In the liver, this can usually be distinguished by the observation that a fatty lesion is low signal on a 2-min postgadolinium fat-suppressed sequence, while isointense or hyperintense on both the immediate and the 1-min nonsuppressed portal venous phase SGE sequences. Generally, if a liver lesion washes out at 2 min, it has most often shown evidence of washout already by 1 min on the portal venous phase non-fat-suppressed SGE images. Further supportive information of a fat effect is evidence that the lesion appears fatty on any of the other sequences employed in the imaging protocol (e.g., out-of-phase or noncontrast fat-suppressed sequences). Figure 1.11 illustrates many of these combined imaging properties in one situation.

With MR imaging, it is possible to acquire images in any desirable anatomic orientation (i.e., transverse, coronal, sagittal, or oblique) without moving the patient. The choice of the plane of data acquisition is influenced by the familiarity of image interpretation using different planes, type of MR equipment used, and the sequence employed. In general terms, the majority of the imaging is acquired in the transverse plane, which can be explained for a number of reasons, including lesser problems with partial volume effects and general familiarity of radiologists with this plane from experience with CT. In the upper abdomen, we routinely supplement the transverse plane by one or two (or more) acquisitions in the coronal plane, and in the pelvis with sagittal plane imaging. Additional planes may be obtained, but as a general principle, our view is to maintain as few possible data acquisitions to achieve the balanced effect of sufficient redundancy but not excessive data acquisition (mainly for time and patient cooperation reasons). In some organ systems, our routine practice of acquiring the primary sequences in the transverse plane and supplementing them with an additional plane is modified when employing the thin-section data acquisition capability of 3D-GE, which facilitates reconstruction in different planes from a single acquired data set. As an example, with imaging of the kidneys using SD-SGE sequences, our approach has been to acquire transverse images and supplement them with sagittal plane images. Using 3D-SGE, our tendency has been to acquire data in the coronal plane, which also facilitates simultaneous assessment of the renal arteries. In the end, since studies often must be viewed at other facilities, radiologists are generally familiar with transverse plane from CT, and comparison must often be made with CT studies, it seems prudent to use the transverse plane as the primary imaging plane.

SIGNAL INTENSITY OF VESSELS

Inhomogeneous signal intensity of vessels is a diagnostic problem not infrequently encountered on MR images. In general, we have found that image acquisition between 1 and 2 min postgadolinium using GE results in consistently high signal of patent arteries and veins. Unfortunately, data acquisition often falls beyond this range, particularly in the setting of acquiring images of the pelvis after images of the abdomen. If patency of vessels is a particular diagnostic concern, then we employ sequences that consistently show high signal in patent vessels, often by combining intrinsic in-flow effects and gadolinium effects. Sequences we employ include gadolinium-enhanced slice-selective 180° MP-RAGE (particularly useful for noncooperative patients), gadolinium-enhanced water excitation SGE, and gradient echo sequences with gradient echo refocusing (without gadolinium) (e.g., true FISP, GRASS). Acquisition of additional planes is also useful, for example, coronal plane of the liver postgadolinium and sagittal plane of the pelvis postgadolinium.

IMAGING STRATEGIES

High diagnostic accuracy can be achieved by describing the T1-, T2-, capillary and interstitial phase gadolinium-enhanced T1-weighted sequence appearance of various disease processes. In practice, it is also important to recognize which technique is the most consistent in demonstrating various lesions in order to target these lesions in an imaging protocol. Table 1.1 lists the MR sequences on which certain disease processes are consistently shown.

A major strength of MRI is the variety of types of information that the modality is able to generate. As a result, MRI is able to provide comprehensive information on organ systems and disease entities. The use of a diverse group of sequences, acquired in multiple planes, minimizes the likelihood of not detecting disease or misclassifying disease. This is a reflection of the fact that the more different information that is acquired, the less likely it is that disease will escape detection. Attention to length of examination is critical because longer examinations result in fewer patients who can be examined and a decrease in patient cooperation. Ideally, many of the different sequences employed should be of short duration and breath hold or breathing-independent. An attempt should be made to achieve

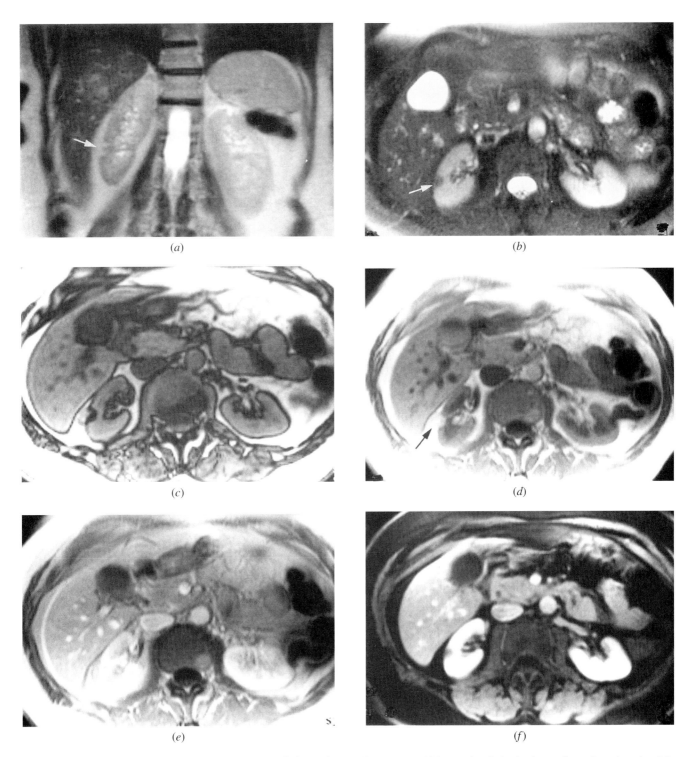

(a) *(b)*

(c) *(d)*

(e) *(f)*

F I G . 1.11 Fat effects, gadolinium effects, and their distinction. Coronal T2-weighted single-shot echo-train spin-echo (*a*), T2-weighted fat suppressed single-shot echo-train spin-echo (*b*), T1-weighted out-of-phase SGE (*c*), T1-weighted in-phase SGE (*d*), 1-min postgadolinium SGE (*e*), and 1.5-min gadolinium-enhanced fat-suppressed SGE (*f*) images. It is always useful to compare noncontrast nonsuppressed (*a*) and fat suppressed (*b*) sequences to ascertain whether high-signal structures observed on nonsuppressed sequences represent fat, or lower-signal structures observed on fat-suppressed sequences represent fat and not low-fluid-content solid masses. Comparing out-of-phase (*c*) to in-phase (*d*) sequences also permits characterization of fatty tumors. In this patient, a right renal angiomyolipoma is present that on the basis of the fat-suppressed T2-weighted sequence alone (arrow, *b*) may be considered a possible renal cancer or hemorrhagic cyst because of its low signal. Comparison with the non-fat-suppressed sequence (*a*) reveals that the tumor is high signal intensity in the absence of suppression (arrow, *a*), showing that it represents fat. Another approach is to show that the high-signal mass on the in-phase image (arrow, *d*) develops a phase cancellation black ring interface with renal parenchyma on the out-of-phase image (*c*). By noting that the mass is fatty, then high signal on early postgadolinium images (arrow, *d*) can be recognized as a fat effect, and not enhancement, and loss of signal on the 1.5-min gadolinium-enhanced fat-suppressed image is not misinterpreted as washout, but correctly observed as a fat suppression effect.

T a b l e 1.1   MR Imaging Sequences That Show Consistent Display of Various Disease Processes

Sequences	Disease Process	Appearance
T1	Fluid	↓↓
T1 out of phase	Adrenal adenoma, fatty liver	↓
T1 fat suppressed	Normal pancreas Subacute hematoma Endometriosis (subacute blood)	↑
T2	Fluid	↑↑
T2	Iron (including hemosiderin)	↓↓
T2	Uterine cervix, prostate	Zonal anatomy, cancer
Capillary phase Gad	Focal lesions of liver, spleen, pancreas	Distinctive patterns
Capillary phase? Gad	Inflammatory disease	↑
Capillary phase Gad	Arterial compromise	↓
Capillary phase? Gad	Portal vein compromise	↑
Interstitial phase Gad	Inflammatory disease, peritoneal metastases, bone metastases, lymphadenopathy	↑

this goal in protocol design. Another consideration is reproducibility of examination protocols. Efficient operation of an MRI system requires the use of set protocols, which serves to speed up examinations, render exams reproducible, and increase utilization by familiarity with a standard approach. A useful approach is to have sufficient redundancy in sequences that if one or two sequences are unsatisfactory there still is enough information for the study to be diagnostic, while at the same time not to have too much redundancy that study times are long and patient cooperation diminishes towards the latter part of the study. The diminishing patient cooperation toward the latter part of the study also implies that the most important sequences should be acquired as early as possible in the exam. MRI techniques are in continuous evolution, and when new sequences are developed it is important to replace older sequences with newer sequences, rather than simply adding new sequences onto an existing protocol. Speed of data acquisition, image quality, disease display, and consistency of image quality are all important considerations when evaluating new sequences. For example, it is well-accepted that the image quality of contrast-enhanced 3D T1-weighted GE imaging has exceeded the point that it is now superior to 2D imaging. Hence, for dynamic contrast imaging, all SGE sequences in our protocols have been replaced with 3D imaging. It is anticipated that this transition may also extend to opposed-phase imaging, with 3D acquisitions being the preferred imaging method. On older MR systems, one may still want to implement SGE technique because of its robustness. On the newest MR systems, the rationale to utilize 3D imaging includes thinner-section data acquisition, lesser problems with motion and phase

artifact, and the ability to use the same data set to generate an MRA exam [11, 12].

The protocoling of MRI studies that investigate the abdomen and pelvis in the same setting may be rendered most efficient by acquiring a complete study of the upper abdomen initially, using precontrast SGE and FS 3D-GE and/or FS SGE, T2-weighted single shot ETSE and single shot FS-ETSE, and serial postgadolinium FS 3D-GE or SGE and FS-SGE images, then acquiring the pelvis study, including postgadolinium FS-SGE or FS 3D-GE followed by T2-weighted sequences (fig. 1.12). Comprehensive examination of all organs and tissues in the abdomen and pelvis can be achieved with this approach, which permits detection of a full range of disease, including unsuspected disease (fig. 1.13). This strategy minimizes table motion and repositioning of the phased-array coil, which are time-consuming procedures. Newer MR systems now allow simultaneous planning of abdomen and pelvis regions, such that each acquisition can be conducted in series. With this capability, all precontrast T2 and T1 imaging can be acquired together without disrupting the specifically-timed T1 postcontrast images. This strategy allows increased exam efficiency, since one can migrate specific T2-weighted precontrast sequences, such as SSFP or MRCP, to postcontrast slots, especially between the portal venous phase (1–2 min post) and delayed interstitial phase (3+ min post). Although it is not generally desired to acquire T2-weighted images after gadolinium, we have not observed significant degradation of T2-weighted images of the pelvis after gadolinium. The presence of concentrated low-signal-intensity gadolinium in the bladder on T2-weighted images may in fact be beneficial by increasing conspicuity of bladder

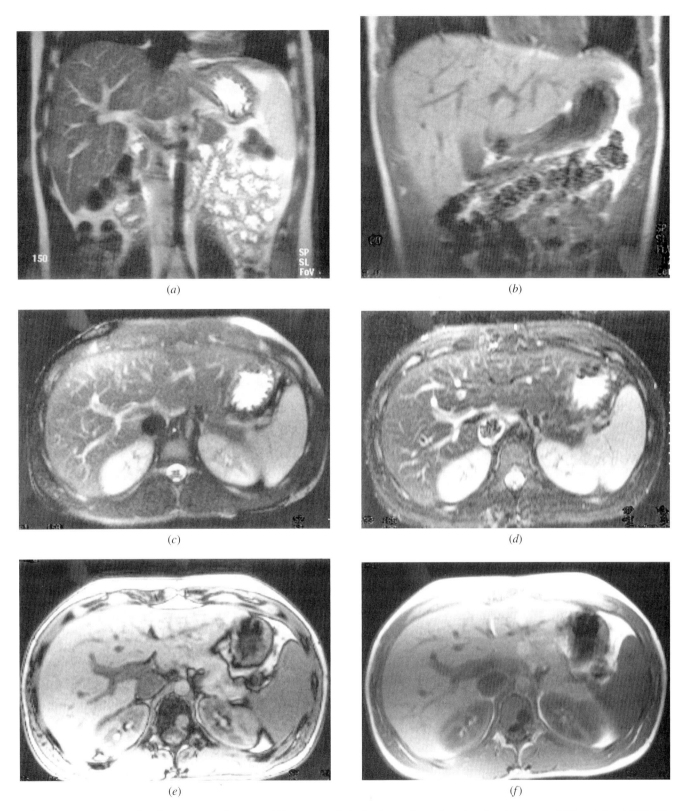

F I G . 1.12 Liver and pelvis protocol. Coronal T2-weighted single-shot echo-train spin-echo (*a*), coronal T1-weighted SGE (*b*), T2-weighted fat-suppressed single-shot echo-train spin-echo (*c*), T2-weighted breath-hold STIR (*d*), T1-weighted out-of-phase SGE (*e*), T1-weighted in-phase SGE (*f*), hepatic arterial dominant phase SGE (*g*), 1-min postgadolinium SGE (*h*), 1.5-min postgadolinium

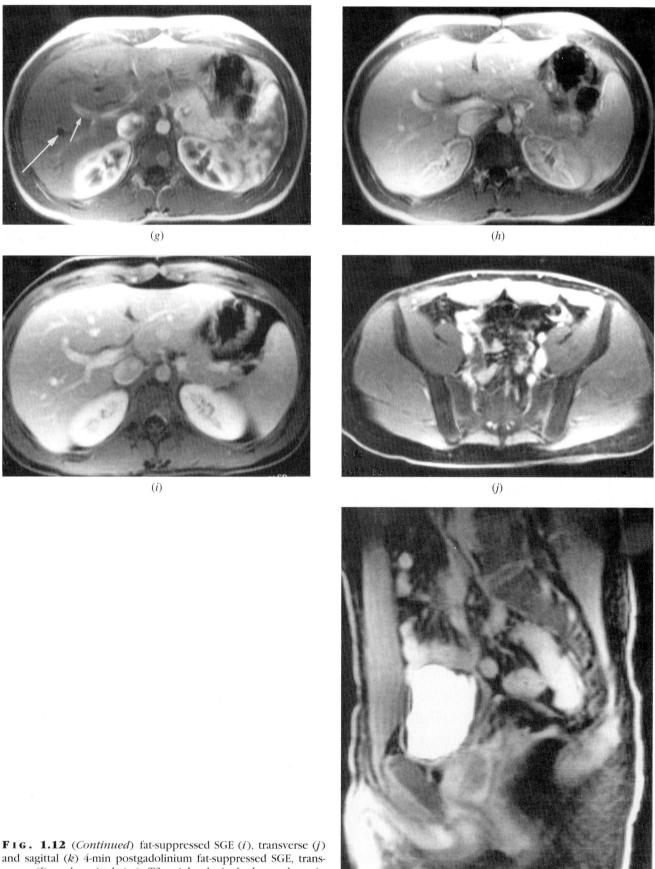

FIG. 1.12 (*Continued*) fat-suppressed SGE (*i*), transverse (*j*) and sagittal (*k*) 4-min postgadolinium fat-suppressed SGE, transverse (*l*) and sagittal (*m*) T2-weighted single-shot echo-train spin-echo images. Pre- and postgadolinium multiplanar T1- and

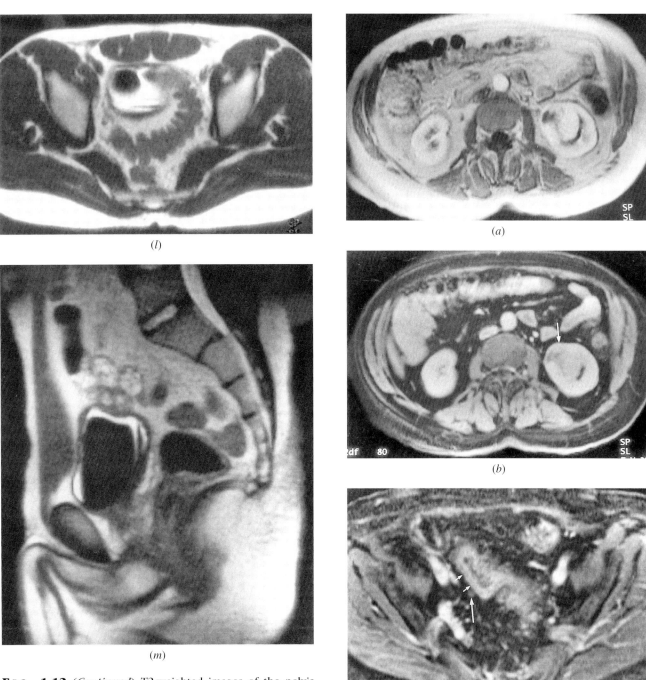

(l)

(m)

(a)

(b)

(c)

F I G . 1.12 (*Continued*) T2-weighted images of the pelvis (*j–m*). A combination of breath-hold (*b, d, e–k*) and breathing-independent (*a, c, l, m*) sequences are used to ensure consistent image quality in cooperative patients, combined with short study duration, typically 30–40 min. On the hepatic arterial dominant phase image, note the presence of gadolinium in portal veins (short arrow, *g*) and not hepatic veins (long arrow, *g*).

F I G . 1.13 Concurrent renal cell cancer and colon cancer. Immediate postgadolinium SGE (*a*), 90-s postgadolinium fat-suppressed SGE (*b*), and 3-min postgadolinium fat-suppressed SGE (*c*) images. Selected images from a liver pelvis protocol in a patient evaluated for colon cancer demonstrate an incidental left renal tumor that enhances intensely on immediate postgadolinium images (*a*) and washes out (arrow, *b*) on the fat-suppressed image, diagnostic for renal cell cancer. Thickening of the sigmoid colon representing cancer (small arrows, *c*) is appreciated on images acquired of the pelvis. A small regional involved lymph node (long arrow, *c*) is well shown on the gadolinium-enhanced fat-suppressed image.

involvement from malignant pelvic diseases. The liver is the organ that benefits the most from immediate postgadolinium imaging, and imaging protocols should be designed in a fashion to image the liver immediately after gadolinium administration. If, however, liver metastases are unlikely and the pelvis is the major focus of investigation, studies can be structured to acquire immediate postgadolinium images of the pelvis (e.g., for the evaluation of bladder tumors).

Patient setup can be performed as follows. The phased-array coil is initially placed over the upper abdomen, and image acquisition is centered over the liver. After precontrast sequences, with the patient positioned in the bore of the magnet, gadolinium is injected as a forceful hand bolus injection over 5s, followed by injection of a normal saline flush over 3s. Image acquisition is initiated immediately after the normal saline flush with the SGE sequence. Another approach, using a power injector, is to administer contrast at 2ml/s and to initiate the scan 17s after the start of contrast injection. Other researchers have also recommended using a timing bolus to increase the reproducibility of data acquisition in a correct phase of enhancement [12].

Accuracy and reproducibility of arterial-phase acquisition is of vital importance, as discussed earlier in this section. It is reasonable to assert that individual arterial transit times from the point of contrast administration to hepatic arteries vary in patients with a range of liver disease. Therefore, customized arterial timing is preferred to fixed timing methods, assuming it also provides efficient implementation for users. To this end, a real-time ("on-the-fly") bolus-tracking method for liver imaging has been utilized by some centers to eliminate the need for test-bolus timing injections. This timing method incorporates a strategy similar to MRA timing, in which a fast (~0.5s), single-slice SGE, with real-time reconstruction, is used to image the arrival of contrast medium into a region-of-interest, whereupon the user performs a breath-hold command and triggers the next acquisition. Extension of real-time bolus tracking to liver timing application involves redefining the specific elements of execution, namely, 1) the trigger point-of-interest to stop bolus tracking and 2) subsequent time delay to commence arterial-phase acquisition with 3D GE. Current clinical implementation utilizes the descending aorta at the level of the diaphragm (celiac axis) as an appropriate stopping point, since it is easily visualized and occurs upstream enough from the hepatic arterial dominant phase to allow adequate delay for breath-hold commands. The precise time for this delay is a matter of continued investigation. In a strict sense, the delay should signify the duration from celiac axis to peak tumor signal contrast in liver. Preliminary perfusion MR data have shown an average duration of approximately 10s [13]. Using this strategy, it is intended

to time 3D GE at peak tumor contrast, which refers to the center of k-space, not the start of the scan. Therefore, the delay following bolus detection in the descending aorta must be adapted according to the pulse sequence (i.e., 6s). For certain 3D GE configurations, the effective center of k-space may not occur near the beginning of the acquisition, as seen with 3D MRA sequences. This may limit the capacity to perform adequate breath-hold commands. In this scenario, the user may choose a vascular reference trigger point further upstream to compensate. It should be emphasized, however, that "optimal delay of 10s" refers to the duration to "peak" tumor contrast, which can be tempered by realizing there naturally exists a finite window of "high tumor contrast," allowing the user a margin of error in 3D GE timing acquisition. The real-time bolus-tracking strategy has been shown to be a highly efficient and reproducible method for capturing the time-sensitive arterial phase over fixed-timing techniques, and without the need for multiple injections, as with a separate timing bolus. Additionally, a separate timing bolus will inevitably result in a small amount of contrast enhancement characteristic of the interstitial phase, which will contaminate the desired perfusion information of the earlier phases.

On the most recent MR systems, remote table motion, performed at the imaging console, and the ability to use either two phased-array torso coils overlying the abdomen and pelvis or one extended-coverage torso coil covering the abdomen and pelvis, are available. This permits time-efficient imaging of the abdomen and pelvis such that precontrast imaging of the pelvis can be performed as well, if needed.

A number of authors have described the use of oral contrast in evaluating the abdomen and pelvis, especially when the primary organ of interest is the small bowel [14]. Reflecting our overall view of wanting to keep MR studies simple to perform, we have generally not routinely advocated or used oral contrast agents, with the one exception that if one knows in advance that the organ of primary interest is the stomach, it is useful to distend the stomach (water suffices for this purpose) and to use a parenteral injection of a hypotonic agent. This is not, however, to say that the use of oral contrast may not be helpful, especially if the interpreting radiologists do not have much experience with bowel studies on MRI. Also, if one is to perform MR colonography, it is likely important to distend the colon with rectally administered fluid.

Tables 1.2–1.11 show the current protocols that are useful for the investigation of abdominopelvic disease when imaging at 1.5T with a phased-array multicoil.

The sequence protocols are designed for a Siemens system. However, the terms used are generic, as current systems produced by all manufacturers can generate

Table 1.2 General Abdomen

Sequence	Plane	TR	TE	Flip	Thickness/Gap	FOV	Matrix
Localizer	3-plane						
SS-ETSE	Coronal	1500*	85	170	8–10mm/20%	350–400	192 × 256
SS-ETSE	Axial	1500*	85	170	8–10mm/20%	350–400	192 × 256
SS-ETSE fat-suppressed	Axial	1500*	85	170	8–10mm/20%	350–400	192 × 256
T1 SGE in/out-of-phase	Axial	170	2.2/4.4	70	7mm/20%	350–400	192 × 320
SS-ETSE MRCP	Coronal	5000	700	180	50mm	300	224 × 384
T1 3D GE FS pre	Axial	3.8	1.7	10	3mm	350–400	160 × 256
Contrast							
T1 3D GE FS arterial	Axial	3.8	1.7	10	3mm	350–400	160 × 256
T1 3D GE FS venous	Axial	3.8	1.7	10	3mm	350–400	160 × 256
T1 3D GE FS delayed	Axial	3.8	1.7	10	3mm	350–400	160 × 256

*TR between slice acquisitions.

Table 1.3 Motion-Resistant Abdomen

Sequence	Motion	Plane	TR	TE	Flip	Thickness/Gap	FOV	Matrix
Localizer		3-plane						
SS-ETSE	FB or RT	Coronal	1500*	85	170	8–10mm/20%	350–400	192 × 256
SS-ETSE	FB or RT	Axial	1500*	85	170	8–10mm/20%	350–400	192 × 256
SS-ETSE fat-suppressed	FB or RT	Axial	1500*	85	170	8–10mm/20%	350–400	192 × 256
T1 SGE in/out-of-phase	RT	Axial	170	2.2/4.4	70	7mm/20%	350–400	192 × 320
SS-ETSE MRCP	FB	Coronal	5000	700	180	50mm	300	224 × 384
SSFP	FB	Axial	3.5	1.2	60	8mm/0%	350–400	224 × 256
2D MP-RAGE fat suppressed	FB	Axial	3.5	1.2	15	8mm/20%	350–400	150 × 256
Contrast								
2D MP-RAGE 15s post	FB	Axial	3.5	1.2	15	8mm/20%	350–400	150 × 256
2D MP-RAGE 1 min	FB	Axial	3.5	1.2	15	8mm/20%	350–400	150 × 256
2D MP-RAGE 5 min	FB	Axial	3.5	1.2	15	8mm/20%	350–400	150 × 256

*TR between slice acquisitions; FB = free breathe; RT = respiratory triggered; SSFP = steady-state free precession.

Table 1.4 Pelvis

Sequence	Plane	TR	TE	Flip	Thickness/Gap	FOV	Matrix
Localizer	3-plane						
SS-ETSE	Coronal	1500*	85	170	8–10mm/20%	350–400	192 × 256
SS-ETSE	Axial	1500*	85	170	8–10mm/20%	350–400	192 × 256
SS-ETSE	Sagittal	1500*	85	170	8–10mm/20%	350	192 × 256
SS-ETSE fat-suppressed	Axial	1500*	85	170	8–10mm/20%	350–400	192 × 256
T1 SGE in/out-of-phase	Axial	170	2.2/4.4	70	7mm/20%	350–400	192 × 320
T2 3D ETSE	Axial	1200	120	150	1.5mm	250	256 × 256
T1 3D GE FS pre	Axial	3.8	1.7	10	3mm	350–400	160 × 256
Contrast							
T1 3D GE FS 30s	Axial	3.8	1.7	10	3mm	350–400	160 × 256
T1 3D GE FS 1 min	Axial	3.8	1.7	10	3mm	350–400	160 × 256
T1 2D ETSE fat suppressed	Axial	600	11	180	5mm/20%	250	224 × 256

*TR between slice acquisitions.

T a b l e 1.5 General Abdomen-Pelvis

Sequence	Coverage	Plane	TR	TE	Flip	Thickness/Gap	FOV	Matrix
Localizer		3-plane						
SS-ETSE	Abd-Pel	Coronal	1500*	85	170	8–10 mm/20%	350–400	192 × 256
SS-ETSE	Abd-Pel	Axial	1500*	85	170	8–10 mm/20%	350–400	192 × 256
SS-ETSE	Pelvis	Sagittal	1500*	85	170	8–10 mm/20%	350	192 × 256
SS-ETSE fat-suppressed	Abd-Pel	Axial	1500*	85	170	8–10 mm/20%	350–400	192 × 256
T1 SGE in/out-of-phase	Abd	Axial	170	2.2/4.4	70	7 mm/20%	350–400	192 × 320
SS-ETSE MRCP	Abd	Coronal	5000	700	180	50 mm	300	224 × 384
T2 3D ETSE	Pel	Axial	1200	120	150	1.5 mm	250	256 × 256
T1 3D GE FS pre	Abd-Pel	Axial	3.8	1.7	10	3 mm	350–400	160 × 256
Contrast								
T1 3D GE FS arterial	Abd	Axial	3.8	1.7	10	3 mm	350–400	160 × 256
T1 3D GE FS 1 min	Abd-Pel	Axial	3.8	1.7	10	3 mm	350–400	160 × 256
T1 3D GE FS 3 min	Abd-Pel	Axial	3.8	1.7	10	3 mm	350–400	160 × 256
T1 2D ETSE fat suppressed	Pel	Axial	600	11	180	5 mm/20%	250	224 × 256

*TR between slice acquisitions.

T a b l e 1.6 Gastric Bowel

Sequence	Coverage	Plane	TR	TE	Flip	Thickness/Gap	FOV	Matrix
Localizer		3-plane						
SS-ETSE	Abd-Pel	Coronal	1500*	85	170	8–10 mm/20%	350–400	192 × 256
SS-ETSE	Abd-Pel	Axial	1500*	85	170	8–10 mm/20%	350–400	192 × 256
SS-ETSE fat-suppressed	Abd-Pel	Coronal	1500*	85	170	8–10 mm/20%	350–400	192 × 256
SS-ETSE	Pelvis	Sagittal	1500*	85	170	8–10 mm/20%	350	192 × 256
SS-ETSE fat-suppressed	Abd-Pel	Axial	1500*	85	170	8–10 mm/20%	350–400	192 × 256
T1 SGE in/out-of-phase	Abd	Axial	170	2.2/4.4	70	7 mm/20%	350–400	192 × 320
SS-ETSE MRCP	Abd	Coronal	5000	700	180	50 mm	300	224 × 384
T2 3D ETSE	Pel	Axial	1200	120	150	1.5 mm	250	256 × 256
T1 3D GE FS pre	Abd-Pel	Axial	3.8	1.7	10	3 mm	350–400	160 × 256
Contrast								
T1 3D GE FS arterial	Abd	Axial	3.8	1.7	10	3 mm	350–400	160 × 256
T1 3D GE FS 1 min	Abd-Pel	Axial	3.8	1.7	10	3 mm	350–400	160 × 256
T1 3D GE FS 3 min	Abd-Pel	Axial	3.8	1.7	10	3 mm	350–400	160 × 256

*TR between slice acquisitions.

T a b l e 1.7 Chest

Sequence	Plane	TR	TE	Flip	Thickness/Gap	FOV	Matrix
Localizer	3-plane						
SS-ETSE	Coronal	1500*	85	170	8–10 mm/20%	350–400	192 × 256
SS-ETSE	Axial	1500*	85	170	8–10 mm/20%	350–400	192 × 256
SS-ETSE fat suppressed	Axial	1500*	85	170	8–10 mm/20%	350–400	192 × 256
bSSFP	Axial	3.5	1.2	60	8 mm/0%	350–400	224 × 256
T1 3D GE FS pre	Axial	3.8	1.7	10	3 mm	350–400	160 × 256
Contrast							
T1 3D GE FS 20 s	Axial	3.8	1.7	10	3 mm	350–400	160 × 256
T1 3D GE FS 1 min	Axial	3.8	1.7	10	3 mm	350–400	160 × 256
T1 3D GE FS 3 min	Coronal	3.8	1.7	10	3 mm	350–400	160 × 256

*TR between slice acquisitions; SSFP = steady-state free precession.

Table 1.8 Chest/Abd/Pel

Sequence	Coverage	Plane	TR	TE	Flip	Thickness/Gap	FOV	Matrix
Localizer		3-plane						
SS-ETSE	Chest-Abd-Pel	Coronal	1500*	85	170	8–10 mm/20%	350–400	192 × 256
SS-ETSE	Chest-Abd-Pel	Axial	1500*	85	170	8–10 mm/20%	350–400	192 × 256
SS-ETSE	Pelvis	Sagittal	1500*	85	170	8–10 mm/20%	350	192 × 256
SS-ETSE fat-suppressed	Chest-Abd-Pel	Axial	1500*	85	170	8–10 mm/20%	350–400	192 × 256
T1 SGE in/out-of-phase	Abd	Axial	170	2.2/4.4	70	7 mm/20%	350–400	192 × 320
bSSFP	Chest	Axial	3.5	1.2	60	8 mm/0%	350–400	224 × 256
SS-ETSE MRCP	Abd	Coronal	5000	700	180	50 mm	300	224 × 384
T2 3D ETSE	Pel	Axial	1200	120	150	1.5 mm	250	256 × 256
T1 3D GE FS pre	Chest-Abd-Pel	Axial	3.8	1.7	10	3 mm	350–400	160 × 256
Contrast								
T1 3D GE FS arterial	Abd	Axial	3.8	1.7	10	3 mm	350–400	160 × 256
T1 3D GE FS 1 min	Chest-Abd-Pel	Axial	3.8	1.7	10	3 mm	350–400	160 × 256
T1 3D GE FS 3 min	Chest-Abd-Pel	Axial	3.8	1.7	10	3 mm	350–400	160 × 256
T1 3D GE FS 5 min	Chest-Abd	Coronal	3.8	1.7	10	3 mm	350–400	160 × 256
T1 2D ETSE fat suppressed	Pel	Axial	600	11	180	5 mm/20%	250	224 × 256

*TR between slice acquisitions; SSFP = steady-state free precession.

Table 1.9 Whole Body (Brain/Chest/Abd/Pel)

Sequence	Coverage	Plane	TR	TE	Flip	Thickness/Gap	FOV	Matrix
Localizer		3-plane						
T2 ETSE (FLAIR)	Brain	Axial	8000	120	180	4 mm/20%	230	192 × 256
3D GE (COW)	Brain	Axial	40	7.0	20	0.9 mm	200	256 × 512
SS-ETSE	Chest-Abd-Pel	Coronal	1500*	85	170	8–10 mm/20%	350–400	192 × 256
SS-ETSE	Chest-Abd-Pel	Axial	1500*	85	170	8–10 mm/20%	350–400	192 × 256
SS-ETSE	Pelvis	Sagittal	1500*	85	170	8–10 mm/20%	350	192 × 256
SS-ETSE fat-suppressed	Chest-Abd-Pel	Axial	1500*	85	170	8–10 mm/20%	350–400	192 × 256
T1 SGE in/out-of-phase	Abd	Axial	170	2.2/4.4	70	7 mm/20%	350–400	192 × 320
bSSFP	Chest	Axial	3.5	1.2	60	8 mm/0%	350–400	224 × 256
SS-ETSE MRCP	Abd	Coronal	5000	700	180	50 mm	300	224 × 384
T1 3D GE FS pre	Chest-Abd-Pel	Axial	3.8	1.7	10	3 mm	350–400	160 × 256
Contrast								
T1 3D GE FS arterial	Abd	Axial	3.8	1.7	10	3 mm	350–400	160 × 256
T1 3D GE FS 1 min	Chest-Abd-Pel	Axial	3.8	1.7	10	3 mm	350–400	160 × 256
T1 3D GE FS 3 min	Chest-Abd-Pel	Axial	3.8	1.7	10	3 mm	350–400	160 × 256
T1 3D GE FS 5 min	Chest-Abd	Coronal	3.8	1.7	10	3 mm	350–400	160 × 256
T1 3D GE fat suppressed	Neck-Brain	Axial	3.8	1.7	10	3 mm	250–275	224 × 256

similar sequences. Vendor specific sequence names are indicated in Table 1.12, and vendor-specific variations in imaging parameters should be employed as needed. Variations in TR/TE/flip angle for SGE sequences, especially in the same patient study, should generally be avoided. Imaging parameters of ETSE sequences are more flexible, with minor changes resulting in no substantial loss of diagnostic information. With the use of phased-array multicoils both slice thickness and FOV can be substantially modified for many protocols (e.g., slice thickness of 5 mm for the pancreas, adrenals, and pelvis and FOV of 200 mm for the pelvis).

Table 1.10 3T General Abdomen

Sequence	Plane	TR	TE	Flip	Thickness/Gap	FOV	Matrix
Localizer	3-plane						
SS-ETSE	Coronal	1500*	70	170	6–8 mm/20%	350–400	192 × 256
SS-ETSE	Axial	1500*	70	170	6–8 mm/20%	350–400	192 × 256
SS-ETSE fat-suppressed	Axial	1500*	70	170	6–8 mm/20%	350–400	192 × 256
T1 SGE in/out-of-phase	Axial	170	1.1/2.2	60	6 mm/20%	350–400	192 × 320
SS-ETSE MRCP	Coronal	5000	700	180	50 mm	300	224 × 384
T1 3D GE FS pre	Axial	3.3	1.2	10	2.5 mm	350–400	180 × 288
Contrast							
T1 3D GE FS arterial	Axial	3.3	1.2	10	2.5 mm	350–400	180 × 288
T1 3D GE FS venous	Axial	3.3	1.2	10	2.5 mm	350–400	180 × 288
T1 3D GE FS delayed	Axial	3.3	1.2	10	2.5 mm	350–400	180 × 288

*TR between slice acquisitions.

Table 1.11 3T Motion-Resistant Abdomen

Sequence	Motion	Plane	TR	TE	Flip	Thickness/Gap	FOV	Matrix
Localizer		3-plane						
SS-ETSE	FB or RT	Coronal	1500*	70	160	6–8 mm/20%	350–400	192 × 256
SS-ETSE	FB or RT	Axial	1500*	70	160	6–8 mm/20%	350–400	192 × 256
SS-ETSE fat-suppressed	FB or RT	Axial	1500*	70	160	6–8 mm/20%	350–400	192 × 256
T1 SGE in/out-of-phase	RT	Axial	170	1.1/2.2	60	6 mm/20%	350–400	192 × 320
SS-ETSE MRCP	FB	Coronal	5000	700	170	50 mm	300	224 × 384
bSSFP	FB	Axial	3.5	1.2	60	6 mm/0%	350–400	224 × 256
2D WE SS-SGE	FB	Axial	3.2	1.1	12	8 mm/20%	350–400	150 × 256
Contrast								
2D WE SS-SGE 15 s	FB	Axial	3.2	1.1	12	8 mm/20%	350–400	150 × 256
2D WE SS-SGE 1 min	FB	Axial	3.2	1.1	12	8 mm/20%	350–400	150 × 256
2D WE SS-SGE 3 min	FB	Axial	3.2	1.1	12	8 mm/20%	350–400	150 × 256

*TR between slice acquisitions; bSSFP = balanced steady-state free precession; WE SS-SGE = water-excited single-shot spoiled gradient echo.

Table 1.12 Vendor-Specific Terms for Common Abdominal Pulse Sequences

Sequence		Siemens	GE	Philips
ETSE	Echo train spin echo	TSE	FSE	TSE
SS-ETSE	Single-shot echo train spin echo	HASTE	SS-FSE	SS-TSE
SGE	Spoiled gradient echo	FLASH	SPGR	T1-FFE
3D GE	3D spoiled gradient echo	VIBE	LAVA	THRIVE
SSFP	Steady-state free precession	FISP	GRASS	FFE
bSSFP	Balanced steady-state free precession	TrueFISP	FIESTA	Balanced FFE
MP-RAGE	Magnetization-prepared rapid acquisition gradient echo	TurboFLASH	Fast SPGR	TFE

SERIAL MRI EXAMINATION

MRI is currently considered the most expensive imaging modality, which has hampered its appropriate utilization. The expense of MRI studies can be dramatically reduced by decreasing study time and the number of sequences employed. This may be done most reasonably in the setting of follow-up examinations. Depending on the amount of information needed, a follow-up study that employs coronal SS-ETSE, transverse pre-contrast 2D or 3D gradient echo, immediate and 45-s postgadolinium 2D or 3D GE, and 2-min postgadolinium fat-suppressed 2D or 3D gradient echo provides relatively comprehensive information in a 10-min study time [5]. Even more curtailed examination can be performed if the only indication is the change in size. An adrenal mass or lymphadenopathy may be adequately followed by precontrast SGE alone or, in the case of an adrenal adenoma, in combination with out-of-phase SGE.

NONCOOPERATIVE PATIENTS

It is crucial to recognize that separate protocols are required for noncooperative patients. In general, noncooperative patients fall into two categories: 1) those who cannot suspend respiration but can breathe in a regular fashion and 2) those who cannot suspend respiration and cannot breathe in a regular fashion. The most common patient population that fits into the first group are sedated pediatric patients. Agitated patients are the most commonly encountered who fit into the second group. Optimal imaging strategies differ for each.

In sedated patients, substitution of breath-hold images (e.g., SGE) can be made readily with breathing-averaged ETSE images, the image quality of which is improved by using fat suppression. Both 2D SGE and ETSE have the ability to be gated to respiration. Since SGE utilizes spoiling gradients within each TR interval, T1 information is preserved between respiratory periods, while T2 ETSE exploits the respiratory period into its inherent T2-weighting. With sedation, breathing is in a more regular pattern than that observed for all other patients. Additionally, breathing-independent T2-weighted SS-ETSE is useful, as is T1-weighted MP-RAGE, if dynamic gadolinium-enhanced images are required (fig. 1.14).

In patients who are agitated, only single-shot techniques should be used, including breathing-independent T2-weighted SS-ETSE and T1-weighted MP-RAGE pre- and postgadolinium administration (fig. 1.15).

EMERGING DEVELOPMENTS IN MRI

There are several emerging developments in MR imaging that are important for body MR imaging. These include 1) recent technical developments, 2) parallel MR imaging, 3) introduction of 3.0 T MR systems as whole body magnets; and 4) whole body MR imaging for screening. MR imaging has undergone major improvements in its diagnostic capability and clinical applications since its introduction in the clinical setting in the 1980s. These developments have mainly occurred in the following areas:

1. Increased main magnetic field strength (from less than 0.3 T to more than 3.0 T)
2. Improved radiofrequency coil design (from large single body or a single surface coil to arrays of multiple smaller (phased-array) coils containing 4–8 elements now, and 16–32 elements or higher in the near future):
3. Improved bandwidth per receiver channel (3 MHz) with advances in digital electronics for faster readouts and faster reconstructions of k-space data sets
4. Increased gradient performance (from gradients of <10 mT/m with switching rates of >1 ms to gradients with >50 mT/m and with switching rates in the order of 100 μs; these gradients can achieve lower TR and TE values, allow better spatial and temporal coverage, and drastically reduce the dead time periods during which no MR signal is acquired.
5. Newer and faster acquisition methods and sequences, like SGE; SS-SGE; bSSFP; ETSE; and SS-ETSE; EPI; and parallel imaging.

As a consequence of these technical improvements, most state-of-the-art MR systems (3.0 T and lower) currently operate just below the physiological barriers of dB/dt, acoustic noise, specific absorption rate (SAR), and perhaps also main magnetic field strength. Beyond these boundaries, regulations on patient safety will limit acquisition speed. For instance, negligible further improvements of imaging speed can be achieved by decreasing interecho spacing or repetition time through gradient performance alone. In this respect, the development and implementation of parallel MR imaging methods in combination with multiple coil arrays provides important means to further improve the diagnostic capability of MR imaging without violating physiological barriers.

Parallel MR Imaging

Parallel MR imaging is comprised of a number of methods that can be used in combination with the majority of the MR imaging sequences to reduce scan time by acquiring less data than would otherwise be necessary to avoid aliasing. Currently, several vendor-specific terms are in use for parallel imaging (Table 1.13). Since 1987, several authors have proposed ideas to reduce scan time in MR imaging by using some form of parallel imaging [15–24]. The first successful in vivo implementation of parallel imaging was demonstrated by Sodickson and colleagues in 1997 based on the simultaneous acquisition of spatial harmonics (SMASH) and coil sensitivities. Currently, sensitivity encoding

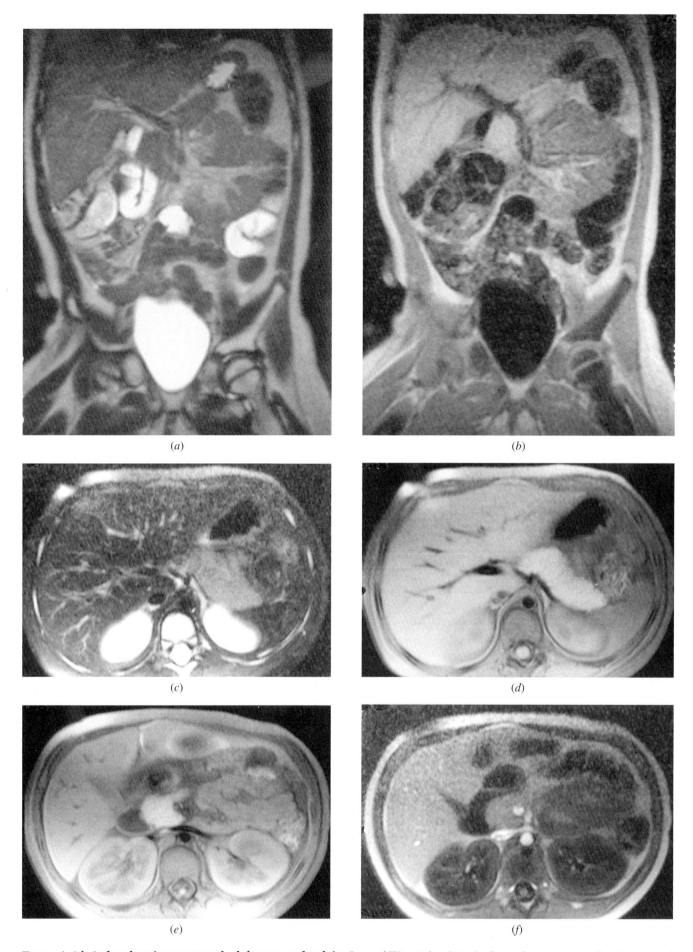

F I G . 1.14 Sedated patient protocol, abdomen and pelvis. Coronal T2-weighted single-shot echo-train spin-echo (*a*), coronal T1-weighted single-shot non-slice-selective 180° magnetization-prepared gradient echo (*b*), T2-weighted fat-suppressed echo-train spin-echo (*c*), T1-weighted fat-suppressed spin-echo (*d*, *e*), immediate postgadolinium T1-weighted slice-selective 180° magnetization-prepared gradient-echo (*f*), 1-min postgadolinium T1-weighted slice-selective 180° magnetization-prepared gradient-echo (*g*),

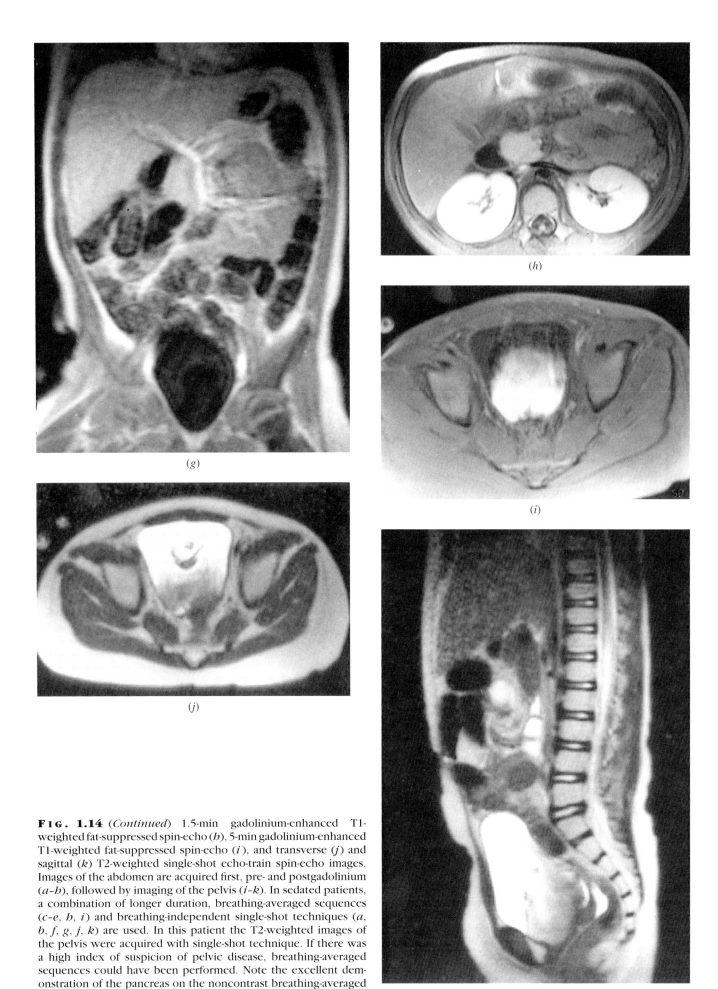

(g)

(h)

(i)

(j)

FIG. 1.14 (*Continued*) 1.5-min gadolinium-enhanced T1-weighted fat-suppressed spin-echo (*h*), 5-min gadolinium-enhanced T1-weighted fat-suppressed spin-echo (*i*), and transverse (*j*) and sagittal (*k*) T2-weighted single-shot echo-train spin-echo images. Images of the abdomen are acquired first, pre- and postgadolinium (*a–h*), followed by imaging of the pelvis (*i–k*). In sedated patients, a combination of longer duration, breathing-averaged sequences (*c–e, h, i*) and breathing-independent single-shot techniques (*a, b, f, g, j, k*) are used. In this patient the T2-weighted images of the pelvis were acquired with single-shot technique. If there was a high index of suspicion of pelvic disease, breathing-averaged sequences could have been performed. Note the excellent demonstration of the pancreas on the noncontrast breathing-averaged fat-suppressed T1-weighted spin-echo images (*d, e*).

(k)

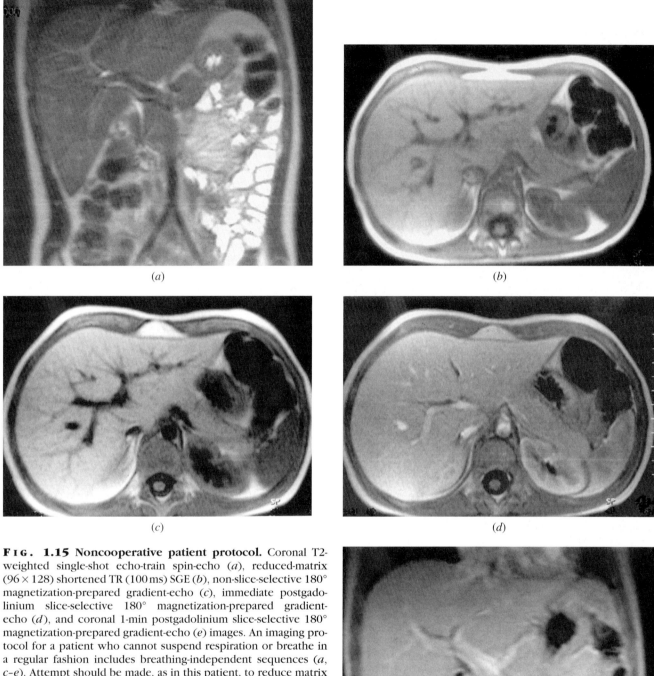

(a)

(b)

(c)

(d)

(e)

F I G . 1.15 Noncooperative patient protocol. Coronal T2-weighted single-shot echo-train spin-echo (*a*), reduced-matrix (96 × 128) shortened TR (100 ms) SGE (*b*), non-slice-selective 180° magnetization-prepared gradient-echo (*c*), immediate postgadolinium slice-selective 180° magnetization-prepared gradient-echo (*d*), and coronal 1-min postgadolinium slice-selective 180° magnetization-prepared gradient-echo (*e*) images. An imaging protocol for a patient who cannot suspend respiration or breathe in a regular fashion includes breathing-independent sequences (*a, c–e*). Attempt should be made, as in this patient, to reduce matrix size, field of view, and TR time on the SGE sequence to render it a 10-s breath hold. In this patient, this reduced-parameter SGE sequence (*b*) resulted in acceptable image quality for this acquisition, but was not reproducible. The study was switched to perform only breathing-independent sequences (*c–e*). Note the comparison between SGE (*b*) and non-slice-selective 180° magnetization-prepared gradient-echo (*c*) images. The former sequence has mirror artifacts from the aorta (arrow, *b*); the latter sequence has very nice signal void in vessels, no mirror artifacts, and strong T1 weighting, as evidenced by excellent liver-spleen contrast. Drawbacks of non-slice-selective 180° magnetization-prepared gradient echo include low signal-to-noise ratio, lengthy total imaging time, and variable image quality outside the liver.

Table 1.13 Vendor-Specific and Other Terms Used for Various Parallel MR Imaging Methods

ASSET	= Array Spatial Sensitivity Encoding Technique (GE Medical Systems)
GRAPPA	= Generalized Auto-calibrating Partially Parallel Acquisition
iPAT	= integrated Parallel Acquisition Technique (Siemens Medical Systems)
SENSE	= SENSitivity Encoding (Philips Medical Systems)
SMASH	= SiMultaneous Acquisition of Spatial Harmonics
SPACE RIP	= Sensitivity Profiles from an Array of Coils for Encoding and Reconstruction In Parallel

(SENSE), which was introduced in 1999 by Pruessmann and colleagues, is the most versatile method of parallel imaging. There are several differences in SMASH and SENSE types of methods. SMASH is considered a k-space-based method, whereas SENSE is an image-domain method. Parallel imaging methods are still evolving, and improvements in the existing and new methods are published on a regular basis. With the introduction of higher-field (>1.5 T) MR systems as well as multiple coil arrays (>8 coils), the role of parallel imaging will become even more important in the near future. One or a combination of several of the current parallel imaging methods may evolve, and eventually the original concept of Hutchinson and colleagues of "massive" parallel MR imaging [in which the number of coil elements equals the number of k-space lines (15)], may become a reality.

In general, parallel imaging methods require the use of suitable phased-array coils, a "reference" or a "calibration" scan, and vendor-specific software to reduce scan time. Each element of the phased-array coil has its own sensitivity profile, which can be measured based on the "reference" scan data. Parallel MR imaging exploits the calculated sensitivities of the coils and allows acquisition of less k-space data than otherwise necessary to avoid aliasing. The undersampling results in heavily aliased k-space data sets that can then be unfolded, using spatial sensitivity maps of the coils (SENSE method).

In the SMASH method, the same field of view (FOV) with the same spatial resolution as in conventional MRI can be obtained with reduced number of phase-encoding steps based—in part—on the sensitivity profiles of the coils and—in part—on the simultaneous acquisition of spatial harmonics.

The key feature of parallel imaging methods is the application of multiple independent receiver coils with distinct sensitivities across the object being imaged. In conventional MR imaging, the role of phased-array coils is merely to improve the signal-to-noise ratio (SNR), whereas in parallel imaging the phased-array coils are also used to reduce the scan time. The application of parallel imaging allows 1) higher temporal resolution (faster imaging; e.g., MRI exams in noncooperative patients, time-resolved MR angiography, and perfusion studies), 2) higher spatial resolution (larger matrices, thinner slices; e.g., high-resolution MRA) (fig. 1.16), 3) reduced effective interecho spacing (less image blurring and image distortion in ETSE and echo planar imaging; e.g., high-quality MRCP and single-shot EPI of the abdomen), and/or 4) reduced specific absorption rate (SAR) due to shorter echo trains (important for optimization of body MRI sequences at 3 T).

There are several limitations of parallel imaging, including

1. Decreased signal-to-noise ratio (SNR): As SNR is proportional to the square root of the total sampling time, there is an intrinsic loss of SNR with the square root of the acceleration factor. Advances in receiver technology, e.g., scanning with torso phased-array coils with eight or higher number of receivers, can significantly improve the SNR. In contrast-enhanced studies (i.e., dynamic imaging of the liver or MR angiography), an increase in the rate of contrast injection can also compensate for the loss of SNR. In contrast to the iodine-contrast media for CT exams, gadolinium-based contrast media have much lower viscosity. Therefore, unlike CT, the higher injection rates of MR contrast media, for instance with 4 ml/s, do not require the use of larger-bore intravenous catheters.

2. Parallel MR imaging foldover artifact: It should be emphasized that parallel imaging does not correct for foldover artifacts that occur if the FOV is chosen too small for the anatomy. In conventional abdominal MR imaging, a slightly smaller FOV, often in combination with a rectangular FOV, improves the spatial resolution in the phase encoding direction without significant increase in scan time. In such cases, the aliased body part projects on the opposite side of the patient, generally outside of the region of interest. With the application of parallel imaging, such artifacts are projected in the center of the image (fig. 1.17), resulting in severely degraded image quality. To avoid such artifacts, a full FOV should always be applied for any parallel imaging acquisition.

3. Reliability of parallel imaging in daily clinical practice: Depending on the imaging sequence and application, the reliability of the parallel imaging is reduced (for instance, with the appearance of artifacts due to image reconstruction errors) if the acceleration factor reaches an assigned value. Therefore

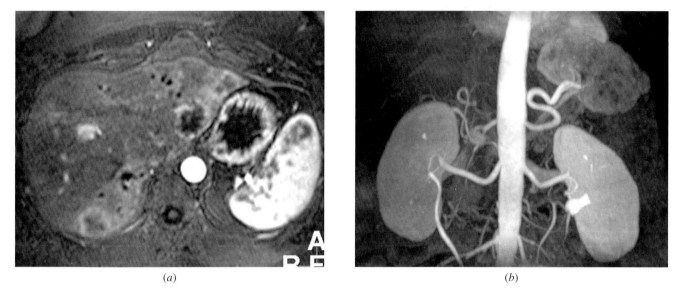

(a)   *(b)*

FIG. 1.16 Application of parallel imaging (acceleration factor 2) at 1.5 T. Axial fat-suppressed arterial dominant (*a*) image of a 3D gradient-echo image (2-mm sections interpolated to 1-mm sections; parallel imaging acceleration factor of 2; scan time 15 s to cover the entire liver). Based on the thin sections of the arterial dominant phase data set, a MR angiography was additionally reconstructed (*b*). This "free" MRA was used to determine the vasculature of the liver for planning chemoperfusion of the liver, which is the choice of treatment at our hospital for patients with colorectal liver metastases who cannot be treated with surgery or other minimally invasive therapies, such as radiofrequency ablation.

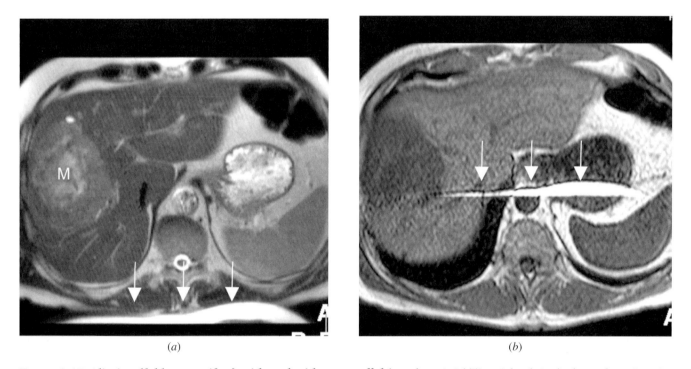

(a)   *(b)*

FIG. 1.17 Aliasing (foldover artifact) with and without parallel imaging. Axial T2-weighted single-shot echo-train spin-echo image without pMRI (*a*) shows the foldover artifact originating from the anterior abdominal wall projected on the opposite side of the image (arrows). A large metastasis is present in the liver (M). Axial SGE image with parallel imaging acceleration factor 2 (*b*) shows the foldover artifact projected in the center of the image (arrows).

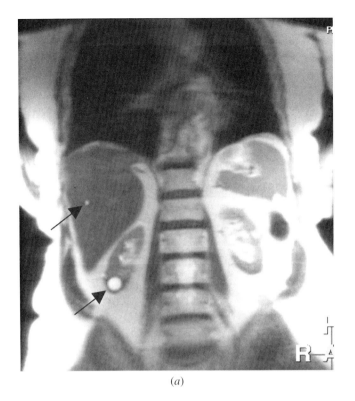

(a)

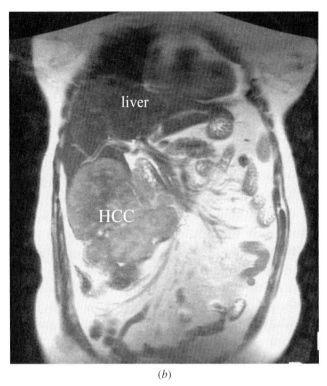

(b)

F I G . 1.18 **8-Channel phased-array torso coil at 3T.** Coronal T2-weighted single-shot echo-train spin-echo images in a patient with liver and renal cysts (arrows) (*a*) and in a patient with a large hepatocellular carcinoma (HCC) (*b*). In both cases, the large coverage with sufficient SNR over the entire anatomy was possible with the use of the 8-channel phased-array torso coil.

caution needs to be exercised when applying parallel imaging protocols with the highest acceleration factor possible. In particular, if the individual sequences are not robust, the examination may have to be repeated. This is especially critical for contrast-enhanced exams, where repeating the sequence (e.g., hepatic arterial dominant phase sequence) may not be feasible in the same MR study sessions.

Body MR Imaging at 3 T: General Considerations Compared to 1.5 T

A major advantage of a 3 T system compared to 1.5 T is that the signal-to-noise ratio (SNR) at 3 T is approximately two times higher. At the present time, research is ongoing to develop imaging approaches that take advantage of the higher SNR. In exploring the use of body imaging at 3 T, reference must be made to the image quality of state-of-the-art abdominal MR imaging that is achievable at 1.5 T, in order to determine the future role of 3 T imaging.

Currently, in several centers state-of-the-art 3 T MR imaging systems are equipped with eight-channel torso phased-array coils and parallel MR imaging capability. The availability of parallel imaging at 3 T is essential for reducing SAR. The eight-channel torso phased-array coils facilitate larger FOV and anatomic coverage in combination with better SNR distribution as compared to four-channel phased-array torso coils at 1.5 T (fig. 1.18). Several issues must be considered when developing body MRI for a 3 T system:

- **Radio-frequency (RF) power deposition is ~4×:** This follows from the following equation: $v = \gamma B_o$ [i.e., frequency (v) is equal to the product of the gyromagnetic ratio (γ) and the main magnetic field (B_o)]. If B_o increases with a factor of 2, the frequency at which the protons can be excited will also be doubled. Therefore, at 3 T RF pulses with 4× higher energy are needed to excite the protons. This results in increased RF heating and higher specific absorption rate (SAR). The limitation of SAR will be greatest for RF-intensive sequences, such as ETSE sequences. At 3 T, these limitations result in a lower number of slices per TR and hence smaller anatomic coverage.
- **Chemical shift and susceptibility artifact is ~2×:** The higher chemical shifts and susceptibility may result in artifacts on the gradient-echo and echo planar imaging. For equivalent imaging bandwidth, the fat-water spatial shift is doubled at 3 T. These artifacts can be reduced by using higher bandwidths than at 1.5 T. At 3 T, bandwidths with a value two

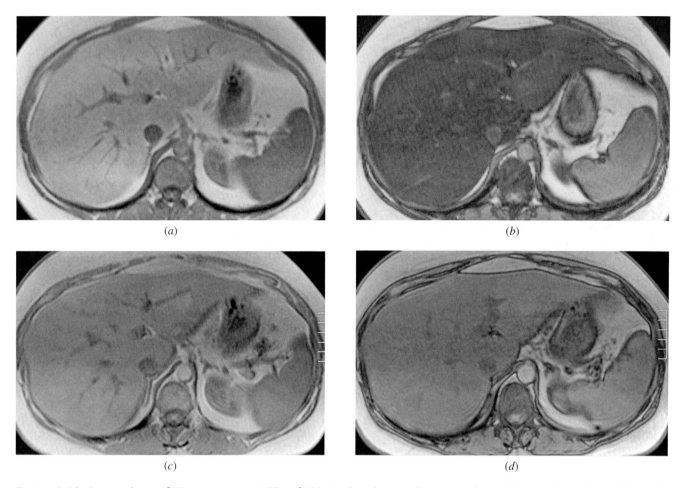

F I G . 1.19 Comparison of T1 contrast at 1.5T and 3T. Axial in-phase and opposed-phase SGE at 1.5T (*a, b*) and 3T (*c, d*). The inherent prolongation of T1 values at 3T reduces T1 contrast between soft tissues, as seen by comparing in-phase images (*a, c*) and opposed-phase images (*b, d*). This assumes identical flip angle and TR between field strengths. However, modifications of pulse sequence parameters, such as lengthening TR or decreasing flip angle, may alleviate low T1 contrast at 3T.

times higher than at 1.5T may be required. Higher chemical shift is also an advantage, for instance, for MR spectroscopy. Spectra with resolution similar to that at 1.5T may be acquired in shorter times, and spectrally selective fat suppression techniques also require less time at 3T.

- **T1 relaxation times are longer (e.g., liver has 30% longer T1):** This leads to increased signal saturation effects, especially for rapid GE imaging, which ultimately decreases T1 contrast on T1-weighted images (fig. 1.19). T1 weighting could be improved by different combinations of repetition times (TR), echo time (TE), and flip angle from those at 1.5T. But it is also noteworthy that T1 information can be constrained at 3T, such that alternative methods need to be employed to reveal contrast similar to 1.5T. On some 3T systems, for instance, dual echo SGE allows the shortest in-phase TE of 2.2ms but, because of SAR, gradient capabilities, and other issues, the

systems may only allow an opposed-phase TE of 5.8ms (which is the fourth opposed-phase TE value at 3T). The shortest in- and opposed-phase TE values (i.e., 1.1ms and 2.2ms) with less susceptibility and inflow effects are possible if the imaging bandwidth is increased, and one employs asymmetric echoes. Despite an SNR trade-off, this latter strategy is recommended at 3T, in order to distinguish between iron and fat effects, which may compete on later echoes. In addition to the decreased T1 weighting, inflow effects in abdominal vessels are more pronounced, which has a detrimental effect on the image quality of GE at 3T. The ability of gadolinium-based contrast agents to reduce T1 (known as the relaxivity, r1) is slightly lower at 3T [25]. However, the impact may not be observable with typical administered doses, stemming from the inherent difficulty of distinguishing very low T1 (<150ms) from one another. The intrinsic differences in T1 between 1.5T and 3T are lessened postcontrast, such that a greater change in T1, and therefore greater contrast enhancement, is expected at 3T, especially in the blood pool [26].

- **T2* of tissues and other structures is shorter (T2 remains practically unchanged):** This can be solved by echo trains with shorter effective interecho spacing or shorter echo trains. This can be achieved by applying parallel MR imaging. The use of parallel imaging has the additional advantage of reducing SAR.

- **3T safety concerns for body imaging:** Increased magneto-hydrodynamic effect results in a peaked T-wave of the electrocardiograms (ECG) during rapid systolic blood flow. In addition, there are 1) increased risk of RF burns from ECG leads, RF coils, and implanted wires, 2) increased torque on ferromagnetic implants, and 3) 6-dB intrinsic increase in acoustic noise.

- **B1 field inhomogeneities, dielectric resonances, RF penetration, and shape of the torso and abdomen have impact at 3T:** B1 inhomogeneities are particularly problematic, and they result in variations in the signal distribution over the region of interest, which appear to be related to the shape and size of the anatomy. For instance, at the level of the pelvis, B1 inhomogeneities cause darkening in the anterior and posterior parts of the abdomen and pelvis. This is evidence of a "field-focusing" effect, which becomes more prevalent as the RF wavelength becomes on the order of the human torso, as seen

at 3T. B1 inhomogeneities, in combination with the intrinsic properties of fat suppression and refocusing pulses in ETSE sequences (Shinnar–Le Roux pulses), may also be responsible for poor quality of fat suppression (fig. 1.20). To reduce SAR and acquire T2-weighted sequences with better fat suppression, alternative fat suppression techniques and T2-weighted imaging sequences must be optimized at 3T (fig. 1.21). The use of spectral-selective adiabatic inversion pulses for fat suppression, such as with SPAIR, has been effective at 3T (fig. 1.21)

Ultimately, the general framework and objectives for abdominal imaging at 3T should remain consistent with 1.5T. At a basic level, the sequence-types depicted in Table 1.2 should be transferred to 3T; however, from a sequence parameter perspective, adjustments must be made. Currently, it seems that the greatest advantage of the higher SNR of 3T, eight-channel torso phased-array coils, and the possibility of higher (>2) parallel imaging acceleration factors is observed in 3D GE gadolinium-enhanced sequences (fig. 1.22). It is highly anticipated that the newly available 32-channel coil will further accelerate 3D GE. This is of great importance at 3T, not only because inherent signal sensitivity increase allows increase in parallel imaging factors with less SNR loss (relative to 1.5T), but it also aids in achieving ultrashort dynamic 3D imaging following bolus contrast administration. This creates new possibilities for acquiring multi-dynamic phases within a single breath hold, or

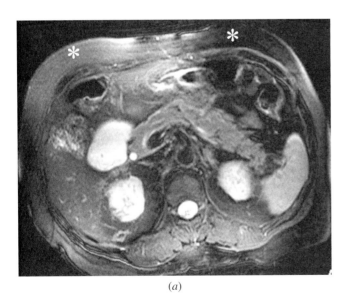
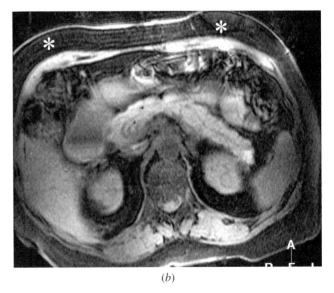

(a)   (b)

F I G. 1.20 Fat suppression in echo-train spin-echo versus SGE sequences at 3T. Axial fat-suppressed T2-weighted echo-train turbo spin-echo sequence (*a*) with inhomogenous fat suppression (*), probably due to multiple refocusing pulses and the MR physics nature of these pulses. Axial fat-suppressed T1-weighted SGE (*b*) shows homogenous fat suppression (*) at the same anatomic level.

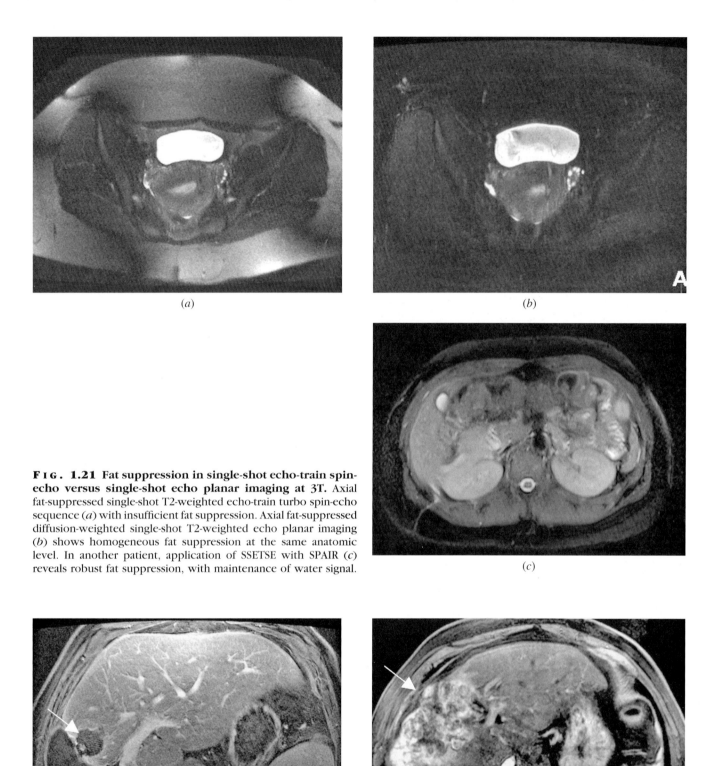

F I G . 1.21 Fat suppression in single-shot echo-train spin-echo versus single-shot echo planar imaging at 3T. Axial fat-suppressed single-shot T2-weighted echo-train turbo spin-echo sequence (*a*) with insufficient fat suppression. Axial fat-suppressed diffusion-weighted single-shot T2-weighted echo planar imaging (*b*) shows homogeneous fat suppression at the same anatomic level. In another patient, application of SSETSE with SPAIR (*c*) reveals robust fat suppression, with maintenance of water signal.

F I G . 1.22 4-Channel versus 8-channel torso phased-array coil at 3T. Axial fat-suppressed 3D gradient echo (4-channel torso phased-array coil; 4-mm section zero-interpolated to 2-mm sections; matrix 320 × 384; parallel imaging acceleration factor 2; scan time 25 s) (*a*) in a patient with status post right liver resection and a radiofrequency ablation of the recurrent metastasis at the resection plane (arrow). Axial fat-suppressed 3D gradient echo (8-channel torso phased-array coil; matrix 512 × 512; parallel imaging acceleration factor 3; other parameters were similar to the previous image) (*b*) in a patient with a recurrent gallbladder carcinoma (arrow).

investigating signal change behavior in the liver. Similarly, the promise of SNR gains at 3T implies the use of thinner sections and higher in-plane resolution with standard single-phase 3D GE. It is often apparent at 1.5T that artifacts due to lower through- and in-plane resolution impair visualization of subtle features of liver disease. This improvement in resolution costs time, effectively negating reasonable breath hold acquisitions. Parallel imaging with multichannel coils will be integral to reducing scan times under 20s. For individuals who still may be stressed from lengthy breath holds, parallel imaging can be further exploited to obtain diagnostic 3D GE at breath hold times between 10 and 15s depending on acceleration factors. As with 1.5T, robust motion insensitivity is vital for maximal diagnostic accuracy (fig. 1.23). Even in extreme cases, 3T still provides comparable, if not superior, robustness to breathing artifacts by utilizing rapid magnetization-prepared single-shot GE, which can eliminate the need for breath holding in noncooperative patients. Figure 1.23 shows clear depiction of a renal cyst on water-excited single-shot GE, in comparison to conventional breath-held 3D GE, which suffers from motion artifact.

For non-fat-suppressed and fat-suppressed T2-weighted MR imaging sequences, the best image quality is currently possible with SS-ETSE and diffusion-weighted single-shot echo planar imaging, respectively (fig. 1.24). Imaging of the pancreas and biliary tree in

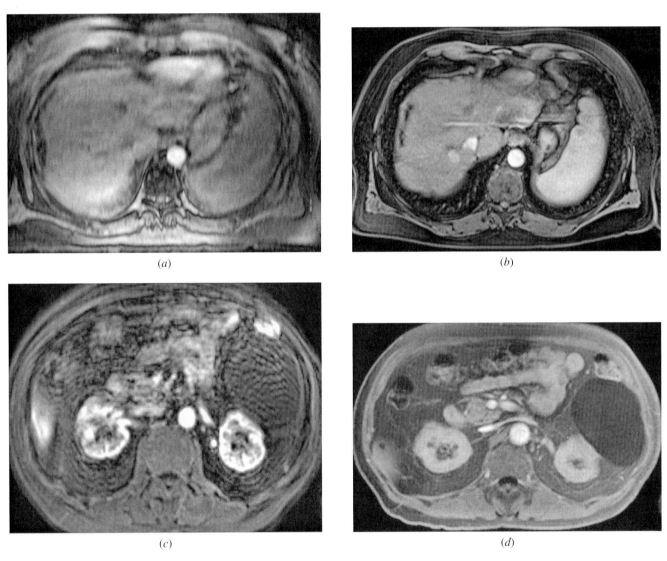

(a)   (b)

(c)   (d)

F I G . 1.23 Motion sensitivity at 1.5T and 3T. The importance of patient breath holding is revealed in two 3D GE acquisitions obtained on separate imaging days (a, b). The initial exam shows the impact of motion on an arterial acquisition, in which no lesion is visible (a). On subsequent repeat scanning, proper breath holding reveals a small arterial-enhancing liver lesion (b). When patient noncooperation is extreme, a water-excited SS-SGE is utilized, as shown in the depiction of a renal cyst at 3T, with conventional breath-held 3D GE (c) and with water-excited SS-SGE (d).

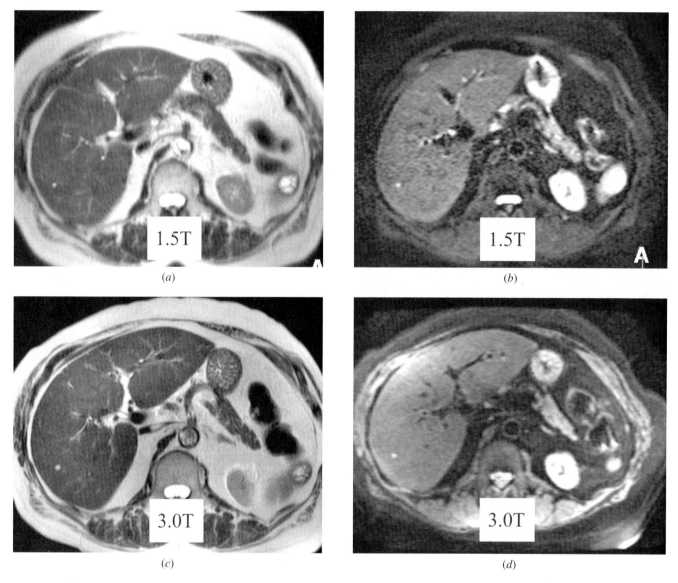

FIG. 1.24 1.5T versus 3.0T. Axial single-shot T2-weighted echo-train spin-echo (*a*) and fat-suppressed diffusion-weighted single-shot echo planar imaging (*b*) sequences at 1.5 T (acquired with 4-channel torso phased-array coil and parallel imaging acceleration factor of 2 for echo planar imaging) show a small cyst in the right liver. Axial single-shot T2-weighted echo-train spin-echo (*c*) and fat-suppressed diffusion-weighted single-shot echo planar imaging (*d*) sequences at 3 T (acquired with 8-channel torso phased-array coil and parallel imaging acceleration factor of 2 for both sequences) show a slightly better image quality with improved SNR and reduced image blurring.

particular may benefit from the use of eight-channel torso coil and parallel imaging (figs. 1.25 and 1.26). SS-ETSE sequences require parallel imaging, for the reduction of SAR and image blurring (by reducing the effective interecho spacing), whereas echo planar imaging mainly requires parallel imaging for the reduction of anatomic distortion (27). In the near future, a greater number of coil elements may allow higher (>2) parallel imaging acceleration factors that might be advantageous for T2-weighted sequences for better anatomic coverage, less image blurring, and less image distortion. At present, noncontrast T1-weighted sequence such as 2D SGE, as

well as T2-weighted ETSE sequences, especially with fat suppression, need further optimization.

Whole Body MRI: Faster and Better

Whole body MRI is a fast, reliable, safe, and accurate means of detecting disease throughout the entire body (figs. 1.27–1.31). This has been well shown in a recent article [28] in which the authors demonstrated that a screening MR protocol showed various disease processes with almost equal accuracy to a variety of comparison "gold standard" diagnostic tests. That article

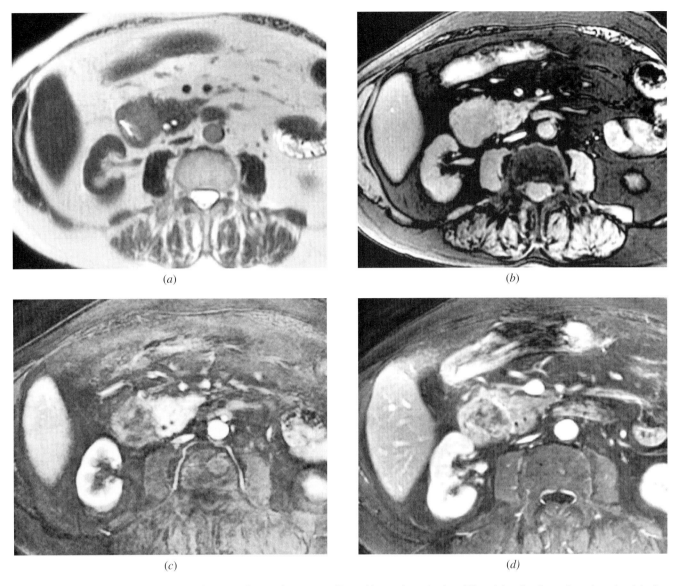

(a)

(b)

(c)

(d)

F I G . 1.25 Pancreas imaged with an 8-channel torso coil at 3T. Axial single-shot T2-weighted echo-train spin-echo (*a*), fat-suppressed 2D spoiled gradient echo (*b*), and gadolinium-enhanced 3D gradient echo (parallel imaging acceleration factor 3) in the arterial (*c*) and delayed (*d*) phases shows clearly the pancreas, the pancreatic duct, the peripancreatic vessels, as well as a duodenal tumor, because of the unique combination of a high in-plane spatial (matrix 512 × 512) and the intrinsic tissue-contrast of MRI at 3 T.

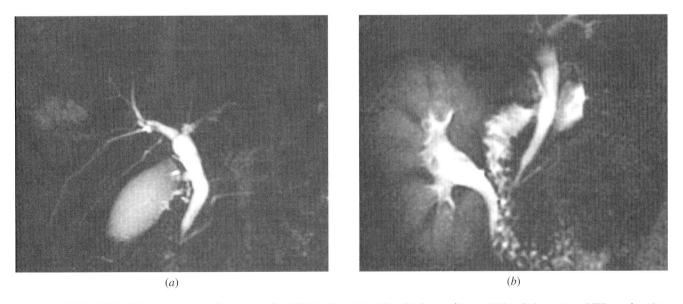

(a)

(b)

F I G . 1.26 MRCP with an 8-channel torso coil at 3 T. A thick-slab (slice thickness 40 mm; 512 × 512 matrix; pMRI acceleration factor 2) shows an overview of the biliary tree (*a*) and a detailed view of the papillary region and the renal collecting system (*b*).

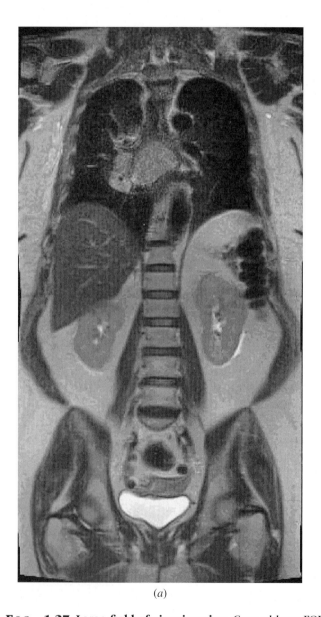

(a)

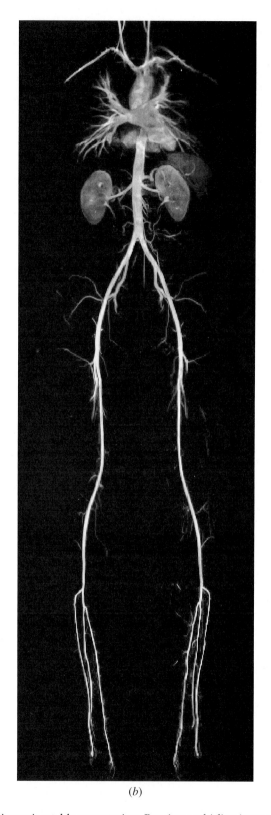

(b)

FIG. 1.27 Large field-of-view imaging. Coronal large FOV acquisition using table recentering. Routine multislice inspection of the chest through pelvis using T2 single-shot ETSE is possible in one acquisition (*a*). The technique can be modified to acquire axial slices over the same regions of interest, with user-specified automatic table movements. Similar strategies can be used to perform whole body MRA using a single bolus injection (*b*).

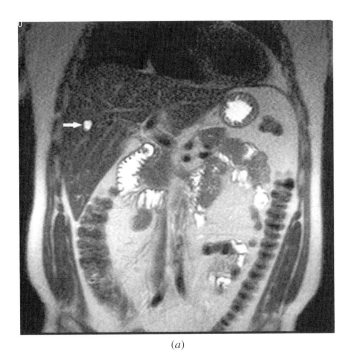
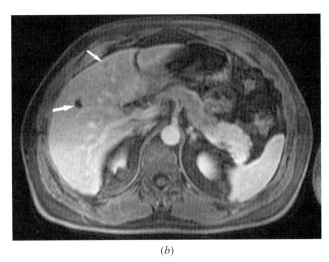

(a) (b)

F I G . 1.28 Liver. Coronal T2-weighted single-shot echo-train spin-echo image (*a*) shows a high-signal-intensity lesion consistent with biliary hamartoma (arrow). Axial T1-weighted fat-suppressed postgadolinium 3D gradient echo image (*b*) shows the biliary hamartomas with low signal intensity (arrows).

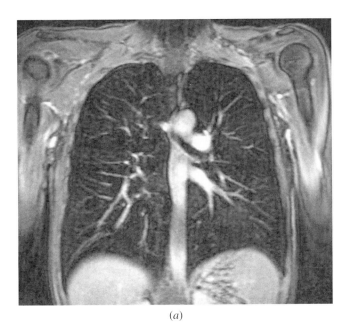
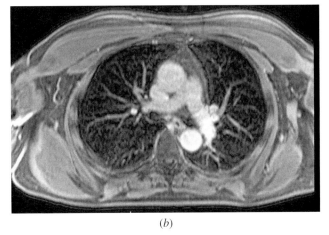

(a) (b)

F I G . 1.29 Chest. Coronal (*a*) and axial (*b*) T1-weighted fat-suppressed 3D gradient-echo postgadolinium (b) images clearly show enhanced pulmonary vessels that can be traced into the periphery of both lungs.

emphasized one component of whole body MRI, which is the use of gadolinium enhanced 3D GE. There are, however, five major technical advances that have rendered whole body screening with MRI a viable method, which include:

1. Remote movement of the imaging table from the imaging console
2. Multiple input channels that allow simultaneous use of multiple localized, specialized surface coils that generate high-spatial-resolution images of multiple

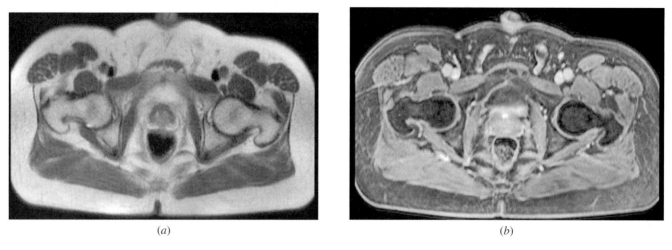

(a)   (b)

FIG. 1.30 Pelvis. Axial T2-weighted single-shot echo-train spin-echo (*a*) and axial T1-weighted fat suppressed 3D gradient echo postgadolinium (*b*) images clearly show the pelvic anatomy.

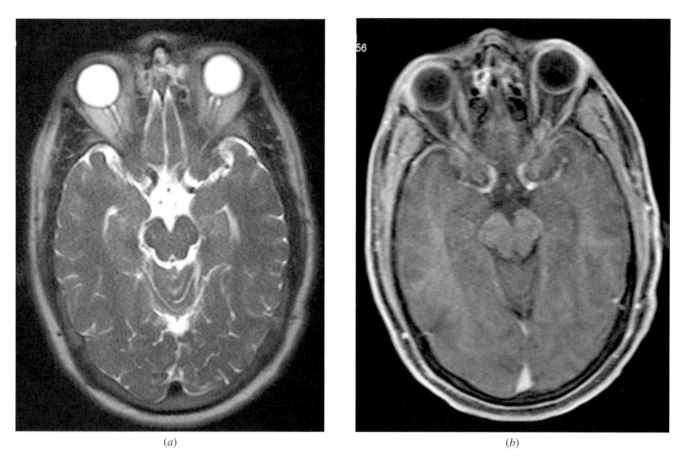

(a)   (b)

FIG. 1.31 Brain. Axial T2-weighted fat-suppressed single-shot echo-train spin-echo (*a*) and axial T1-weighted fat-suppressed 3D gradient-echo postgadolinium (*b*) images provide a detailed view of the intra- and extracranial anatomic structures.

regions of the body, without the delay of coil exchange and setup

3. Specialized surface coils that are designed for independent operation of the individual coil elements

4. Concurrent development of sequence (data acquisition) technology that operates in conjunction with the new specialized coils, such as parallel imaging

5. Development of high-image-quality 3D T1-weighted gradient echo with short echo time (TE) that facilitates acceptable imaging quality of various organ systems, most notably the lungs

The combined effect of all these above innovations has allowed, among other things, full body imaging to be performed more rapidly (because of remote table movement and new short data acquisitions), with maintenance of high image quality (simultaneous use of multiple specialized coils), and with the ability to image the lungs with adequate image quality (3D T1-weighted gradient echo imaging). The result is that the entire body can be imaged in a matter of 10–15 min, with high image quality maintained (Table 1.9).

To use an imaging study to screen for disease, it must be able to detect disease accurately and reliably while avoiding describing normal parts of the body as diseased. Since whole body CT and MRI screening are relatively new procedures, limited data have been collected comparing the two methods. There is growing concern in the medical community that whole body CT screening leads to a large number of questionable findings, requiring additional procedures, including surgery, and creating added risks and costs for the individual (29). Most of the information comparing the performance of CT and MRI has been gathered through diagnostic studies, that is, imaging studies ordered for the detection of suspected disease. Overall, MRI has been found to discover more lesions and correctly characterize more disease, whether benign or malignant, than CT. In these capacities, MRI has been shown to be superior to CT for examining specific regions of the body, for example, head, spine, musculoskeletal, abdomen, and pelvis [30–36]. In the past, the sole exception to this rule has been imaging of the lungs, which is performed better by CT than MRI, although new MRI techniques show promising results [28, 37].

Cost of the imaging study is also an important consideration. Because of the nature of the complexity of the imaging system and intrinsic maintenance costs, MRI is unavoidably a more expensive test than CT. The machinery has many more components, and the requirement for liquid helium and liquid nitrogen to be continuously replenished renders it intrinsically more expensive. The real cost of MRI is greater than that of CT: An approximate estimate is that studies are about 20% more expensive.

Regarding safety, MRI is a safer modality than CT, both the imaging system itself and the intravenous contrast agent employed [38–42]. The powerful magnetic field and radiofrequency energy of MRI has not been shown to cause cancer or fetal abnormalities, unlike the ionizing radiation used in CT that is a known cause of cancer and fetal anomalies. It is important to note that although X-rays are known to cause cancer, the exact risk of cancer from receiving CT scans, and even repeat CT exams, is unknown. A more in-depth discussion on cancer risks from radiation exposure in CT and other X-ray procedures has recently been published [43]. The

intravenous contrast agents used routinely in MRI, gadolinium-containing agents, are also considerably safer than the analogous intravenous agents employed in contrast-enhanced CT, which are iodine-based agents. There is a much lesser association with kidney injury with the MRI contrast agents, and much lesser association with allergic reactions, including severe allergic reactions that can lead to death [44–46]. That is why in general individuals who are undergoing diagnostic imaging studies will have an MRI study rather than CT if they have poor kidney function or a history of allergies. Other very compelling aspects of the use of intravenous contrast agents with MRI are that the diameter of the intravenous catheter inserted is much smaller with MRI, the volume of contrast material that is injected intravenously is 10 times less than with CT (the rapid injection of the large volume of contrast with CT can create a strong sense of nausea), and the injection rate is slower with MRI than with CT. Additionally, the chance of the injected contrast agent not going into the vein but into the surrounding tissues is also greater with CT, which is a problem compounded by the large volume of the fluid injected.

Therefore, if MRI is superior to CT for finding small-volume disease, correctly classifying disease, demonstrating that normal structures are intact and not diseased, and safer and less painful (smaller needle stick with MRI), then why is MRI still not considered the method of choice for whole body screening? Historically, the primary reason for this is that MRI is much slower to perform than CT, and imaging of the lungs was suboptimal. Recently, the MR systems that are manufactured have imaging capability that allows them to image the entire body much faster, while maintaining high image quality that even machines made in 2003 did not possess. Basically new designs of transmit-receiver coils, easier movement of the imaging table, and new data acquisition techniques have allowed rapid imaging of the entire body, and also acceptable image quality of the lungs. High-quality whole body MRI imaging that would take 2 hours even in 2003, now can be done in 10–15 min, making the technique very suitable for rapid, highly accurate whole body imaging in an easily tolerable time frame.

Although at present reliability and accuracy of MR imaging at detecting diseases of certain organs including liver, brain, spine, pancreas, and kidneys is extremely high and imaging of the lungs is reasonable, optimal imaging of the heart, breast, and colon still requires further development to achieve consistent image quality and consistent accurate display of small-volume disease. Nonetheless, imaging of all the latter mentioned organs is currently at a diagnostically acceptable level.

Currently manufactured MR systems have evolved to the point that the equipment can image through the entire body with good image quality and sensitivity to detect disease within a 15-min period. Whole body, high-quality, MRI screening is now feasible.

REFERENCES

1. Brown MA, Semelka RC. *MRI: Basic Principles and Applications.* Second Edition. New York: Wiley-Liss, 1999.
2. Semelka RC, Willms AB, Brown MA, Brown ED, Finn JP. Comparison of breath-hold T1-weighted MR sequences for imaging of the liver. *J Magn Reson Imaging* 4: 759–765, 1994.
3. Semelka RC, Kelekis NL, Thomasson D, Brown MA, Laub GA. HASTE MR imaging: description of technique and preliminary results in the abdomen. *J Magn Reson Imaging* 6: 698–699, 1996.
4. Gaa J, Hutabu H, Jenkins RL, Finn JP, Edelman RR. Liver masses: replacement of conventional T2-weighted spin echo MR imaging with breath-hold MR imaging. *Radiology* 200: 459–464, 1996.
5. Semelka RC, Balci NC, Op de Beeck B, Reinhold C. Evaluation of a 10-minute comprehensive MR imaging examination of the upper abdomen. *Radiology* 211: 189–195, 1999.
6. Semelka RC, Helmberger T. Contrast enhanced MRI of the liver: state-of-the-art. *Radiology* 2001.
7. Low RN, Semelka RC, Worawattanakul S, Alzate GD. Extrahepatic abdominal imaging in patients with malignancy: comparison of MR imaging and helical CT in 164 patients. *J Magn Reson Imaging* 12: 269–277, 2001.
8. Low RN, Semelka RC, Worawwattanakul S, Alzate GD, Sigeti JS. Extrahepatic abdominal imaging in patients with malignancy: comparison of MR imaging and helical CT, with subsequent surgical correlation. *Radiology* 210: 625–632, 1999.
9. Altun E, Semelka RC, Dale BM, Elias J Jr.. Water excitation MPRAGE: an alternative sequence for postcontrast imaging of the abdomen in noncooperative patients at 1.5 Tesla and 3.0 Tesla MRI. *J Magn Reson Imaging* 27: 1146–1154, 2008.
10. Lauenstein TC, Sharma P, Hughes T, Heberlein K, Tudorascu D, Martin DR. Evaluation of optimized inversion-recovery fat-suppression techniques for T2-weighted abdominal MR imaging. *J Magn Reson Imaging* 27(6): 1448–1454, 2008.
11. Rofsky NM, Lee VS, Laub G, Pollack MA, Krinsky GA, Thomasson D, Ambrosino MM, Weinreb JC. Abdominal MR imaging with a volumetric interpolated breath-hold examination. *Radiology* 212: 876–884, 1999.
12. Lee VS, Lavelle MT, Rofsky NM, Laub G, Thomasson DM, Krinsky GA, Weinreb JC. Hepatic MR imaging with a dynamic contrast-enhanced isotropic volumetric interpolated breath-hold examination: feasibility, reproducibility, and technical quality. *Radiology* 215: 365–372, 2000.
13. Sharma P, Salman K, Burrow B, Lauenstein T, Martin D. Quantification of arterial-phase perfusion kinetics in the liver. In: *Proceedings of the 15th Annual Meeting of ISMRM*, Berlin, 2007 (abstract 2980).
14. Low RN, Francis IR, Politoske D, Bennett M. Crohn's disease evaluation: comparison of contrast-enhanced MR imaging and single-phase helical CT scanning. *J Magn Reson Imaging* 11: 127–135, 2000.
15. Hutchinson M, Raff U. Fast MRI data acquisition using multiple detectors. *Magn Reson Med* 6: 87–91, 1988.
16. Kelton JR, Magin RL, Wright SM. An algorithm for rapid image acquisition using multiple receiver coils. In: *Proceedings 8th Annual Meeting of SMRM*, p. 1172.
17. Ra JB, Rim CY. Fast imaging using subencoding data sets from multiple detectors. *Magn Reson Med* 30: 142–145, 1993.
18. Carlson JW, Minemura T. Imaging time reduction through multiple receiver coil data acquisition and image reconstruction. *Magn Reson Med* 29: 681–688, 1993.
19. Kwiat D, Einav S. Preliminary experimental evaluation of an inverse source imaging procedure using a decoupled coil detector array in magnetic resonance imaging. *Med Eng Phys* 17: 257–263, 1995.
20. Sodickson DK, Manning WJ. Simultaneous acquisition of spatial harmonics (SMASH): fast imaging with radio-frequency coil arrays. *Magn Reson Med* 38: 591–603, 1997.
21. Jakob PM, Griswold MA, Edelman RR, Sodickson DK. AUTO-SMASH, a self-calibrating technique for SMASH imaging. *MAGMA* 7: 42–54, 1998.
22. Pruessmann KP, Weiger M, Scheidigger MB, Boesiger P. SENSE: sensitivity encoding for fast MRI. *Magn Reson Med* 42: 952–962, 1999.
23. Kyriakos WE, Panych LP, Kacher DK et al. Sensitivity profiles from an array of coils for encoding and reconstruction in parallel (SPACE RIP). *Magn Reson Med* 44: 301–308, 2000.
24. Griswold MA, Jakob PM, Heidemann RM et al. Generalized auto-calibrating partially parallel acquisition (GRAPPA). *Magn Reson Med* 47: 1202–1210, 2002.
25. Ramalho M, Altun E, Heredia V, Zapparoli M, Semelka R. Liver MR imaging: 1.5T versus 3T. *Magn Reson Imaging Clin N Am* 15: 321–347, 2007.
26. Goncalves Neto JA, Altun E, Elazzazi M, Vaidean G, Chaney M, Semelka RC. Enhancement of abdominal organs on hepatic arterial phase: quantitative comparison between 1.5T and 3.0T MRI. *Magn Reson Imaging* 2009, In press.
27. Hussain SM, De Becker J, Hop WCJ, Dwarkasing S, Wielopolski PA. Can a single-shot black-blood T2-weighted spin-echo echo planar imaging sequence with sensitivity encoding replace the respiratory-triggered turbo spin-echo sequence for the liver? An optimization and a feasibility study. *J Magn Reson Imaging* 21: 219–229, 2005.
28. Lauenstein TC, Goehde SC, Herborn CU, Goyen M, Oberhoff C, Debatin JF, Ruehm SG, Barkhausen J. Whole-body MR imaging: evaluation of patients for metastases. *Radiology* 233: 139–148, 2004.
29. Ko J, Casola G. Whole Body MR Screening Found Feasible. Whole Body CT Screening. http://www.rsna.org/publications/rsnanews/febo4/mri-1.html
30. Gillman S. Imaging the brain: second of two parts. *N Engl J Med* 338(13): 889–896, 1998.
31. Semelka R, Martin D, Balci C, Lance T. Focal liver lesions: comparison of dual-phase CT and multisequence multiplanar MR imaging including dynamic gadolinium enhancement. *J Magn Reson Imaging* 13: 397–401, 2001.
32. Low R, Semelka R, Woranwattanakul S, Alzate G, Sigeti J. Extrahepatic abdominal imaging in patients with malignancy: comparison of MR imaging and helical CT, with subsequent surgical correlation. *Radiology* 210: 625–632, 1999.
33. Low R, Semelka R, Woranwattanakul S, Alzate G. Exrahepatic abdominal imaging in patients with malignancy: comparison of MR imaging and helical CT in 164 patients. *J Magn Reson Imaging* 12: 269–277, 2000.
34. Semelka RC, Kelekis NL, Molina PL, Sharp TJ, Calvo B. Pancreatic masses with inconclusive findings on spiral CT: Is there a role for MRI? *J Magn Reson Imaging* 6: 585–588, 1996.
35. Sheridan MB, Ward J, Guthrie JA, Spencer JA, Craven CM, Wilson D, Guillou P, Robinson P. Dynamic contrast-enhanced MR imaging and dual-phase helical CT in the preoperative assessment of suspected pancreatic cancer: a comparative study with receiver operating characteristic analysis. *AJR Am J Roentgenol* 173: 583–590, 1999.
36. Semelka RC, Martin D, Balci C, Lance T. Focal liver lesions: comparison of dual-phase CT and multisequence multiplanar MR

imaging Including dynamic gadolinium enhancement. *J Magn Reson Imaging* 13: 397–401, 2001.

37. Bader T, Semelka R, Pedro M, Armao D, Brown M, Molina P. Magnetic resonance imaging of pulmonary parenchymal disease using a modified breath-hold 3D gradient-echo technique: Initial observations. *J Magn Reson Imaging* 15: 31–38, 2002.

38. Budinger TF. Nuclear magnetic resonance (NMR) in vivo studies: known thresholds for health effects. *J Comp Assist Tomogr* 5: 800–811, 1981.

39. Reid A, Smith FW et al. Nuclear magnetic resonance imaging and its safety implications: follow-up of 181 patients. *Br J Radiol* 55: 784–786, 1982.

40. McRobbie D, Foster MA. Pulsed magnetic field exposure during pregnancy and implications for NMR fetal imaging: a study with mice. *Magn Reson Imaging* 3: 231–234, 1985.

41. Heinrichs WL, Fong P et al. Midgestational exposure of pregnant BALB/c mice to magnetic resonance imaging conditions. *Magn Reson Imaging* 6: 305–313, 1988.

42. Terens WL, Gluck R, Golimbu M, Rofsky NM. Use of gadolinium-DTPA-enhancement MRI to characterize renal masses in patient with renal insufficiency. *Urology* 40: 152–154, 1992.

43. Berrington de González A, Darby S. Risk of cancer from diagnostic X-rays: estimates for the UK and 14 other countries. *Lancet* 363: 345–351, 2004.

44. Brezis M, Epsetein FH. A closer look at radiocontrast-induced nephropathy. *N Engl J Med* 323: 179–181, 1989.

45. Berns AS. Nephrotoxicity of contrast media. *Kidney Int* 35: 730–740, 1989.

46. Parfrey PS, Griffths SM, Barrett BJ et al. Contrast material-induced renal failure in patients with diabetes mellitus, renal insufficiency or both; a prospective controlled study. *N Engl J Med* 323: 143–149, 1989.

LIVER

LARISSA BRAGA, DIANE ARMAO, MOHAMED ELAZZAZI,
AND RICHARD C. SEMELKA

NORMAL ANATOMY

The liver is the most massive of the viscera and commands the right upper quadrant of the abdomen. The current classification system of liver segmental anatomy, as refined by Couinaud [1], describes the liver as divided into eight independent functioning units or segments, each of which is served by its own vascular pedicle (arterial, portal venous, and lymphatic) and biliary drainage. This improved understanding of the intrahepatic architecture has fueled technical progress in liver surgery and transplantation. Vessels are clearly discernible with MRI, which makes this technique ideally suited to the study of the functional segmental anatomy of the liver (fig. 2.1).

With respect to the imaging features of liver, there are three fissures that help define functional right and left hepatic lobes and the major hepatic segments. The interlobar fissure, located on the inferior liver margin, is oriented along a line passing through the gallbladder fossa inferiorly and the middle hepatic vein superiorly. Although well defined in some patients, the interlobar fissure is usually difficult to identify. The left intersegmental fissure (fissure for the ligamentum teres) forms a well-defined sagitally oriented cleft in the caudal aspect of the left hepatic lobe, serving to divide the lobe into medial and lateral segments. The ligamentum teres, or obliterated vestige of the left umbilical vein, normally ensconced in a small amount of fat, runs through this fissure after entering it via the free margin of the falciform ligament. The third fissure, or fissure for the ligamentum venosum, is oriented in a coronal or oblique plane between the posterior aspect of the left lateral hepatic segment and the anterior aspect of the caudate lobe. This fissure forms a continuum with the intersegmental fissure. The fissure for the ligamentum venosum cuts deeply anterior to the caudate lobe and contains the two layers of the lesser omentum.

The porta hepatis is a deep transverse fissure situated between the medial segment anteriorly and the caudate process posteriorly. At the porta hepatis, the portal vein, hepatic artery, and hepatic nerve plexus enter the liver and the right and left hepatic ducts and lymphatic vessels emerge from it. The caudate lobe stands at the watershed between right and left portobiliary arterial territories. Because the caudate lobe drains directly into the inferior vena cava, it may escape injury from venous outflow obstruction [2]. Whereas branches of the hepatic artery, the portal vein, and

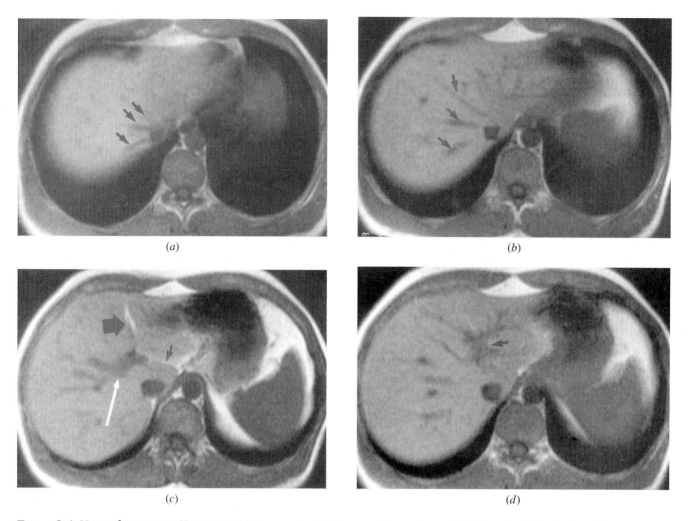

(a)   (b)

(c)   (d)

F I G . 2.1 Normal anatomy. Transverse SGE images (*a–d*). The vascular anatomy of the liver includes the hepatic venous system—superior, middle, and inferior hepatic veins (arrows, *a*, *b*) and portal venous system—right portal vein(long white arrow, *c*) and left portal vein (arrow, *d*). Note the caudate lobe, the fissure for the ligamentum venosum (small black arrow, *c*), and the fissure for the ligamentum teres (large black arrow, *c*).

tributaries of the bile ducts travel together serving segments of the liver, hepatic veins run independently and are intersegmental (fig. 2.2). The close relationship of the hepatic artery portal vein and bile ducts on a macroscopic level is mirrored on a microscopic level by the presence of portal triads comprising hepatic arterioles, portal venules, and interlobular bile ducts.

MRI TECHNIQUE

The current standard MRI examination of the liver includes a T2-weighted sequence, a T1-weighted sequence, and a dynamic contrast-enhanced sequence (fig. 2.3). The most comprehensive contrast administration approach is the use of gadolinium chelate, as a rapid bolus injection with serial imaging using spoiled gradient echo (SGE), 3D gradient echo, or a combination of both. A variety of sequences exist that generate

T2- and T1-weighted images. Field strength and gradient factors of the MRI machine generally dictate the type of sequences employed. At lower field strength (<1.0 T) spin-echo sequences are generally used because of gradient strength and signal-to-noise ratio (SNR) limitations. At high field strength (3.0 T) echo-train sequences are used for T2-weighted sequences, and gradient-echo sequences are generally used for T1-weighted sequences. At 3.0 T the higher SNR significantly improves the image quality of postcontrast 3D-GE sequences, mainly to depict and characterize small liver nodules in chronic disease. However, new sequences are needed to improve image quality before contrast and reduce artifacts [3]. See Chapter 1 for a more complete description of standard liver imaging protocols. The vast majority of liver diseases can be characterized by the combined information provided by T2, T1, and early (hepatic arterial dominant) and late (hepatic venous) gradient echo images (figs. 2.4–2.6). A recent study [4] stressed that

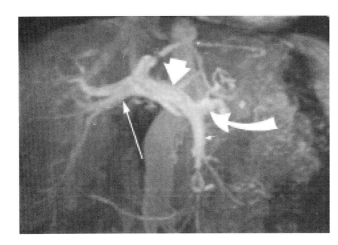

FIG. 2.2 Portal venous system. Anteroposterior projection from 3D MIP reconstruction of a set of coronal gadolinium-enhanced 2-mm 3D MRA source images. Superior mesenteric vein (small arrow), splenic vein (curved arrow), main portal vein (large arrow), and intrahepatic portal veins (long arrow) are well defined on this gadolinium-enhanced 3D MRA source image.

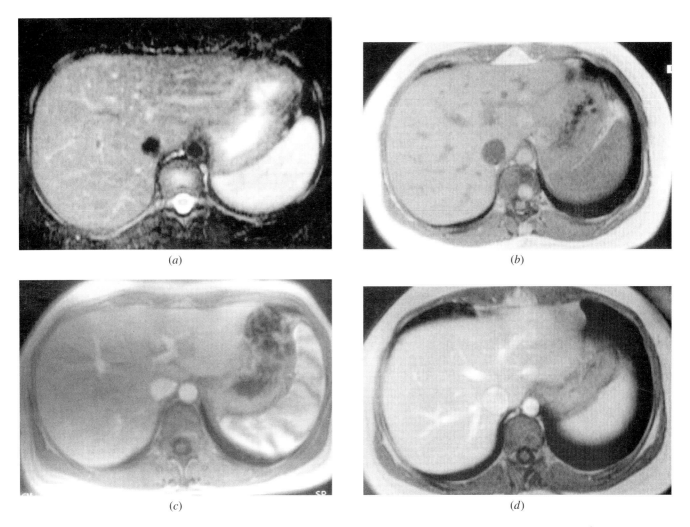

(a)

(b)

(c)

(d)

FIG. 2.3 Normal liver and sequences. T2-weighted fat-suppressed SS-ETSE (*a*), SGE (*b*), and immediate (*c*), 45-s (*d*), and 90-s fat-suppressed (*e*) postgadolinium SGE images. Liver is lower in signal than normal, non-iron-deposited spleen on the T2-weighted (*a*) and higher in signal intensity than spleen on the T1-weighted (*b*) images. A liver imaging protocol should include noncontrast T2-weighted (*a*) and T1-weighted (*b*) sequences and hepatic arterial dominant phase (*c*), early hepatic venous phase (*d*), and hepatic venous phase fat-suppressed (*e*) sequences.

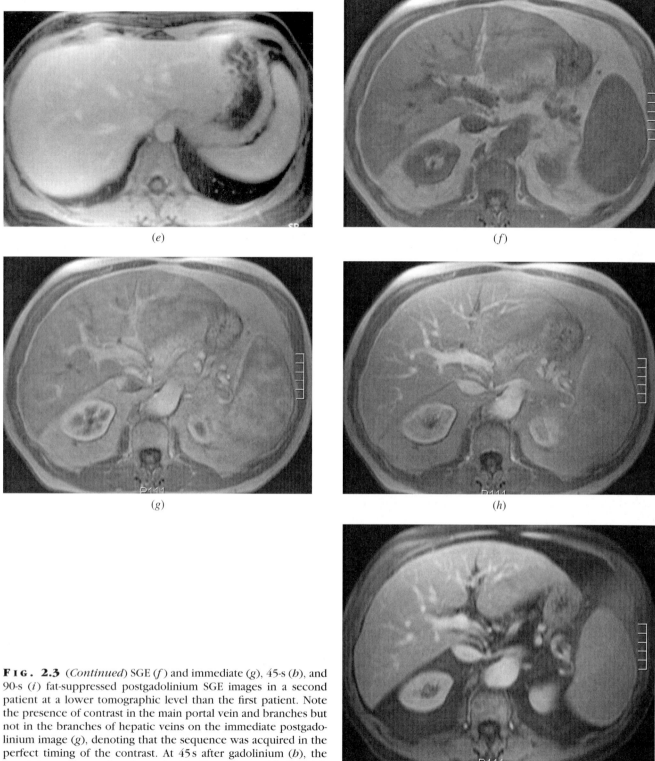

(e)

(f)

(g)

(h)

(i)

FIG. 2.3 (*Continued*) SGE (*f*) and immediate (*g*), 45-s (*h*), and 90-s (*i*) fat-suppressed postgadolinium SGE images in a second patient at a lower tomographic level than the first patient. Note the presence of contrast in the main portal vein and branches but not in the branches of hepatic veins on the immediate postgadolinium image (*g*), denoting that the sequence was acquired in the perfect timing of the contrast. At 45 s after gadolinium (*h*), the liver is homogeneously enhanced with all vessels opacified, which persists on 90-s images (*i*).

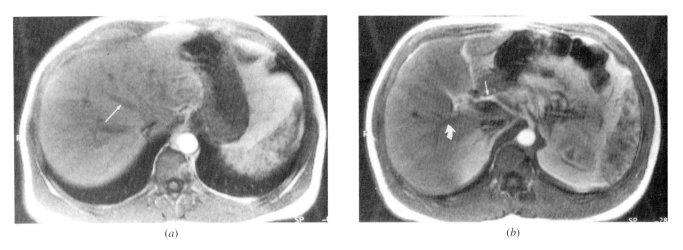

(a)   (b)

F I G . 2.4 Hepatic arterial-phase gadolinium-enhanced SGE images. Transverse hepatic arterial-phase images from the level of the hepatic veins (*a*) and portal vein (*b*). The hepatic artery (thin arrow, *b*) is enhanced. Hepatic veins (arrow, *a*) and portal vein (curved arrow, *b*) are not enhanced. Some enhancement is appreciated in the splenic parenchyma and superior aspect of the left kidney, showing that these images were acquired in approximately the middle of the hepatic arterial enhancement phase.

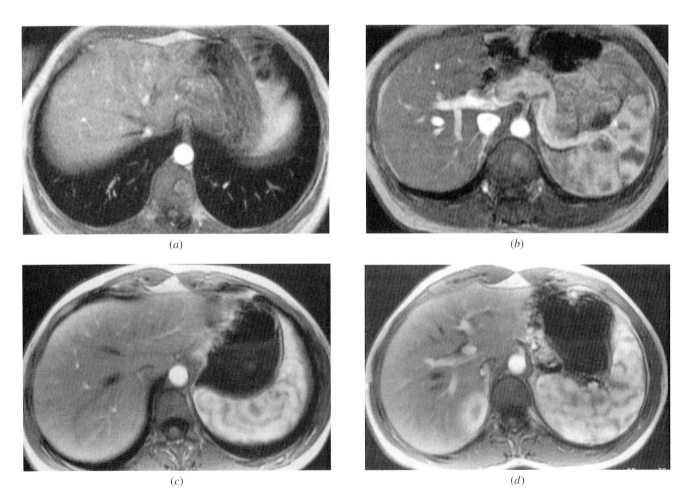

(a)   (b)

(c)   (d)

F I G . 2.5 Hepatic arterial dominant-phase gadolinium-enhanced SGE images. Immediate postgadolinium SGE images in 2 patients (*a* and *b*, and *c* and *d*, respectively). Images acquired from the higher tomographic sections (*a*, *c*) demonstrate absence of gadolinium in hepatic veins and images acquired from the more inferior tomographic sections (*b*, *d*) demonstrate presence of gadolinium in hepatic arteries and portal veins.

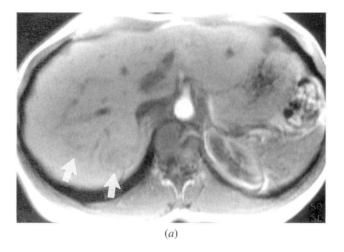

(a)

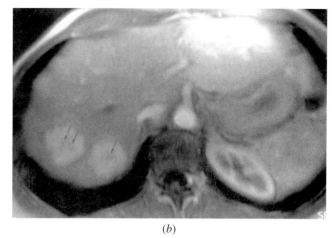

(b)

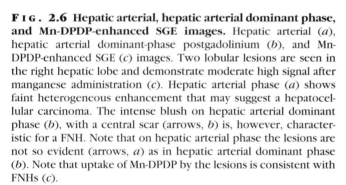

FIG. 2.6 Hepatic arterial, hepatic arterial dominant phase, and Mn-DPDP-enhanced SGE images. Hepatic arterial (*a*), hepatic arterial dominant-phase postgadolinium (*b*), and Mn-DPDP-enhanced SGE (*c*) images. Two lobular lesions are seen in the right hepatic lobe and demonstrate moderate high signal after manganese administration (*c*). Hepatic arterial phase (*a*) shows faint heterogeneous enhancement that may suggest a hepatocellular carcinoma. The intense blush on hepatic arterial dominant phase (*b*), with a central scar (arrows, *b*) is, however, characteristic for a FNH. Note that on hepatic arterial phase the lesions are not so evident (arrows, *a*) as in hepatic arterial dominant phase (*b*). Note that uptake of Mn-DPDP by the lesions is consistent with FNHs (*c*).

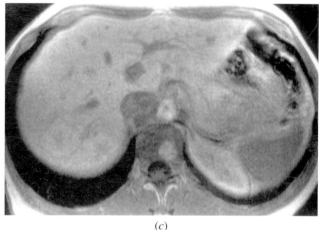

(c)

the arterial phase can be divided in five subgroups as follows: early hepatic arterial phase, mid-hepatic arterial phase, late hepatic arterial phase, splenic-vein-only hepatic arterial dominant phase, and hepatic arterial dominant phase, based on the presence of contrast in major abdominal vessels, as well as renal cortex, spleen, pancreas, and liver parenchyma. The importance of this subdivision is the impact of detection of hypervascular liver lesions based upon the phase where images were acquired. Table 2.1 describes the appearance of common focal liver lesions with this approach.

LIVER CONTRAST AGENTS

Intravenously administered contrast agents have been used in clinical magnetic resonance imaging of the liver since 1988. The need for more accurate detection and characterization of the full spectrum of liver pathology has been the major impetus for continued development in intravenous contrast agents [4, 5]. The first category of contrast agents to be used in clinical practice was that of nonspecific extracellular gadolinium chelates.

Since then, other classes of contrast agents have been developed for liver MR studies. There are two histologically and functionally distinct populations of cells in the liver. Liver epithelial cells, or hepatocytes, carry out the major metabolic activities. Hepatocyte function is assisted by another major class of cells, the reticuloendothelial system (RES), which possess storage, phagocytic, and mechanically supportive functions. In recent years, hepatocyte-selective contrast agents and RES-specific contrast agents have targeted these cell populations and added a new dimension to hepatic MR imaging. Clinically available liver contrast agents can be categorized as follows: 1) nonspecific extracellular contrast: gadolinium chelates; 2) hepatocyte-selective: Mn-DPDP (mangafodipir trisodium); 3) agents with combined early nonspecific extracellular and late hepatocyte-selective properties: Gd-EOB-DTPA (gadolinium ethoxybenzyl diethylenetriaminepentaacetic acid) and Gd-DTPA-BOPTA (gadolinium benzyloxypropionictetraacetate); 4) RES-specific: superparamagnetic iron oxide particles (SPIO); 5) agents with combined early blood pool and late RES-specific properties: ultrasmall paramagnetic iron oxide particles.

Table 2.1 Liver lesion pattern recognition

	T1	T2	EARLY GD	LATE GD	OTHER FEATURES
Cyst	↓↓	↑↑	○	○	Well defined
Hamartoma	↓↓	↑↑	Thin rim	Thin rim	<1 cm
Hemangioma	↓↓	↑↑	Peripheral nodules	Nodules coalesce, retain contrast	<1.5-cm lesion may enhance homogeneously
FNH	↓–Ø	Ø–↑	Homogeneous intense, negligible scar enhancement	Homogeneous washout, late scar enhancement	Central scar, liver is commonly fatty
Adenoma	↓–↑	Ø–↑	Homogeneous intense	Homogeneous washout	Uniform signal loss on out-of-phase T1, hemorrhage not uncommon
Metastases	↓	↑	Ring	Progressive with heterogeneous washout	<1.5-cm lesion may enhance homogeneously
HCC	↓–↑	Ø–↑	Diffuse heterogeneous	Heterogeneous late washout, capsule enhancement	<1.5-cm lesion may enhance homogeneously
Bacterial abscess	↓↓	↑–↑↑	Perilesional enhancement, capsule enhancement	Perilesional enhancement fades, capsule remains enhanced	Resemble metastases but no progressive lesion enhancement
Lymphoma, secondary	↓	↑	Ring	Progressive mild enhancement	Resemble metastases
Lymphoma, primary	↓	↑	Diffuse heterogeneous	Progressive with heterogeneous washout	Resemble HCC
Regenerative nodule	↓–Ø	↓–Ø	Negligible	Negligible	Lesions generally <1.5 cm and homogeneous
Mildly dysplastic nodule	↓–↑	—	Minimal	Minimal	Lesions generally <1.5 cm and homogeneous
Severely dysplastic nodule	↓–↑	—	Homogeneous intense	Fade to isointensity with liver	Lesions generally <1.5 cm, homogeneous, and no capsule

↓↓ Moderately decreased signal intensity, ↓ Mildly decreased signal intensity, Ø Isointense, ↑ Mildly increased signal intensity, ↑↑ Moderately increased signal intensity, ○ No enhancement

Nonspecific extracellular gadolinium chelates are the standard contrast agents to image liver and other organs and tissues in patients evaluated with MR imaging for a diverse range of indications. These paramagnetic contrast agents provide important information about tumor perfusion, which is a key factor in the assessment of liver masses [6–8]. Gadolinium chelates are optimally used when they are administered as a rapid bolus and imaging is performed with a T1-weighted gradient-echo sequence that is repeated in a dynamic serial fashion. This is best achieved at high field strength. The elimination is 100% renal. The most important phase of enhancement may be termed the hepatic arterial dominant phase, with contrast present in hepatic arteries and portal veins and before contrast appears in hepatic veins (figs. 2.5 and 2.6). The hepatic arterial phase has contrast present only in the hepatic arteries (see fig. 2.4). See Chapter 1 for a more complete description.

Hepatocyte-selective contrast agents undergo uptake by hepatocytes and are eliminated through the renal and biliary system [9–11]. This category of contrast agents—Mn-DPDP (mangofodipir), Gd-EOB-DTPA (primivist), and Gd-BOPTA (multiHance)—are all T1-relaxation-enhancing agents that are taken up by and result in an increase in the signal intensity of normal liver tissue and hepatocyte-containing tumors. Gd-EOB-DTPA and Gd-BOPTA exhibit early perfusional information as well. These contrast agents are not taken up by non-hepatocyte-containing masses (e.g., hemangioma, metastases) on late, >10-min, postcontrast images; therefore, they leave signal unchanged in these entities on T1-weighted images. Non-hepatocyte-containing masses are rendered more conspicuous by the increase in signal of background liver tissue. Advantages of T1 relaxation agents include the following: 1) Use of gradient echo (as 2D or 3D sequences with or without fat suppression) results in robust, reproducible image quality with complete liver coverage in one breath hold, and 2) they do not result in artifacts, such as susceptibility artifact, that can mask small lesions. Mangofodipir and multiHance are licensed by the FDA for use in humans. Mangofodipir is administered as a slow (1 min) intravenous infusion, and the maximal imaging window is between 15 min and 4h [5, 12, 13]. Dynamic images cannot be obtained with this agent, and therefore it is not necessary that the MR machine have high field strength. At this stage of clinical use, this agent appears to be safe and well tolerated. At present, the best clinical role for Mn-DPDP is to improve detection of the number and extension of focal liver metastases from colon cancer in patients in whom hepatic resection is being contemplated [5, 13, 14]. The combined use of conventional gadolinium chelates and Mn-DPDP has been described [13]. This approach combines the perfusional information of gadolinium with the hepatocyte uptake information of Mn-DPDP (fig. 2.7). In selected cases, the combination of gadolinium chelates and liver-specific contrast agents may provide additional information. This combined-agent approach may not be necessary any more since multiHance, which possesses

both early perfusional and late hepatocellular activity, is now licensed for use.

Gd-EOB-DTPA (fig. 2.8) and Gd-BOPTA are combined extracellular/hepatocyte agents that can be used to acquire early perfusional information similar to standard gadolinium chelates. Gd-EOB-DTPA demonstrates diagnostically useful hepatocyte enhancement at 10–15 min after injection, whereas Gd-BOPTA requires a delay of 1 h after injection for hepatocyte selection enhancement [15–21]. The early perfusional information is very important for lesion characterization, with the additional benefit of improved detection, particularly for hypervascular lesions. The late images may be used for lesion detection with some additional information to distinguish hepatocyte-containing from non-hepatocyte-containing tumors. Although hepatocyte-specific agents

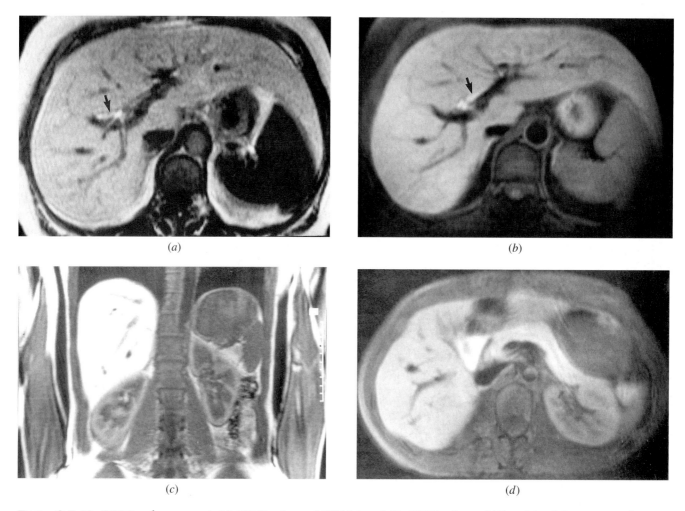

(a)   (b)

(c)   (d)

F I G . 2.7 Mn-DPDP-enhancement. Mn-DPDP-enhanced SGE (*a*) and Mn-DPDP-enhanced T1-weighted fat-suppressed SE (*b*) images in a normal patient. Normal liver homogeneously enhances with Mn-DPDP because of its T1-shortening effect. Excretion of Mn-DPDP in the biliary system is shown as high-signal-intensity fluid in biliary ducts (arrow, *a*, *b*).
    Coronal Mn-DPDP-enhanced SGE (*c*) and transverse Mn-DPDP-enhanced T1-weighted fat-suppressed spin-echo (*d*) images in a second patient. Note the increased signal intensity of normal liver tissue after administration of Mn-DPDP.

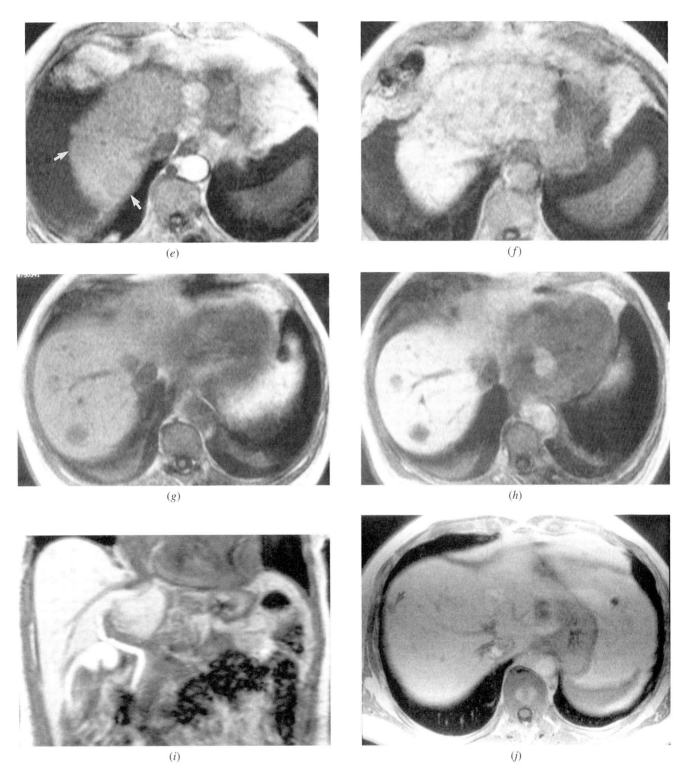

F I G . 2.7 (*Continued*) SGE (*e*) and 30-min post-Mn-DPDP SGE (*f*) images in a third patient. Subtle low-signal-intensity mass lesions are apparent on the precontrast image (arrows, *e*). After Mn-DPDP enhancement (*f*) the HCCs enhance slightly more intensely than background liver, rendering the tumors minimally hyperintense. A pseudocapsule is appreciated around the more posterior tumor on both the precontrast and postcontrast images.

Transverse noncontrast SGE (*g*) and 10-min post-Mn-DPDP-enhanced SGE (*h*) and coronal 10-min Mn-DPDP-enhanced SGE (*i*) images in a fourth patient with liver metastases. The liver increases in signal from pre (*g*)- to post (*h*)-Mn images, increasing the conspicuity of the metastases. Note the excretion of Mn-DPDP into the biliary system (*i*).

Mn-DPDP-enhanced 512-resolution SGE image (*j*) in a fifth patient who has a liver metastasis (arrow, *j*). The liver detail is greater than usual, reflecting the use of 512 matrix.

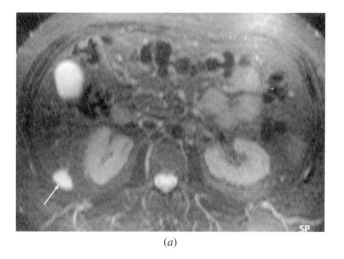

(a)

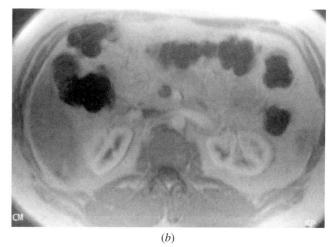

(b)

F I G . 2.8 Hemangioma, Gd-EOB-DTPA-enhanced. Echo-train STIR (*a*) and immediate (*b*) and 10-min post-Gd-EOB-DTPA (*c*) images. There is a lobular lesion in the tip of the right lobe (arrow, *a*) that is high signal intensity on the T2-weighted image (*a*) and exhibits peripheral nodular enhancement immediately after the administration of contrast (*b*) and hepatocellular uptake and washout of the lesion at 5 min. This lesion is consistent with a hemangioma based on the well-defined lobular margins, high signal on T2, and early peripheral nodular enhancement.

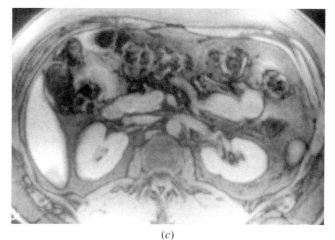

(c)

permit distinction between hepatocyte-containing tumors (e.g., adenoma, focal nodular hyperplasia, hepatocellular carcinoma) and non-hepatocyte-containing tumors (e.g., hemangioma, metastases), it is generally more important to distinguish between benign and malignant tumors. Early perfusional information generally achieves this goal. Gd-BOPTA provides distinction between FNH, which demonstrates delayed 1-h enhancement, and hepatic adenoma and moderately poorly differentiated HCC, which do not exhibit late enhancement (fig. 2.9).

Iron oxide particle agents are selectively taken up by RES in the liver, spleen, and bone marrow. This class of contrast agent is also termed superparamagnetic iron oxide (SPIO), and the first of these agents licensed for use in the United States are the ferumoxides. RES cell-specific contrast agents are T2 relaxation-enhancing agents that lower the signal intensity of normal RES cell-containing liver tissue on T2-weighted images and do not alter the signal intensity of mass lesions that do not contain RES cells (e.g., metastases) [22–24]. Blood pool effects may be observed with hemangiomas, which

can result in T1 shortening on T1-weighted sequences [25, 26]. This results in an increase in detection and in the conspicuity of liver tumors that are moderately high in signal intensity on T2-weighted images [25] (fig. 2.10). The patient group in which this role for SPIO may be the most applicable is patients with liver metastases from colon cancer and HCC who are considered to be candidates for hepatic resection or liver transplant [5, 27, 28]. Studies have shown that SPIO-enhanced T2-weighted MR imaging has performance comparable to that of CT during arterial portography for the demonstration of liver metastases [29, 30]. However, other reports demonstrated that SPIO-enhanced MRI has a higher sensitivity and accuracy to detect hepatic malignancies than helical CT [31–34]. A cautionary note for this agent is that susceptibility artifact may potentially interfere with detection of sub-centimeter lesions such as metastases. A number of sequences have been employed to improve image quality, including gradient-echo sequences with a longer TE (≥6 ms), single-shot or breath-hold echo-train spin echo, and breathing-averaged proton density echo-train spin echo. Combined

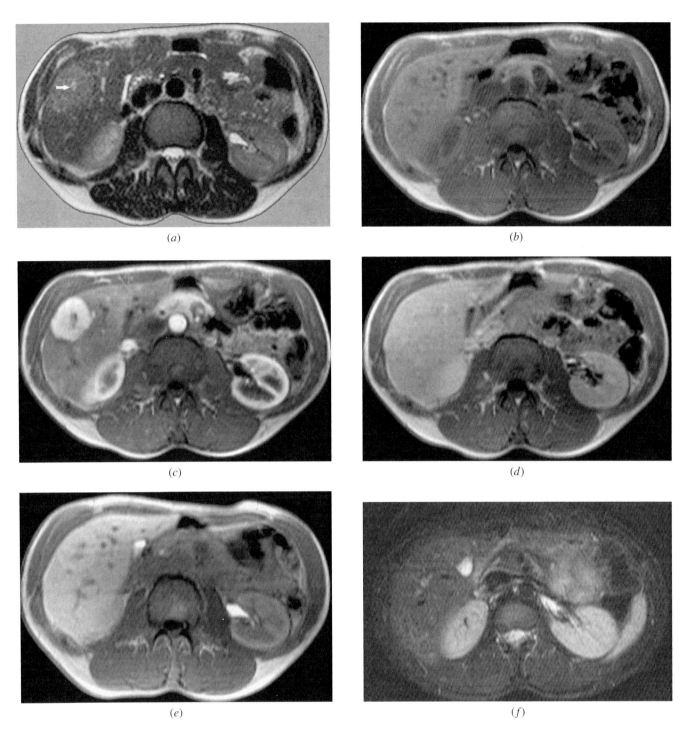

F I G . 2.9 FNH, Gd-BOPTA-enhanced. SS-ETSE (*a*), SGE (*b*), and immediate (*c*), 90-s (*d*), and 1-h (*e*) postinjection Gd-BOPTA contrast images. There is a lesion in the right hepatic lobe that exhibits slightly high signal intensity on T2-weighted image (*a*), isointensity on T1-weighted image (*b*), and intense enhancement on immediate post contrast image (*c*) and fades as the background parenchyma on 90-s postcontrast image (*d*). This lesion has a central scar that is well seen on the T2-weighted image (arrow, *a*) and on the immediate postcontrast image (*c*). On 90-s postcontrast image (*d*) the scar enhances and acquires signal intensity comparable to the lesion. The lesion shows higher signal intensity than the background parenchyma 1 h after administration of contrast (*e*), and the scar demonstrates lower signal intensity than the lesion, consistent with lesional contrast uptake in this phase. (Courtesy of Guenther Schneider, M.D., Ph.D., Dept. of Diagnostic and Interventional Radiology, University Hospital Homburg/Saar, Germany.)

T2-weighted SS-ETSE (*f*), SGE (*g*), and immediate (*h*), 90-s fat-suppressed (*i*), and 1-h (*j*) postcontrast SGE images in a second patient show similar findings. The tumor enhances intensely on immediate postcontrast images (arrow, *h*) and shows 1-h delayed

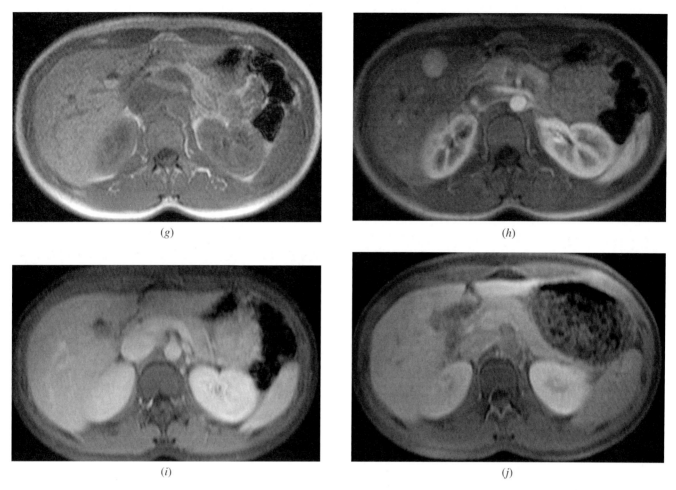

(g)

(h)

(i)

(j)

F I G . 2.9 (*Continued*) enhancement, consistent with and FNH. The central scar is not as well defined as in the first patient.

use of SPIO and conventional gadolinium chelates has been described [35]. This approach combines the perfusional information of gadolinium with the RES information of SPIO. It may be expected that their combined use would be more effective for detection and characterizing focal lesions than either contrast agent alone [35]. The long infusion period (30 min) is an inconvenient aspect of this agent, which necessitates two imaging sessions for nonenhanced and enhanced images. Attractive features of the agent include the long imaging window (1–4 h), no need for precise dynamic image acquisition related to contrast material administration, and acceptable image quality with machines of various field strengths. Although serious adverse events are rare, approximately 3% of patients will experience severe back pain while the contrast agent is being administered. This back pain appears to be a side effect of particulate agents in general and develops in patients in whom the contrast agent is administered too rapidly

[35]. This agent can also be administered as a small-volume rapid bolus, which is greatly advantageous over the larger particulate agent superparamagnetic iron oxide.

Ultrasmall paramagnetic iron oxide particles have blood pool effects that may be helpful in detecting or characterizing vascular lesions such as hemangiomas [36] and provide bright vessel enhancement in the vascular phase, which can be used for MR angiography [5].

Other tissue-specific contrast agents are under development such as those targeted to cell membrane antigens [37]. The application and role of new contrast agents will ultimately depend on how they compare with nonspecific extracellular gadolinium chelates. Prior studies have compared contrast agents in an attempt to define clinical uses [12, 17, 38–42]. Defined clinical roles are under development for these new agents. It is likely that the majority of these agents cannot replace extracellular gadolinium entirely because of its broad applicability.

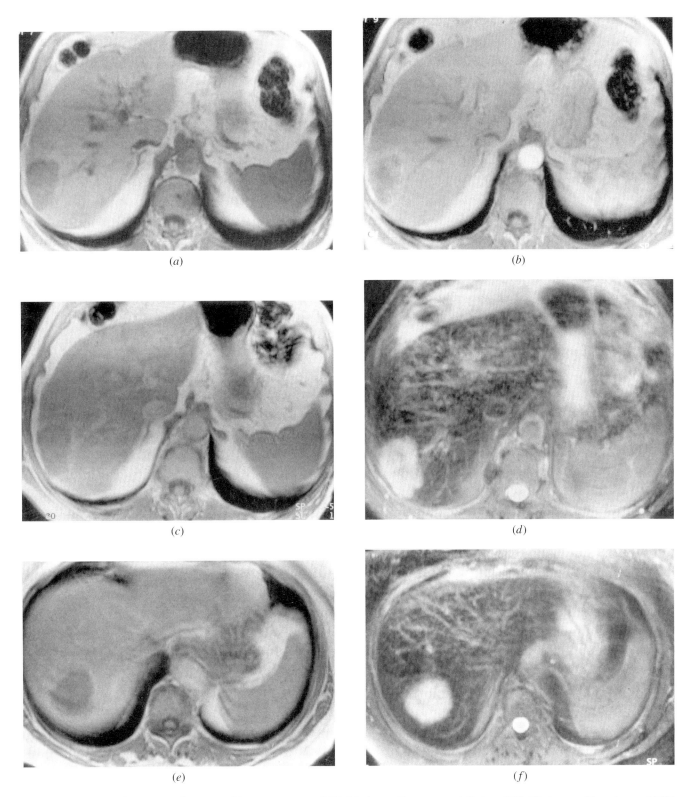

(a)

(b)

(c)

(d)

(e)

(f)

FIG. 2.10 Gadolinium and iron oxide. Noncontrast SGE (*a*), immediate postgadolinium SGE (*b*), iron oxide-enhanced SGE (*c*), and iron oxide-enhanced T2-weighted fat-suppressed (*d*) images in a patient with colon carcinoma imaged with a gadolinium study performed 19 days before an iron oxide study. A 3-cm metastasis is seen in the right hepatic lobe, which is moderately low signal on the noncontrast SGE image (*a*) and demonstrates a peripheral ring enhancement on the immediate postgadolinium SGE image (*b*), consistent with metastasis. On the iron oxide-enhanced SGE image (*c*), a lowered signal intensity in the liver and spleen is noted, diminishing the conspicuity of the metastasis. On the iron oxide-enhanced T2-weighted image (*d*), the signal intensity of the liver and spleen are markedly lower, increasing the conspicuity of the metastasis.

Iron oxide-enhanced SGE (*e*), iron oxide-enhanced T2-weighted fat-suppressed (*f*), and immediate postgadolinium iron oxide-enhanced SGE (*g*) images in a second patient with colon carcinoma imaged with iron oxide and gadolinium contrast agents, with iron oxide imaged first in a combined protocol. A lesion is present in the right hepatic lobe, which is low signal intensity on the iron oxide-enhanced SGE image (*e*) and high signal intensity on the iron oxide-enhanced T2-weighted image (*f*). The lesion enhances

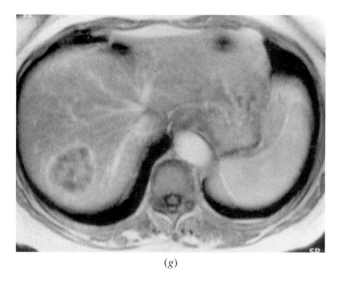

(g)

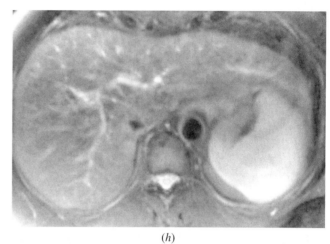

(h)

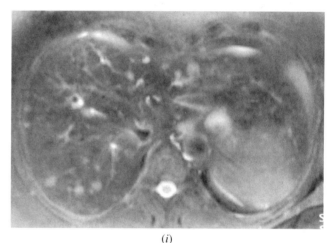

(i)

FIG. 2.10 (*Continued*) with a peripheral ring pattern consistent with a metastasis on the immediate postgadolinium iron oxide-enhanced SGE image (*g*). Lesion conspicuity is high on the postgadolinium iron oxide-enhanced image because of the lowered signal intensity of the background liver parenchyma and intense early enhancement of the neoplasm. (Reproduced with permission from Semelka RC, Lee JKT, Worawattanakul S, Noone TC, Patt RH, Asher SM. Sequential use of ferumoxide particles and gadolinium chelate for the evaluation of focal liver lesions on MRI. *J Magn Reson Imaging* 8: 670–674, 1998).

Nonenhanced (*h*) and iron oxide particulate-enhanced (*i*) T2-weighted fat-suppressed ETSE images in a third patient, who has liver metastases. After contrast administration (*i*), a greater number of <1-cm metastases are identified in the liver.

NORMAL VARIATIONS

A number of normal variations in liver size and shape occur. Common variations include horizontal elongation of the lateral segment of the left lobe, hypoplasia of the left lobe, and vertical elongation of the right lobe, termed the Riedel lobe. The Riedel lobe is fairly common and is characterized by a downward tonguelike projection of the right lobe. This anatomic variation is more frequent in women [43]. Correct identification of a Riedel lobe is necessary to avoid confusion with hepatomegaly. Transverse and coronal images are effective at demonstrating this variant, and coronal images are useful for excluding an exophytic mass lesion such as hepatic adenoma or HCC (fig. 2.11).

An elongated lateral segment may wrap around the anterior aspect of the upper abdomen and extend laterally to the spleen. This variation is also more common in women. A clear distinction between liver and spleen may be made with T2-weighted images, in which normal spleen is high in signal intensity and distinct from the lower-signal-intensity liver (fig. 2.12). Hypoplasia of the left lobe does not generally result in diagnostic difficulties, although it may simulate a left hepatectomy, which clinical history readily establishes.

Diaphragmatic insertions are not an uncommon finding along the lateral aspect of the liver. They tend to be multiple and closely related to overlying ribs, having wedge-shaped margins with the capsular surface of the liver (fig. 2.13). Insertions are low in signal on T2- and T1-weighted images. These features help to distinguish diaphragmatic insertions from peripheral mass lesions.

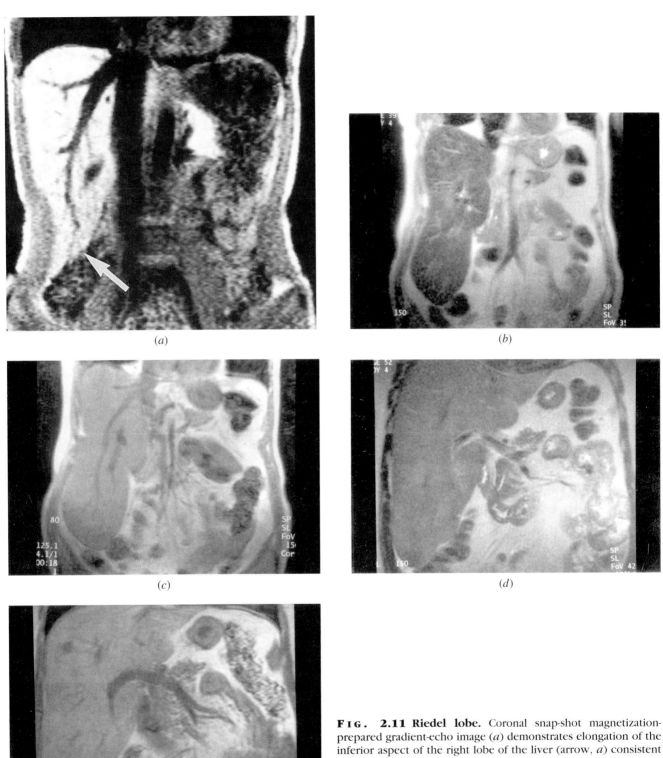

(a)

(b)

(c)

(d)

(e)

F I G . 2.11 Riedel lobe. Coronal snap-shot magnetization-prepared gradient-echo image (*a*) demonstrates elongation of the inferior aspect of the right lobe of the liver (arrow, *a*) consistent with Riedel lobe.

Coronal T2-weighted SS-ETSE (*b*) and SGE (*c*) images in a second patient exhibit a Riedel lobe with bulbous inferior aspect.

Coronal T2-weighted SS-ETSE (*d*) and SGE (*e*) images in a third patient demonstrate hypertrophy of the Riedel lobe, with a convex medial border.

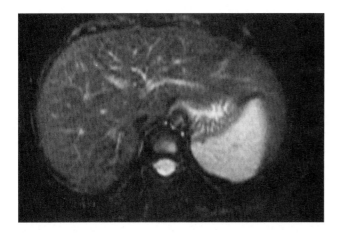

FIG. 2.12 Elongated lateral segment of the left lobe. T2-weighted fat-suppressed ETSE image demonstrates an elongated lateral segment that extends lateral to the spleen. Clear distinction is made between lower-signal-intensity liver and moderately high-signal-intensity spleen on T2-weighted images.

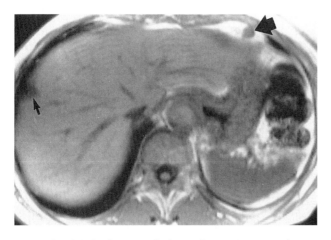

FIG. 2.13 Diaphragmatic insertion. SGE image demonstrates a wedge-shaped defect along the lateral superior margin of the liver (arrow). Diaphragmatic insertions are usually multiple but may be single as in this case. Incidental note is made of a subdiaphragmatic lymph node (large arrow).

DISEASE OF THE HEPATIC PARENCHYMA

Benign Masses

Solitary (Nonparasitic) Cysts

Hepatic cysts are common lesions and are usually divided into unilocular (95 %) or multilocular varieties. Although the pathogenesis of these cysts is not clear, developmental and acquired causes are postulated. Acquired cysts are thought to represent retention cysts of bile ductule derivation [44]. Pathologically, the lining of the cyst shows a single layer of cuboidal to columnar epithelial cells. Lining epithelium rests on an underlying fibrous stroma.

On imaging, cysts are homogeneous, well-defined lesions that possess a sharp margin with liver. Although slight variations are common, cysts are usually oval-shaped [45]. Occasionally, cysts are so closely grouped that they resemble a multicystic mass. Simple cysts are low in signal intensity on T1-weighted images and high in signal intensity on T2-weighted images, and thus retain signal intensity on longer echo time (e.g. >120 ms) T2-weighted images. Because cysts do not enhance with gadolinium on MR images, delayed postgadolinium images (up to 5 min) may be useful to ensure that lesions are cysts and not poorly vascularized metastases that show gradual enhancement (figs. 2.14–2.17) [46]. Rarely, a simple cyst may bleed because of trauma or malformation within or nearby the cyst wall. On T2- and T1-weighed precontrast images, the hemorrhagic cysts may show variable findings according to the age of hemorrhage (see trauma section) (fig. 2.18). Fluid-fluid level within the cyst cavity and a thickened and irregular wall are often observed in the hemorrhagic cyst [47]. Negligible enhancement of the cyst walls is generally present when the cysts do not exhibit inflammatory or fibrotic changes.

An advantage of MRI over computed tomography (CT) imaging in the characterization of cysts is that on gadolinium-enhanced MR images cysts are nearly signal void, whereas cysts on contrast-enhanced CT images are a light gray in attenuation. Single-shot breathing-independent T2-weighted sequences (e.g., SS-ETSE) are especially effective at showing small (≤5 mm) cysts. MRI is particularly valuable when lesions are small and the patient has a known primary malignancy.

Ciliated Hepatic Foregut Cysts

Foregut cysts are an uncommon type of solitary unilocular cyst. These congenital lesions are believed to arise from the embryonic foregut and to differentiate toward bronchial tissue in the liver. Pathologically, the cyst wall consists of four layers: pseudostratified ciliated columnar epithelium with mucous cells, subepithelial connective tissue, abundant smooth muscle, and an outermost fibrous capsule. These cysts are most frequently located at the anterosuperior margin of the liver, but may be situated elsewhere, superficially along the external surface of the liver, typically at intersegmental locations.

On MRI, foregut cysts characteristically bulge the liver contour and show hyperintensity on T2-weighted images and range from hypo- to hyperintense on T1-weighted images [48, 49]. The presence of mucin in these cysts results in high signal intensity on T1-weighted images, with the extent of increase in signal intensity dependent on the concentration of mucin (fig. 2.19).

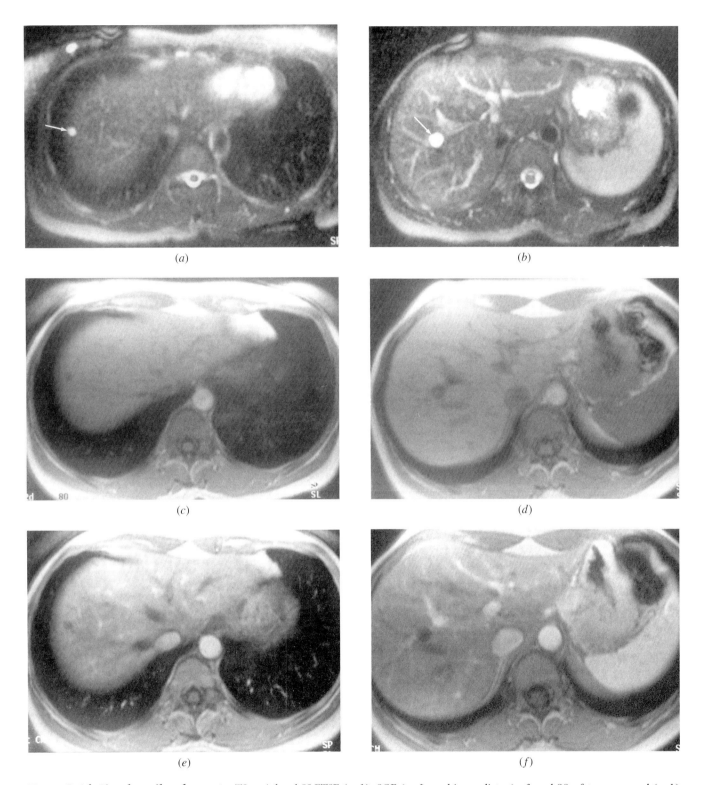

F I G . 2.14 Simple unilocular cysts. T2-weighted SS-ETSE (*a, b*), SGE (*c, d*), and immediate (*e, f*) and 90-s fat-suppressed (*g, h*) postgadolinium SGE images in the same patient but at different levels. There are two well-defined lesions (arrow, *a, b*) that are homogeneously high signal on T2-weighted images (*a, b*) and homogeneously low signal on T1-weighted images (*c, d*) and show no enhancement after administration of gadolinium (*e–h*), consistent with simple liver cysts.

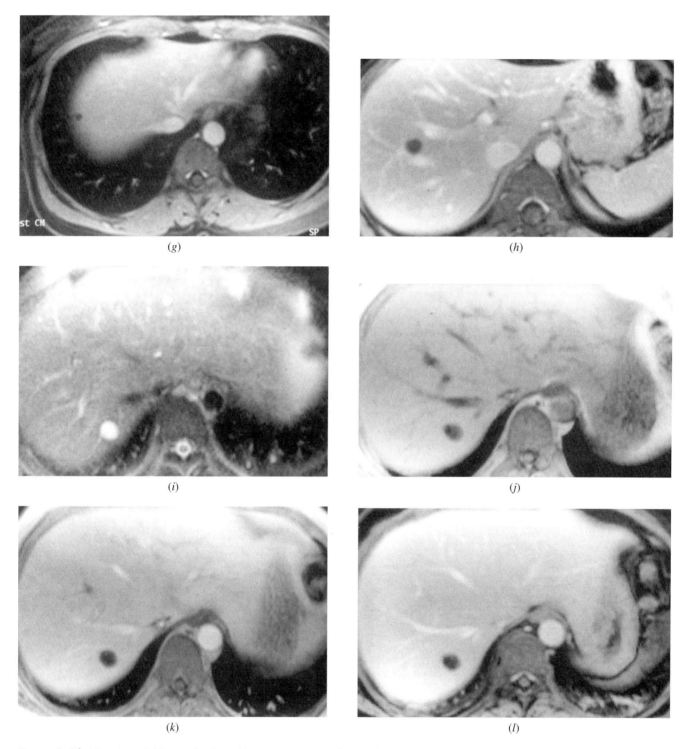

(g)

(h)

(i)

(j)

(k)

(l)

FIG. 2.14 (*Continued*) T2-weighted SS-ETSE (*i*), SGE (*j*), and immediate (*k*) and 90-s fat-suppressed (*l*) postgadolinium images in a second patient that demonstrate a small cyst in the right hepatic lobe with the same MRI characteristics as described above.

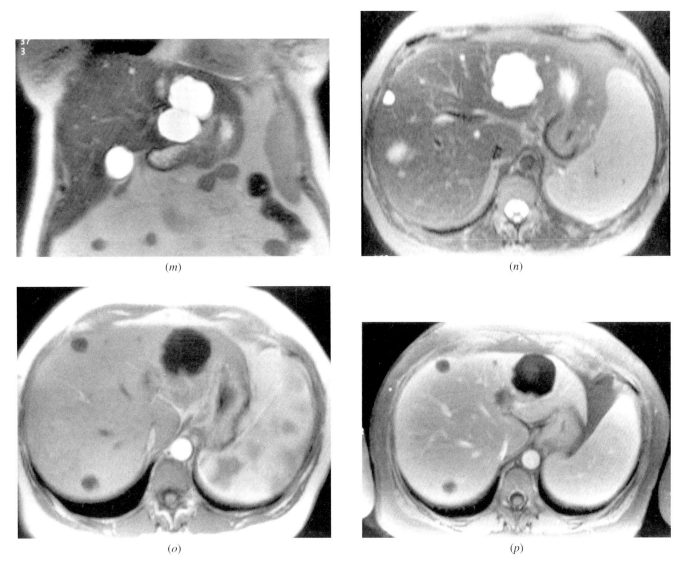

(m)

(n)

(o)

(p)

F I G . 2.14 (*Continued*) Coronal T2-weighted SS-ETSE (*m*), transverse echo train-STIR (*n*), and immediate (*o*) and 90-s fat-suppressed (*p*) postgadolinium SGE images in a third patient. Multiple simple cysts of different sizes are scattered throughout the hepatic parenchyma.

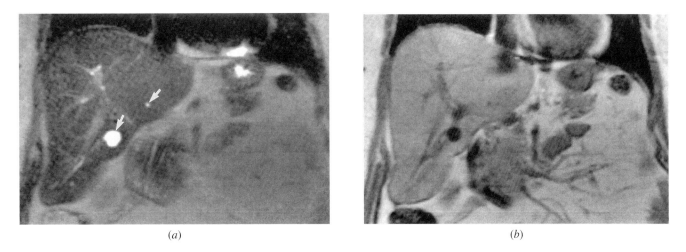

(a)

(b)

F I G . 2.15 Small simple cysts. Coronal T2-weighted SS-ETSE (*a*), SGE (*b*), and immediate (*c*) and 90-s fat-suppressed (*d*) post-gadolinium SGE images. Two cysts, 2 mm and 10 mm, are present in this patient. Cysts measuring <5 mm are most clearly shown

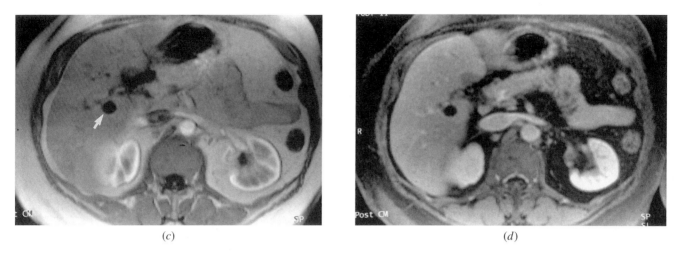

(c)   (d)

FIG. 2.15 (*Continued*) on T2-weighted images (arrows, *a*). The 10-mm cyst is signal void on early (arrow, *c*) and late (*d*) postgadolinium images.

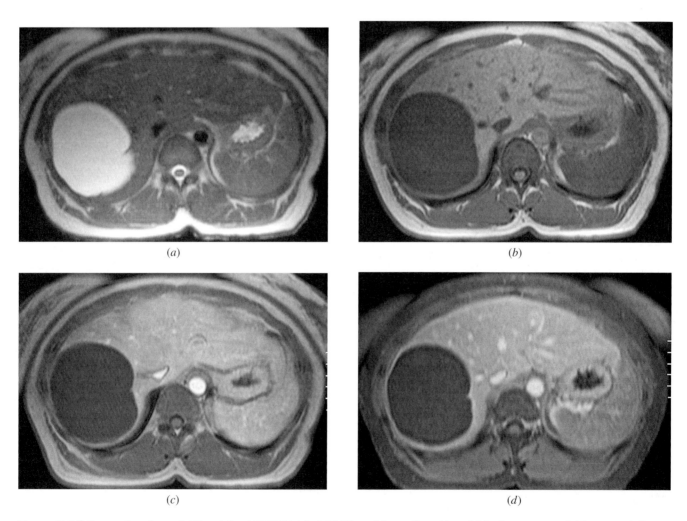

(a)   (b)

(c)   (d)

FIG. 2.16 Large simple cyst. T2-weighted SS-ETSE (*a*), SGE (*b*), and immediate (*c*) and 90-s fat-suppressed (*d*) postgadolinium SGE images. A large cyst is seen in the right hepatic lobe, which shows high signal intensity on the T2-weighted image (*a*), low signal intensity on the T1-weighted image (*b*), and lack of enhancement on early (*c*)- and late (*d*)-phase images.

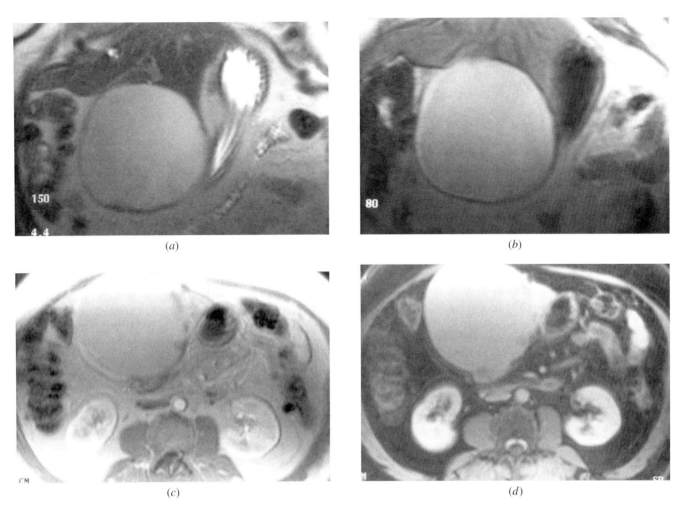

F I G. 2.17 Hemorrhagic cyst. Coronal T2-weighted SS-ETSE (*a*), transverse SGE (*b*), and transverse immediate (*c*) and 90-s fat-suppressed(*d*) postgadolinium images. A large cystic mass with thickened and irregular wall arises from the lateral segment of the liver and demonstrates high signal on both T2-weighted (*a*) and T1-weighted (*b*) images and lack of enhancement on early (*c*) and late (*d*) postcontrast images. A blood-filled cyst was proven by histopathology.

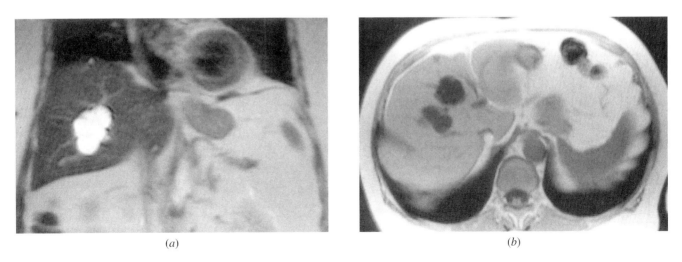

F I G. 2.18 Multilocular cyst. Coronal T2-weighted SS-ETSE (*a*), transverse SGE (*b*), and immediate (*c*) and 90-s fat-suppressed (*d*) postgadolinium SGE images. Multiple cystic lesions, some with internal septations, are present in the liver parenchyma.

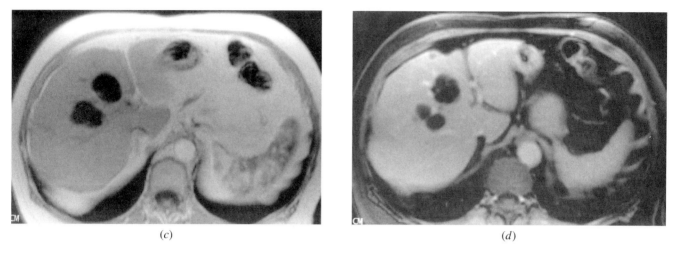

(c)   (d)

F I G . 2.18 (*Continued*)

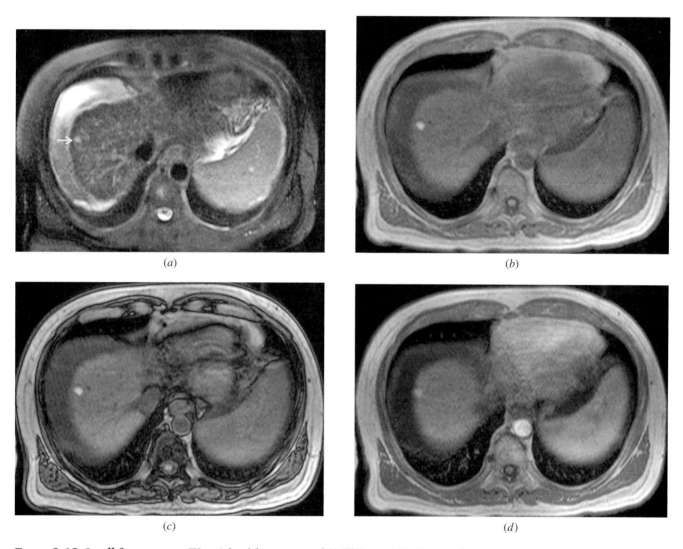

(a)   (b)

(c)   (d)

F I G . 2.19 Small foregut cyst. T2-weighted fat-suppressed SS-ETSE (*a*), SGE (*b*), out-of-phase SGE (*c*), and immediate postgado-linium SGE (*d*) images. A small lesion is seen superiorly in the liver (arrow, *a*) that exhibits high signal intensity on all sequences (*a–d*). Note that on the out-of-phase image (*c*) the lesion signal intensity does not drop, confirming that the high signal intensity on the in-phase T1-weighted image represents mucin (proteinaceous material) rather than fat within the lesion.

On the serial dynamic enhanced images, there is a lack of lesional enhancement but a subtle perceptible enhancing cyst wall is noticed (figs. 2.20 and 2.21). The presence of a cystic lesion with an enhancing wall and extension beyond the contour of the liver may also be observed in some forms of metastatic disease such as hepatic metastasis from ovarian malignancies. For this reason, a diagnosis of foregut cyst on imaging studies should only be made in the absence of peritoneal disease and a clinical history of malignancy.

Autosomal Dominant Polycystic Kidney Disease

In autosomal dominant polycystic kidney (ADPKD) disease, the liver is the most common extrarenal organ in which cysts occur. It is estimated that up to 75% of patients with ADPKD have hepatic involvement. Although these cysts vary in number and size, they tend to be multiple and smaller than the renal cysts, measuring up to 4 cm [50]. However, extensive hepatic replacement with large cysts has been described [51]. Liver cysts in ADPKD generally do not distort hepatic architecture or undergo hemorrhage, in contrast to kidney cysts in this entity. Liver cysts in the setting of ADPKD exhibit the same MR features as simple cysts, mentioned above in this section (figs. 2.22 and 2.23). Occasionally, hemorrhage may be observed in cysts. Massive involvement of the liver with large cysts, which are sometimes hemorrhagic, may result in right upper quadrant pain [50].

Biliary Hamartoma

Biliary hamartomas (or von Meyenburg complexes) are benign biliary malformations, which are currently considered as part of the spectrum of fibropolycystic diseases of the liver due to ductal plate malformation [52]. This entity is common and estimated to be present in approximately 3% of patients. Tumors may be solitary or multiple, and multiple tumors can be extensive.

Histopathologically biliary hamartomas consist of a collection of small, sometimes dilated, irregular and branching bile ducts embedded in a fibrous stroma. A few of the ducts may contain inspissated bile. In general, biliary hamartomas contain no or few vascular channels.

On MR images, lesions are small (usually <1 cm) and well defined. The high fluid content renders these lesions high signal on T2-weighted images, low signal on T1-weighted images, and negligible lesional enhancement on early and late postgadolinium images. Although this appearance resembles simple cysts, biliary hamartomas demonstrate a subtle thin rim of enhancement on early and late postcontrast images (figs. 2.24 and 2.25). The major potential diagnostic error is to misclassify these lesions as metastases because of the presence of the rim enhancement. The thin enhancing rim of biliary hamartomas, visualized on imaging, may be cor-

related histopathologically with the presence of compressed hepatic parenchyma bordering the lesion [52]. In contrast, the pattern of ring enhancement displayed by metastases relates histopathologically with the outer, most vascularized portion of the tumor. Peritumoral enhancement is also observed in some metastases as described in the next section. MR imaging further corroborates the different histologic profiles of the two processes through the observation that enhancement in biliary hamartoma does not progress centrally, whereas enhancement in metastases most often progresses centrally (fig. 2.26).

Biliary Cystadenoma/Cystadenocarcinoma

Although rare, benign and malignant cystic tumors of biliary origin may arise in the liver. There is a peak incidence of these lesions in the fifth decade, with a great predominance in women. Pathologically, on gross inspection, tumors are typically large and multiloculated and filled with clear or mucinous fluid. Mural nodules may be a component of some cysts. Histologically, cystic and stromal components are present to variable degrees. Malignant lesions will exhibit pronounced cytologic atypia with evidence of stromal invasion [53–56].

On imaging, these tumors frequently have solid nodules associated with cystic components (fig. 2.27) [57]. Occasionally, mucin content renders these tumors high in signal intensity on T1-weighted images [53, 56]. Solid components of the tumor demonstrate early heterogeneous enhancement in a pattern consistent with tumors of hepatic origin. Enhancement is often minimal in intensity, distinguishing these tumors from the extensive enhancement of HCC [58].

Extramedullary Hematopoiesis

Focal intrahepatic extramedullary hematopoiesis (EH) is an unusual condition that may appear as focal hepatic masses in the setting of hereditary disorders of hematopoiesis or in longstanding hematologic malignancies. EH is a compensatory phenomenon that occurs when erythrocyte production is diminished or destruction is accelerated [59]. EH is usually microscopic and commonly involves the liver, spleen, and lymph nodes. Rarely, the involvement may be macroscopic [59]. The focal hepatic disease can manifest as solitary or multiple lesions [60]. The masses tend to be homogeneously moderate high signal intensity on T2- and T1-weighted images and usually enhance in a diffuse homogeneous fashion on immediate postgadolinium images (fig. 2.28). A histopathological specimen is required for definitive diagnosis.

Angiomyolipomas

Angiomyolipomas of the liver are uncommon benign mesenchymal tumors. Histologically, the tumor is

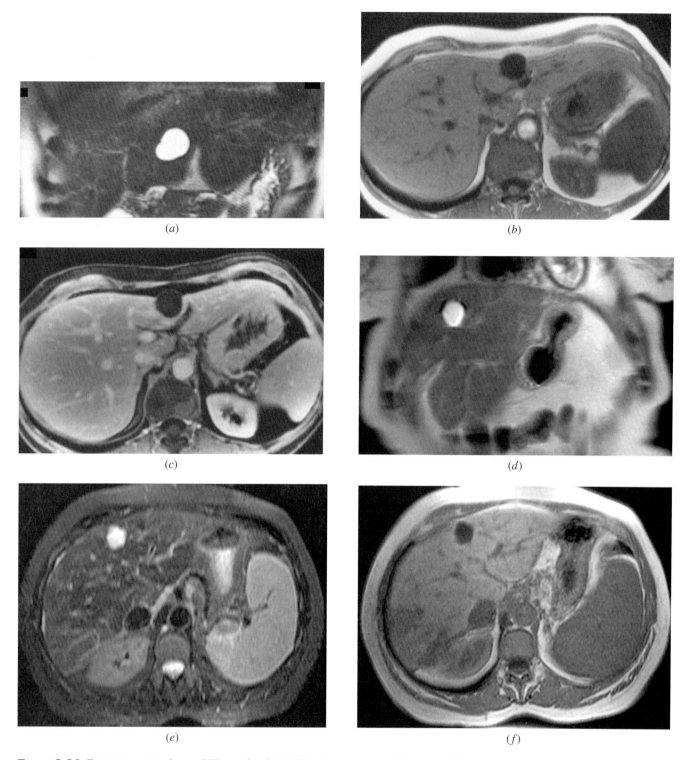

(a)   *(b)*

(c)   *(d)*

(e)   *(f)*

FIG. 2.20 Foregut cysts. Coronal T2-weighted SS-ETSE (*a*), transverse SGE (*b*), and 90-s fat-suppressed postgadolinium SGE (*c*) images. A 3-cm cystic lesion is noted superiorly on the border between medial and lateral segments. The lesion extends beyond the contour of the liver and has a thin perceptible wall, features that are characteristic of foregut cysts.

Coronal T2-weighted SS-ETSE (*d*), transverse T2-weighted fat-suppressed SS-ETSE (*e*), SGE (*f*), and immediate (*g*) and 90-s fat-suppressed (*h*) postgadolinium SGE images in a second patient. A cystic lesion is seen in segment 4 of the liver, consistent with a foregut cyst. Note faint enhancement of the cyst wall best appreciated on the late-phase image (*h*).

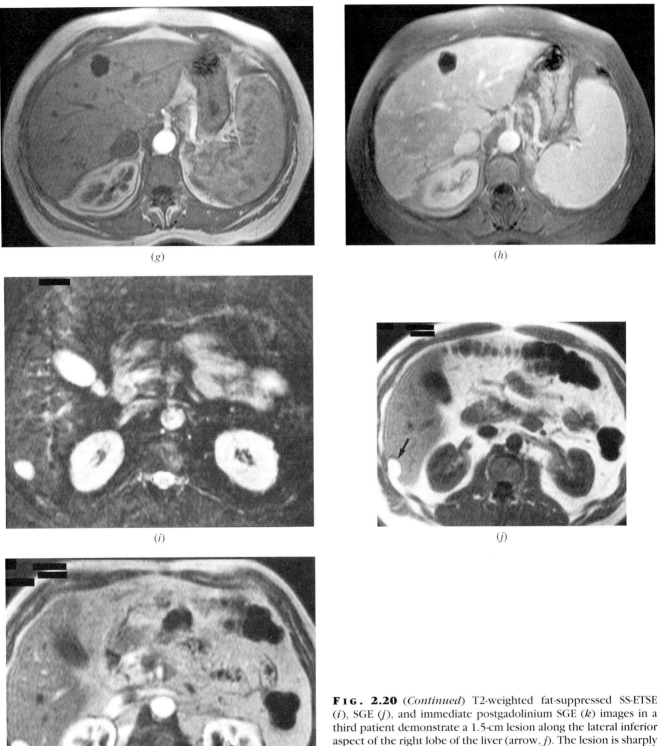

(g)

(h)

(i)

(j)

(k)

FIG. 2.20 (*Continued*) T2-weighted fat-suppressed SS-ETSE (*i*), SGE (*j*), and immediate postgadolinium SGE (*k*) images in a third patient demonstrate a 1.5-cm lesion along the lateral inferior aspect of the right lobe of the liver (arrow, *j*). The lesion is sharply demarcated, is high in signal intensity on the T2-weighted (*i*) and T1-weighted (*j*) images, and does not change in shape or appearance after gadolinium administration (*k*). The high concentration of mucin in the cyst accounts for the high signal intensity on the T1-weighted (*j*) images. Note also that the lesion extends beyond the contour of the liver, which is characteristic of foregut cysts.

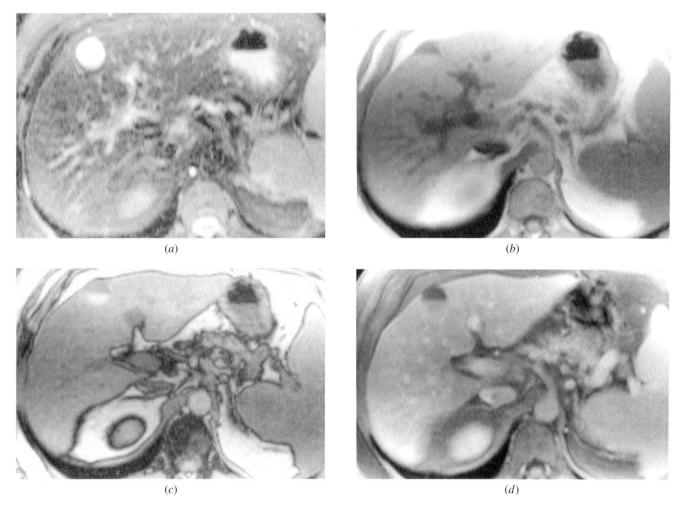

(a)   (b)

(c)   (d)

F I G . 2.21 Foregut cyst with layering. Echo train-STIR (*a*), SGE (*b*), out-of-phase SGE (*c*), and 90-s fat-suppressed postgado-linium SGE (*d*) images. A cystic lesion is identified in segment 4 and distorts the anterior liver contour. The lesion is homogeneously high signal on T2-weighted image (*a*) and shows layering with high signal intensity on T1-weighted image (*b*), which does not lose signal on out-of-phase image (*c*), consistent with proteinaceous material (mucin) observed in these cysts.

composed of mature fat, blood vessels, and smooth muscle. Some tumors may contain foci of extramedullary hematopoiesis (angiomyomyelolipomas). Some patients have tuberous sclerosis [61], although the association is less strong than with renal angiomyolipomas.

Angiomyolipomas are well-defined, sharply margin-ated masses that frequently have a high fat content, and therefore are high in signal intensity on T1-weighted images and low in signal intensity on fat-suppressed images. Angiomyolipomas may also have a low fat content and appear moderately high in signal on T2-weighted images and low in signal intensity on T1-weighted images and exhibit a diffuse heterogeneous enhancement on immediate postgadolinium SGE images (figs. 2.29 and 2.30) [62]. A similar enhancement pattern is observed in well-differentiated hepatocellular carci-noma, and this enhancement reflects the appearance of well-defined tumors of hepatic origin. The pattern of enhancement of angiomyolipomas tends to be much more orderly than well-differentiated hepatocellular carcinomas.

Lipomas
Hepatic lipomas are rarer than angiomyolipomas. On imaging, tumors are commonly multiple and appear as fatty tumors that are high in signal intensity on T1-weighted sequences and low in signal intensity with fat-suppressed techniques [63]. These lesions show negligible enhancement on postgadolinium images (fig. 2.31).

Hemangiomas
Hemangiomas are the most common benign hepatic neoplasm, with an autopsy incidence between 0.4 and 20% [64, 65]. Hemangiomas are more frequent in females, rarely produce symptoms, and are usually detected incidentally.

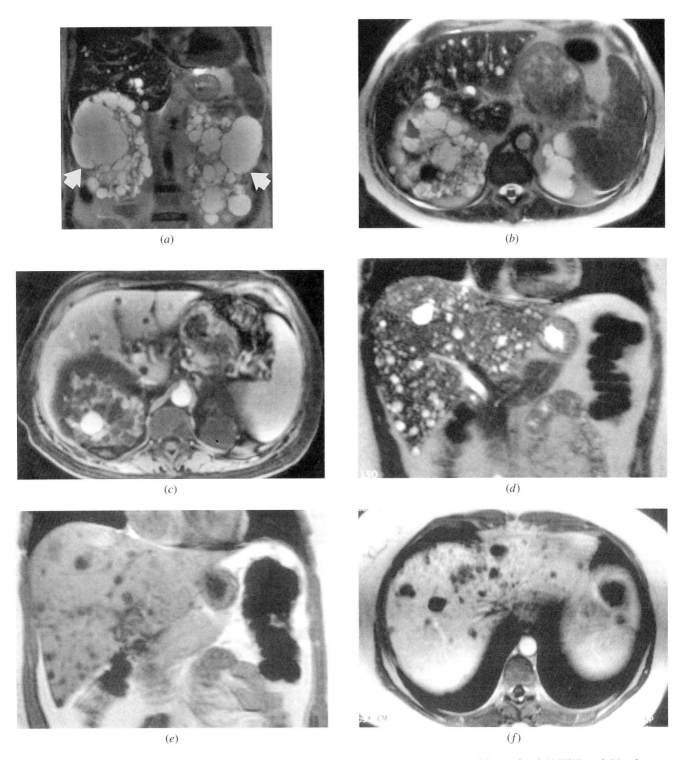

F I G . 2.22 Liver cysts in polycystic kidney disease. Coronal (*a*) and transverse (*b*) T2-weighted SS-ETSE and 90-s fat-suppressed postgadolinium SGE (*c*) images. The kidneys are massively enlarged and contain multiple cysts of varying size with no definable renal parenchyma (arrows, *a*). Multiple <1-cm cysts are present and scattered throughout the liver that are high in signal intensity on T2-weighted images (*a, b*) and do not enhance after gadolinium administration (*c*).

Coronal T2-weighted SS-ETSE (*d*) and SGE (*e*) and transverse 1-min postgadolinium SGE (*f*) images in a second patient show cysts scattered throughout the liver parenchyma with no evidence of hemorrhage or distortion of hepatic architecture.

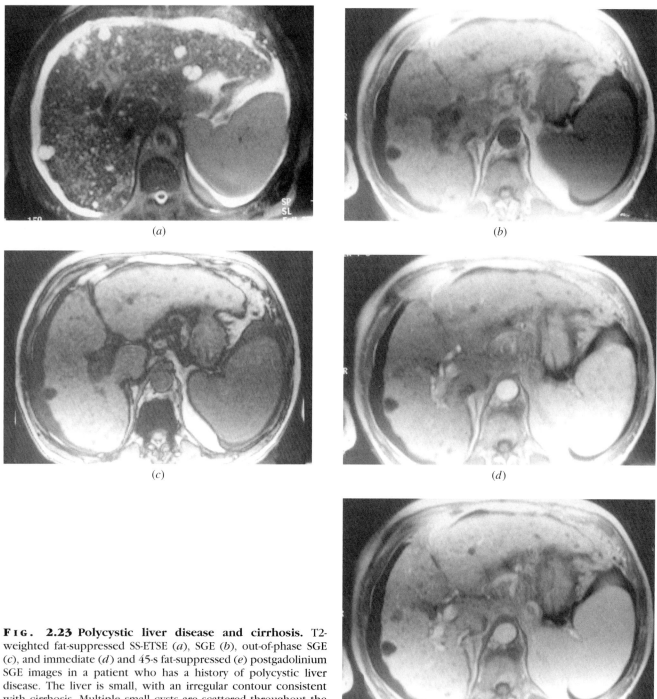

(a)

(b)

(c)

(d)

(e)

F I G . 2.23 Polycystic liver disease and cirrhosis. T2-weighted fat-suppressed SS-ETSE (*a*), SGE (*b*), out-of-phase SGE (*c*), and immediate (*d*) and 45-s fat-suppressed (*e*) postgadolinium SGE images in a patient who has a history of polycystic liver disease. The liver is small, with an irregular contour consistent with cirrhosis. Multiple small cysts are scattered throughout the liver, compatible with liver cysts seen in autosomal dominant polycystic kidney disease.

Pathologically, hemangiomas are characterized grossly as well-circumscribed, spongelike blood-filled mesenchymal tumors. Microscopically, hemangiomas reveal numerous large vascular channels lined by a single layer of flat endothelial cells, separated by slender fibrous septa. Foci of thrombosis, extensive fibrosis, and calcification may be present. The great majority of these benign vascular lesions are cavernous hemangiomas, but in rare instances they may represent capillary telangiectasias. Cavernous hemangiomas are composed primarily of large vascular lakes and channels. Some of the vascular channels undergo thrombosis and fibrous organization [66].

Hemangiomas are usually multiple (fig. 2.32). Small hemangiomas typically appear round, whereas larger

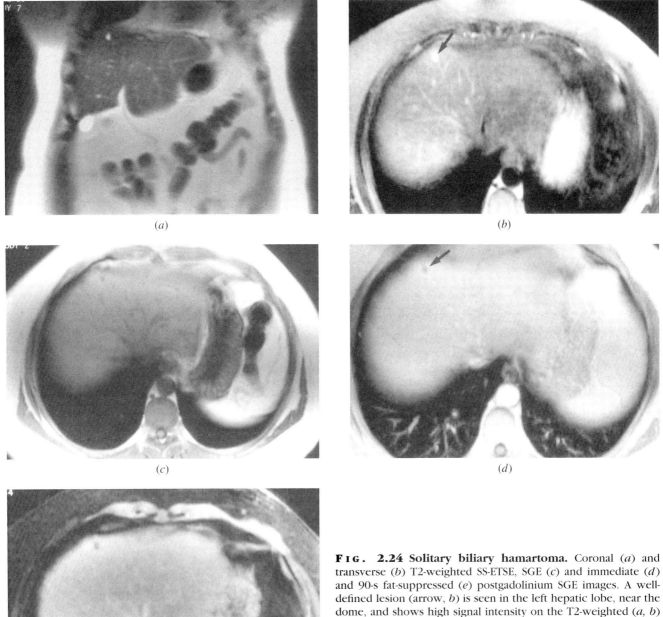

FIG. 2.24 Solitary biliary hamartoma. Coronal (*a*) and transverse (*b*) T2-weighted SS-ETSE, SGE (*c*) and immediate (*d*) and 90-s fat-suppressed (*e*) postgadolinium SGE images. A well-defined lesion (arrow, *b*) is seen in the left hepatic lobe, near the dome, and shows high signal intensity on the T2-weighted (*a, b*) and low signal intensity on the T1-weighted (*c*) images. On the immediate postgadolinium image (*d*), the lesion does not enhance with gadolinium, but a thin perilesional rim of enhancement is appreciated (arrow, *d*). (Reproduced with permission from Semelka RC, Hussain SM, Marcos HB, Woosley JT. Biliary hamartomas: solitary and multiple lesions shown on current MR techniques including gadolinium enhancement. *J Magn Reson Imaging* 10: 196–201, 1999).

lesions have either a well-defined round or lobular margin.

On MRI, hemangiomas have long T2 and T1 values, so they are high in signal intensity on T2-weighted images and low in signal intensity on T1-weighted images, maintaining signal intensity on longer echo times (e.g., >120 ms) [67, 68]. T2 measurements are less than those of cysts. On dynamic serial postcontrast images, hemangiomas typically enhance on a peripheral nodular fashion, which enlarge, coalesce, and slowly progress centripetally to complete or nearly complete fill-in of the entire lesion by 10 min [69–72]. Hemangiomas may fade

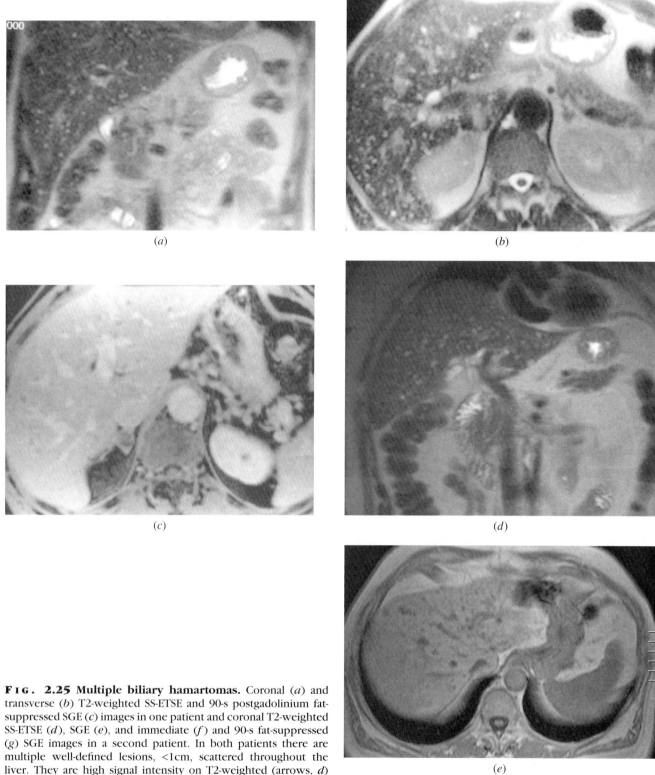

(a)

(b)

(c)

(d)

(e)

FIG. 2.25 Multiple biliary hamartomas. Coronal (*a*) and transverse (*b*) T2-weighted SS-ETSE and 90-s postgadolinium fat-suppressed SGE (*c*) images in one patient and coronal T2-weighted SS-ETSE (*d*), SGE (*e*), and immediate (*f*) and 90-s fat-suppressed (*g*) SGE images in a second patient. In both patients there are multiple well-defined lesions, <1cm, scattered throughout the liver. They are high signal intensity on T2-weighted (arrows, *d*)

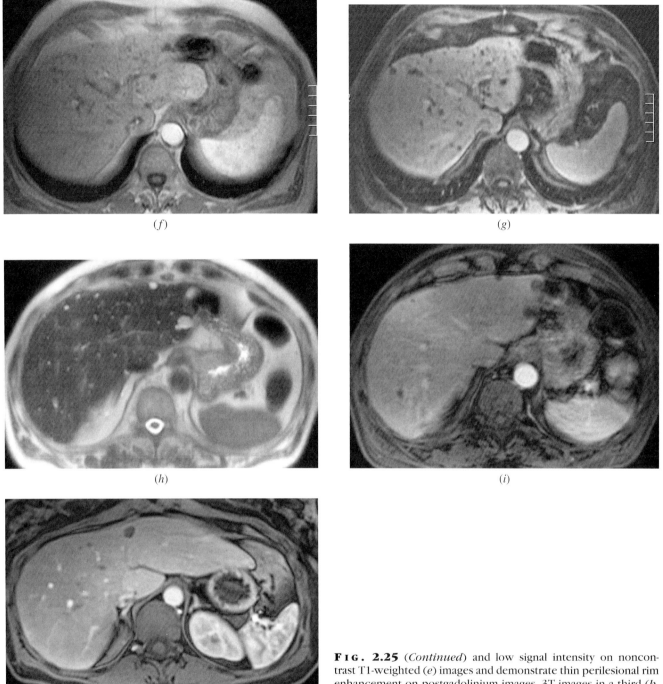

(f)

(g)

(h)

(i)

(j)

FIG. 2.25 (*Continued*) and low signal intensity on noncontrast T1-weighted (*e*) images and demonstrate thin perilesional rim enhancement on postgadolinium images. 3T images in a third (*h, i*) and a fourth (*j*) patient with biliary hamartoma, with imaging features similar to those previously described.

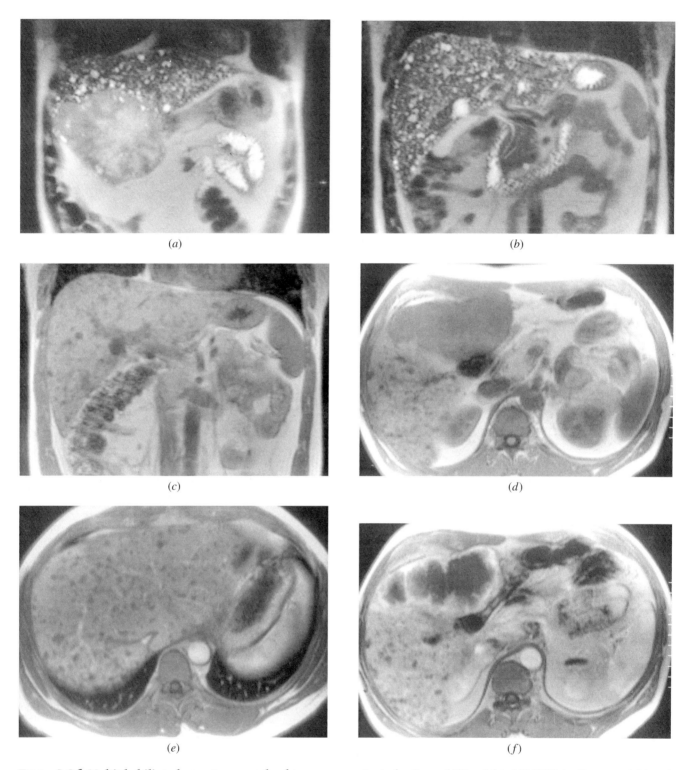

Fig. 2.26 Multiple biliary hamartomas and colon cancer metastasis. Coronal T2-weighted SS-ETSE (*a, b*), coronal (*c*) and transverse (*d*) SGE, and immediate (*e, f*) and 90-s fat-suppressed (*g, h*) postgadolinium SGE images in a patient who has a history of colon cancer. There is a large hepatic mass in segments 4/5 that demonstrates heterogeneous and moderately high signal on

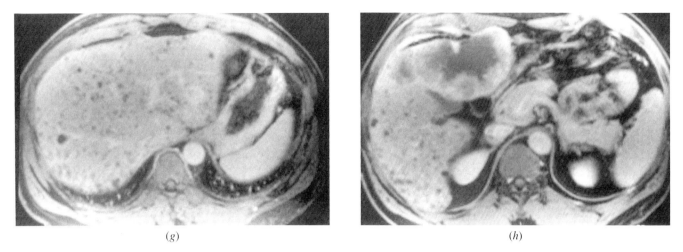

(g)   (h)

F I G. 2.26 (*Continued*) T2-weighted image (*a*) and moderately low signal on T1-weighted image (*d*) and ring enhancement after administration of contrast (*f, h*), consistent with a metastasis. The liver is riddled with many small well-defined lesions, measuring <1 cm, that also demonstrate ring enhancement after contrast, consistent with biliary hamartomas. Note that the metastasis progresses in enhancement from early (*f*) to late (*h*) images, whereas biliary hamartomas show identical ring enhancement on early and late images with no progressive enhancement.

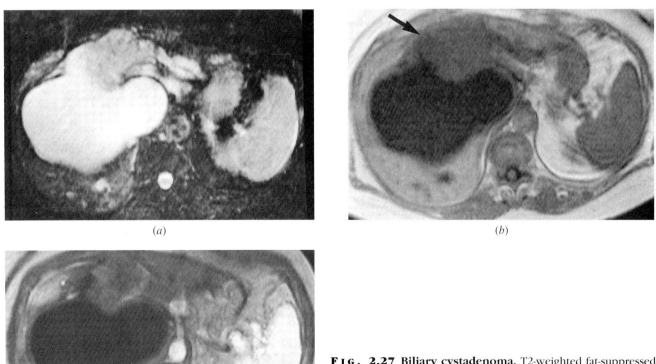

(a)   (b)

(c)

F I G. 2.27 Biliary cystadenoma. T2-weighted fat-suppressed ETSE (*a*), SGE (*b*), and immediate postgadolinium SGE (*c*) images. A large cystic mass with a 5-cm solid nodular component (arrow, *b*) is present in the liver. The nodular component is moderately hyperintense on the T2-weighted image (*a*) and slightly hypointense on the T1-weighted image (*b*) and enhances in a diffuse heterogeneous fashion on the immediate postgadolinium image (*c*). Diffuse heterogeneous enhancement on immediate postgadolinium images is a feature of tumors of hepatic origin.

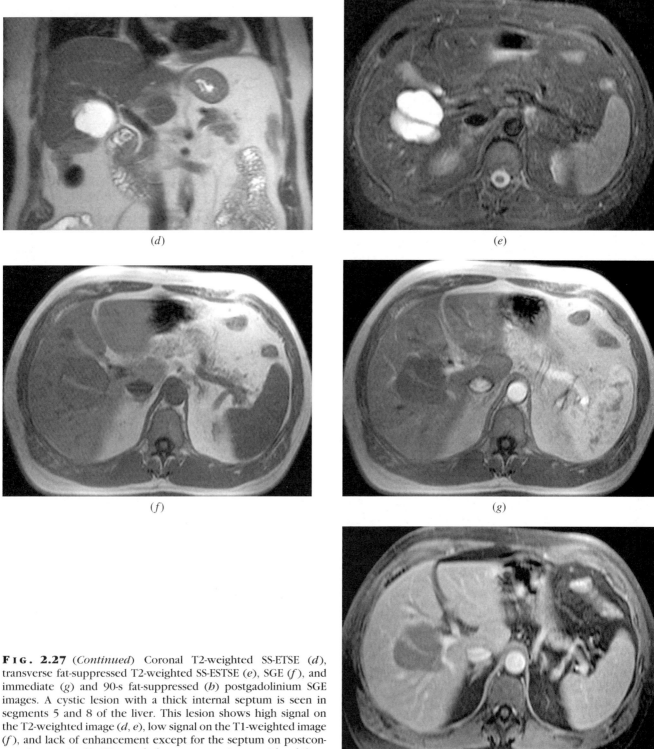

(d)

(e)

(f)

(g)

(h)

FIG. 2.27 (*Continued*) Coronal T2-weighted SS-ETSE (*d*), transverse fat-suppressed T2-weighted SS-ESTSE (*e*), SGE (*f*), and immediate (*g*) and 90-s fat-suppressed (*h*) postgadolinium SGE images. A cystic lesion with a thick internal septum is seen in segments 5 and 8 of the liver. This lesion shows high signal on the T2-weighted image (*d, e*), low signal on the T1-weighted image (*f*), and lack of enhancement except for the septum on postcontrast images (*g, h*). Histopathology was consistent with a biliary cystadenoma.

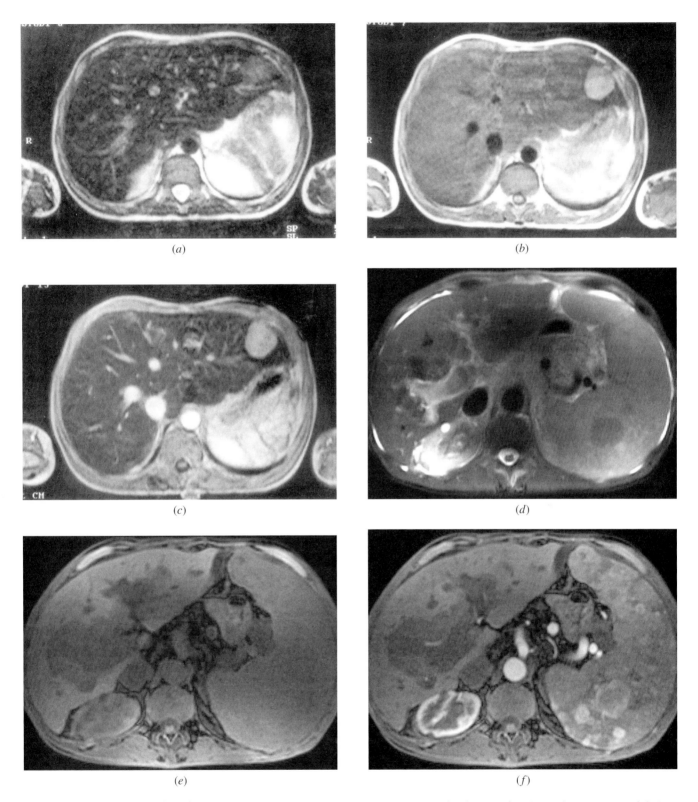

F I G . 2.28 Extramedullary hematopoiesis. T2-weighted SS-ETSE (*a*), T1-weighted spin-echo (*b*), and 1-min postgadolinium SGE (*c*) images. A rounded lesion is present in the left lobe that demonstrates moderate increase in signal intensity on T2-weighted (*a*) and T1-weighted (*b*) images and mild diffuse homogeneous enhancement after administration of gadolinium (*c*). (Courtesy of Cem Balci, M.D).

T2-weighted SS-ETSE fat-suppressed (*d*), T1-weighted SGE (*e*), and immediate (*f*) and 90-s fat-suppressed (*g*) postgadolinium SGE 3T images in a second patient with the diagnosis of extramedullary hematopoiesis. The liver is irregular in contour with

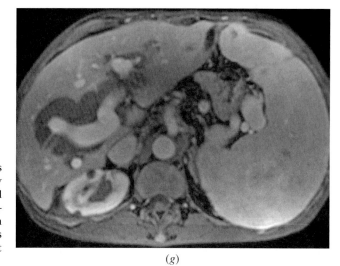

(g)

FIG. 2.28 (*Continued*) prominence of periportal area that is intermediate signal intensity on T2-weighted images (*d*) and low signal intensity on T1-weighted images (*e*) and shows minimal enhancement after contrast administration (*f*, *g*), reflecting infiltration by hypovascular tissue which is well-demarcated. The spleen is massively enlarged in size with multiple hypervascular lesions on immediate postcontrast images (*f*). This patient has coexistent cirrhosis and periportal extramedullary hematopoiesis.

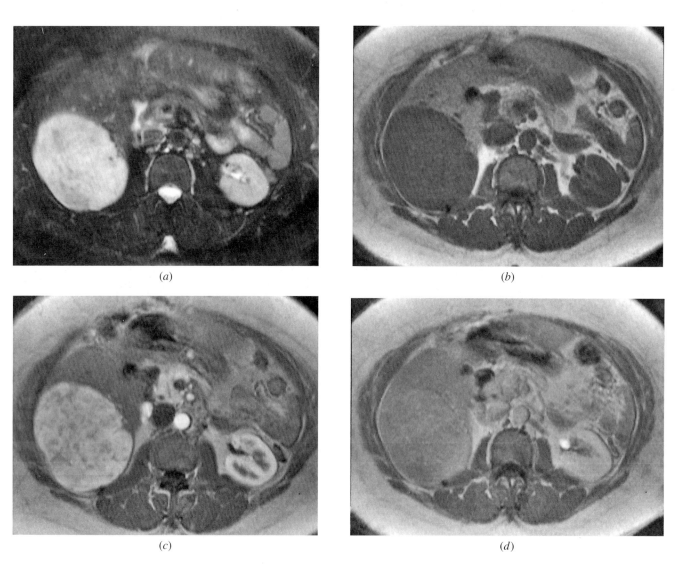

(a)

(b)

(c)

(d)

FIG. 2.29 **Angiomyolipoma with minimal fat.** T2-weighted fat-suppressed ETSE (*a*), SGE (*b*), and immediate (*c*) and 90-s (*d*) postgadolinium SGE images. The angiomyolipoma is moderately hyperintense with slight heterogeneity on the T2-weighted image (*a*) and moderately hypointense on the T1-weighted image (*b*) and enhances intensely in a diffuse heterogeneous fashion on the immediate postgadolinium image (*c*). On the 90-s image (*d*), the lesion has faded in signal intensity to slightly higher than background liver. This angiomyolipoma is unusual in that it contains minimal fat. The diffuse heterogeneous enhancement is typical of tumors of hepatic origin.

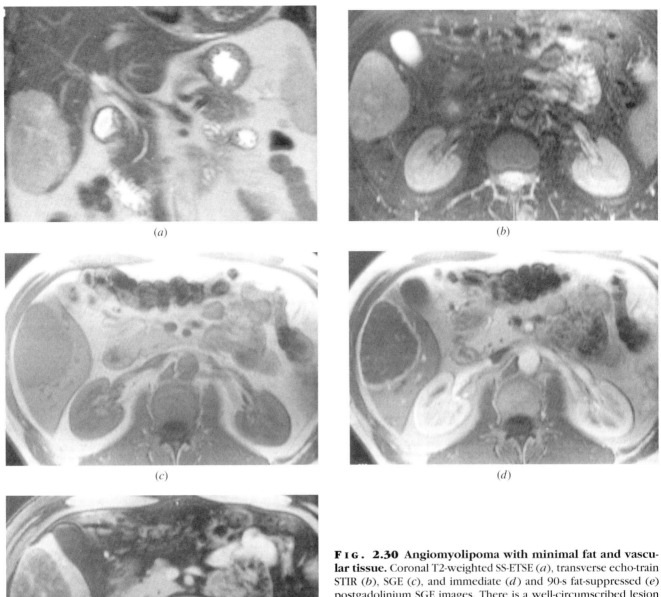

FIG. 2.30 Angiomyolipoma with minimal fat and vascular tissue. Coronal T2-weighted SS-ETSE (*a*), transverse echo-train STIR (*b*), SGE (*c*), and immediate (*d*) and 90-s fat-suppressed (*e*) postgadolinium SGE images. There is a well-circumscribed lesion in the right hepatic lobe that demonstrates moderately high signal intensity on T2-weighted image (*a, b*), low signal intensity on T1-weighted image (*c*), and capsular enhancement on immediate postgadolinium (*d*) images that fades by 90 s (*e*). On the early (*d*) and late (*e*) images there is a fine regular network of vessels apparent within the lesion. Angiomyolipoma with minimal fat was present at histopathology. Blood vessels are well organized throughout the tumor, unlike the irregular pattern observed in HCC. There is also a paucity of vascular tissue in this tumor.

away in signal intensity toward parenchyma isointensity over time, but they will fade in a homogeneous fashion with no evidence of peripheral or heterogeneous lesional washout [73].

The most distinctive imaging feature of hemangiomas is the demonstration of a discontinuous ring of nodules immediately after contrast administration [73]. Nodular enhancement is most frequently eccentric in location and

may originate from the superior or inferior aspect of the hemangioma, simulating central enhancement on transverse images (fig. 2.33). True central enhancement may rarely occur. The appearance of central enhancement is rare for all histologic types of tumors and occurs by early filling of a large central lake by a narrow feeding vessel.

The MRI appearances of small (<1.5 cm), medium (1.5–5.0 cm), and large (>5.0 cm) hemangiomas have

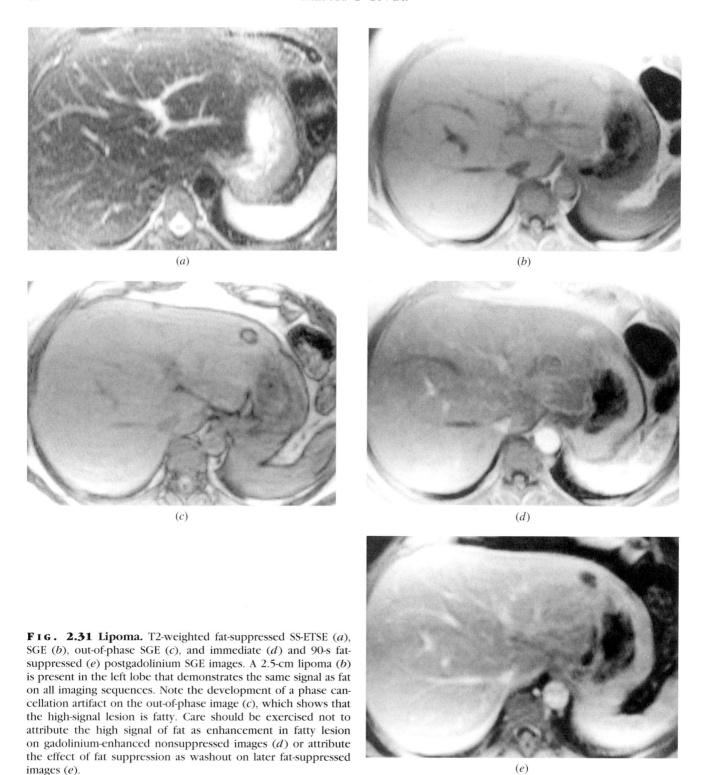

FIG. 2.31 Lipoma. T2-weighted fat-suppressed SS-ETSE (*a*), SGE (*b*), out-of-phase SGE (*c*), and immediate (*d*) and 90-s fat-suppressed (*e*) postgadolinium SGE images. A 2.5-cm lipoma (*b*) is present in the left lobe that demonstrates the same signal as fat on all imaging sequences. Note the development of a phase cancellation artifact on the out-of-phase image (*c*), which shows that the high-signal lesion is fatty. Care should be exercised not to attribute the high signal of fat as enhancement in fatty lesion on gadolinium-enhanced nonsuppressed images (*d*) or attribute the effect of fat suppression as washout on later fat-suppressed images (*e*).

been reported in a multi-institutional study [73]. Among the 154 hemangiomas in 66 patients, 52.6 % (81/154) lesions were small, 36.4% (56/154) medium, and 11% (17/154) large. Hemangiomas were multiple in 68% of patients. All lesions were high in signal intensity on T2-weighted images. Three types of enhancement patterns were observed: uniform high signal intensity immediately after contrast (Type 1); peripheral nodular enhancement with centripetal progression to uniform high signal intensity (Type 2); and peripheral nodular enhancement with centripetal progression and a persistent central scar (Type 3). Type 1 enhancement was observed only in

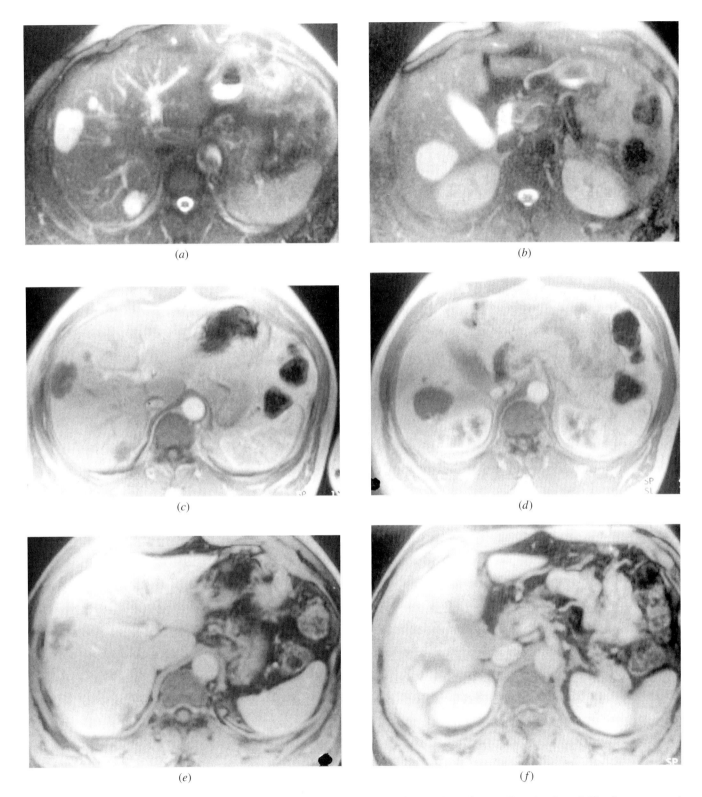

(a)

(b)

(c)

(d)

(e)

(f)

F I G . 2.32 Multiple hemangiomas. T2-weighted fat-suppressed SS-ETSE (*a*, *b*) and immediate (*c*, *d*) and 90-s fat-suppressed (*e*, *f*) postgadolinium images. Multiple hemangiomas are appreciated throughout the liver. All of these lesions show increased signal intensity on T2-weighted images (*a*, *b*), peripheral nodular enhancement after contrast administration (*c*, *d*), and enlargement and coalescence of nodules on delayed postcontrast images (*e*, *f*), consistent with multiple hemangiomas.

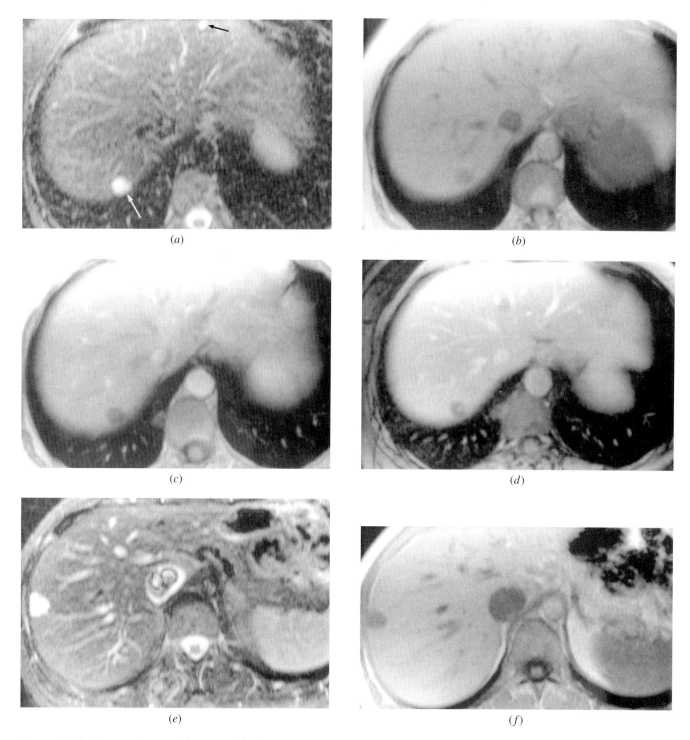

FIG. 2.33 Hemangioma with central filling. T2-weighted fat-suppressed SS-ETSE (*a*), SGE (*b*), and immediate (*c*) and 90-s fat-suppressed (*d*) postgadolinium SGE images. There are two lesions (arrows, *a*) located in the left and right hepatic lobe. The lesion in the right lobe shows increased signal intensity on T2-weighted image (*a*) and decreased signal intensity on T1-weighted image (*b*). On both early (*c*)- and late (*d*)-phase images the lesion demonstrates peripheral and central enhanced nodules. The small left lobe lesion lobe is hyperintense on the T2-weighted image (black arrow, *a*) and is barely perceptible on any of the other sequences. This is not uncommon with <1-cm hemangiomas with type 1 enhancement, in which enhancement may be minimally greater comparable in intensity to background liver on immediate postgadolinium images and lesions fade to isointensity by 1-2 min. Note the presence of a phase encoding mirror artifact from the IVC, which should not be mistaken for a lesion (*c*).

Echo train-STIR (*e*), SGE (*f*), and immediate (*g*) and 90-s fat-suppressed (*h*) postgadolinium SGE images in a second patient.

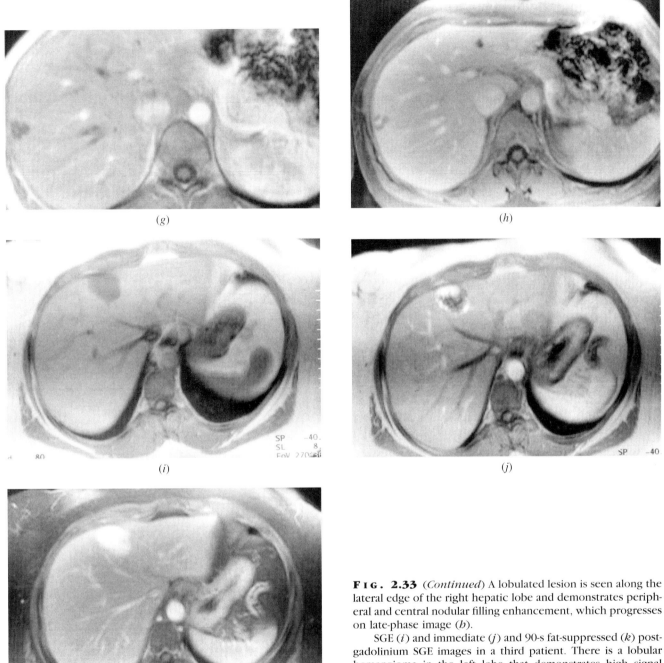

(g)

(h)

(i)

(j)

(k)

FIG. 2.33 (*Continued*) A lobulated lesion is seen along the lateral edge of the right hepatic lobe and demonstrates peripheral and central nodular filling enhancement, which progresses on late-phase image (*h*).

SGE (*i*) and immediate (*j*) and 90-s fat-suppressed (*k*) post-gadolinium SGE images in a third patient. There is a lobular hemangioma in the left lobe that demonstrates high signal intensity on T2-weighted image (not shown) and low signal on T1-weighted image (*i*), enhances in a peripheral nodular pattern on early-phase image (*j*), and fills in completely on late-phase image (*k*).

small tumors. Type 2 and Type 3 enhancements were observed in all size categories. Type 3 enhancement was observed in 16 of 17 large tumors.

Small hemangiomas most commonly demonstrate Type 2 enhancement. The peripheral nodules of enhancement are typically very small (fig. 2.34). Type 1 enhancement is the next most common pattern (fig.

2.35), whereas Type 3 enhancement is uncommonly noted (fig. 2.36). Small hemangiomas are difficult to distinguish from other types of liver lesions, specifically hypervascular liver metastases, and MRI follow-up is generally required.

The great majority of medium-sized hemangiomas exhibit Type 2 enhancement (fig. 2.37 and 2.38) and

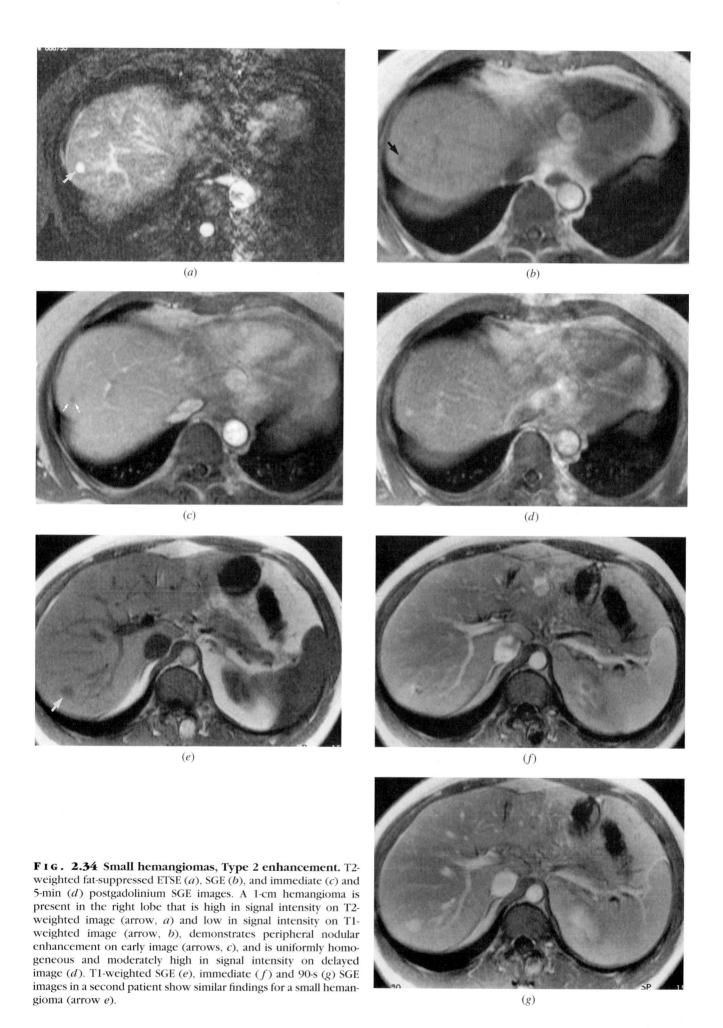

F I G . 2.34 Small hemangiomas, Type 2 enhancement. T2-weighted fat-suppressed ETSE (*a*), SGE (*b*), and immediate (*c*) and 5-min (*d*) postgadolinium SGE images. A 1-cm hemangioma is present in the right lobe that is high in signal intensity on T2-weighted image (arrow, *a*) and low in signal intensity on T1-weighted image (arrow, *b*), demonstrates peripheral nodular enhancement on early image (arrows, *c*), and is uniformly homogeneous and moderately high in signal intensity on delayed image (*d*). T1-weighted SGE (*e*), immediate (*f*) and 90-s (*g*) SGE images in a second patient show similar findings for a small hemangioma (arrow *e*).

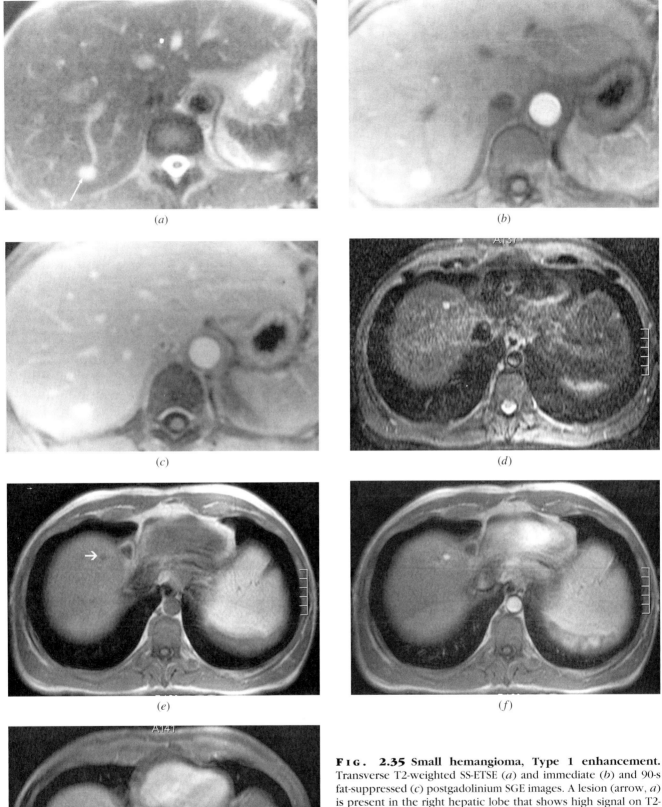

(a)

(b)

(c)

(d)

(e)

(f)

(g)

FIG. 2.35 Small hemangioma, Type 1 enhancement.
Transverse T2-weighted SS-ETSE (*a*) and immediate (*b*) and 90-s
fat-suppressed (*c*) postgadolinium SGE images. A lesion (arrow, *a*)
is present in the right hepatic lobe that shows high signal on T2-
weighted image (*a*), low signal on T1-weighted image (not shown),
and intense uniform enhancement immediately after administration of gadolinium (*b*) that persists at 90-s image (*c*). These findings represent a Type 1 hemangioma.

T2-weighted fat-suppressed SS-ETSE (*d*), SGE (*e*), and immediate (*f*) and 90-s fat-suppressed (*g*) postgadolinium SGE image in a
second patient. A tiny lesion is seen in segment 4 of the liver that
shows high signal intensity on the T2-weighted image, low signal
intensity on the T1-weighted image (arrow, *e*), and homogeneous
enhancement on early phase (*f*) that remains on the late phase
image (*g*), consistent with Type 1 hemangioma.

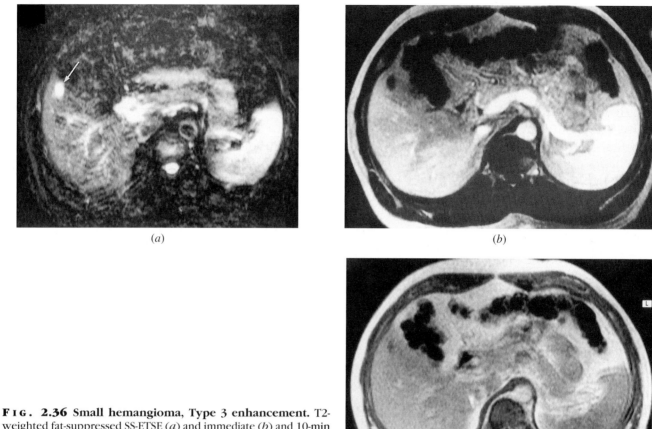

(a)

(b)

FIG. 2.36 Small hemangioma, Type 3 enhancement. T2-weighted fat-suppressed SS-ETSE (*a*) and immediate (*b*) and 10-min (*c*) postgadolinium SGE images. A 1.5-cm lesion is present in the right lobe that is high in signal intensity on the T2-weighted image (arrow, *a*) and nearly signal void with subtle small peripheral nodules on the early image (*b*) and shows peripheral enhancement with persistence of central low signal intensity on the late image (*c*), consistent with a central scar.

(c)

represent the classic hemangiomas. Type 3 enhancement is the next most common enhancement pattern (figs. 2.39–2.41), whereas Type 1 enhancement is exceedingly rare. Lesions > 1.5 cm with Type 1 enhancement represent either well-differentiated tumors of hepatocellular origin or hypervascular liver metastases.

Giant hemangiomas most frequently have a central scar, and virtually all giant hemangiomas have Type 3 enhancement (fig. 2.42) [73–75]. Absence of a central scar should raise the concern that the mass may represent another lesion. Giant hemangiomas often have a multiloculated appearance with mildly complex signal intensity on T2-weighted images and the common presence of low-signal strands, which reflects the internal network of fibrous stroma that is observed histologically (fig. 2.43) [75]. In rare instances, large hemangiomas may compress adjacent portal veins, resulting in transient segmental increased enhancement on immediate postgadolinium images secondary to autoregulatory increased hepatic arterial supply (fig. 2.44). On rare

occasions, large hemangiomas may also undergo hemorrhage.

Hemangiomas vary in the rate and completeness of tumor enhancement. A variation in the Type 2 or 3 enhancement pattern consists of enhancement that spreads at a fairly rapid rate with complete enhancement at 1–2 min [73]. Rapidity of enhancement has been determined on 90-s images as slow (approximately 25% of tumor enhancement at the maximum transverse diameter), medium (approximately 50% enhancement), and fast (approximately 75% enhancement) [73, 76]. Tumors at all sizes may enhance very slowly to very quickly, and enhance minimally to complete enhancement, with the exception that >5-cm tumors almost invariably demonstrate lack of central enhancement [73].

Slow enhancement of hemangiomas permits distinction from most tumors. The only other neoplasm that may show comparable slow enhancement is chemotherapy-treated metastases (as described below). Fast-enhancing hemangiomas show enhancement

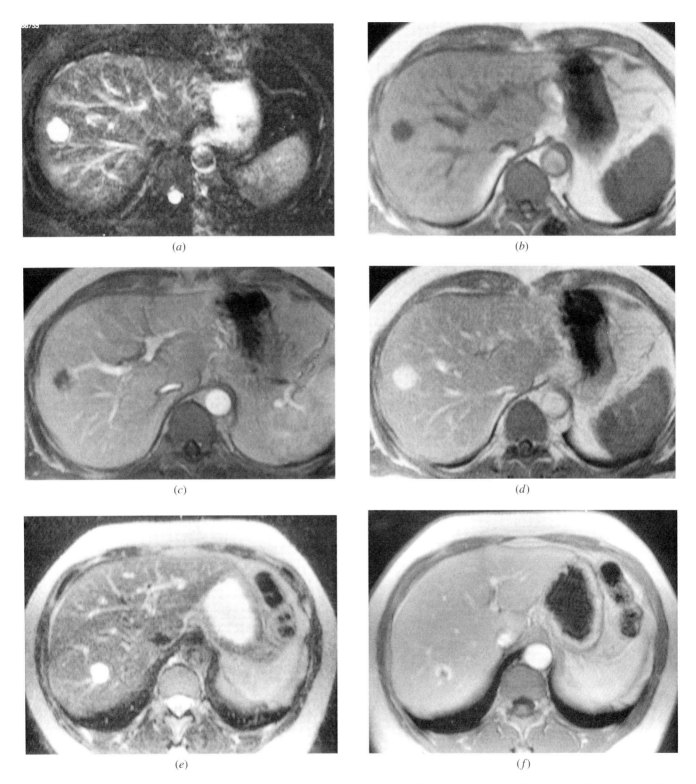

FIG. 2.37 Medium-sized hemangioma, Type 2 enhancement. T2-weighted fat-suppressed ETSE (*a*), SGE (*b*), and immediate (*c*) and 5-min (*d*) postgadolinium SGE images demonstrate a well-defined, round lesion that is high signal on T2-weighted image (*a*) and moderately low signal on T1-weighted image (*b*) and enhances in a peripheral nodular fashion on early image (*c*) with complete filling of the entire lesion on the late image (*d*), consistent with hemangioma.

T2-weighted fat-suppressed ETSE (*e*) and immediate (*f*) and 90-s fat-suppressed (*g*) postgadolinium SGE images in a second patient. A 2.1-cm hemangioma is present in the right hepatic lobe, and it shows high signal intensity on T2-weighted image (*e*) and

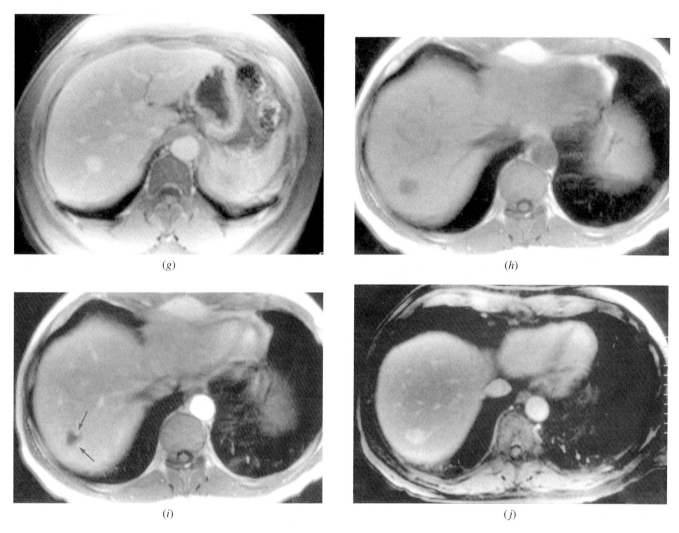

(g)   (h)

(i)   (j)

F I G . 2.37 (*Continued*) low signal intensity on T1-weighted image (not shown) and enhances in a peripheral nodular fashion on early image (*f*), which fills in on late image (*g*).

SGE (*h*) and immediate (*i*) and 90-s fat-suppressed (*j*) postgadolinium SGE images in a third patient showing the same findings as the second patient.

patterns that can resemble other tumors, with metastases being the most difficult to distinguish. Transient increased perilesional enhancement may occur, and is seen most often in small capsule-based hemangiomas (fig. 2.45). This phenomenon may reflect recruitment of capsular vessels. These findings are rare in hemangiomas and are more commonly observed in metastases, especially colon cancer metastases. A study [77] correlated the temporal parenchyma enhancement surrounding hepatic cavernous hemangiomas with the rapidity of intratumoral contrast material enhancement and tumor volume. Thirty-two of the 167 (19%) hemangiomas had temporal peritumoral enhancement, and this was more common in hemangiomas with rapid enhancement (41%). However, there was no statistically significant relationship between peritumoral enhancement and tumor volume. The mean diam-

eter of hemangiomas with peritumoral enhancement was not significantly different from that of hemangiomas without peritumoral enhancement.

Hemangiomas not uncommonly coexist with focal nodular hyperplasia (FNH) lesions, particularly in the setting of the multiple FNH syndrome [78]. Hemangiomas are a common finding in patients with breast cancer. An early report [79] showed that among all benign liver lesions observed in patients with breast cancer who underwent screening examinations, hemangiomas were the most frequent type. This is important information since small metastases from breast cancer are hypervascular and may mimic the appearance of type 1 hemangiomas on early-phase postgadolinium images. However, late-phase demonstrates distinction between these entities: small hypervascular metastases tend to

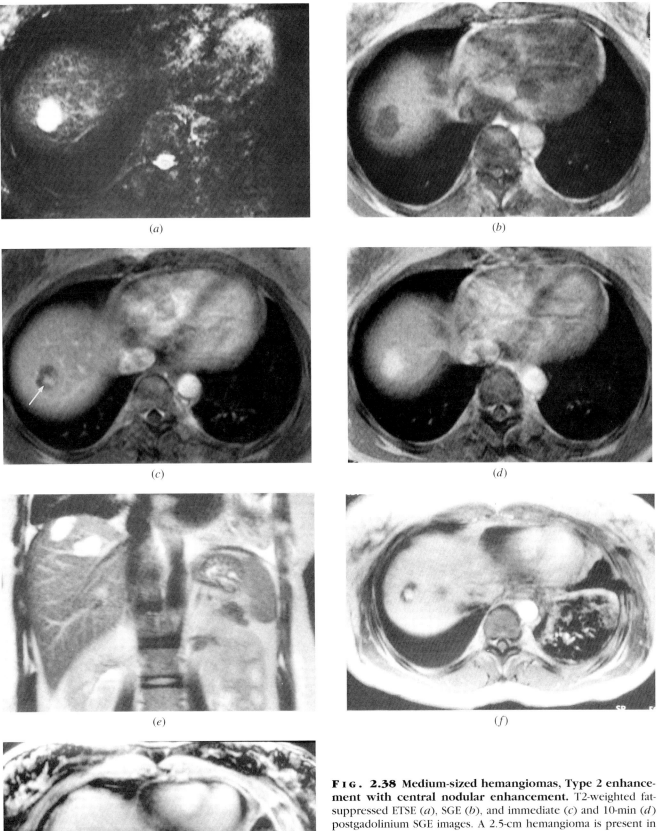

(a)

(b)

(c)

(d)

(e)

(f)

(g)

FIG. 2.38 Medium-sized hemangiomas, Type 2 enhancement with central nodular enhancement. T2-weighted fat-suppressed ETSE (*a*), SGE (*b*), and immediate (*c*) and 10-min (*d*) postgadolinium SGE images. A 2.5-cm hemangioma is present in segments 8 and 7 of the liver, and it demonstrates high signal on T2-weighted image (*a*), moderately low signal on T1-weighted image (*b*), and nodular progressive enhancement after contrast administration (*c*) with complete fill in with contrast on the late image (*d*). The early image (arrow, *c*) demonstrates one predominant enhancing nodule that is almost central in location.

Coronal T2-weighted SS-ETSE (*e*) and transverse immediate (*f*) and 90-s fat-suppressed (*g*) postgadolinium SGE images in a second patient demonstrate two hemangiomas with the same features described in the first patient. Note that on early image (*f*) one of the hemangiomas has a central enhancing nodule.

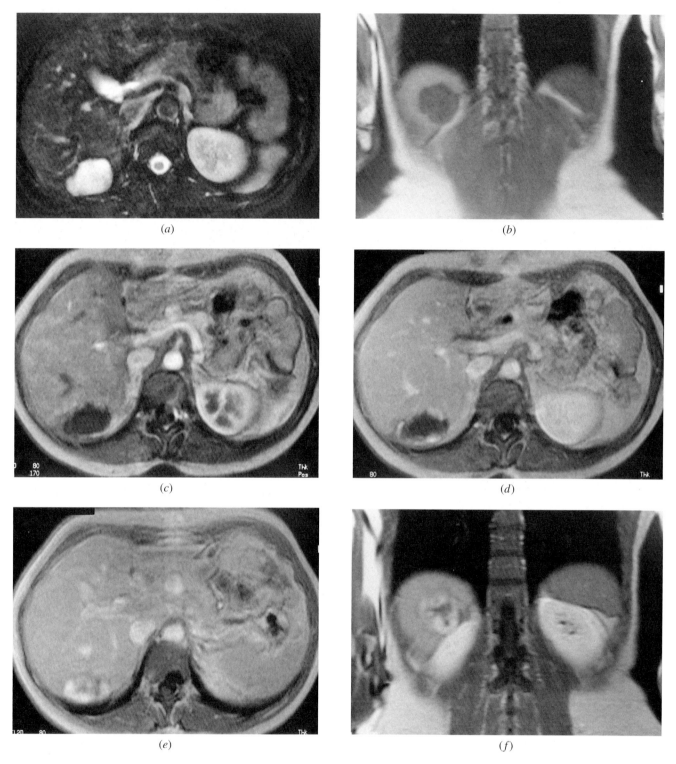

(a)

(b)

(c)

(d)

(e)

(f)

F i g . 2.39 Medium-sized hemangioma, Type 3 enhancement. T2-weighted fat-suppressed ETSE (*a*), coronal SGE (*b*), immediate (*c*) and 45-s (*d*) postgadolinium SGE images, and transverse (*e*) and coronal (*f*) 10-min postgadolinium SGE images. The hemangioma is high in signal intensity on the T2-weighted image (*a*) and moderately low in signal intensity on the T1-weighted image (*b*) and demonstrates peripheral nodular enhancement (*c*) that progresses centripetally (*d*). Note the persistence of a central scar on delayed images (*e, f*).

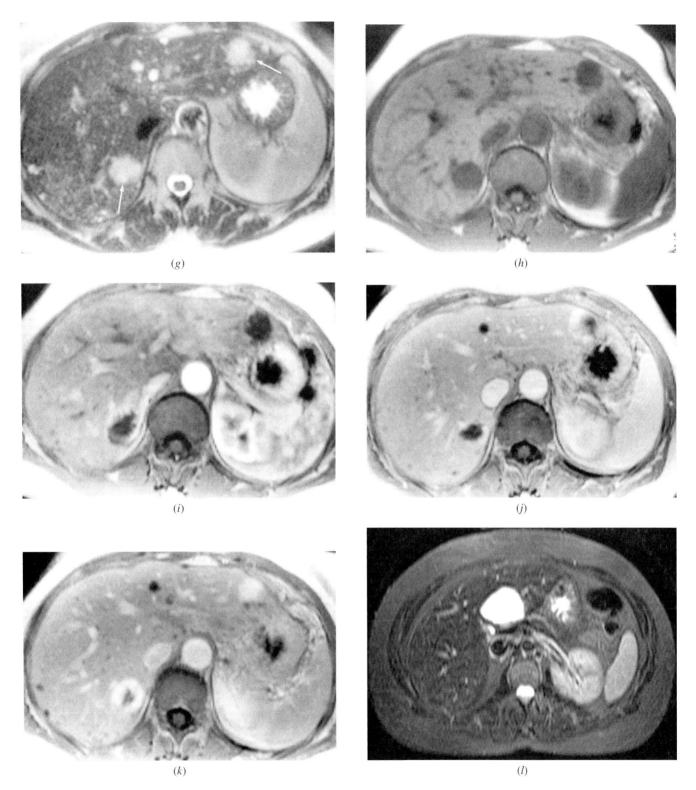

F I G . 2.39 (*Continued*) Transverse T2-weighted SS-ETSE (*g*), SGE (*h*), and immediate (*i*), 45-s (*j*), and 5-min (*k*) postgadolinium SGE images in a second patient. There are two lobular lesions that appear high in signal intensity on T2-weighted image (arrows, *g*) and low in signal intensity on T1-weighted (*h*) images. The first lesion is situated in the left lobe, demonstrates peripheral nodular enhancement after administration of gadolinium, and gradually fills in completely on delayed images (*k*), consistent with a Type 2 hemangioma. The other lesion is situated in the right hepatic lobe and shows peripheral nodular enhancement that progresses centripetally but with persistence of a central scar on the delayed image consistent with a Type 3 hemangioma. Note also multiple tiny lesions throughout the hepatic parenchyma consistent with biliary hamartomas.

T2-weighted fat-suppressed SS-ETSE (*l*), SGE (*m*), and immediate (*n*), 45-s (*o*), and 90-s fat-suppressed (*p*) postgadolinium SGE images in a third patient with a Type 3 hemangioma in the left lobe.

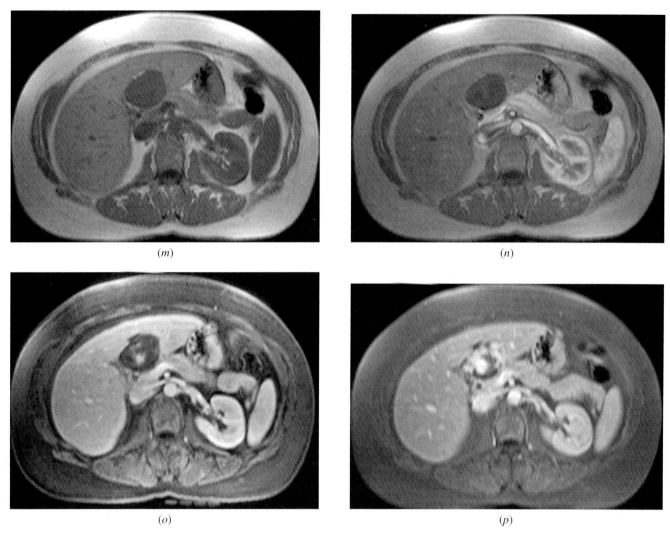

(m)

(n)

(o)

(p)

FIG. 2.39 (*Continued*)

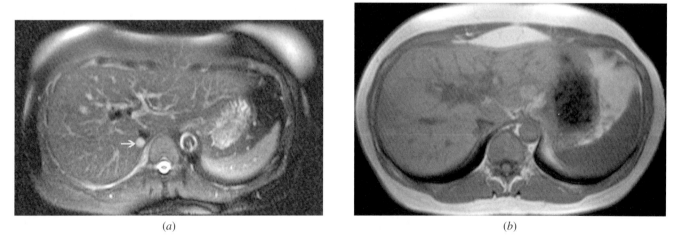

(a)

(b)

FIG. 2.40 Small-sized slow-enhancing hemangioma. T2-weighted fat-suppressed SS-ETSE (*a*), SGE (*b*), and immediate (*c*) and 90-s fat-suppressed (*d*) postgadolinium SGE images. There is a small hepatic lesion adjacent to the inferior vena cava that shows

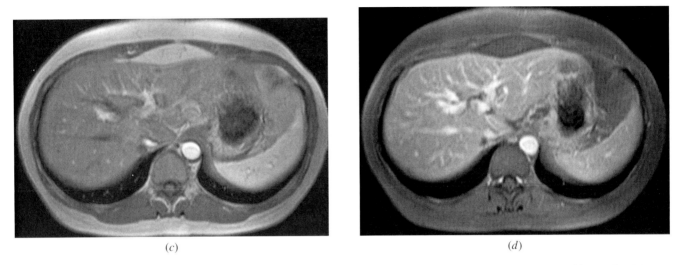

(c)   (d)

F I G . 2.40 (*Continued*) high signal intensity on the T2-weighted image (arrow, *a*), low signal intensity on T1-weighted image (*b*), a lack of enhancement on early image (*c*) and peripheral globular enhancement on late image (*d*) compatible with a slow-enhancing hemangioma. Slow enhancement is a feature that suggests the diagnosis of a hemangioma.

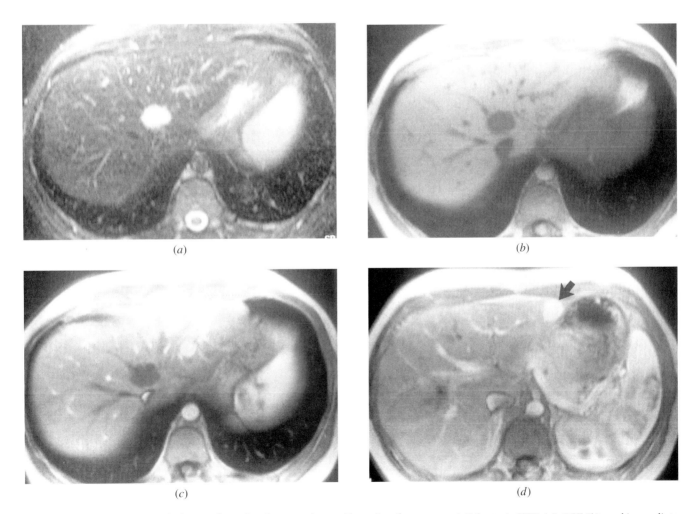

(a)   (b)

(c)   (d)

F I G . 2.41 Medium-sized slow-enhancing hemangioma, Type 3 enhancement. Echo train-STIR (*a*), SGE (*b*), and immediate (*c*, *d*) and 90-s fat-suppressed (*e*) postgadolinium SGE images. A lobular lesion is present that demonstrates moderately high signal intensity on the T2-weighted image (*a*) and moderately low signal intensity on the T1-weighted image (*b*), small peripheral nodules

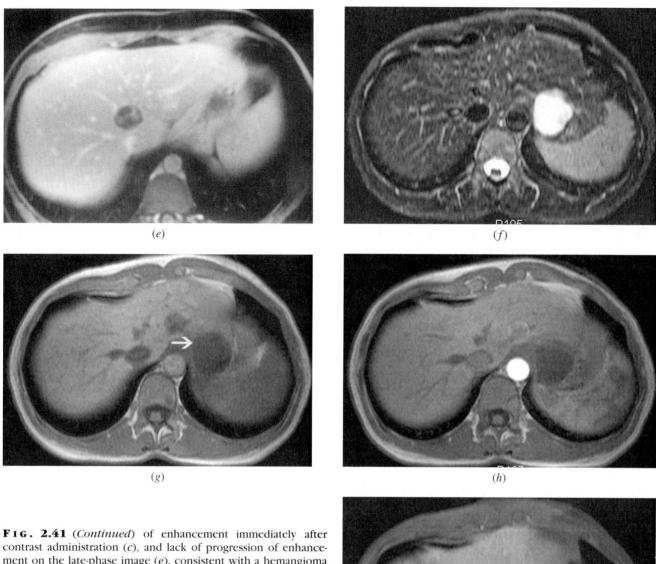

(e)   (f)

(g)   (h)

(i)

FIG. 2.41 (*Continued*) of enhancement immediately after contrast administration (*c*), and lack of progression of enhancement on the late-phase image (*e*), consistent with a hemangioma Type 3 enhancement. There is another rounded lesion in the tip of the left lobe that shows intense enhancement on the immediate postgadolinium image (arrow, *d*), consistent with focal nodular hyperplasia.

Echo train-STIR (*f*), SGE (*g*), and immediate (*h*) and 90-s fat-suppressed (*i*) SGE images in a second patient. A hemangioma is seen in the left hepatic lobe that appears moderately high signal intensity on the T2-weighted image (*f*), moderately low signal intensity on T1-weighed image (arrow, *g*), a lack of enhancement on early phase (*h*), and a globular focus of enhancement on the late postcontrast image (*i*), consistent with a slow-enhancing hemangioma.

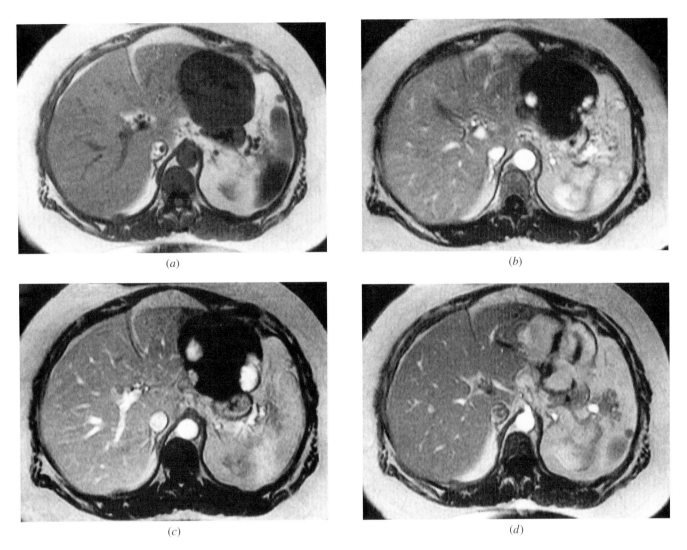

F I G . 2.42 Giant hemangioma. SGE (*a*) and immediate (*b*), 90-s (*c*), and 10-min (*d*) postgadolinium SGE images. A hemangioma is present in the left lobe that is moderately low in signal intensity on T1-weighted image (*a*), demonstrates peripheral nodular enhancement in a discontinuous ring on the early image (*b*), and gradually enhances in a centripetal fashion (*c*) with persistent low signal intensity central scar on delayed image (*d*).

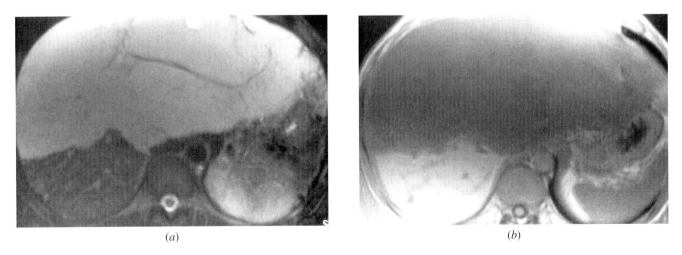

F I G . 2.43 Massive hemangiomas. Echo train-STIR (*a*), SGE (*b*), and immediate (*c*) and 90-s fat-suppressed (*d*) postgadolinium SGE images. A massive tumor replaces the majority of the liver, with sparing of segments 6 and 7 in the right hepatic lobe. After administration of gadolinium, this lesion demonstrates discontinuous peripheral nodular enhancement with enlargement and coalescence of the nodules. The appearance is consistent with a massive hemangioma.

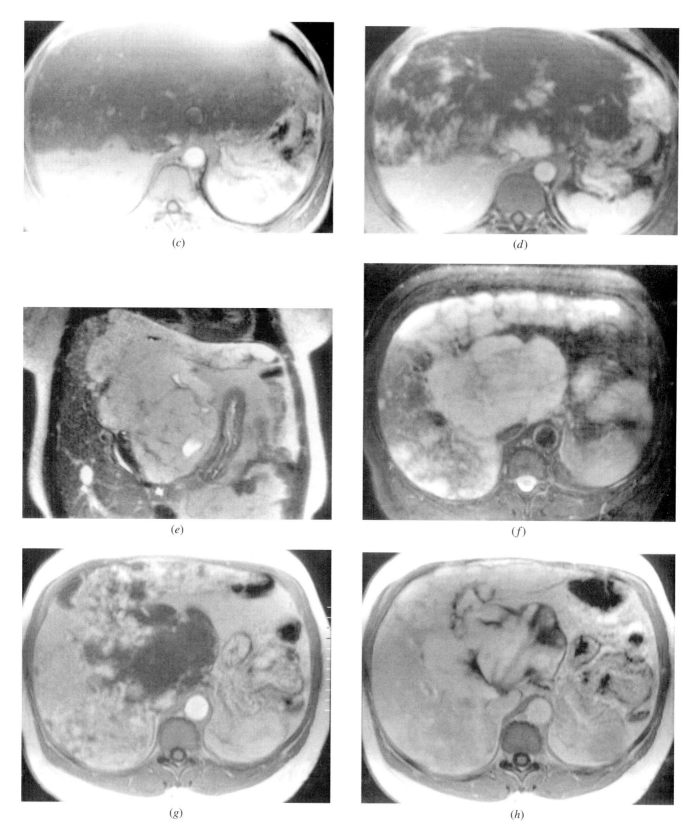

(c)

(d)

(e)

(f)

(g)

(h)

F I G . 2.43 (*Continued*) Coronal T2-weighted SS-ETSE (*e*), transverse echo-train STIR (*f*), and immediate (*g*) and 5-min (*h*) post-gadolinium SGE images in a second patient. A massive lobulated lesion is present in the liver parenchyma that is predominantly high signal intensity on T2-weighted images (*e, f*), but with multiple low-signal strands, and demonstrates discontinuous nodular enhancement (*g*) with centripetal progression (*h*) after the administration of gadolinium. Regions of hypointense central scar persist on the late images (*h*). Low-signal-intensity linear strands are common on T2-weighted images in giant hemangiomas and represent bands of collagenous tissue. This patient underwent liver transplantation because of the extensive hepatic replacement by hemangiomas.

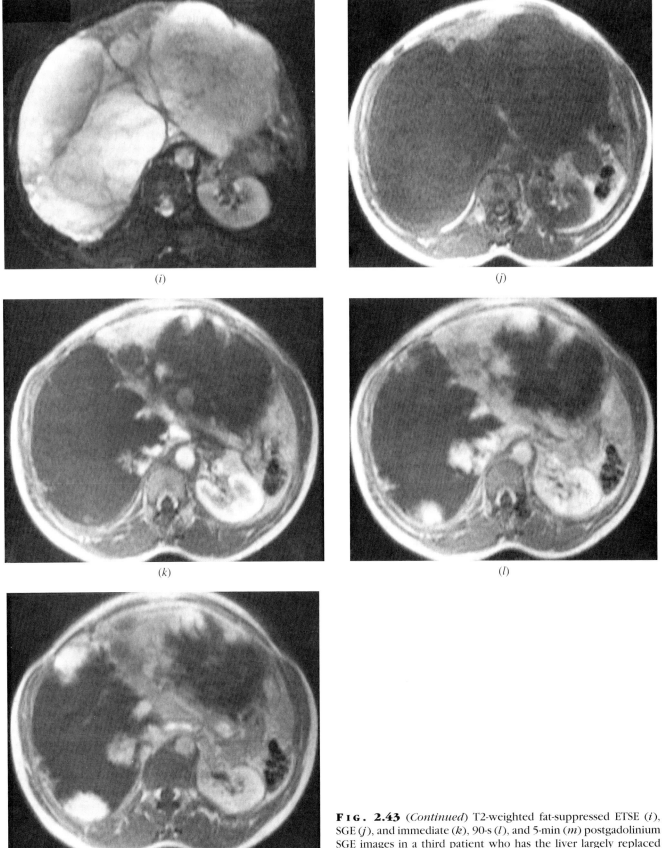

FIG. 2.43 (*Continued*) T2-weighted fat-suppressed ETSE (*i*), SGE (*j*), and immediate (*k*), 90-s (*l*), and 5-min (*m*) postgadolinium SGE images in a third patient who has the liver largely replaced by massive hemangiomas. The findings appreciated in this patient are similar to those in the second patient.

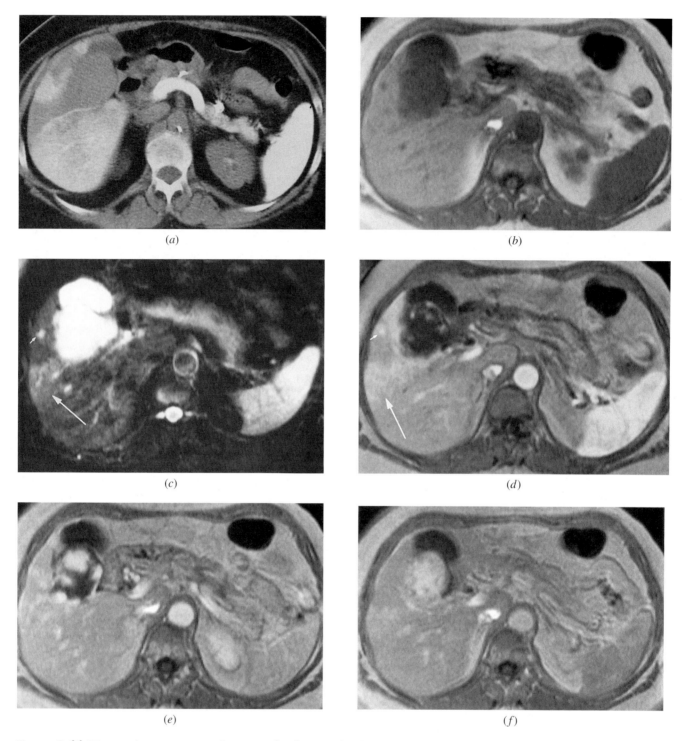

(a)

(b)

(c)

(d)

(e)

(f)

FIG. 2.44 Hemangioma compressing portal vein. Spiral CTAP (*a*), SGE (*b*), T2-weighted fat-suppressed ETSE (*c*), and immediate (*d*), 90-s (*e*), and 10-min (*f*) postgadolinium SGE images. A 6-cm lesion is present in the anterior segment of the right lobe that causes distal wedge-shaped diminished portal venous perfusion on the CTAP image (*a*), findings that were considered consistent with a malignant tumor. The tumor is moderately low in signal intensity on T1-weighted image (*b*) and high in signal intensity on T2-weighted image (*c*) and has perilesional and peripheral nodular enhancement on early-phase image (*d*) that progressively fills in a centripetal fashion on late and delayed images (*e, f*). The perfusion defect observed on the CTAP image (*a*) is noted to be wedge-shaped and mildly hyperintense on T2-weighted image (long arrow, *c*) and enhances in a transient fashion greater than adjacent liver on the early-phase image (long arrow, *d*), findings consistent with portal vein compression. Additional note is made of a 6-mm hemangioma lateral to the large hemangioma (small arrow, *c*), which enhances intense and homogeneously on early-phase image (small arrow, *d*), compatible with a Type 1 pattern of enhancement.

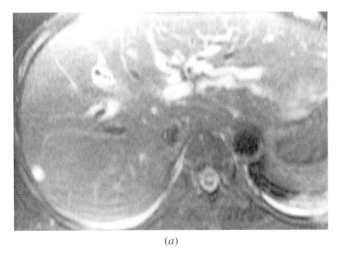

(a)

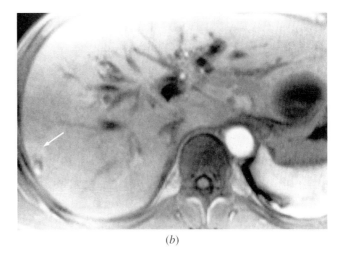

(b)

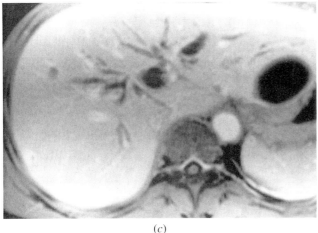

(c)

FIG. 2.45 Hemangioma with perilesional enhancement. T2-weighted SS-ETSE (*a*) and immediate (*b*) and 90-s fat-suppressed (*c*) postgadolinium SGE images. This patient, who has an inflammatory pseudotumor arising in the common hepatic duct that causes dilatation of the biliary tree, also demonstrates a round, well-defined lesion, which is hyperintense on T2-weighted image (*a*) and shows peripheral nodular enhancement on the immediate postcontrast image (*b*) with nearly complete fill-in of the lesion on the delayed image (*c*). Note the transient ill-defined increased perilesional enhancement (arrow, *b*) on the immediate postcontrast image (*b*). Perilesional enhancement.

washout and the type 1 hemangioma are more likely to maintain the signal intensity or to fade away toward background isointensity. In this setting, a large lesion is usually present that will exhibit the enhancement features of either a hemangioma or a metastasis, so that the histology of the small lesions may be inferred. Reports have shown that hemangiomas may be reliably distinguished from metastases on T2-weighted images based on the smooth lobular margins and the higher calculated T2 values of hemangiomas (mean of 140 ms) [80]. Although this may be true in the majority of patients, cumulative experience from many centers has shown that T2-weighted images alone may not allow characterization of small tumors or allow reliable distinction between hemangiomas and metastases from hypervascular malignant tumors. For this reason, long-TE T2-weighted sequences for hemangiomas are not performed at our institution because some diagnostically difficult lesions, such as hypervascular metastases, may also show long T2 values. The routine combination of T2-weighted information with serial gadolinium-

enhanced SGE is useful to increase observer confidence for establishing the correct diagnosis and also to maximize evaluation of other hepatic and extrahepatic diseases (fig. 2.46) [72, 81].

Chemotherapy-treated liver metastases may resemble the appearance of hemangiomas when chemotherapy treatment has occurred within a 2- to 12-month period before MRI. A less aggressive enhancement pattern that develops in chemotherapy-treated liver metastasis may be reflective of underlying histologic changes associated with a salutary response to chemotherapy, that is, antiangiogenic effect with altered vascularity [82].

Few studies to date have reported the imaging findings of hemangiomas in the setting of cirrhosis or chronic liver disease. It is suggested that the incidence of hemangiomas in patients with chronic liver disease is up to 9% [83]. Hemangiomas in this setting are more likely to be solitary and subcapsular [84, 85]. It has been suggested that hemangiomas tend to decrease in size with the progression of liver disease due to fibrotic

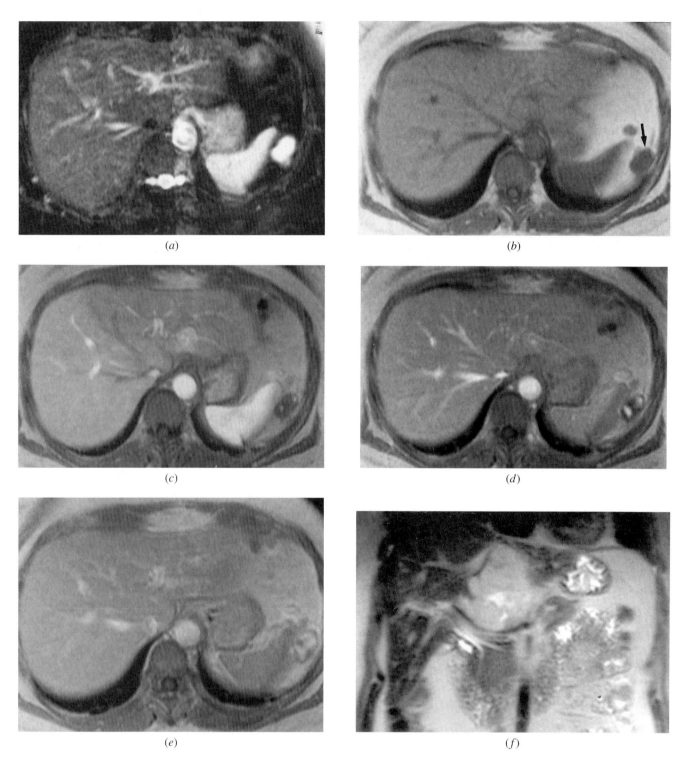

(a)

(b)

(c)

(d)

(e)

(f)

FIG. 2.46 Exophytic hemangioma. T2-weighted fat-suppressed ETSE (*a*), SGE (*b*), and immediate (*c*), 90-s (*d*), and 10-min (*e*) postgadolinium SGE images. A pedunculated 2.5-cm hemangioma (arrow, *b*) arises from the tip of the lateral segment of the liver. The hemangioma is high in signal intensity on T2-weighted image (*a*) and moderately low in signal intensity on T1-weighted image (*b*), enhances in a peripheral nodular fashion on the early-phase image (*c*), and shows centripetal progression on late (*d*) and delayed (*e*) images. Despite the thin stalk of the hemangioma, it exhibits circumlesional peripheral nodular enhancement, comparable to standard intraparenchymal hemangiomas.

Coronal (*f, g*) and transverse (*h*) T2-weighted SS-ETSE, T1-weighted fat-suppressed SGE (*i*), and immediate (*j*) and 90-s fat-suppressed (*k*) postgadolinium SGE images in a second patient. There is a mass arising from segment 1 of the liver, with extension

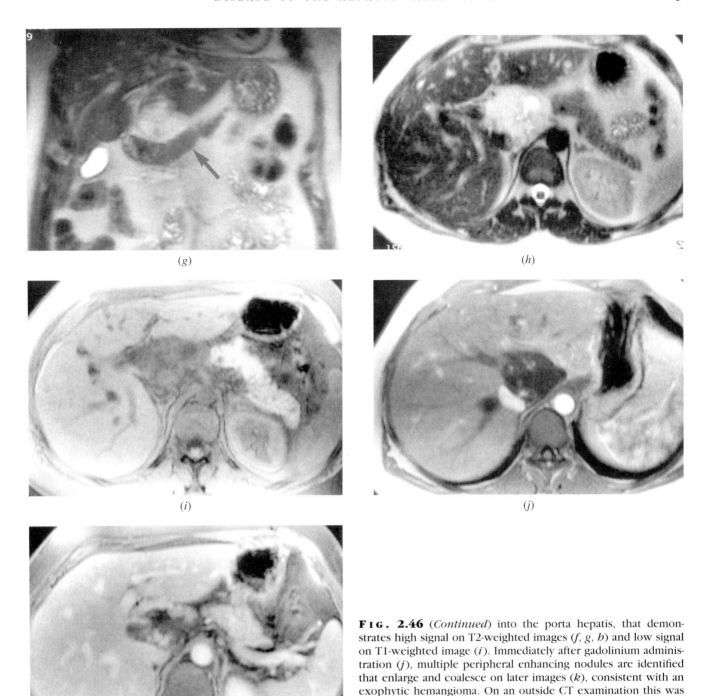

(g)

(h)

(i)

(j)

(k)

FIG. 2.46 (*Continued*) into the porta hepatis, that demonstrates high signal on T2-weighted images (*f, g, h*) and low signal on T1-weighted image (*i*). Immediately after gadolinium administration (*j*), multiple peripheral enhancing nodules are identified that enlarge and coalesce on later images (*k*), consistent with an exophytic hemangioma. On an outside CT examination this was thought to arise from the pancreas. The coronal T2-weighted image (*g*) demonstrates inferior displacement of an intact pancreas (arrow, *g*). Additionally, the pancreas distal to the mass exhibits normal high signal on the T1-weighted fat-suppressed image (*i*), which essentially excludes a pancreatic adenocarcinoma.

degeneration, thrombosis, or hemorrhage [83–85]. Mastropasqua and colleagues [84] also have shown that there is no statistically significant difference between the size of small and medium hemangiomas in unaffected livers and in cirrhotic or chronic liver disease, although there was a tendency for cirrhotic livers to have small hemangiomas and no giant hemangiomas

were observed in cirrhosis (fig. 2.47). This observation may reflect the fact that, in severely fibrotic livers, these is a paucity of vascular tissue available to support the growth of hemangiomas to a large size. On MRI, the signal intensity of hemangiomas on T2- and T1-weighted images pre- and postcontrast in patients with cirrhosis or chronic liver disease is similar to that in patients with

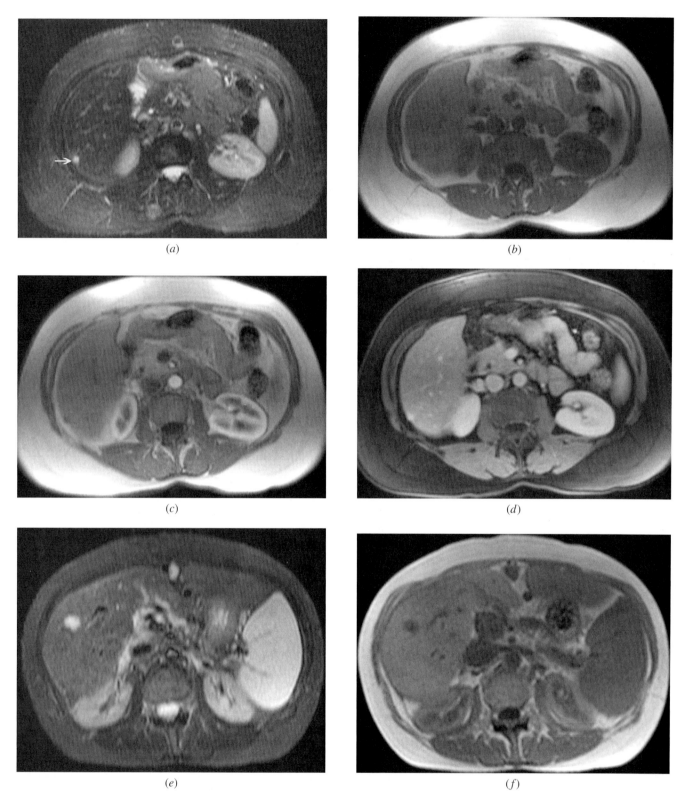

(a)

(b)

(c)

(d)

(e)

(f)

FIG. 2.47 Hemangioma in the setting of chronic liver disease. T2-weighted SS-ETSE (*a*), SGE (*b*), and immediate (*c*) and 90-s fat-suppressed (*d*) postgadolinium SGE images in a patient with chronic liver disease patient. There is an hepatic lesion in segment 6 that demonstrates moderately high signal intensity on the T2-weighted image (arrow, *a*), moderately low signal intensity on the T1-weighted image (*b*), and enhancement of a peripheral focus on the early-phase image (*c*) that fills in on the late-phase image (*d*), consistent a with Type 2 hemangioma.

T2-weighted SS-ETSE (*e*), SGE (*f*), and immediate (*g*) and 90-s fat-suppressed (*h*) postgadolinium SGE images in a second patient with a history of acute on chronic hepatitis. There is a hemangioma in segment 5 of the liver that shows high signal intensity on

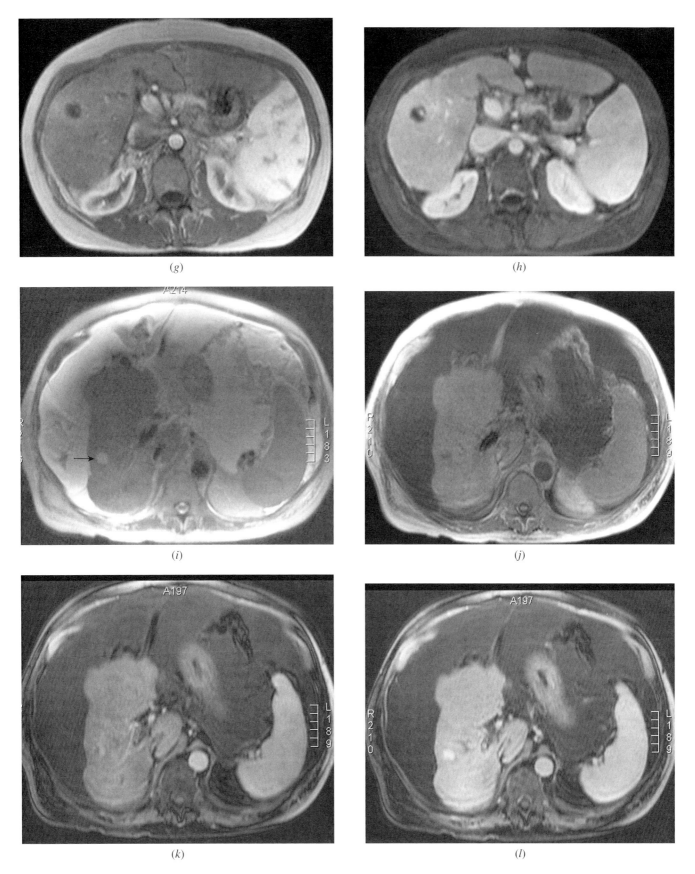

FIG. 2.47 (*Continued*) the T2-weighted image, low signal intensity on the T1-weighted image (*f*), and globular enhancement on early-phase image (*g*) that persists on late-phase (*h*) images. Increased perilesional enhancement surrounding the hemangioma is appreciated on the early-phase image (*g*). Additionally, the parenchyma enhances in a patchy fashion on early- and late-phase images, consistent with acute on chronic hepatitis.

T2-weighted SS-ETSE (*i*), SGE (*j*), and immediate (*k*) and 90-s fat-suppressed (*l*) postgadolinium SGE images in a third patient with end-stage chronic liver disease and a Type 2 hemangioma (arrow, *i*).

nonaffected livers. Regardless of the size, hemangiomas are more likely to show a fast lesional fill-in after contrast. The recognition of the MR features of hemangioma type 1 is useful since it may be indistinguishable from HCC in early phase because both entities exhibit homogeneous moderately intense enhancement. The signal intensity on T2-weighted images may help in this differentiation, because small HCCs are often near isointensity in contrast to the moderately high signal of hemangiomas.

Advantages of MRI over CT imaging in the evaluation of hemangiomas include: 1) the greater ability to image the entire liver in the same phase of contrast enhance-

ment, which is particularly useful when multiple lesions are present; 2) greater lesion enhancement on contrast-enhanced images such that lesions are comparatively brighter than background liver (fig. 2.48); 3) superior detection of small hemangiomas; and 4) effective lesion detection and characterization with T2-weighted images, which CT does not have an analogous technique.

Infantile Hemangioendothelioma

Infantile hemangioendotheliomas (IHE) are congenital lesions and the most common mesenchymal tumor of the liver in childhood [86]. Although infantile heman-

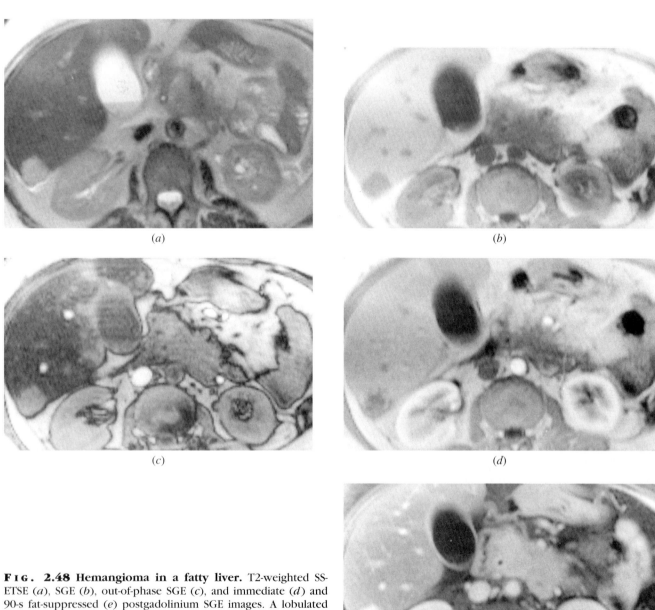

FIG. 2.48 Hemangioma in a fatty liver. T2-weighted SS-ETSE (*a*), SGE (*b*), out-of-phase SGE (*c*), and immediate (*d*) and 90-s fat-suppressed (*e*) postgadolinium SGE images. A lobulated hemangioma is present in the right hepatic lobe, which shows peripheral nodular enhancement on early-phase image (*d*) and gradually fills with contrast on late-phase image (*e*) but with the persistence of a central scar. The liver is diffusely fatty infiltrated (*c*), which renders the lesion relatively high signal on out-of-phase sequence.

gioendotheliomas are histologically benign, they may lead to death within months secondary to heart or liver failure. Spontaneous regression of the lesions tends to occur after 8 months of age [87, 88]. Pathologic examination shows a multinodular tumor involving both lobes. Microscopically, numerous dilated vascular channels are lined by multiple layers of plump endothelial cells. Cavernous vascular channels are frequent.

On imaging, these lesions tend to be numerous similar-size tumors that are uniformly moderately to markedly hyperintense on T2-weighted images and hypointense on T1 weighted images and enhance homogeneously on interstitial-phase gadolinium-enhanced images (fig. 2.49) [89].

Hepatocellular Adenoma

Hepatocellular adenomas (HCA) are benign epithelial neoplasms [2]. Approximately 90% of HCAs occur in young women [90]. These lesions are associated with the use of oral contraceptive steroids [2]. Tumors will involute spontaneously after patients withdraw from birth control pill. Other much less frequent associations include the use of anabolic steroids and disorders associated with abnormal carbohydrate metabolism, such as familial diabetes mellitus, galactosemia, and glycogen storage disease type Ia [91–93]. Patients may present with acute abdominal pain, related to hemorrhage into the tumor [94]. Rarely, rupture into the peritoneal cavity may occur that requires emergency intervention. Malignant transformation is sporadic [95].

Pathologically, HCA are most commonly solitary tumors characterized as a bulging mass with dilated blood vessels traversing the surface. HCA are partially or completely enclosed by a pseudocapsule derived from compressed and collapsed hepatic parenchyma. Sectioning reveals a spherical, well-demarcated, richly vascular lesion, frequently with areas of hemorrhage or necrosis. Focal scar formation is indicative of remote infarction. The histologic hallmark consists of clusters of benign hepatocytes arranged in slender plates of two- to three-cell thickness. Steatosis may be prominent. Neoplastic hepatocytes are separated by slitlike sinusoids and numerous thin-walled veins. Bile ducts are absent [87].

The typical MR appearance of HCA is homogeneously mild hyperintensity on T2-weighted images, homogeneously mild hypointensity or isointensity on T1-weighted images, and transient homogeneous blush immediately after contrast that uniformly fades to isointensity with liver parenchyma by 1 min. The intensity and heterogeneity of signal on T2- and T1-weighted images may vary and reflect the quantity of fat, hemorrhage, and necrosis within the tumor (figs. 2.50 and 2.51) [53, 96, 97]. The arrangement of vessels and stroma in HCA may result in an intense marbled pattern of enhancement that may be difficult to distinguish from HCC on arterial dominant phase. However, the presence of lesional washout and complete capsule enhancement on late phase suggest the diagnosis of HCC. HCA may decrease homogeneously in signal intensity on out-of-phase or fat-suppressed images because of their fat content, which is commonly uniform (fig. 2.52).

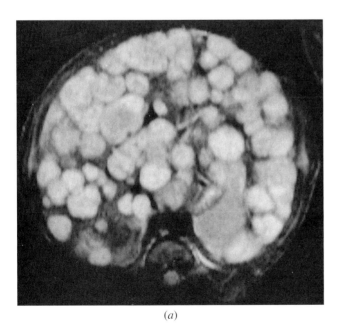

(a)

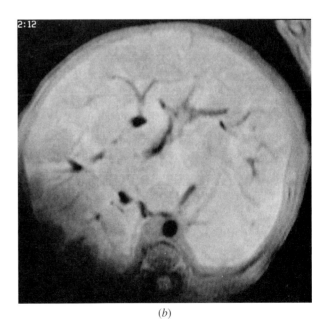

(b)

F I G. 2.49 Infantile hemangioendothelioma. T2-weighted fat-suppressed ETSE (*a*), T1-weighted fat-suppressed SE (*b*), and T1-weighted interstitial-phase fat-suppressed gadolinium-enhanced SE (*c*) images. The liver in this 9-month-old boy is extensively replaced with focal mass lesions, smaller than 1 cm, that are high in signal intensity on the T2-weighted image (*a*) and mildly low in signal intensity on the T1-weighted image (*b*) and enhance homogeneously on the interstitial-phase gadolinium-enhanced image (*c*). This appearance is characteristic for hemangioendothelioma in neonatal patients.

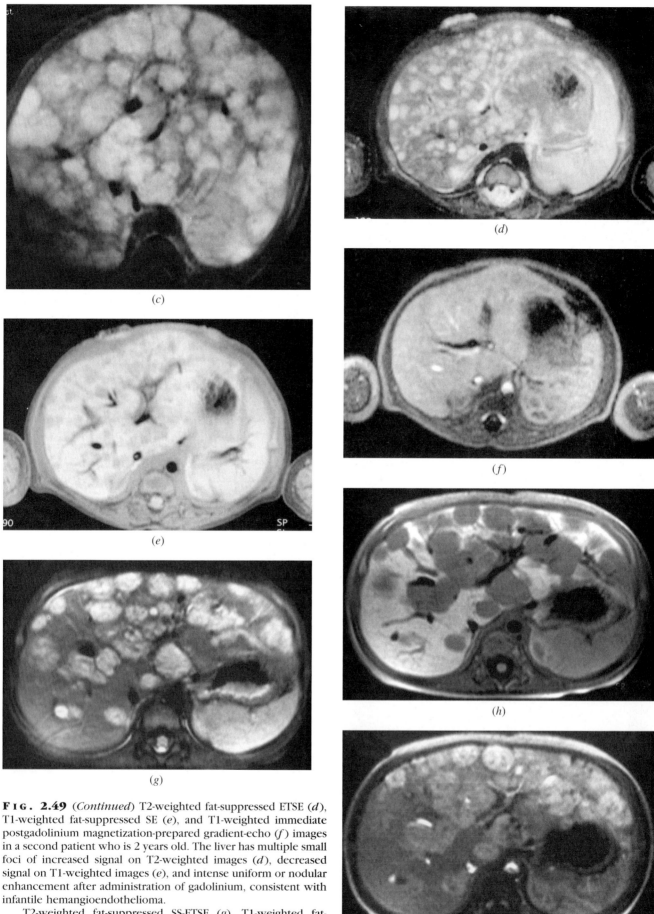

FIG. 2.49 (*Continued*) T2-weighted fat-suppressed ETSE (*d*), T1-weighted fat-suppressed SE (*e*), and T1-weighted immediate postgadolinium magnetization-prepared gradient-echo (*f*) images in a second patient who is 2 years old. The liver has multiple small foci of increased signal on T2-weighted images (*d*), decreased signal on T1-weighted images (*e*), and intense uniform or nodular enhancement after administration of gadolinium, consistent with infantile hemangioendothelioma.

T2-weighted fat-suppressed SS-ETSE (*g*), T1-weighted fat-suppressed SGE (*b*), and immediate (*i*) and 90-s (*j*) postgadolinium SGE images in a third patient show findings similar to those in the second patient.

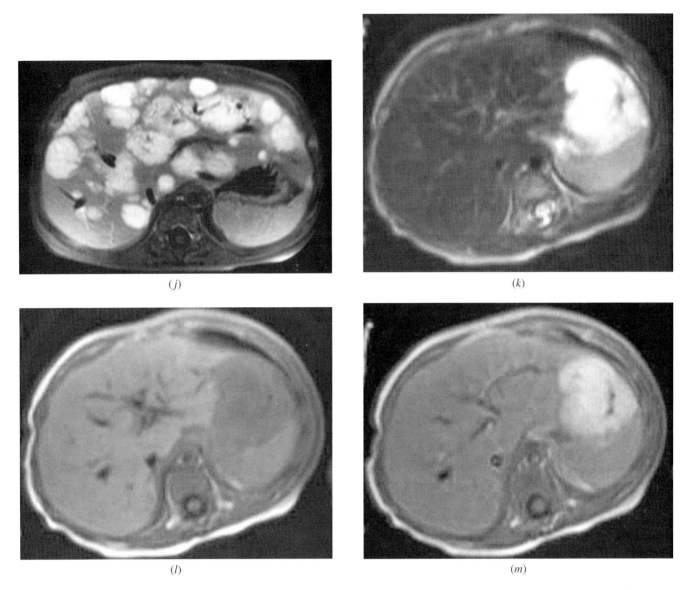

(j)

(k)

(l)

(m)

FIG. 2.49 (*Continued*) T2-weighted SS-ETSE (*k*), SGE (*l*), and immediate postgadolinium SGE (*m*) images in a fourth patient demonstrate a lobular lesion in the tip of the left lobe that shows moderately high signal intensity on the T2-weighted image (*k*), low signal on the T1-weighted image (*l*), and intense enhancement after administration of contrast (*m*). Histopathology was consistent with infantile hemangioendothelioma.

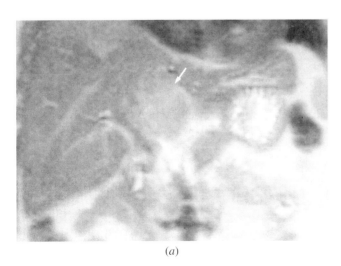

(a)

FIG. 2.50 Hepatic adenoma. Coronal T2-weighted SS-ETSE (*a*), SGE (*b*), out-of-phase SGE (*c*), and immediate (*d*) and 90-s fat-suppressed (*e*) postgadolinium SGE images. There is a lesion in

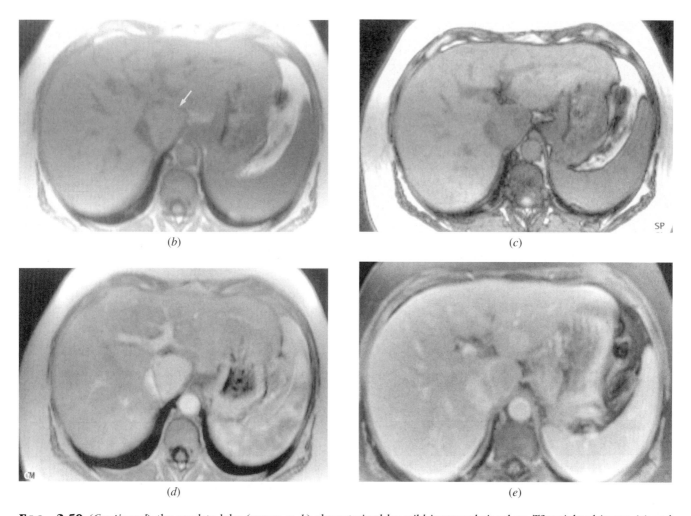

(b)

(c)

(d)

(e)

F I G . 2.50 (*Continued*) the caudate lobe (arrow, *a, b*) characterized by mild increased signal on T2-weighted image (*a*) and T1-weighted image (*b*), drop in signal on out-of-phase images (*c*), diffuse intense homogeneous enhancement on early-phase image (*d*), and fading to near isointensity on late-phase image (*e*). Loss of signal on out-of-phase image (*c*) is characteristic of hepatic adenoma. Late capsular enhancement (*e*), as observed in this case, may be occasionally observed in hepatic adenomas.

F I G . 2.51 Hepatic adenoma complicated by hemorrhage. T2-weighted fat-suppressed ETSE (*a*), SGE (*b*), and immediate post-gadolinium SGE (*c*) images. An 8-cm mass arises from the inferior aspect of the right hepatic lobe. Regions within the mass possess high signal intensity on T2-weighted image (*a*) and high signal intensity peripheral rims on T1-weighted image (arrows, *b*) consistent with blood. Heterogeneous enhancement of the nonhemorrhagic portions of the mass is identified on early phase image (*c*). The patient discontinued birth control pills and on the 3-month follow-up study the mass had decreased in size to 3.5-cm (not shown).

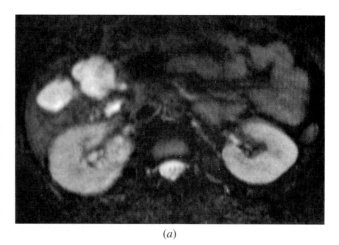

(a)

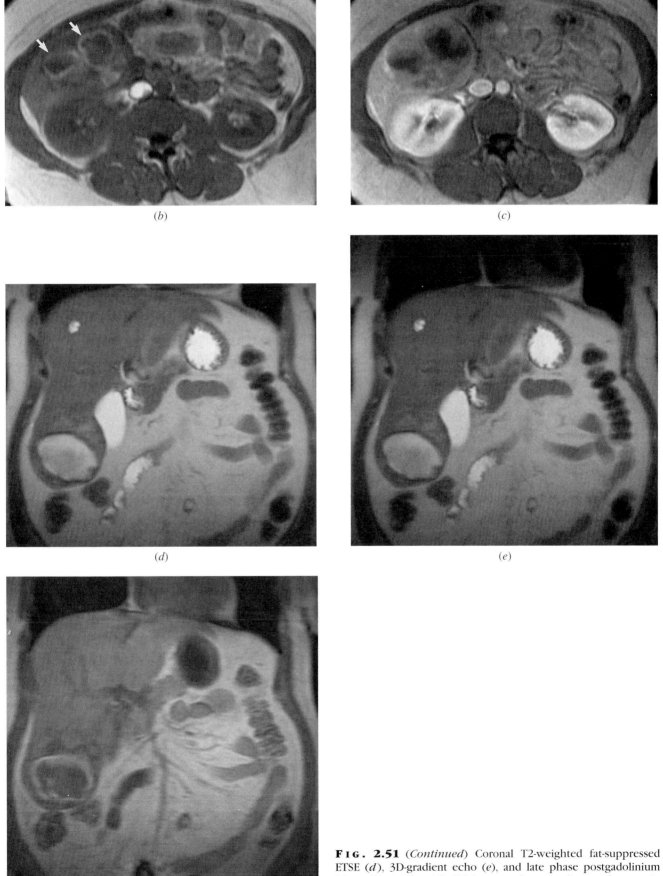

(b)

(c)

(d)

(e)

(f)

FIG. 2.51 (*Continued*) Coronal T2-weighted fat-suppressed ETSE (*d*), 3D-gradient echo (*e*), and late phase postgadolinium 3D-gradient echo (*f*) 3T images of a complicate adenoma in segment 6 of the liver **at 3T** in a second patient. Note the heterogeneous signal intensity on T2-weighted (*d*) and high signal intensity on T1-weighted (*e*) consistent with various age hemorrhage.

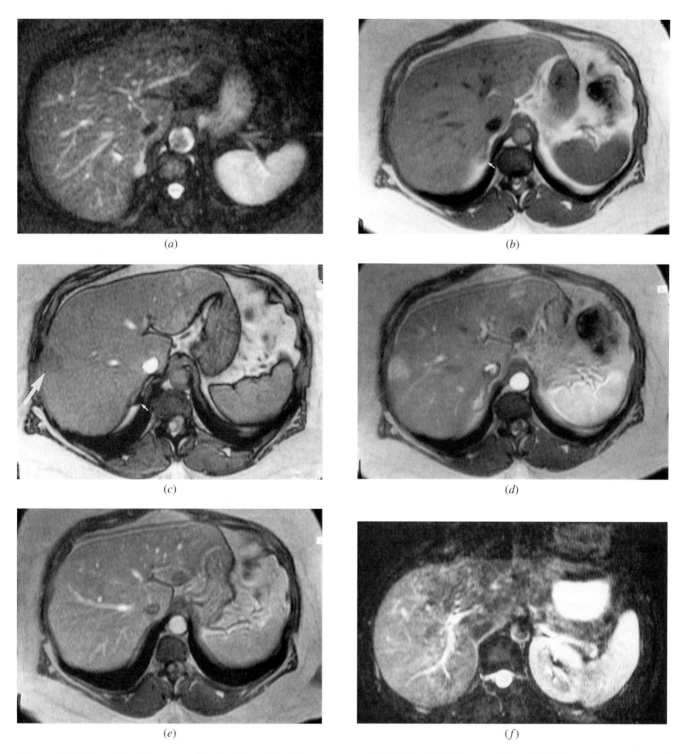

(a)

(b)

(c)

(d)

(e)

(f)

F I G . 2.52 Hepatic adenoma with fat. T2-weighted fat-suppressed ETSE (*a*), SGE (*b*), out-of-phase SGE (*c*), and immediate (*d*) and 90-s (*e*) postgadolinium SGE images. No focal liver lesions are apparent on the T2-weighted image (*a*) or the T1-weighted image (*b*). On out-of-phase image the adenoma is shown as a low-signal mass (arrow, *c*) because of signal drop caused by the presence of fat within the tumor. The adenoma enhances with a characteristic uniform hepatic arterial dominant-phase blush (*d*), which rapidly fades, rendering the tumor isointense with liver by 90 s. Incidental note is made of a right adrenal mass (small arrow, *b*, *c*) that drops in signal intensity from in-phase (*b*) to out-of-phase (*c*) images, which is diagnostic for adrenal adenoma.

T2-weighted fat-suppressed ETSE (*f*), SGE (*g*), out-of-phase SGE (*h*), and immediate postgadolinium SGE (*i*) images in a second patient. A 4-cm hepatic adenoma is nearly isointense on T2-weighted (*f*) and T1-weighted (*g*) images, drops in signal intensity on

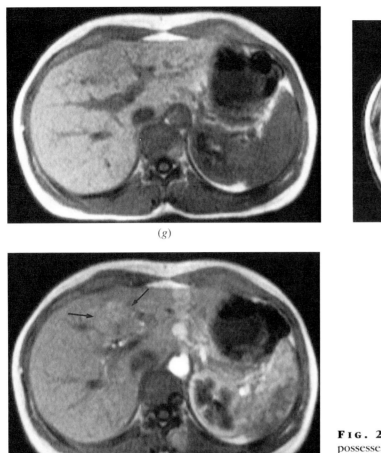

(g)

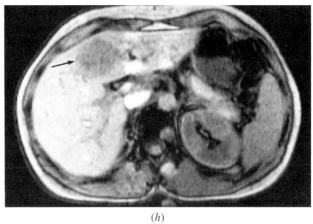

(h)

(i)

FIG. 2.52 (*Continued*) out-of-phase image (arrow, *h*), and possesses a faint blush on early-phase image (arrows, *i*) greater than that of adjacent liver. The uniform hepatic arterial dominant-phase blush of adenomas permits distinction from focal fatty infiltration, which enhances less than or equal to adjacent liver.

The drop in signal intensity is a relatively common feature of fat-containing HCA and is rarely observed in HCC. Occasionally, the presence of central fibrosis may cause diagnostic confusion with FNH. Although the signal intensity on T2- and T1-weighted precontrast images and the pattern of enhancement of both entities may be quite similar, the presence of fat or hemorrhage within the lesion is suggestive of HCA. Moreover, FNH rarely contains fat or blood, and is more likely to exist in the setting of fatty liver.

Similar to FNH, hepatic adenomas tend to involute with age. In part, this may reflect age-related changes, but this may also reflect hormone-related changes. Unlike FNH, which maintain a well-organized, nonaggressive rounded configuration as they involute, hepatic adenomas tend to have more irregular margins and more irregular signal on all sequences, which mimics the appearance of more aggressive tumors such as metastases and HCC. The explanation for the more heterogenous signal and irregular morphology of these lesions is that they presumably have more fibrosis and perhaps internal hemorrhage as they involute, rendering

a more aggressive appearance. A lesion with strikingly irregular spiculated margins within the liver suggests the presence of fibrosis, which may be either spontaneous or the result of therapy. Hence, if a lesion has this appearance, but the patient has no history of chemotherapy for primary malignancy or local therapy for malignant liver lesion, then spontaneous fibrosis should be considered. The lesions with the greatest propensity for spontaneous fibrosis are myofibroblastic tumor (see *Inflammatory Myofibroblastic Tumor* below) and hepatic adenoma.

Rarely, HCA may arise in men, often related to the use of anabolic steroids or an underlying genetic disorder, although sporadic cases with no underlying cause may be observed. The majority of these HCA are asymptomatic and are discovered incidentally during a routine examination. The MR findings of HCA in men are not well established because of their rarity. Preliminary reports suggest that only 25% of the cases will demonstrate the typical findings of HCA as observed in women; notably, in most cases of HCA in men, uniform fat content is not present [98]. The presence

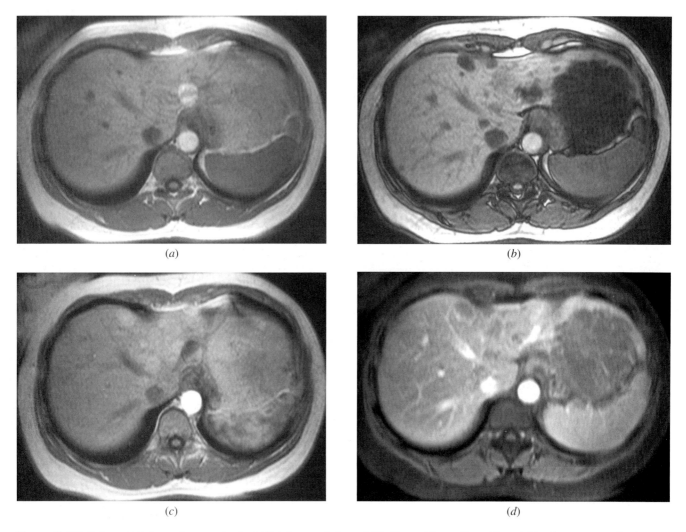

F I G . 2.53 Fat containing adenomatosis. SGE (*a*), out-of-phase SGE (*b*), and immediate (*c*) and 90-s fat-suppressed (*d*) post-gadolinium SGE images. Multiple lesions with varying sizes are seen predominantly present in the left hepatic lobe that show isointensity on T1-weighted images (*a*) and drop in signal intensity on out-of-phase images (*b*) and show a faint homogeneous enhancement on early-phase images (*c*) compatible with fat-containing adenomatosis. On the late-phase image (*d*) some lesions show lower signal intensity than background parenchyma, which may reflect a fat suppression effect, lesion washout, or a combination of both.

and extent of fat, hemorrhage, and necrosis are responsible for the variation in the signal intensity on MRI. The major differential diagnosis to be considered in this setting is HCC. Histopathology is crucial to distinguish these entities. Because hepatocellular adenomas contain hepatocytes, hepatocyte-specific contrast agents (e.g., Mn-DPDP) will be taken up by these tumors [5, 13, 99, 100].

Liver adenomatosis is an uncommon condition first described by Flejou and colleagues in 1985 [101]. As a separate clinical entity, liver adenomatosis may be distinguished from liver cell adenoma by the presence, in the former, of numerous adenomas (>10), lack of correlation with steroid medication, equal involvement in men and women, abnormal liver function tests, and a

higher incidence of hemorrhage and malignant transformation. HCAs in the setting of adenomatosis tend to exhibit a more heterogeneous appearance on all MR sequences and more variable enhancement on arterial dominant-phase images when compared to solitary HCAs (figs. 2.53–2.56) [102–104].

Peliosis Hepatis
Peliosis hepatis is characterized by the presence of grossly visible cystic blood-filled spaces in the liver [2, 3]. Peliosis occurs most commonly in the liver, but can occasionally occur in other parts of the reticuloendothelial system including the spleen or bone marrow [105]. Risk factors for peliosis include chronic wasting illnesses such as AIDS, tuberculosis, and cancer [106]

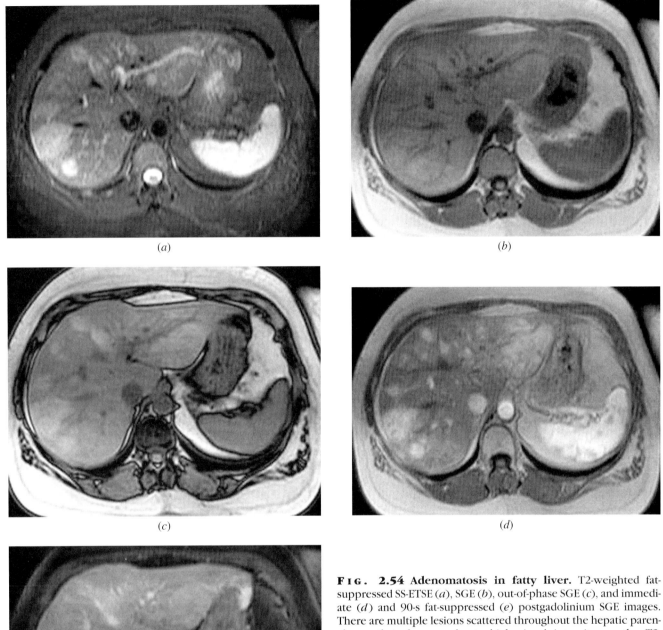

(a)

(b)

(c)

(d)

(e)

F I G . 2.54 Adenomatosis in fatty liver. T2-weighted fat-suppressed SS-ETSE (*a*), SGE (*b*), out-of-phase SGE (*c*), and immediate (*d*) and 90-s fat-suppressed (*e*) postgadolinium SGE images. There are multiple lesions scattered throughout the hepatic parenchyma that show moderate high signal intensity on the T2-weighted image (*a*), mild high signal intensity on the T1-weighted image (*b*), no signal loss on the out-of-phase image (*c*), and intense enhancement on the early-phase image (*d*) that fades on the late-phase image (*e*). On out-of-phase image (*c*), these lesions do not drop in signal but the background parenchyma does, showing a convergence in the signal intensity of the liver and spleen compared to the in-phase image (*b*). Background fatty liver in the setting of focal lesions is commonly seen with FNH, but not solitary adenomas. Adenomatosis is a different condition than solitary adenomas, and greater variability in the appearance of the lesions and liver is observed.

and drugs such as androgenenic anabolic steroids and oral contraceptives. The term was originally ascribed to macroscopic lesions (*peliosis* = dusky or purple), which may be several centimeters in diameter. The ectatic blood-filled spaces lack an endothelial lining when viewed microscopically. Peliosis hepatis may occur within hepatic neoplasms, including adenomas and hepatocellular carcinoma [2, 3].

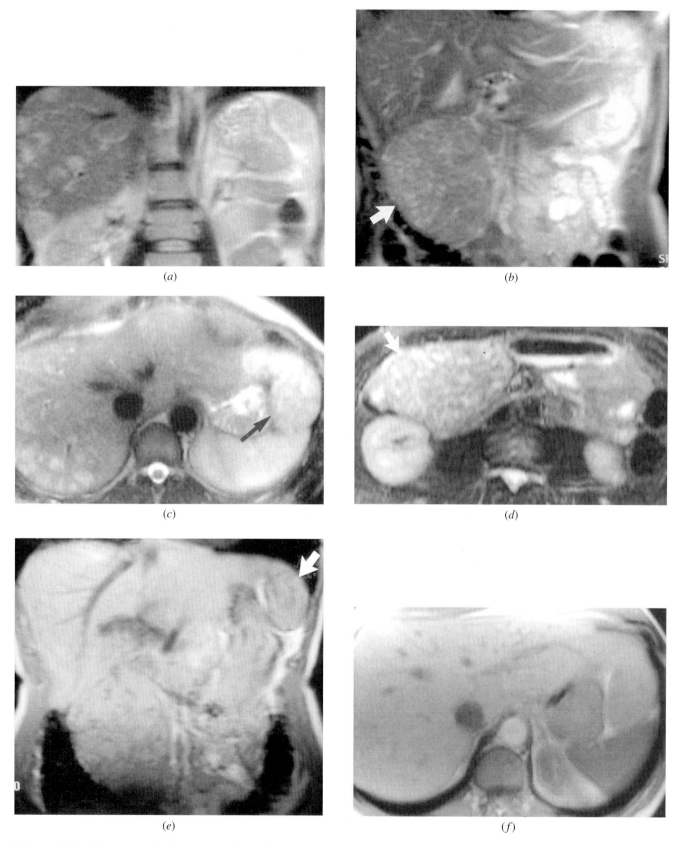

F I G . 2.55 Adenomatosis. Coronal (*a*, *b*) and transverse (*c*, *d*) T2-weighted SS-ETSE, coronal (*e*) and transverse (*f*, *g*) SGE, out-of-phase SGE (*h*, *i*), and immediate (*j*, *k*) and 90-s fat-suppressed (*l*, *m*) postgadolinium SGE images. Multiple small lesions are

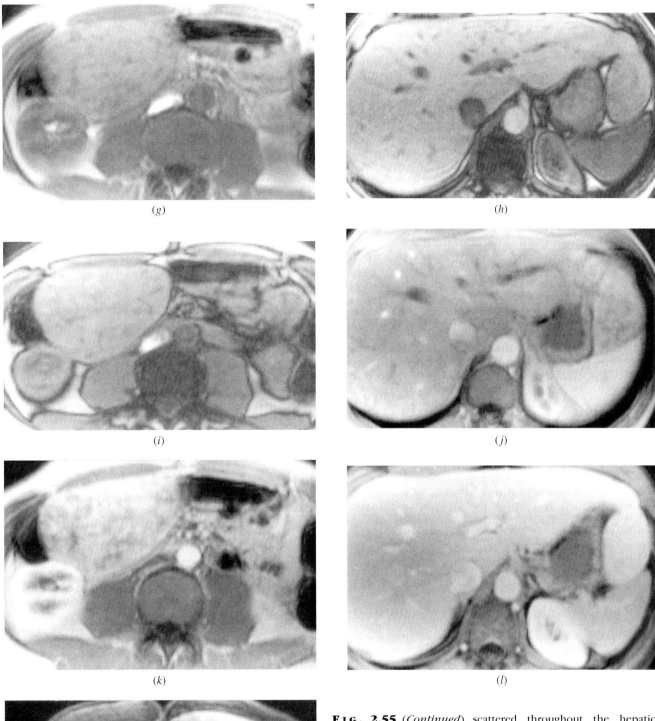

(g)

(h)

(i)

(j)

(k)

(l)

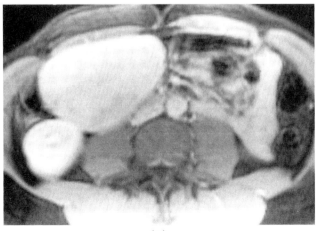

(m)

FIG. 2.55 (*Continued*) scattered throughout the hepatic parenchyma, predominantly in the right lobe, that demonstrate slight high signal on T2-weighted images (*a, c*), near isointensity on T1-weighted image (*f*), and mildly intense homogeneous enhancement immediately after administration of contrast (*j, k*) and become isointense with the liver by 90 s (*l, m*). Two exophytic lesions are seen, one of them in the tip of the left lobe (arrow, *c, e*) and the other an 8-cm tumor (arrow, *b, d*), in the right lobe. Both lesions demonstrate mildly heterogeneous signal intensity on T2-weighted images (*a–d*) and T1-weighted images (*e–g*). On early-phase images (*j, k*) the lesions enhance in a heterogeneous variegated fashion and become homogeneous on late-phase images (*l, m*). The intense heterogeneous variegated regular pattern on the early-phase images is rare for adenomas and raises the suspicious of hepatocellular carcinoma. It may be that adenomas in the setting of adenomatosis may be more heterogeneous than standard adenomas.

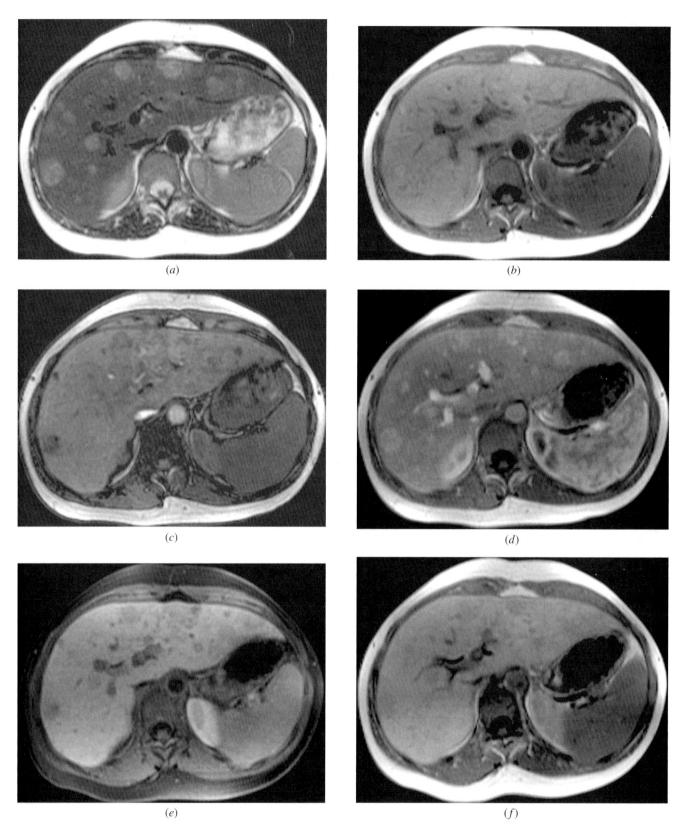

(a)   (b)

(c)   (d)

(e)   (f)

FIG. 2.56 Adenomatosis, Gd-BOPTA. T2-weighted SS-ETSE (*a*), SGE (*b*), out-of-phase SGE (*c*), and immediate (*d*), 90-s fat-suppressed (*e*), and 1-h (*f*) SGE after administration of Gd-BOPTA. Multiple lesions with varying sizes are seen in the hepatic parenchyma. These lesions demonstrate moderately high signal intensity on the T2-weighted image (*a*), isointensity on the T1-weighted image (*b*), drop in signal intensity on the out-of-phase image (*c*), and intense enhancement on the early phase image (*d*). On the late-phase image (*e*) these lesions show low signal intensity partially due to the fat suppression effect of this sequence. One hour (*f*) after administration of contrast, the lesions are low signal relative to liver, suggesting that there is no uptake of the contrast by the hepatocytes. This finding is consistent with adenomatosis and rules against multiple FNHs. (Courtesy of Guenther Schneider, M.D., Ph.D., Dept. of Diagnostic and Interventional Radiology, University Hospital Homburg/Saar, Germany).

The MR imaging appearance of peliosis hepatis is not well established. It has been described that peliosis hepatis may demonstrate varying signal intensity on T2-weighted and T1-weighted images according to the stage of hemorrhage. After contrast administration, peliosis hepatis may show moderate to intense enhancement on arterial dominant-phase images [107–111]. It is not clear to date whether the MR findings reflect this entity itself or the appearance of coexistent focal lesions, such as hepatic adenomas (fig. 2.57).

Focal Nodular Hyperplasia

Focal nodular hyperplasia (FNH) is an uncommon lesion defined by a localized region of hyperplasia within otherwise normal liver [2]. Although the lesion may occur in all age groups and both sexes, FNH predominantly is found in women during the third to fifth decades of life; after that age they tend to show progressive involution and are rarely observed in individuals beyond age 60, reflecting the frequency of this age-related involution. In contrast to hepatocellular adenomas (HCA), FNH does not appear to have a clear-cut association with oral contraceptive use [92]. Generally, FNH is a solitary lesion and tends to involute while maintaining its rounded configuration. Multicentric lesions may be encountered as part of the multiple FNH syndrome including other lesions such as liver hemangioma, meningioma, astrocytoma, telangiectasias of the brain, berry aneurysm, dysplastic systemic arteries, and portal vein atresia [78]. FNH does not exhibit malignant potential [93].

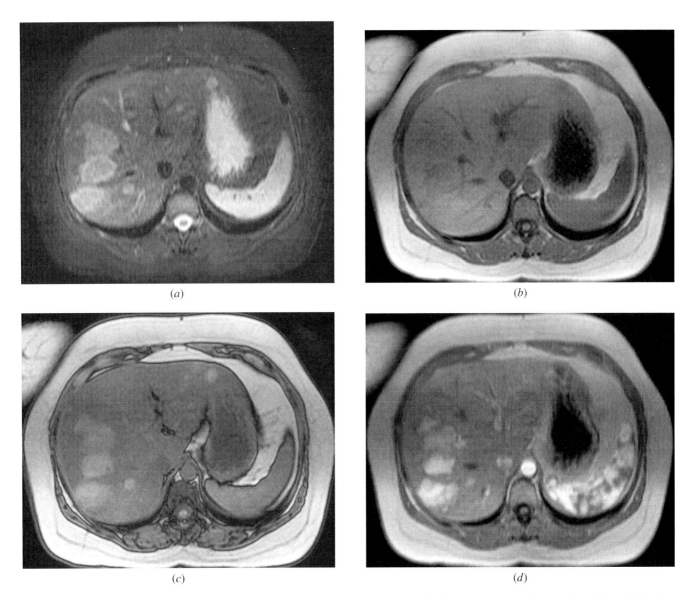

(a)   (b)   (c)   (d)

F I G . 2.57 Peliosis. Fat-suppressed T2-weighted SS-ETSE (*a*), SGE (*b*), out-of-phase SGE (*c*), and immediate (*d*) and 90-s fat-suppressed (*e*) postgadolinium SGE images. There are multiple liver lesions that demonstrate moderately high signal intensity on

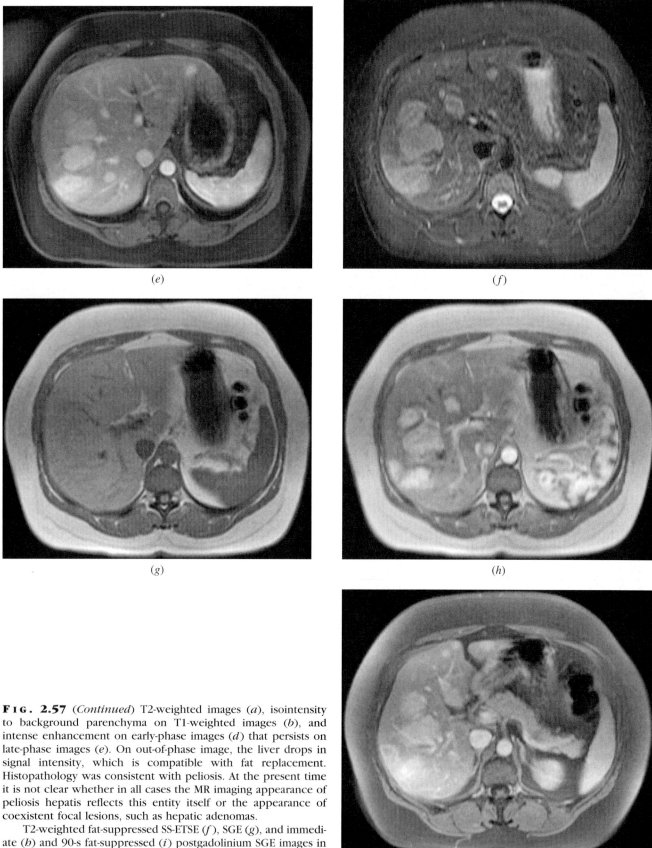

(e)

(f)

(g)

(h)

(i)

FIG. 2.57 (*Continued*) T2-weighted images (*a*), isointensity to background parenchyma on T1-weighted images (*b*), and intense enhancement on early-phase images (*d*) that persists on late-phase images (*e*). On out-of-phase image, the liver drops in signal intensity, which is compatible with fat replacement. Histopathology was consistent with peliosis. At the present time it is not clear whether in all cases the MR imaging appearance of peliosis hepatis reflects this entity itself or the appearance of coexistent focal lesions, such as hepatic adenomas.

T2-weighted fat-suppressed SS-ETSE (*f*), SGE (*g*), and immediate (*h*) and 90-s fat-suppressed (*i*) postgadolinium SGE images in a second patient showing features similar to those previously described.

Although the pathoetiology of FNH is incompletely understood, it has been proposed that the lesion is developmental in origin, consisting of a hyperplastic response of hepatic parenchyma to a preexisting arterial malformation [112]. From a pathologic perspective, FNH is characterized grossly as a sharply circumscribed, but unencapsulated, rounded or lobulated mass. The cut surface reveals a central stellate scar, often containing large, malformed blood vessels. It is postulated that the spiderlike branches of the anomalous vessels provide excellent blood supply to the component nodules; hence these tumors arc usually homogeneous (with internal necrosis and hemorrhage being rare events) [113]. Microscopically, fibrous septa radiating from the central scar contain vascular channels, exuberant bile duct proliferation, and intense inflammation. Parenchyma between the septa shows benign hepatocytes.

Two subtypes of FNH have been described: 1) solid type, which is most common and is characterized by the presence of a central fibrous scar containing enlarged malformed arteries that may be inconspicuous or absent in lesions <1 cm, and 2) telangiectatic type, which is characterized by the presence of centrally located multiple dilated blood-filled spaces. This subtype is enriched with more abundant and smaller arteries than the solid type. The telangiectatic type of FNH is more commonly associated with the multiple FNH syndrome [78, 93].

The most common appearance on noncontrast MR images is mild hyperintensity on T2-weighted images and mild hypointensity on T1-weighted images, although tumors may be nearly isointense on both of these sequences. Unlike HCA, FNH rarely has higher signal intensity than liver on T1-weighted images; hemorrhage is uncommon, encountered most often in large lesions [92, 114–116]. FNH enhances with an intense uniform blush on immediate postgadolinium images and fades rapidly to near isointensity (typically at 1 min after contrast) (fig. 2.58). Commonly, small (<1.5 cm) FNH is isointense on all precontrast images and may be appreciated only on the immediate postgadolinium SGE images.

The central scar in FNH has a typical appearance of a relatively small size with sharp angular margins. Thin radial septations are also often present. High signal intensity on T2-weighted images of the central scar is a characteristic feature of FNH but is observed in only 10–49% of patients [114, 117–121]. The hyperintense appearance of the central scar on T2-weighted images may correlate with the presence of vascular channels, bile ducts, fibrosis, chronic inflammation, and edema noted histopathologically. When observed, the central scar exhibits lack of enhancement on immediate postgadolinium images, and the majority show gradual enhancement to hyperintensity over time (figs. 2.59 and 2.60). This enhancement pattern is that of scar tissue

independent of location. In small FNH (<1.5 cm), the central scar is often not apparent. Larger FNH has a tendency to have central scars that show only partial enhancement on delayed images, which may reflect more mature, less vascularized scar tissue.

On imaging, background fatty liver may be more common in FNH than that observed with other focal liver lesions, except metastases. A collar of higher-concentration perilesional fatty infiltration may rarely be present [122], which differs from the perilesional fatty sparing of metastasis. In the setting of diffuse fatty liver the tumor may be mildly hypointense on in-phase T1-weighted images and hyperintense on out-of-phase images (figs. 2.61 and 2.62). Fatty infiltration of FNH is rare and only sporadically mentioned in the literature [115, 116]. Unlike the situation with HCA, we have not observed signal drop of FNH on out-of-phase images. In previous reports describing the presence of fat in FNH, fatty infiltration of the lesion was interpreted as an extension of the patient's underlying disease, that is, hepatic steatosis. In theory, intralesional steatosis in FNH may be encountered in several types of hepatic injury associated with steatosis, including alcoholic toxicity, obesity, diabetes, and malnutrition [114].

FNH may also occur as exophytic lesions and the attachment to liver may be a thin stalk. Even exophytic tumors possess the characteristic imaging appearance (fig. 2.63) [103].

There are several imaging features that help to distinguish between FNA and HCA. A central scar that shows delayed enhancement is typical for FNH, whereas pseudocapsule, internal hemorrhage, focal necrosis, and intralesional fat are features more commonly noted in HCA. Both lesions have an uniform transient tumor blush on early gadolinium enhanced images that fades away toward parenchyma isointensity on late images. Also, both lesions may take up Mn-DPDP [96, 99, 121, 123, 124].

Hepatocyte-selective contrast agents may distinguish between hypervascular metastases and atypical FNHs. However, a uniform capillary blush and uptake of Mn-DPDP must be cautiously interpreted because they are features of well-differentiated tumors of hepatocellular origin, including well-differentiated or small HCC. On Gd-EOB-DTPA- and Gd-BOPTA-enhanced images, FNH will show an early capillary blush and late hepatocellular uptake, and the late uptake is not observed with HCA (figs. 2.64 and 2.65) [5, 125].

Malignant Masses

Liver Metastases

Metastases are the most common malignant tumors of the liver in western countries. The most common primary tumors metastatic to the liver originate from the

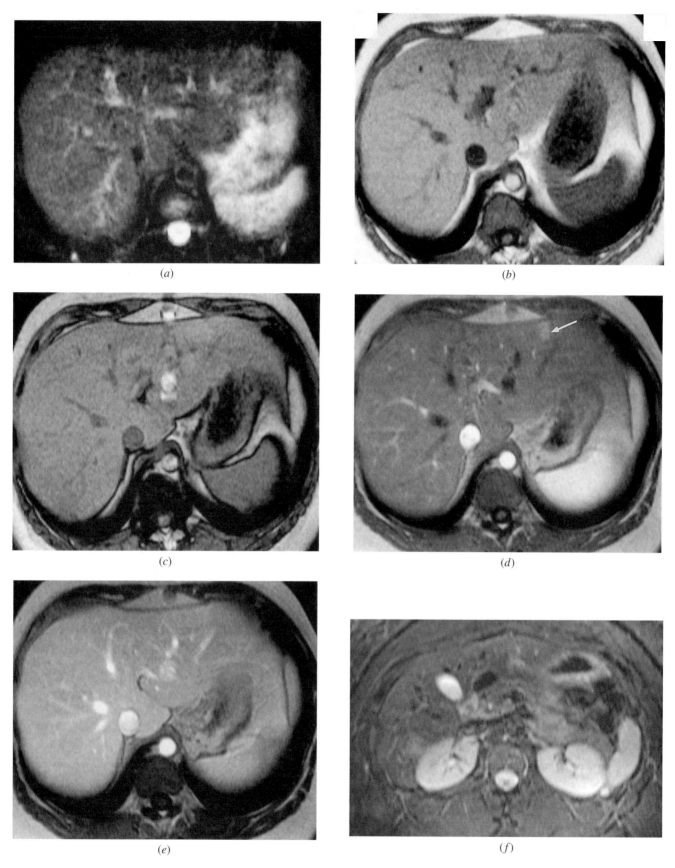

(a)

(b)

(c)

(d)

(e)

(f)

FIG. 2.58 Small-sized FNH. T2-weighted fat-suppressed ETSE (*a*), SGE (*b*), out-of-phase SGE (*c*), and immediate (*d*) and 90-s (*e*) postgadolinium SGE images. A 1.5-cm FNH is present in the lateral hepatic segment, and it is isointense on T2-weighted image (*a*) and near isointense on T1-weighted image (*b*) and does not drop in signal on out-of-phase images (*c*). The tumor is only visualized on the immediate postgadolinium SGE image by the presence of a hepatic arterial dominant blush (arrow, *d*). The tumor fades by 90 s to isointensity with background liver (*e*).

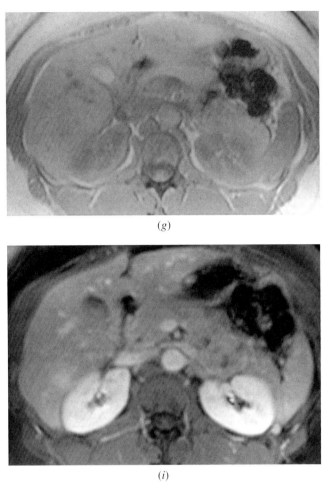

(g)

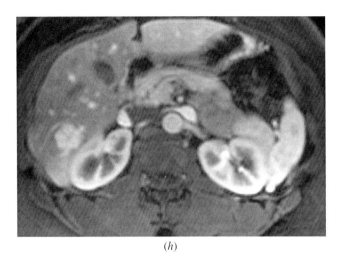

(h)

(i)

FIG. 2.58 (*Continued*) T2-weighted fat-suppressed SS-ETSE (*f*), 3D-gradient echo (*g*), and immediate (*h*) and 90-s fat-suppressed (*i*) postgadolinium 3D-gradient echo images obtained **at 3T** in a third patient with an FNH showing findings similar to those previously described.

Small, 1-cm, FNH may be only visible on hepatic arterial dominant-phase images. A central scar is often not visualized in small FNHs.

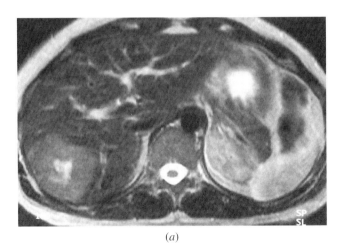

(a)

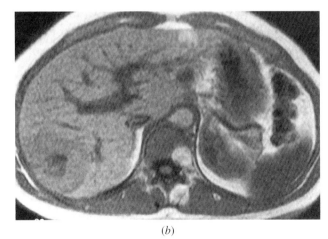

(b)

FIG. 2.59 Medium-sized FNH. T2-weighted ETSE (*a*), SGE (*b*), and immediate (*c*) and 5-min (*d*) postgadolinium SGE images.

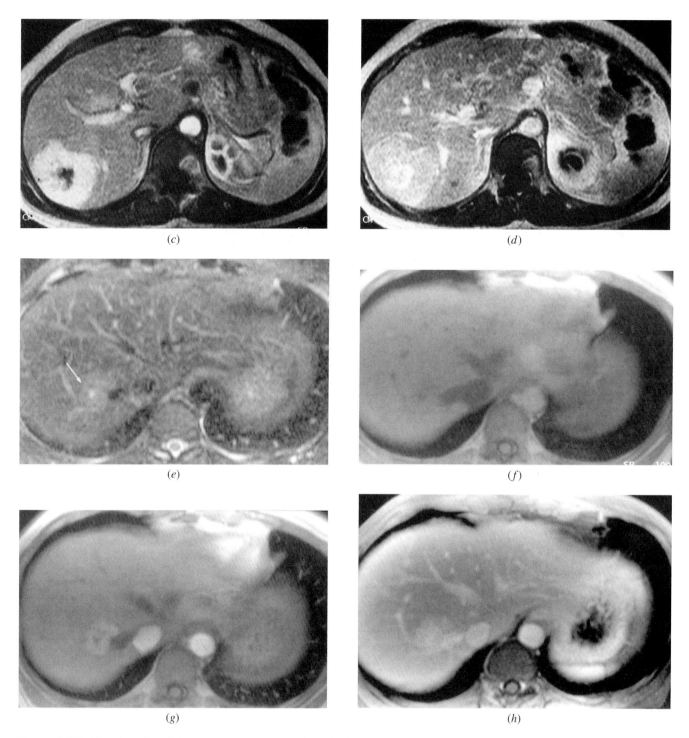

FIG. 2.59 (*Continued*) A 5.5-cm mass is present in the right hepatic lobe, and it shows mildly hyperintense on T2-weighted image (*a*) and mildly hypointense on the T1-weighted image (*b*). A central scar is present that is high in signal intensity on T2 (*a*) and low in signal intensity on T1 (*b*). On the immediate postgadolinium image (*c*), the tumor enhances with a uniform capillary blush, whereas the central scar remains low in signal intensity. On the late-phase image (*d*), the tumor fades to near isointensity with background parenchyma, whereas the central scar shows delayed enhancement (Courtesy of Susan M. Ascher, M.D., Department of Radiology, Georgetown University Medical Center.)

Echo train-STIR (*e*), SGE (*f*), and immediate (*g*) and 90-s (*h*) postgadolinium SGE images in a second patient. There is a lesion in the right hepatic lobe (arrow, *e*) that demonstrates minimally high signal on the T2-weighted image (*e*) and isointensity on the T1-weighted image (*f*), enhances with a uniform blush on early-phase image (*g*), and fades to near isointensity on the late-phase image (*h*). Note the small central scar that is high signal on T2-weighted image (*e*) and low signal intensity on T1-weighted image (*f*) and demonstrates negligible enhancement on early-phase image (*g*) and moderate enhancement over time (*h*).

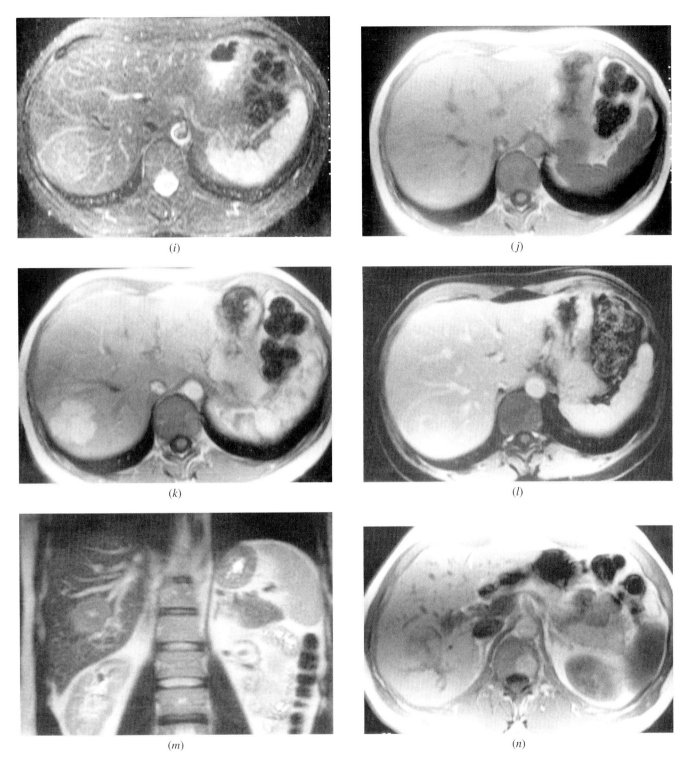

(i)

(j)

(k)

(l)

(m)

(n)

F I G . 2.59 (*Continued*) Echo train-STIR (*i*), SGE (*j*), and immediate (*k*) and 90-s fat-suppressed (*l*) postgadolinium SGE images in a third patient. There is a lobular lesion in the right hepatic lobe that has minimally increased signal on T2-weighted image (*i*) and near isointensity on T1-weighted image (*j*), demonstrates intense uniform enhancement on the early-phase image (*k*), and fades to near isointensity on the late-phase image (*l*). There is a small central scar best seen as a low-signal linear structure on the immediate postcontrast image (*k*).

Coronal T2-weighted SS-ETSE (*m*), SGE (*n*), and immediate (*o*) and 90-s fat-suppressed (*p*) postgadolinium SGE images in a fourth patient. The 3.5-cm FNH has a partial pseudocapsule (arrow, *o*). The pseudocapsule and central scar show partial enhancement on the late-phase image (*p*). The lesion otherwise has a typical MRI appearance for a FNH.

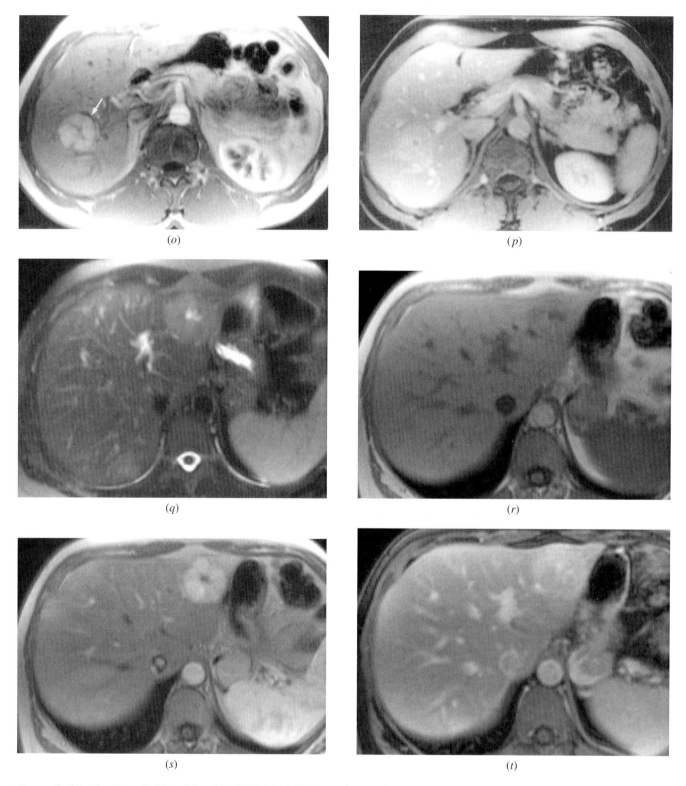

(o)

(p)

(q)

(r)

(s)

(t)

FIG. 2.59 (*Continued*) T2-weighted SS-ETSE (*q*), SGE (*r*), and immediate (*s*) and 90-s fat-suppressed (*t*) postgadolinium SGE images in a fifth patient with a typical FNH in the left lobe.

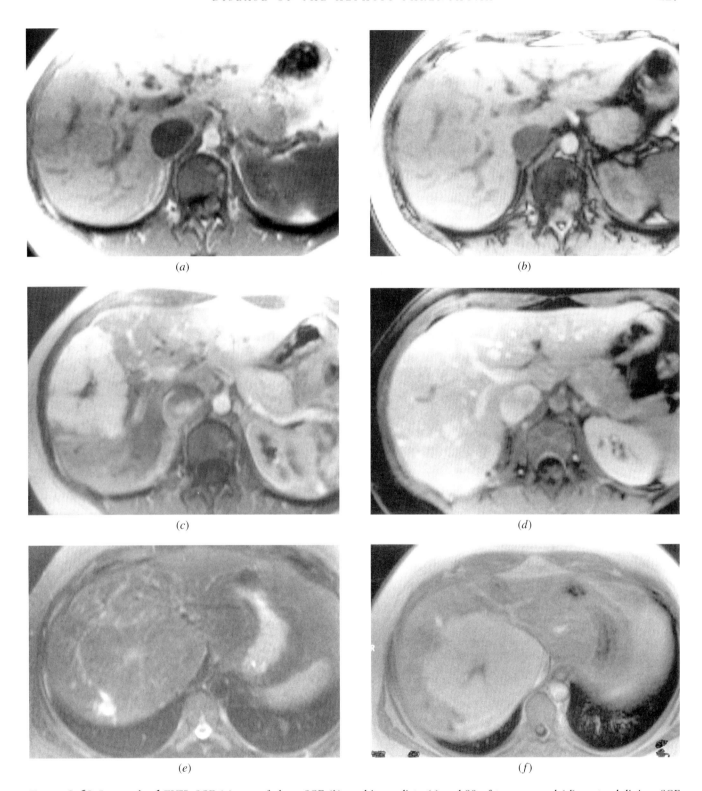

F I G . 2.60 Large-sized FNH. SGE (*a*), out-of-phase SGE (*b*), and immediate (*c*) and 90-s fat-suppressed (*d*) postgadolinium SGE images. A large lesion is seen in the right hepatic lobe that is mildly hypointense on T1-weighted image (*a*), does not drop in signal intensity on out-of-phase image (*b*), and shows intense homogeneous enhancement on early-phase image (*c*) that fades away on late-phase image (*d*). The central scar exhibits lack of enhancement on early-phase image (*c*) but enhances partially on late-phase image (*d*). The central scar in FNH is commonly small in size with angular margins. FNH almost never drop in signal on out-of-phase images, unlike adenomas, which commonly do.

Echo-train STIR (*e*) and immediate (*f*) and 90-s fat-suppressed (*g*) postgadolinium SGE images in a second patient. There is a

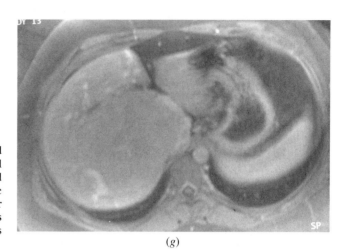

(g)

FIG. 2.60 (*Continued*) FNH with a small central scar and lobular margins in the right hepatic lobe. The tumor has signal comparable to surrounding liver on T2-weighted image (*e*) and shows moderate homogeneous enhancement on early-phase image (*f*) that fades away on late-phase image (*g*). The central scar is slightly hyperintense on the T2-weighted image (*e*), exhibits negligible enhancement on the early-phase image (*f*), but enhances over time (*g*).

lung, gastrointestinal tract, and breast [2, 3]. Pathologically, liver metastases usually appear as solitary or multiple nodules, with rare appearances including confluent masses or small, infiltrative lesions mimicking cirrhosis. Lesion shape is influenced by its size. Small metastases tend to be round or oval, and large metastases may adopt a more irregular morphology. Borders are commonly ill defined but may be sharp. Metastasis may be complicated by hemorrhage, central necrosis, or cystic change.

Role of MRI in the Detection and Characterization of Liver Metastases. Optimal hepatic imaging evaluation involves both detection and characterization of focal lesions [69, 124, 126, 127]. The detection of focal liver lesions by imaging is achieved through signal intensity differences between the lesion and the surrounding parenchyma. Detection involves identification of the presence of lesions and the segmental extent of liver involvement [126]. Demonstration that malignant disease has limited hepatic involvement may have a substantial impact on patient management. Survival of patients with colorectal metastases may be improved by partial hepatectomy, if metastases are localized to three or fewer segments [128, 129]. Tantamount to detection by imaging is characterization of lesions as benign or malignant, and in cases where initial imaging assessment is uncertain, histologic diagnosis or follow-up imaging.

An imaging protocol including T2-weighted images, T1-weighted gradient-echo precontrast images, and dynamic serial gadolinium-enhanced gradient-echo images acquired with whole liver coverage per acquisition achieves good lesion detection (T2-weighted and immediate postgadolinium gradient echo images) and characterization (T2-weighted and serial postgadolinium gradient echo images) (fig. 2.66).

The use of fat suppression on T2-weighted sequences is advisable because it facilitates detection of subcapsu-

lar lesions [130]. Fat suppression is especially important to apply on echo-train spin-echo sequences, because fatty liver results in a bright liver on nonsuppressed T2-weighted echo-train sequences that can obscure liver metastases. In addition to histologic features of the metastases themselves, histologic changes often occur in uninvolved portions of liver.

Dynamic serial gadolinium-enhanced MR images are particularly important for lesion detection and characterization in patients with known hypervascular primary tumors (fig. 2.67). The hepatic arterial dominant phase of enhancement is the most important phase of image acquisition both for detection and characterization.

On out-of-phase gradient echo images, liver metastases may appear high in signal intensity because of signal drop of background liver parenchyma (fig. 2.68). On occasion, this may facilitate lesion detection, particularly if lesions are intrinsically high in signal intensity on T1-weighted images (fig. 2.69). More often, however, lesions are rendered less conspicuous on short TE because the lowered signal of the liver reduces the contrast with low-signal focal liver lesions on in-phase images. Pathologically, in the setting of liver metastasis, surrounding parenchyma may show compression or atrophy of hepatocyte cords, scattered foci of chronic inflammation replacing lost hepatocytes, and the absence of fatty change. On out-of-phase images, this zone of compressed liver parenchyma bordering on the metastasis appears as a moderately bright rim. This finding is relatively common in the setting of colon cancer metastases with background fatty liver, and may occasionally be seen in other lesions including hemangiomas.

The acquisition of at least one sequence in the coronal plane may be of value in evaluating the superior and inferior margins of the liver, particularly the infracardiac portion of the left lobe [131]. Short-duration techniques such as SS-ETSE, T1-weighted gradient echo, or both are useful for this purpose (fig. 2.70).

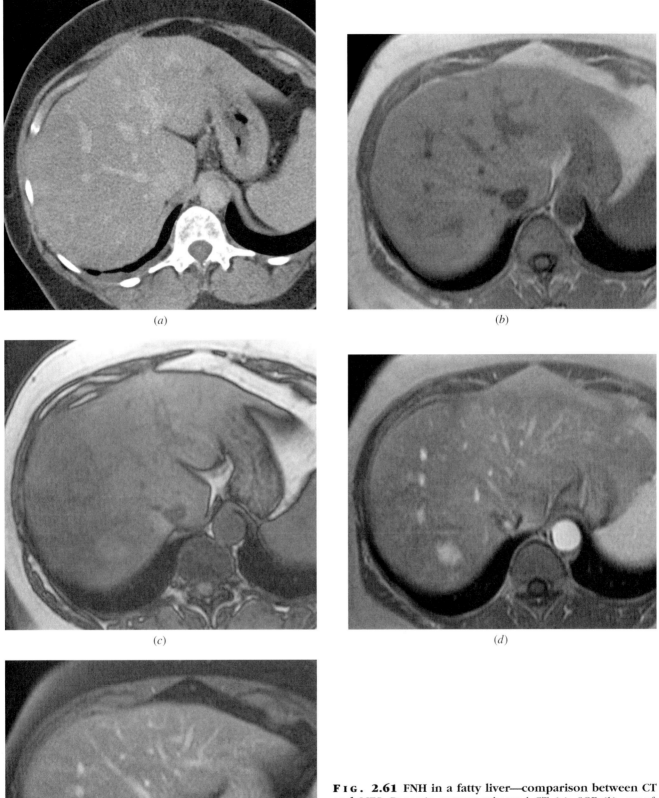

FIG. 2.61 FNH in a fatty liver—comparison between CT and MRI. Dynamic contrast-enhanced CT (*a*), SGE (*b*), out-of-phase SGE (*c*), and immediate (*d*) and 90-s fat-suppressed (*e*) postgadolinium SGE images. A FNH is situated in segment 6 of the liver and demonstrates isointensity with the background paren-chyma on T1-weighted image (*b*) and intense and homogeneous enhancement on the immediate post contrast image (*d*) and remains enhanced on late-phase image (*e*). Note that the signal intensity of the liver parenchyma is isointense to the signal intensity of the spleen on out-of-phase image (*c*), suggesting the presence of moderate fat liver replacement, but the lesion does not drop in signal. In contrast to MRI, the CT examination is unremarkable.

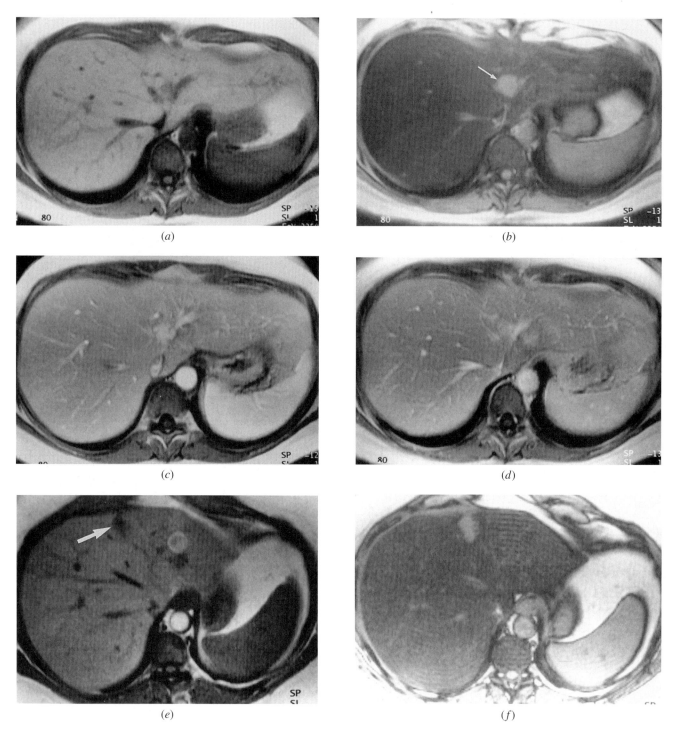

(a)

(b)

(c)

(d)

(e)

(f)

FIG. 2.62 FNH with surrounding fatty infiltration. SGE (*a*), out-of-phase SGE (*b*), and immediate (*c*) and 90-s (*d*) postgadolinium SGE images. A 2-cm focal nodular hyperplasia is present in the medial segment that is hypointense on in-phase (*a*) and hyperintense on out-of-phase (arrow, *b*) images because of signal dropout of the fatty liver. The tumor enhances with a uniform blush on the early-phase image (*c*) and fades in signal intensity on the late-phase image (*d*).

SGE (*e*), out-of-phase SGE (*f*), and immediate (*g*) and 90-s (*h*) postgadolinium SGE images in a second patient, who has diffuse fatty infiltration of the liver and a 2-cm FNH in the medial segment (arrow, *e*). Imaging findings identical to those shown in the first patient are present.

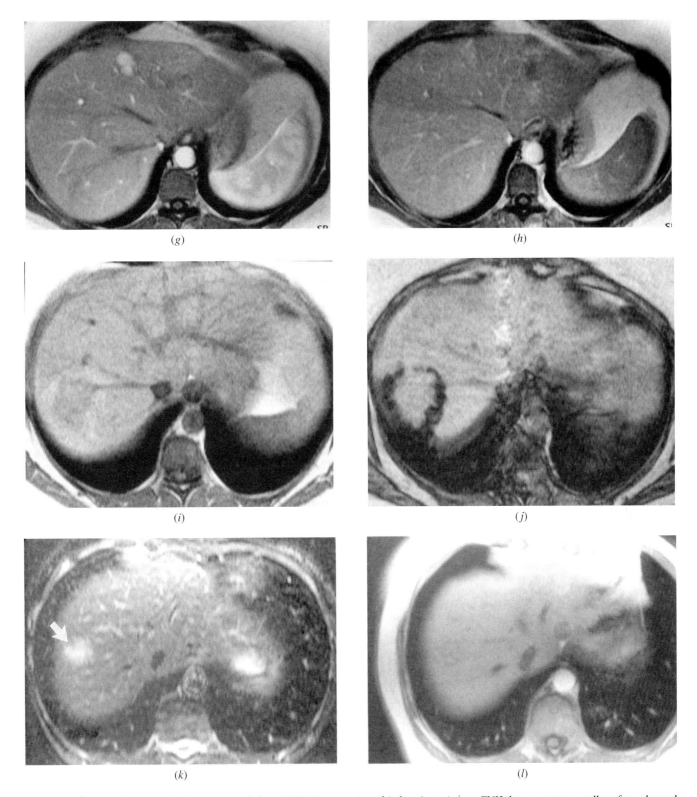

FIG. 2.62 (*Continued*) SGE (*i*) and out-of-phase SGE (*j*) images in a third patient. A 4-cm FNH demonstrates a collar of condensed fatty infiltration. The perilesional fat is moderately high in signal intensity on in-phase image (*i*) and drops to nearly signal void on out-of-phase image (*j*).

Echo-train STIR (*k*), SGE (*l*), out-of-phase SGE (*m*), and immediate (*n*) and 90-s (*o*) postgadolinium SGE images in a fourth patient, who has minimal fatty liver infiltration. The FNH in the right hepatic lobe (arrow, *k*) has mildly high signal intensity on T2-weighted image (*k*) and mildly low signal intensity on T1-weighted image (*l*) and becomes near isointense on the out-of-phase image (*m*), reflecting slight drop in signal of background liver. Note that the pseudocapsule appears slightly hyperintense on out-of-phase image. This lesion exhibits a central scar more evident, as a low-signal linear structure, on early-phase image (*n*).

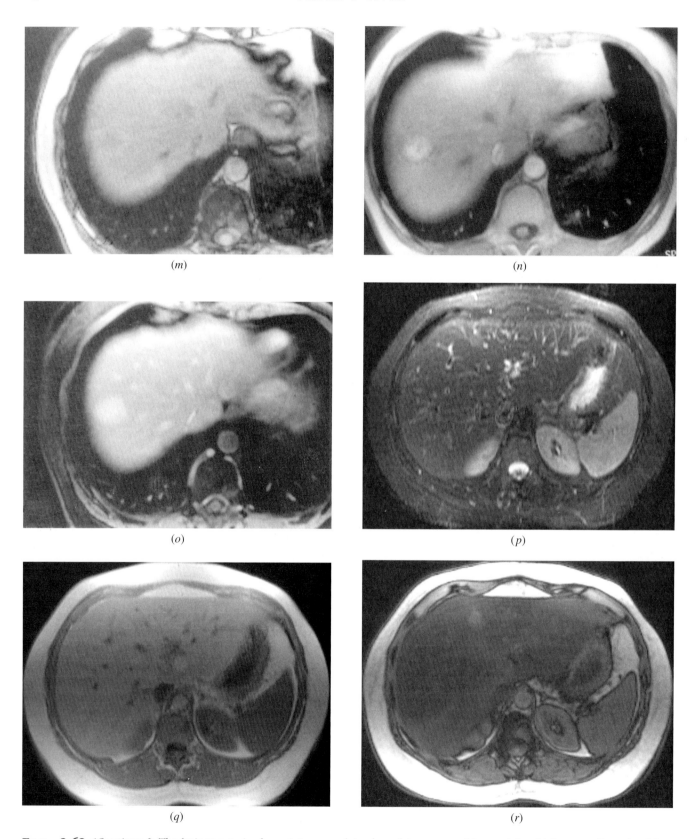

(m)

(n)

(o)

(p)

(q)

(r)

FIG. 2.62 (*Continued*) The lesions remains hyperintense on late-phase fat-suppressed image (*o*), which may reflect signal loss in background liver more than retention of contrast in the lesion.

T2-weighted fat-suppressed SS-ETSE (*p*), SGE (*q*), out-of-phase SGE (*r*), and immediate (*s*) and 90-s fat-suppressed (*t*) post-gadolinium images in a fifth patient show a FNH in a fatty liver.

These cases illustrate that fatty infiltration of background liver is not uncommon in the setting of focal nodular hyperplasia.

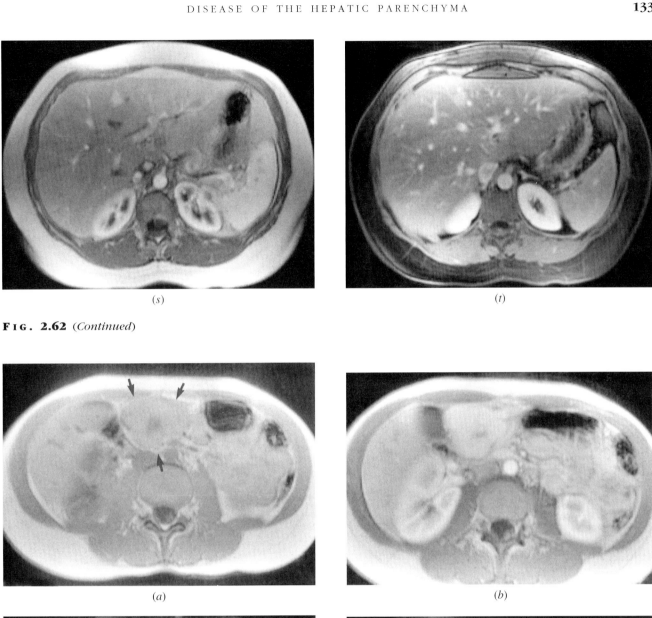

(s) (t)

F I G . 2.62 (*Continued*)

(a) (b)

(c) (d)

F I G . 2.63 Exophytic FNH. SGE (*a*), immediate (*b*, *c*) and 3-min (*d*) postgadolinium SGE images. There is a lobular mass with a central scar in the anterior upper abdomen, which abuts the left hepatic lobe. This lesion is isointense on T1-weighted image (arrows, *a*) and demonstrates a transient blush on the immediate postgadolinium image with lack of enhancement of the central scar (*b*). Note early filling of the left hepatic vein (arrow, *c*) that drains the tumor, confirming its hepatic origin. Transverse (*d*)

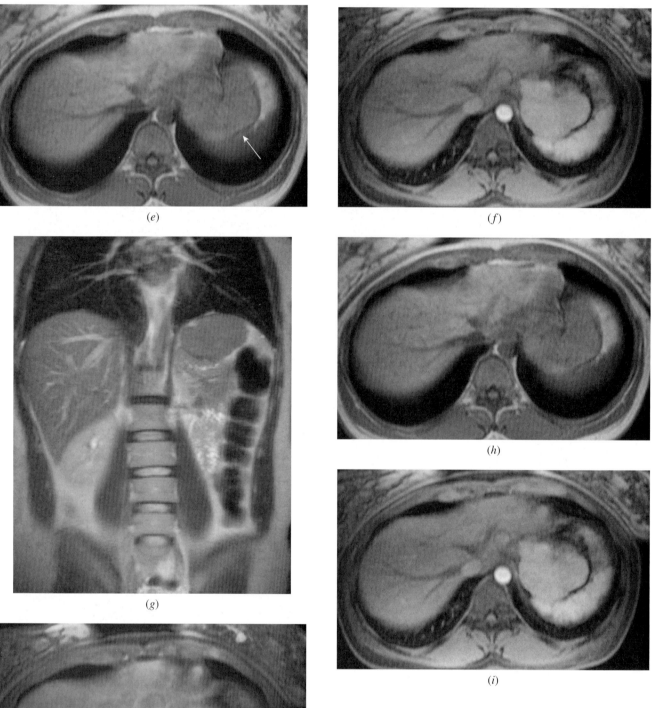

(e)

(f)

(g)

(h)

(i)

(j)

FIG. 2.63 (*Continued*) delayed image demonstrates late enhancement of the central scar. Despite its completely exophytic origin to the liver, the tumor exhibits the classic imaging features of FNH, which establishes the diagnosis.

Immediate (*e*) and 90-s fat-suppressed (*f*) postgadolinium SGE images in a second patient with an exophytic FNH (arrow, *e*). No central scar is appreciated in this lesion.

Coronal SS-ETSE (*g*), 3D-gradient echo (*h*), and immediate (*i*) and 90-s (*j*) fat-suppressed 3D-gradient echo images obtained **at 3T** reveal an exophytic FNH arising from the left lobe, adjacent to the spleen, in another patient.

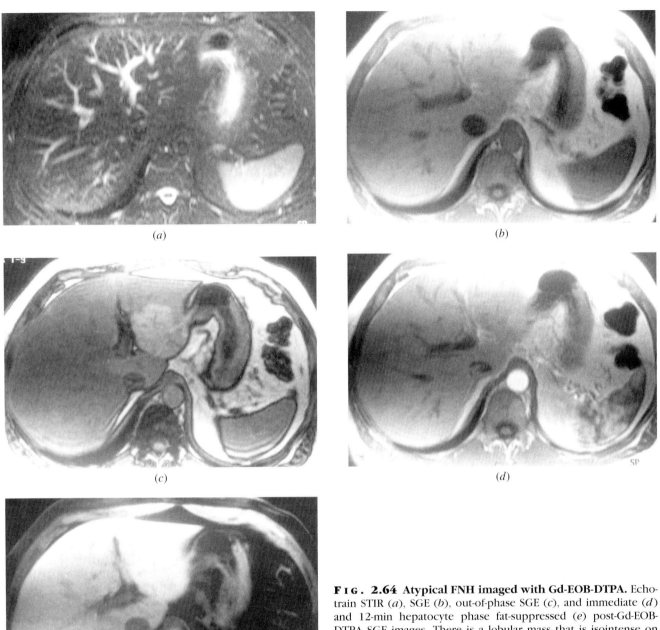

(a)

(b)

(c)

(d)

(e)

FIG. 2.64 Atypical FNH imaged with Gd-EOB-DTPA. Echo-train STIR (a), SGE (b), out-of-phase SGE (c), and immediate (d) and 12-min hepatocyte phase fat-suppressed (e) post-Gd-EOB-DTPA SGE images. There is a lobular mass that is isointense on T2-weighted image (a) and T1-weighted image (b), but it is well seen on out-of-phase image (c) as a high-signal mass because of signal drop of surrounding fatty liver. Atypical for FNH is negligible enhancement immediately after gadolinium administration (d). Note the high signal of the mass on the hepatocyte phase fat-suppressed image (e) that reflects both signal loss in the fatty liver and Gd-EOB-DTPA uptake in the hepatocytes of the FNH.

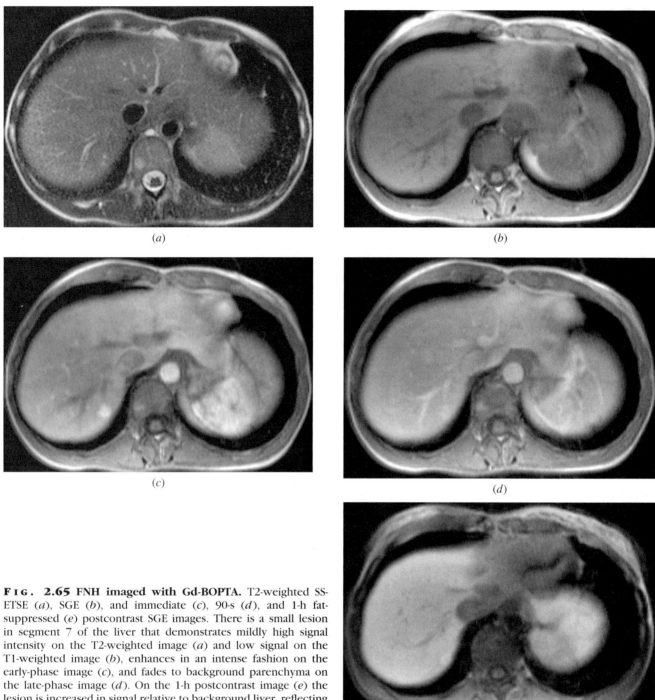

(a) (b)

(c) (d)

(e)

F IG . 2.65 FNH imaged with Gd-BOPTA. T2-weighted SS-ETSE (*a*), SGE (*b*), and immediate (*c*), 90-s (*d*), and 1-h fat-suppressed (*e*) postcontrast SGE images. There is a small lesion in segment 7 of the liver that demonstrates mildly high signal intensity on the T2-weighted image (*a*) and low signal on the T1-weighted image (*b*), enhances in an intense fashion on the early-phase image (*c*), and fades to background parenchyma on the late-phase image (*d*). On the 1-h postcontrast image (*e*) the lesion is increased in signal relative to background liver, reflecting hepatocyte uptake and retention of Gd-BOPTA (Courtesy of Guenther Schneider M.D., Ph.D.; Dept. of Diagnostic and Interventional Radiology, University Hospital Homburg/Saar, Germany).

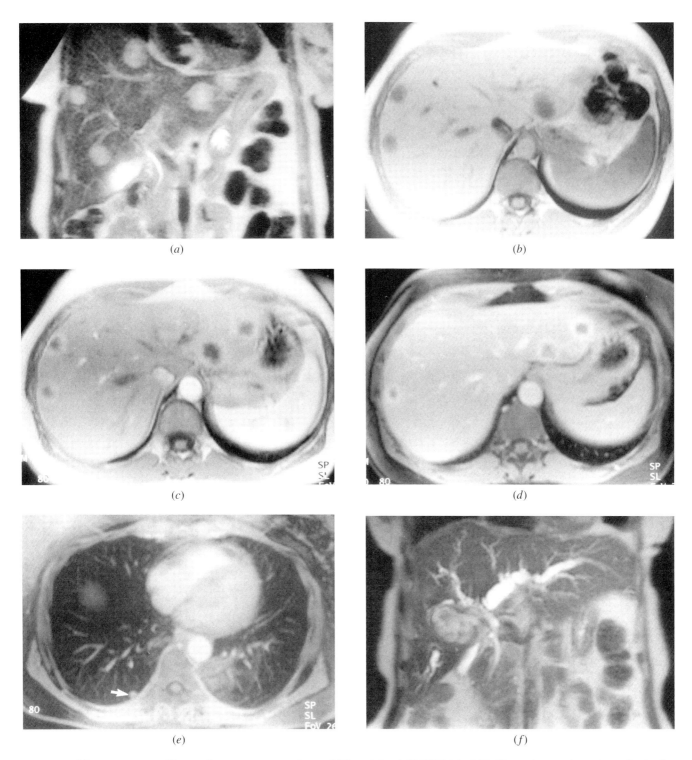

FIG. 2.66 Metastases—illustrating sequences. Coronal T2-weighted SS-ETSE (*a*), SGE (*b*), and immediate (*c*) and 90-s fat-suppressed (*d, e*) postgadolinium images in a patient with metastases from cloacogenic carcinoma. A MR study of the liver should include coronal (*a*) in addition to transverse plane images, T2 (*a*), T1 (*b*), and immediate (*c*) and 90-s fat-suppressed (*d*) images. Multiple metastases are present throughout the liver. Well-defined ring enhancement is appreciated on immediate postgadolinium images (*c*). Attention to lung bases must be made to evaluate for lung metastases (arrow, *e*).

Coronal T2-weighted SS-ETSE (*f*) and transverse echo-train STIR (*g*), SGE (*h*), and immediate (*i*) and 90-s fat-suppressed (*j*) postgadolinium SGE images in a second patient with capsule-based metastases who has colon cancer. Two capsule-based metastases are present that demonstrate scalloping of the liver margin. A large metastasis in segment 5 is also present, which obstructs the common hepatic duct (*f*).

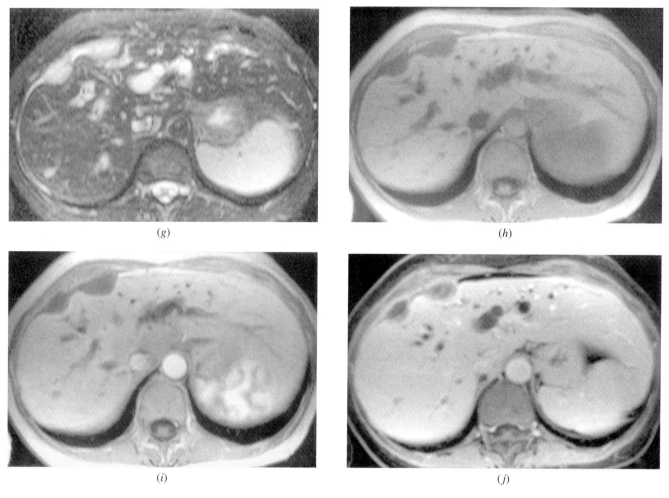

(g)   (h)

(i)   (j)

FIG. 2.66 (*Continued*)

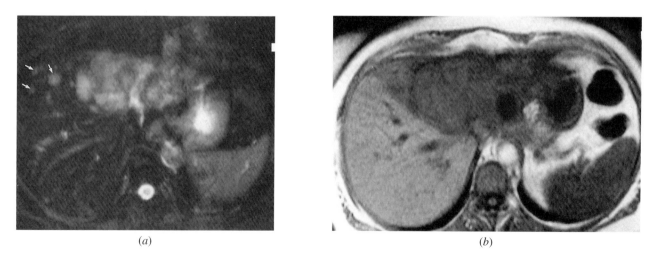

(a)   (b)

FIG. 2.67 Hypervascular liver metastases. Fat-suppressed T2-weighted ETSE (*a*), SGE (*b*), and immediate (*c*) and 90-s (*d*) postgadolinium SGE images. A 7-cm metastasis is identified in the left lobe of the liver (*a–d*). Several metastases smaller than 1 cm

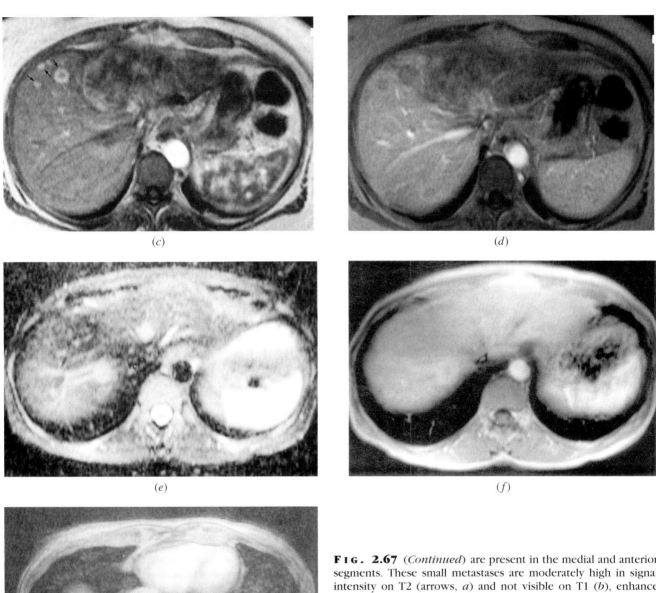

(c)

(d)

(e)

(f)

(g)

FIG. 2.67 (*Continued*) are present in the medial and anterior segments. These small metastases are moderately high in signal intensity on T2 (arrows, *a*) and not visible on T1 (*b*), enhance intensely on immediate postgadolinium images (arrows, *c*), and wash out to lower signal intensity than liver on 90-s postgadolinium images (*d*). On the immediate postgadolinium image (*c*) the smallest lesions enhance homogeneously, whereas the 1-cm metastasis has ring enhancement.

Echo-train STIR (*e*) and immediate (*f*) and 90-s fat-suppressed (*g*) postgadolinium SGE images in a second patient, who has a history of thyroid cancer. Two lesions are seen in the liver that are high signal on T2 (*e*) and enhance intensely on immediate postgadolinium images (*f*), consistent with hypervascular metastases. Note also the presence of lung metastases (arrows, *g*).

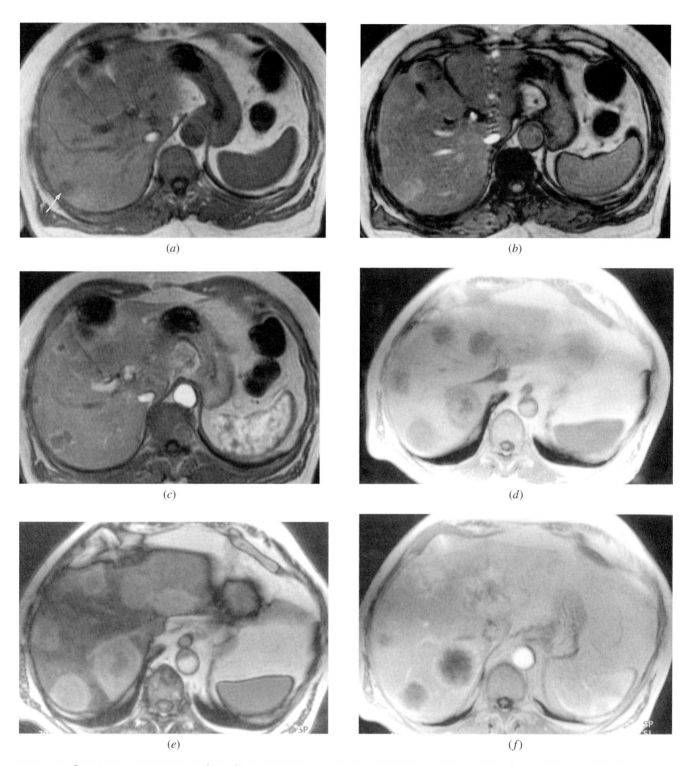

(a)   (b)

(c)   (d)

(e)   (f)

FIG. 2.68 Liver metastases in fatty liver. SGE (*a*), out-of-phase SGE (*b*), and immediate postgadolinium SGE (*c*) images. Multiple low-signal-intensity metastases are present in the liver on the in-phase T1-weighted image (arrow, *a*). On the out-of-phase T1-weighted image (*b*), the liver diminishes in signal intensity, rendering the metastases mildly high in signal intensity relative to liver. The immediate postcontrast image (*c*) shows that the lesions enhance in a peripheral ring fashion, consistent with metastases.

SGE (*d*), out-of-phase SGE (*e*), and immediate postgadolinium SGE (*f*) images in a second patient with colon cancer liver metastases. Fatty liver may arise as a response to the presence of liver metastases or also as a response to the chemotherapy directed at the metastases.

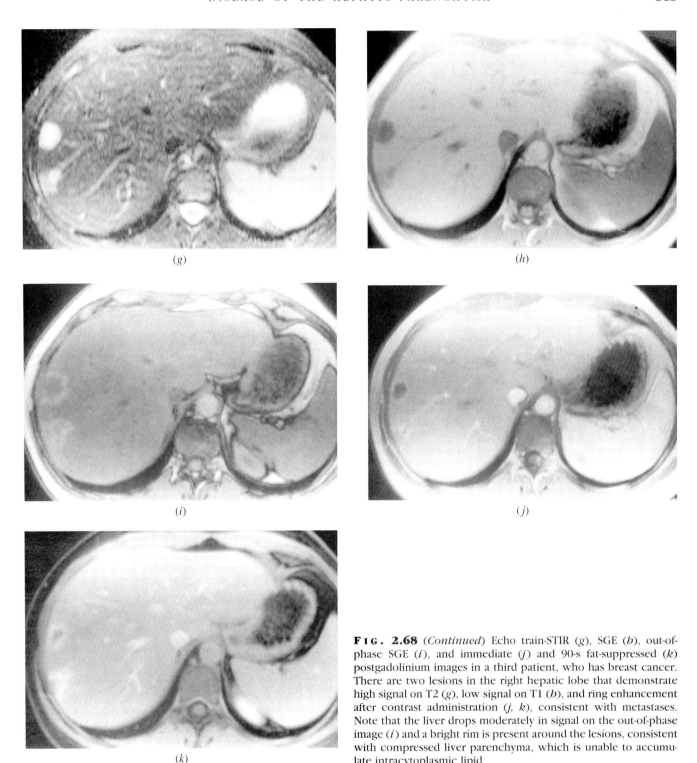

FIG. 2.68 (*Continued*) Echo train-STIR (*g*), SGE (*h*), out-of-phase SGE (*i*), and immediate (*j*) and 90-s fat-suppressed (*k*) postgadolinium images in a third patient, who has breast cancer. There are two lesions in the right hepatic lobe that demonstrate high signal on T2 (*g*), low signal on T1 (*h*), and ring enhancement after contrast administration (*j, k*), consistent with metastases. Note that the liver drops moderately in signal on the out-of-phase image (*i*) and a bright rim is present around the lesions, consistent with compressed liver parenchyma, which is unable to accumulate intracytoplasmic lipid.

MRI versus CT. MRI is superior to CT imaging in the evaluation of the liver [69, 132–136]. The current challenge is whether the superior performance of MRI translates into a beneficial effect on patient management, disease outcome, and health care costs. New MR sequences, phased-array surface coils, and tissue-specific MR contrast agents suggest that MRI may further exceed the diagnostic ability of CT imaging.

An earlier study [69] compared the efficacy of non-spiral dynamic contrast-enhanced CT imaging and MRI employing T2-weighted fat-suppressed spin-echo, T1-weighted precontrast gradient-echo, and dynamic serial

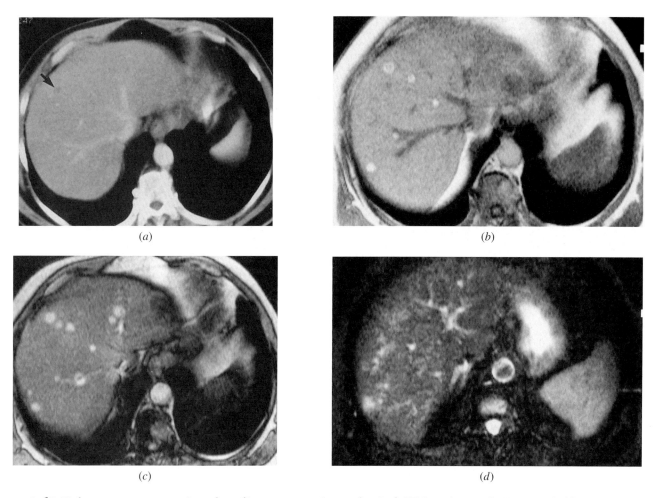

(a)   (b)

(c)   (d)

F I G . 2.69 Melanoma metastases in a fatty liver—comparison of spiral CT imaging and MRI. Spiral CT (*a*), SGE (*b*), out-of-phase SGE (*c*), and fat-suppressed T2-weighted ETSE (*d*) images. A solitary melanoma metastasis is apparent on the spiral CT image (arrow, *a*). Multiple mildly hyperintense metastases smaller than 1 cm are identified on the SGE image (*b*), and these high-signal-intensity lesions become more conspicuous on the out-of-phase image (*c*). Lesions are apparent on the T2-weighted images (*d*) but are not as clearly shown as on the out-of-phase images (*c*). The presence of fatty infiltration of the liver has resulted in a signal drop on out-of-phase images (*c*), which has increased the conspicuity of the high T1-weighted signal intensity liver metastases.

postgadolinium gradient-echo images in 73 patients with clinically suspected liver disease. The results demonstrated a statistically significant difference in lesion detection ($P < 0.03$) and characterization ($P < 0.01$) by dynamic MRI (fig. 2.71). A follow-up study [133] compared these MRI sequences to dynamic nonspiral contrast-enhanced CT images in 20 patients with solitary hepatic metastases detected by CT imaging and demonstrated that MRI depicted more than one lesion in 30% (6 of 20) of patients.

The authors reported [137] a comparison between MRI using T2-weighted fat-suppressed echo-train spin echo and immediate postgadolinium spoiled gradient echo with single-phase spiral CT for the detection and characterization of hepatic lesions in 89 patients. The results demonstrated a statistically significant difference in the detection ($P < 0.001$) and characterization ($P<$

0.001) of lesions by MR images on a patient-by-patient basis. No patients had true-positive lesions shown on spiral CT that were not shown on MRI. Regarding effect on patient management, findings on MRI provided information that altered care compared to findings on spiral CT in 64% of patients. A follow-up study [138] comparing dual-phase spiral CT and the above-described MRI sequences in 22 patients also showed the superiority of MR over dual-phase spiral CT in the detection and characterization of lesions. Our current clinical experience with 16-row multidetector CT and MRI shows similar findings that reveal the superiority of MRI in liver imaging. As MRI and CT both evolve as modalities, MRI has consistently shown superiority over CT, including comparison to current CT techniques. In fact, our impression is that with increasing numbers of rows of detectors, although spatial resolution may improve,

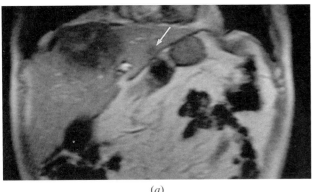

(a)

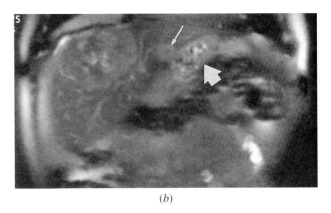

(b)

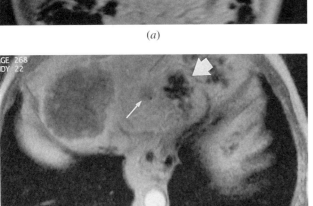

(c)

F I G . 2.70 Liver metastases, coronal images. Coronal magnetization-prepared gradient-echo (a), coronal T2-weighted SS-ETSE (b), and 45-s postgadolinium SGE (c) images. A 6-cm colon cancer metastasis is present in the medial segment that is heterogeneous and low in signal intensity on the T1-weighted image (a) and heterogeneous and mildly hyperintense on the T2-weighted image (b). A 1-cm capsule-based metastasis is identified in the lateral segment (arrows a, b) that has signal intensity features similar to those of the larger metastasis. Close proximity to the stomach (large arrow, b) is appreciated. The transverse postgadolinium image (c) demonstrates ring enhancement around the large heterogeneously low-signal-intensity metastasis. Ring enhancement is also appreciated around the small lesion (arrow, c). This lesion could easily be mistaken for a partial volume artifact with the nearby stomach (large arrow, c) on transverse sections. At least one coronal acquisition is recommended to minimize potential errors of ascribing lesions on the superior and inferior edges of the liver as partial volume effects.

contrast resolution, which is essential to detect small malignant tumors, may actually suffer.

MRI versus CTAP. Comparison between spiral CT arterial portography (CTAP) and current MRI techniques for diagnostic accuracy, cost, and effect on patient management has been studied using a population of 26 patients referred for hepatic surgery with suspected malignant liver lesions [139]. Regarding lesion detection, CTAP and MRI, respectively, showed 185 and 176 true-positive malignant lesions, 15 and 0 false-positive malignant lesions, 0 and 18 true-negative malignant lesions, and 13 and 22 false-negative malignant lesions. Regarding segmental involvement, CTAP and MRI, respectively, showed 107 and 105 true-positive segments, 11 and 0 false-positive segments, 80 and 91 true-negative segments, and 4 and 6 false-negative segments. A statistically significant difference in specificity of segmental involvement was observed between MRI and CTAP ($P < 0.03$). Total procedural charges were twofold higher for CTAP than for MRI. Findings at MR imaging altered patient treatment in seven patients, whereas findings at CTAP did not impact on patient treatment in any of the cases; this result was statistically

significant ($P = 0.015$). The results of this study demonstrated that MRI has higher diagnostic accuracy and greater effect on patient management than spiral CTAP and is 64% less expensive. A follow-up study [140] comparing spiral CTAP and MRI in 20 surgically staged patients showed a trend that MR was superior for lesion detection and segmental involvement. CTAP and MR images demonstrated, respectively, 54 and 60 true-positive lesions, six and one false-positive lesions, 15 and 22 true-negative (i.e., benign) lesions, and eight and two false-negative lesions. CTAP and MR images demonstrated, respectively, 57 and 62 true-positive segmental involvement, six and one false-positive segmental involvement, 89 and 95 true-negative segmental involvement, and eight and two false-negative segmental involvement. A major problem with CTAP is the frequent occurrence of perfusion defects that can resemble a focal mass or can mask the presence of metastases on CTAP images. Perfusion defects are rarely problematic on MR images (figs. 2.72 and 2.73).

MR Features of Liver Metastases. Metastases vary substantially in appearance on T2- and T1-weighted images. Generally, they are moderately high in signal

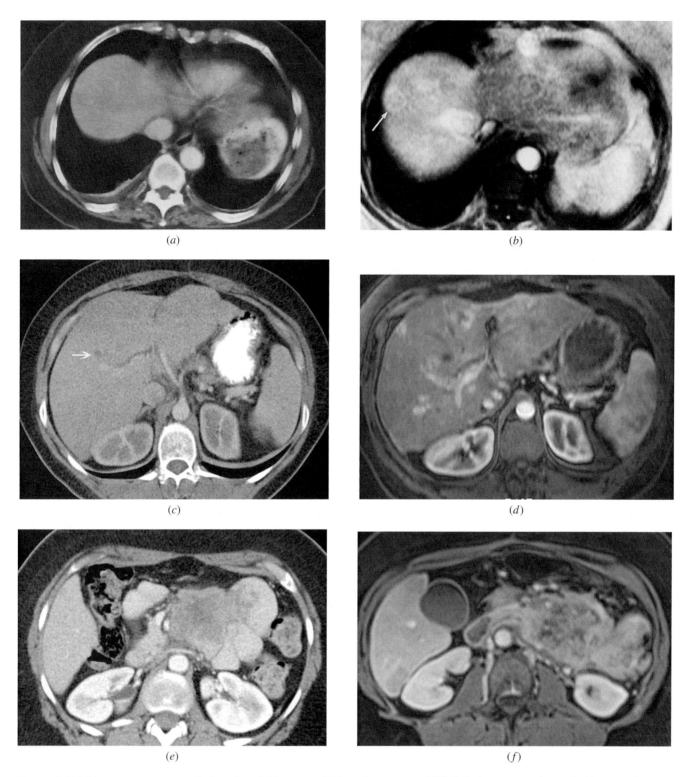

FIG. 2.71 Liver metastases, spiral and multidetector CT imaging versus MRI. Spiral contrast-enhanced CT (*a*), and immediate post gadolinium SGE (*b*) image. No lesions in the liver dome are apparent on the spiral CT image, while uniform ring enhancing lesions are evident on the immediate postgadolinium SGE image (arrow, *b*).

Multidetector contrast-enhanced CT (*c*) and immediate fat-suppressed postgadolinium SGE (*d*) images in a patient with liver metastases from carcinoid tumor. Note that extensive metastases are observed on the early-phase postcontrast MR image (*d*), while only one lesion (arrow, *c*) is appreciated on the multidetector CT image.

Multidetector contrast-enhanced CT (*e*) and immediate postgadolinium fat-suppressed 3D-gradient obtained **at 3T** (*f*) images in a patient with a large pancreatic tumor. No liver lesion is detected on CT (*e*), but on the MR image a metastasis is apparent in segment 6.

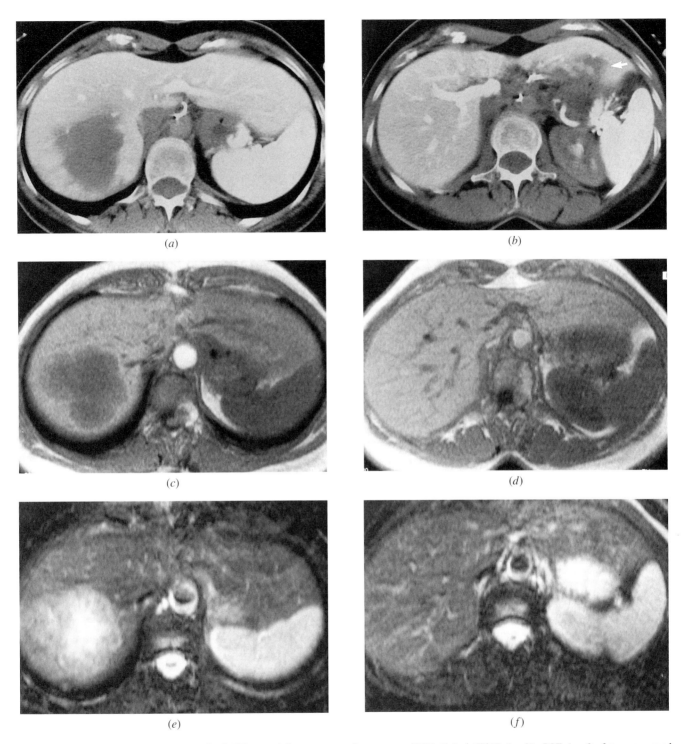

FIG. 2.72 Liver metastases—spiral CT arterial portography versus MRI. Spiral CTAP (*a, b*), SGE (*c, d*), fat-suppressed T2-weighted SS-ETSE (*e, f*) and immediate postgadolinium SGE (*g, h*) images from superior (*a, c, e, g*) and more inferior (*b, d, f, h*) tomographic sections. A large metastasis is present in the right lobe of the liver shown on all imaging techniques (*a, c, e, g*). A second metastasis was suspected on the CTAP image (arrow, *b*) in the lateral segment. No lesion was identified in this location on any MRI sequence. CTAP findings would have precluded surgery. However, the decision to operate was based on MRI findings. No liver metastasis was identified in the lateral segment by surgical palpation or intraoperative sonography. The patient is disease-free for more than 5 years since right hepatectomy. MRI was more accurate and had a greater impact on patient management and outcome than CTAP.

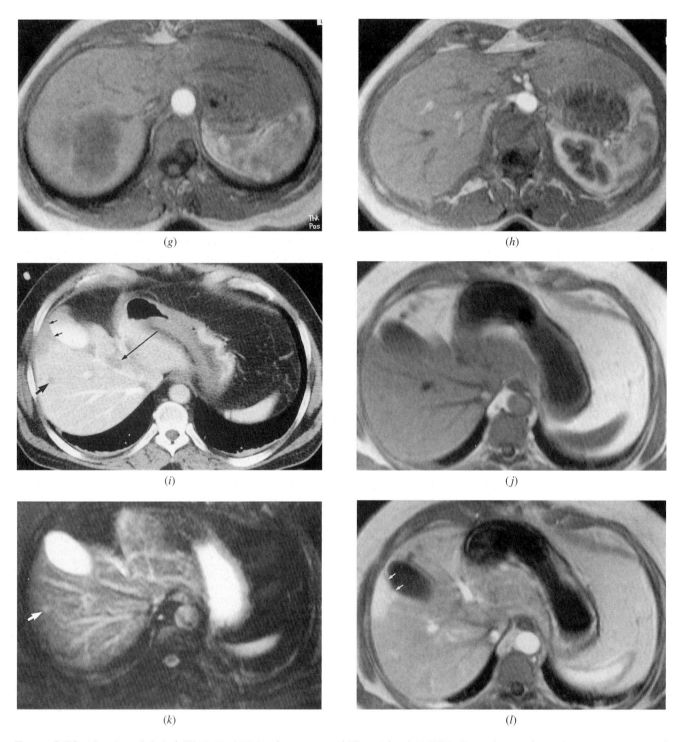

(g)   (h)

(i)   (j)

(k)   (l)

F I G . 2.72 (*Continued*) Spiral CTAP (*i*), SGE (*j*), fat-suppressed T2-weighted SS-ETSE (*k*), and immediate (*l*) images in a second patient with liver metastases from colon cancer. Spiral CTAP and MR images demonstrate an 8-mm metastasis in the anterior segment of the right lobe (arrow, *i, k*) and a perfusional abnormality related to a metastasis in the anterior segment of the right lobe (short arrows, *i, l*). A focal defect interpreted as metastasis on the CTAP image (long arrow, *i*) is apparent in the medial segment, but is not identified on any of the MR images (*j–l*). No metastasis in this location was identified at surgery and intraoperative sonography.

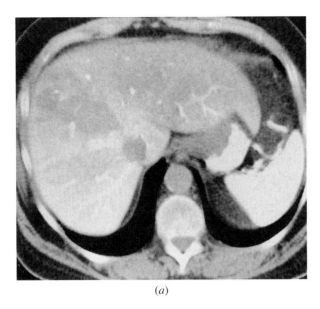
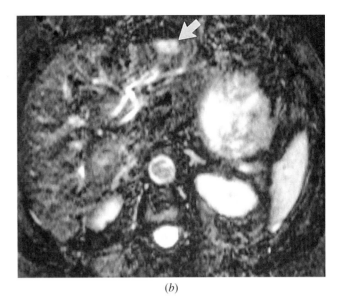

(a)   (b)

F I G . 2.73 Liver metastases—perfusional defect. Spiral CTAP (*a*) and fat-suppressed T2-weighted SS-ETSE (*b*) images. Multiple large perfusional defects are present on the CTAP image (*a*), with the entire left lobe exhibiting diminished perfusion. A 1.5-cm liver metastasis is present on the T2-weighted image (arrow, *b*), which was masked by the perfusion defect on the CTAP image.

intensity on T2-weighted images and moderately low in signal intensity on T1-weighted images.

Lesional and Perilesional Enhancement.

Enhancement is considered lesional when the size of the metastases on T1-weighted precontrast images and on arterial dominant-phase images is equal, and generally the outer margin of enhancement is well defined. Perilesional enhancement is described when the enhancement occurs beyond the margins of the lesion delineated on precontrast images, and the outer margin of enhancement is generally ill defined or wedge shaped.

The pattern of lesional enhancement of liver metastases has a strong association with the size of the lesion. Liver metastases can be classified according to the following features based on the pattern of enhancement on arterial dominant-phase images and the size of metastases: 1) homogeneous, usually when the lesion is ≤1.5-cm in the transverse diameter; 2) heterogeneous (uncommon), usually when the lesion is >1.5 cm in the transverse diameter; and 3) ring enhancement, commonly when the lesion is >1.5 cm in transverse diameter [141, 142]. It should be noted that homogeneity of enhancement occurring in lesions >1.5 cm is not rare, particularly when the primary tumor is hypervascular. Heterogeneity observed on early-phase images may reflect necrosis within the metastases. Diffuse heterogeneous enhancement observed in >1.5-cm hypervascular metastases may possess a radial spoke-wheel appearance with thin radial strands of lesser enhancement.

The ring enhancement pattern on early-phase images is the most characteristic appearance of liver metastases (fig. 2.74) [72, 81, 141, 143–145]. On arterial dominant-phase images, the outer margin of the metastasis enhances prominently and the inner portion has negligible enhancement, reflecting the underlying pathophysiology that the most vascularized outer portion of the tumor enhances more intensely. On interstitial-phase images there is an equilibration of enhancement as the less vascularized central tumor gradually receives its blood supply. The outer margin demonstrates a decrease in the degree of enhancement that may appear as heterogeneous fading to near isointensity or washout, and the inner area shows an increase in the degree of enhancement. The centripetal enhancement with the washout of the outer margin observed in the interstitial phase is highly suggestive of malignancy [145]. It is suggested that the lesional washout occurs because the peripheral margin of the metastasis is more vascularized, and therefore contrast enters and leaves this region more rapidly, while the inner portion is less well vascularized, ischemic, and fibrotic and thus receives a decreased amount of contrast but retains it to a longer extent [145–149]. The outer margin has a high ratio between intravascular and interstitial space, but the inner portion has a decreased intravascular space and an increased interstitial space [145, 146]. As a consequence, the blood supply is decreased in the inner portion of the metastases [145] and the clearance of the gadolinium is slower [150]. Well-defined peripheral washout with centripetal enhancement is most typical of hypervascular metastases, with gastrinoma being the most common.

Perilesional enhancement can be classified based on the shape of parenchymal enhancement as follows:

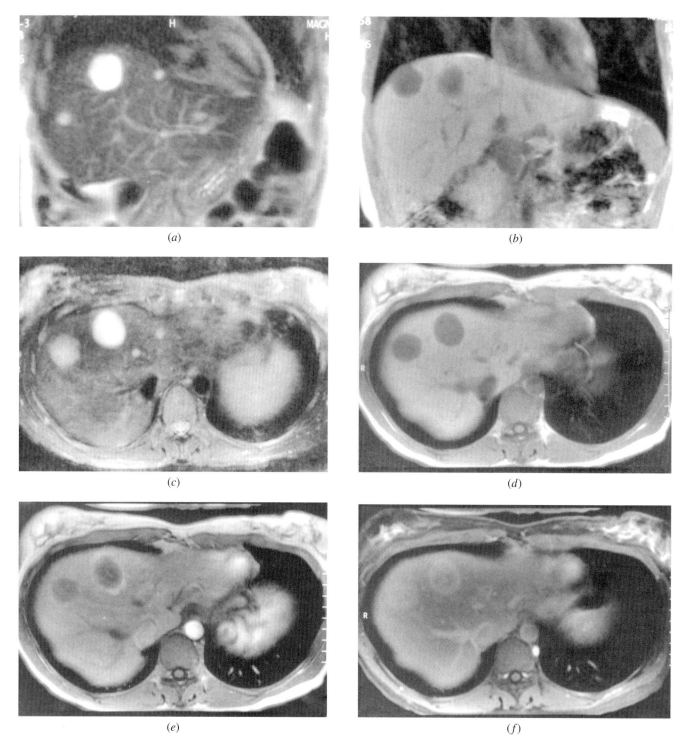

FIG. 2.74 Gastrointestinal stromal sarcoma—metastases that mimic hemangiomas on T2. Coronal T2-weighted SS-ETSE (*a*), coronal SGE (*b*), fat-suppressed T2-weighted ETSE (*c*), SGE (*d*), and immediate (*e*) and 90-s (*f*) fat-suppressed postgadolinium SGE images. There are two lesions that are well-defined and demonstrate high signal on T2-weighted images (*a*, *c*) and low signal on T1-weighted images (*b*, *d*). The high signal on T2-weighted images (*a*, *c*) resembles hemangiomas. Ring enhancement is shown on immediate postgadolinium images (*e*), diagnostic for metastases.

1) Circumferential enhancement is more typically ill-defined and better demonstrated on the arterial dominant phase with fading on interstitial-phase images; commonly observed in colon cancer metastases, and 2) wedge-shaped enhancement that is more sharply demarcated and often observed on metastases from pancreatic ductal adenocarcinoma [151].

Perilesional enhancement is uncommonly observed in other metastases apart from colorectal and pancreatic ductal adenocarcinoma [141, 151–153]. Perilesional enhancement is uncommon in hypervascular tumors such as islet cell tumors or renal cell carcinomas, implying that increased hepatic arterial supply is not the cause of perilesional enhancement. A study [151] reported that microscopic examination of liver tissue surrounding metastases showed variable degrees of hepatic parenchyma compression, desmoplastic reaction, inflammatory infiltrates, and neovascularization. This histopathologic zone, surrounding the metastasis, was termed the tumor border. Tumors with more extensive perilesional enhancement had a thicker tumor border. The area of perilesional enhancement observed on imaging was, however, broader than the tumor border noted on histopathologic inspection, suggesting the possibility that vascular changes extended beyond the outer confines of compressed liver tissue. Hypothetically, hepatocellular damage induced by the presence of nearby tumor or secretion of tumor metabolites into the vicinity adjacent to tumor may have incited an inflammatory response and neovascularization, contributing to the perilesional enhancement seen on MR images (fig. 2.75).

Association Between Vascularity of Liver Metastases and Degree of Enhancement. Liver metastases are fed primarily by arterial blood supply. The degree of enhancement of liver metastases on arterial dominant-phase images is determined by the size and number of vessels and the capillary permeability within the lesion. Moreover, the presence of fibrosis, necrosis, or confluent dense cellularity may also influence the degree of enhancement of liver metastases (fig. 2.76).

On the basis of the degree of enhancement of both arterial dominant- and interstitial-phase images, and on the lesion conspicuity on the interstitial-phase images, liver metastases by MRI may be categorized as follows: 1) avascular when there is a lack of lesional enhancement on arterial dominant- and interstitial-phase images; 2) hypovascular when the lesion demonstrates a lack of or faint enhancement on arterial dominant phase, comparable with the signal intensity of the pancreas and/or renal cortex, and becomes more conspicuous on interstitial-phase images; 3) isovascular when the lesion demonstrates similar enhancement as the background parenchyma on arterial dominant-phase images and

may become more conspicuous on interstitial phase; and 4) hypervascular when the lesion shows moderate or intense enhancement on arterial dominant-phase images more accentuated than the background parenchyma and similar to the signal intensity of the pancreas and/or renal cortex and less conspicuous on interstitial phase [5, 142].

To analyze the degree of enhancement on arterial dominant-phase images, it is crucial to determine whether the sequence was acquired in the "perfect timing of enhancement." Perfect timing of enhancement is considered when contrast is seen in hepatic arteries and portal veins but not in hepatic veins [5]. Normal pancreas and/or renal cortex are used as referent organs to establish the degree of lesional enhancement on arterial dominant-phase images. These structures are highly vascularized and are located in close proximity to the liver, facilitating this analysis.

Avascular metastases appear as completely cystic or necrotic metastases. They are characterized by high signal intensity on T2-weighted images, low signal intensity on T1-weighed images, and lack of enhancement on arterial dominant- and interstitial-phase images. A thin lesional or perilesional enhancement in the margin of the metastases is often demonstrated in one of the phases postcontrast. Metastases from ovarian cancer and after treatment (chemotherapy, chemoembolization, or ablation) may demonstrate avascularity on dynamic postcontrast images (fig. 2.77). Avascular metastases may mimic the appearance of benign cysts (fig. 2.78). Sometimes, the delayed postgadolinium images demonstrate indistinct borders of metastatic lesions and a decrease in size due to peripheral enhancement. This feature distinguishes avascular metastases from true cysts since the latter lesions remain sharply circumscribed with no change in size on late postcontrast images.

Hypovascular metastases are characterized by near isointensity or high signal intensity on T2-weighted images and low signal on T1-weighted images. After contrast, hypovascular metastases demonstrate minimal enhancement on arterial dominant-phase images that tends to be more conspicuous on interstitial-phase images [154]. Primary tumors that commonly result in hypovascular metastases include colorectal carcinoma (fig. 2.79), transitional cell carcinoma (fig. 2.80) [5], pancreatic ductal adenocarcinoma, small bowel adenocarcinoma, pulmonary carcinoma, bladder carcinoma, and prostate carcinoma [141, 152].

Isovascular metastases are characterized by lesional enhancement similar to background parenchyma on arterial dominant-phase images. On interstitial-phase images, isovascular metastases often, but not always, show decrease in the degree of enhancement (washout), becoming more conspicuous. Isovascular metastases are

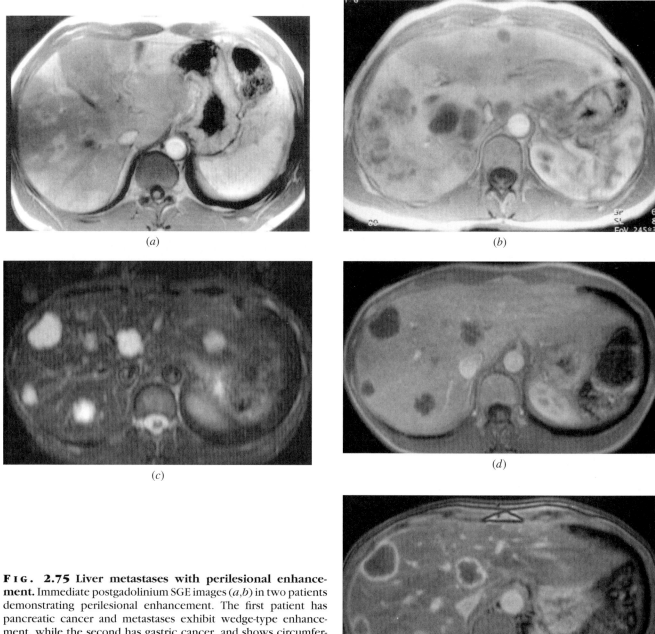

(a)

(b)

(c)

(d)

(e)

F I G . 2.75 Liver metastases with perilesional enhancement. Immediate postgadolinium SGE images (*a,b*) in two patients demonstrating perilesional enhancement. The first patient has pancreatic cancer and metastases exhibit wedge-type enhancement, while the second has gastric cancer, and shows circumferential perilesional enhancement.

T2-weighted fat-suppressed SS-ETSE (*c*) and T1-weighted fat-suppressed immediate- (*d*) and 90-s-phase (*e*) postgadolinium images obtained **at 3T** in a third patient demonstrate perilesional enhancement on delayed phase images that is characteristic for colon cancer metastases.

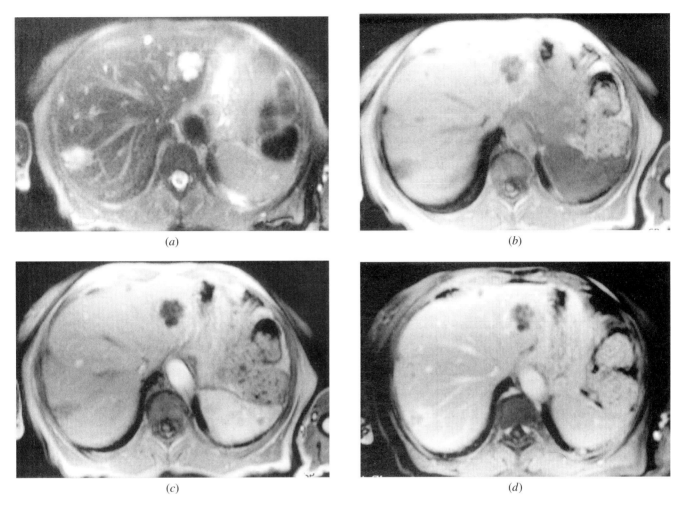

(a)   (b)

(c)   (d)

F I G . 2.76 Endometrial cancer with liver metastases. Echo-train STIR (a), SGE (b), and immediate (c) and 90-s fat-suppressed postgadolinium SGE(d) images in a patient who has endometrial cancer. There are multiple lesions that demonstrate high signal on T2 (a)- and low signal on T1 (b)-weighted images and exhibit ring enhancement and perilesional enhancement on immediate postgadolinium images (c). Ring enhancement persists on interstitial-phase images (d).

generally well-demonstrated on precontrast images as high signal intensity on T2-weighted images, low signal on T1-weighted images, or both. This appearance is most often observed in metastases after chemotherapy, presumably reflecting an antiangiogenic effect. Most commonly, metastases from colon, thyroid, and endometrium may demonstrate isovascularity [5, 150].

Hypervascular metastases are generally high in signal intensity on T2-weighted images and low in signal intensity on T1-weighted images and possess a moderate or intense peripheral ring of enhancement on early-phase images, comparable with the extent of enhancement of the pancreas and/ or renal cortex. On interstitial-phase images these metastases are the most likely to show centripetal enhancement and peripheral washout (figs. 2.81–2.84) [72, 143, 144]. Hypervascular metastases are more conspicuous on arterial dominant-phase images because of the great signal difference

between intensely enhanced lesions and minimal enhancement of the background parenchyma.

Small (<1.5 cm) hypervascular metastases are commonly homogeneously high in signal intensity on T2-weighted images and homogeneously low in signal intensity on T1-weighted images and show either fading to background or washout. Often, small hypervascular metastases (especially those <1.0 cm) are only evident on hepatic arterial dominant-phase images; that is, the lesion is isointense on T2- and T1-weighed images and interstitial-phase postcontrast images [143].

The malignancies that most commonly result in hypervascular liver metastases include breast cancer, renal cell carcinoma, carcinoid tumor, islet cell tumor, thyroid carcinoma, adenocarcinoma of unknown primary site, leiomyosarcoma, and malignant melanoma. Other malignancies that occasionally result in hypervascular liver metastases include colon carcinoma, pancreatic

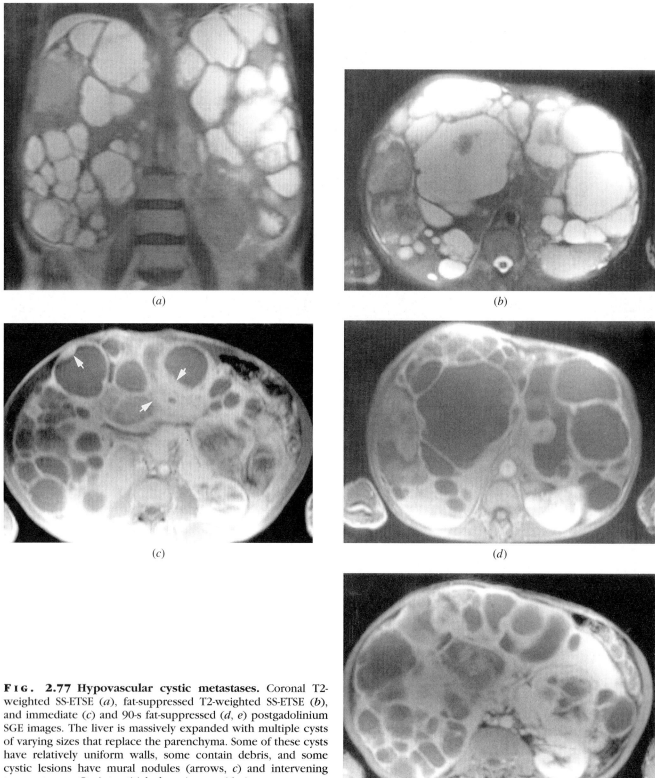

(a)

(b)

(c)

(d)

(e)

FIG. 2.77 Hypovascular cystic metastases. Coronal T2-weighted SS-ETSE (*a*), fat-suppressed T2-weighted SS-ETSE (*b*), and immediate (*c*) and 90-s fat-suppressed (*d, e*) postgadolinium SGE images. The liver is massively expanded with multiple cysts of varying sizes that replace the parenchyma. Some of these cysts have relatively uniform walls, some contain debris, and some cystic lesions have mural nodules (arrows, *c*) and intervening tumor stroma. On interstitial phase images (*d, e*), some progressive enhancement of tumor stroma is appreciated. The metastases are from epithelioid stromal tumor.

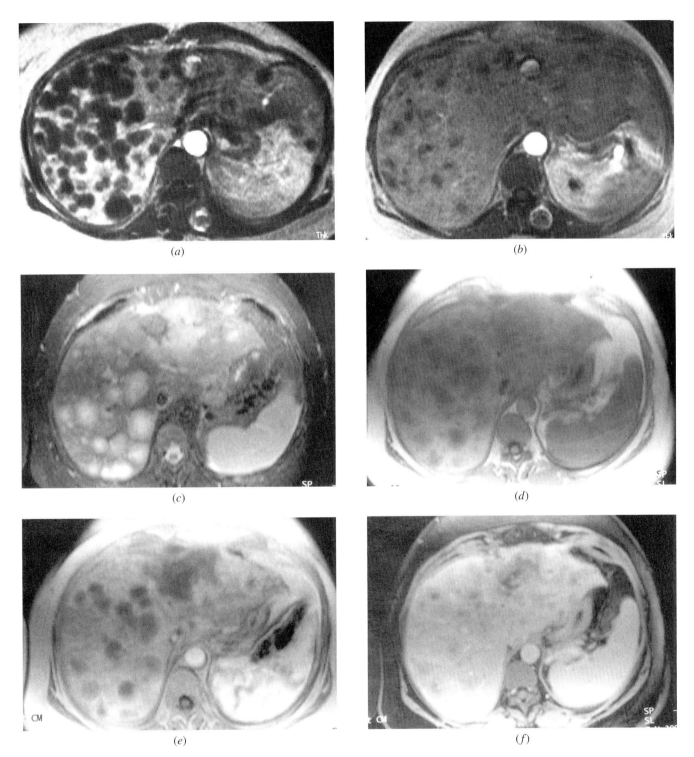

F I G . 2.78 Hypovascular liver metastases with high fluid content from adenocarcinoma of unknown primary.
Immediate (*a*) and 10-min (*b*) postgadolinium SGE images. Hypovascular liver metastases with a high fluid content are low in signal intensity on T1 (not shown) and high in signal intensity on T2 (not shown) images. On immediate postgadolinium images (*a*), they may appear well defined and nearly signal void, mimicking the appearance of cysts. On delayed postgadolinium images (*b*) these lesions will partially enhance and decrease in size, permitting correct characterization (Reproduced with permission from Semelka RC, Shoenut JP, Greenberg HM, Micflikier AB. The liver. In: Semelka RC, Shoenut JP, eds. *MRI of the Abdomen with CT Correlation*. New York: Raven Press, 1993. p.13–41).

Echo-train STIR (*c*), SGE (*d*), and immediate (*e*) and 90-s fat-suppressed (*f*) postgadolinium SGE images in a second patient with adenocarcinoma of unknown primary. There are multiple metastases scattered throughout the liver that exhibit high signal on T2-weighted images (*c*), low signal on T1-weighted images (*d*), and mild ring enhancement on immediate postgadolinium images (*e*) with progressive enhancement of the lesions on delayed images (*f*).

As these cases illustrate, patients with adenocarcinoma of unknown primary often have extensive liver metastases that also may be of relatively low vascularity.

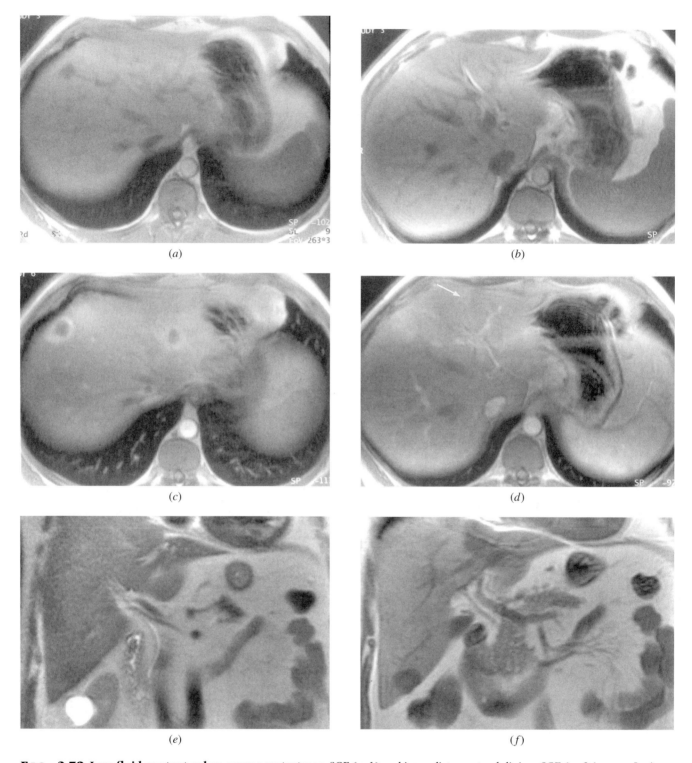

(a)

(b)

(c)

(d)

(e)

(f)

FIG. 2.79 Low-fluid-content colon cancer metastases. SGE (*a*, *b*) and immediate postgadolinium SGE (*c*, *d*) images. Lesions, especially small lesions, are difficult to discern on noncontrast T2 (not shown)- and T1 (*a*, *b*)-weighted images. On immediate postgadolinium images (*c*, *d*), lesions are rendered conspicuous because of ring enhancement. Lesions <1 cm in size may be detected and characterized with this technique.

Coronal fat-suppressed T2-weighted SS-ETSE (*e*), coronal SGE (*f*), transverse T2-weighted SS-ETSE (*g*), and transverse immediate postgadolinium SGE (*h*) images in a second patient. There are multiple metastases in the liver that are near isointense on T2 (*e*, *g*)

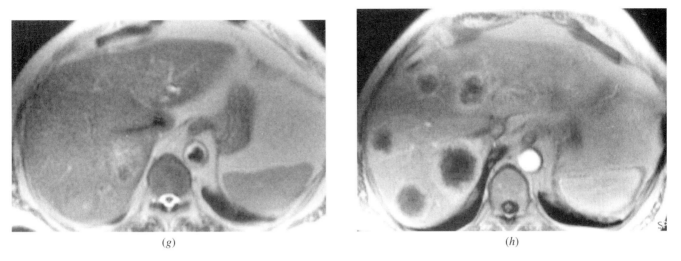

(g)   (h)

FIG. 2.79 (*Continued*) and hypointense on T1-weighted images (*f*), and demonstrate ring enhancement on postgadolinium images (*h*). These liver metastases are poorly seen on T2 (*e*, *g*), well seen on T1 (*f*), and very well shown on immediate postgadolinium images (*h*).

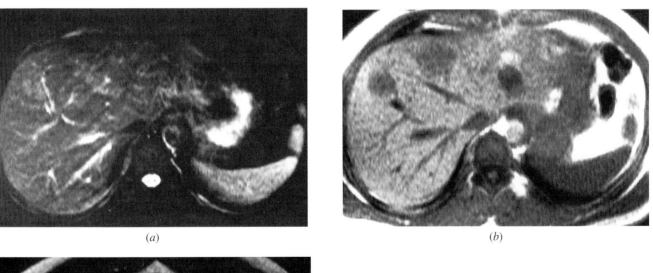

(a)   (b)

(c)

FIG. 2.80 Hypovascular liver metastases with low fluid content. Fat-suppressed T2-weighted ETSE (*a*), SGE (*b*), and immediate postgadolinium SGE (*c*) images. Hypovascular liver metastases with low fluid content are usually low in signal intensity on T2- and T1-weighted images, which renders them isointense to minimally hyperintense in signal intensity relative to liver on T2-weighted images (*a*) and low in signal relative to liver on T1-weighted images (*b*). Hypovascular liver metastases with low fluid content possess imaging features comparable to those of fibrous tissue. Despite their hypovascularity, these metastases exhibit faint peripheral rim enhancement on the immediate image (*c*) (Reproduced with permission from Semelka RC, Shoenut JP, Greenberg HM, Micflikier AB. The liver. In: Semelka RC, Shoenut JP, eds. *MRI of the Abdomen with CT Correlation.* New York: Raven Press, 1993, p.13–41).

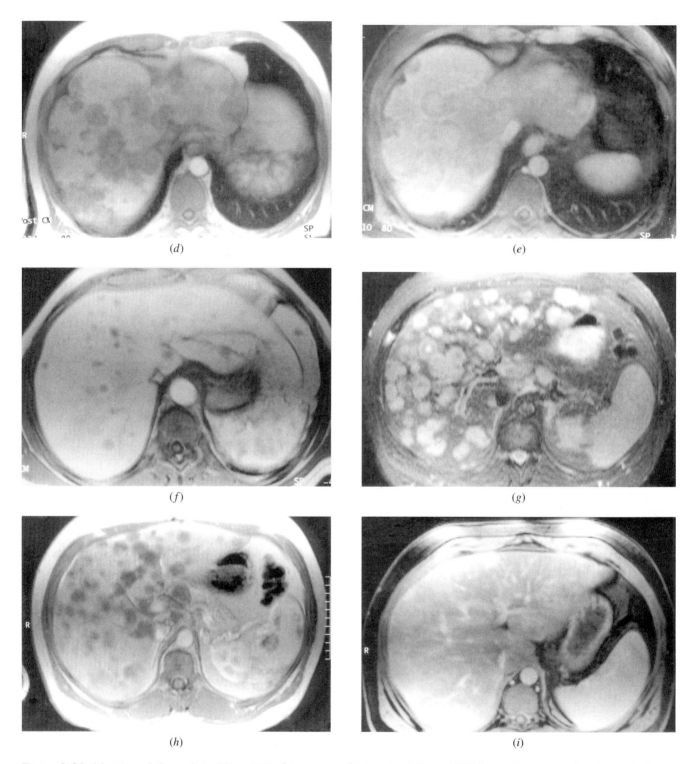

(d)

(e)

(f)

(g)

(h)

(i)

F I G . 2.80 (*Continued*) Immediate (*d*) and 90-s fat-suppressed (*e*) postgadolinium SGE images in a second patient, who has a history of bladder carcinoma. On the immediate postgadolinium image (*d*), the lesions exhibit negligible enhancement, and on the interstitial-phase image (*e*), they become heterogeneously isointense with liver.

Immediate postgadolinium SGE (*f*) image in a third patient. Multiple hypointense lesions with faint ring enhancement are seen in the hepatic parenchyma, consistent with metastases.

Echo-train STIR (*g*) and immediate (*h*) and 90-s fat-suppressed (*i*) postgadolinium SGE images in a fourth patient. Extensive metastases are scattered throughout the liver that appear moderately high signal on T2 (*g*) and moderately low signal on T1 (not shown), show ring enhancement on immediate postgadolinium images (*h*), and enhance to near isointensity on late images (*i*).

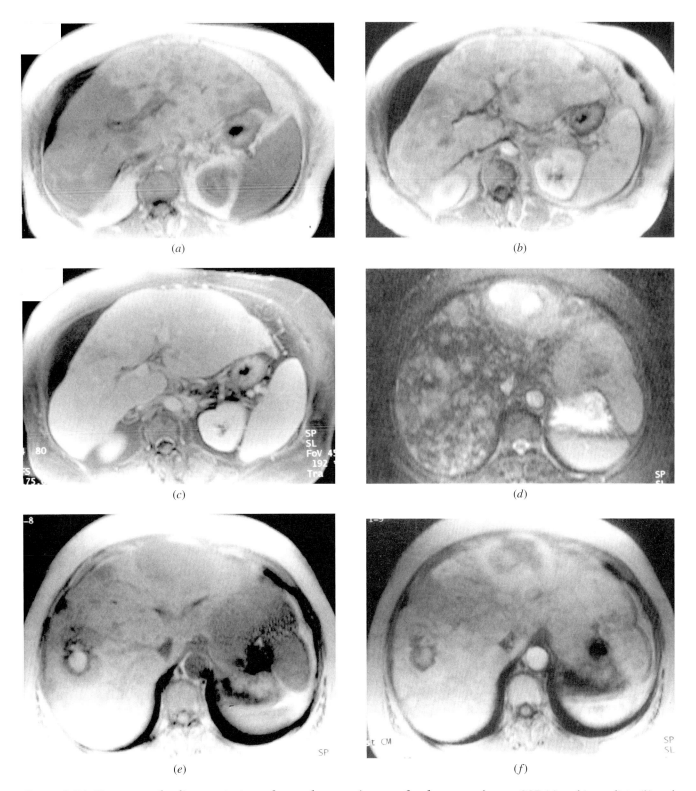

FIG. 2.81 Hypervascular liver metastases from adenocarcinoma of unknown primary. SGE (*a*) and immediate (*b*) and 90-s fat-suppressed postgadolinium SGE (*c*) images. There are numerous lesions scattered throughout the hepatic parenchyma, which are low signal on T1-weighted image (*a*), exhibit ring enhancement immediately after gadolinium administration (*b*), and enhance to near isointensity with liver on interstitial-phase images (*c*).

Echo-train STIR (*d*), SGE (*e*) and immediate postgadolinium SGE (*f*) images in a second patient. There are numerous metastases in the liver. One lesion has mildly increased signal on T2-weighted image (*d*) and high signal on T1-weighted image (*e*), consistent with hemorrhage. Note that many of the <1-cm metastases exhibit moderately intense uniform enhancement (*f*).

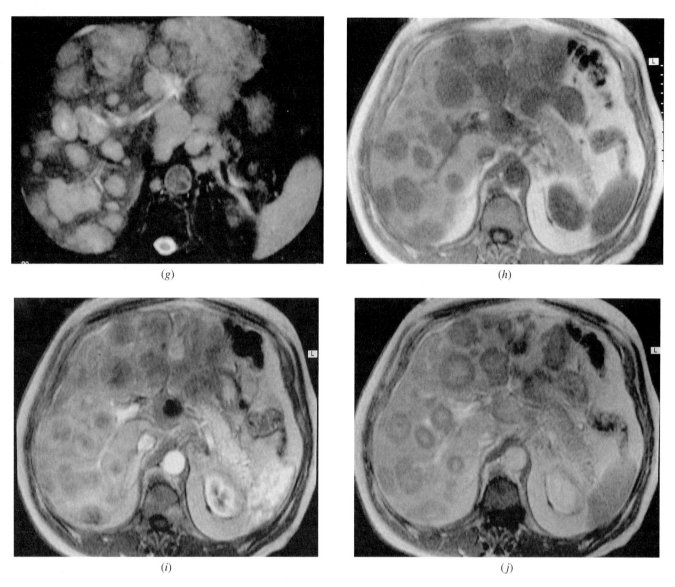

F I G . 2.81 (*Continued*) Fat-suppressed T2-weighted ETSE (*g*), SGE (*h*), and immediate (*i*) and 2-min (*j*) postgadolinium SGE images. The liver contains numerous metastases scattered throughout all segments that are moderately high in signal intensity on T2 (*g*) and well defined and moderately low in signal intensity on T1 (*h*) and have prominent thick uniform rings of enhancement on immediate postgadolinium images (*i*). Peripheral washout with centripetal progression of enhancement is noted on the delayed postcontrast image (*j*). Peripheral washout is common in hypervascular tumors that possess uniform intense rings of enhancement on immediate postgadolinium images.

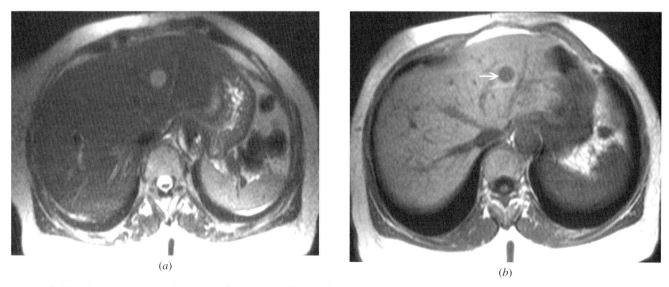

F I G . 2.82 Liver metastases from ovarian cancer. T2-weighted SS-ETSE (*a*), SGE (*b*), and immediate (*c*) and 90-s fat-suppressed (*d*) SGE images. A rounded lesion is seen in the left hepatic lobe that shows high signal intensity on the T2-weighted image (*a*),

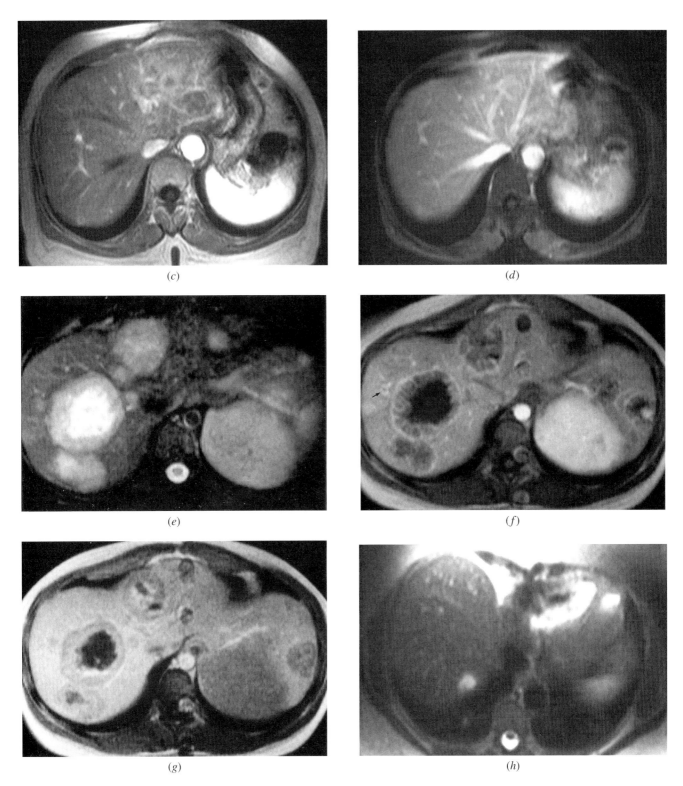

(c)

(d)

(e)

(f)

(g)

(h)

F I G . 2.82 (*Continued*) low signal intensity on the T1-weighted image (arrow, *b*), and faint ring enhancement and perilesional enhancement on the early-phase image (*c*) that become less conspicuous on the late-phase image (*d*), consistent with a metastasis.

Fat-suppressed T2-weighted ETSE (*e*) and immediate (*f*) and 10-min (*g*) postgadolinium SGE images in a second patient with ovarian cancer. Multiple varying-sized metastases are scattered throughout the liver. The largest metastasis is high in signal intensity centrally on the T2-weighted image (*e*) because of central necrosis. Metastases are better shown on the immediate postgadolinium image and appear as multiple hypervascular lesions with ring enhancement. Ring enhancement is appreciated in metastases as small as 6 mm (arrow, *f*). Peripheral washout of metastases is apparent on the 10-min postgadolinium image (*g*).

T2-weighted SS-ETSE (*h*) and immediate (*i*) and 90-s fat-suppressed (*j*) postgadolinium SGE images in a third patient demonstrates a liver metastasis that is high signal intensity on the T2-weighted image (*h*) and low signal intensity on the T1-weighted image (not shown) and shows a faint thin ring enhancement on the early-phase image (*i*) that becomes more conspicuous on the late-phase image (*j*).

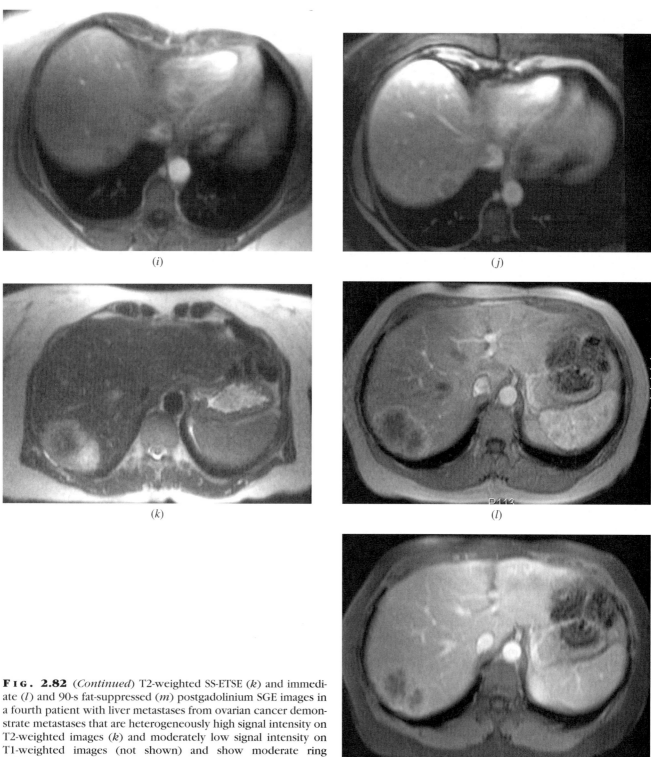

(i)

(j)

(k)

(l)

(m)

FIG. 2.82 (*Continued*) T2-weighted SS-ETSE (*k*) and immediate (*l*) and 90-s fat-suppressed (*m*) postgadolinium SGE images in a fourth patient with liver metastases from ovarian cancer demonstrate metastases that are heterogeneously high signal intensity on T2-weighted images (*k*) and moderately low signal intensity on T1-weighted images (not shown) and show moderate ring enhancement on early-phase images (*l*) that becomes less conspicuous on late-phase images (*m*).

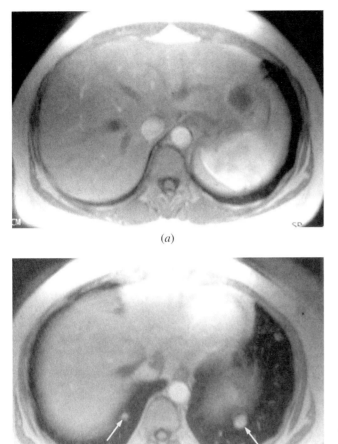

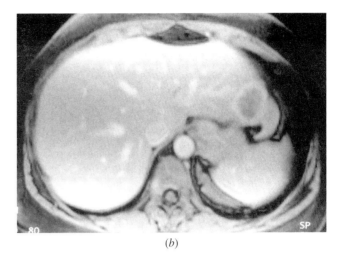

(a)

(b)

(c)

F I G . 2.83 Lung and liver metastases. Immediate (*a*, *c*) and 90-s fat-suppressed (*b*) postgadolinium SGE images in a patient who has a history of carcinoma of the sphenoid sinus. A metastasis in the left hepatic lobe is present, which demonstrates peripheral rim enhancement following administration of contrast (*a*) that persists on the late image (*b*), consistent with a metastasis. Note that lung metastases are also present (arrows, *c*).

ductal carcinoma, and lung cancer [143, 155]. The most commonly observed extremely hypervascular metastases are of neuroendocrine origin (i.e., carcinoid and islet cell tumor).

Enhancement of hypervascular metastases is better shown on MR than on CT images because of the higher sensitivity of MRI for gadolinium chelates, the more compact bolus of contrast delivered to the hepatic parenchyma, and the better temporal resolution for dynamic image acquisition (fig. 2.85).

MR Features of Liver Metastases According to Primary Site. Certain histologic types of metastases may display distinctive morphology or patterns of enhancement (figs. 2.86–2.88).

Metastases from colon cancer are commonly hypovascular. As a characteristic histopathologic finding, these tumors have a thin zone of fibrous tissue and inflammatory cells that translates in a thin peripheral ring of enhancement on MR images that enhances on early-phase images and remains enhanced on late-phase images [141]. When tumors exceed 3 cm in diameter,

metastases from colorectal cancer typically develop a cauliflower-type appearance. It is suggested that this appearance is due to the presence of fibrous tissue strands and inflammatory cells that extend into the lesions, surrounded by islets of tumoral cells that arise with tumor growth and bulge through portions of the fibrous encapsulation [141]. This creates areas of peripheral enhancement that extend into the periphery of the tumor, creating the cauliflower-type appearance. Large solitary metastases are most commonly observed in colon carcinoma. This imaging observation may in part reflect the fact that colon cancer is the most frequently encountered liver metastasis. Minimal involvement of the liver with metastatic disease explains why colon cancer is one of the few malignancies amenable to curative surgical resection of liver metastases. Colorectal metastases may exhibit coagulative necrosis, which may produce central low signal intensity on T2-weighted images surrounded by higher-signal-intensity viable tumor [156].

Multiple small subcapsular metastases are observed in approximately one-third of patients with liver metastases from colon cancer. These metastases may only

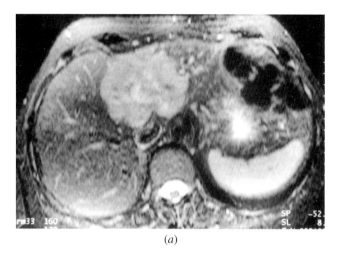

(a)

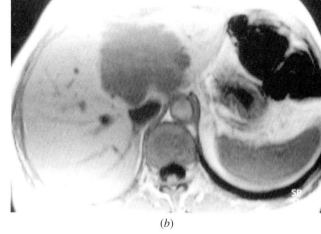

(b)

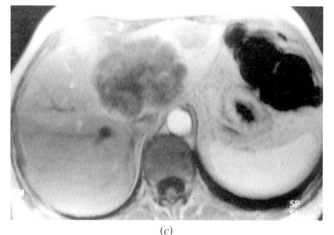

(c)

FIG. 2.84 Cauliflower-shaped metastasis from ovarian cancer. Echo-train STIR (*a*), SGE (*b*), and immediate postgadolinium SGE (*c*) images. A large mass is seen in the left hepatic lobe, which demonstrates high signal on T2-weighted (*a*), low signal on T1-weighted (*b*), and ring and perilesional enhancement on immediate postgadolinium images (*c*). Note that the lesion resembles a colon cancer metastasis because of its cauliflower shape.

be apparent on immediate postgadolinium images (fig. 2.89).

Metastases from breast cancer are characterized as hypervascular. Breast cancer liver metastases have a greater range of MR findings than other common types of liver metastases. These patterns include ring, miliary, and confluent segmental (figs. 2.90–2.92). Confluent segmental involvement is more typical of breast cancer than of any other cancer. [141, 142].

Metastases from pancreatic ductal adenocarcinoma are commonly hypovascular, but hypervascularity is not rare. Lesions tend to be multiple and scattered throughout the parenchyma or capsule based. Circumferential or wedge-shaped perilesional enhancement is not uncommon. On T2-weighted images, lesions show moderately high signal intensity, and on T1-weighted images lesions exhibit mildly low signal intensity or isointensity, particularly when ≤1.5 cm. In approximately 20% of patients, the only liver metastases present are small (<1.5 cm) and capsule based and are only seen transiently on hepatic arterial dominant-phase images as hypervascular lesions [152].

Metastases from squamous cell lung cancer are generally characterized as well-defined rounded masses that have a high-signal-intensity rim and a low-signal-intensity center on T2-weighted images and show intense enhancement of the outer rim on early postcontrast images (fig. 2.93). Squamous cell carcinomas from other sites of origin also tend to be rounded and have uniform ring enhancement on immediate postcontrast SGE images (fig. 2.93).

Metastases from unknown primary site are commonly hypervascular and multiple. However, hypovascular lesions and solitary lesions are not uncommon [152]. Hypervascular metastases appear high in signal intensity on T2-weighted images and moderately low signal intensity on T1-weighted images and show intense enhancement on immediate postgadolinium images that becomes less evident on interstitial-phase images.

Poorly differentiated adenocarcinomas frequently demonstrate numerous metastases <2 cm scattered throughout the entire liver. These metastases are typically high in signal intensity on T2-weighted images and

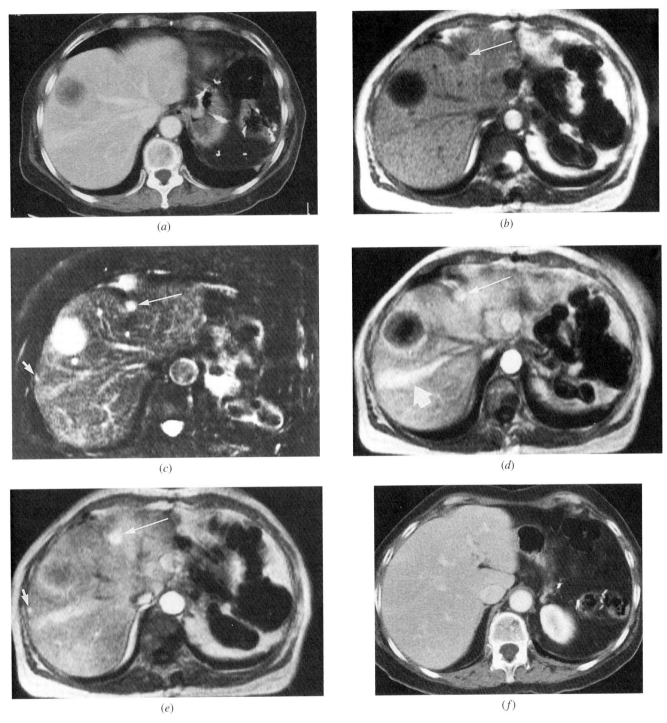

FIG. 2.85 Hypervascular liver metastases from small bowel leiomyosarcoma. Dynamic contrast-enhanced CT (*a*), SGE (*b*), fat-suppressed T2-weighted SE (*c*), and immediate postgadolinium SGE (*d, e*) images. A 4-cm metastasis was appreciated on the CT imaging study (*a*). The SGE image (*b*) demonstrated a second 8-mm lesion in the lateral segment (arrow, *b*). The fat-suppressed T2-weighted SE image (*c*) demonstrated the lesion in the lateral segment (long arrow, *c*) and a 5-mm subcapsular lesion in the anterior segment (short arrow, *c*). Immediate images (*d, e*) demonstrate ring enhancement around the 4-cm metastases and uniform enhancement of the 8-mm metastases in the lateral segment (long arrow, *d, e*) and of the 5-mm subcapsular metastases (short arrow, *e*). Wedge-shaped transient increased enhancement is present in the posterior segment (large arrow, *d*), which is also faintly apparent on the CT image (*a*). Dynamic contrast enhanced CT (*f*), SGE (*g*), fat-suppressed T2-weighted SE (*h*), and immediate (*i*) and 45-s (*j*) postgadolinium SGE images from the midhepatic level in the same patient. A 7-mm metastasis is present in the right lobe

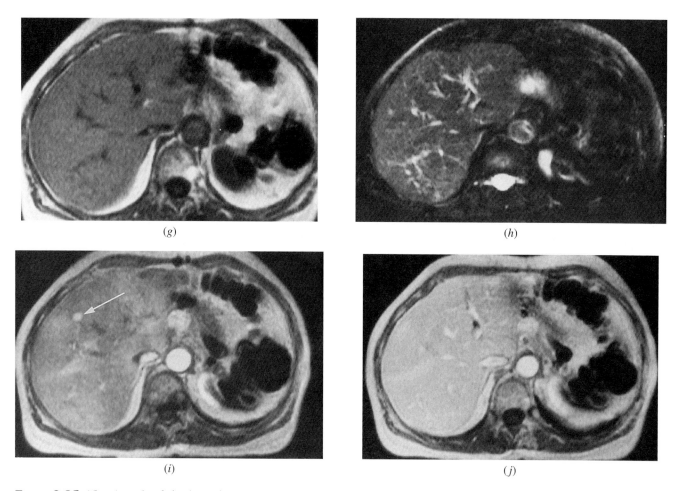

(g)   *(h)*

(i)   *(j)*

F I G . 2.85 *(Continued)* of the liver that is not visualized on the CT (*f*) or noncontrast T1-weighted (*g*) or T2-weighted (*h*) images, but is well shown as a uniformly enhancing lesion (arrow, *i*) on the immediate image (*i*). The metastasis washes out rapidly and becomes isointense with liver by 45 s (*j*). Small hypervascular malignant lesions commonly are shown only on hepatic arterial dominant-phase images.

show peripheral ring enhancement on immediate post-gadolinium images. These metastases range from hypovascular to very hypervascular. Small cell and other aggressive nonsquamous cell lung cancers have similar imaging findings (figs. 2.94 and 2.95).

Metastases from gastrinomas exhibit a uniform moderately intense peripheral ring pattern of enhancement on arterial dominant-phase images and have a particular propensity to washout peripherally on late-phase images (fig. 2.96). Gastrinoma metastases often appear as a relatively uniform population of lesions. Metastases may also be extremely extensive despite relatively mild patient symptomatology.

Metastases from melanoma may represent a mixture of high- and low-signal-intensity lesions on T2- and T1-weighted images because of the paramagnetic property of melanin (fig. 2.97). Melanoma metastases must be highly pigmented, well-differentiated lesions to produce this paramagnetic effect. Amelanocytic malignant melanomas or poorly-differentiated tumors do not contain melanin and therefore will not produce the paramagnetic effect and will appear mildly hyperintense on T2-weighted images and mildly hypointense on T1-weighted images. Melanoma metastases may be hypervascular and may also be very extensive.

Metastases from carcinoid tumor commonly demonstrate high signal intensity on T2-weighted images, low signal intensity on T1-weighted images, and moderate or intense enhancement after contrast administration, suggesting hypervascularity (fig. 2.98) [157]. On late-phase images, metastases from carcinoid tumor either wash out or fade to isointensity. Not uncommonly, they are only appreciated on immediate postgadolinium images. In addition, carcinoid metastases may resemble HCC as they can also be high signal intensity on noncontrast T1-weighed images (reflecting protein synthesis) and can show washout with capsule enhancement on late-phase images. In approximately 90% of patients with liver metastases, the lesions are hypervascular, and in 10% they can be hypovascular [158].

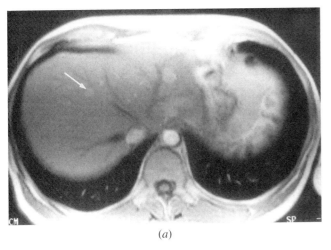

(a)

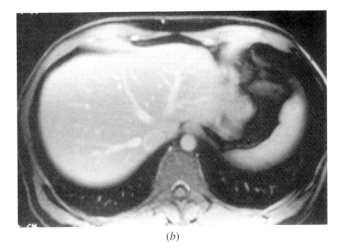

(b)

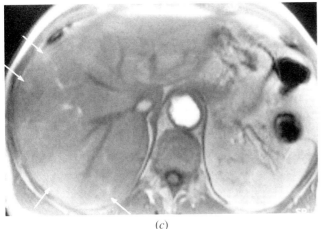

(c)

FIG. 2.86 Small colon cancer metastases. Immediate (*a*) and 90-s fat-suppressed postgadolinium SGE (*b*) images. On the immediate postgadolinium SGE image (*a*), a 1-cm ring enhancing metastasis is identified in segment 8 (arrow, *a*) that equilibrates with background liver on the interstitial-phase image (*b*)

Immediate postgadolinium SGE image (*c*) in a second patient shows multiple small subcapsular metastases (arrows) from colon cancer.

Metastases from mucin-producing tumors such as ovarian cancer or mucinous cystadenocarcinoma of the pancreas may result in liver metastases that are high in signal intensity on T1-weighted images because of the protein content (fig. 2.99).

Metastases that are active in protein synthesis, such as in the production of enzymes or hormones (e.g., carcinoid tumors) may also be high in signal intensity on T1-weighted images because of the presence of a high concentration of protein (fig. 2.100).

Capsule-based metastases frequently occur in the setting of tumors that metastasize by intraperitoneal spread (fig. 2.101). Ovarian cancer most commonly results in capsule-based metastases (fig. 2.102) followed by colon cancer. A prior study [152] reported that 81% (13/16) of patients with liver metastases from pancreatic ductal adenocarcinoma showed capsule-based metastases, among them, 19% (3/16) exhibit only capsule-based metastases. A variety of other malignancies can also produce capsule-based metastases (fig. 2.103).

Hemorrhagic metastases result in varying high- and low-signal-intensity lesions on T2- and T1-weighted images.

Distinction Between Liver Metastases and Benign Lesions.

METASTASES VERSUS HEMANGIOMAS. On T2-weighted images small (≤1.5 cm) hypervascular liver metastases, particularly from islet cell tumors, leiomyosarcoma, gastrointestinal stromal tumors, pheochromocytoma and renal cell carcinoma, and small avascular metastases, necrotic or cystic metastases from ovarian cancer, may mimic the appearance of hemangiomas [67, 132, 144, 159].

Small (<1.5 cm) hypervascular metastases often enhance in an intense homogeneous fashion on arterial dominant-phase images and tend to wash out below the signal intensity of the background parenchyma on interstitial-phase images [144]. Type I hemangiomas may enhance in similar fashion on arterial dominant-phase images; however, they tend to retain contrast or fade to isointensity with the background parenchyma on interstitial-phase images. Often at least one lesion greater than 2 cm in diameter is present that possesses the typical enhancement features of a metastasis or hemangioma, allowing inference of the nature of the smaller lesions.

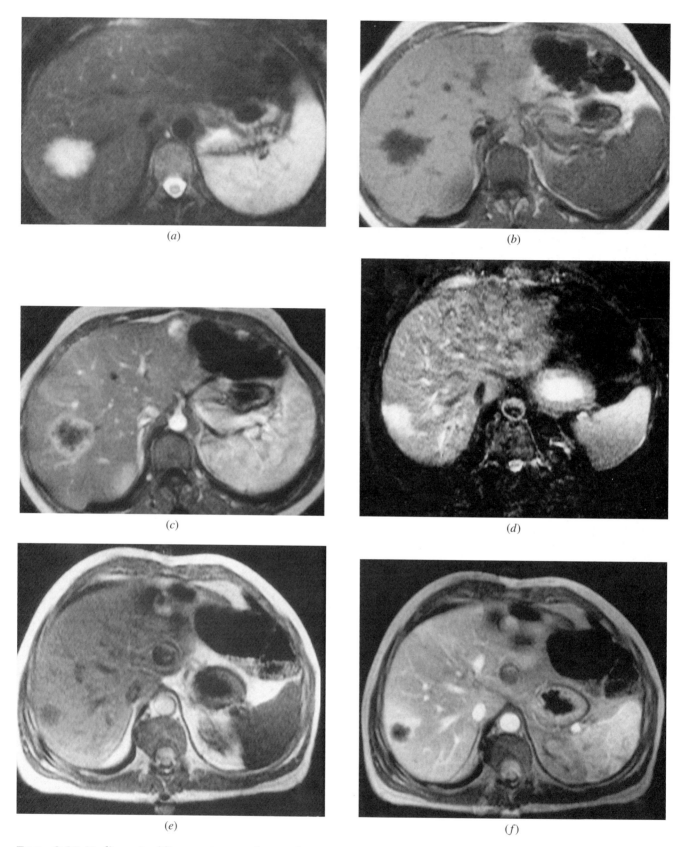

F I G . 2.87 Medium-sized liver metastases from colon cancer. Fat-suppressed T2-weighted ETSE (*a*), SGE (*b*), and immediate postgadolinium SGE (*c*) images. An irregularly marginated mass is present in the right lobe that is moderately high in signal intensity on the T2-weighted image (*a*) and moderately low in signal intensity on the T1-weighted image (*b*) and demonstrates intact ring enhancement on the immediate postgadolinium image (*c*) with an irregular inner margin to the ring. A faint region of ill-defined transient increased enhancement is present on the immediate postgadolinium image (*c*).

Fat-suppressed T2-weighted SS-ETSE (*d*), SGE (*e*), and immediate (*f*) and 90-s (*g*) postgadolinium SGE images in a second patient.

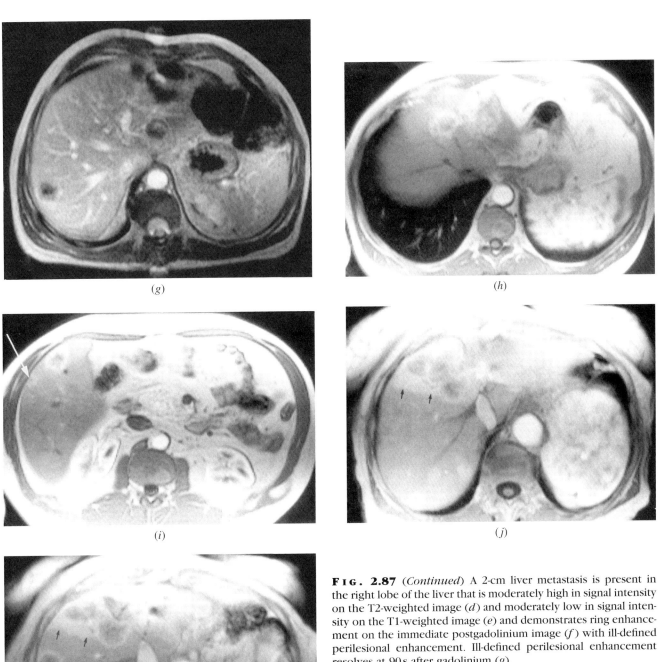

(g)

(h)

(i)

(j)

(k)

FIG. 2.87 (*Continued*) A 2-cm liver metastasis is present in the right lobe of the liver that is moderately high in signal intensity on the T2-weighted image (*d*) and moderately low in signal intensity on the T1-weighted image (*e*) and demonstrates ring enhancement on the immediate postgadolinium image (*f*) with ill-defined perilesional enhancement. Ill-defined perilesional enhancement resolves at 90 s after gadolinium (*g*).

Immediate images (*h, i*) in a third patient demonstrate irregular ring enhancement lesions consistent with metastases. Even metastases <1 cm often exhibit ring enhancement (arrow, *i*).

Immediate postgadolinium SGE images (*j, k*) in a fourth patient with colon cancer demonstrate multiple metastatic foci, several small rounded masses, and one large cauliflower-shaped lesion, all with ring enhancement. Note ill-defined perilesional enhancement (arrows, *j, k*) around the cauliflower-shaped metastasis, characteristic for colon cancer metastases.

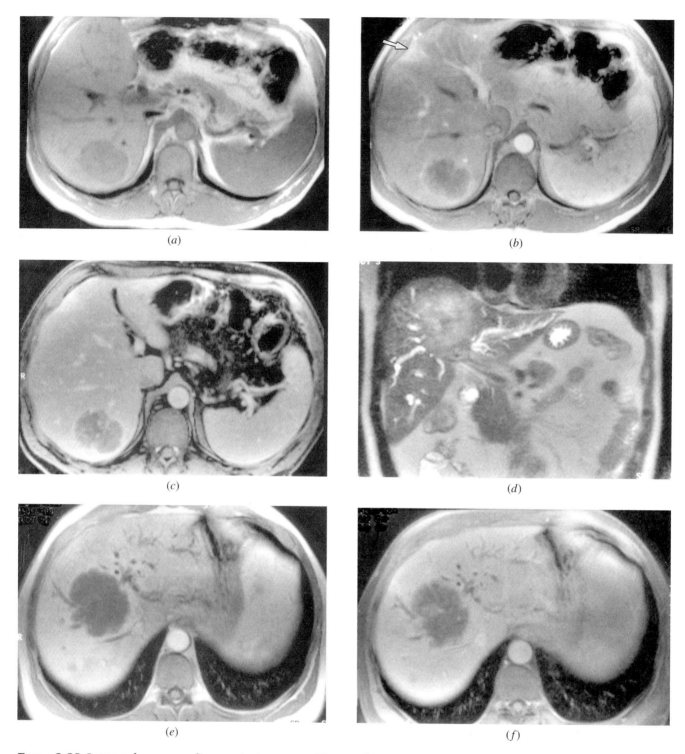

(a)

(b)

(c)

(d)

(e)

(f)

F I G . 2.88 Large colon cancer liver metastases—cauliflower shape. SGE (*a*) and immediate (*b*) and 90-s (*c*) fat-suppressed postgadolinium SGE images demonstrate a colon cancer metastasis with a cauliflower shape. A small peripheral metastasis with intense wedge-shaped perilesional enhancement (arrow, *b*) is present.

Coronal T2-weighted SS-ETSE (*d*) and transverse immediate (*e*) and 90-s fat-suppressed (*f*) postgadolinium SGE images in a second patient demonstrate a large, centrally located metastasis that has a cauliflower shape. Note that the central location of the metastases has resulted in bile duct obstruction (*d*).

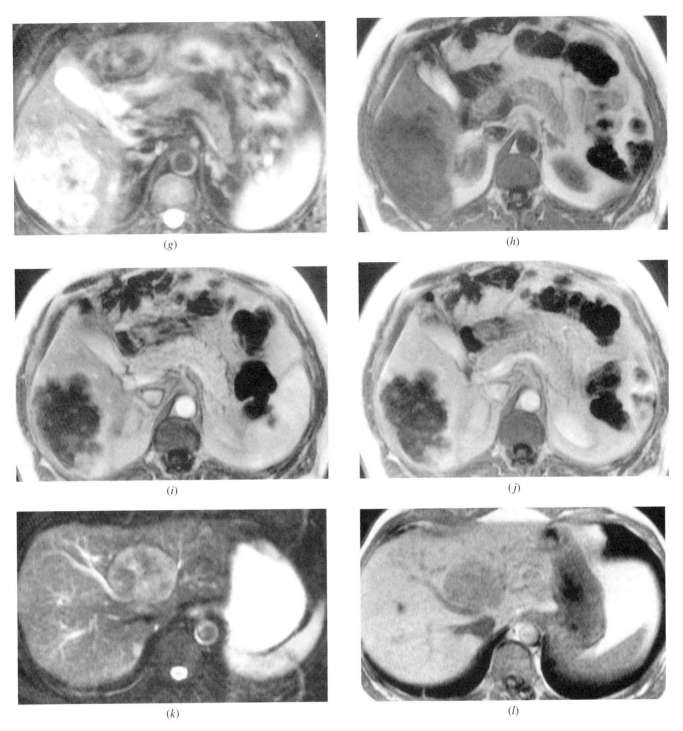

(g)

(h)

(i)

(j)

(k)

(l)

FIG. 2.88 (*Continued*) Fat-suppressed T2-weighted SS-ETSE (*g*), SGE (*h*), and immediate (*i*) and 45-s (*j*) postgadolinium SGE images in a third patient demonstrate a large cauliflower-shaped metastasis that has ring enhancement with perilesional enhancement. Note that arcs of peripheral enhancement extend into the lesion.

Fat-suppressed T2-weighted SS-ETSE (*k*), SGE (*l*), and immediate postgadolinium SGE (*m*) images in a fourth patient. This lesion possesses the typical imaging features of a colon cancer metastasis. The metastasis is heterogeneous and moderately hyperintense on the T2-weighted image (*k*) and mildly hypointense on the T1-weighted image (*l*) and has ring enhancement with perilesional enhancement on the immediate postgadolinium SGE image (*m*).

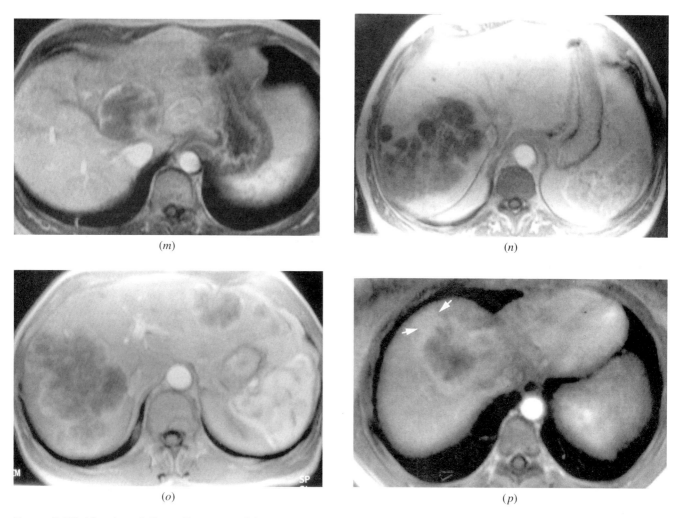

(m)

(n)

(o)

(p)

FIG. 2.88 (*Continued*) Immediate postgadolinium SGE images (*n–p*) in three additional patients with large metastases that exhibit the characteristic cauliflower shape of colon cancer metastases. Ill-defined perilesional enhancement (arrows, *p*) is observed in the last of these patients.

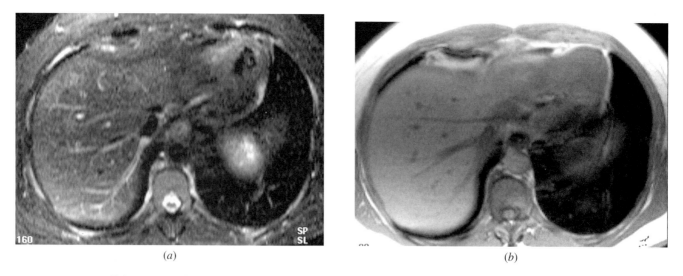

(a)

(b)

FIG. 2.89 Small hypervascular colon cancer metastases. T2-weighted SS-ETSE (*a*), SGE (*b*), and immediate (*c*) and 90-s fat-suppressed (*d*) postgadolinium SGE images. Multiple small lesions are seen scattered throughout the parenchyma that show

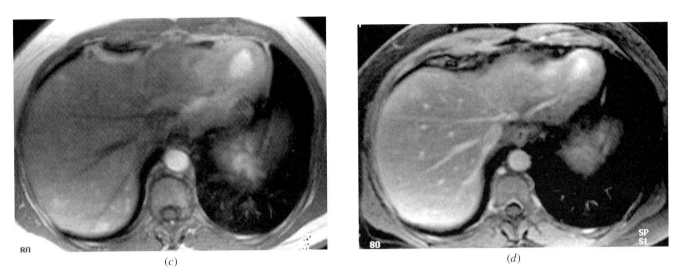

(c)   (d)

F I G . 2.89 (*Continued*) isointensity on T2-weighted (*a*) and T1-weighted (*b*) images and intense enhancement on early-phase images (*c*) that fade to background parenchyma on late-phase images (*d*).

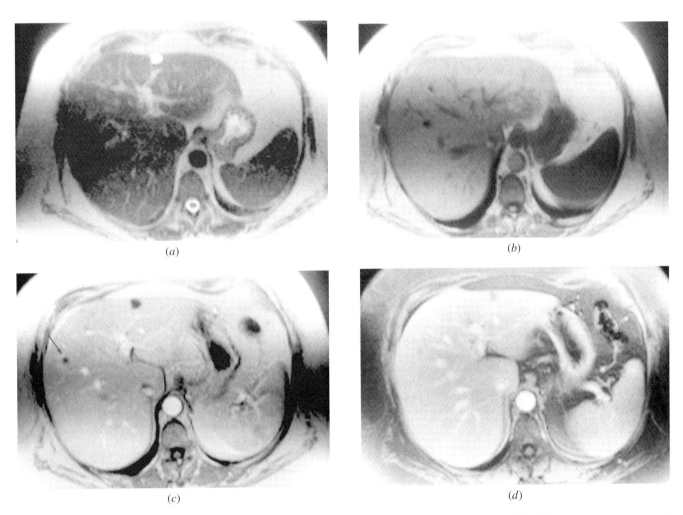

(a)   (b)

(c)   (d)

F I G . 2.90 Breast cancer liver metastases—ring enhancement. T2-weighted SS-ETSE (*a*), SGE (*b*), and immediate (*c*) and 90-s fat-suppressed (*d*) postgadolinium SGE images. There is a small lesion in the right lobe that is almost imperceptible on T2 (*a*) and T1 (*b*) images. The metastasis exhibits mild ring enhancement (arrow, *c*) on immediate postgadolinium images that renders it conspicuous. The metastasis fades on the interstitial-phase image (*d*). This lesion was not seen on spiral CT (not shown). Note also a ciliated hepatic foregut cyst between segments 4 and 2 anteriorly.

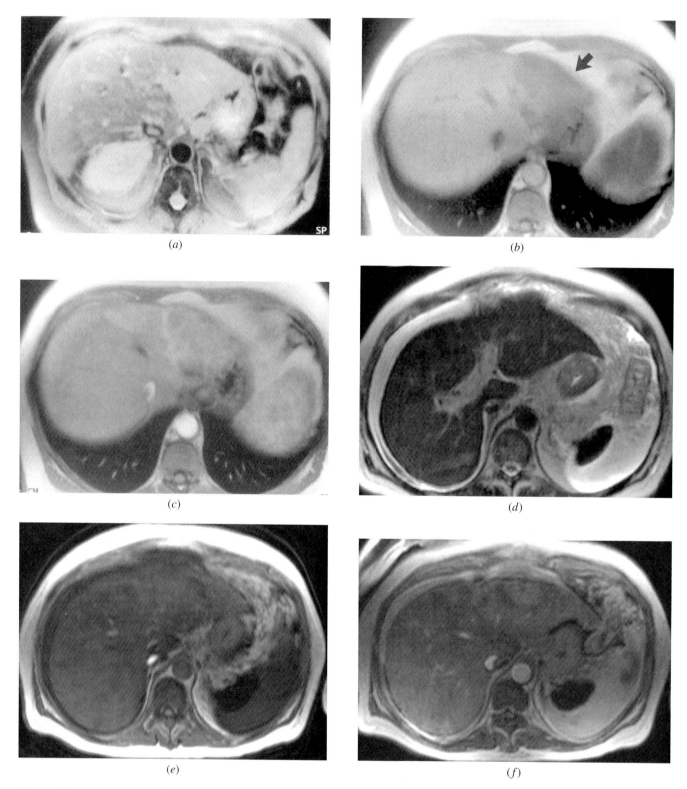

(a)   (b)   (c)   (d)   (e)   (f)

F I G . 2.91 Breast cancer liver metastases—infiltrative pattern. Fat-suppressed T2-weighted SS-ETSE (*a*), SGE (*b*), and imme-diate postgadolinium SGE (*c*) images. There is a mass (arrow, *b*) in the left hepatic lobe that demonstrates slightly increased signal on T2-weighted (*a*), decreased signal on T1-weighted (*b*), and heterogeneous enhancement on immediate postgadolinium SGE (*c*) images, consistent with metastatic disease. The confluent involvement of a segment, as in this case, is characteristic of breast cancer but represents an uncommon pattern.

T2-weighted SS-ETSE (*d*), SGE (*e*) and immediate postgadolinium SGE (*f*) images in a second patient. The liver shows normal signal intensity on both T2 (*d*)- and T1 (*e*)-weighted images, but diffuse increased parenchymal enhancement in a heterogeneous fashion on early-phase images (*f*) reflects infiltrative metastatic disease. The liver signal intensity becomes more homogeneously enhanced on late-phase images (not shown).

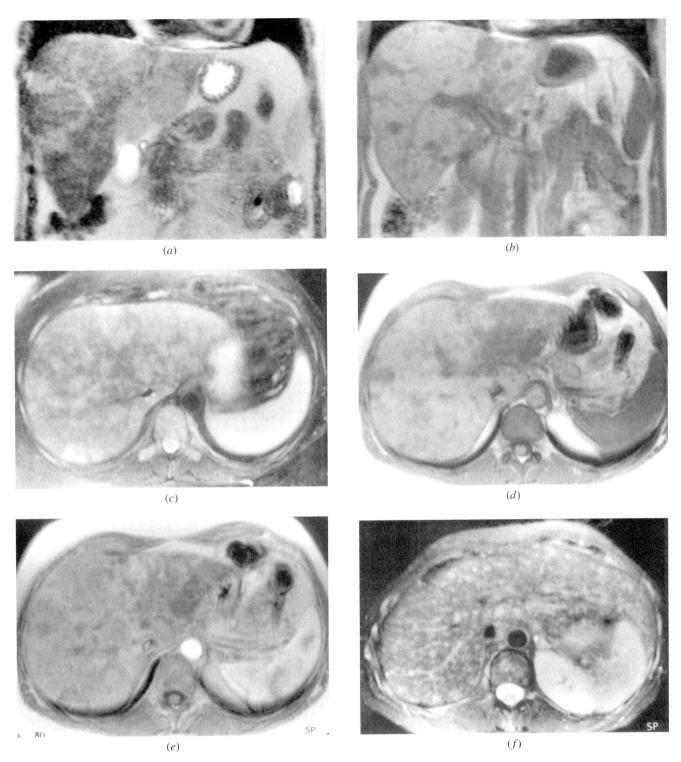

FIG. 2.92 Breast cancer liver metastases—miliary pattern. Coronal T2-weighted SS-ETSE (*a*), coronal SGE (*b*), transverse fat-suppressed T2-weighted ETSE (*c*), SGE (*d*), and immediate postgadolinium SGE (*e*) images. There are numerous lesions scattered throughout the hepatic parenchyma that demonstrate moderate signal on T2 (*a, c*) and moderately low signal on T1 (*b, d*) and show mild ring enhancement on immediate postgadolinium (*e*) images, consistent with metastases.

Fat-suppressed T2-weighted SS-ETSE (*f*), SGE (*g*), and immediate (*h*) and 90-s fat-suppressed (*i*) postgadolinium SGE images in a second patient. Extensive liver metastases, <5 mm in size, are present throughout the liver with a miliary pattern of involvement. The lesions show high signal on T2-weighted images (*f*), low signal on T1-weighted images (*g*), and a mild ring enhancement

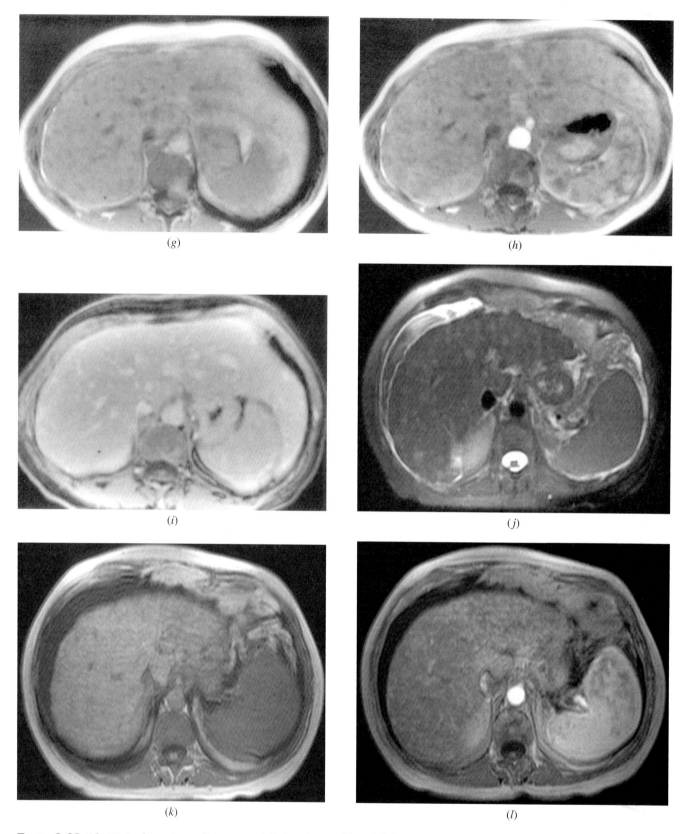

(g)

(h)

(i)

(j)

(k)

(l)

FIG. 2.92 (*Continued*) on immediate postgadolinium image (*h*) and fades on late image (*i*). Note that the metastases are best seen on T2-weighted images (*f*) and not definable on late phase (*i*).

T2-weighted SS-ETSE (*j*), SGE (*k*), and immediate (*l*) and 90-s fat-suppressed (*m*) postgadolinium SGE images in a third patient demonstrate similar findings.

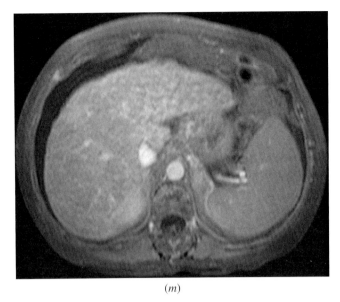

(*m*)

FIG. 2.92 (*Continued*) Miliary involvement of the liver with metastases is an uncommon but characteristic appearance for breast cancer liver metastases. Note that coexistent bone metastases are common in vertebral bodies, and they appear as high-signal small foci on fat-suppressed T2 and exhibit uniform enhancement on interstitial-phase fat-suppressed SGE images. If the liver metastases in patients with miliary involvement respond to chemotherapy, the liver develops extensive fibrosis with an appearance that resembles cirrhosis.

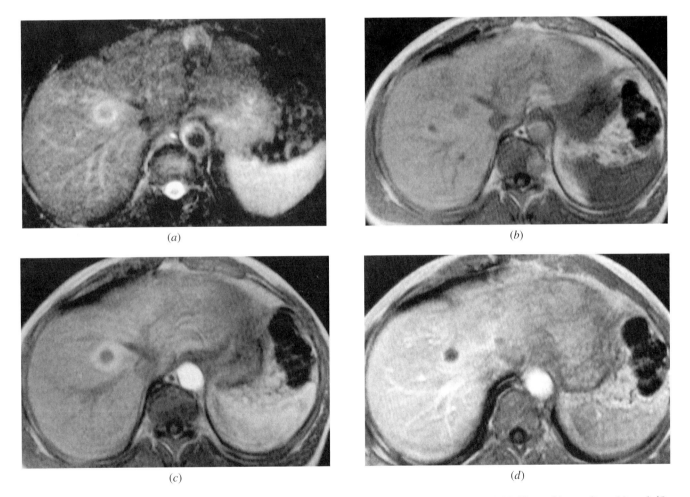

(*a*)   (*b*)

(*c*)   (*d*)

FIG. 2.93 Liver metastases, squamous cell type. Fat-suppressed T2-weighted ETSE (*a*), SGE (*b*), and immediate (*c*) and 45-s (*d*) postgadolinium SGE images. A well-defined 2-cm metastasis is present in the anterior segment of the right lobe that appears as a moderately high-signal intensity ring with central isointensity on the T2 (*a*) and mildly low in signal intensity on the T1 (*b*) images, has a uniform ring enhancement on the immediate image (*c*), and fades over time with negligible central enhancement (*d*). The enhancing ring on the immediate postgadolinium image (*c*) corresponds to the high-signal-intensity rim on the T2-weighted image (*a*). This is a typical appearance for liver metastases from squamous cell lung cancer.

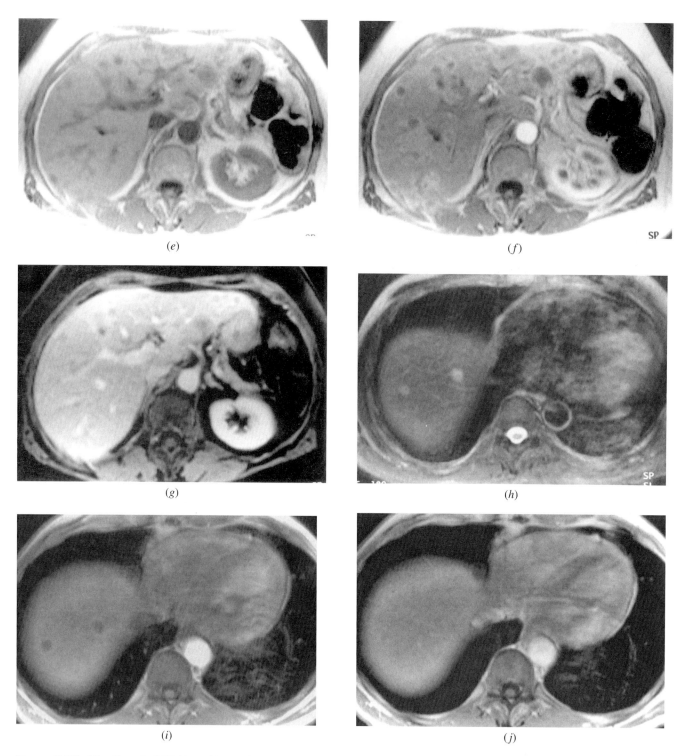

(e)

(f)

(g)

(h)

(i)

(j)

FIG. 2.93 (*Continued*) SGE (*e*) and immediate (*f*) and 90-s fat-suppressed (*g*) postgadolinium SGE images in a second patient with squamous cell lung cancer. There are multiple rounded lesions scattered throughout the liver that demonstrate low signal on T1-weighted images (*e*) and ring enhancement immediately after gadolinium administration (*f*), consistent with metastases.

Fat-suppressed T2-weighted SS-ETSE (*h*) and immediate (*i*) and 90-s (*j*) postgadolinium SGE images in a third patient, who has liver metastases from esophageal squamous cell cancer. The metastases are round, well-defined, and high in signal on the T2-weighted image (*h*), enhance with uniform rings on the early-phase image (*i*), and become isointense with liver on the late-phase image (*j*).

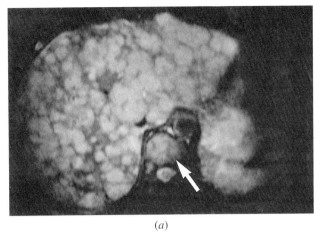

(a)

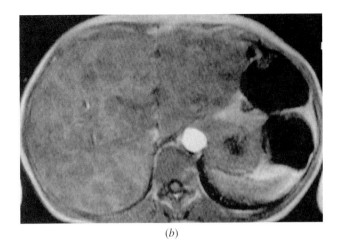

(b)

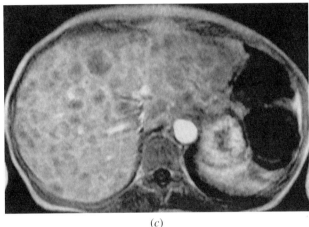

(c)

FIG. 2.94 Liver metastases, poorly-differentiated small cell type. Fat-suppressed T2-weighted ETSE (*a*), SGE (*b*), and immediate postgadolinium SGE (*c*) images. The liver is extensively replaced by numerous metastatic lesions smaller than 2 cm. Lesions are high in signal intensity on the T2-weighted image (*a*) and mildly low in signal intensity on the T1-weighted image (*b*) and demonstrate ring enhancement on the immediate postgadolinium images (*c*). High signal intensity is also apparent in the bone marrow on the T2-weighted image (arrow, *a*), which represents bone metastases. Poorly-differentiated or anaplastic malignancies not uncommonly result in this pattern of liver metastases. This patient has small cell lung cancer.

The distinction between liver metastases treated with systemic chemotherapy and rapid-enhancing type II or III hemangiomas is challenging. Chemotherapy-treated metastases demonstrate high signal intensity on T2-weighted images and peripheral irregular enhancement that may resemble globular enhancement [82]. Clinical history of liver metastases with recent initiation of chemotherapy is critical. Attention should be paid to unusual features such as partial washout pattern of enhancement and jagged rather than nodular inner margin of enhancement.

We reported [79] the occurrence of benign liver lesions in a consecutive population of women with newly diagnosed breast cancer and suspected liver metastases who were referred to MRI. A total of 32% (11 of 34) patients had benign lesions; 62% (21 of 34) had malignant lesions, two of whom had coexistent benign lesions. Characterization of focal liver lesions as benign or malignant is important because patients with known primary malignancies commonly have small hepatic lesions that are benign cysts or hemangiomas. The whole organ coverage per acquisition of spoiled gradient echo permits optimal evaluation of the entire liver in distinct phases of enhancement with serial image acquisition after gadolinium administration. In the presence of multiple liver lesions, the distinction of benign and malignant lesions is of critical importance and is well performed by MRI (fig. 2.104).

Lesion characterization is critical in assessing and staging patients with primary nonhepatic malignancies, as benign liver lesions are common, even in these patients. One previous report [160] described the detection of small (<15 mm) lesions in 254 of 1454 patients who underwent CT examination. The majority of patients (82%) with liver lesions in this study had a known primary tumor, yet lesions in 51% of these patients were benign. Another report [161] described a large series of cancer patients in whom 41.8% of detected focal liver lesions were benign.

METASTASIS VERSUS FNH AND HCA. Hypervascular metastases may demonstrate a homogeneous intense enhancement on arterial dominant-phase images similar to FNH and HCA. Small hypervascular metastases (<1.5 cm) may also be isointense on noncontrast T2- and T1-weighted images. Large hypervascular metastases

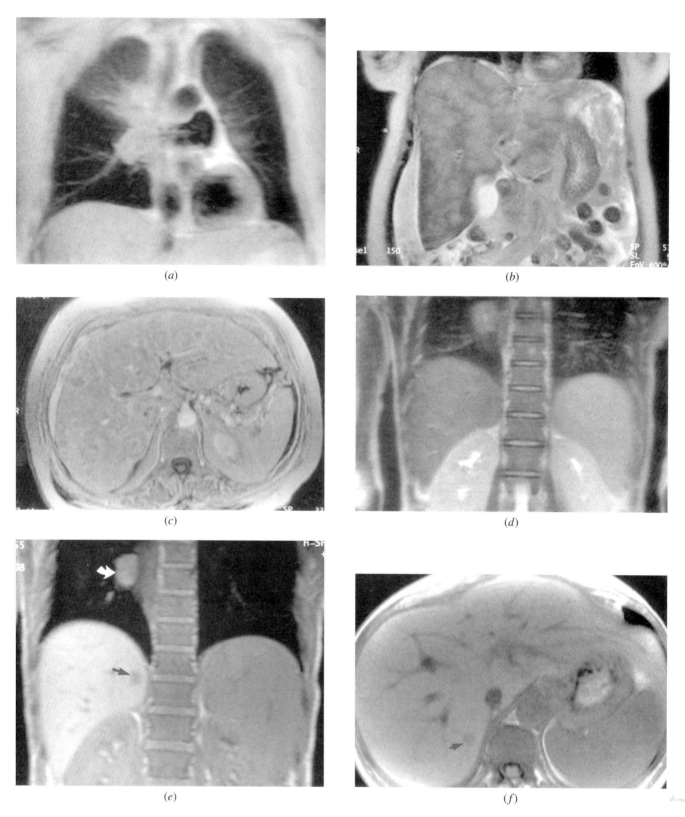

(a)

(b)

(c)

(d)

(e)

(f)

FIG. 2.95 Metastases from lung cancer. Coronal T2-weighted SS-ETSE (*a, b*) and transverse immediate postgadolinium magnetization-prepared gradient-echo (*c*) images. Multiple lesions are scattered throughout the liver, which appear high signal on T2-weighted images (*b*) and show ring enhancement on immediate postgadolinium images (*c*). Note the right hilar mass associated with an alveolar infiltrate due to postobstructive pneumonia (*a*).

Coronal T2-weighted SS-ETSE (*d*), coronal SGE (*e*), SGE (*f*), and immediate postgadolinium (*g*) images in a second patient. A small lesion is seen in the right hepatic lobe (arrow, *e, f*) and demonstrates low signal on T1-weighted image (*e, f*) and thin ring enhancement immediately after contrast administration (*g*), consistent with a metastasis. Note the right infrahilar mass in the lung (curved arrow, *e*).

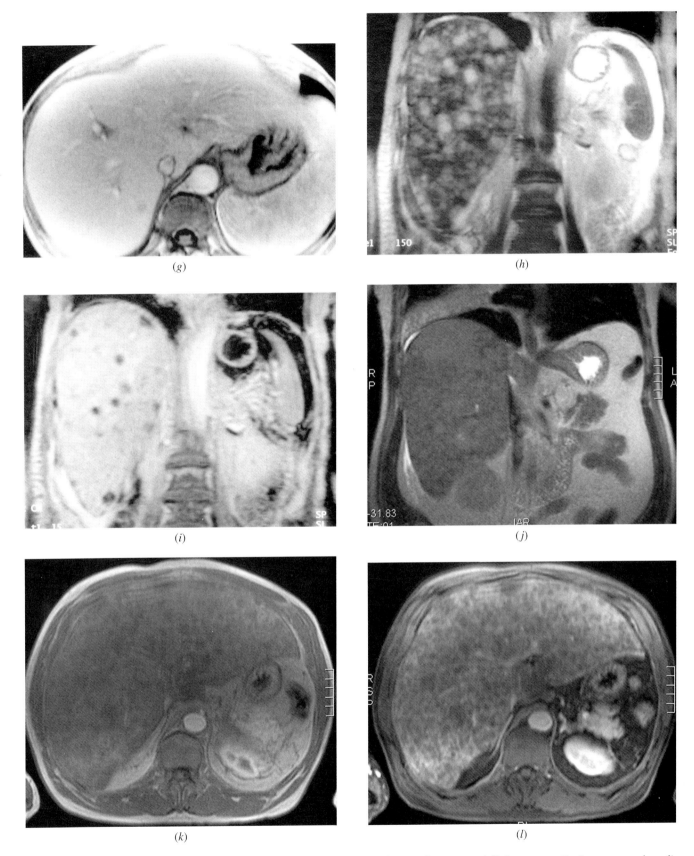

FIG. 2.95 (*Continued*) Coronal T2-weighted SS-ETSE (*h*) and coronal immediate postgadolinium magnetization prepared gradient-echo (*i*) images in a third patient. There are numerous metastases scattered throughout the liver, which exhibit high signal on T2-weighted image (*h*) and ring enhancement after gadolinium administration (*i*), consistent with metastases from non-small cell carcinoma.

Coronal T2-weighted SS-ETSE (*j*) and immediate (*k*) and 90-s fat-suppressed (*l*) postgadolinium SGE images in a fourth patient that show similar findings.

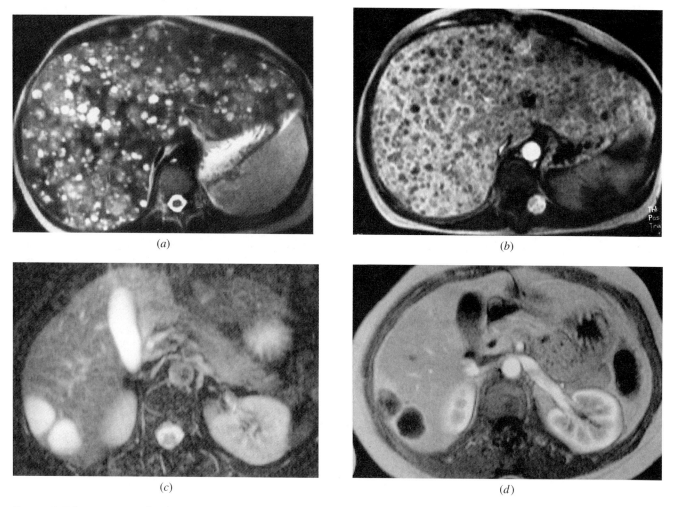

(a)

(b)

(c)

(d)

F I G . 2.96 Hypervascular liver metastases from islet cell tumors. Transverse 512-resolution ETSE (a) and immediate post-gadolinium SGE (b) images in a patient with gastrinoma. Numerous metastases smaller than 1 cm are scattered throughout all segments, many of which are well defined and high in signal intensity on the T2-weighted image (a). The immediate postgadolinium image (b) demonstrates that the metastases have intact ring enhancement.

Fat-suppressed T2-weighted ETSE (c) and immediate postgadolinium SGE (d) images in a second patient who has an untyped islet cell tumor. The metastases are well-defined round masses that are high in signal intensity on the T2-weighted image (c) and have calculated T2 values of 160 ms. On the immediate postgadolinium image (d), the lesions possess intact rings of enhancement that are a feature of metastases and not of hemangiomas. Prior outside MRI performed with conventional spin-echo techniques and original outside interpretation of percutaneous biopsy specimen suggested the diagnosis of hemangiomas. On the gadolinium-enhanced images, hypervascular cystic liver metastases and a 2-cm islet cell tumor in the head of the pancreas were shown. The histology specimen was re-examined, and the diagnosis of islet cell tumor was confirmed.

(>1.5 cm) often possess a radial spoke-wheel appearance with thin radial strands of lesser enhancement on arterial-phase images. Also, FNH and HCA, independent of lesion size, almost invariably show isointensity or mild hyperintensity on T2-weighted images and isointensity or mild hypointensity on T1-weighted images. Larger hypervascular metastases are generally moderately high in signal on T2-weighted images. On interstitial-phase images, FNH and HCA show enhancement that fades to isointensity with surrounding parenchyma. Hypervascular metastases commonly show lesion washout, although small lesions may fade on late post-

contrast images [69, 72, 81, 113, 121, 132, 162]. Clinical history of a primary hypervascular tumor is usually present, facilitating the correct diagnosis.

Secondary Infection of Liver Metastases. Secondary infection of metastases may occur and is most commonly observed with colon cancer metastases. It is postulated that the high content of intraluminal bacteria within the colon may be conducive to embolization of coliform bacteria with tumor cells. Experimental data suggests that certain anaerobic bacteria grow selectively in tumor nodules but not in the

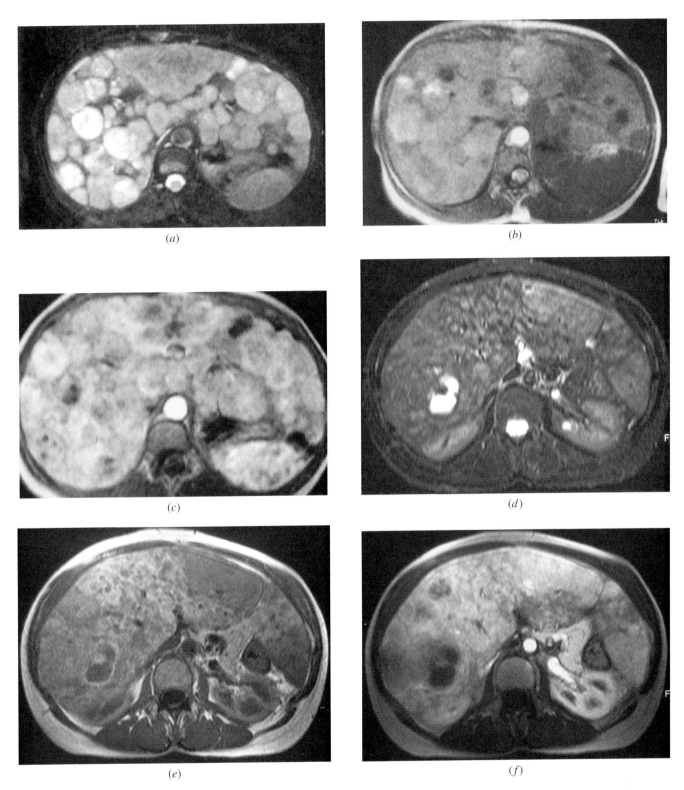

F I G . 2.97 Melanoma metastases. Fat-suppressed T2-weighted ETSE (*a*), SGE (*b*), and immediate postgadolinium SGE (*c*) images. Melanoma metastases are a mixed population of low- to high-signal intensity lesions on T2 (*a*)- and T1 (*b*)-weighted images. This reflects the paramagnetic properties of melanin. Intense ring enhancement is present on the immediate postgadolinium SGE image (*c*), demonstrating the hypervascularity of these metastases.

Fat-suppressed T2-weighted SS-ETSE (*d*), SGE (*e*), and immediate (*f*) and 90-s fat-suppressed (*g*) postgadolinium SGE images in a second patient. There are multiple lesions scattered throughout hepatic parenchyma that show heterogeneous high signal on the

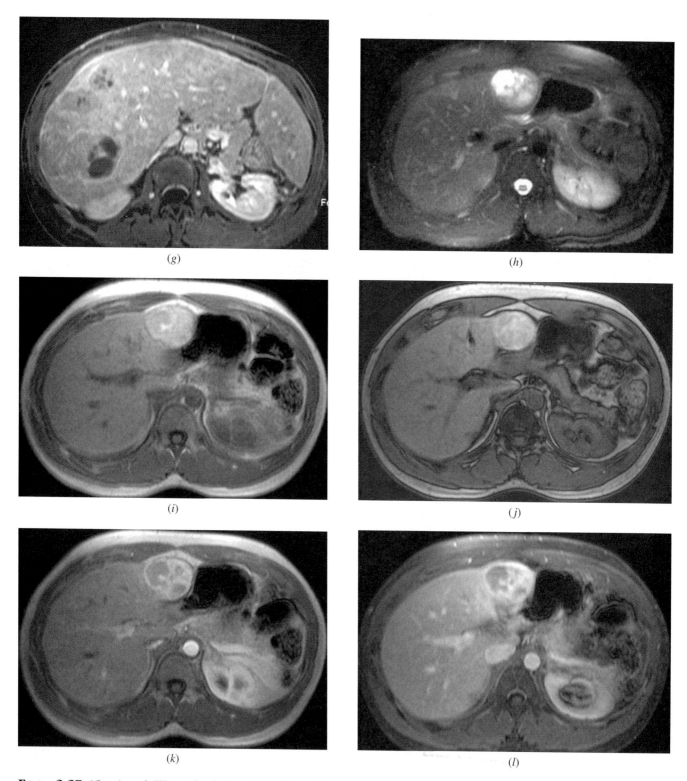

(g)

(h)

(i)

(j)

(k)

(l)

F I G . 2.97 (*Continued*) T2-weighted (*d*) and the T1-weighted (*e*) images and intense heterogeneous enhancement on the early-phase image (*f*) that becomes more homogeneous on the late-phase image (*g*). The high signal intensity on both the T2- and T1-weighted images reflects the presence of melanin.

Fat-suppressed T2-weighted SS-ETSE (*h*), SGE (*i*), out-of-phase SGE (*j*), and immediate (*k*) and 90-s fat-suppressed (*l*) SGE images in a third patient show similar features.

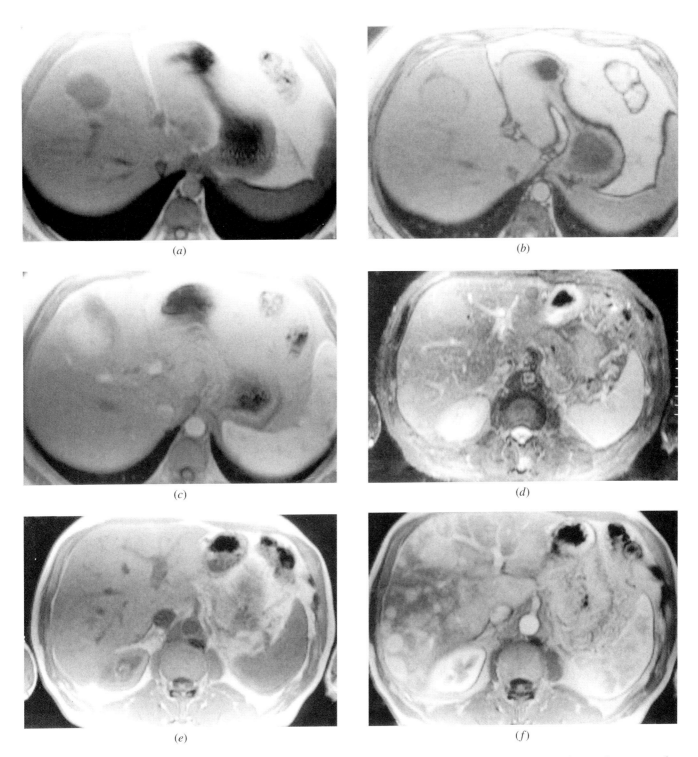

F I G . 2.98 Hypervascular liver metastases from carcinoid tumor. SGE (*a*), out-of-phase SGE (*b*), and immediate postgadolinium SGE (*c*) images. There is a rounded lesion in the right hepatic lobe that demonstrates low signal intensity on T1-weighted image (*a*), the lesion and liver become comparable in signal on out-of-phase image (*b*) due to signal loss in background fatty liver—note the rim of greater fat content. The lesion shows intense and homogeneous enhancement after gadolinium administration (*c*), consistent with a hypervascular metastasis. Carcinoid tumor was present at histopathology.

Echo train-STIR (*d*), SGE (*e*), and immediate (*f*) and 90-s fat-suppressed (*g*) postgadolinium SGE images in a second patient. Numerous metastases are scattered throughout the hepatic parenchyma that demonstrate near-isointense signal on T2 (*d*)- and T1 (*e*)-weighted images and intense enhancement on immediate postgadolinium images (*f*) that wash out on later images (*g*), consistent with hypervascular metastases. The difference in lesion conspicuity between immediate postgadolinium images and other sequences, including noncontrast T2- and T1-weighted images and late postgadolinium images, is particularly impressive in the setting of hypervascular malignant disease.

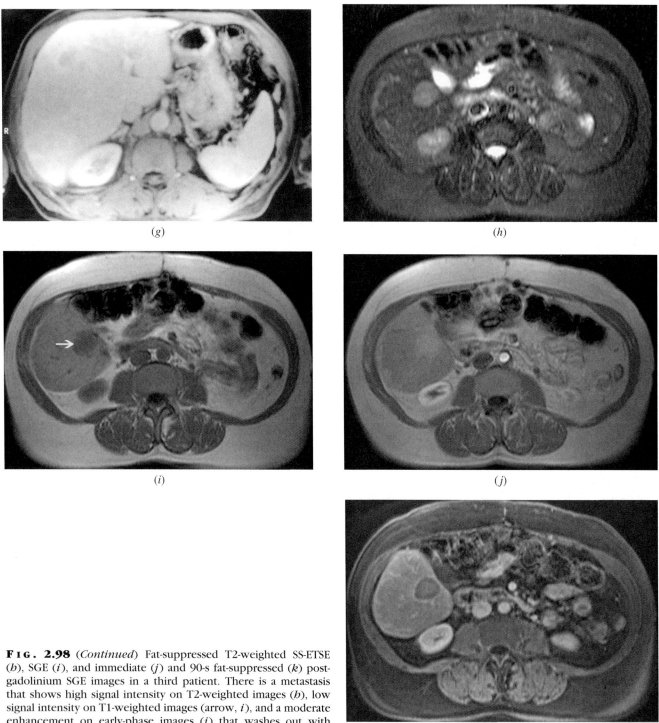

(g)

(h)

(i)

(j)

(k)

FIG. 2.98 (*Continued*) Fat-suppressed T2-weighted SS-ETSE (*h*), SGE (*i*), and immediate (*j*) and 90-s fat-suppressed (*k*) post-gadolinium SGE images in a third patient. There is a metastasis that shows high signal intensity on T2-weighted images (*h*), low signal intensity on T1-weighted images (arrow, *i*), and a moderate enhancement on early-phase images (*j*) that washes out with persistent ring enhancement on late-phase images (*k*).

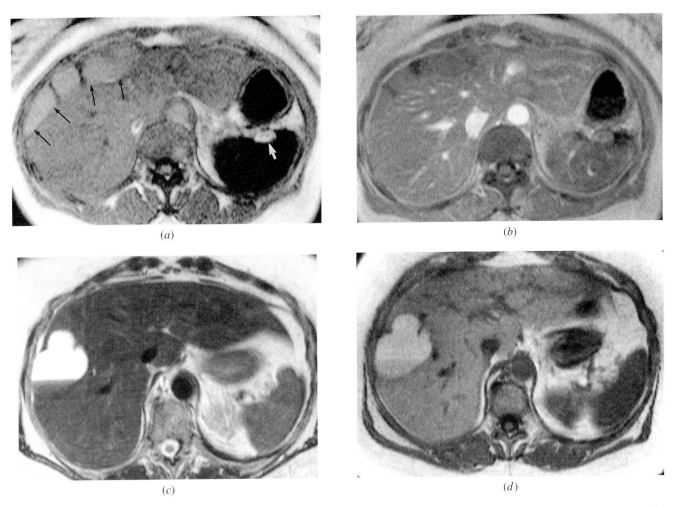

(a)

(b)

(c)

(d)

F I G . 2.99 High T1 signal mucin-producing liver metastases, ovarian cancer. SGE (*a*) and 90-s postgadolinium SGE (*b*) images. A large capsule-based metastasis is present along the lateral margin of the liver (black arrows, *a*), and a smaller subcapsular metastasis is present in the spleen (white arrow, *a*). The metastases are high in signal intensity on T1-weighted image, reflecting high mucin content. Enhancement of cyst walls is present on postgadolinium images (*b*). The spleen is nearly signal void on these T1-weighted images because of transfusional hemosiderosis.

T2-weighted ETSE (*c*) and SGE (*d*) images in a second patient demonstrate a cystic ovarian metastasis located superficially in the right lobe of the liver. On the T2-weighted image (*c*), low-signal-intensity material layers in the dependent portion of the metastasis. The high mucin content of the cystic metastasis renders it high in signal intensity on the T1-weighted image (*d*).

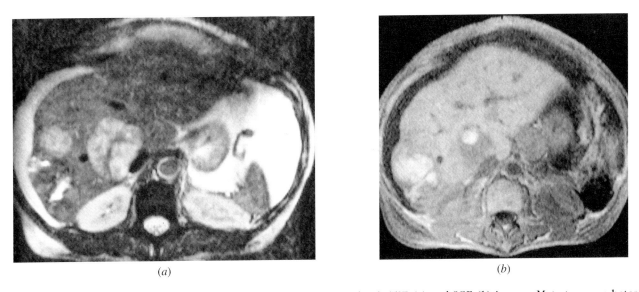

(a)

(b)

F I G . 2.100 Carcinoid liver metastases. Fat-suppressed T2-weighted ETSE (*a*) and SGE (*b*) images. Metastases are heterogeneous with mixed high-signal intensity on T2 (*a*) and T1 (*b*) images. The high signal intensity on the T1-weighted image (*b*) reflects a high protein concentration due to protein synthesis from hormone production. The high signal on T1-weighted image (*b*) is an uncommon appearance for carcinoid metastases.

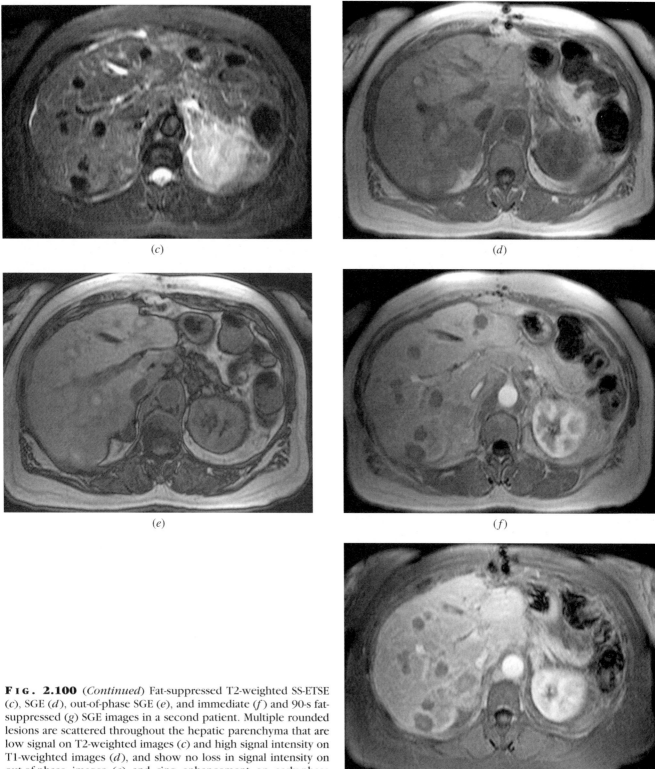

FIG. 2.100 (*Continued*) Fat-suppressed T2-weighted SS-ETSE (*c*), SGE (*d*), out-of-phase SGE (*e*), and immediate (*f*) and 90-s fat-suppressed (*g*) SGE images in a second patient. Multiple rounded lesions are scattered throughout the hepatic parenchyma that are low signal on T2-weighted images (*c*) and high signal intensity on T1-weighted images (*d*), and show no loss in signal intensity on out-of-phase images (*e*) and ring enhancement on early-phase images (*f*), with persistent appearance on late-phase images (*g*).

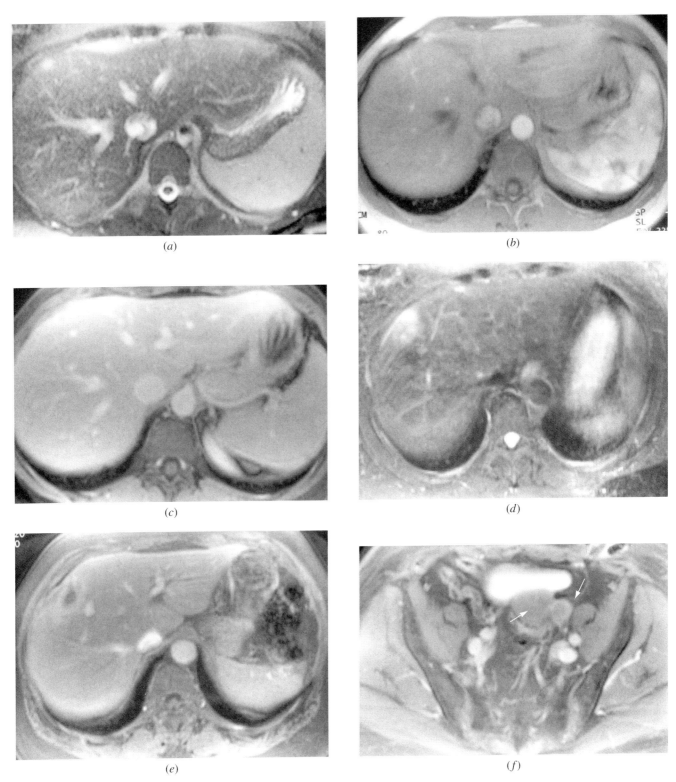

F I G . 2.101 Liver and peritoneal metastases from ovarian tumor. Echo-train STIR (*a*) and immediate (*b*) and 90-s fat-suppressed (*c*) postgadolinium SGE images in one patient and echo-train STIR (*d*) and 90-s fat-suppressed postgadolinium SGE (*e*, *f*) images in a second patient, both of whom have ovarian cancer and peritoneal metastases. Both patients demonstrate liver metastases characterized by high signal on T2-weighted images (*a*, *d*) and ring enhancement on early (*b*) and late (*c*, *e*) postgadolinium images. Note the presence of recurrent pelvic tumor (arrows, *f*) in the second patient.

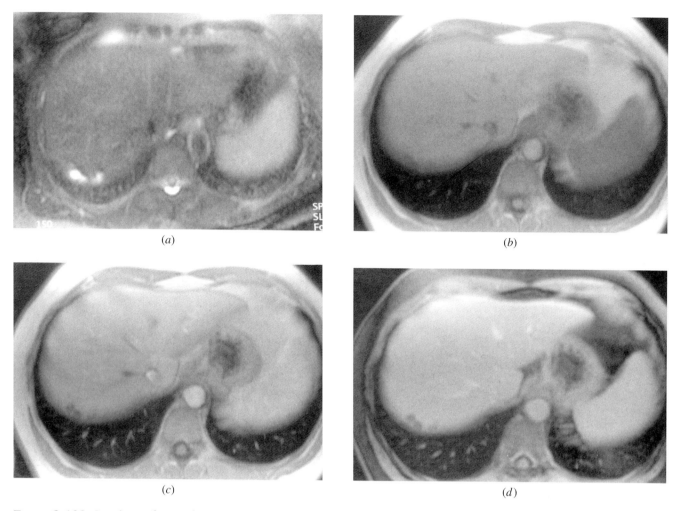

(a)   (b)

(c)   (d)

FIG. 2.102 Ovarian subcapsular metastases. Echo-train STIR (*a*), SGE (*b*), and immediate (*c*) and 90-s fat-suppressed (*d*) postgadolinium SGE images. There is a cluster of small lesions in a subcapsular location along the dome of the liver, which demonstrate high signal on T2 (*a*), low signal on T1 (*b*), and faint ring enhancement on early (*c*) and late (*d*) postgadolinium images consistent with capsule-based metastatic implants. This is the most common pattern of involvement of the liver with ovarian cancer and represents part of the generalized process of intraperitoneal seeding and spread.

normal tissues of a tumor-bearing host [163]. Secondary infection of liver metastases after chemoembolization of these lesions has been reported [164]. Infected metastases may simulate both the clinical and imaging features of liver abscesses.

On MRI, infected metastases tend to have thickened, irregular walls and heterogeneous intermediate signal intensity on T2-weighted images and show some progressive central stromal enhancement on delayed images (fig. 2.105). Abscesses tend to have thinner walls and higher signal intensity on T2-weighted images and do not demonstrate progressive central lesion stromal enhancement over time, even in abscesses with thick walls and internal septations. Both types of lesions will show transient, ill-defined perilesional enhancement reflecting an inflammatory hyperemic response in the liver.

Hepatocellular Carcinoma

Hepatocellular carcinoma (HCC) is the most common primary malignancy of the liver and usually develops in patients with cirrhosis [165]. It should be recognized that HCC does occur in the noncirrhotic liver as well. HCC is the fifth most common cancer in the world and accounts for up to 1 million deaths annually worldwide [166]. Incidence of HCC is particularly high in patients with cirrhosis from chronic hepatitis C infection, chronic hepatitis B infection, and alcoholic liver disease [165]. Men are affected three times more frequently than women [167]. The 5-year survival rate for untreated symptomatic HCC is <5% [167]. This statistic is in sharp contrast to the survival rate in patients with cirrhosis with small (<2 cm) HCC who have undergone liver transplantation, where the 5-year survival is 80% [165]. Thus detection of small HCC is imperative for improved

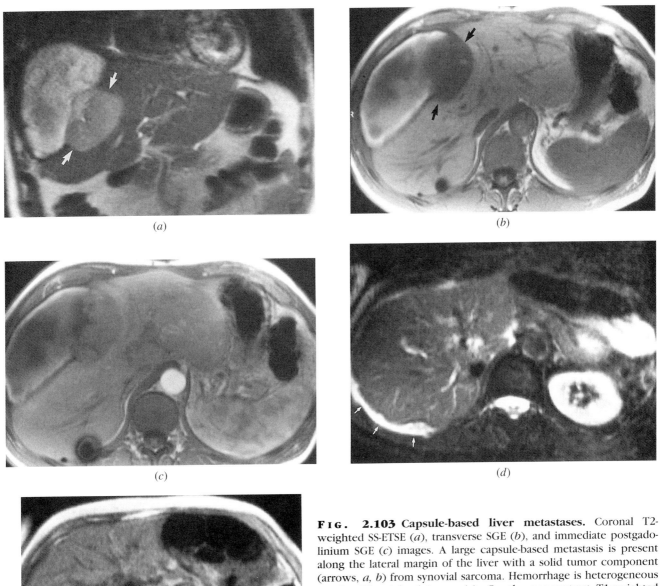

(a)

(b)

(c)

(d)

(e)

FIG. 2.103 Capsule-based liver metastases. Coronal T2-weighted SS-ETSE (*a*), transverse SGE (*b*), and immediate postgadolinium SGE (*c*) images. A large capsule-based metastasis is present along the lateral margin of the liver with a solid tumor component (arrows, *a, b*) from synovial sarcoma. Hemorrhage is heterogeneous on the T2-weighted image (*a*). On the noncontrast T1-weighted image (*b*), a peripheral rim of high signal intensity is present from recent hemorrhage. On the immediate postgadolinium image (*c*), the solid tumor component enhances uniformly.

Fat-suppressed T2-weighted SS-ETSE (*d*) and SGE (*e*) images in a second patient with capsule-based metastases from colon cancer. Capsule-based metastases are very conspicuous on the fat-suppressed T2-weighted image (arrows, *d*) because of the intrinsic high signal intensity of the masses and removal of the competing signal of fat. They are subtle on the T1-weighted image (*e*).

outcomes. In North America, most HCCs are large at the time of diagnosis, although with increasing surveillance of patients with liver cirrhosis and/or chronic hepatitis, detection of earlier stage neoplasms appears to be occurring more often [168].

Hepatocarcinogenesis is attributed to genetic predisposition and epigenetic changes that accumulate over time [169]. Liver cancer is considered a linear process beginning with the development of benign, hyperplastic foci of hepatocytes, or regenerative nodules (RNs), then evolving through premalignant stages of dysplastic nodules (DNs), and finally culminating in malignant HCC [169]. Continuous inflammation and hepatocyte regeneration provide the optimal setting for

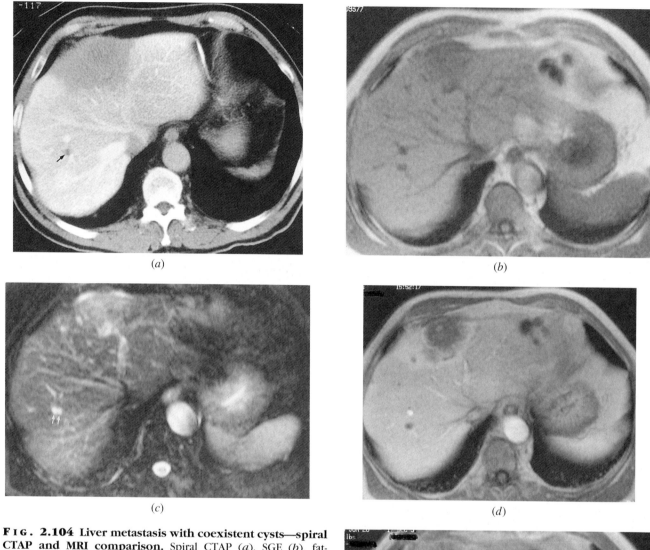

(a)

(b)

(c)

(d)

F I G . 2.104 Liver metastasis with coexistent cysts—spiral CTAP and MRI comparison. Spiral CTAP (*a*), SGE (*b*), fat-suppressed T2-weighted ETSE (*c*), and immediate (*d*) and 5-min (*e*) postgadolinium SGE images. The CTAP image (*a*) demonstrates a large perfusional defect in the medial segment related to a colon cancer metastasis. A 6-mm lesion in the anterior segment (arrow, *a*) was interpreted as one of several similar-appearing small lesions consistent with metastases scattered throughout the remainder of the liver. The MR images demonstrate a 4-cm mass in the medial segment with the imaging features of a colon cancer metastasis, including transient ill-defined perilesional enhancement on the immediate postgadolinium image (*d*). The lesion in the anterior segment represents two 3-mm juxtaposed cysts (arrows, *c*) that are small, sharply marginated, low in signal intensity on the T1-weighted image (*b*), and high in signal intensity on the T2-weighted image (*c*). Lack of enhancement on early (*d*) and later (*e*) postgadolinium-enhanced images is diagnostic for cysts. The remaining small liver lesions scattered throughout the liver were all shown to be cysts on MR images. The patient was operated on based on the MRI findings of a solitary liver metastases and multiple coexistent cysts. Intraoperative sonography-guided aspiration demonstrated that these small lesions were cysts. MRI was more diagnostically accurate than CTAP and had a greater effect on patient management.

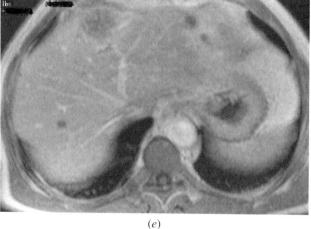

(e)

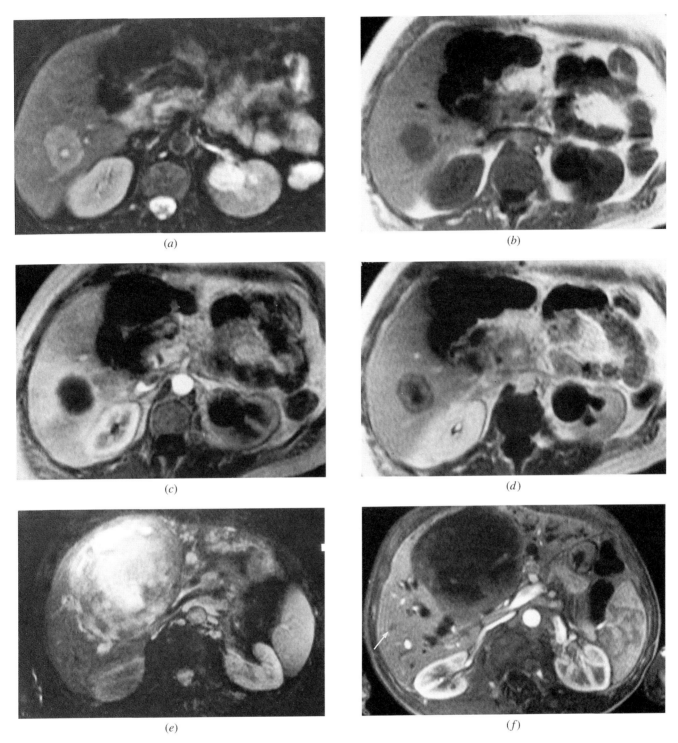

F I G . 2.105 Infected liver metastases. Fat-suppressed T2-weighted SE (*a*), SGE (*b*), and immediate (*c*) and 10-min (*d*) post-gadolinium SGE images. This patient with colon cancer and clinical findings of sepsis has a 4-cm infected metastasis in the right lobe of the liver. The tumor has ill-defined margins and is minimally hyperintense on T2 (*a*) with a small central focus of high signal intensity and moderately low in signal intensity on T1 (*b*), and on the immediate postgadolinium image (*c*) the infected metastasis shows ring enhancement with prominent ill-defined perilesional enhancement. The 10-min postcontrast image (*d*) shows some centripetal enhancement with peripheral washout resulting in a low-signal-intensity outer border. Chronic obstruction of the left renal collecting system is caused by entrapment of the ureter in the pelvis by the carcinoma arising in the sigmoid colon.

Fat-suppressed T2-weighted ETSE (*e*) and immediate (*f*) and 2-min (*g*) postgadolinium SGE images in a second patient. A 14-cm

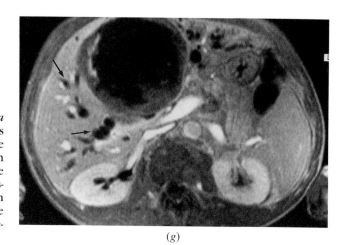

(g)

F i g . 2.105 (*Continued*) metastasis superinfected by *Listeria* is present in the left lobe of the liver. The infected metastasis is heterogeneous and high in signal intensity on T2-weighted image (*e*) and demonstrates enhancement of the thick irregular wall on the immediate postgadolinium image (*f*), with progressive enhancement on the interstitial-phase image (*g*). Additional metastases <1 cm are evident only on the immediate postgadolinium images (arrow, *f*). The mass causes obstruction of the biliary tree at the level of the porta hepatis, resulting in substantial intrahepatic biliary dilatation (arrows, *g*).

critical molecular alterations to become established in the genome [170]. Therefore, HCC is much more common in individuals with chronic liver disease, such as chronic viral hepatitis and cirrhosis, than it is in the population at large [169].

Statistics from the National Liver Cancer Network reveal that 87% of patients with HCC have underlying chronic liver disease and 52% have hepatitis C virus [171]. In part because of the increasing incidence of hepatitis C infection, HCC is the fastest growing malignancy in the U.S. [171]. Although cirrhosis of any etiology increases the risk of developing HCC, cirrhosis from viral hepatitis, alcohol, or hereditary hemochromatosis carries significantly more increased risk [170, 172, 173].

From a pathologic perspective, HCC forms soft, hemorrhagic, occasionally bile-stained nodules and masses with a propensity for necrosis [2]. On gross inspection, HCC may present as a single mass, as multiple nodules, as diffuse liver involvement, or as a large mass replacing most of the liver. In our experience, on MRI HCC is solitary in approximately 50% of cases (fig. 2.106), multifocal in approximately 40% (figs. 2.107 and 2.108), and diffuse in less than 10% of cases.

Histologically, malignant cells usually form trabeculae or plates of varying thickness, separated by a rich network of sinusoidal spaces filled with arterial blood. HCCs are fed by the hepatic arterial blood supply, but both hepatic and portal veins proliferate alongside tumors and cavernous structures develop in collaterals. As a consequence of these intrahepatic vascular changes, intra- and extrahepatic spread may occur by a number of routes including hepatic veins, inferior vena cava, and portal system (figs. 2.109–2.112).

Detection and characterization of focal liver lesions by imaging examination are closely related to the tumor size. Several reports describe the sensitivity and specificity of CT and MRI in the depiction of HCCs. The results vary widely, presumably because of the high frequency of bias in these studies, including the bias of greater experience with one or other modality. In general, there is a consensus that MRI is superior to CT in the detection of HCC, especially tumors that are <2.0 cm. (figs. 2.113 and 2.114) [174–179]. The superiority of MR imaging to detect and characterize liver lesions is due to its inherent excellent contrast resolution, combination of multiplanar T2- and T1-weighted images, and serial dynamic imaging after gadolinium administration. All sequences are necessary because tumors vary in signal intensity on noncontrast images [143, 180, 181], and this combination of sequences increases observer confidence.

A retrospective analysis examined the rate of HCC undetected by MRI in a large medical center transplant service over a 1-year period [182]. After review of imaging studies and pathologic diagnoses in explanted livers, there were 4 cases out of 279 MRI examinations in which HCC was not detected by MRI. Explanations for the presence of HCC undetected by MRI included patient motion, the misclassification of HCC as high-grade dysplastic nodules, and isovascular HCC. These results show the outstanding performance of MRI in detecting HCC.

Small HCCs (<2 cm) are frequently isointense on T2-weighted images [183–187]. Isointensity on T2-weighted images may correlate with a more favorable histology for well-differentiated HCC (fig. 2.115) [188]. Signal intensity on T1-weighted image varies from moderately low to moderately high signal. High signal intensity on T1-weighted images may reflect the presence of fat or protein (figs. 2.116 and 2.117) [185, 188, 189]. The majority of HCCs do not contain fat, and high protein content is most commonly responsible for the high signal intensity of these lesions (fig. 2.118) [189]. The most sensitive sequence for detecting small HCCs is hepatic arterial dominant-phase images, in which the majority of small tumors will enhance moderately; and not uncommonly these tumors may only be apparent

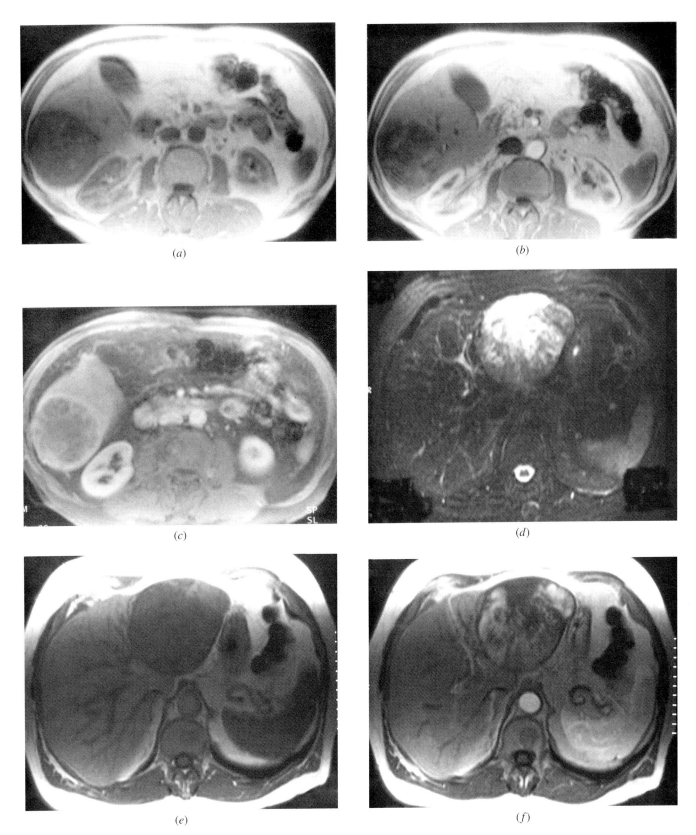

F I G . 2.106 Hepatocellular carcinoma, solitary hypovascular tumor. SGE (*a*) and immediate (*b*) and 90-s fat-suppressed (*c*) postgadolinium SGE images. There is an 8-cm mass arising from the inferior aspect of the right lobe that is low signal on the T1-weighted image (*a*) and demonstrates minimal heterogeneous enhancement immediately after gadolinium administration (*b*) and late mild and heterogeneous enhancement with a pseudocapsule (*c*) consistent with hypovascular HCC.

Fat-suppressed T2-weighted SS-ETSE (*d*), SGE (*e*), and immediate (*f*) and 90-s fat-suppressed (*g*) SGE images in a second patient with a small HCC that shows minimal tumor enhancement after contrast administration (*f*), consistent with hypovascular HCC.

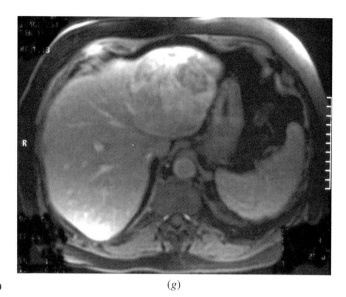

FIG. 2.106 (*Continued*)   (*g*)

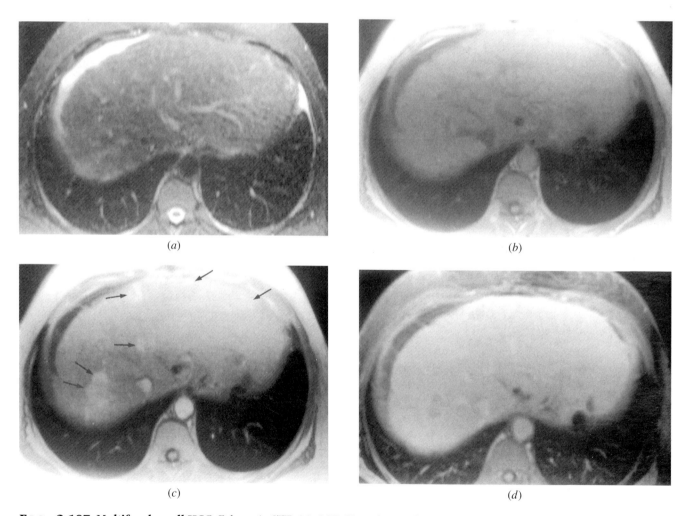

FIG. 2.107 Multifocal small HCC. Echo-train STIR (*a*), SGE (*b*), and immediate (*c*) and 90-s fat-suppressed (*d*) postgadolinium SGE images. There are multiple small HCCs (arrows, *c*) scattered throughout the hepatic parenchyma. These lesions are isointense on T2 (*a*)- and T1 (*b*)-weighted images and show homogeneous moderate enhancement after contrast administration (*c*) and lesion washout with pseudocapsule enhancement on late images (*d*).

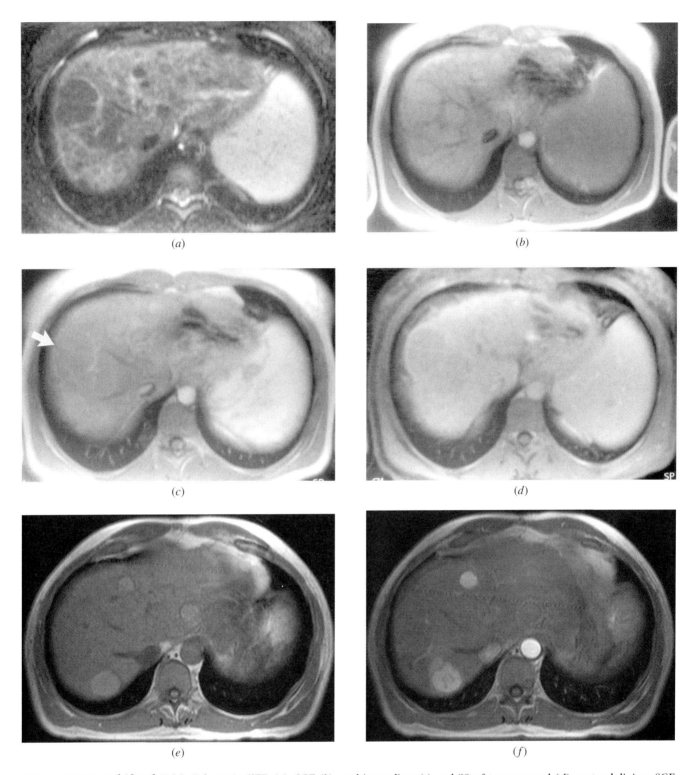

F I G. 2.108 Multifocal HCC. Echo-train STIR (*a*), SGE (*b*), and immediate (*c*) and 90-s fat-suppressed (*d*) postgadolinium SGE images. Multiple HCCs are present that are moderately hypointense on T2 (*a*)- and mildly hyperintense on T1 (*b*)-weighted images. The smaller lesions possess mildly intense homogeneous enhancement, and the 4-cm tumor (arrow, *c*) shows isointense enhancement immediately after gadolinium administration (*c*). Lesional washout along with pseudocapsule enhancement is observed on interstitial-phase images (*d*).

SGE (*e*) and immediate (*f*) and 90-s fat-suppressed (*g*) postgadolinium SGE images in a second patient. There are multiple rounded lesions that show mildly high signal intensity on T1-weighted images (*e*), intense enhancement on early-phase images (*f*),and washout with capsular enhancement on late-phase images (*g*), compatible with mutifocal HCC.

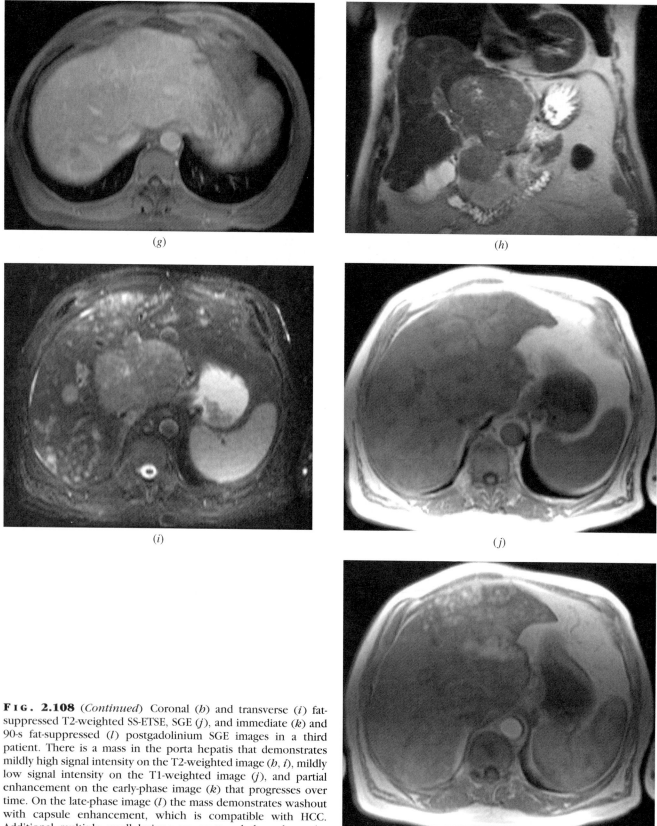

(g)

(h)

(i)

(j)

FIG. 2.108 (*Continued*) Coronal (*h*) and transverse (*i*) fat-suppressed T2-weighted SS-ETSE, SGE (*j*), and immediate (*k*) and 90-s fat-suppressed (*l*) postgadolinium SGE images in a third patient. There is a mass in the porta hepatis that demonstrates mildly high signal intensity on the T2-weighted image (*h, i*), mildly low signal intensity on the T1-weighted image (*j*), and partial enhancement on the early-phase image (*k*) that progresses over time. On the late-phase image (*l*) the mass demonstrates washout with capsule enhancement, which is compatible with HCC. Additional multiple small lesions are scattered throughout the hepatic parenchyma, consistent with multifocal HCCs.

(k)

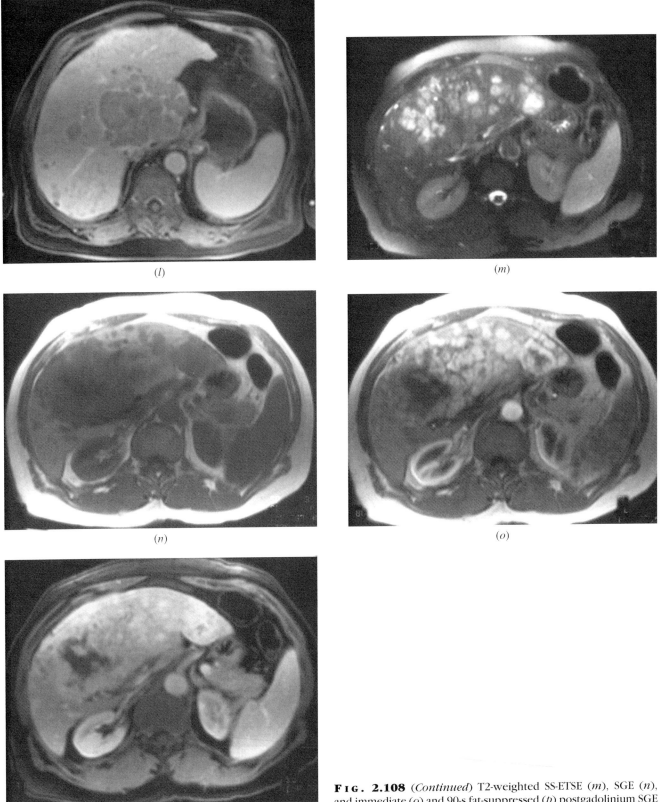

FIG. 2.108 (*Continued*) T2-weighted SS-ETSE (*m*), SGE (*n*), and immediate (*o*) and 90-s fat-suppressed (*p*) postgadolinium SGE images in a fourth patient show similar findings.

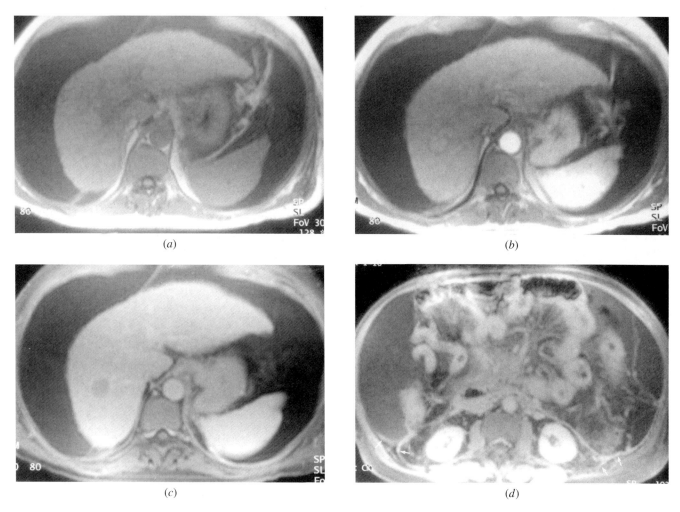

(a)   (b)

(c)   (d)

F I G . 2.109 HCC and microvarices in peritoneum. SGE (*a*) and immediate (*b*) and 90-s fat-suppressed (*c, d*) postgadolinium images. There is a 2-cm tumor centrally located in the right hepatic lobe that is not seen on the precontrast image (*a*) and demonstrates homogeneous moderate enhancement on the immediate postcontrast image (*b*) with washout and capsular enhancement on the late image (*c*), consistent with a small HCC. Note extensive varices throughout the peritoneal cavity (arrows, *d*). Varices typically show extension of small curvilinear structures deep to the peritoneum, as observed in this patient. Peritoneal metastases stay confined to the peritoneal surface and within the peritoneal cavity. A small well-defined central HCC, as in this patient, would also not be expected to have peritoneal metastases. Note the micronodular contour of the liver and the large volume of ascites.

on this set of images[183, 190, 191]. Intense enhancement revealed on early-phase images is not specific to HCC as high-grade DNs may also show similar findings. Rarely, small HCCs may be hypovascular, shown by minimal extent of enhancement on arterial dominant-phase images (fig. 2.119) [181, 183]. Isovascular HCCs on arterial-phase images have been reported, and attention should be paid to interstitial-phase images that may show washout of the tumors with capsule enhancement [182, 192]. At present it is not known how often washout and late capsule enhancement are observed in small hypo- or isovascular HCCs.

The distinction between small hypovascular HCC with washout and late capsule enhancement on interstitial-phase images must be made from regenerative liver surrounded by fibrosis. Late enhancement of fibro-

sis generally appears as reticular stromal with more angular margins and is also part of an extensive pattern in the liver of similar findings, whereas the capsule of HCCs is more rounded, and the appearance is distinctly different from surrounding bands of fibrous tissue (if fibrosis is present); for example, the capsule may be thicker or enhance more intensely.

Large HCC (≥2-cm) may range from hypo- to hyperintensity on T2- and T1-weighted images. The most frequent appearance is mildly high signal intensity on T2-weighted images and minimally low signal intensity on T1-weighted images [180, 181, 184–186, 193–196]. The hyperintensity on T2-weighted images and hypointensity on T1-weighted images are highly suggestive of moderately differentiated HCC [188]. The primary hepatic origin of HCC presumably results in a blood

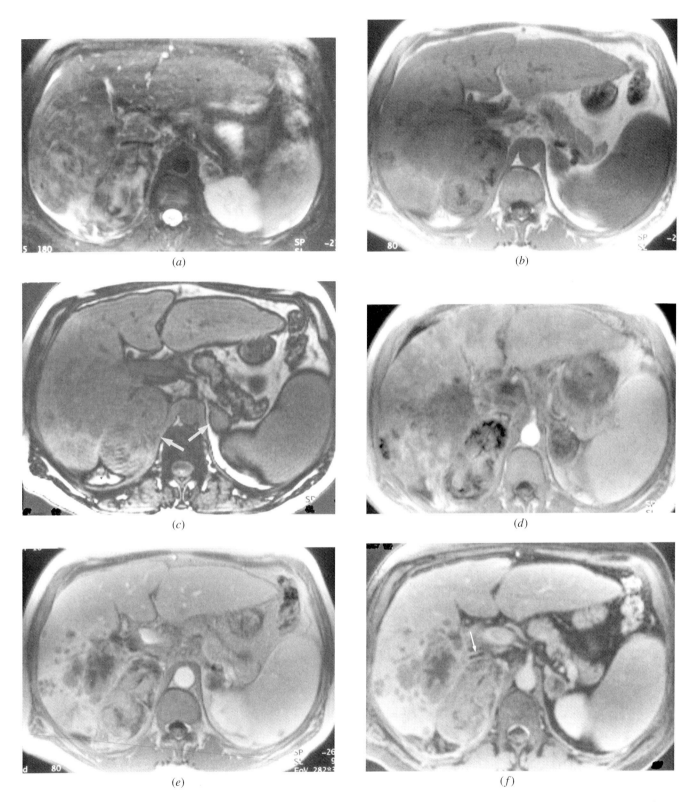

F I G . 2.110 HCC and adrenal metastases. Fat-suppressed T2-weighted ETSE (*a*), SGE (*b*), out-of-phase SGE (*c*), and immediate (*d*), 45-s (*e*), and 90-s fat-suppressed postgadolinium SGE (*f*) images. There are multiple lesions throughout the liver, which are high signal on T2 (*a*) and low signal on T1 (*b*) and demonstrate a mixed population of lesions that enhance in a diffuse heterogeneous or peripheral ring fashion on immediate postgadolinium images (*d*), consistent with multifocal HCC. Ring enhancement in many of these lesions presumably represents intrahepatic metastases. Bilateral adrenal masses (arrows, *c*) are present that demonstrate mixed signal intensity on T1 (*b*), do not drop in signal on out-of-phase (*c*), and enhance heterogeneously after contrast administration (*d-f*) consistent with metastases. Abnormal signal in the IVC (arrow, *f*) represents thrombus.

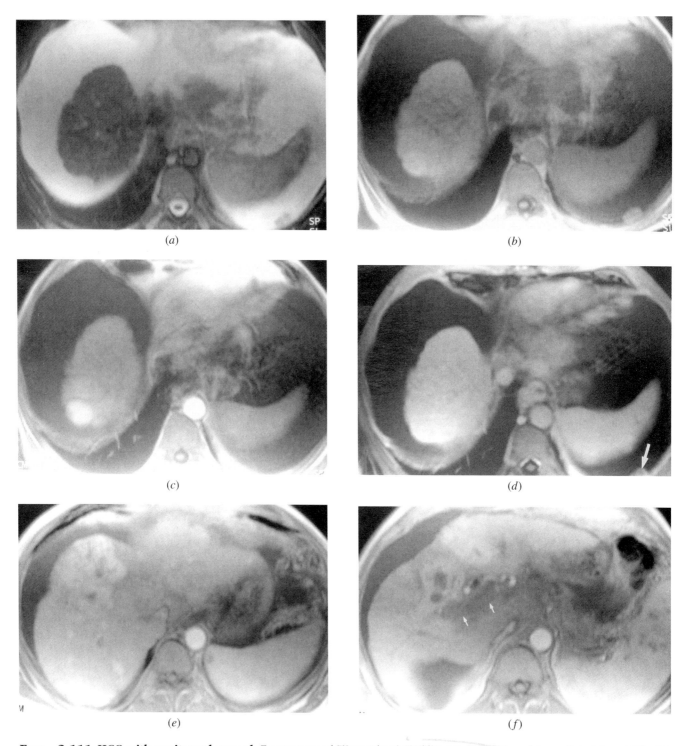

(a)

(b)

(c)

(d)

(e)

(f)

F I G . 2.111 HCC with peritoneal spread. Fat-suppressed T2-weighted SS-ETSE (*a*), SGE (*b*), and immediate (*c*) and 90-s fat-suppressed postgadolinium SGE (*d*) images. The liver is small and irregular in contour, compatible with cirrhosis. There is a small exophytic HCC in the right hepatic lobe that demonstrates isointensity on T2 (*a*), slight hyperintensity on T1 (*b*), intense enhancement immediately after contrast administration (*c*), and washout with capsular enhancement on the late image (*d*), consistent with HCC. Note the peritoneum-based mass (arrow, *d*) in the left upper abdomen, near the spleen, consistent with a peritoneal metastasis from HCC.

Immediate (*e, f*) and 90-s fat-suppressed postgadolinium SGE (*g*) images in a second patient. The liver is nodular in contour and demonstrates a reticular pattern of enhancement compatible with cirrhosis. There is a large HCC in the dome of the liver that bulges the liver contour and shows intense heterogeneous enhancement immediately after gadolinium (*e, f*). Other smaller HCCs are also identified. Note that the main portal vein is expanded with tumor thrombus (arrows, *f*). Peritoneal thickening and enhancement is observed within the paracolic gutters (arrows, *g*), consistent with peritoneal metastases.

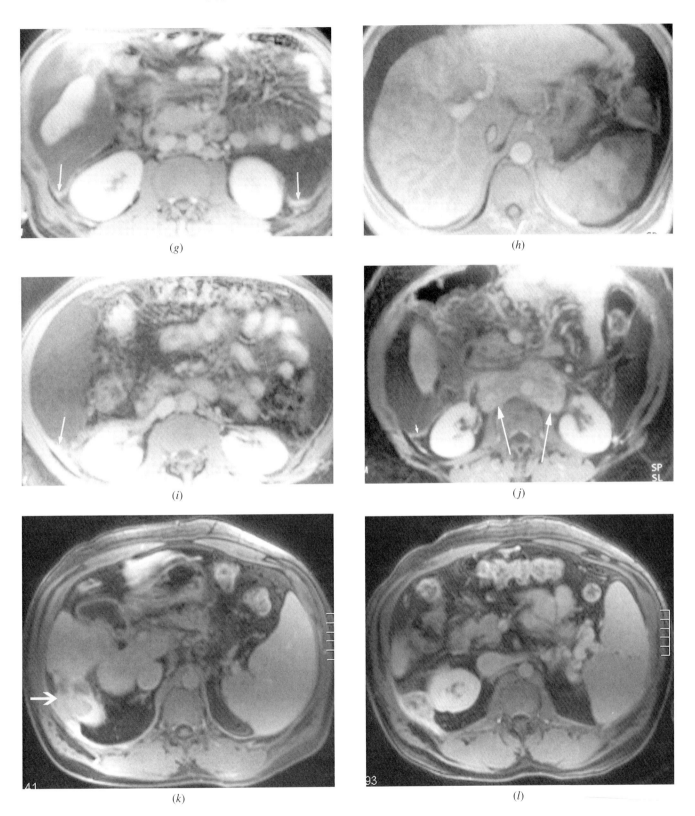

FIG. 2.111 (*Continued*) Immediate (*h*) and 90-s fat-suppressed postgadolinium SGE (*i*) images in a third patient. There is heterogeneous mottled enhancement of the hepatic parenchyma after the administration of gadolinium, consistent with diffuse HCC. Note the infiltrative peritoneal thickening and enhancement compatible with small tumoral implants (arrow, *i*).

Transverse 90-s fat-suppressed postgadolinium SGE image (*j*) in a fourth patient. This patient with HCC has thickening of the peritoneum in the right paracolic gutter (small arrow, *j*) and multiple, enlarged aortocaval and retroaortic lymph nodes (long arrows, *j*).

90-s fat-suppressed postgadolinium SGE images (*k*, *l*) in a fifth patient show nodular peritoneal metastases from HCC.

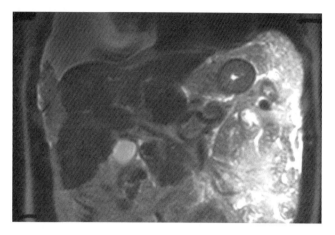

FIG. 2.112 HCC with pleural metastases. Coronal T2-weighted SS-ETSE image shows tumor extension through the diaphragm resulting in pleural metastases.

supply similar to and in continuity with background liver, explaining the diffuse heterogeneous enhancement on arterial dominant-phase images [143, 197, 198]. In the interstitial phase, large HCCs tend to demonstrate washout below the signal intensity of background parenchyma, and capsule enhancement, which may only be apparent around some portions of the tumor (fig. 2.120) [183].

It is postulated that small well-differentiated HCCs are vascularized by a mixture of arterial and portal blood supply, with predominance of arterial supply, while moderate and poorly differentiated HCCs are supplied only by hepatic arteries [199–201]. In a previous study [202], the authors demonstrated a correlation between the presence of vascular endothelial growth factor (VEGF) in hepatic nodules and high signal intensity on T2- and T1-weighted images, but a similar relationship was not shown with the degree of enhancement on arterial dominant-phase and interstitial-phase images. The authors postulated that VEGF is present in highest concentration early in the process of transformation of large regenerative or dysplastic hepatic nodules into well-differentiated HCCs in order to stimulate vessel growth. VEGF may then be downregulated at the last stages of development into hypervascular HCC (fig. 2.121–2.123).

Important ancillary features of HCC include late capsule enhancement and venous thrombosis [203]. In histopathologic analysis, 60–87% of large HCC have a fibrosis tumor capsule [204]. The typical signal intensity of a capsule is mild hyperintensity on T2-weighted images, hypointensity on T1-weighted images, and negligible mild enhancement on immediate postgadolinium images that becomes more intense on interstitial phase images (fig. 2.124).

Tumor extension occurs most commonly into portal veins (figs. 2.125 and 2.126); however, hepatic venous extension also occurs (fig. 2.127). Although tumor thrombus is observed in fewer than 50% of cases, it is common in the setting of large and advanced tumors. The appearance on hepatic arterial dominant-phase gadolinium-enhanced images often permits distinction between HCC and metastatic disease when tumors are ≥1.5 cm in diameter, because HCCs typically demonstrate enhancing stroma throughout the entire tumor, whereas metastases have ring enhancement [143]. However, there is an overlap of MR features between small HCCs (<1.5 cm) and hypervascular metastases. Both entities commonly show homogeneous moderate or intense enhancement on arterial dominant phase and lesional washout on late phase. The presence of capsule enhancement on late phase and the presence of underlying chronic hepatic disease or cirrhosis are supportive features of HCC. Ring enhancement observed on hepatic arterial dominant-phase images in HCCs, especially in patients with underlying hepatitis C, may represent an aggressive appearance of the neoplasm. Explosive growth has been observed in some of these tumors. The ring enhancement is a pattern of enhancement most typical for metastases, and its presence in HCCs may reflect a more aggressive blood supply, with recruitment of additional surrounding vessels to the tumor (fig. 2.128).

In the setting of viral hepatitis, the hepatic architecture tends to be less distorted than in patients with cirrhosis. As livers may not appear cirrhotic, a high index of suspicion for HCC is recommended in patients with focal liver masses and underlying viral hepatitis.

Higher doses of gadolinium or higher flow rates may improve visualization of HCCs that may possess minimal increased vascularity [5]. Newer contrast agents with higher T1 relaxivity may aid in lesion detection of hypovascular, isovascular, or minimally hypervascular tumors. Also, new techniques such as parallel imaging may improve detection of HCCs in debilitated patients unable to suspend breathing for 20 s with conventional spoiled gradient echo sequences [205, 206].

Overlap exists between the appearance of high-grade dysplastic nodules and HCC, as HCC may also exhibit the classic appearance described for high-grade dysplastic nodules; which is near isointense on T2-weighted and noncontrast T1-weighted images and moderately intense enhancement on early postgadolinium images that fades to isointensity on late postgadolinium images. The great majority of these lesions can be correctly classified using the following ancillary features: 1) in the presence of a coexistent large HCC, the small lesions are more likely satellite HCCs; 2) interval growth of lesion by greater than 30% in transverse dimension in a 3-month interval is consistent with HCC;

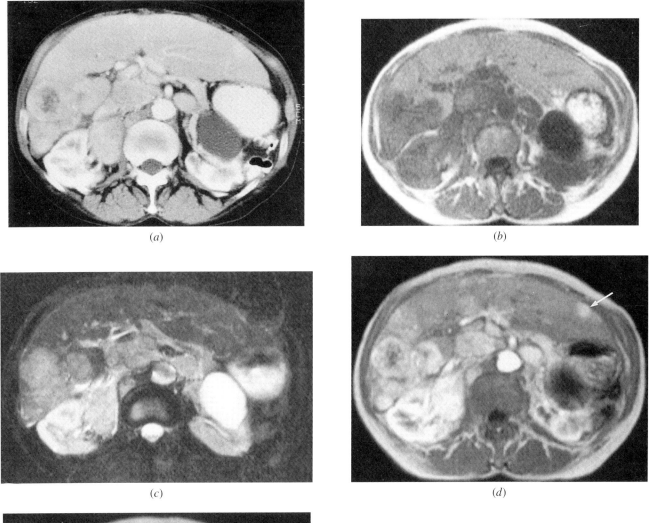

(a)   (b)

(c)   (d)

(e)

F I G . 2.113 Multifocal HCC with adenopathy—spiral CT imaging and MRI comparison. Spiral CT (*a*), SGE (*b*), fat-suppressed T2-weighted ETSE (*c*), and immediate (*d*) and 45-s (*e*) postgadolinium SGE images. On the CT image (*a*), an HCC is identified in the right lobe with multiple nodes in the porta hepatis and retroperitoneum. Precontrast SGE image (*b*) demonstrates the HCC as a moderately low-signal-intensity mass in the right lobe and the lymph nodes as moderately low in signal intensity. The T2-weighted image (*c*) demonstrates the tumor and lymph nodes as moderately high in signal intensity. On the immediate image (*d*), the HCC in the right lobe demonstrates intense diffuse heterogeneous enhancement. Multiple additional HCCs smaller than 1 cm are also apparent (arrow, *d*) that were not visible on spiral CT images (*a*) or on noncontrast T1 (*b*)- and T2 (*c*)-weighted images. The small HCCs wash out to isointensity with the liver by 45 s (*e*), at a time when renal CMD is still pronounced. Intense enhancement of the associated adenopathy is also present on the immediate postgadolinium image (*d*).

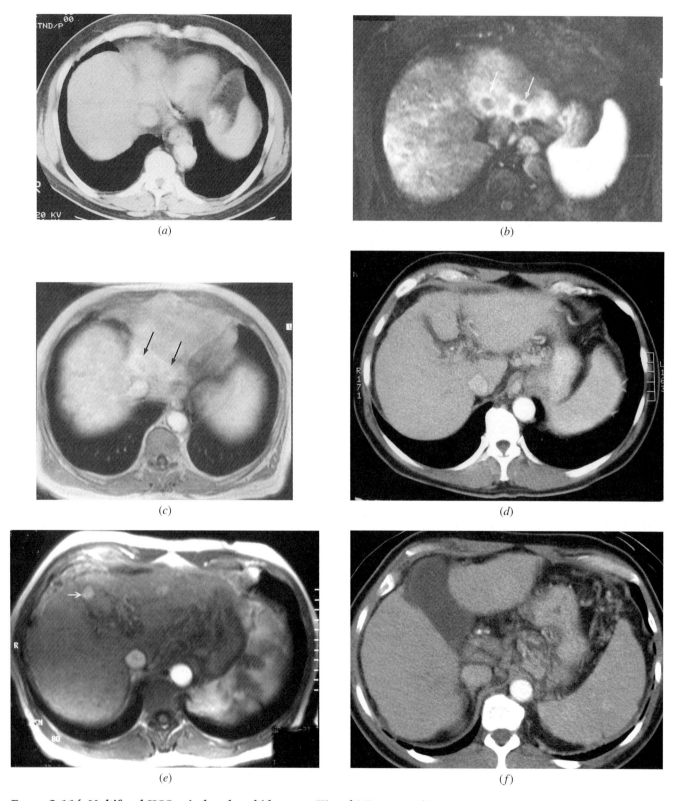

(a) *(b)* *(c)* *(d)* *(e)* *(f)*

FIG. 2.114 Multifocal HCC-spiral and multidetector CT and MR comparison. Spiral CT (*a*), fat-suppressed T2-weighted ETSE (*b*), and immediate postgadolinium SGE (*c*) images. The spiral CT image demonstrates a solitary HCC in a patient with 8 HCCs shown on MRI tumors. No tumors are evident on CT at this tomographic level (*a*). The T2-weighted image (*b*) demonstrates two 1.8-cm HCCs at this level that have high-signal-intensity peripheral rims and are isointense centrally (arrows, *b*). On immediate postgadolinium image (*c*), these tumors enhance in a predominantly ring fashion (arrows, *c*).

Multidetector CT (*d*, *f*) and immediate postgadolinium SGE (*e*, *g*) images in a second patient at two tomographic levels. Note

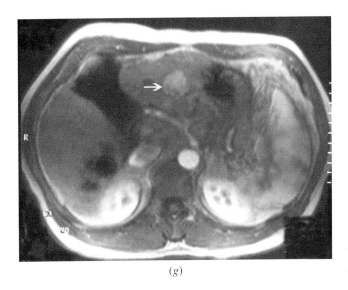

(g)

FIG. 2.114 (*Continued*) that the HCCs are more evident on early-phase postgadolinium MR images (arrow, *e, g*) than on the multidetector CT images.

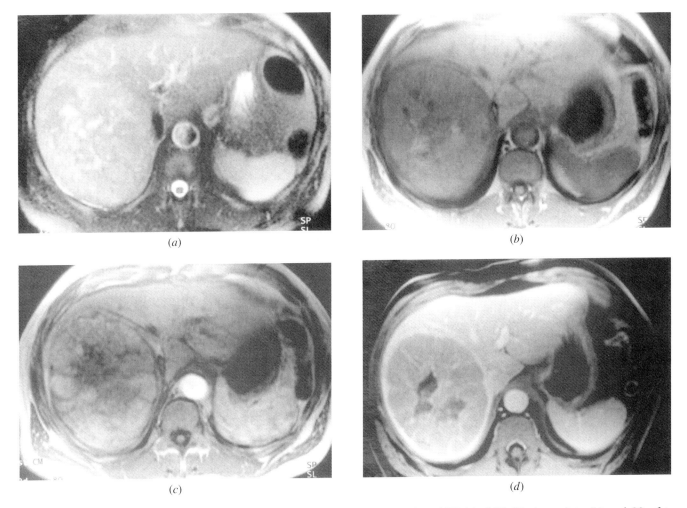

(a)

(b)

(c)

(d)

FIG. 2.115 Large well-differentiated HCC. Fat-suppressed T2-weighted SS-ETSE (*a*), SGE (*b*), immediate (*c*) and 90-s fat-suppressed (*d*) postgadolinium SGE images. There is a large well-defined mass in the right hepatic lobe that demonstrates slightly increased and heterogeneous signal intensity on T2 (*a*), moderately decreased signal intensity on T1 (*b*), heterogeneous enhancement on immediate postgadolinium images (*c*), and heterogeneous washout with late enhancement of a pseudocapsule (*d*).

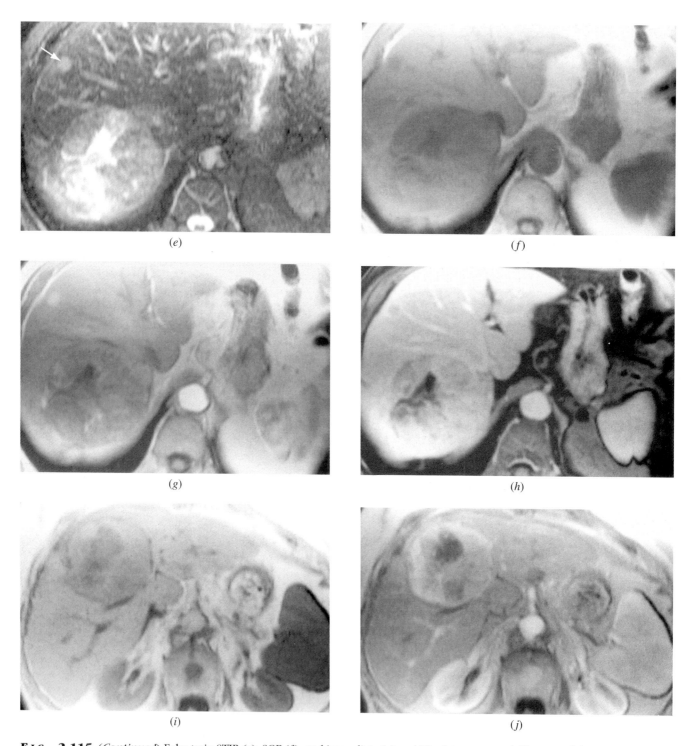

(e)   (f)

(g)   (h)

(i)   (j)

FIG. 2.115 (*Continued*) Echo-train STIR (*e*), SGE (*f*), and immediate (*g*) and 90-s fat-suppressed (*h*) postgadolinium SGE images in a second patient. There is a large mass in the right hepatic lobe that is moderately and heterogeneously hyperintense on T2-weighted image (*e*) and mildly hypointense on T1-weighted image (*f*) and demonstrates heterogeneous enhancement on immediate postgadolinium images (*g*) and washout with pseudocapsular enhancement on late image (*h*). Note a small satellite lesion (arrow, *e*) that exhibits high signal on T2 (*e*), low signal on T1 (*f*), homogeneous intense enhancement on hepatic arterial dominant phase (*g*), and washout with pseudocapsule enhancement on late image (*h*). Both lesions are consistent with HCC.

SGE (*i*) and immediate (*j*) and 90-s fat-suppressed (*k*) postgadolinium SGE images in a third patient. There is a large HCC that demonstrates heterogeneous mainly hypo- to isointense signal on T1 (*i*), heterogeneous enhancement immediately after contrast administration (*j*), and washout with an enhanced pseudocapsule on late images (*k*), consistent with HCC.

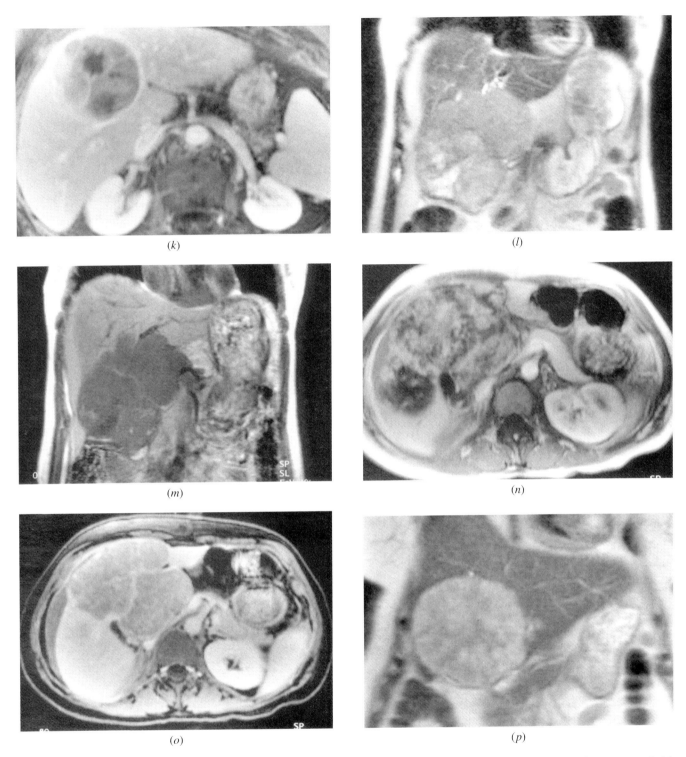

F I G . 2.115 (*Continued*) Coronal T2-weighted SS-ETSE (*l*), coronal SGE (*m*), and immediate (*n*) and 90-s fat-suppressed (*o*) postgadolinium SGE images in a fourth patient. A large mass is present that demonstrates heterogeneous moderately high signal intensity on T2 (*l*), moderate low signal intensity on T1 (*m*), heterogeneous enhancement immediately after contrast administration (*n*), and washout with an enhanced pseudocapsule on interstitial-phase image (*o*).

Coronal T2-weighted SS-ETSE (*p*), transverse fat-suppressed T2-weighted ETSE (*q*), SGE (*r*), and immediate (*s*) and 5-min (*t*) postgadolinium SGE images in a fifth patient. An 8-cm mass is present in the right hepatic lobe with heterogeneous and moderately

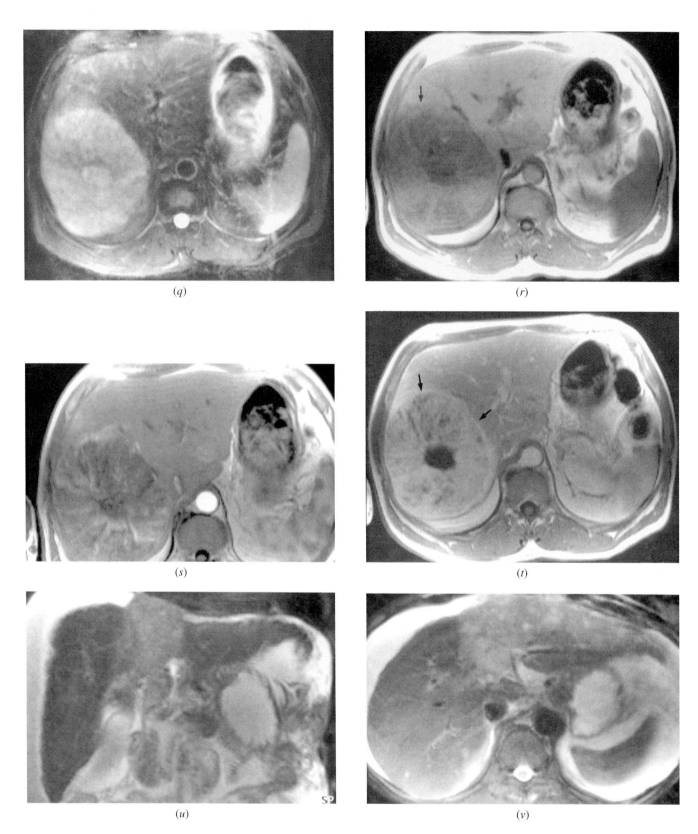

(q)

(r)

(s)

(t)

(u)

(v)

F IG . 2.115 (*Continued*) high signal on T2 (*p, q*), heterogeneous low signal intensity on T1-weighted images (*r*), and diffuse heterogeneous enhancement on immediate (*s*) and late (*t*) postgadolinium images. A tumor capsule is evident, which is hypointense on SGE (arrow, *r*) and immediate postgadolinium images, and enhances on late images (arrows, *t*). A large and dark central scar is best seen on late image (*t*) (Reproduced with permission from Kelekis NL, Semelka RC, Worawattanakul S, Lange EE, et al. Hepatocellular carcinoma in North America: a multiinstitutional study of appearance on T1-weighted, T2-weighted, and serial gadolinium-enhanced gradient-echo images. *AJR Am J Roentgenol* 170: 1005–1013, 1998).

Coronal T2-weighted SS-ETSE (*u*), transverse fat-suppressed T2-weighted ETSE (*v*), SGE (*w*), and immediate (*x*) and 90-s fat-suppressed (*y*) postgadolinium SGE images in a sixth patient. There is a large tumor mass occupying the majority of the left lobe

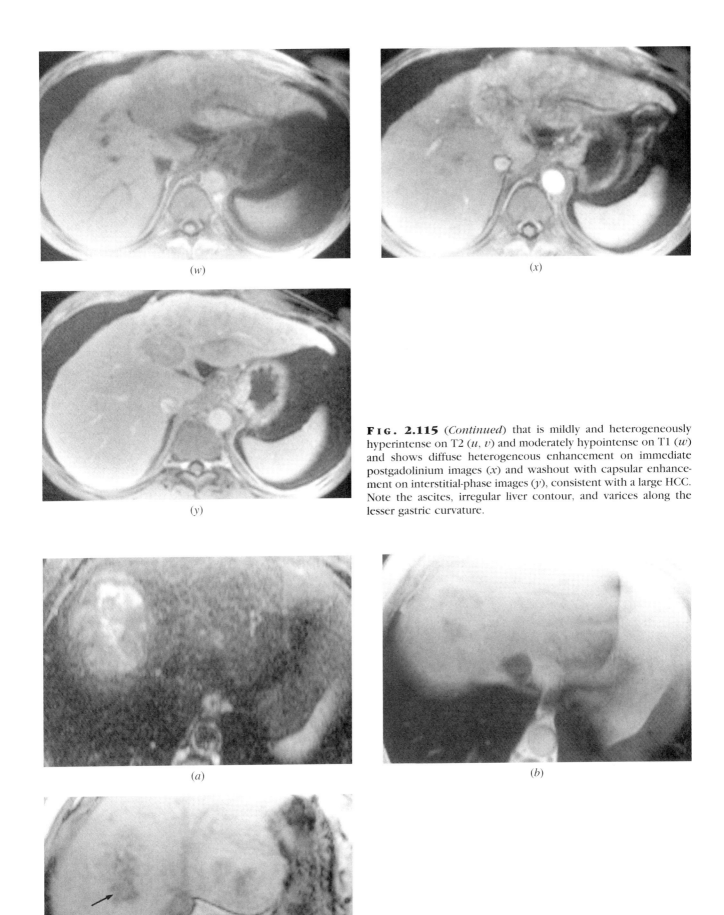

FIG. 2.115 (*Continued*) that is mildly and heterogeneously hyperintense on T2 (*u*, *v*) and moderately hypointense on T1 (*w*) and shows diffuse heterogeneous enhancement on immediate postgadolinium images (*x*) and washout with capsular enhancement on interstitial-phase images (*y*), consistent with a large HCC. Note the ascites, irregular liver contour, and varices along the lesser gastric curvature.

FIG. 2.116 Fat-containing well-differentiated HCC. Echo-train STIR (*a*), SGE (*b*), out-of-phase SGE (*c*), and immediate (*d*) and 90-s fat-suppressed (*e*) postgadolinium SGE images. There is

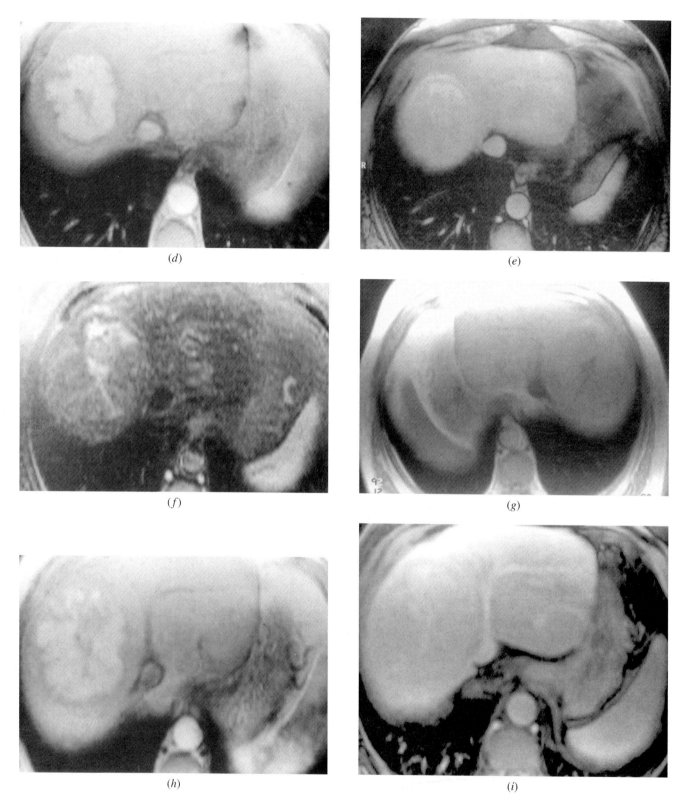

(d)

(e)

(f)

(g)

(h)

(i)

FIG. 2.116 (*Continued*) a lobular mass in the right hepatic lobe that demonstrates high signal on T2 (*a*), isointensity on T1 (*b*), partial loss of signal on out-of-phase image (*c*), intense immediate enhancement after contrast (*d*), and washout (*e*). On late images (*e*), the pseudocapsule is high signal and well visualized. Note a small central scar that is high signal on T2 (*a*), and hypointense immediately after gadolinium (*d*) and shows late enhancement (*e*). Superficially this well-differentiated HCC resembles an FNH. A distinguishing feature is the regions of signal heterogeneity on all MR sequences; FNH should be homogeneous on all sequences. Note also that the lesion demonstrates a peripheral region of signal loss (arrow, *c*) on the out-of-phase sequence consistent with fat. Presence of fat is a feature of well-differentiated HCC and not FNH, and irregular regions of fatty infiltration distinguish it from adenoma, which most commonly shows uniform fatty infiltration. Echo train-STIR (*f*), SGE (*g*), and immediate (*h*) and 90-s fat-suppressed postgadolinium SGE (*i*) images in the same patient, 4 months later. The lesion has increased in size, reflecting its malignant behavior.

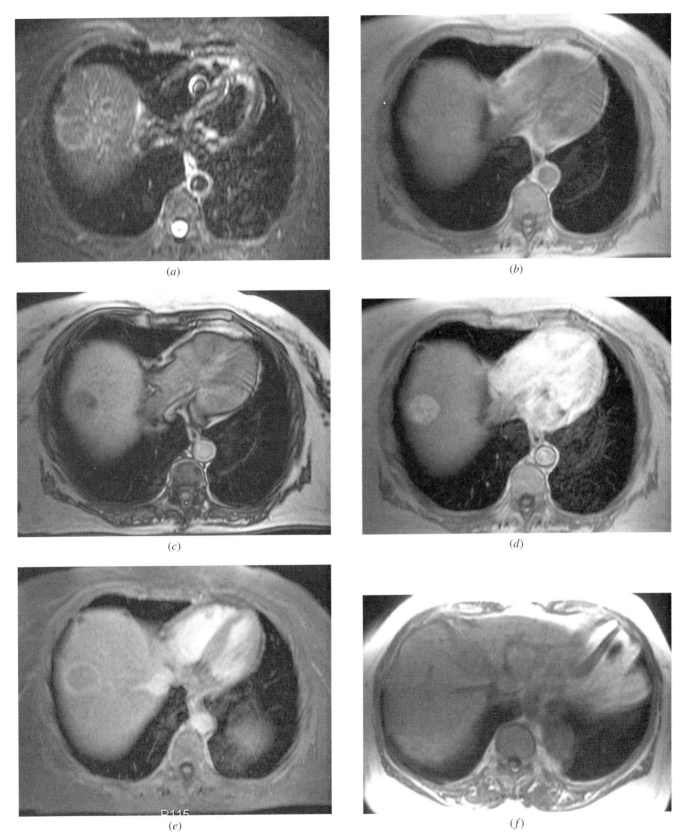

FIG. 2.117 Fat-containing well-differentiated HCC. T2-weighted SS-ETSE (*a*), SGE (*b*), out-of-phase (*c*), and immediate (*d*) and 90-s fat-suppressed (*e*) postgadolinium SGE images. A mass is present in the segment 8 of the liver that shows signal intensity similar to background parenchyma on the T2-weighted image (*a*), slightly higher signal intensity on the T1-weighted image (*b*), heterogeneous loss in signal intensity on the out-of-phase image (*c*), intense enhancement the on the early-phase image (*d*), and washout with late capsule enhancement on the late-phase image (*e*), but with the persistence of the capsule enhancement.

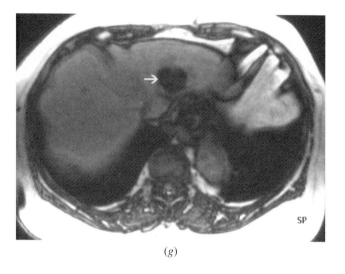

(g)

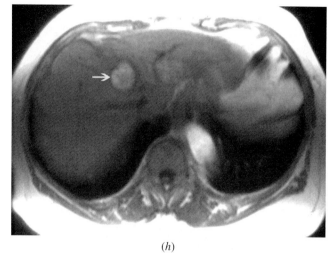

(h)

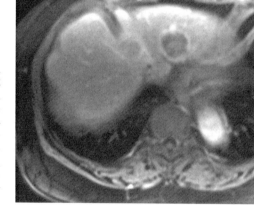

(i)

FIG. 2.117 (*Continued*) SGE (*f*), out-of-phase SGE (*g*), and immediate (*h*) and 90-s fat-suppressed (*i*) postgadolinium SGE image in a second patient. There are two rounded lesions situated side by side in the left hepatic lobe. The nodule adjacent to the middle hepatic vein demonstrates low signal intensity on T1-weighted image, intense enhancement on early-phase image (arrow, *h*), and washout with capsule enhancement on late-phase image (*i*). This HCC does not show drop in signal intensity on out-of-phase image (*g*). The tumor located near the left hepatic vein has similar imaging features, but it drops in signal intensity on the out-of-phase image (arrow, *g*), consistent with the presence of fat within the HCC.

3) stability of lesion over a 1-year period is suggestive of high-grade dysplastic nodule, although HCC can still develop; 4) regression of lesion on follow-up MR studies is suggestive of dysplastic nodule; 5) size of nodule <1.5 cm (in combination with absence of a large coexistent HCC) is consistent with high-grade dysplastic nodule; and 6) size of nodule >2 cm is worrisome for HCC.

The most reliable feature that raises the concern for high likelihood of HCC is interval growth. It may be prudent to identify the presence of all nodules, even those <1 cm, that show moderately intense early enhancement, even though recognizing that many lesions <1 cm will diminish in enhancement or resolve on serial follow-up MR studies. At the present time, it may not be possible to predict which <1-cm lesions will resolve, and patients with chronic liver disease at high risk for development of HCC (e.g., hepatitis C or alcohol related) may have a greater tendency for these lesions to continue to grow into HCCs.

Diffuse HCC

The diffuse type of HCC is a permeative hepatic tumor that involves at least 50% of the hepatic parenchyma and occurs in approximately 13% of patients with HCC [207]. The most common appearance of diffuse infiltrative HCC is extensive hepatic parenchymal involvement with mottled, punctate mildly to moderate high signal intensity on T2-weighted images and mildly to moderate low signal on T1-weighted images. The MR features on unenhanced images are nonspecific, that is, similar to those in cirrhotic livers without tumor involvement. Patchy or miliary pattern of enhancement is often observed on immediate postgadolinium images with tumor washout and segments of late capsule enhancement on late images (fig. 2.129). Miliary enhancement on early phase is a relatively specific MR finding of diffuse HCCs and may represent the enhancement of extensive micronodules as shown on histopathology [207, 208].

Diffuse HCC may also appear as irregular linear strands that are iso- to moderately hyperintense on

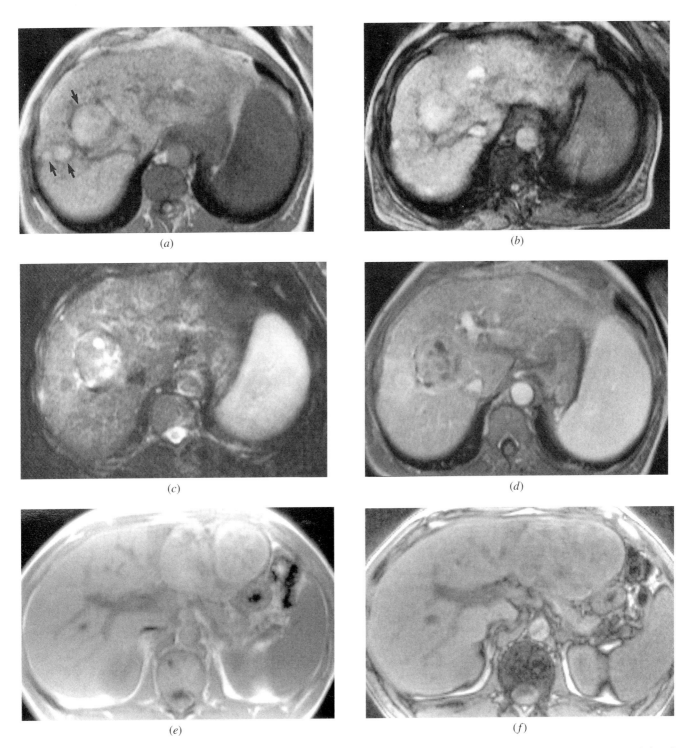

FIG. 2.118 Hepatocellular carcinoma, multifocal with high signal intensity, not representing fat, on T1-weighted images. SGE (*a*), out-of-phase SGE (*b*), fat-suppressed T2-weighted ETSE (*c*), and immediate (*d*) postgadolinum SGE images. Multiple HCCs are present that are high in signal intensity on T1 in-phase images (arrows, *a*) and do not drop in signal or develop a phase-cancellation artifact on the out-of-phase image (*b*), which excludes the presence of fat. The small HCCs are isointense with liver on T2 (*c*), whereas the large tumor is heterogeneous and mildly hyperintense. On the immediate postgadolinium image (*d*), the small HCCs exhibit predominantly peripheral enhancement, whereas the larger HCC has diffuse heterogeneous enhancement. A low-signal-intensity pseudocapsule is appreciated around the larger HCC on all imaging sequences.

SGE (*e*), out-of-phase SGE (*f*), and immediate postgadolinium SGE (*g*) images in a second patient. There is a large HCC with high signal intensity on T1-weighted image (*e*), which does not drop in signal on out-of-phase images (*f*) and shows diffuse hetero-geneous enhancement on immediate postcontrast images (*g*). This lesion is consistent with a nonfatty HCC.

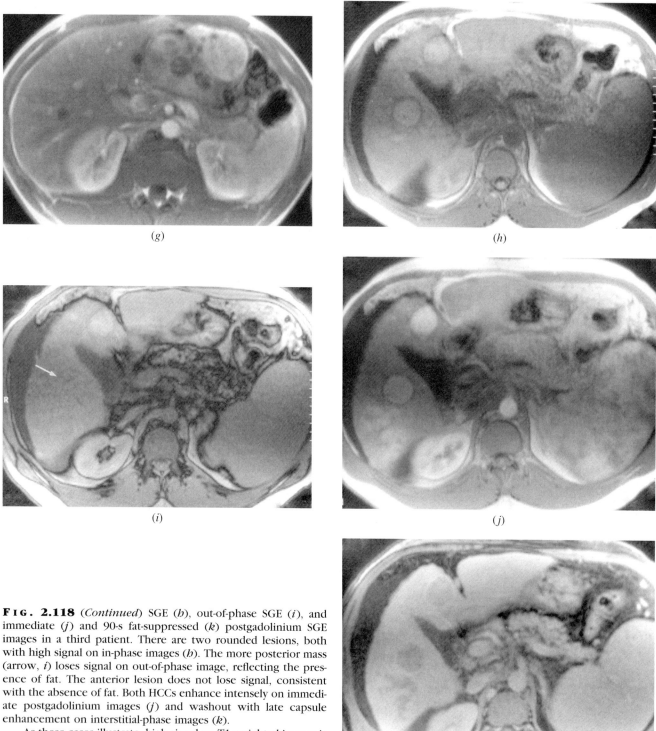

(g)

(h)

(i)

(j)

(k)

FIG. 2.118 (*Continued*) SGE (*h*), out-of-phase SGE (*i*), and immediate (*j*) and 90-s fat-suppressed (*k*) postgadolinium SGE images in a third patient. There are two rounded lesions, both with high signal on in-phase images (*h*). The more posterior mass (arrow, *i*) loses signal on out-of-phase image, reflecting the presence of fat. The anterior lesion does not lose signal, consistent with the absence of fat. Both HCCs enhance intensely on immediate postgadolinium images (*j*) and washout with late capsule enhancement on interstitial-phase images (*k*).

As these cases illustrate, high signal on T1-weighted images is relatively common in HCC, but in the majority of cases it does not reflect the presence of fat. The high signal is most often on the basis of high protein content.

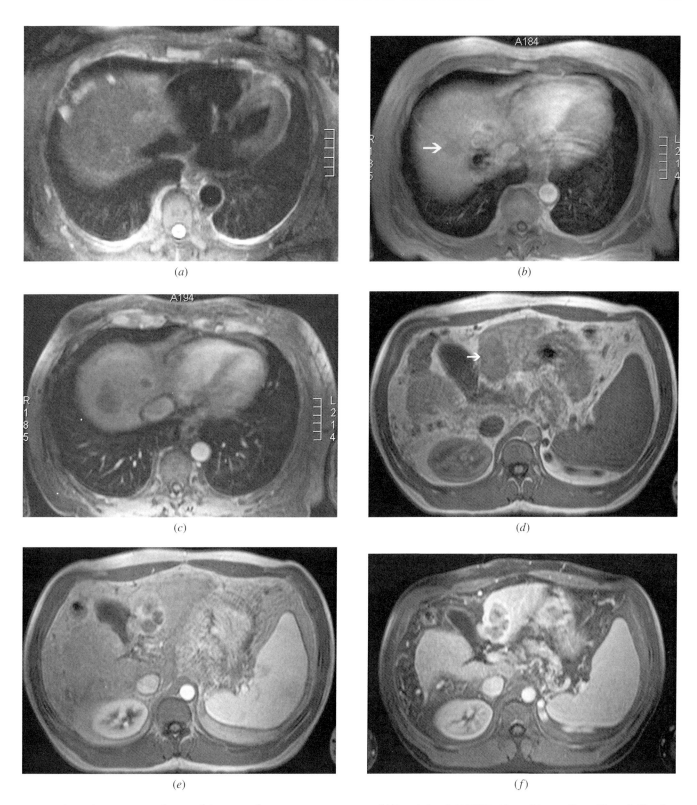

F I G . 2.119 Hypovascular and isovascular HCC. Fat-suppressed T2-weighted SS-ETSE (*a*) and immediate (*b*) and 90-s fat-suppressed (*c*) postgadolinium SGE images. There are two nodular lesions in the top of the liver. The largest one (arrow, *b*) shows low signal intensity on T2-weighted image (*a*) and minimal enhancement on early-phase image (*b*) that decreases over time (*c*), compatible with hypovascular HCC. Nearby the hypovascular HCC, there is a smaller lesion that shows high signal intensity on T2-weighted image (*a*) and ring and perilesional enhancement on early-phase image (*b*) that becomes more conspicuous on late-phase image (*c*), consistent with metastasis from the HCC.

SGE (*d*) and immediate (*e*) and 90-s fat-suppressed (*f*) postgadolinium SGE images in a second patient. A HCC is present in the liver that is moderately low signal intensity on the T1-weighted image (arrow, *d*), shows partial faint enhancement on the early-phase image (*e*) and partially washes out on late-phase image (*f*), consistent with hypovascular HCC.

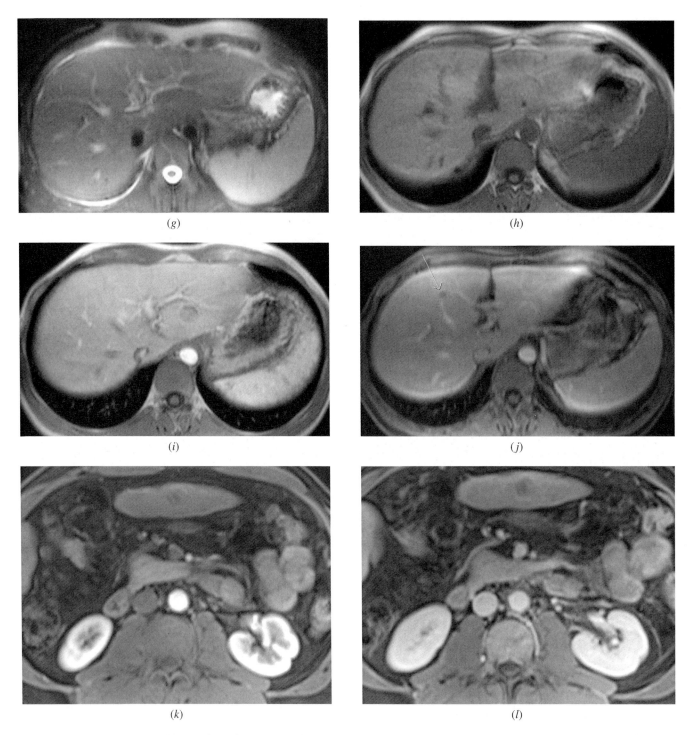

(g)

(h)

(i)

(j)

(k)

(l)

FIG. 2.119 *(Continued)* T2-weighted fat-suppressed SS-ETSE (*g*), SGE (*h*), and immediate (*i*, *k*) and 90-s (*j*, *l*) postgadolinium fat-suppressed 3D-gradient echo images obtained **at 3T** show similar findings with multiple hypovascular HCCs.

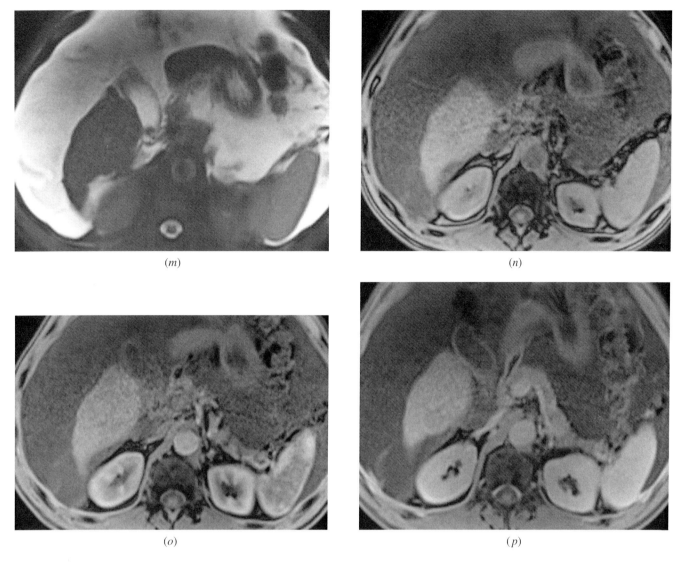

F I G . 2.119 (*Continued*) T2-weighted SS-ETSE fat-suppressed (*m*), SGE (*n*), and immediate (*o*) and 90-s (*p*) postgadolinium fat-suppressed 3D gradient echo images obtained **at 3T** show a hypointense lesion on T2 (*m*)- and T1 (*n*)-weighted images, that enhances in an isointense fashion on early phase (*o*) and demonstrates washout with capsular enhancement on late phase (*p*), compatible with isovascular HCC.

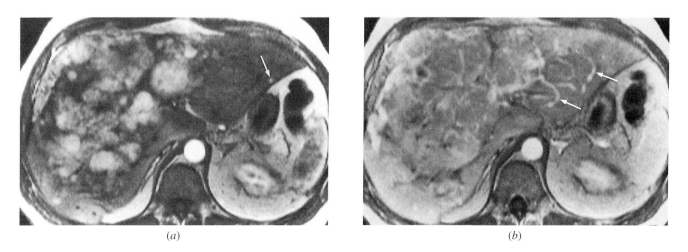

F I G . 2.120 Hypervascular HCC with small satellite tumors. Immediate (*a*) and 90-s (*b*) postgadolinium SGE images. Intense diffuse heterogeneous enhancement of a 15-cm HCC is present on the immediate postgadolinium image (*a*). Multiple additional small HCCs are apparent, including tumors as small as 3 mm (arrow, *a*). By 90 s after gadolinium (*b*), the large tumor has washed out in a heterogeneous fashion with prominent abnormal curvilinear hepatic veins apparent (arrows, *b*). The small HCC has become isointense with liver at this time.

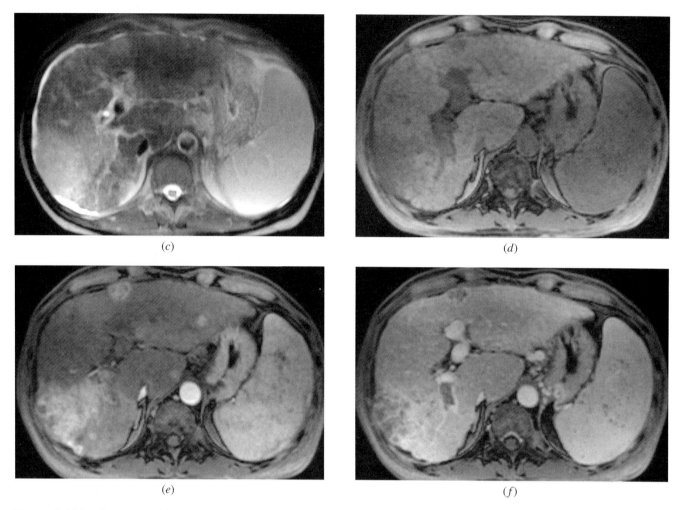

(c)   (d)

(e)   (f)

FIG. 2.120 (*Continued*) T2-weighted fat-suppressed SS-ETSE (*c*), SGE (*d*), and immediate (*e*) and 90-s postcontrast (*f*) fat suppressed 3D gradient echo images obtained **at 3T** show multiple hypervascular lesions on early phase image (*e*) with washout and
capsular enhancement on late phase (*f*) compatible with HCCs in a second patient. Note tumor thrombosis of the right branch of
the portal vein (*f*).

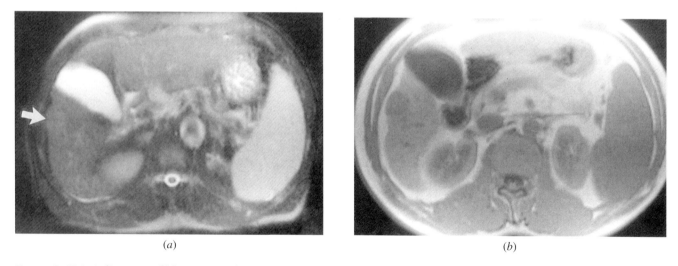

(a)   (b)

FIG. 2.121 Solitary small hypervascular HCC. Fat-suppressed T2-weighted SS-ETSE (*a*), SGE (*b*), and immediate (*c*) and 90-s
fat-suppressed postgadolinium SGE (*d*) images. There is a 2-cm mass that bulges the liver contour slightly in the right lobe. The
mass is minimally hyperintense on T2 (*a*) and mildly hypointense on T1 (*b*), demonstrates intense uniform enhancement on the
immediate postgadolinium image (*c*), and fades to hypointensity by 90 s (*d*) with late enhancement of a pseudocapsule. Intense
hepatic arterial dominant-phase enhancement is the most sensitive technique for the detection of small HCCs. Washout to hypointensity with late capsular enhancement is the most specific.

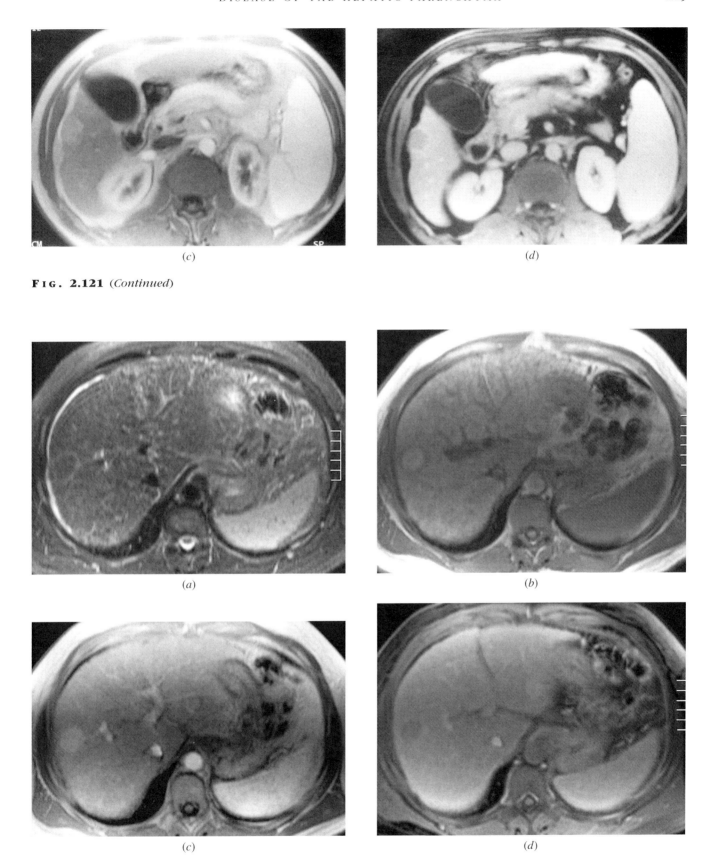

F i g . 2.121 (*Continued*)

F i g . 2.122 Small hypervascular HCC. T2-weighted SS-ETSE (*a*), SGE (*b*), immediate (*c*) and 90-s fat-suppressed (*d*) post-gadolinium SGE in one patient; T2-weighted SS-ETSE (*e*), SGE (*f*), out-of-phase SGE (*g*), and immediate (*b*) and 90-s fat-suppressed

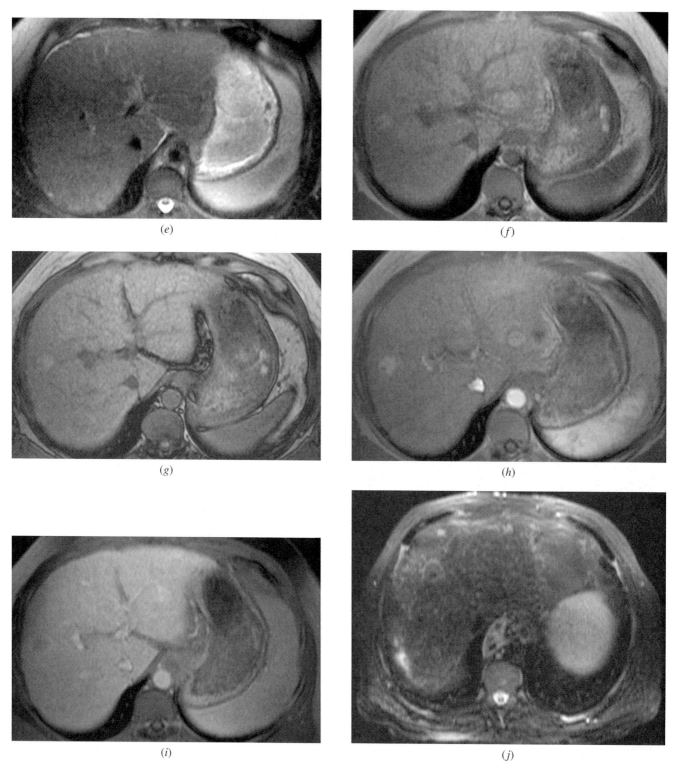

(e)

(f)

(g)

(h)

(i)

(j)

F IG . 2.122 (*Continued*) (*i*) postgadolinium SGE in a second patient; and T2-weighted SS-ETSE (*j*), SGE (*k*), out-of-phase SGE (*l*), and immediate (*m*) and 90-s fat-suppressed (*n*) postgadolinium SGE in a third patient, all with a small hypervascular HCC. Note that in all cases the tumor has intense enhancement on early-phase images and washout with late capsule enhancement on late-phase images.

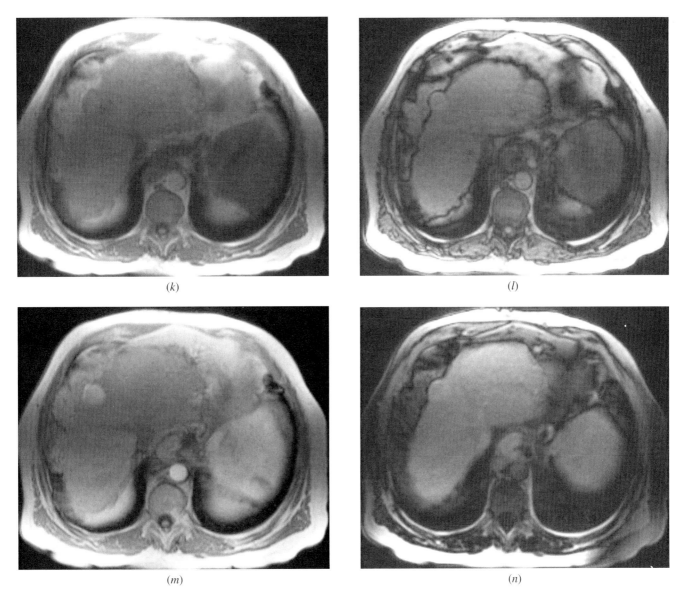

(k)

(l)

(m)

(n)

F I G . 2.122 (*Continued*)

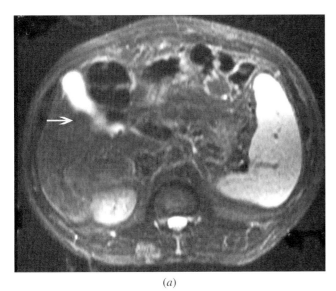

(a)

F I G . 2.123 Hypervascular HCC. Fat-suppressed T2-weighted SS-ETSE (*a*), SGE (*b*), and immediate (*c*) and 90-s fat-suppressed (*d*) postgadolinium SGE images. There is a lesion that bulges into the gallbladder fossa that appears mildly low signal intensity on the T2-weighted image (arrow, *a*), mildly high signal intensity on the T1-weighted image (*b*), intense enhancement on the early-phase image (*c*), and washout with capsule enhancement on the late-phase image (*d*), consistent with an HCC.

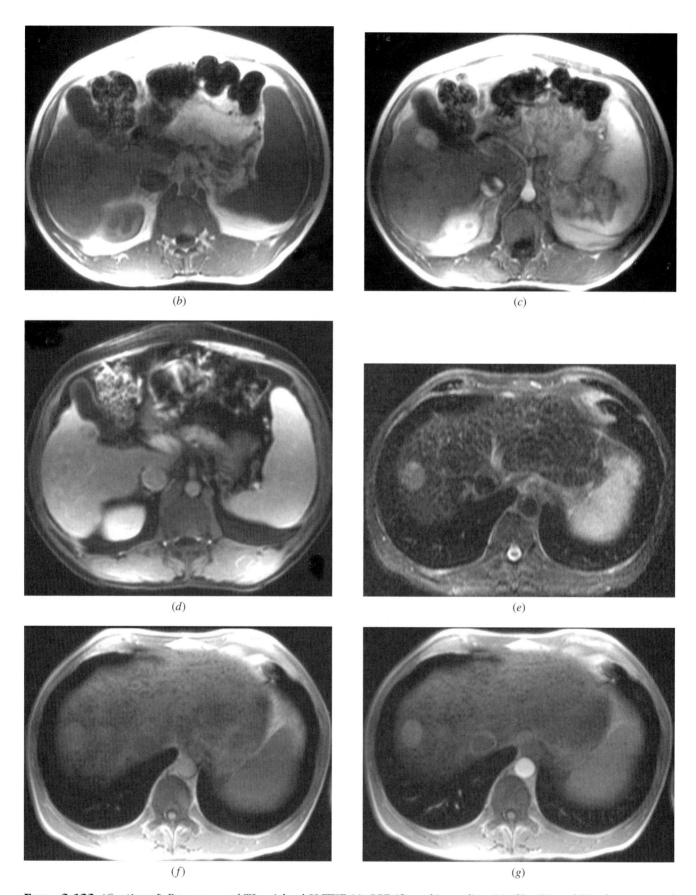

F IG. 2.123 (*Continued*) Fat-suppressed T2-weighted SS-ETSE (*e*), SGE (*f*), and immediate (*g*), 45-s (*h*), and 90-s fat-suppressed (*i*) postgadolinium SGE images in a second patient with a tumor located in segment 8. This mass shows mildly high signal intensity on the T2-weighted image (*e*), mildly high signal intensity on the T1-weighted image (*f*), moderate enhancement on the early phase (*g*), and washout and capsule enhancement on 45-s image (*h*) that persist on late-phase image (*i*), consistent with HCC. Note that washout occurs by 1 min postgadolinium for HCCs, and excellent renal corticomedullary enhancement is still present when the tumor has washed out.

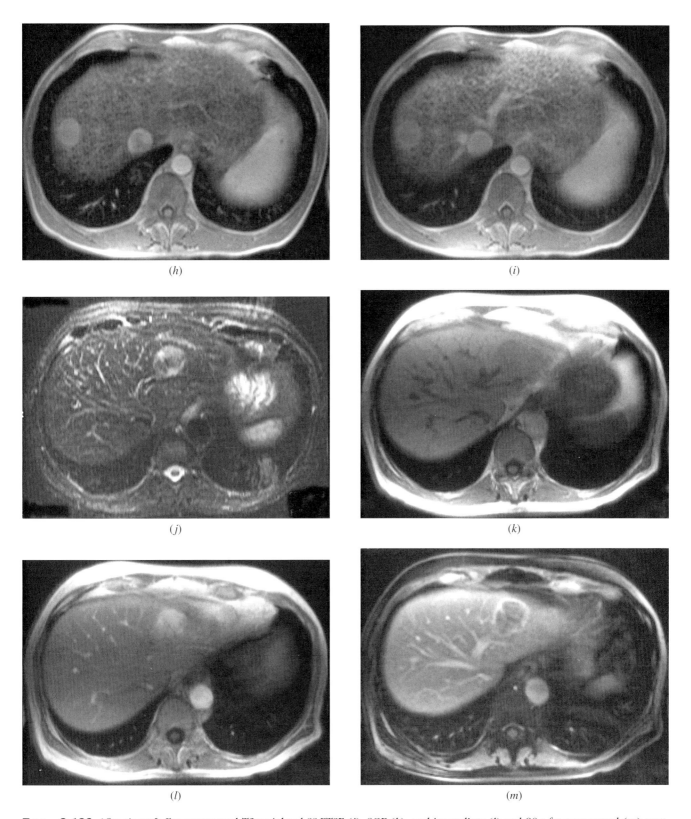

(h)   *(i)*

(j)   *(k)*

(l)   *(m)*

F I G . 2.123 (*Continued*) Fat-suppressed T2-weighted SS-ETSE (*j*), SGE (*k*), and immediate (*l*) and 90-s fat-suppressed (*m*) post-gadolinium SGE images in an additional patient with HCC shows similar findings.

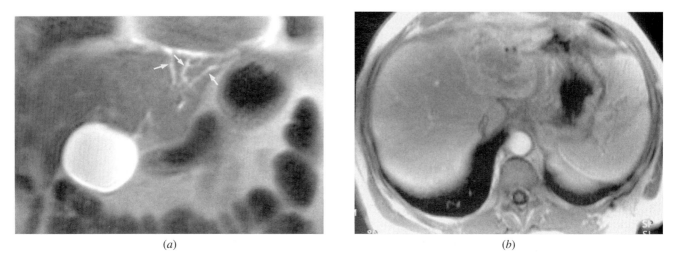

(a)   (b)

F I G . 2.124 Focal HCC with bile duct obstruction. Coronal T2-weighted SS-ETSE (*a*) and immediate postgadolinium SGE (*b*) images. There is a large lesion in the left hepatic lobe that demonstrates minimally hyperintense signal on T2-weighted images (*a*) and moderate heterogeneous enhancement immediately after gadolinium administration (*b*), consistent with a large HCC. Note that the mass causes ductal obstruction (arrows, *a*) of the biliary tree in segment 2 of the left lobe.

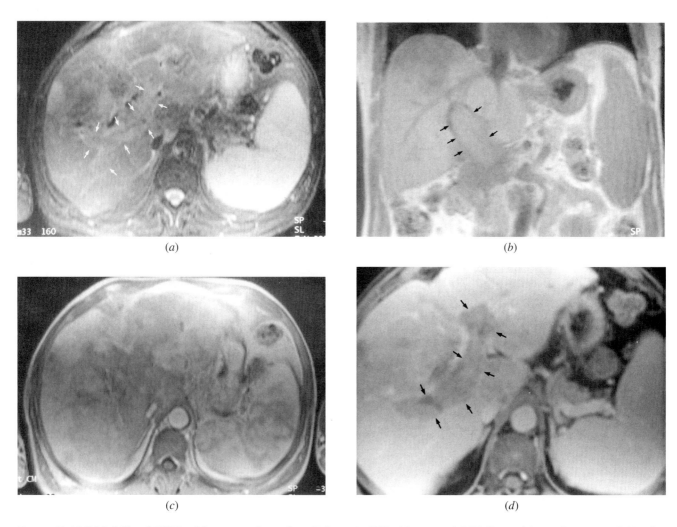

(a)   (b)

(c)   (d)

F I G . 2.125 Multifocal HCC with tumor thrombus. Echo-train STIR (*a*), coronal SGE (*b*), and immediate (*c*) and 90-s fat-suppressed postgadolinium SGE (*d*) images. There are multiple irregular, ill-defined multifocal HCCs scattered throughout all hepatic segments that demonstrate mildly decreased signal on T1 (*a*), mildly increased signal on T2 (*b*), and heterogeneous moderate enhancement on hepatic arterial dominant-phase images (*c*), with late washout and capsular enhancement (*d*). The portal vein is expanded with tumor thrombus (arrows, *a, b, d*). The thrombus is not well seen on the immediate postgadolinium image (*c*), as it enhances in a comparable fashion to background liver. Portions of tumor show late washout and capsule enhancement as observed in focal HCC.

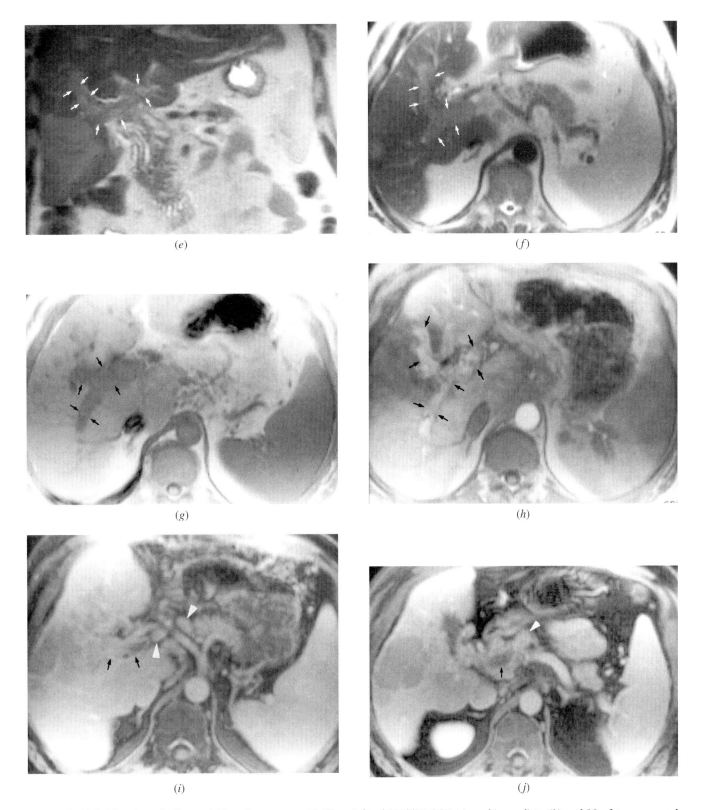

(e)

(f)

(g)

(h)

(i)

(j)

FIG. 2.125 (*Continued*) Coronal (*e*) and transverse (*f*) T2-weighted SS-ETSE, SGE (*g*), and immediate (*h*) and 90-s fat-suppressed (*i-l*) postgadolinium SGE images in a second patient. There is a large irregular mass occupying the majority of segments 5 and 6 of the right hepatic lobe, with tumor thrombus (small arrows, *e-j*) extending into the right, left, and main portal veins. Interstitial-phase gadolinium-enhanced images clearly depict multiple lymph nodes (arrowheads, *i-l*).

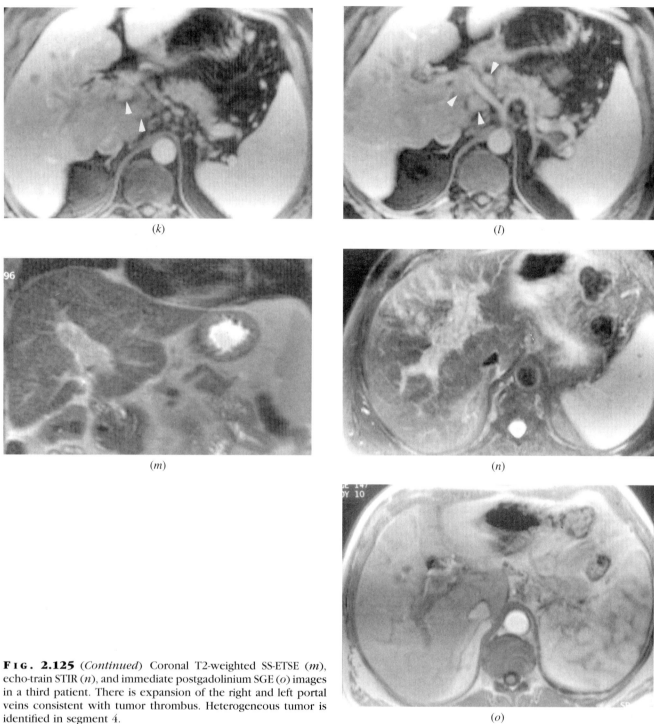

(k)

(l)

(m)

(n)

(o)

F I G . 2.125 (*Continued*) Coronal T2-weighted SS-ETSE (*m*), echo-train STIR (*n*), and immediate postgadolinium SGE (*o*) images in a third patient. There is expansion of the right and left portal veins consistent with tumor thrombus. Heterogeneous tumor is identified in segment 4.

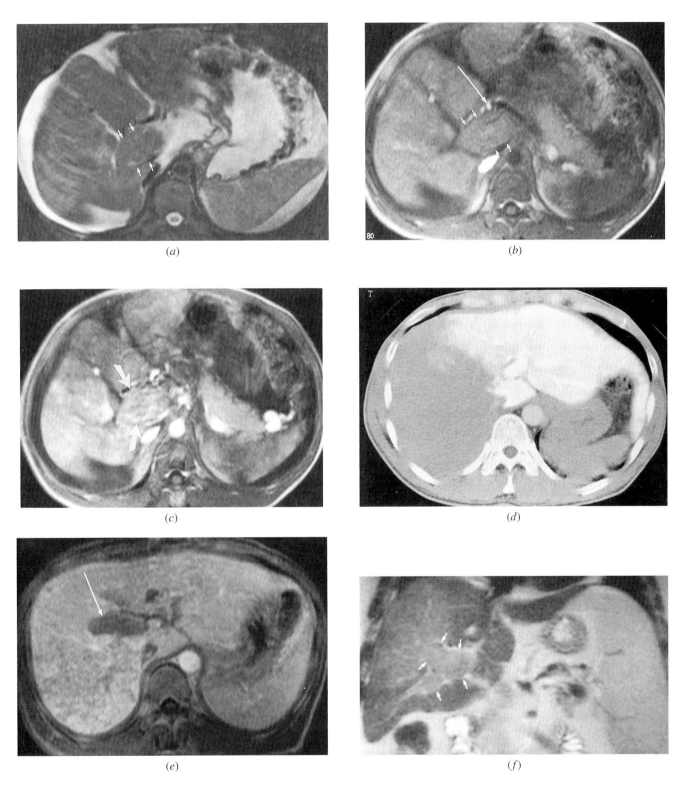

(a)

(b)

(c)

(d)

(e)

(f)

F I G . 2.126 Diffuse hepatocellular carcinoma with portal vein thrombosis. Fat-suppressed T2-weighted ETSE (*a*), SGE (*b*), and immediate postgadolinium SGE (*c*) images. The portal vein is expanded with tumor thrombus (small arrows, *a, b*), which is nearly isointense with liver on T2 (*a*) and T1(*b*) images. Tumor thrombus enhances in a diffuse heterogeneous fashion (arrows, *c*) on the immediate postgadolinium image (*c*). The hepatic artery is identified as a small high-signal tubular structure on the precontrast and immediate images (long arrow, *b*). Heterogeneous enhancement of the liver on the immediate postgadolinium image (*c*) reflects a combination of vascular abnormality from portal vein thrombosis and heterogeneous enhancement of diffusely infiltrative HCC. A substantial volume of ascites is present that is high in signal intensity on T2-weighted images (*a*) and low in signal intensity on pre- and postcontrast T1-weighted images (*b, c*).

Portal vein thrombosis in a second patient with diffuse HCC shown on spiral CTAP (*d*) and immediate postgadolinium SGE (*e*) images. On the CTAP image (*d*), nonopacification of the right hemiliver because of thrombosis of the right portal vein is noticed. The immediate postgadolinium image demonstrates a tumor thrombus that expands the right portal vein (arrow, *e*). Diffuse heterogeneous mottled enhancement of the right lobe of the liver is present on the MR image (*e*), which is a typical appearance for diffusely infiltrative HCC.

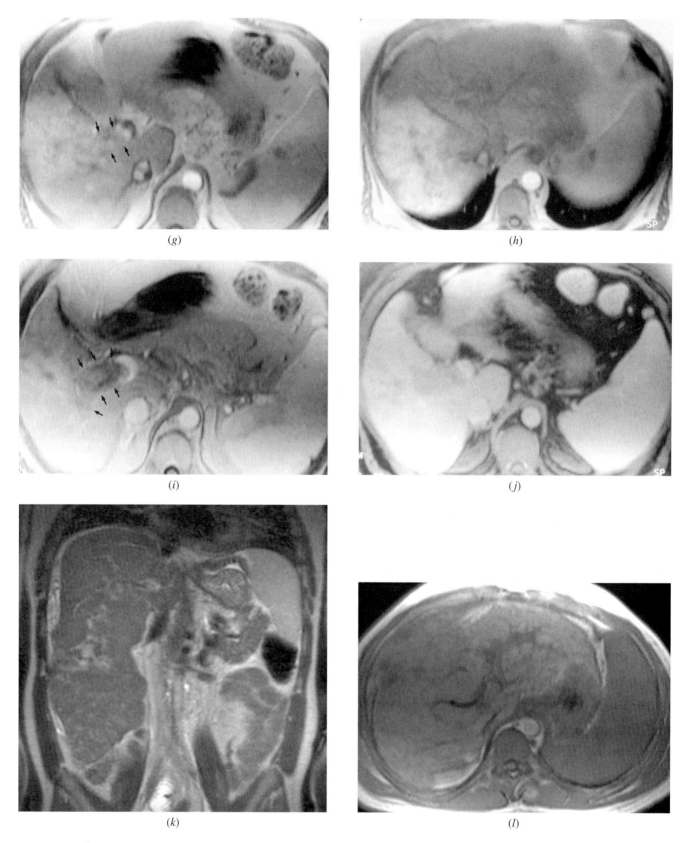

(g)

(h)

(i)

(j)

(k)

(l)

FIG. 2.126 (*Continued*) Coronal T2-weighted SS-ETSE (*f*), transverse immediate (*g, h*) and 45-s postgadolinium SGE (*i*) and 90-s fat-suppressed postgadolinium SGE (*j*) images in a second patient. There is an infiltrative HCC in the right hepatic lobe that demonstrates mild high signal intensity on the T2-weighted image (*f*) and heterogeneous intense enhancement immediately after gadolinium administration (*g, h*). The portal vein is expanded with tumor thrombus (arrows, *f, g, i*), which enhances in a diffuse fashion after contrast.

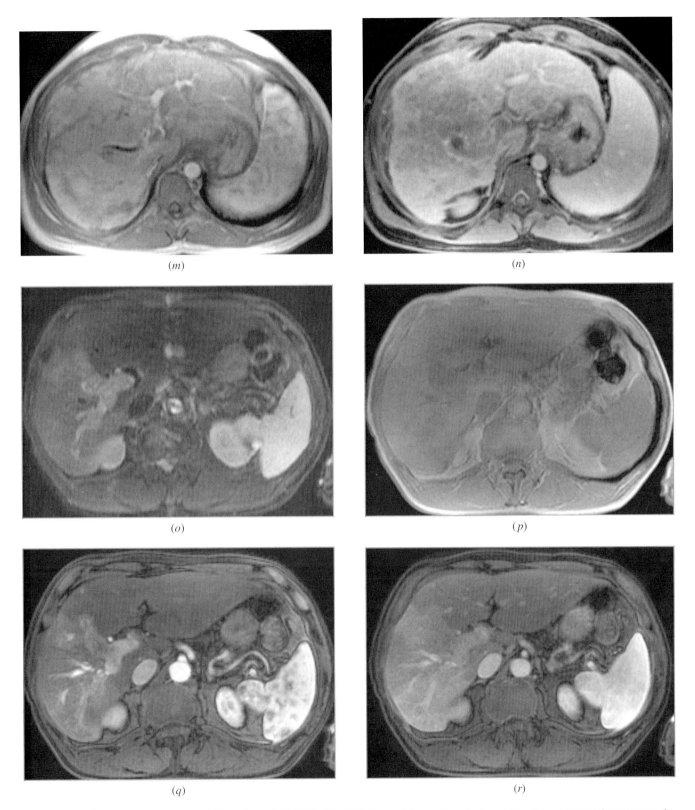

F I G . 2.126 (*Continued*) Coronal T2-weighted SS-ETSE (*k*), SGE (*l*), and immediate (*m*) and 90-s fat-suppressed (*n*) postgado-linium SGE images in a third patient with a diffuse HCC and tumor thrombus of the right portal vein. T2-weighted fat-suppressed SS-ETSE (*o*), SGE (*p*) and immediate (*q*) and 90s postcontrast fat-suppressed 3D-gradient echo images **at 3T** demonstrate poorly defined diffuse HCC in the right lobe. Note intense early enhancement of the tumor thrombus (*q*).

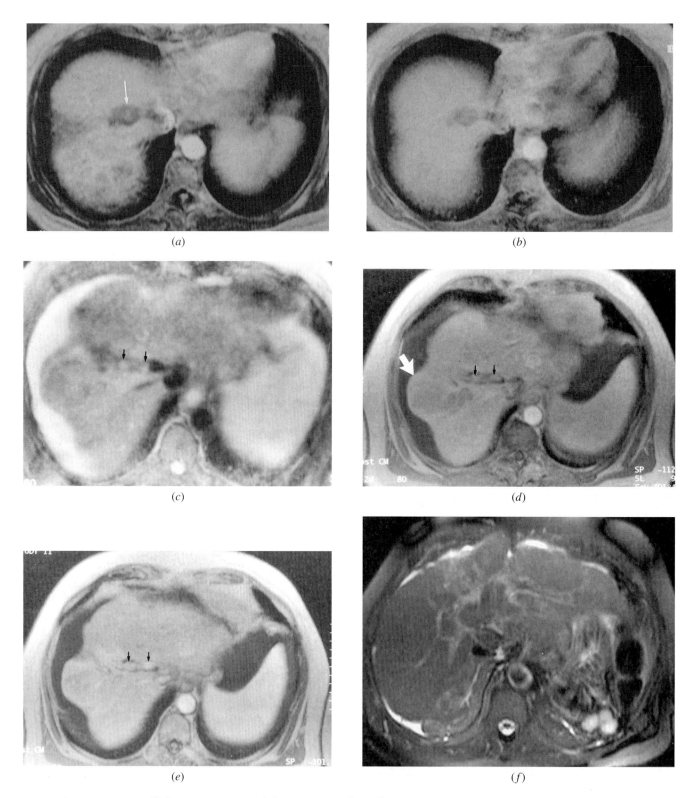

(a)

(b)

(c)

(d)

(e)

(f)

F I G . 2.127 Hepatocellular carcinoma with hepatic-vein thrombosis. Transverse 45-s (*a*) and 90-s (*b*) postgadolinium SGE images. On the 45-s postgadolinium image (*a*) tumor thrombus is apparent in the middle hepatic vein as low-signal-intensity material that expands the vein (arrow, *a*). Diffuse heterogeneous enhancement is noted in the right lobe that represents diffuse infiltrative HCC. Distal to the thrombosed hepatic vein, a wedge-shaped perfusion defect is identified. On the 90-s image (*b*) the tumor thrombus maintains low signal intensity compared to liver. However, the perfusion defect resolved, and the diffuse HCC is more isointense with background liver.

Fat-suppressed T2-weighted ETSE (*c*), SGE (*d*), and immediate postgadolinium SGE (*e*) images in a second patient. A 5-cm HCC (large arrow, *d*) is present in the right hepatic lobe that appears isointense on T2 (*c*)- and mildly hypointense on T1 (*d*)-weighted images and exhibits mild enhancement on hepatic dominant-phase image (*e*). A thin tumor capsule is identified on the precontrast T1-weighted image (*d*). In the middle hepatic vein there is an abnormal soft tissue with isointense signal intensity on T1- and T2-weighted images (arrows, *c, d, e*) and moderate enhancement after gadolinium administration (arrow, *e*). A perfusional abnormality adjacent to middle hepatic vein is related to the presence of tumor thrombus.

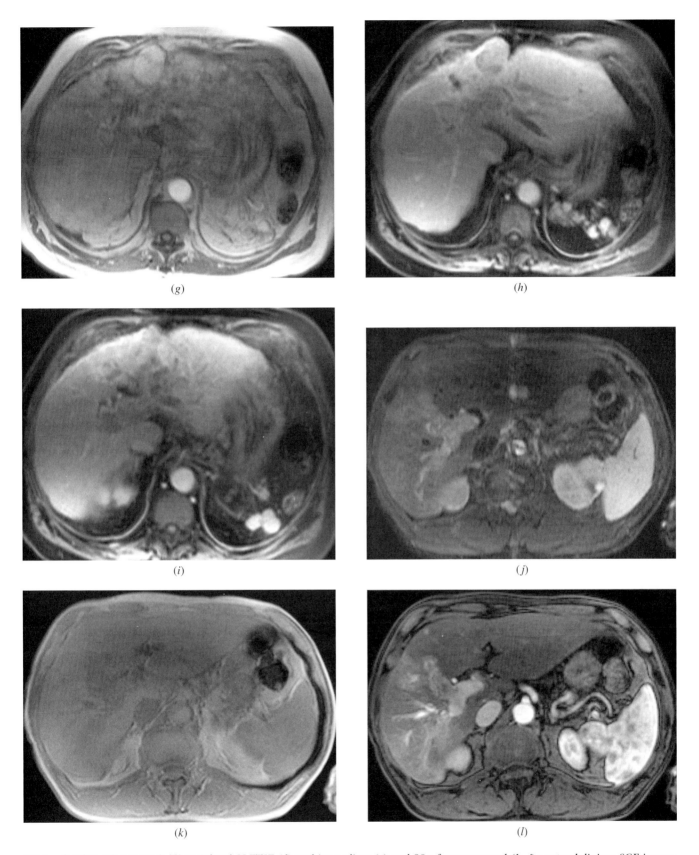

(g)

(h)

(i)

(j)

(k)

(l)

F I G . 2.127 (*Continued*) T2-weighted SS-ETSE (*f*) and immediate (*g*) and 90-s fat-suppressed (*h, i*) postgadolinium SGE images in a third patient. The left hepatic lobe and part of the right hepatic lobe show irregularity of the contour and distortion of the normal architecture due to the presence of a large tumor. On T2-weighted image (*f*), this tumor demonstrates mildly high signal intensity, on T1-weighted images (not shown) it shows low signal intensity, and after administration of contrast there is a moderate and heterogeneous enhancement on early-phase images (*g*) that fades to background signal intensity on late-phase images (*h, i*). Tumor thrombus is present in the main branches of the portal vein, which enhances on late-phase images. Note the biliary dilatation due to tumor compression.

T2-weighted SS-ETSE fat-suppressed (*j*), SGE (*k*), and immediate (*l*) and 90-s (*m*) fat-suppressed postgadolinium fat-suppressed 3D-gradient echo images **at 3T** images in a fourth patient. Tumor thrombus is apparent in the main portal vein as well right and left branches with features similar to those previously described. Note the perfusional parenchymal abnormality adjacent to the right portal vein.

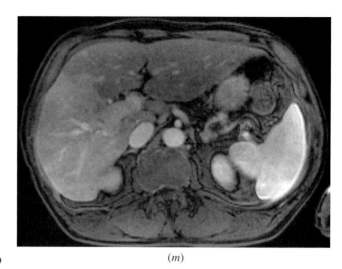

FIG. 2.127 (*Continued*)

(*m*)

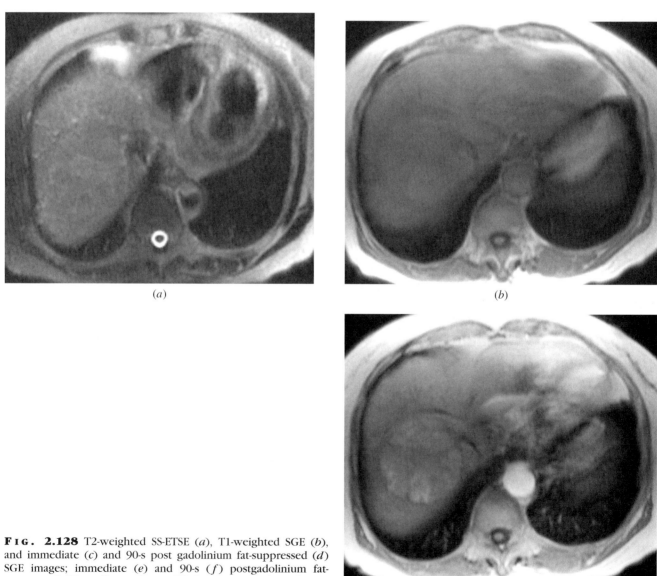

(*a*)

(*b*)

FIG. 2.128 T2-weighted SS-ETSE (*a*), T1-weighted SGE (*b*), and immediate (*c*) and 90-s post gadolinium fat-suppressed (*d*) SGE images; immediate (*e*) and 90-s (*f*) postgadolinium fat-suppressed 3D gradient-echo **at 3T** demonstrate a large hypervascular HCC.

(*c*)

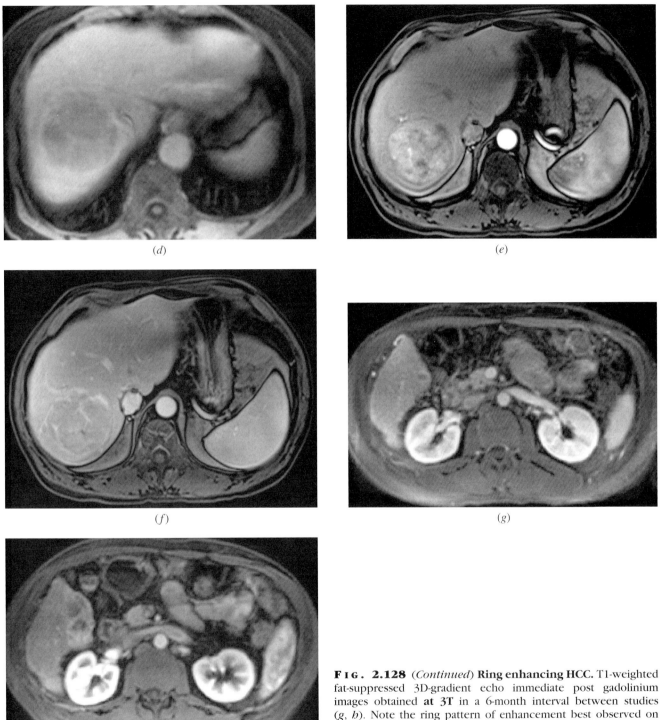

(d)

(e)

(f)

(g)

(h)

F I G . 2.128 (*Continued*) **Ring enhancing HCC.** T1-weighted fat-suppressed 3D-gradient echo immediate post gadolinium images obtained **at 3T** in a 6-month interval between studies (*g, b*). Note the ring pattern of enhancement best observed on 6-month follow-up exam, which mimics the enhancement pattern of metastases. Ring enhancement may be a sign of a more aggressive HCC.

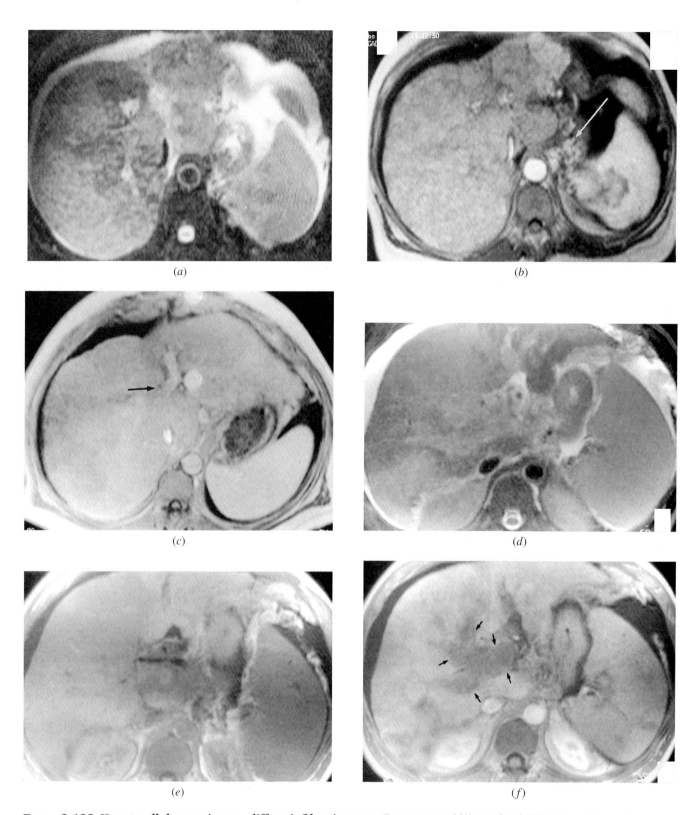

(a)

(b)

(c)

(d)

(e)

(f)

F I G . 2.129 Hepatocellular carcinoma, diffuse infiltrative type. Fat-suppressed T2-weighted ETSE (*a*) and immediate post-gadolinium SGE (*b*) images. Mottled diffuse high signal intensity is present throughout the liver on the T2-weighted image (*a*). Diffuse mottled heterogeneous enhancement is appreciated on the immediate postgadolinium image (*b*). These findings represent diffuse infiltrative HCC. Mottled signal intensity is the most common MRI appearance for diffuse infiltrative HCC. Occasionally, diffuse infiltrative HCC will appear as low in signal intensity on T2-weighted images and very low in signal intensity on postgado-linium images. Prominent varices are present along the lesser curvature of the stomach (arrow, *b*).

Transverse 45-s postgadolinium SGE (*c*) in a second patient. There is a large heterogeneous region of mottled enhancement throughout the right lobe of the liver, consistent with an infiltrating HCC. Note the irregularity of liver contour. Tumor thrombus of the right portal vein (arrow, *c*) is also present.

Transverse fat-suppressed T2-weighted SS-ETSE (*d*), SGE (*e*), and immediate postgadolinium SGE (*f*) images in a third patient. The liver is diffusely heterogeneous in appearance on both T2 (*d*)- and T1 (*e*)-weighted images and shows mild diffuse heteroge-neous enhancement after contrast (*f*), consistent with infiltrative HCC. The main, right, and left portal veins are distended with tumor thrombus (arrows, *f*). Note ascites and splenomegaly.

These cases illustrate the mottled heterogeneity of infiltrative HCC and illustrate that tumor thrombus in veins is almost invari-ably present. A third important feature is that α-fetoprotein is frequently extremely high.

T2-weighted images and hypo isointense on T1-weighted images. Immediate postcontrast images, tumor strands enhance variably. Late imperceptible enhancement or increased enhancement of tumor strands may reflect a high fibrous composition (fig. 2.130).

Venous thrombosis, almost always portal veins, sometimes in combination with hepatic venous thrombosis, is virtually invariably present. Very high serum α-fetoprotein (AFP) levels are commonly observed with diffuse HCC, with 78% of patients reported as presenting with increased AFP levels. AFP levels can be normal or near normal in a sizable minority of patients. A prior study [207] reported that 100% (22 of 22) of patients with diffuse HCC presented with portal vein thrombosis. Tumor thrombus is commonly high signal intensity on T2-weighted images and enhances with gadolinium;

meanwhile, bland thrombus is low in signal intensity on T2-weighted images and does not enhance after gadolinium.

Diffuse HCC may simulate the appearance of acute on chronic hepatitis or recent-onset fibrosis on imaging studies. Acute on chronic hepatitis tends to fade to background parenchyma rather than washing out on late postcontrast images and does not have expansive thrombus. AFP levels for acute on chronic hepatitis are usually relatively low. Major differential diagnoses to be considered are cholangiocarcinoma and metastases. Commonly, cholangiocarcinoma has better defined margins and does not exhibit tumor venous thrombus. Infiltrative metastases such as from breast cancer also have a more clearly focal pattern of involvement than diffuse HCC, and the primary tumor is almost always

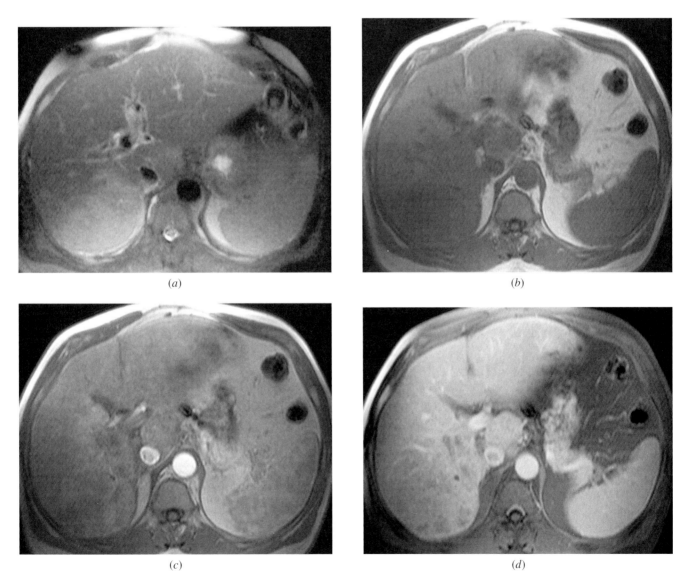

(a)   (b)   (c)   (d)

F I G . 2.130 Diffuse Infiltrative HCC. Fat-suppressed T2-weighted SS-ETSE (*a*), SGE (*b*), and immediate (*c*) and 90-s fat-suppressed (*d*) postgadolinium SGE images; fat-suppressed T2-weighted SS-ETSE (*e*) and immediate (*f*) and 90-s fat-suppressed (*g*)

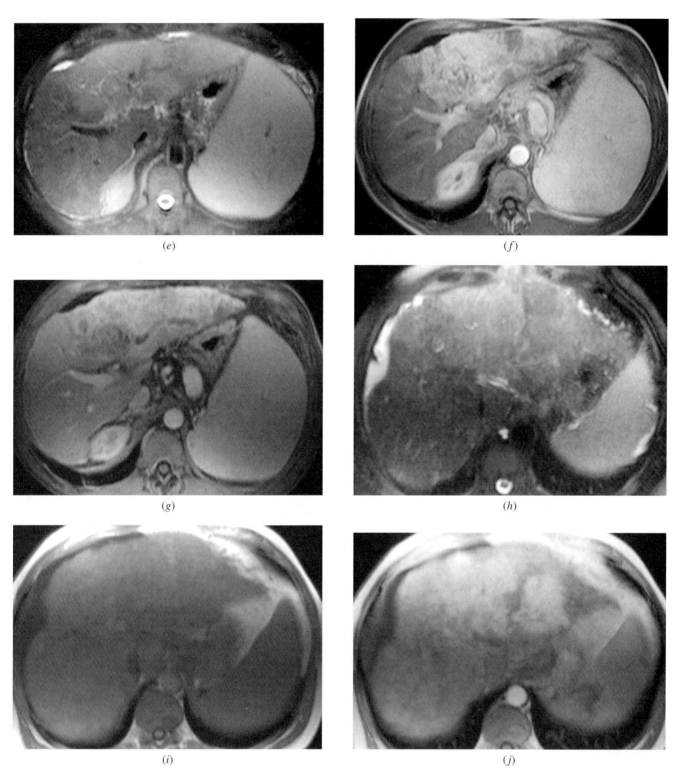

(e)

(f)

(g)

(h)

(i)

(j)

F I G . 2.130 (*Continued*) postgadolinium SGE images; fat-suppressed T2-weighted SS-ETSE (*h*), SGE (*i*), and immediate (*j*) and 90-s fat-suppressed (*k*) postgadolinium SGE images.

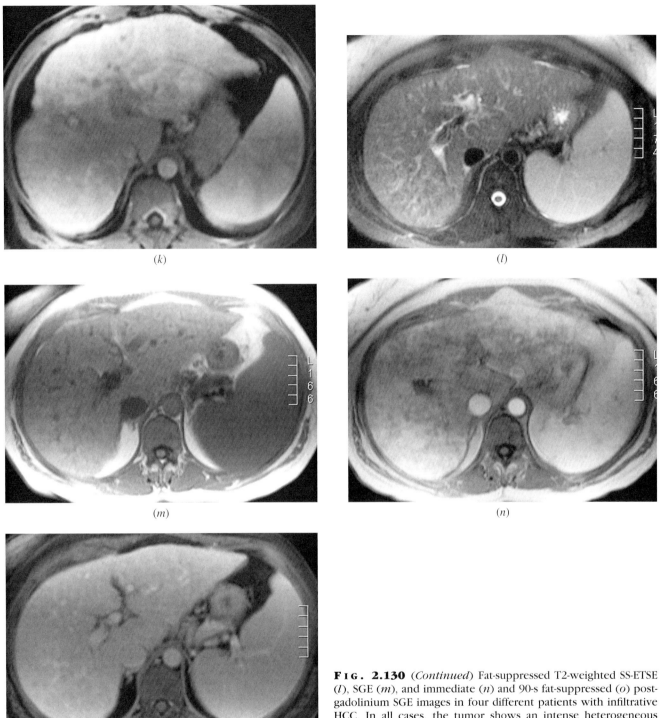

(k)

(l)

(m)

(n)

(o)

F I G . 2.130 (*Continued*) Fat-suppressed T2-weighted SS-ETSE (*l*), SGE (*m*), and immediate (*n*) and 90-s fat-suppressed (*o*) post-gadolinium SGE images in four different patients with infiltrative HCC. In all cases, the tumor shows an intense heterogeneous enhancement on early-phase images (*e, f, j, n*) that becomes less evident but with persistent enhancement (*d, g, k*) or imperceptible (*o*) on late-phase images.

known [207]. Venous tumor thrombus rarely may occur in the setting of metastases.

Fibrolamellar Carcinoma

Fibrolamellar carcinoma is a distinct morphologic subtype of liver cell carcinoma. This tumor occurs in younger patients, frequently females, without underlying cirrhosis or chronic liver disease. Fibrolamellar carcinoma is biologically distinct from other HCCs because it exhibits slow growth and is associated with a favorable prognosis [209]. From a pathologic viewpoint, the tumor is oftentimes large, usually solitary and well defined [2]. Macroscopically, the tumor shows a lobular architecture with intervening fibrous septa or a central stellate scar. Microscopically, tumor cells are polygonal, large, and eosinophilic. An extensive meshwork of collagenous stroma surrounding nests of tumor cells is the sine qua non for pathologic diagnosis. The rich fibrous network that incarcerates tumor has been credited for the slow, indolent growth of fibrolamellar carcinoma in contrast with ordinary HCC, which has a richly vascularized stroma permissive for intra- and extrahepatic spread [2].

On imaging, fibrolamellar carcinomas are generally large, solitary tumors that are heterogeneous and moderately high in signal intensity on T2-weighted images and heterogeneous and moderately low in signal intensity on T1-weighted images. Enhancement of the tumor is diffuse heterogeneous and moderately intense on immediate postgadolinium images. A huge central scar with radiating appearance is present. The central scar is variable in signal and has large low-signal components on T2-weighted images that enhance negligibly on delayed gadolinium-enhanced images (fig. 2.131) [210, 211]. On MR imaging, the scar is characterized by a complex arborizing pattern, radiating from a central focus and extending out to the tumor periphery. This profile is distinctly different from the appearance of FNH, in which the scar occupies a small central portion of the tumor and exhibits more uniform signal enhancement characteristics on late images [210].

Lymphoma

Secondary involvement of the liver by Hodgkin and non-Hodgkin lymphoma is common in stage IV disease [212]. On imaging, non-Hodgkin lymphoma more frequently results in focal hepatic lesions than Hodgkin disease. Lesions vary in signal intensity from low to moderately high on T2-weighted images and are typically low in signal intensity on T1-weighted images. Enhancement on immediate postgadolinium images tends to parallel the signal intensity on T2-weighted images; lesions that are low in signal intensity on T2-weighted images tend to enhance minimally (fig. 2.132), whereas lesions that are high in signal intensity tend to enhance in a substantial fashion (fig. 2.133) [213]. As with liver metastases, enhancement on immediate postgadolinium images usually is predominantly peripheral. Lesions of malignant lymphoma may possess transient, ill-defined perilesional enhancement on immediate postgadolinium images independent of the degree of enhancement of the lesions themselves (fig. 2.134). Rarely tumors may directly invade vessels producing an angiotropic pattern of involvement (fig. 2.135). Histopathologically, secondary involvement of the liver by malignant lymphoma is heralded by tumor deposits within the portal tracts. A clinical correlate with this microscopic appearance may be reflected on MR imaging with the appearance of periportal tumor tracking. This particular pattern may be very difficult to diagnose but is best visualized on a combination of T2-weighted fat-suppressed images and hepatic venous-phase gadolinium-enhanced fat-suppressed images. On both techniques, periportal tumor is moderately high in signal intensity (fig. 2.136).

Primary hepatic lymphoma is considerably rarer than secondary involvement, and histologically the majority are non-Hodgkin lymphomas. Most tumors are characterized grossly as a large solitary mass, but they may vary in appearance from multiple nodules to diffuse involvement. Tumors are mild to moderately high in signal on T2-weighted images and moderately low in signal intensity on T1-weighted images and show relatively diffuse heterogeneous enhancement on immediate postgadolinium gradient-echo images (figs. 2.137 and 2.138), analogous to primary hepatic tumors of other histologic types.

Multiple Myeloma

Focal deposits of multiple myeloma rarely occur in the liver and most often in the setting of disseminated disease. Pathologically, hepatic lesions are characterized by tumor cell infiltration of sinusoids and portal tracts. Focal hepatic lesions are observed most commonly in light-chain multiple myeloma. Lesions are often small, measuring approximately 1 cm in diameter. They are moderately hyperintense on T2-weighted images and iso- to mildly hyperintense on T1-weighted images [214]. The hyperintensity on T1-weighted images may reflect the increased production of monoclonal protein. Multiple myeloma lesions are sufficiently rare that is difficult to establish their enhancement characteristics; many, however, appear to be hypervascular (fig. 2.139).

Intrahepatic or Peripheral Bile Duct Carcinoma (Cholangiocarcinoma)

Intrahepatic or peripheral cholangiocarcinoma are terms applied to lesions that originate in the ducts proximal to (i.e., above) the hilum of the liver. Malignant tumors arising from intrahepatic bile ducts are much less

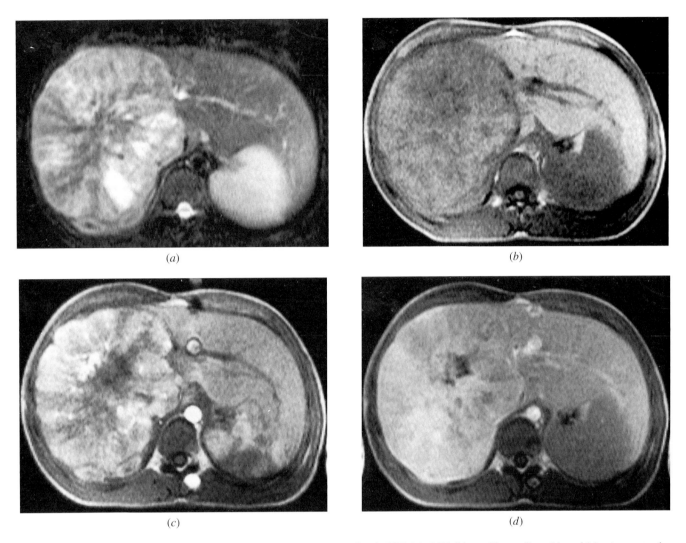

(a)

(b)

(c)

(d)

FIG. 2.131 Fibrolamellar carcinoma. Fat-suppressed T2-weighted ETSE (*a*), SGE (*b*), and immediate (*c*) and 10-min postgado-linium SGE (*d*) images. A 14-cm fibrolamellar hepatocellular carcinoma is present in this adolescent male with no history of liver disease and 1-yr duration of gynecomastia. The tumor is heterogeneously hyperintense on the T2-weighted image (*a*) with the central radiating scar largely low in signal intensity and hypointense on the T1-weighted image (*b*) with the central scar also low in signal intensity. On the immediate image (*c*), the tumor exhibits diffuse moderate heterogeneous enhancement with negligible enhancement of the radiating scar. On the 10-min image (*d*), the bulk of the tumor has become isointense with background liver. Portions of the central scar are higher in signal intensity than surrounding tissue, whereas other parts remain low in signal. In contrast to FNH, the scar in fibrolamellar HCC is much larger and exhibits more heterogeneous signal on T2 and early and late postgadolinium images.

common than those arising from hepatocytes and have no direct association with cirrhosis [215]. Most cases of cholangiocarcinoma occur after the age of 60 years. Pathologically, the tumor is generally better circum-scribed and of firmer consistency than hepatocellular carcinoma. The microscopic picture is characterized by glandular configurations surrounded by abundant, dense fibrous stroma. The prominent sinusoidal pattern of HCC is not present [22].

The tumor is frequently large at presentation [216]. Cholangiocarcinoma resembles HCC with moderate high signal intensity on T2-weighted images and low

signal intensity on T1-weighted images. High signal on T1-weighted images, pseudocapsule, and invasion into portal and hepatic veins are common with HCC and rarely seen with cholangiocarcinoma. Also, biliary and extrinsic portal vein obstruction are more common with cholangiocarcinoma. Enhancement with gadolinium varies from minimal to intense diffuse heterogeneous enhancement immediately after contrast administration (fig. 2.140). Minimal enhancement is most commonly observed. Persistent enhancement on delayed images is relatively common [217]. The intrahepatic origin of the tumor likely explains the early diffuse heterogeneous

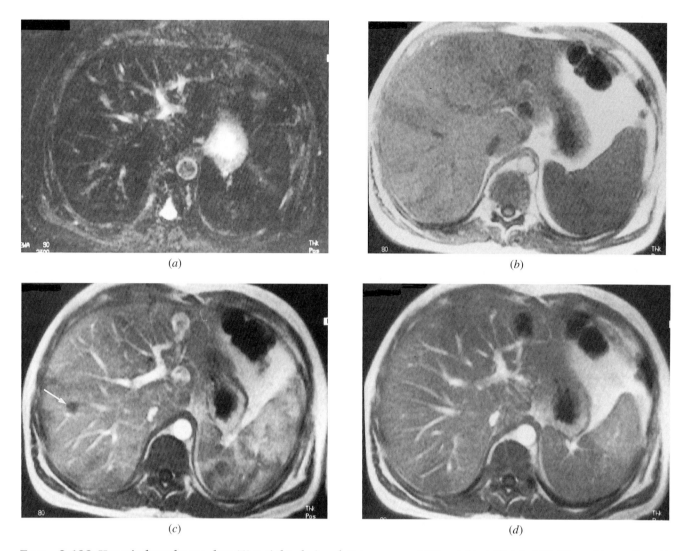

(a)

(b)

(c)

(d)

FIG. 2.132 Hepatic lymphoma, low T2-weighted signal. Fat-suppressed T2-weighted SE (*a*), SGE (*b*), and immediate (*c*) and 90-s (*d*) postgadolinium SGE images. On the T2-weighted image (*a*), the liver and spleen demonstrate transfusional siderosis with low signal intensity of the liver and spleen. The SGE image (*b*) demonstrates wedge-shaped regions of low signal intensity representing increased iron deposition. On the immediate postgadolinium image (*c*), focal low-signal intensity masses (arrow, *c*) of diffuse histiocytic lymphoma are shown. These masses enhance to isointensity with hepatic parenchyma on interstitial-phase images.

enhancement. (For a more complete description of cholangiocarcinoma see Chapter 3, *Gallbladder and Biliary System*).

Malignant tumors of mixed liver cell and bile duct differentiation are rare. Mixed HCC-cholangiocarcinoma may occur, and the imaging appearance is generally indistinguishable from that of HCC (fig. 2.141). These tumors tend to be multifocal and hypervascular.

Angiosarcoma

Angiosarcoma is the most common sarcoma arising in the liver and accounts for 1.8% of all liver cancers. An increased risk for the development of this tumor in adults has been documented in the following settings:

1) cirrhosis; 2) vinyl chloride exposure; 3) thorium dioxide exposure (Thorotrast) for radiographic purposes; and 4) arsenic exposure. This tumor is usually encountered in middle-aged patients and occurs more commonly in men. Pathologically, angiosarcomas appear most commonly as multicentric nodules diffusely involving the liver. Occasionally, tumor may present as a solitary, large mass. Microscopically, angiosarcoma is characterized by ill-defined clusters of malignant endothelial cells lining and expanding the sinusoids. Internal hemorrhage is relatively common [218].

On MRI, angiosarcoma usually appears as a multifocal process, but an infiltrative pattern is also described [219, 220]. Angiosarcoma may be high signal intensity

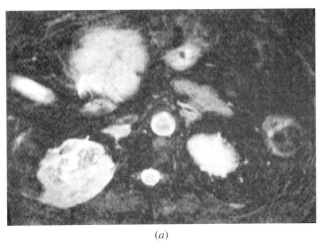

(a)

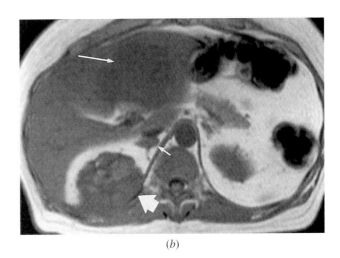

(b)

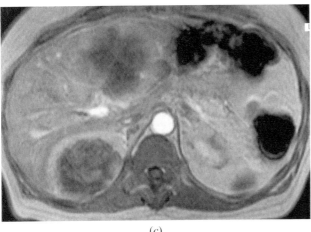

(c)

FIG. 2.133 Hepatic lymphoma, after transplant. Fat-suppressed T2-weighted SE (*a*), SGE (*b*), and immediate postgadolinium SGE (*c*) images. In this patient with post-heart transplant lymphoma, and 8-cm hepatic mass (long arrow, *b*), a 1-cm adrenal mass (short arrow, *b*), and a 6-cm peritoneum-based mass (large arrow, *b*) are present. The hepatic mass is moderately hyperintense on the T2-weighted image (*a*) and moderately hypointense on the T1-weighted image (*b*) and demonstrates predominantly peripheral enhancement on the immediate postgadolinium image (*c*). Minimal heterogeneous enhancement of the peritoneal and adrenal masses is present on the immediate postgadolinium image (*c*).

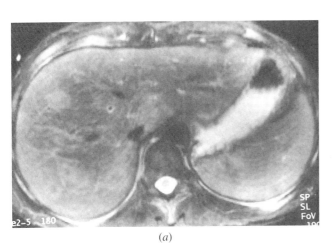

(a)

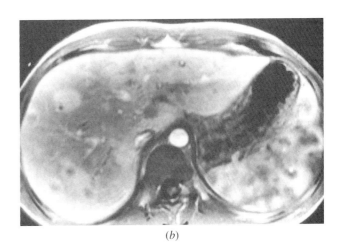

(b)

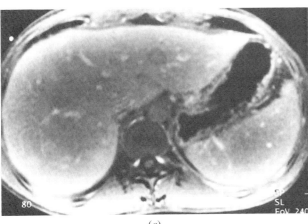

(c)

FIG. 2.134 Hodgkin lymphoma. Fat-suppressed T2-weighted ETSE (*a*) and immediate (*b*) and 90-s fat-suppressed postgadolinium SGE (*c*) images. Multiple focal mass lesions smaller than 2 cm are present throughout the liver, many of which show mildly hyperintense tumor periphery on T2 (*a*) and demonstrate ring enhancement with ill-defined perilesional enhancement on immediate postgadolinium images (*b*). Arciform enhancement of the spleen is present on the immediate postgadolinium image, with no evidence of focal low-signal-intensity masses (*b*). By 90 s after gadolinium (*c*), many of the hepatic masses have become isointense with the liver.

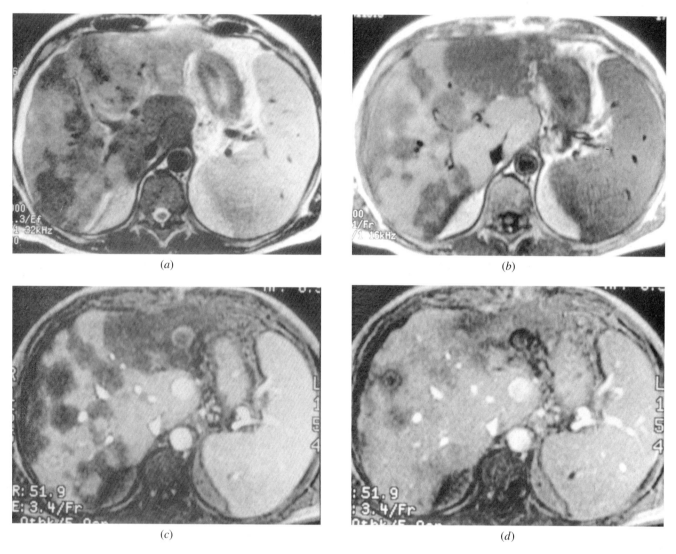

(a)   (b)

(c)   (d)

FIG. 2.135 Angiotropic intravascular lymphoma. T2-weighted ETSE (*a*), SGE (*b*), and immediate (*c*) and 90-s (*d*) postgadolinium SGE images. There is an irregular geographic pattern of liver involvement that represents angiotropic intravascular lymphoma. The vascular involvement causes moderately high signal on T2 (*a*), moderately low signal on T1 (*b*), and negligible early enhancement (*c*) with delayed enhancement (*d*) (Courtesy of Evan Siegelman, M. D., Dept. Radiology, Hospital of the University of Pennsylvania.)

on T2-weighted images and low signal on T1-weighted images. The frequent presence of hemorrhage results in focal areas of low signal intensity on T2-weighted images and high signal on T1-weighted images. After contrast, angiosarcoma may demonstrate peripheral nodular enhancement with centripetal progression, mimicking the appearance of hemangioma (fig. 2.142) [220]. The frequent presence of hemorrhage, which results in low signal intensity on T2-weighted images, high signal on T1-weighted images, and lack of central enhancement due to hemorrhage, fibrosis, or necrosis are distinguishing features [219, 220]. Mild to moderate heterogeneous enhancement on arterial dominant phase that increases in the extent of enhancement on delayed-phase images has also been reported [219].

Malignant Mesothelioma

Malignant mesothelioma of the liver is a rare soft tissue tumor that occurs most commonly in men, with peak incidence beginning in the fifth decade of life. Asbestos exposure is suggested to be a risk factor. Malignant mesotheliomas of the liver are large tumors, oftentimes greater than 10 cm, solid and well-circumscribed. The cut surface shows cystic areas with interlacing septations [221].

Malignant mesothelioma exhibits heterogeneous high signal intensity on T2-weighted images and heterogeneous low signal on T1-weighted images. Heterogeneity on both T2- and T1-weighted images usually reflects the presence of hemorrhage. Diffuse heterogeneous enhancement is commonly observed (fig. 2.143).

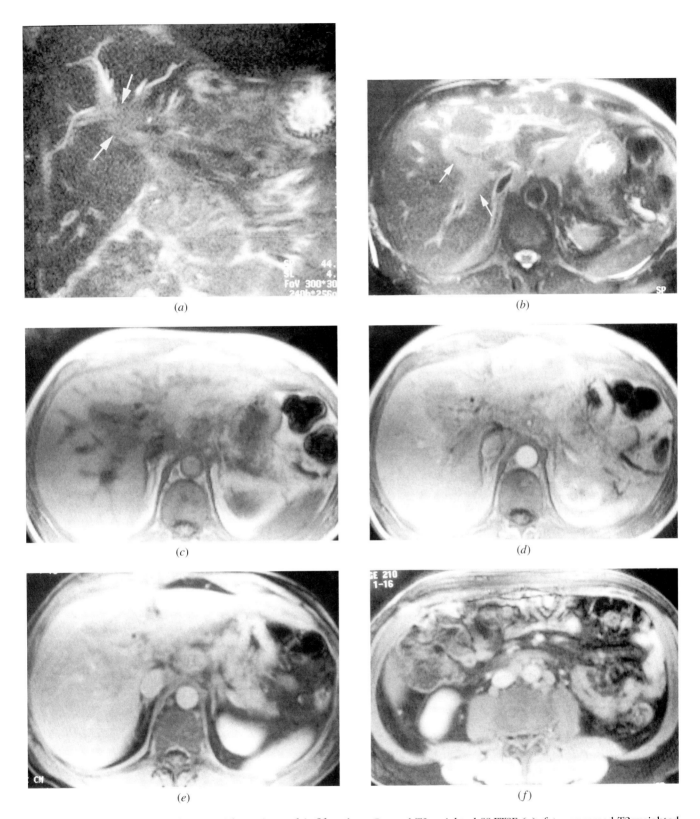

FIG. 2.136 Burkitt lymphoma with periportal infiltration. Coronal T2-weighted SS-ETSE (*a*), fat-suppressed T2-weighted SS-ETSE (*b*), SGE (*c*), and immediate (*d*) and 90-s fat-suppressed postgadolinium SGE (*e, f*) images. There is extensive soft tissue infiltration in the porta hepatis with periportal extension (arrows, *a, b*). Periportal tumor infiltration is more common with lymphoma than with other forms of malignant disease. Retroperitoneal nodes are also present (*f*).

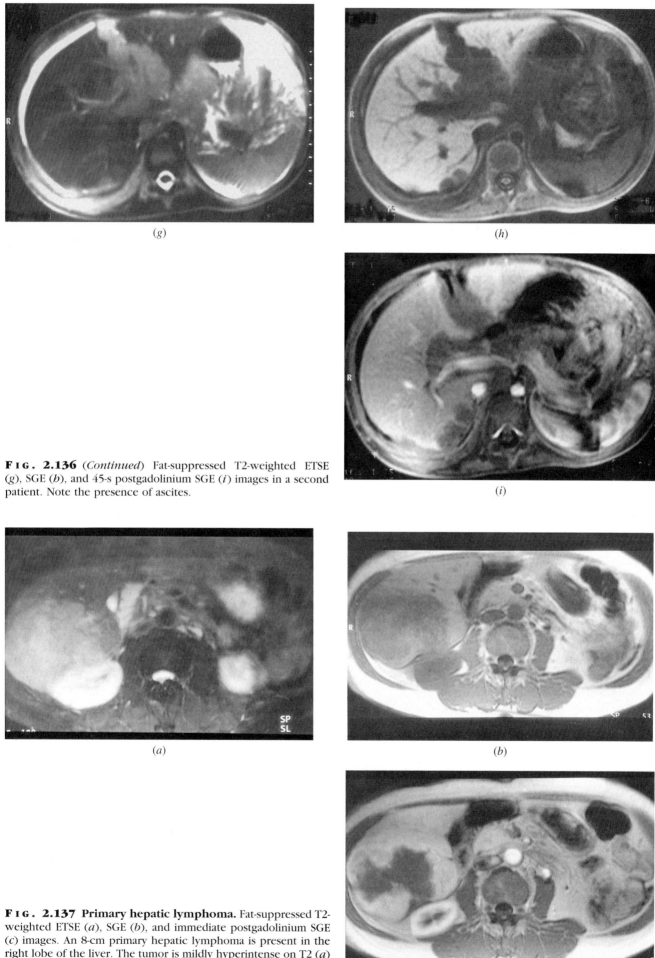

(g)

(h)

FIG. 2.136 (*Continued*) Fat-suppressed T2-weighted ETSE (*g*), SGE (*b*), and 45-s postgadolinium SGE (*i*) images in a second patient. Note the presence of ascites.

(i)

(a)

(b)

FIG. 2.137 **Primary hepatic lymphoma.** Fat-suppressed T2-weighted ETSE (*a*), SGE (*b*), and immediate postgadolinium SGE (*c*) images. An 8-cm primary hepatic lymphoma is present in the right lobe of the liver. The tumor is mildly hyperintense on T2 (*a*) and moderately hypointense on T1 (*b*) and demonstrates thick, irregular multilayered peripheral enhancement on immediate postgadolinium images (*c*).

(c)

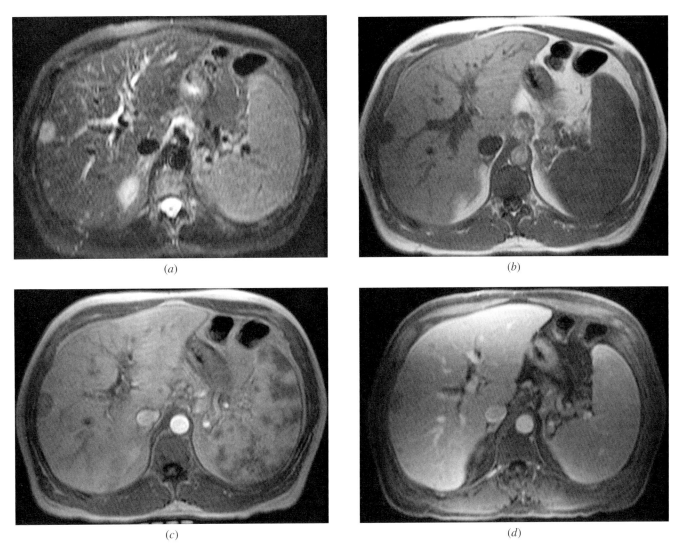

FIG. 2.138 Liver lymphoma in a HIV patient. T2-STIR (*a*), SGE (*b*), immediate postgadolinium SGE (*c*), and 90-s fat-suppressed postgadolinium SGE (*d*) images in a patient with HIV. Multiple focal lesions are present throughout the liver that are mildly hyperintense on T2 (*a*) and moderately hypointense on T1 (*b*) and demonstrate minimal early enhancement with perilesional enhancement (*c*), with mild progression of lesion enhancement and fading of the perilesional enhancement. A variety of etiologies of liver disease occurs in HIV patients in greater frequency than in patients with normal immune systems, including infectious and neoplastic disease. In this patient, multiple foci of lymphoma are present throughout the liver. Note also abnormal signal intensity of the bone marrow of the spine consistent with disease involvement in this location as well.

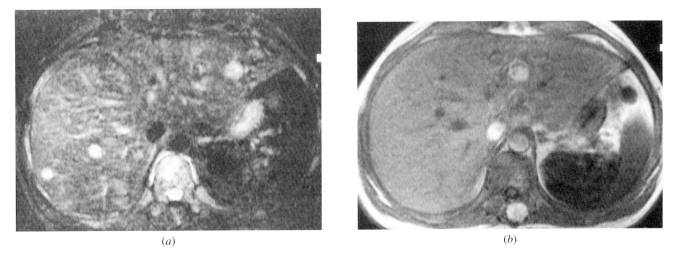

FIG. 2.139 Multiple myeloma. Fat-suppressed T2-weighted ETSE (*a*), SGE (*b*), and T1-weighted fat-suppressed spin-echo (*c*) images. Multiple focal masses <1.5 cm are present in the liver that are moderately hyperintense on T2 image (*a*), nearly isointense

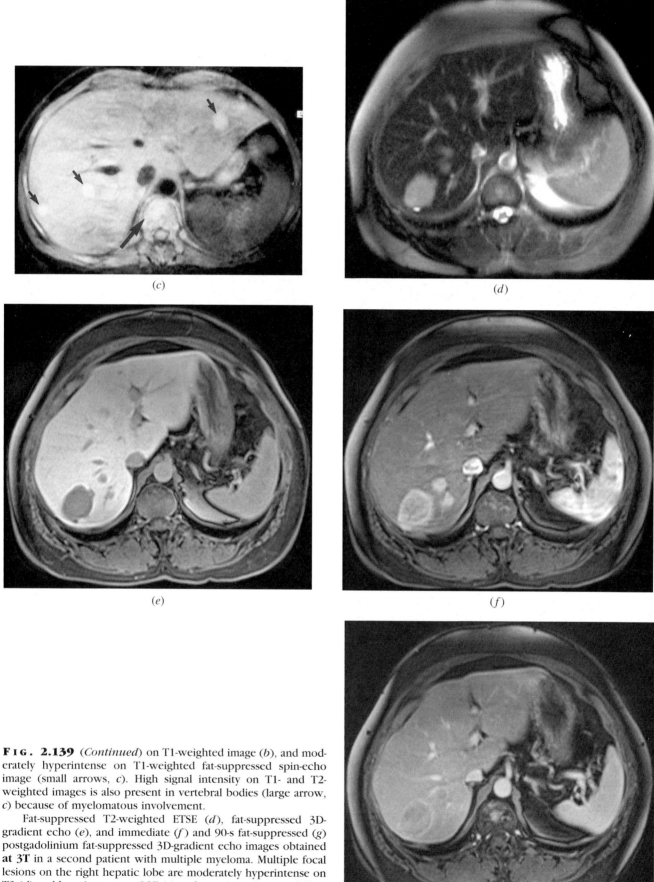

(c)

(d)

(e)

(f)

FIG. 2.139 (*Continued*) on T1-weighted image (*b*), and moderately hyperintense on T1-weighted fat-suppressed spin-echo image (small arrows, *c*). High signal intensity on T1- and T2-weighted images is also present in vertebral bodies (large arrow, *c*) because of myelomatous involvement.

Fat-suppressed T2-weighted ETSE (*d*), fat-suppressed 3D-gradient echo (*e*), and immediate (*f*) and 90-s fat-suppressed (*g*) postgadolinium fat-suppressed 3D-gradient echo images obtained **at 3T** in a second patient with multiple myeloma. Multiple focal lesions on the right hepatic lobe are moderately hyperintense on T2 (*d*) and hypointense on SGE (*e*), enhance in an intense diffuse heterogeneous fashion on immediate images (*f*), with lesional washout and thin rim enhancement on delayed images (*g*).

(g)

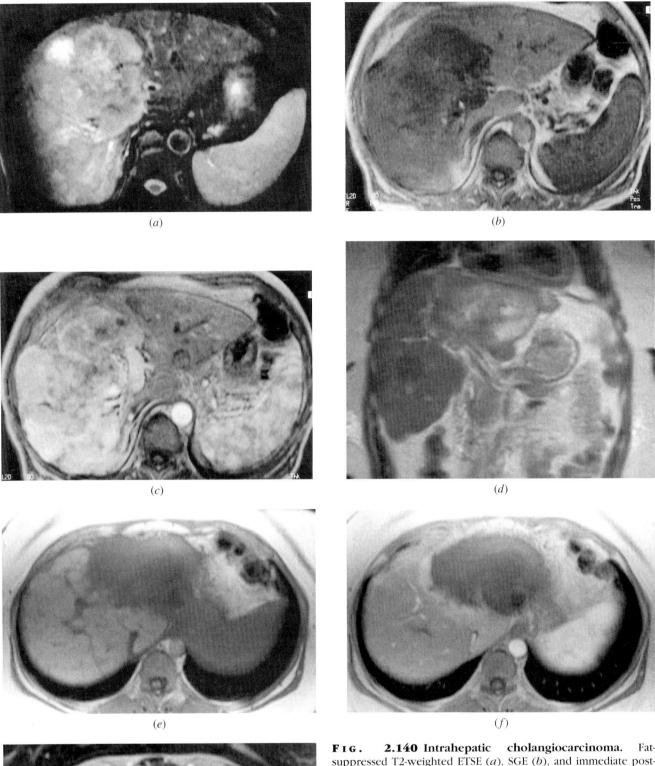

(a)

(b)

(c)

(d)

(e)

(f)

(g)

FIG. 2.140 Intrahepatic cholangiocarcinoma. Fat-suppressed T2-weighted ETSE (*a*), SGE (*b*), and immediate post-gadolinium SGE (*c*) images. A 14-cm tumor is present in the right lobe of the liver that is moderately high in signal intensity on the T2-weighted image (*a*) and moderately low in signal intensity on the T1-weighted image (*b*) and enhances in an intense, diffuse heterogeneous fashion on the immediate image (*c*). The appearance resembles that of an HCC.

Coronal T2-weighted SS-ETSE (*d*), SGE (*e*), and immediate (*f*) and 90-s fat-suppressed (*g*) postgadolinium SGE images in a second patient. There is a mass in the left hepatic lobe that demonstrates heterogeneous high signal intensity on T2-weighted image (*d*), low signal intensity on T1-weighted images (*e*), and perilesional enhancement on early-phase images (*f*) that fades on late phase images (*g*). Minimal lesional enhancement is appreciated in this case. Histopathology was consistent with intrahepatic cholangiocarcinoma.

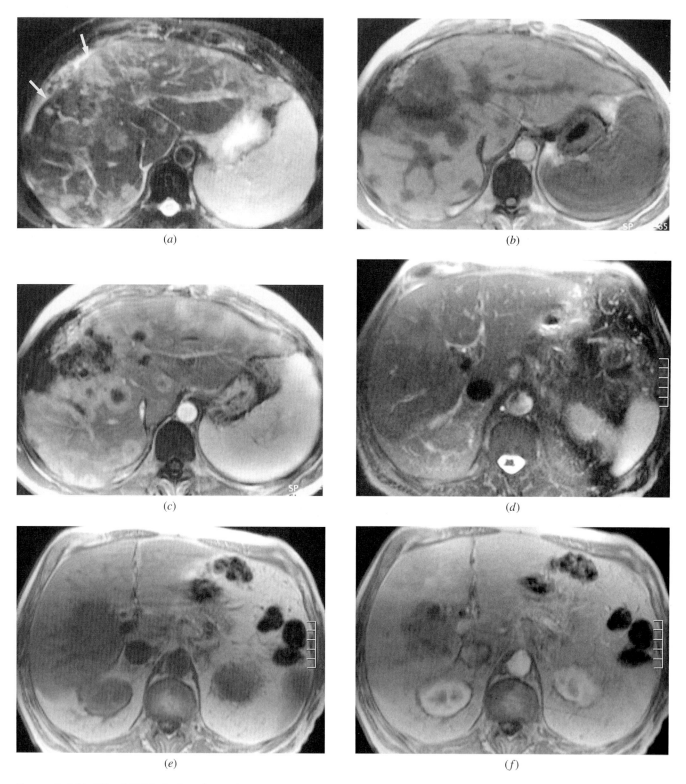

(a)

(b)

(c)

(d)

(e)

(f)

F I G . 2.141 Mixed HCC-cholangiocarcinoma. Fat-suppressed T2-weighted ETSE (*a*), SGE (*b*), and immediate postgadolinium SGE (*c*) images. A large 14-cm tumor is centered in the anterior segments 4/8, and multiple small satellite lesions are scattered throughout the remainder of the liver. The tumors are moderately high in signal on the T2-weighted image (*a*) and moderately low in signal intensity on the T1-weighted image (*b*) and enhance intensely immediately after gadolinium administration (*c*). Capsular retraction is also noted (arrows, *a*).

T2-weighted SS-ETSE (*d*), SGE (*e*), and immediate (*f*) and 90-s fat-suppressed (*g*) postgadolinium SGE images in a second patient. A mass is present adjacent to the porta hepatis. This lesion is isointense with background parenchyma on T2-weighted images (*d*) and moderately low signal intensity on T1-weighted images (*e*), shows moderate heterogeneous enhancement on early-phase images (*f*), and demonstrates washout on late-phase images (*g*).

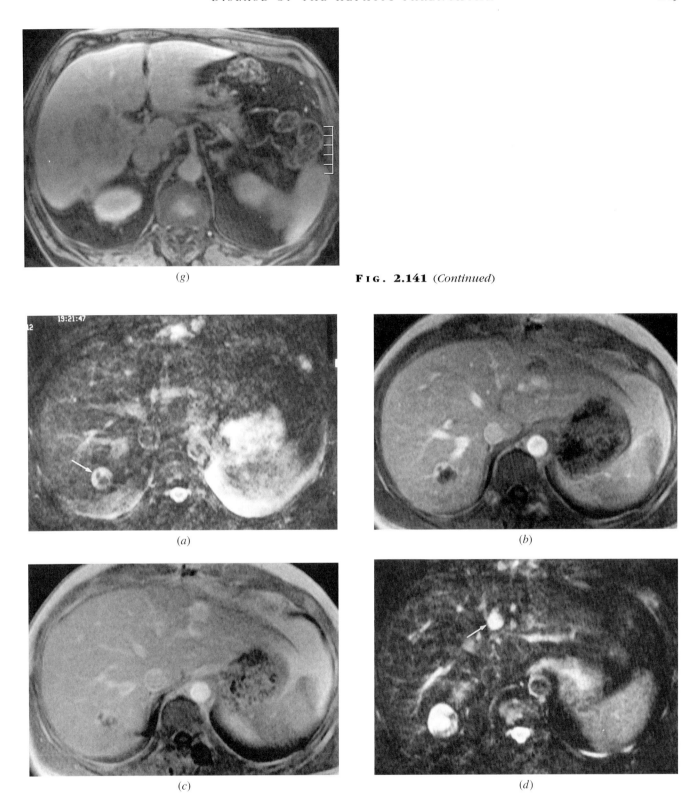

(g)   **F I G . 2.141** (*Continued*)

(a)   (b)

(c)   (d)

F I G . 2.142 Angiosarcoma. Fat-suppressed T2-weighted ETSE (*a*) and 90-s (*b*) and 10-min (*c*) postgadolinium SGE images. A 2-cm angiosarcoma is present in the right lobe of the liver. The mass is well defined and largely hyperintense on the T2-weighted image (arrow, *a*) with a central region of low signal intensity due to hemorrhage. On the 90-s postgadolinium image (*b*), peripheral nodular enhancement is present. By 10 min after contrast (*c*), nodular enhancement has progressed centripetally, with a central nonenhanced area that corresponds to the region of hemorrhage on the T2-weighted image. Angiosarcomas mimic the appearance of hemangiomas. The presence of hemorrhage in this case is a common finding in angiosarcomas and rare in hemangiomas. Interval increase in size of this tumor is identified on a follow-up study obtained 1 month later, shown on fat-suppressed T2-weighted SS-ETSE image (*d*). Increase in size of a second tumor is also present. Rapid growth is compatible with angiosarcomas and not with hemangiomas. A change in the signal intensity of the larger mass on the T2-weighted image (*d*) is also noted between studies because of aging of the central hemorrhage.

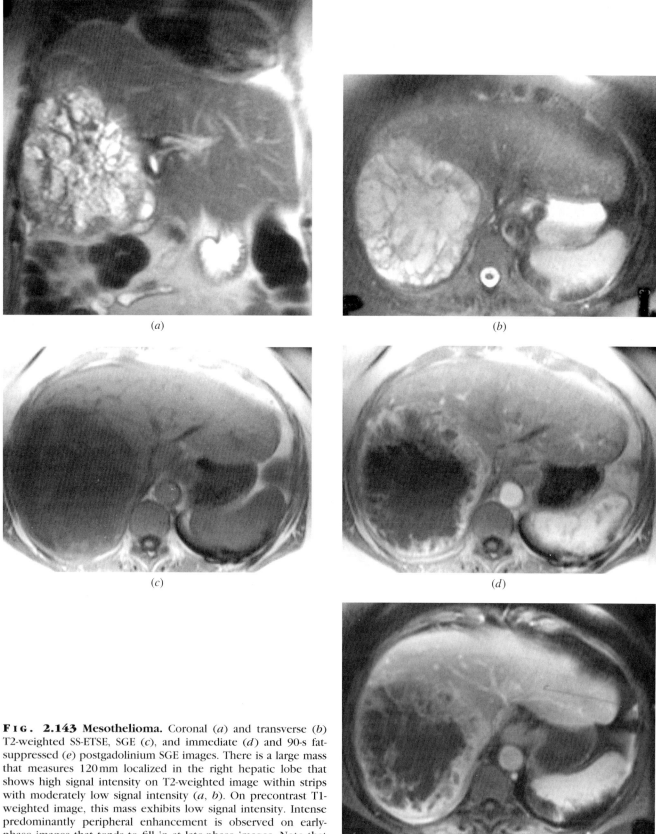

F I G . 2.143 Mesothelioma. Coronal (*a*) and transverse (*b*) T2-weighted SS-ETSE, SGE (*c*), and immediate (*d*) and 90-s fat-suppressed (*e*) postgadolinium SGE images. There is a large mass that measures 120 mm localized in the right hepatic lobe that shows high signal intensity on T2-weighted image within strips with moderately low signal intensity (*a*, *b*). On precontrast T1-weighted image, this mass exhibits low signal intensity. Intense predominantly peripheral enhancement is observed on early-phase images that tends to fill in at late-phase images. Note that multiple septations are well appreciated on late-phase images.

Septations demonstrate mild to moderate enhancement on early phase that tend to be more intense on delayed-phase images. Lack of central enhancement is common, reflecting central necrosis [222]. (See also Chapter 7, *Peritoneal Cavity*, on mesothelioma.)

Epithelioid Hemangioendothelioma

Epithelioid hemangioendothelioma (EHE) is a malignant, slow-growing vascular tumor, usually occurring in middle-aged patients. Females predominate over males in a 2-to-1 ratio, and oral contraceptives have been implicated as possible causative agents in younger patients [223]. Pathologically, lesions tend to be multiple, tough, fibrous masses distributed throughout the liver. Microscopically, there is characteristically abundant stroma with scattered clumps of neoplastic cells invading sinusoids and vessels [2]. Tumors tend to be low-grade malignancies with a much more favorable prognosis than for angiosarcoma. EHE are moderately high signal on T2-weighted images and moderately low signal on T1-weighted images and show a mild heterogeneous enhancement on early-phase images. The MRI findings described above are consistent with the predominance of stroma and relatively less conspicuous areas of sinusoid and blood vessel infiltration by tumor cells [224]. EHE can also appear as moderately high signal intensity on T2-weighted images and moderately intense diffuse heterogeneous enhancement on immediate postcontrast images (fig. 2.144). This appearance is similar to that of hepatocellular carcinoma, particularly in tumors with aggressive growth patterns.

Hepatoblastoma

Hepatoblastoma is the most common primary malignant tumor of the liver in children and may occur from the newborn to adolescent period and rarely older. The tumor is most often detected by 3 years of age, with a median age of 1 year. Hepatoblastoma occurs more often in boys than in girls, with a ratio of 3:2. On gross inspection, hepatoblastoma is a solid, well-defined, occasionally lobulated mass surrounded by a pseudo-capsule. Although it is usually solitary, multiple lesions can be seen in less than 20% of cases. Areas of necrosis and calcifications are frequently present [225].

On MR imaging, hepatoblastoma resembles hepatocellular carcinoma in that the tumor shows diffuse heterogeneous enhancement on immediate postgadolinium images (fig. 2.145).

Undifferentiated Sarcoma of the Liver

Undifferentiated sarcoma of the liver (USL) is a rare mesenchymal tumor occurring most frequently in pediatric patients [226]. Pathologically, USL appears as a solitary, large mass with internal septations, commonly surrounded by a fibrous pseudocapsule. USL is mainly a solid tumor, with large cystic areas consistent with hemorrhage and necrosis. Histologically, USL demonstrates typically a myxoid stroma containing undifferentiated cells similar to embryonic cells [226–228].

On MRI, USL has a cystic appearance due to the presence of hemorrhagic and necrotic portions along with the high water content of myxoid stroma in the solid portion of the tumor [227, 228]. On T2-weighted images, USL is heterogeneously high signal intensity, and on T1-weighted images the tumor is heterogeneously low signal intensity. After gadolinium, solid areas enhance heterogeneously. Areas with lack of enhancement are consistent with hemorrhage or necrosis. Septations may show mild or moderate enhancement on arterial dominant-phase images that persists on late-phase images (fig. 2.146) [227–230].

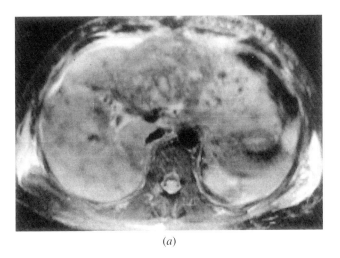

(a)

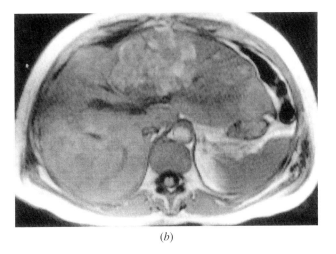

(b)

F I G . 2.144 Epithelioid hemangioendothelioma. Fat-suppressed T2-weighted ETSE (*a*), SGE (*b*), and immediate (*c*) and 90-s fat-suppressed (*d*) postgadolinium SGE images in an adult patient with epithelioid hemangioendotheliosarcoma. Extensive liver

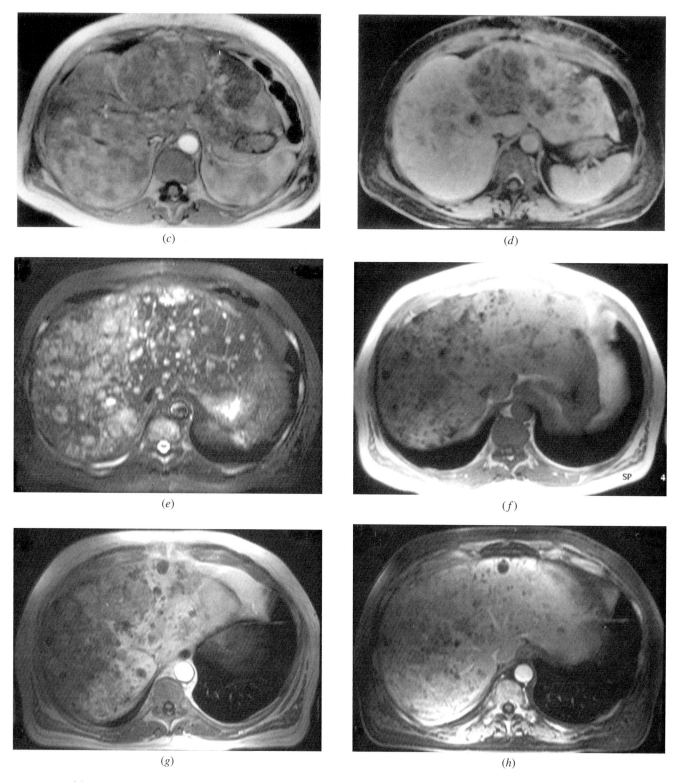

(c)

(d)

(e)

(f)

(g)

(h)

FIG. 2.144 (*Continued*) involvement with a multifocal malignant epithelioid hemangioendotheliosarcoma is present. The tumor is heterogeneous and isointense to minimally hyperintense on the T2-weighted image (*a*). Regions of high signal intensity are present in the largest mass on the T1-weighted image (*b*). Enhancement is diffuse heterogeneous on the immediate postgadolinium image (*c*), with heterogeneous washout on the 90-s postcontrast image (*d*). The MRI appearance of this epithelioid hemangioendothelioma resembles HCC.

Fat-suppressed T2-weighted SS-ETSE (*e*), SGE (*f*), and immediate (*g*) and 90-s fat-suppressed (*h*) postgadolinium SGE images in a second patient. There are multiple focal rounded liver lesions, some of them confluent, that have moderately high signal intensity on T2-weighted images (*e*), moderately low signal intensity on T1-weighed images (*f*), and mild diffuse heterogeneous enhancement on early-phase images (*g*) that remains on late-phase images (*h*). Histopathology was epithelioid hemangioendothelioma.

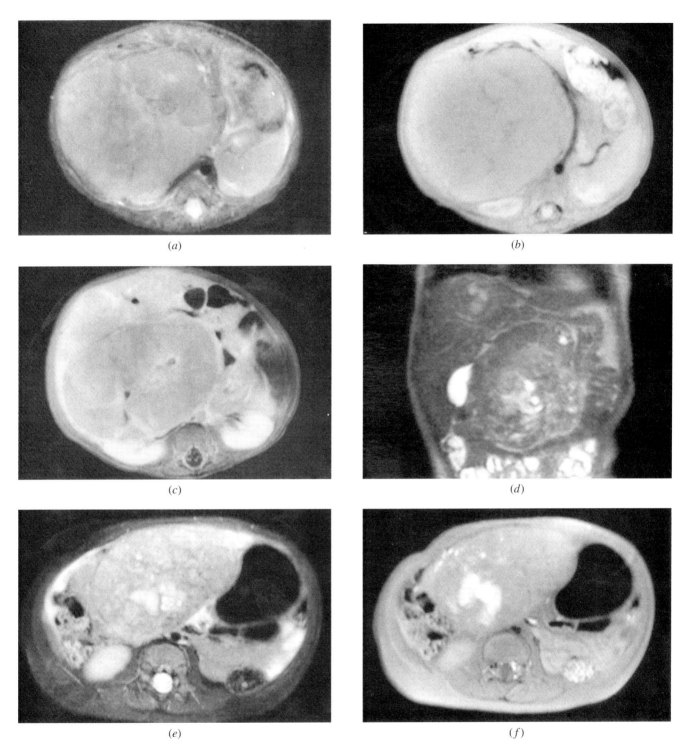

(a)

(b)

(c)

(d)

(e)

(f)

FIG. 2.145 Hepatoblastoma. Fat-suppressed T2-weighted ETSE (a), T1-weighted fat-suppressed SE (b), and T1-weighted 90-s fat-suppressed SE (c) images in a 2-month-old boy. There is a large, slightly lobulated mass arising from the liver, which demonstrates slightly increased signal intensity on T2 (a), mildly decreased signal intensity on T1(b), and mildly heterogeneous enhancement on interstitial-phase gadolinium-enhanced (c) images. Note that the mass displaces the celiac axis, the right kidney, aorta, inferior vena cava, and pancreas.

Coronal T2-weighted SS-ETSE (d), transverse fat-suppressed T2-weighted ETSE (e), T1-weighted fat-suppressed SE (f), and immediate postgadolinium SE (g) images in a second (1-year old) patient with hepatoblastoma. There is a large mass arising from

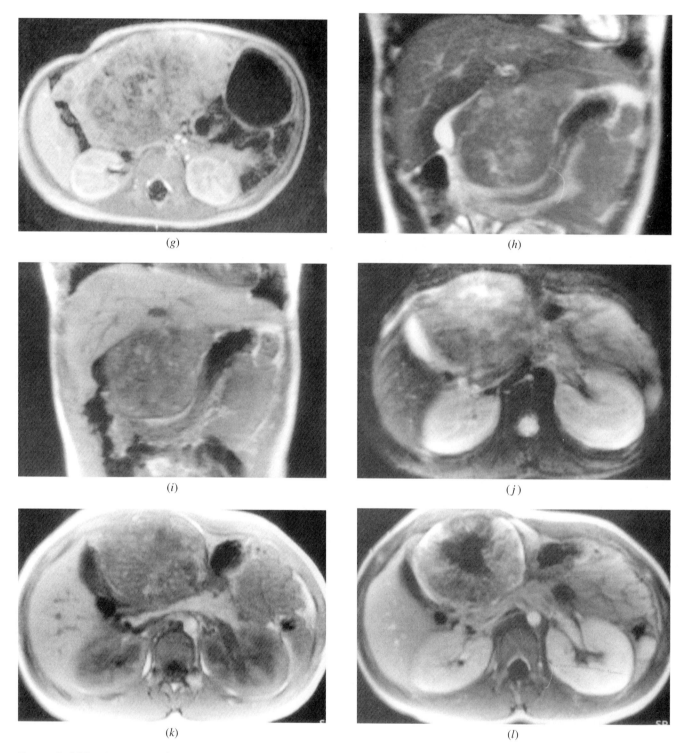

(g)   (h)

(i)   (j)

(k)   (l)

FIG. 2.145 (*Continued*) the left hepatic lobe inferiorly, that demonstrates heterogeneous signal on T2 (*d, e*) and T1 (*f*) images. On the T1-weighted image (*f*) there are also several focal areas of high signal consistent with hemorrhage. The tumor enhances in a diffuse heterogeneous fashion (*g*).

Coronal T2-weighted SS-ETSE (*h*), coronal SGE (*i*), fat-suppressed T2-weighted SS-ETSE (*j*), SGE (*k*), and immediate (*l*) and 90-s fat-suppressed (*m*) postgadolinium SGE in a 14-year-old girl. There is a large tumor that is heterogeneous and moderately

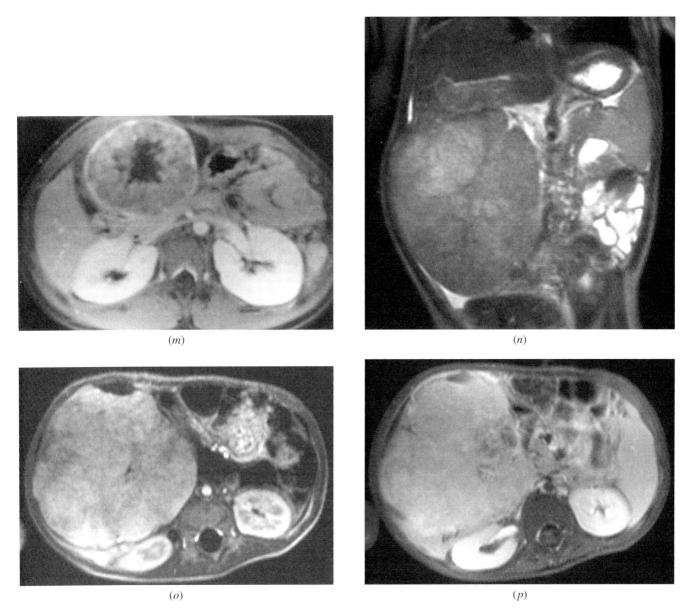

(m)

(n)

(o)

(p)

F I G . 2.145 (*Continued*) hyperintense on T2 (*h, j*). The tumor shows diffuse heterogeneous enhancement on immediate post-gadolinium images (*l*), which fades by 90 s (*m*). The central region does not enhance, consistent with fibrous tissue.

Coronal T2-weighted SS-ETSE fat suppressed (*n*) and immediate (*o*) and 90-s fat-suppressed (*p*) postgadolinium SGE images. There is large exophytic lobular hepatic mass (12 cm in the longest axis) with mildly high signal intensity on T2-weighted images (*n*), moderately high signal intensity on T1-weighted images (not shown), and heterogeneous enhancement on early-phase images (*o*) that becomes more homogeneous on late-phase images (*p*). Note the posterior displacement of the kidney by the mass.

The most common primary liver malignancy changes from hepatoblastoma to hepatocellular carcinoma in the adolescent period between 14 and 16 years of age. This last patient is at the upper age range of hepatoblastoma.

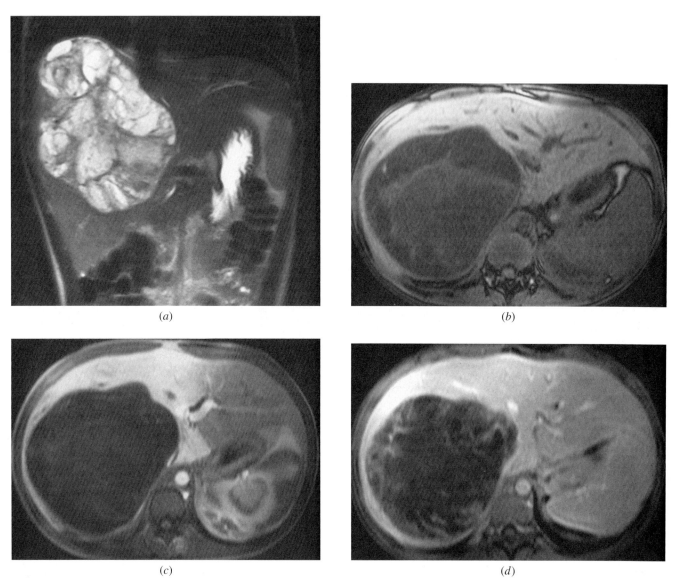

(a)

(b)

(c)

(d)

FIG. 2.146 Undifferentiated sarcoma of the liver. Coronal T2-weighted SS-ETSE (*a*), SGE (*b*), and immediate (*c*) and 90-s fat-suppressed (*d*) postgadolinium SGE images. There is a large mass in the right hepatic lobe that measures 12 cm in the longest axis and demonstrates moderately high signal intensity on T2-weighted images (*a*) and moderately low signal intensity on T1-weighted images (*b*), and shows negligible enhancement on early-phase images (*c*) and moderate enhancement of the outer margin of the tumor on late-phase images (*d*). At histopathology, the mass was undifferentiated sarcoma of the liver.

Posttreatment Lesions

Malignant liver lesions may be treated by a number of interventions, including surgical resection, radiation therapy, systemic chemotherapy, transcatheter arterial chemoembolization, ablative therapy, and liver transplantation [231–251]. The appearance of hepatic parenchyma and malignant liver lesions after therapeutic interventions has been previously described [233–240, 242, 244–248]. In the evaluation of posttreatment liver, the time course of benign posttreatment tissue changes, primarily tissue injury and development and maturation of granulation tissue, and the appearance of persistent or recurrent disease must be ascertained. Certain fea-

tures of treatment-related changes depend on the form of therapy. The following discussion describes many of those features.

Resection. Surgical removal with resection of negative margins remains the optimal therapy for primary and secondary liver tumors. However, only up to 25% of patients are eligible for curative resection [252–254].

Within the first 3–5 months after resection, the parenchyma and surgically resected margins often appear as high signal intensity on T2-weighted images and low signal intensity on T1-weighted images and display homogeneously mild to moderately increased enhancement on arterial dominant-phase images that fades to background parenchyma on interstitial-phase images [231, 255] (fig. 2.147). These focal areas reflect edema and granulation tissue in the liver parenchyma, and they may appear linear, circular, oval, or serpiginous in configuration [255].

Hyperplasia of the remaining liver may be appreciated as early as 3 months after surgery. Within 1 year, general enlargement of the remaining liver occurs. After right hepatectomy, hypertrophy of the medial segment may create the appearance of a pseudo-right lobe (fig. 2.148). Magnetic susceptibility artifact, related to surgical clips, is often present along the resection margin of the liver.

After surgery, malignancy may recur along the margin of resection or separate focal lesions may develop in the remainder of the liver (figs. 2.149 and 2.150) [239]. Tumor recurrence has an appearance similar to untreated malignant lesions.

Postradiation Therapy. As with postradiation changes in other tissues and organ systems, the distinction between benign and malignant disease usually can be made with certainty beyond 1 year after treatment. At this time point, benign disease usually exhibits regular or linear margins, low signal intensity on T2-weighted image, and mild or negligible enhancement on immediate postgadolinium images. In comparison, malignant disease tends to appear more irregular, nodular, or masslike, with moderately high signal intensity on T2-weighted images and moderate or intense enhancement on hepatic arterial dominant-phase images. Radiation changes generally exhibit linear margins that do not conform to segmental anatomy but rather conform to expected radiation portals. Within the first 3 months, radiation changes generally exhibit features of edema (i.e., moderately high signal on T2-weighted images and moderately low signal on T1-weighted images). Beyond 3 months, radiation changes may show increased granulation tissue progressing to fibrosis (fig. 2.151). Often, immediate postcontrast images effectively define pathophysiological changes that reflect successful response or recurrence.

Systemic Chemotherapy. A number of chemotherapeutic agents are currently utilized in the treatment of focal liver malignancies. The number of agents and their cytotoxic effectiveness continue to progress dramatically. The mechanisms of tumor cell control are complex and probably involve a number of pathways. However, studies have focused on the antiangiogenic activity of some of these agents.

Tumor response after systemic chemotherapy is assessed by evaluating the number and size of the tumors before and after systemic chemotherapy. The time course and variation in imaging appearance of metastases that have responded to chemotherapy have not been fully elucidated. However, it has been reported that in after as little as 2 weeks of therapy there is a decrease in the tumor size and vascularity if tumor shows a good response [256].

We have previously described the appearance of liver metastases 2 to 7 months after initiation of chemotherapy [82]. In that report, liver metastases became better defined and higher in signal intensity on T2-weighted images, showing peripheral nodular enhancement with progressive enhancement that remained on 10-min delayed images (fig. 2.152). The appearance was considered to mimic that of hemangiomas. Explanations for this change in appearance are related to altered physiology and blood supply of metastatic tumors treated with chemotherapy. The less aggressive enhancement patterns of metastasis after chemotherapy might be ascribed to chemo-induced tumor antiangiogenesis (fig. 2.153). Continued resolution of metastatic lesions results in a progressive decrease in signal intensity on T2-weighted images and progressive decrease in contrast enhancement (fig. 2.154). One report described the appearance of liver metastases treated by intravenous chemotherapy in 34 patients on serial MRI studies [234]. In that report, a good prognosis was associated with decreased signal intensity on T2-weighted images and increased signal intensity of the lesions on T1-weighted images, essentially approaching the signal intensity of the liver.

The vascularity of liver metastases, that is, hypervascularity and hypovascularity, can be assessed based on the degree of enhancement on arterial dominant-phase images (fig. 2.155). This is an important imaging feature since evidence points to a close association between tumor vascularity and patients' response to therapy. A prior study [142] demonstrated that breast cancer patients with persistently hypervascular liver metastases after systemic chemotherapy were more likely to have disease progression compared to patients whose liver metastases became hypovascular.

The appearance of chronic healed metastases is comparable to the appearance of treated focal lesions of other causes, such as infection. The chronic healed phase of lesion response usually develops at least 1.5 years after initiation of treatment. Chronic healed lesions possess an irregular, angular, polygonal margin frequently associated with retraction of surrounding liver parenchyma. In superficial lesions, capsule retraction may develop, creating a puckered appearance on imaging studies. Chronic healed lesions contain mature fibrous tissue that has a low fluid content and is hypovascular. These lesions appear as low signal intensity or isointensity on T2-weighted images and moderately

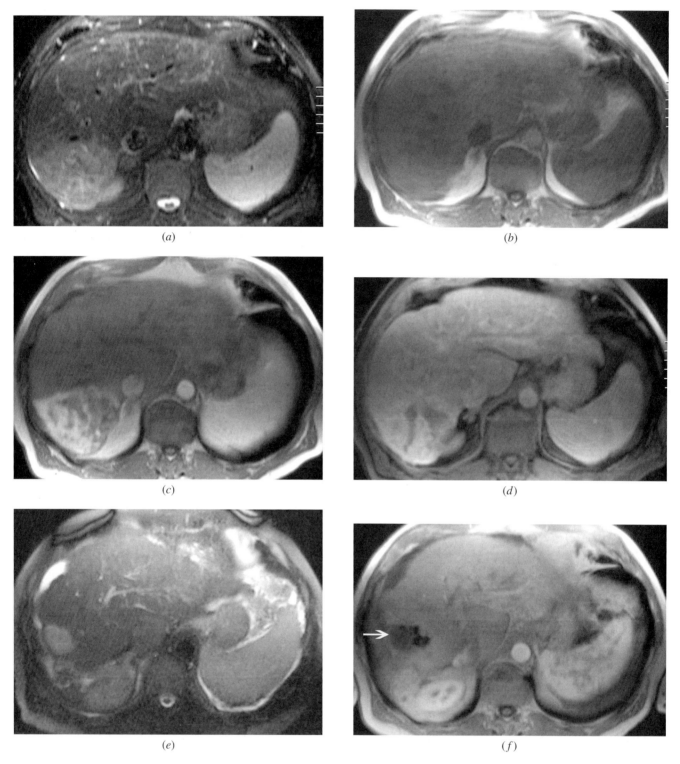

(a)

(b)

(c)

(d)

(e)

(f)

FIG. 2.147 Before and after liver resection. T2-weighted SS-ETSE (*a, e*), SGE (*b*), and immediate (*c, f*) and 90-s fat-suppressed (*d, g*) postgadolinium SGE images. The images before resection (*a–d*) show a 9-cm HCC in the right hepatic lobe. After resection, a small biloma is present (arrow, *f*). Note the heterogeneous mildly increased enhancement along the resection margin on early-phase images (*f*) that fades on late-phase images (*g*), features of early granulation tissue and mild inflammation.

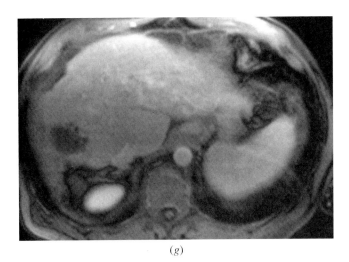

(g)   **FIG. 2.147** (*Continued*)

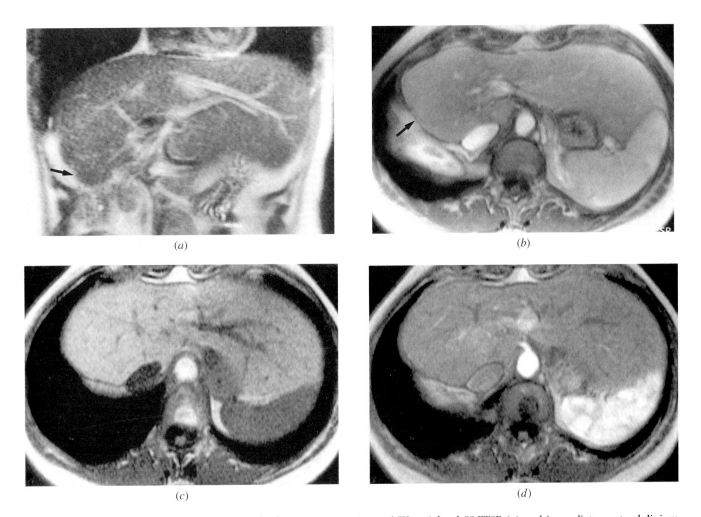

(a)

(b)

(c)

(d)

FIG. 2.148 Liver regeneration after right hepatectomy. Coronal T2-weighted SS-ETSE (*a*) and immediate postgadolinium SGE (*b*) images. The lateral segment of the left lobe is enlarged and rounded in contour (*a*, *b*). Hypertrophy of the medial segment results in an appearance of a pseudo-right lobe (arrow, *a*). A relatively sharp resection margin is noted (arrow, *b*) with no abnormal tissue apparent.

Transverse SGE (*c*) and immediate postgadolinium SGE (*d*) images in a second patient with hypertrophy of the left liver lobe after right lobectomy. Note that the lateral segment of the left lobe is enlarged but there is a clear distinction between the liver and the spleen.

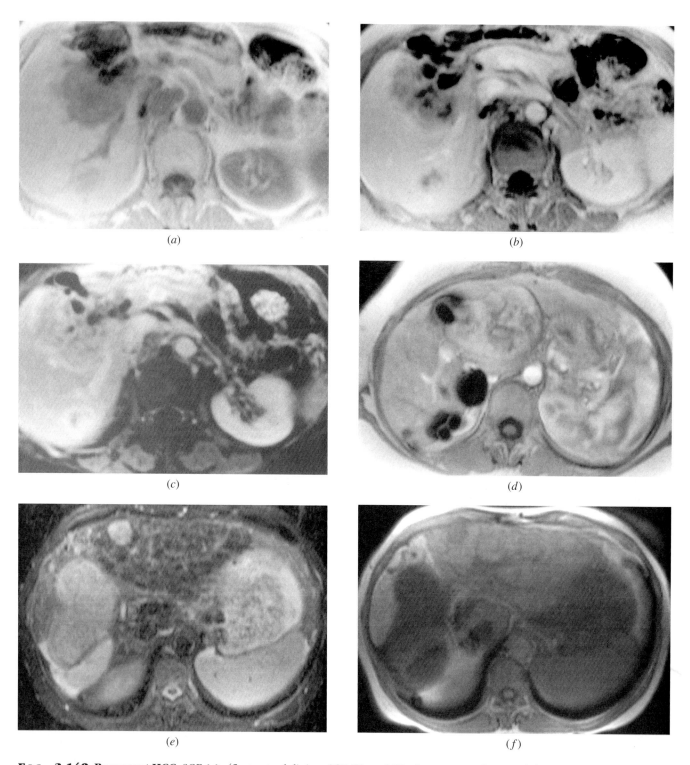

(a)

(b)

(c)

(d)

(e)

(f)

F I G . 2.149 Recurrent HCC. SGE (*a*), 45-s postgadolinium SGE (*b*), and 90-s fat-suppressed postgadolinium SGE (*c*) images. This patient had previously undergone a left hepatic lobe resection for HCC. There are multiple lesions throughout the right lobe, all of which appear low signal on T1-weighted images (*a*) and exhibit lesional enhancement after gadolinium (*b*, *c*), consistent with recurrent disease. Note the large volume of tumor along the resection margin consistent with incomplete excision.

Immediate postgadolinium SGE (*d*) image in a second patient with a history of HCC, and left hepatectomy. There is a large mass that enhances heterogeneously on immediate postgadolinium images, consistent with recurrent HCC. The recurrence is along the resection margin, compatible with incomplete excision. Note the surgical clips along the liver edge from prior resection.

T2-weighted fat-suppressed SS-ETSE (*e*), SGE (*f*), and immediate (*g*) and 90-s fat-suppressed (*h*) postgadolinium SGE images in a third patient with recurrence of HCC after liver resection show similar findings.

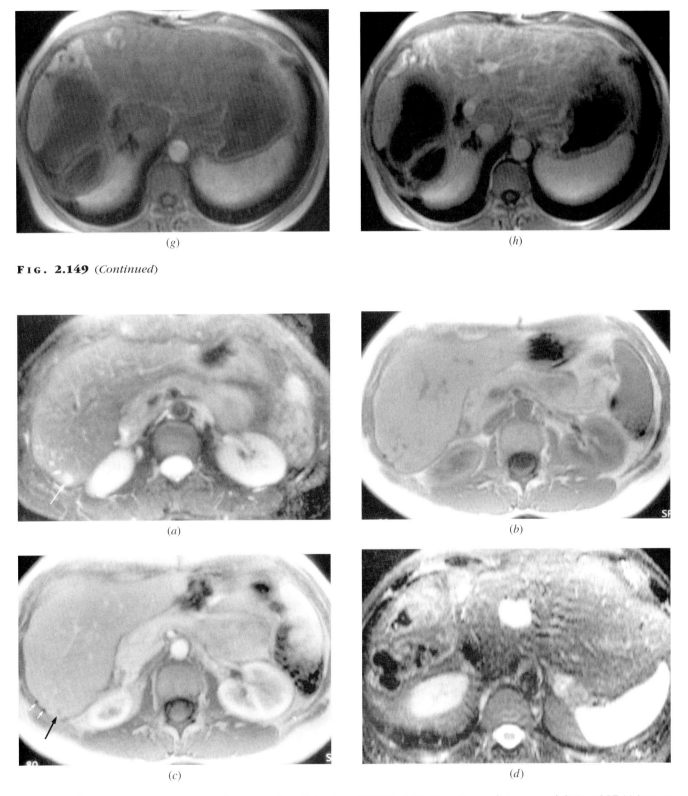

(g)   (h)

F I G . 2.149 (*Continued*)

(a)   (b)

(c)   (d)

F I G . 2.150 Recurrent metastases after resection. Echo-train STIR (*a*), SGE (*b*) and immediate postgadolinium SGE (*c*) images in a patient who has a history of colon cancer and previous resection of liver metastases. There is a small lesion that demonstrates moderately high signal on T2 (arrow, *a*), mildly low signal on T1 (*b*), and ring enhancement (arrow, *c*) after gadolinium administration, consistent with a recurrent metastasis. Note the surgical clips (small arrows, *c*) adjacent to the lesion.

Echo-train STIR (*d*), SGE (*e*), immediate postgadolinium SGE (*f*), and 90-s fat-suppressed postgadolinium SGE (*g*) images in a second patient, who has a history of gastrointestinal stromal sarcoma and right hepatectomy 15 months earlier for liver metastasis.

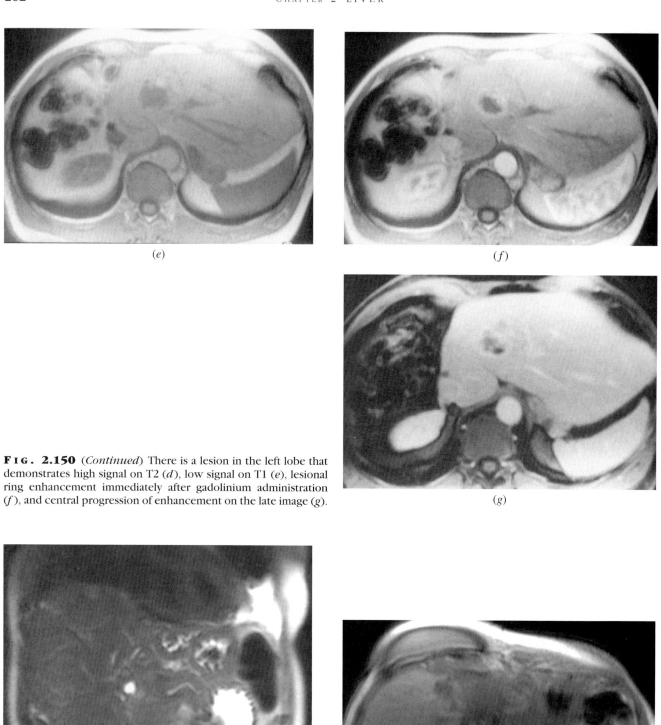

(e)

(f)

(g)

FIG. 2.150 (*Continued*) There is a lesion in the left lobe that demonstrates high signal on T2 (*d*), low signal on T1 (*e*), lesional ring enhancement immediately after gadolinium administration (*f*), and central progression of enhancement on the late image (*g*).

(a)

(b)

FIG. 2.151 Liver metastasis from breast cancer after radiation. Coronal T2-weighted SS-ETSE (*a*), immediate (*b*), 45-s (*c*), and 90-s fat-suppressed (*d*) postgadolinium SGE images, and sagittal 90-s fat-suppressed post gadolinium SGE image (*e*) in a patient with liver and bone metastases from breast cancer after breast radiation therapy. The left lobe of the liver is shrunken, causing

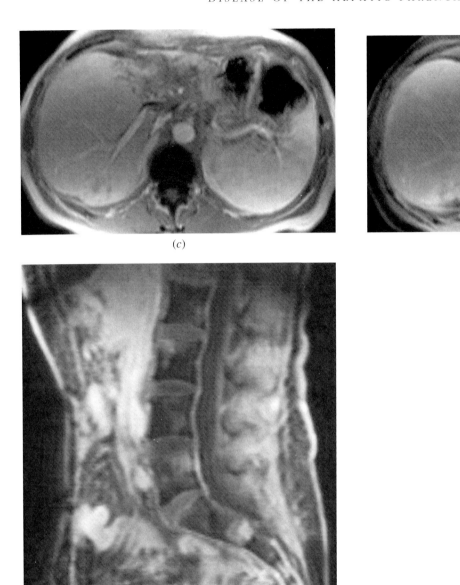

(c)

(d)

(e)

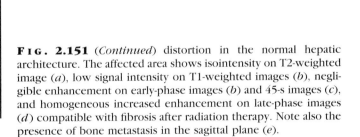

FIG. 2.151 (*Continued*) distortion in the normal hepatic architecture. The affected area shows isointensity on T2-weighted image (*a*), low signal intensity on T1-weighted images (*b*), negligible enhancement on early-phase images (*b*) and 45-s images (*c*), and homogeneous increased enhancement on late-phase images (*d*) compatible with fibrosis after radiation therapy. Note also the presence of bone metastasis in the sagittal plane (*e*).

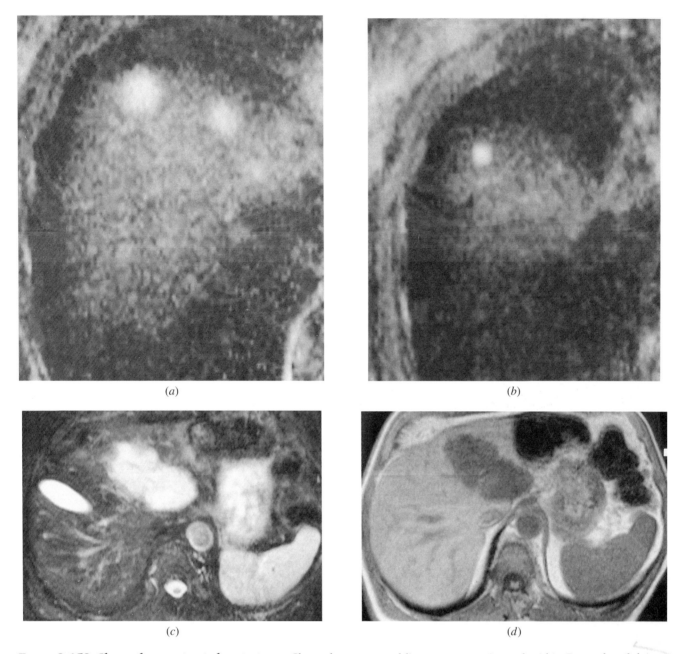

(a)

(b)

(c)

(d)

F I G . 2.152 Chemotherapy-treated metastases. Chemotherapy-treated liver metastases imaged within 7 months of therapy initiation. T2-weighted fat-suppressed ETSE image before (*a*) and 3 months after (*b*) initiation of chemotherapy. On the pretreatment examination (*a*), two metastases (1.5 cm and 1 cm) are evident in the dome of the liver. The metastases have slightly ill-defined margins and are moderately high in signal intensity. Three months after initiation of chemotherapy, the larger metastasis has decreased in size to 4 mm, has well-defined margins, and appears more hyperintense (*b*).

T2-weighted fat-suppressed SS-ETSE (*c*), SGE (*d*), and 90-s (*e*) and 10-min (*f*) postgadolinium SGE images in a second patient demonstrate two 4-cm metastases. The metastases are well-defined, moderately high in signal intensity on T2-weighted images (*c*), and moderately low in signal intensity on T1-weighted image (*d*) and demonstrate peripheral irregular enhancement (*e*) that progresses centripetally. The lesions appear hyperintense relative to liver with a low-signal intensity central scar at 10 min (*f*).

In both patients, the appearance of these subacute treated metastases (2–7 months after initiation of chemotherapy) mimics the appearance of hemangiomas. History of chemotherapy treatment for liver metastasis is critical to obtain in patients with lesions that resemble hemangiomas.

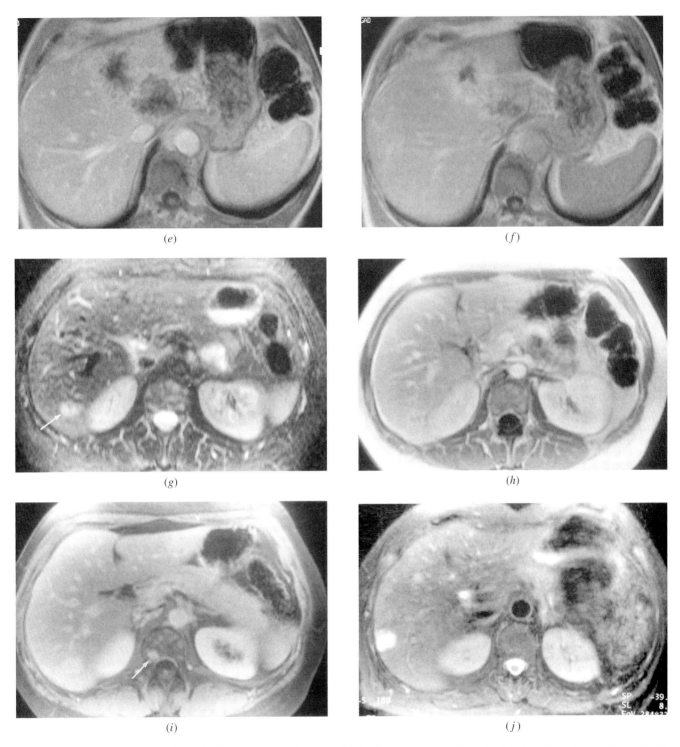

(e)

(f)

(g)

(h)

(i)

(j)

F I G . 2.152 (*Continued*) Echo-train STIR (*g*) and 45-s (*h*) and 90-s fat-suppressed (*i*) postgadolinium SGE images in a patient who has a history of liver metastases from breast cancer, treated with chemotherapy 2 years before this MR study. There is a lesion in the right hepatic lobe that demonstrates high signal on T2 (arrow, *g*), peripheral ring enhancement on the 45-s (*h*), and complete fill-in on the delayed image (*i*), consistent with a subacute chemotherapy-treated metastasis with features suggestive of hemangioma. Note also multiple bone metastases (arrow, *i*).

Echo-train STIR (*j*), SGE (*k*), and immediate (*l*) and 45-s (*m*) postgadolinium SGE images in a patient who has liver metastases from ovarian cancer. A lobular lesion is present in the right hepatic lobe that demonstrates high signal on T2 (*j*), low signal intensity

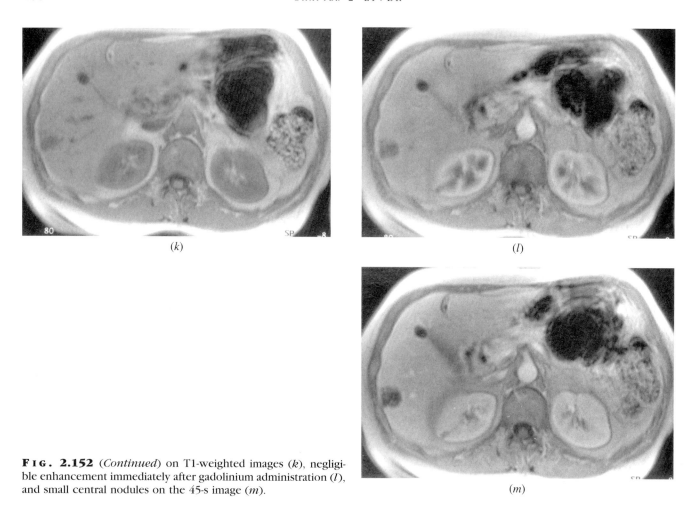

(k)

(l)

(m)

FIG. 2.152 (*Continued*) on T1-weighted images (*k*), negligible enhancement immediately after gadolinium administration (*l*), and small central nodules on the 45-s image (*m*).

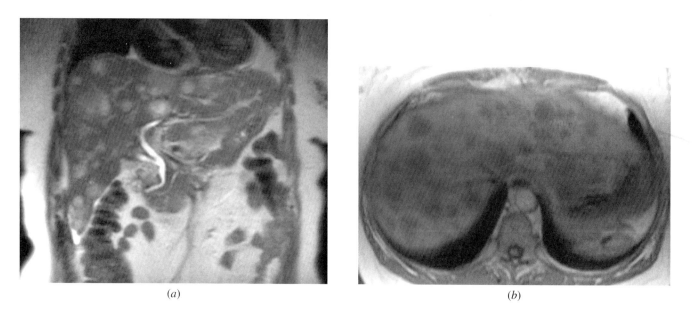

(a)

(b)

FIG. 2.153 Metastases from breast cancer before and after chemotherapy. Coronal T2-weighted SS-ETSE (*a*), SGE (*b*), and immediate (*c*) and 90-s fat-suppressed (*d*) postgadolinium SGE images. Multiple lesions are seen throughout the liver that appear

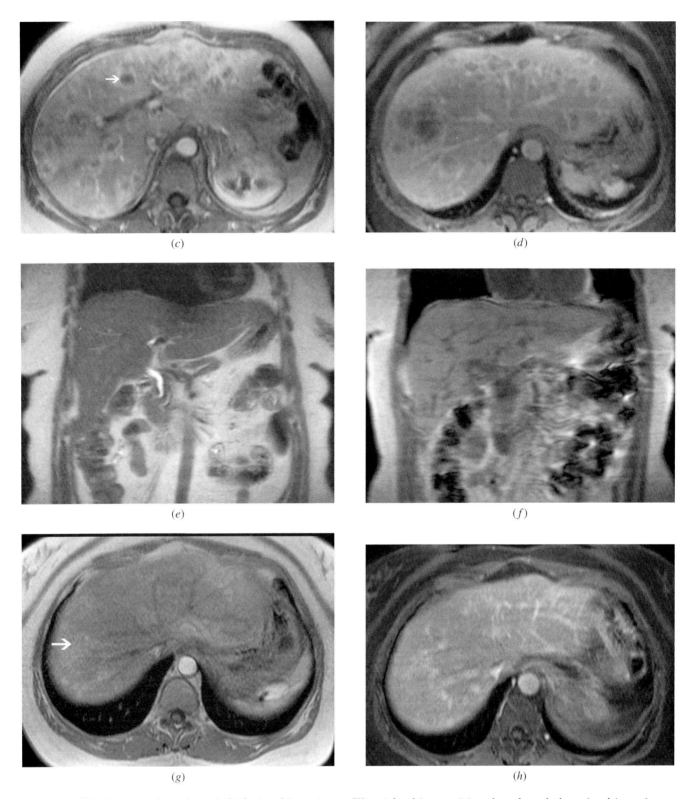

FIG. 2.153 (*Continued*) moderately high signal intensity on T2-weighted images (*a*) and moderately low signal intensity on T1-weighted image (*b*) and show ring enhancement on early-phase image (arrow, *c*) that become less conspicuous on the late-phase image (*d*). Coronal T2-weighted SS-ETSE (*e*) and T1-weighted SGE (*f*) and transverse immediate (*g*) and 90-s fat-suppressed (*h*) postgadolinium SGE images in the same patient after a course of cycles of chemotherapy. Only patchy enhancement on early-phase images can be appreciated (arrow, *g*). The remaining sequences are unremarkable.

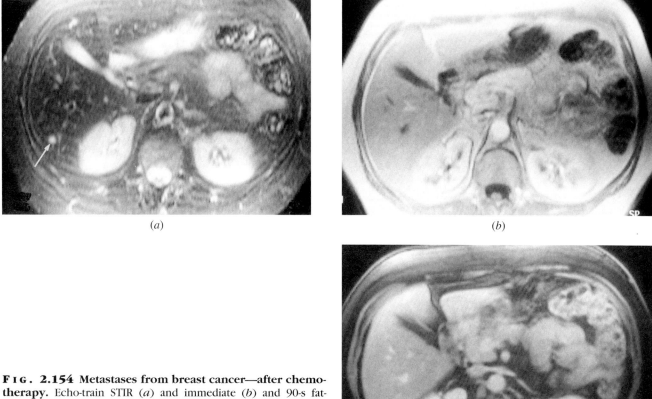

FIG. 2.154 Metastases from breast cancer—after chemo-therapy. Echo-train STIR (*a*) and immediate (*b*) and 90-s fat-suppressed (*c*) postgadolinium SGE images. There is a small lesion in the right lobe that exhibits high signal on T2 (arrow, *a*) and ring enhancement on the immediate postgadolinium image (*b*) that persists on the late image (*c*). High signal on T2-weighted images may be observed as an early response (<1 year) to chemotherapy.

low signal intensity on T1-weighted images. After contrast, these lesions exhibit negligible early enhancement with progressive enhancement on later postcontrast images (fig. 2.156).

The fibrotic process of chronic healed metastases may be very extensive in the presence of numerous liver metastases, such that a cirrhosis-type liver appearance may develop [238, 240]. This appearance is most commonly observed in breast cancer patients with a miliary pattern of hepatic metastases, who have subsequently shown a salutary response to chemotherapy (fig. 2.157).

During the course of chemotherapy, lesions develop acute granulation tissue that may mask the appearance of coexistent viable tumor. Successful resolution of metastases should not be considered until lesions are in the chronic healed phase.

Transcatheter Arterial Chemoembolization. Chemoembolic therapy is based on the pathophysiologic premise that hypervascular malignant tumors receive a disproportionately greater blood supply from hepatic arteries than surrounding intact liver and thus cytotoxic agents are preferentially delivered to malignant cells (figs. 2.158–2.162) [242]. Within 1 month after chemoembolization, complete response is demonstrated by the lack of enhancing tumor stroma. In one report [232], 27 tumors treated with chemoembolization were low in signal on T2-weighted image and showed lack of enhancement after contrast administration. All of these tumors were necrotic at biopsy. Partial response shows increased signal intensity on T2-weighted images and enhancement on immediate postgadolinium images of residual tumor (fig. 2.163). Substantial variation does occur, reflecting variation in the degree of response and the time course of healing. One series correlated serial changes of liver lesions on T2, T1, and dynamic postgadolinium images before and after chemoembolization (figs. 2.158 and 2.160) [257]. On pretreatment MR studies, homogeneous intense enhancement on hepatic arterial dominant-phase images combined with small malignant lesion size were the best predictors of successful response. Lesions that showed good response became low signal on T2-weighted images immediately

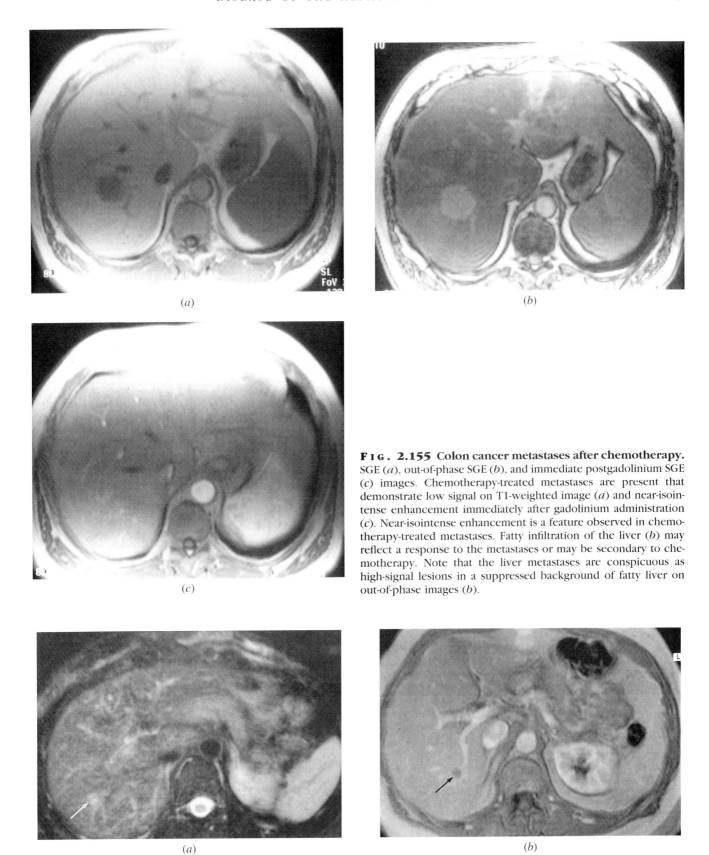

F I G . 2.155 Colon cancer metastases after chemotherapy. SGE (*a*), out-of-phase SGE (*b*), and immediate postgadolinium SGE (*c*) images. Chemotherapy-treated metastases are present that demonstrate low signal on T1-weighted image (*a*) and near-isointense enhancement immediately after gadolinium administration (*c*). Near-isointense enhancement is a feature observed in chemotherapy-treated metastases. Fatty infiltration of the liver (*b*) may reflect a response to the metastases or may be secondary to chemotherapy. Note that the liver metastases are conspicuous as high-signal lesions in a suppressed background of fatty liver on out-of-phase images (*b*).

F I G . 2.156 Liver metastases, chronic (11 years) after chemotherapy treatment. T2-weighted fat-suppressed ETSE (*a*) and immediate postgadolinium SGE (*b*) images. A 7-mm lesion is present in the right lobe of the liver that is minimally hyperintense on the T2-weighted image (arrow, *a*) and demonstrates negligible enhancement on the immediate postgadolinium SGE image (arrow, *b*).

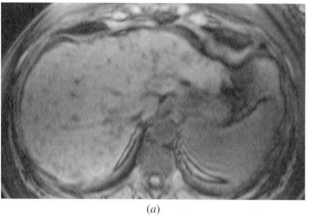

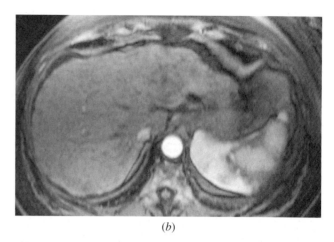

(a)

(b)

FIG. 2.157 Chronic treated metastases simulating cirrhosis. Non-contrast T1-weighted fat-suppressed 3D-gradient echo (*a*), immediate (*b*) and 2 min (*c*) postgadolinium fat-suppressed 3D gradient echo images. The liver has an irregular contour and contains numerous angular-marginated focal lesions, many with adjacent linear stranding, and some associated with capsule retraction. The lesions are low signal intensity on T1-weighted images (*a*) and show negligible enhancement on early (*b*) and late (*c*) postgadolinium images, consistent with focal masses of low biological activity. The appearance of these lesions is diagnostic for chronic fibrotic lesions, in this case, chronically fibrosed breast cancer liver metastases. The background hepatic fibrosis that may develop in patients who have breast cancer with chronically treated liver metastases, reflects a marked fibrogenic response, and may simulate the appearance of hepatic cirrhosis. Clinical history and the presence of numerous larger angular marginated defects (the latter may not always be present) establishes the correct diagnosis.

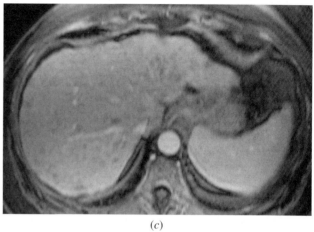

(c)

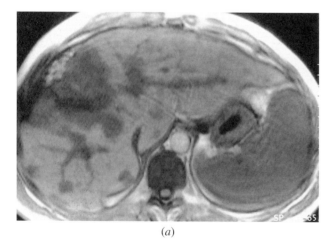

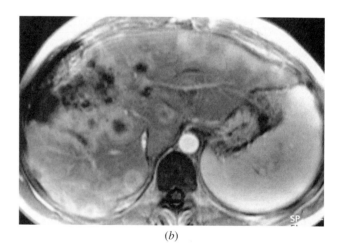

(a)

(b)

FIG. 2.158 Liver metastases, before and after chemoembolization. SGE (*a*) and immediate postgadolinium SGE (*b*) images before chemoembolization and immediate postgadolinium SGE image (*c*) 1 month after chemoembolization. On the pretreatment images (*a*, *b*), an 8-cm tumor and multiple tumors <2.5 cm are present throughout the liver. Prominent ring enhancement is present in these tumors (*b*). One month after chemoembolization (*c*), lesions have decreased in size and number and mural enhancement has markedly diminished.

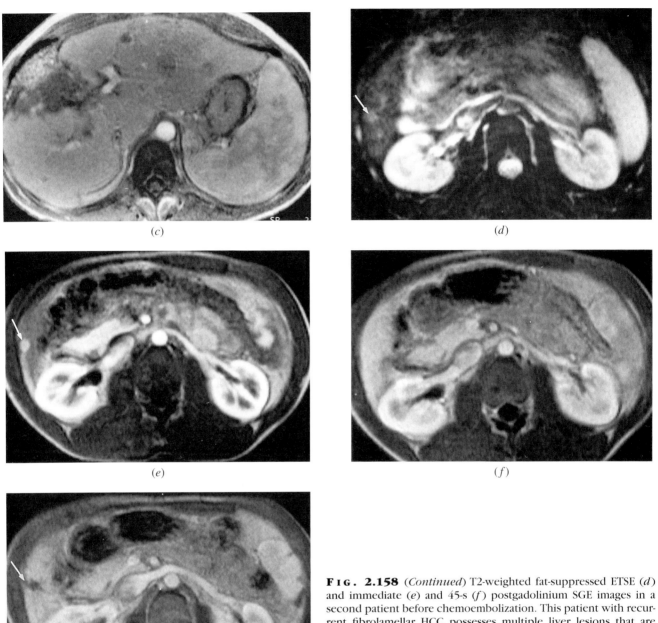

(c)

(d)

(e)

(f)

(g)

FIG. 2.158 (*Continued*) T2-weighted fat-suppressed ETSE (*d*) and immediate (*e*) and 45-s (*f*) postgadolinium SGE images in a second patient before chemoembolization. This patient with recurrent fibrolamellar HCC possesses multiple liver lesions that are moderately high in signal intensity on T2-weighted images (arrow, *d*), show intense uniform enhancement immediately after gadolinium administration (arrow, *e*), and fade rapidly to isointensity with liver by 45 s (*f*). Immediate postgadolinium SGE image acquired 1 month after chemoembolization (*g*) shows complete lack of enhancement of the lesion, which now has polygonal angular margins (arrow, *g*), consistent with scarring.

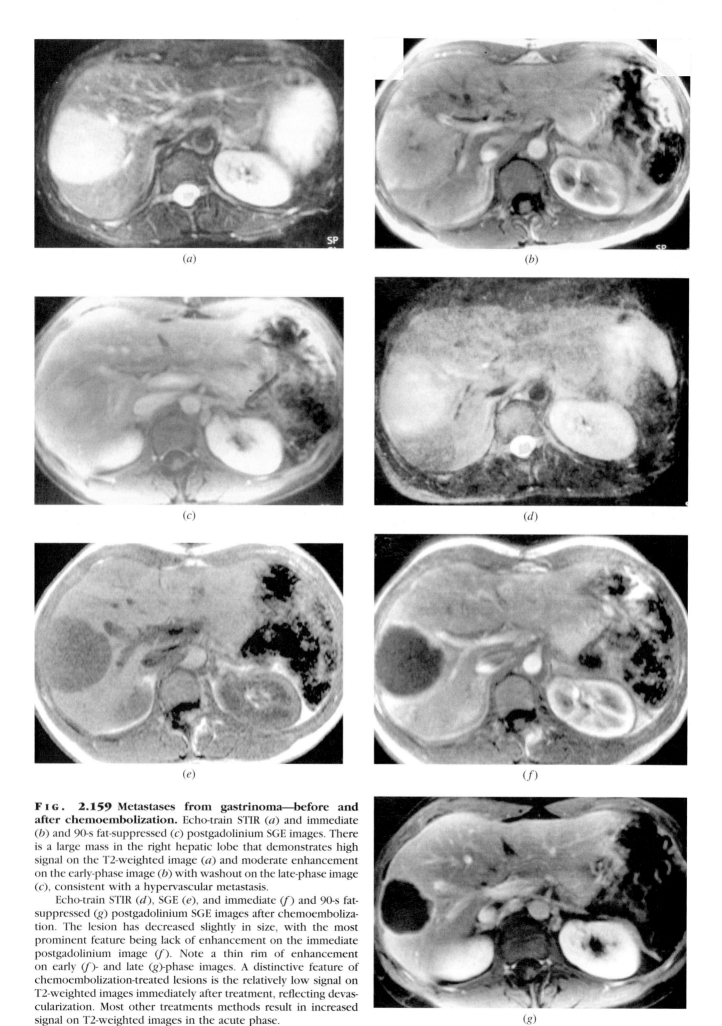

F I G . 2.159 Metastases from gastrinoma—before and after chemoembolization. Echo-train STIR (*a*) and immediate (*b*) and 90-s fat-suppressed (*c*) postgadolinium SGE images. There is a large mass in the right hepatic lobe that demonstrates high signal on the T2-weighted image (*a*) and moderate enhancement on the early-phase image (*b*) with washout on the late-phase image (*c*), consistent with a hypervascular metastasis.

Echo-train STIR (*d*), SGE (*e*), and immediate (*f*) and 90-s fat-suppressed (*g*) postgadolinium SGE images after chemoembolization. The lesion has decreased slightly in size, with the most prominent feature being lack of enhancement on the immediate postgadolinium image (*f*). Note a thin rim of enhancement on early (*f*)- and late (*g*)-phase images. A distinctive feature of chemoembolization-treated lesions is the relatively low signal on T2-weighted images immediately after treatment, reflecting devascularization. Most other treatments methods result in increased signal on T2-weighted images in the acute phase.

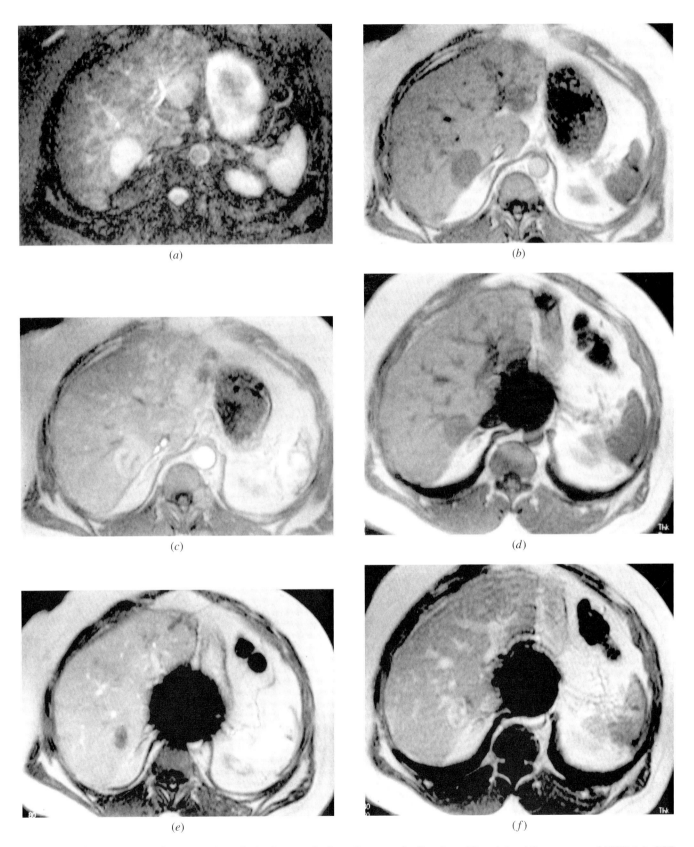

F I G . 2.160 Metastasis from carcinoid—before and after chemoembolization. T2-weighted fat-suppressed ETSE (*a*), SGE (*b*), and immediate postgadolinium SGE (*c*) images. A 4-cm metastasis is present in the right lobe and a second 4-cm lesion in the lateral segment. They appear moderately high signal intensity on T2-weighted image (*a*) and moderately low signal intensity on T1-weighted image (*b*) and show intense enhancement on early-phase image (*c*).

SGE (*d*) and immediate (*e*) and 45-s (*f*) postgadolinium SGE images in the same patient after chemoembolization. Note that the lesion has decreased in size and shows minimal enhancement on the immediate postgadolinium image (*e*), with progressive enhancement on later images. This enhancement pattern is consistent with fibrosis. Note the large metal artifact in the porta hepatis that represents a metal coil placed at the time of chemoembolization.

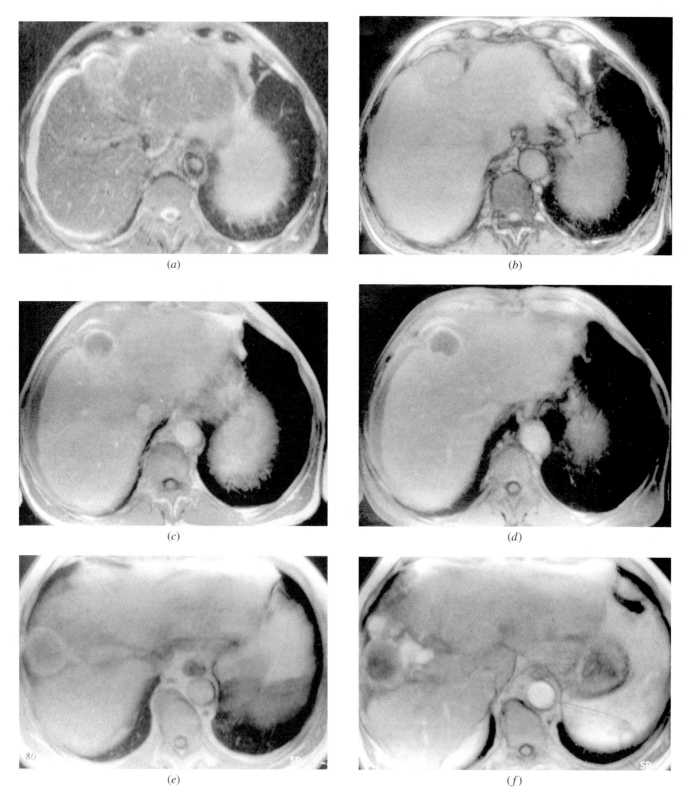

(a)   (b)

(c)   (d)

(e)   (f)

F I G . 2.161 HCC and chemoembolization. Echo-train STIR (*a*), out-of-phase SGE (*b*), and 45-s (*c*) and 90-s fat-suppressed (*d*) postgadolinium SGE images. A rounded lesion is seen in the left hepatic lobe that demonstrates minimal high signal intensity on T2 (*a*), minimal low signal intensity with a high signal rim on T1 (*b*), capsular enhancement after gadolinium (*c, d*) with lack of tumor enhancement. The combination of isointensity on T2 with lack of central enhancement on postgadolinium T1-weighted images is consistent with devascularization of tumor, which occurs after chemoembolization.

SGE (*e*), immediate postgadolinium SGE (*f*), and 90-s fat-suppressed postgadolinium SGE (*g*) images in a second patient. There is an oval lesion located in the right hepatic lobe that shows decreased signal intensity centrally and increased signal intensity

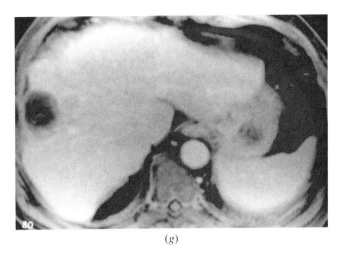

(g)

FIG. 2.161 (*Continued*) peripherally on the noncontrast T1-weighted image (*e*). On the immediate postgadolinium image (*f*), there is intense enhancement with well-defined margins anterior to the ablation site. This persistent tumor washes out and shows late capsule enhancement on interstitial phase images (*g*). The central devascularized ablation site does not enhance on early or late postcontrast images. The high-signal material on the precontrast T1-weighted image (*e*) represents extracellular methemoglobin.

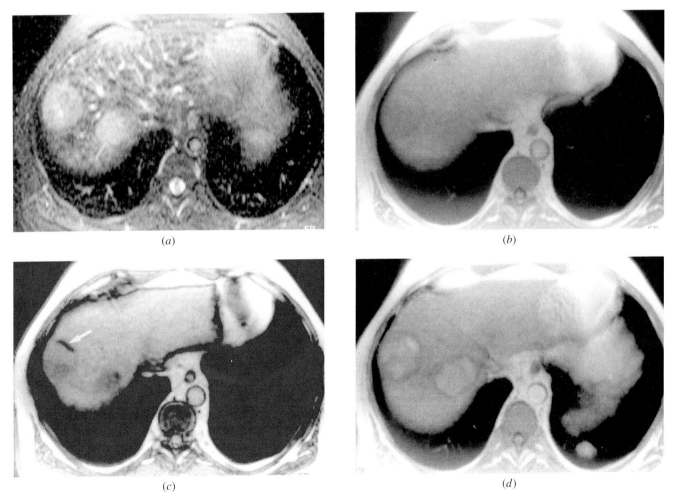

(a)

(b)

(c)

(d)

FIG. 2.162 HCC after chemoembolization—poor response. Echo-train STIR (*a*), SGE (*b*), out-of-phase SGE (*c*), and immediate (*d*) and 90-s fat-suppressed (*e*) postgadolinium SGE images. There are two rounded lesions that are mildly high signal on T2 (*a*) and minimally low signal on T1 (*b*) and demonstrate intense heterogeneous enhancement immediately after gadolinium (*d*), with washout and capsular enhancement on the late image (*e*), consistent with HCC. Note that one of the lesions demonstrates a small focus (arrow, *c*) that exhibits signal drop on the out-of-phase image, consistent with fat.

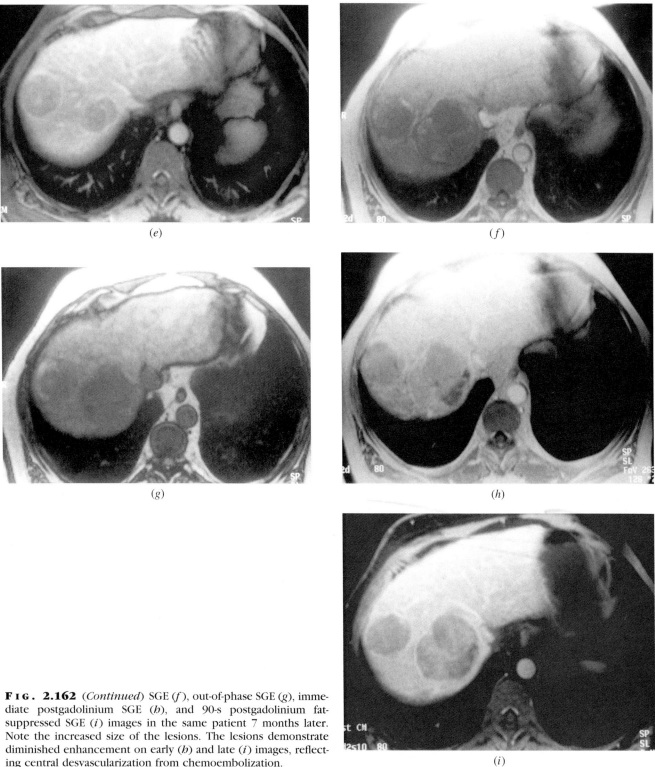

(e)

(f)

(g)

(h)

(i)

F I G . 2.162 (*Continued*) SGE (*f*), out-of-phase SGE (*g*), immediate postgadolinium SGE (*h*), and 90-s postgadolinium fat-
suppressed SGE (*i*) images in the same patient 7 months later.
Note the increased size of the lesions. The lesions demonstrate
diminished enhancement on early (*h*) and late (*i*) images, reflecting central desvascularization from chemoembolization.

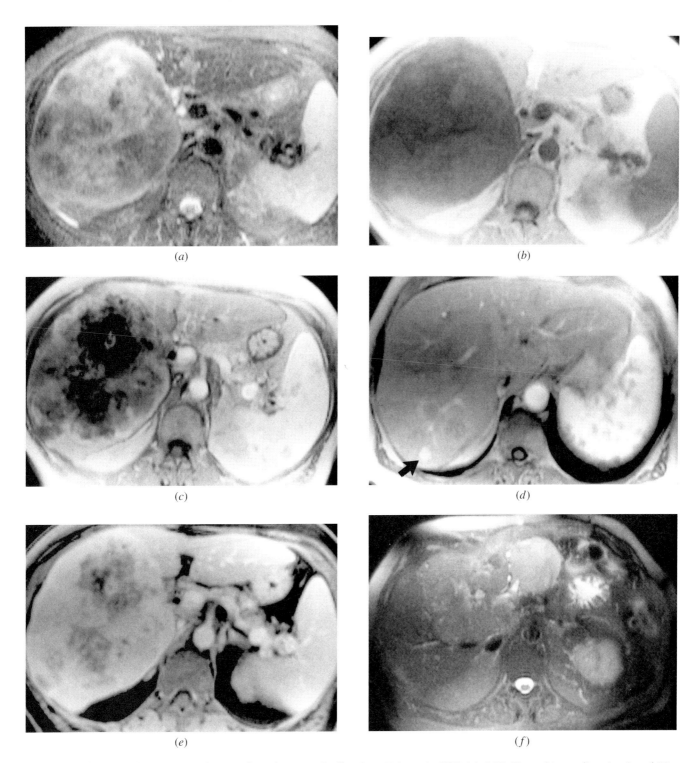

(a)

(b)

(c)

(d)

(e)

(f)

FIG. 2.163 Partial response of HCC after chemoembolization. Echo-train STIR (*a*), SGE (*b*), and immediate (*c, d*) and 90-s fat-suppressed (*e*) postgadolinium SGE images. There is a huge mass that shows high signal intensity on T2-weighted image (*a*) and low signal intensity on T1-weighted image (*b*). Immediately after gadolinium, it shows intense heterogeneous enhancement (*c*) with large regions of low signal centrally within the tumor consistent with necrosis, reflecting a partial response to chemoembolization. On a higher tomographic section, a small satellite HCC (arrow, *d*) is present, which demonstrates intense uniform enhancement.

T2-weighted fat-suppressed SS-ETSE (*f*), SGE (*g*), and immediate (*h*) and 90-s fat-suppressed (*i*) postgadolinium SGE images in a second patient. There is a lesion mainly on the left lobe of the liver that shows moderate high signal intensity on T2-weighted

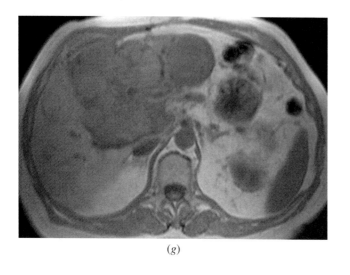

(g)

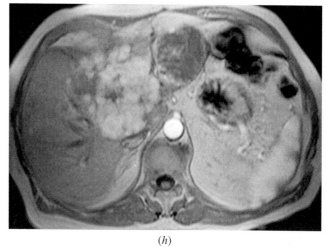

(h)

FIG. 2.163 (*Continued*) image (*f*), low signal intensity on T1-weighted image (*g*), and a partial enhancement on early-phase image (*h*) that washes out on late-phase image (*i*). The enhanced portion corresponds to viable tumor and the nonenhanced area to necrosis.

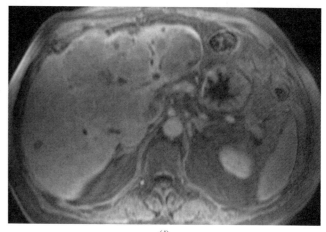

(i)

after treatment, reflecting the devascularization of tumor. Low signal intensity on T2-weighted images early after therapy is distinctive for chemoembolization. This differs from local therapy techniques (e.g., RF ablation), which result in high T2 signal early after therapy. The best indication of good response is negligible enhancement on hepatic arterial dominant-phase images after chemoembolization.

Ablative Therapies. Radiofrequency (RF) ablation, cryoablation, ethanol ablation, microwave ablation, and laser ablation are alternative methods to treat focal liver malignancies when curative resection is not feasible (figs. 2.164–2.166) [235].

Successful treatment occurs when the entire tumor is destroyed with mild injury of the surrounding parenchyma. The best predictor of successful ablation is the size of the necrotic cavity after intervention. The ablated area must exceed the tumor margins by approximately 1.0 cm [258]. Over time, the ablated zone might either regress in dimensions or retain similar size to pretreatment [259, 260]. Small necrotic areas may disappear

completely. Enlargement of the ablated area on follow-up examinations is suggestive of unsuccessful intervention [261, 262].

Up to 1 week after ablation, the signal intensity on T2-weighted and T1-weighted images is determined by the stage of hemorrhage and the presence of either liquefactive or coagulative necrosis [259, 262, 263]. In a successful procedure, lack of contrast enhancement is observed. Initially after intervention, an ill-defined perilesional rim is often observed, measuring up to 1 cm in thickness, that appears mildly high signal intensity on T2-weighted images and exhibits moderate to intense enhancement on arterial dominant-phase images [259, 262, 263]. The thickness of this perilesional rim regresses over time in successfully treated lesions, which additionally shows decrease in the extent of enhancement on early-phase images and gradually disappears by 6 months after ablation (figs. 2.167 and 2.168) [258, 260, 263, 264]. At histopathology, the perilesional rim corresponds to intense inflammatory reaction and hemorrhage, which gradually are replaced by granulation tissue [258, 263, 265].

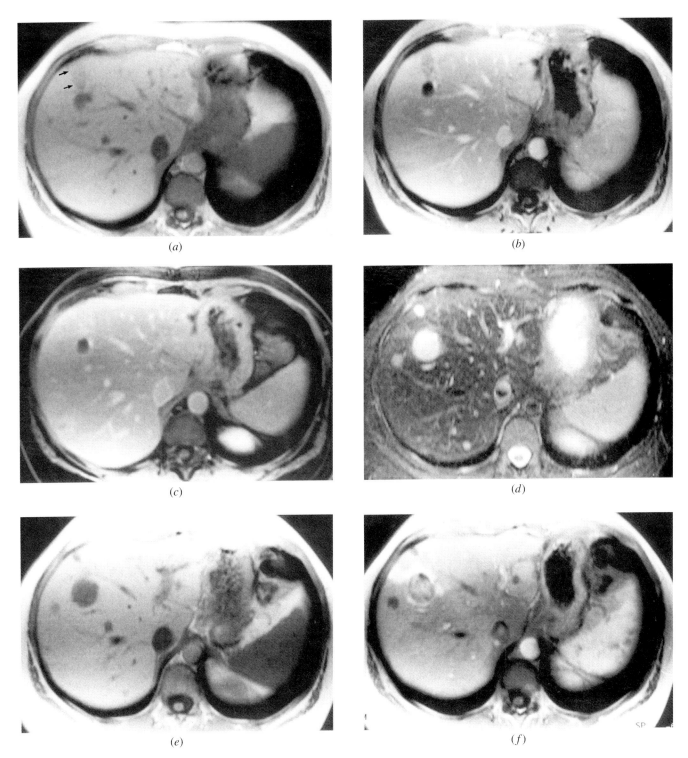

(a)

(b)

(c)

(d)

(e)

(f)

F I G . 2.164 Radiofrequency ablation. SGE (*a*), 45-s postgadolinium SGE (*b*), and 90-s postgadolinium fat-suppressed SGE (*c*) images in a patient, who has a history of a liver metastasis from retroperitoneum leiomyosarcoma that has been treated with radiofrequency ablation. There is a rounded lesion in the right hepatic lobe that demonstrates low signal on T1 (*a*), negligible enhancement immediately after gadolinium administration (*b*), and a thin rim of enhancement on the late image (*c*). Note that the track of the radiofrequency probe is visible as a linear defect extending from the liver surface to the lesion (arrows, *a*).

Echo-train STIR (*d*), SGE (*e*), and immediate (*f*) and 90-s fat-suppressed (*g*) postgadolinium SGE images in the same patient 2 months later. More lesions are appreciated in the hepatic parenchyma. The largest lesion, which was present on the first exam, demonstrates diffuse heterogeneous enhancement on the immediate postgadolinium image (*f*) that persists on the later image (*g*), in comparison to the findings from the earlier study in which no central lesion enhancement was observed. Note the presence of perilesional enhancement on the immediate postgadolinium image (*f*).

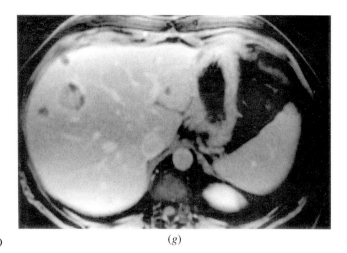

FIG. 2.164 (*Continued*)   (*g*)

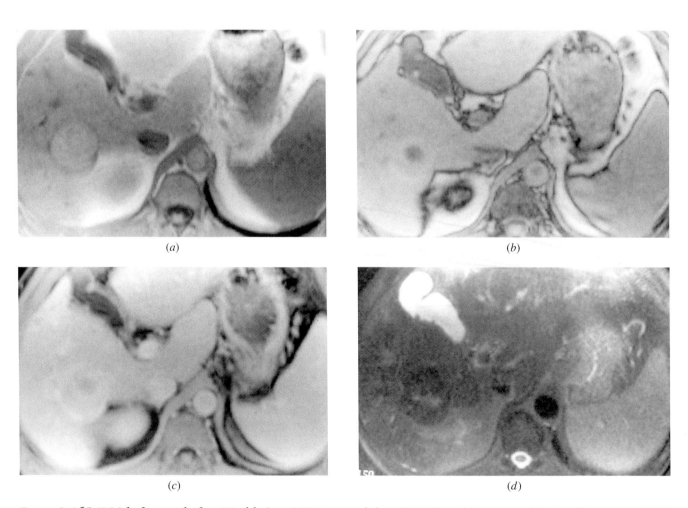

(*a*)   (*b*)

(*c*)   (*d*)

FIG. 2.165 HCC before and after RF ablation. SGE (*a*), out-of-phase SGE (*b*), and 90-s postgadolinium fat-suppressed SGE (*c*) images. There is an HCC in the right hepatic lobe that is isointense on T1 (*a*), contains a central focus that drops in signal on out-of-phase (*b*), and demonstrates heterogeneous enhancement on interstitial-phase images. The central focus that loses signal on out-of-phase represents fat.

T2-weighted fat-suppressed SS-ETSE (*d*), SGE (*e*), out-of-phase SGE (*f*), 45-s postgadolinium SGE (*g*), and 90-s postgadolinium fat-suppressed SGE (*h*) images in the same patient 5 months later, after radiofrequency ablation. The HCC has increased in size, is

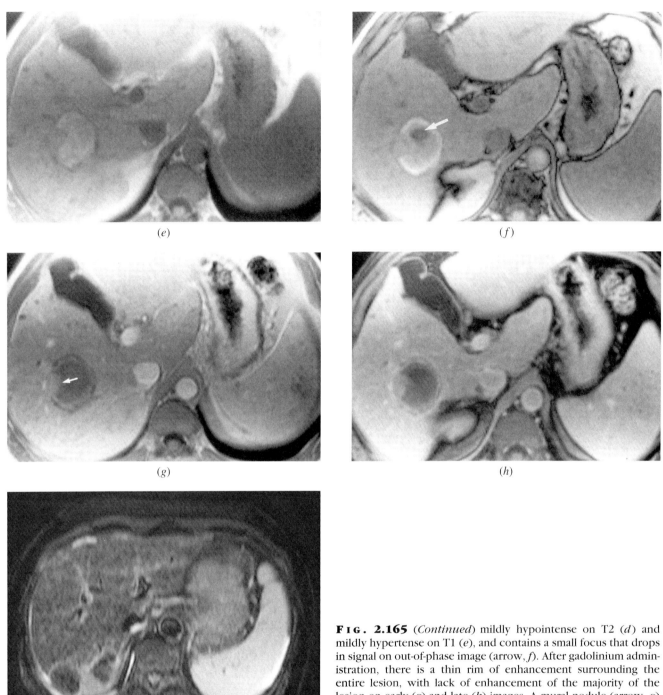

(e)

(f)

(g)

(h)

(i)

F I G . 2.165 (*Continued*) mildly hypointense on T2 (*d*) and mildly hypertense on T1 (*e*), and contains a small focus that drops in signal on out-of-phase image (arrow, *f*). After gadolinium administration, there is a thin rim of enhancement surrounding the entire lesion, with lack of enhancement of the majority of the lesion on early (*g*) and late (*h*) images. A mural nodule (arrow, *g*) is present along the lateral wall of the lesion that demonstrates moderate contrast enhancement consistent with residual tumor.

T2-weighted fat-suppressed SS-ETSE (*i*), SGE (*j*), and immediate (*k*) and 90-s fat-suppressed (*l*) postgadolinium 3D-gradient

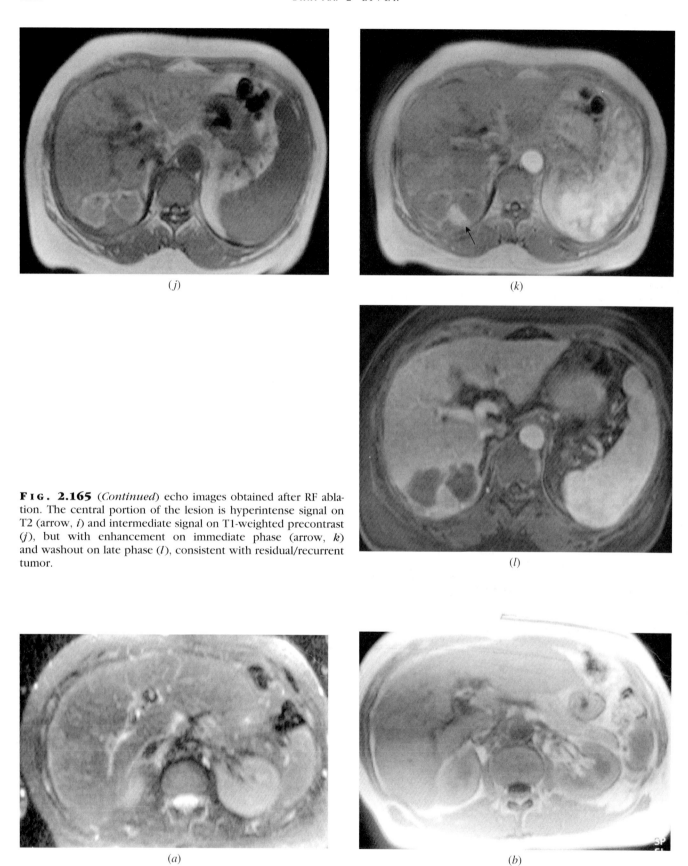

(j)

(k)

FIG. 2.165 (*Continued*) echo images obtained after RF ablation. The central portion of the lesion is hyperintense signal on T2 (arrow, *i*) and intermediate signal on T1-weighted precontrast (*j*), but with enhancement on immediate phase (arrow, *k*) and washout on late phase (*l*), consistent with residual/recurrent tumor.

(l)

(a)

(b)

FIG. 2.166 HCC before and after RF ablation. Echo-train STIR (*a*), SGE (*b*), immediate postgadolinium SGE (*c*), and 90-s postgadolinium fat-suppressed SGE (*d*) images. There is a small lesion in the right hepatic lobe that is near isointense on T2 (*a*)

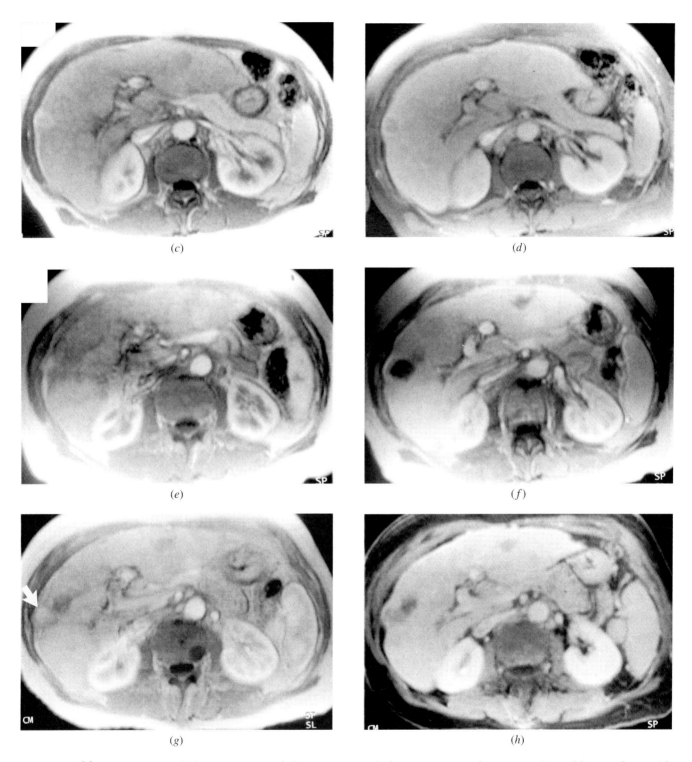

(c)

(d)

(e)

(f)

(g)

(h)

F I G . 2.166 (*Continued*) and T1 (*b*) images and demonstrates early heterogeneous enhancement (*c*) and late washout with capsule enhancement (*d*), consistent with a small HCC. Immediate (*e*) and 45-s (*f*) postgadolinium SGE images in the same patient 1 week after radiofrequency ablation show a necrotic lesion with thick ring enhancement on the 45-s postcontrast administration image (*f*). Immediate postgadolinium SGE (*g*) and 90-s postgadolinium fat-suppressed SGE (*h*) images 2 months after radiofrequency ablation. In the interval, a soft tissue mass (arrow, *g*) has developed on the lateral aspect of the tumor consistent with recurrence. The recurrent nodule shows moderate enhancement on the immediate postgadolinium images (*g*) with heterogeneous washout at 90 s (*h*).

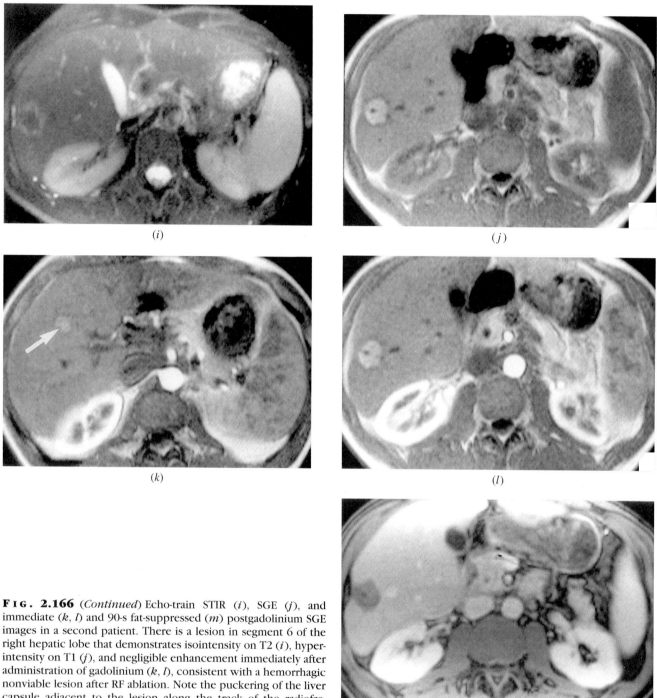

FIG. 2.166 (*Continued*) Echo-train STIR (*i*), SGE (*j*), and immediate (*k*, *l*) and 90-s fat-suppressed (*m*) postgadolinium SGE images in a second patient. There is a lesion in segment 6 of the right hepatic lobe that demonstrates isointensity on T2 (*i*), hyperintensity on T1 (*j*), and negligible enhancement immediately after administration of gadolinium (*k*, *l*), consistent with a hemorrhagic nonviable lesion after RF ablation. Note the puckering of the liver capsule adjacent to the lesion along the track of the radiofrequency probe. A small satellite lesion (arrow, *k*) has developed in the interval between radiofrequency ablation and this MR study.

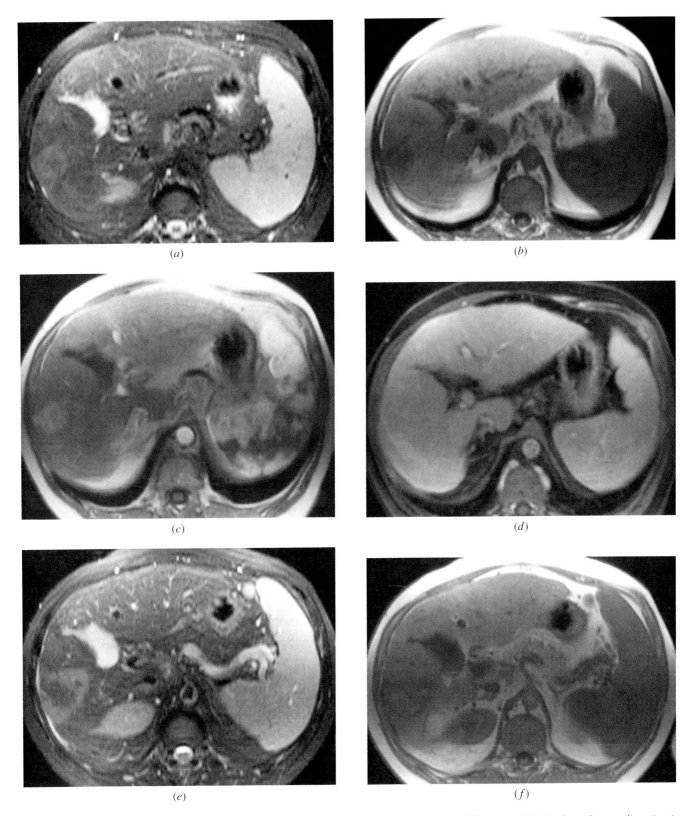

FIG. 2.167 HCC before and after RF ablation—early changes. T2-weighted SS-ETSE (*a, e*), SGE (*b, f*), and immediate (*c, g*) and 90-s fat-suppressed (*d, h*) postgadolinium SGE images. Before RF ablation (*a–d*), a lesion is appreciated in the right hepatic lobe that shows mildly high signal intensity on T2-weighted image (*a*), mildly low signal intensity on T1-weighted image (*b*), and intense enhancement on early-phase image (*d*) that fades with capsule enhancement on late-phase image (*d*), consistent with an HCC. At 1 week after RF ablation (*e–h*), the ablated area demonstrates isointensity on T2-weighted image (*e*), high signal intensity on T1-weighted image (*f*), and lack of enhancement on early (*g*)- and late (*h*)-phase images. Surrounding the ablated area, there is

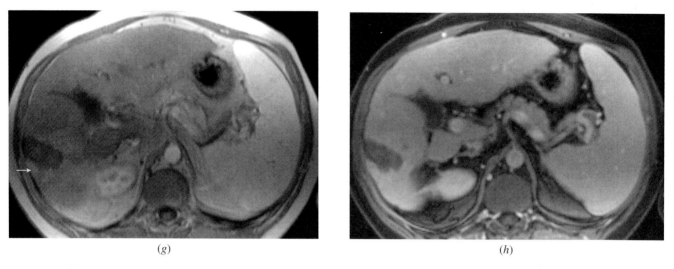

(g)   (h)

FIG. 2.167 (*Continued*) a parenchymal reaction due to the intervention, and it demonstrates high signal intensity on T2-weighted image (*e*), low signal intensity on T1-weighted image (*f*), and moderate enhancement on early-phase image (arrow, *g*) that fades on late-phase image (*h*). This inflammatory reaction is normal early after RF ablation.

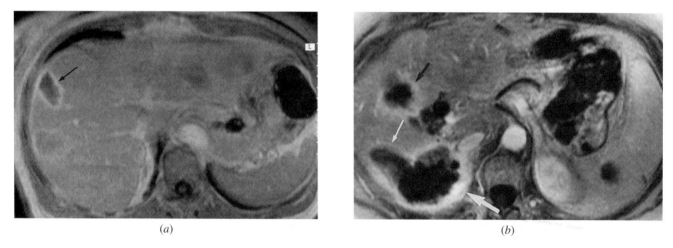

(a)   (b)

FIG. 2.168 Liver metastases after cryotherapy—acute changes. Transverse 90-s postgadolinium SGE images (*a*, *b*) in two patients. In the first patient (*a*), a cryotherapy defect is present in the right lobe (arrow, *a*) that has a uniform-thickness enhancing wall in continuity with enhancing liver capsule of similar thickness. In the acute stage, this appearance is compatible with tumor ablation and formation of acute granulation tissue along the cavity wall. The oblong shape of the defect corresponds to the direction of placement of the cryotherapy device. In the second patient (*b*), a cryotherapy tract (thin white arrow, *b*) is noted in continuity with a necrotic cavity. Portions of the cavity wall are thick and irregular (large white arrow, *b*). A second cryotherapy defect is noted in a more anterior location (black arrow, *b*). The cavity wall is thick and irregular. The presence of thick irregular walls after treatment is consistent with persistent disease.

The presence of a nodular focus distorting the internal contour within the ablated area is indicative of residual or recurrent tumor [258, 259, 263, 266]. Residual or recurrent tumor shows moderately high signal intensity on T2-weighted images and moderate to intense enhancement on arterial dominant-phase images, which may persist on late-phase images (fig. 2.169).

Gas bubbles present within the necrotic cavity immediately after the intervention are a common feature and tend to disappear within the first month [264, 267, 268]. Gas bubbles appear signal void on both T2- and T1-weighted images and show lack of enhancement after contrast administration.

Perfusional parenchymal abnormalities may be seen after ablation, and they may be due to arterial-venous

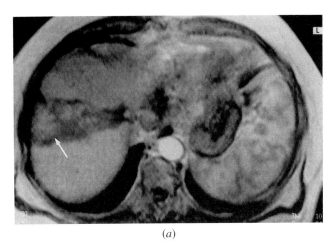
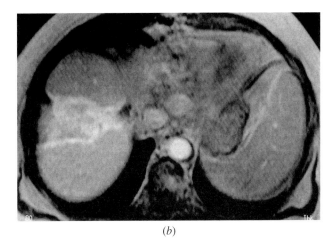

(a)   (b)

F I G . 2.169 Liver metastases after cryotherapy—chronic changes with recurrent disease. Immediate (*a*) and 10-min (*b*) postgadolinium SGE images. A large wedge-shaped defect is present in the superior aspect of the liver that enhances minimally on the immediate postgadolinium image (*a*) and shows delayed enhancement at 10 min (*b*). This enhancement pattern is consistent with fibrosis. Focal irregular regions of soft tissue are identified within the wedge-shaped tissue (arrow, *a*) that represent recurrent adenocarcinoma.

shunts or obstructed vascular structures. Often, the perfusional abnormalities vanish by 1 month after the procedure [264, 269]. On MRI, perfusional abnormalities are seen as wedge-shaped enhancing areas on early-phase images that fade on late-phase images.

HEPATIC TRANSPLANTATION

Liver disease is the tenth leading cause of death in the United States, and transplantation has become the treatment of choice for end-stage disease [270]. Major recent advances and technical progress in liver surgery and transplantation have been based, in large part, on improved understanding of the internal architecture of the liver. Toward this end, MRI provides valuable information for preoperative and postoperative liver evaluation of both donors and recipients. The increased utilization of adult-to-adult living related hemi-liver donation has resulted in an increased role for MRI in the preoperative evaluation, reflecting the comprehensive nature of the information provided by MRI. Donors may undergo a liver MR protocol with MRCP and MRA (figs. 2.170–2.172). The usual surgical procedure involves resecting the right lobe for donation and retaining the left lobe in the donor. The resection plane is approximately 1 cm into the right lobe from the middle hepatic vein and extends inferiorly to the bifurcation between the right and left portal veins [271], so that the donor retains the middle hepatic vein. Evaluation is made of relative size of right and left lobes and anomalies of the biliary or vascular system. Contraindications

for transplant include focal mass lesions, depending on size and type (e.g., malignant), or preexistent diffuse liver disease that may be the same type as that in the recipient (e.g., chronic hepatitis, primary sclerosing cholangitis). After surgery, donors are assessed for surgical complications of transplantation (e.g., abscess, biloma, transection or stenosis of vessels on bile duct) and for hypertrophy of the left lobe (figs. 2.173 and 2.174).

In recipients, preoperatively, patency of the inferior vena cava, portal vein, hepatic artery, and common bile duct are evaluated, and the presence of malignant disease is determined. Patients with malignant tumors evaluated for possible transplantation are evaluated for extent of hepatic involvement and for the presence of porta hepatis nodes or distant disease. Recipients may receive living related partial livers (lateral segment for small pediatric patients, right lobe for adult-to-adult recipients) (fig. 2.175) or cadaveric whole or partial livers (fig. 2.176).

The most common cause of early liver graft failure is rejection. The incidence of rejection is as high as 64% in some published series [272]. Early diagnosis is essential to allow modification of immunosuppressive therapy [273]. The differential diagnosis of rejection includes biliary obstruction, cholangitis, ischemic injury, viral infection, and drug toxicity.

Vascular complications are important causes of graft failure [274, 275]. Hepatic artery thrombosis is the most frequent and severe complication, occurring in up to 12% of adult patients [276, 277]. Hepatic artery patency can be documented by MRI in most cases. Technical

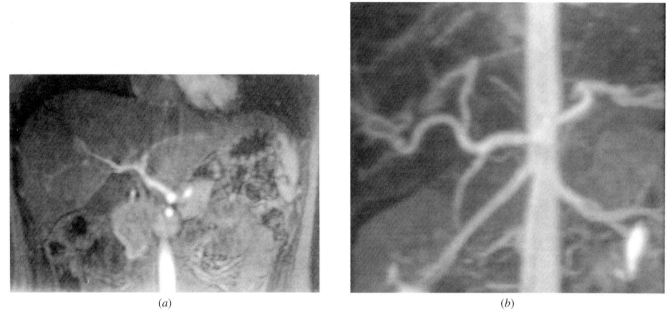

(a)   (b)

F i g . 2.170 Liver donor MRA. Coronal 3D gradient-echo 2-mm source image (*a*) and MIP reconstruction of the 2-mm 3D gradient-echo sections (*b*) in two different patients show the hepatic artery arising from the celiac axis.

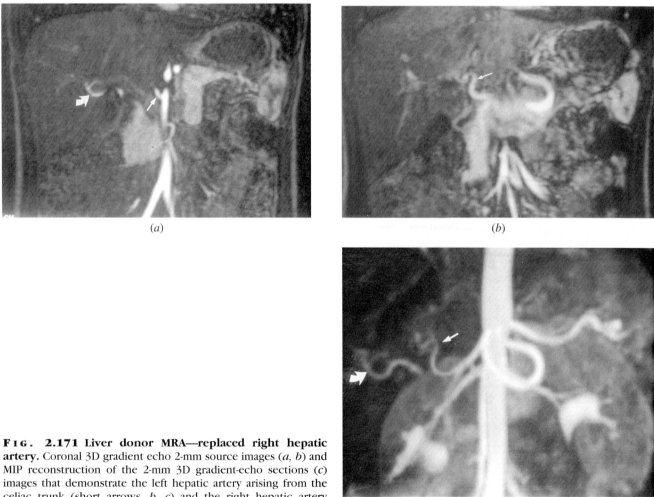

(a)   (b)

(c)

F i g . 2.171 Liver donor MRA—replaced right hepatic artery. Coronal 3D gradient echo 2-mm source images (*a, b*) and MIP reconstruction of the 2-mm 3D gradient-echo sections (*c*) images that demonstrate the left hepatic artery arising from the celiac trunk (short arrows, *b, c*) and the right hepatic artery (curved arrows, *a, c*) arising from the SMA.

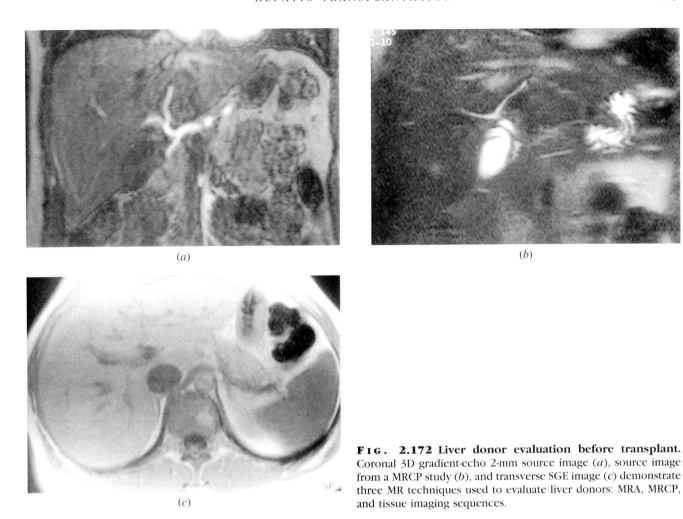

(a)

(b)

(c)

FIG. 2.172 Liver donor evaluation before transplant. Coronal 3D gradient-echo 2-mm source image (a), source image from a MRCP study (b), and transverse SGE image (c) demonstrate three MR techniques used to evaluate liver donors: MRA, MRCP, and tissue imaging sequences.

(a)

(b)

FIG. 2.173 Hemi-liver donor after transplant. Coronal T2-weighted SS-ETSE (a), SGE (b), and immediate (c) and 90-s fat-suppressed (d) postgadolinium SGE images with an unremarkable examination of the retained left lobe after right hemiliver donation.

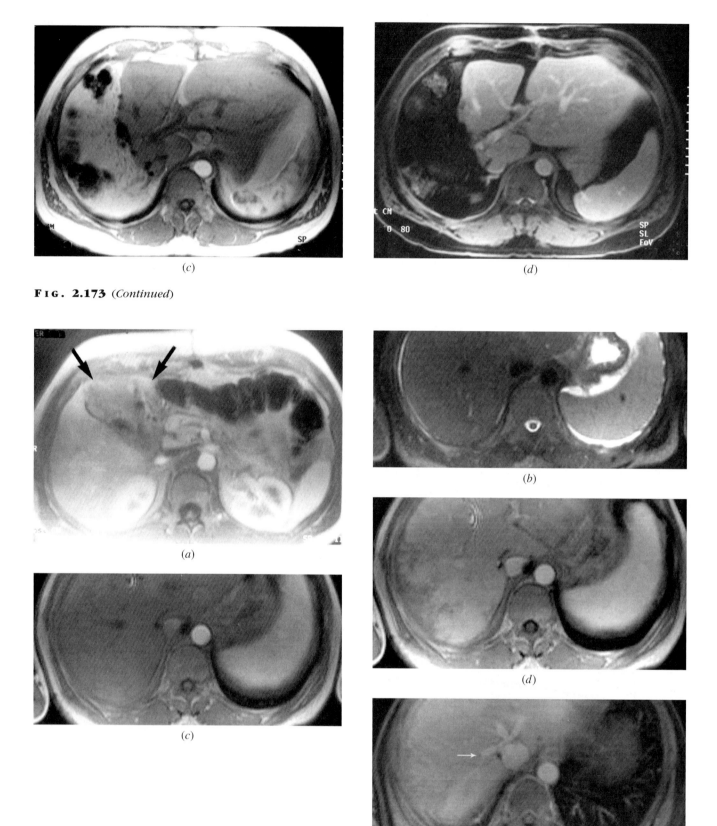

(c)

(d)

FIG. 2.173 (Continued)

(a)

(b)

(c)

(d)

(e)

FIG. 2.174 Ischemic changes. Immediate postgadolinium image (*a*) in a lateral segment liver donor patient demonstrates heterogeneous areas with diminished enhancement in segment 4 (arrows), reflecting postsurgical injury.

T2-weighted fat-suppressed SS-ETSE (*b*), and immediate (*c*), 45-s (*d*), and 90-s fat-suppressed (*e*) postgadolinium SGE images in a second patient. There is an irregular area in the periphery of the right lobe of the liver that is not evident on T2-weighted image (*b*) or on early-phase image (*c*) but becomes evident on 45-s image (*d*), reflecting greater contrast between the enhanced normal parenchyma and the nonenhanced ischemic portion. On late-phase image, a stricture in the right hepatic vein is appreciated (arrow, *e*).

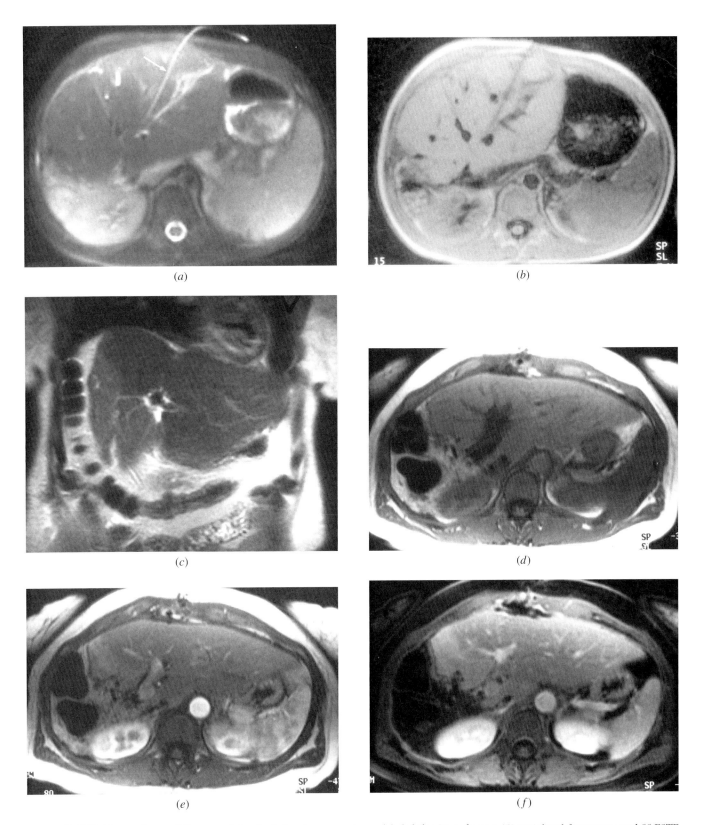

(a)

(b)

(c)

(d)

(e)

(f)

F I G . 2.175 Transplanted liver recipient—lateral segment; and left lobe in a donor. T2-weighted fat-suppressed SS-ESTE (a) and SGE (b) images in a pediatric patient who had undergone liver transplantation of a lateral segment 6 years earlier. The liver has developed a rounded configuration through hyperplasia. Note a percutaneous biliary drain (arrow, a).

Coronal T2-weighted SS-ETSE (c), SGE (d), and immediate (e) and 90-s fat-suppressed (f) SGE images in a second patient. Along the resection margin, there is an abnormal area that shows higher signal intensity on T2-weighted image (c) and demonstrates a faint enhancement after contrast (e, f) compatible with inflamation and granulation tissue.

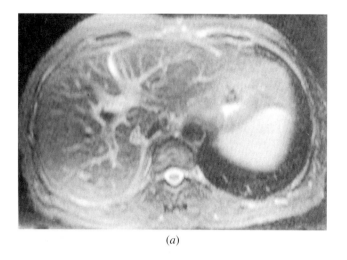

(a)

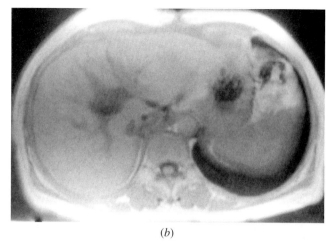

(b)

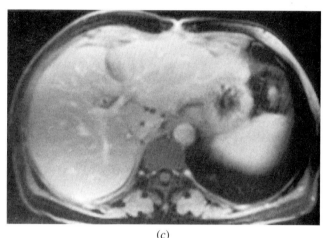

(c)

FIG. 2.176 Cadaveric liver transplant recipient. Echo train-STIR (*a*), SGE (*b*) and 90-s postgadolinium fat-suppressed SGE (*c*) images in a patient after transplant of a cadaveric liver. The liver showed normal signal without evidence for mass lesions or abnormal enhancement. No perihepatic fluid is identified. Note the clip artifacts in the porta hepatis and adjacent to the IVC, which are observed in patients with cadaveric liver transplant.

modifications of the gadolinium-enhanced 3D MRA technique to demonstrate small-vessel stenosis is undergoing continued refinement. One report that compared 3D gadolinium-enhanced MR angiograms with conventional angiography and surgery found that gadolinium-enhanced 3D MRA achieved accurate results in 58 (94%) of the 62 vessels analyzed [278]. Breathing-arrested protocols have recently been developed and show promise in examining for patency of the hepatic artery in patients, especially young children, who are unable to suspend respiration for a high-quality breath-hold MRA examination. High-spatial-resolution noninvasive arterial studies of small vessels are at present best performed with multidetector CT. The incidence of venous complications—portal vein and inferior vena cava thrombosis/stenosis—is lower than that of arterial complication [274–276]. Portal vein and IVC patency can be diagnosed reproducibly on MR images (fig. 2.177) [278, 279].

Fluid collections are commonly observed after hepatic transplantation and include hematomas (figs. 2.178 and 2.179), seromas, bilomas (fig. 2.180), abscesses, and simple ascites. Bile leaks may develop at the anas-

tomosis for technical reasons or may be secondary to bile duct necrosis in those patients with hepatic artery thrombosis [276].

Strictures of the biliary tree are often a late complication of liver transplantation and usually occur at the anastomosis secondary to scar formation. Stenosis or obstruction of the biliary tree (fig. 2.181) may be shown with techniques that render bile low in signal, high in signal (MR cholangiography), or a combination of both. Mucocele of the cystic duct remnant is a rare cause of biliary obstruction and may appear as a focal fluid collection adjacent to the hepatic duct [276, 280]. MRI is able to distinguish between hematomas and other fluid collections in hepatic transplants. In the acute phase (7–72h), deoxyhemoglobin has distinctive very low signal on T2-weighted images. In the period spanning several days to several months after surgery, intra- or extracellular methemoglobin in subacute hematoma is higher in signal on T1-weighted images than other fluid.

Periportal signal abnormalities are frequently present in transplanted livers. The typical appearance is tissue that is low in signal intensity on T1-weighted images and high in signal intensity on T2-weighted

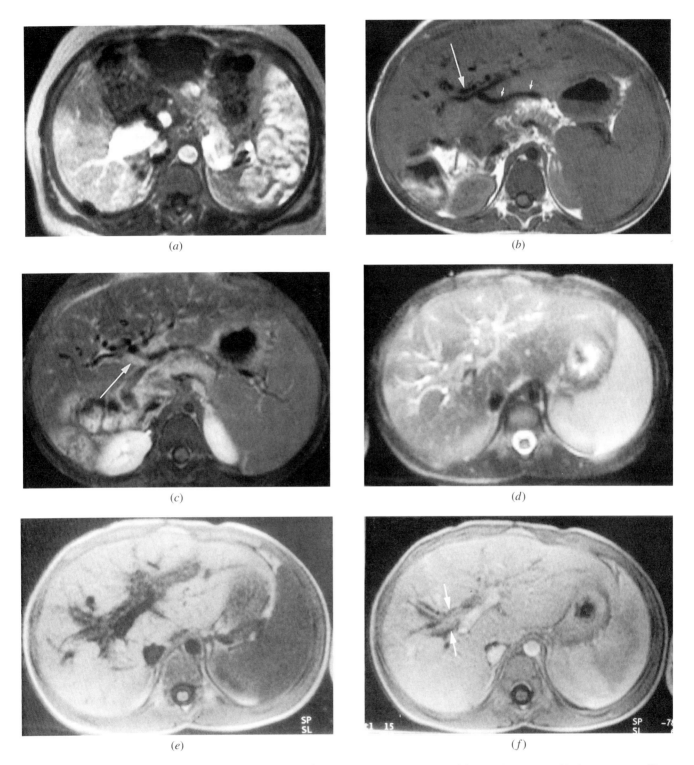

(a) *(b)*

(c) *(d)*

(e) *(f)*

F I G . 2.177 Hepatic transplant—portal vein complications. Immediate postgadolinium SGE image (*a*) demonstrates dilatation of the right portal vein secondary to anastomotic stenosis.

T1-weighted SE (*b*) and interstitial-phase gadolinium-enhanced T1-weighted fat-suppressed SE (*c*) images in a pediatric patient with a trisegmental transplant. Patent hepatic arterial graft (small arrows, *b*) and biliary ducts (long arrow, *b*) are evident. There is no evidence of a patent portal vein. Enhancing inflammatory tissue is present in the porta hepatis and in the expected location of the portal vein (long arrow, *c*).

Echo train-STIR (*d*), SGE (*e*), and immediate postgadolinium SGE (*f*) images in a 6-year-old girl, 14 months after transplant. There is an abnormal decreased signal intensity seen in the distal right portal vein (arrows, *f*) on the post-contrast image with slight expansion of the portal vein and patchy enhancement to this segment of the liver. These features are consistent with thrombosis of the right portal vein. Note also that mild intrahepatic ductal dilatation is present (*d*).

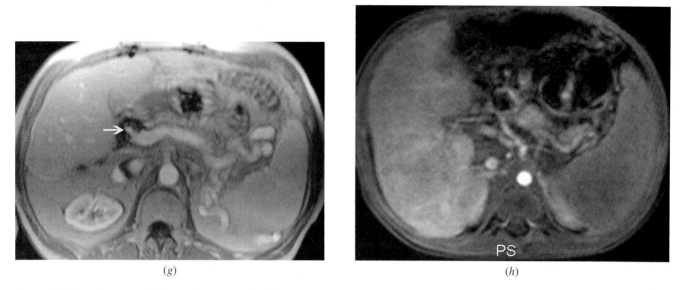

(g)   (h)

F I G . 2.177 (*Continued*) Immediate (*g*) postgadolinium SGE images in a fourth patient who has a stricture of the portal vein distal to its bifurcation (arrow, *g*).

Breathing-arrested postgadolinium 3D-gradient echo **at 3T** in an infant demonstrates extremely narrowed but patent portal vein (*h*).

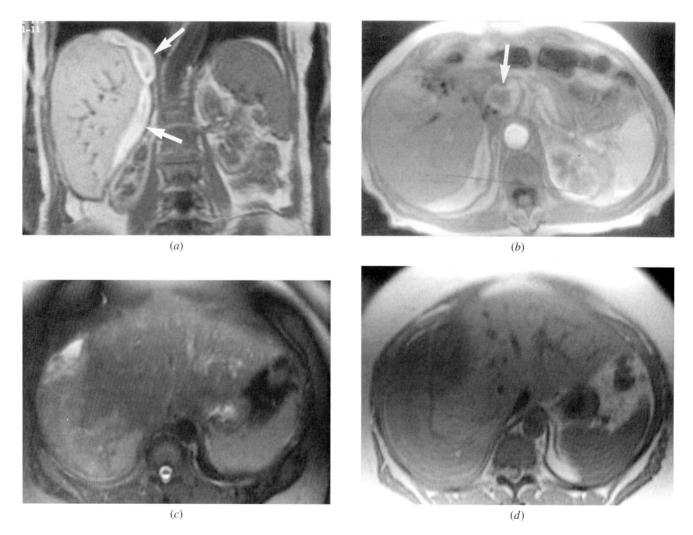

(a)   (b)

(c)   (d)

F I G . 2.178 Hematoma in recipient. Coronal SGE (*a*) and transverse immediate postgadolinium SGE (*b*) images in a patient who is the recipient of a right hepatic lobe transplant. There is a perihepatic fluid collection (arrows, *a, b*) that demonstrates a high-signal peripheral rim on noncontrast T1-weighted images (*a*), consistent with hematoma.

T2-weighted SS-ETSE (*c*), SGE (*d*), and 90-s fat-suppressed (*e*) postgadolinium SGE images in a second patient after liver

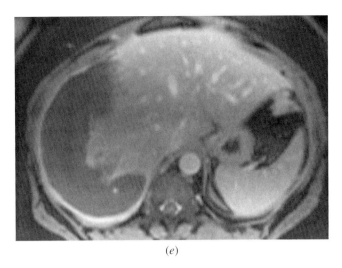

(e)

FIG. 2.178 (*Continued*) transplantation. There is a subcapsular collection characterized by heterogeneous mild/moderate high signal intensity on T2-weighted image (*c*), low signal intensity on T1-weighted image (*d*) and this capsular enhancement on late-phase image (*e*) consistent with a contained hemorrhage.

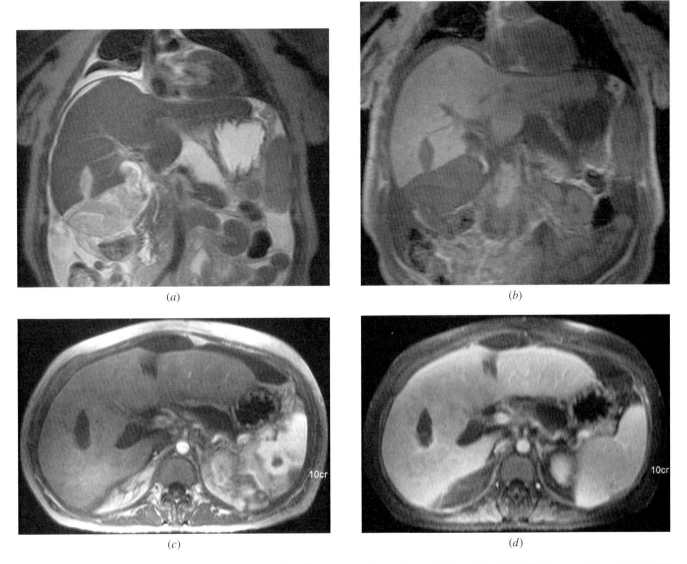

(a)

(b)

(c)

(d)

FIG. 2.179 Liver laceration and hematoma after liver transplant. Coronal T2-weighted SS-ETSE (*a*) and T1-weighted SGE (*b*) and transverse immediate (*c*) and 90-s fat-suppressed (*d*) postgadolinium SGE images. There is a linear laceration in the inferior portion of the liver associated with a hematoma.

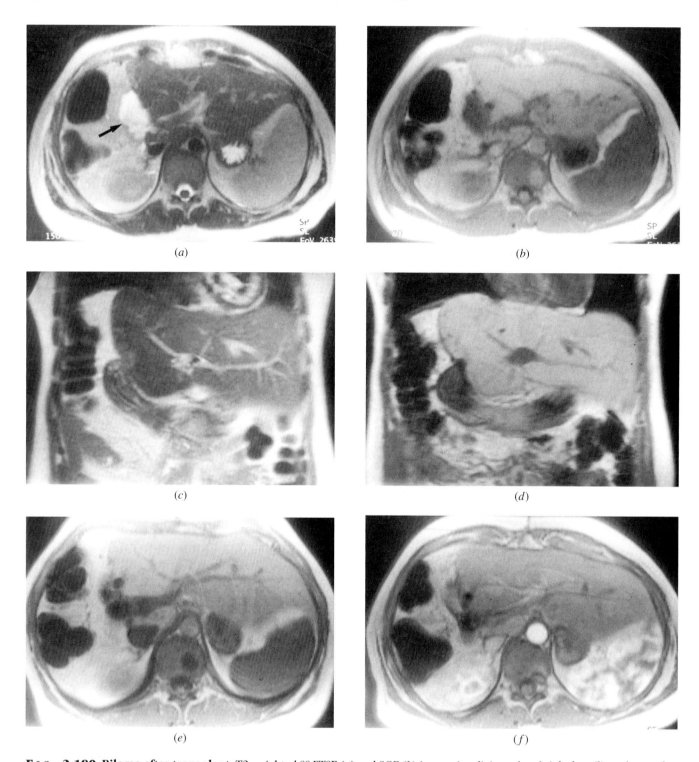

(a)

(b)

(c)

(d)

(e)

(f)

F I G . 2.180 Biloma after transplant. T2-weighted SS-ETSE (*a*) and SGE (*b*) images in a living-related right hemiliver donor after transplant. There is a fluid collection (arrow, *a*) along the resection margin of the liver that demonstrates high signal on T2-weighted (*a*) and low signal on T1-weighted (*b*) images, consistent with biloma.

Coronal T2-weighted SS-ETSE (*c*), coronal SGE (*d*), transverse SGE (*e*), and immediate (*f*) and 90-s fat-suppressed (*g*) post-gadolinium SGE images in the same patient 3 months after the prior exam. Note the resolution of the biloma.

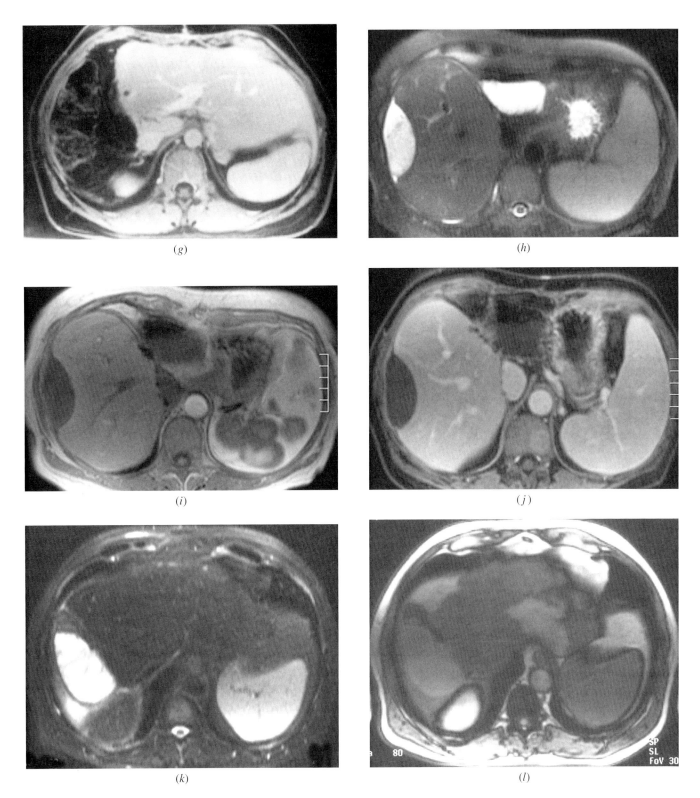

(g) *(h)* *(i)* *(j)* *(k)* *(l)*

FIG. 2.180 *(Continued)* T2-weighted SS-ETSE (*h*), SGE (*i*), and 90-s fat-suppressed (*j*) postgadolinium SGE images in a liver recipient patient demonstrate an elongated subcapsular fluid collection consistent with a biloma.

T2-weighted SS-ETSE (*k*), out-of-phase SGE (*l*), and immediate (*m*) and 90-s fat-suppressed (*n*) postgadolinium SGE images in a liver recipient. A subcapsular biloma along the resection margin is present. Additionally, there are fatty spared regions shown on

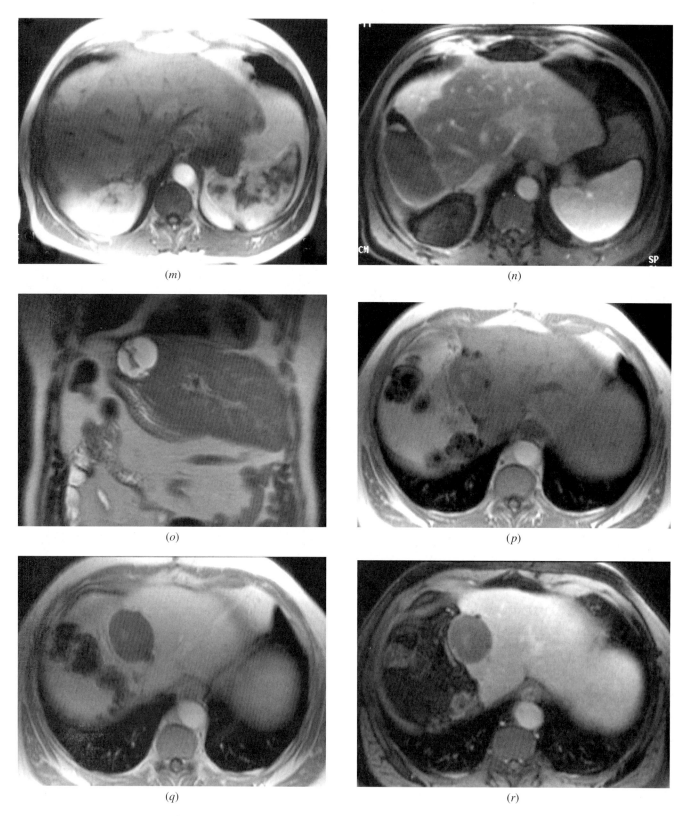

(m)

(n)

(o)

(p)

(q)

(r)

F I G . 2.180 (*Continued*) out-of-phase image that exhibit faint increased enhancement on early-phase image (*m*) and remain slightly higher signal on late-phase image (*n*). Enhancement differences likely reflect fat suppression effects of the fatty liver. Consideration must always be made of whether enhancement variations reflect true enhancement phenomena or reflect the use of concomitant fat suppression on some or all postcontrast sequences.

    Coronal T2-weighted SS-ETSE (*o*), SGE (*p*), and immediate (*q*) and 90-s fat-suppressed (*r*) postgadolinium SGE images in a fourth patient demonstrate a biloma along the resection margin.

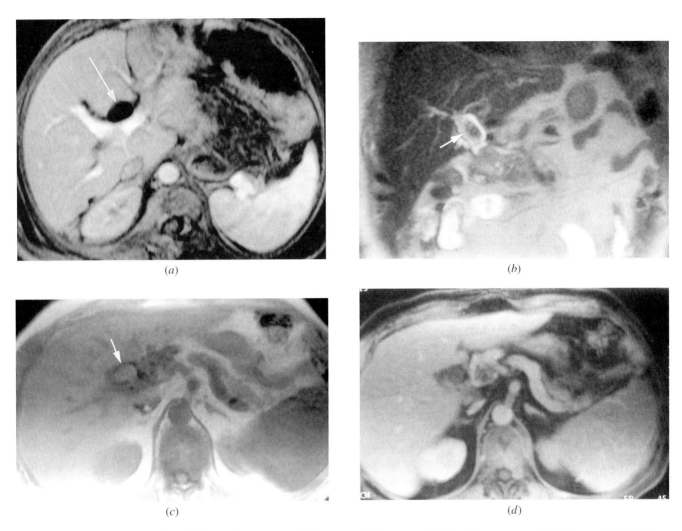

(a)

(b)

(c)

(d)

FIG. 2.181 Liver transplant, biliary duct stenosis. Transverse 90-s postgadolinium fat-suppressed SGE image (*a*). Dilatation of the common hepatic duct (arrow, *a*) is present, secondary to anastomotic stenosis.

Coronal T2-weighted SS-ETSE (*b*), SGE (*c*) and 90-s postgadolinium fat-suppressed SGE (*d*) images in a second patient. There is an anastomotic stricture associated with a filling defect within the common bile duct suggestive of sludge ball or stone (arrow, *b*, *c*). Note the mild intrahepatic biliary ductal dilatation (*b*). The findings were confirmed by ERCP.

images. Abnormal tissue is most substantial in the porta hepatis and extends along the branching portal tracts into the liver parenchyma (fig. 2.182) [281]. In many cases, periportal signal abnormalities may represent lymphocytic infiltration due to rejection; however, other causes such as dilated lymphatics due to impaired drainage after surgery must be considered [282]. Beyond the immediate transplant period, expansion of the periportal tissue in a masslike fashion may be a harbinger of posttransplant lymphoproliferative disorder (PTLD) (fig. 2.183) [283, 284]. PTLD occurs in transplant recipients whose immune systems are compromised. Most cases can be linked to infection with Epstein–Barr virus and may involve any organ in the body [283, 284]. Liver, small bowel, and kidney are the most common extranodal abdominal organs involved with PTLD [283].

PTLD is varied in presentation, ranging from polyclonal (nonmalignant) B cell proliferations to malignant lymphoma, usually B cell [285]. Inflammatory periportal tissue also may be observed in acute hepatitis, after biliary surgery, in various benign or malignant diseases, and in portal adenopathy [286].

Hepatocellular carcinoma may develop in the transplanted liver. This is an important complication in patients who were diagnosed with HCC before transplantation or in whom focal HCC was found incidentally in the pathologic evaluation of the recipient's resected liver (fig. 2.184) [276, 287].

MRI demonstrates a variety of morphologic abnormalities in transplanted livers and is able to identify various causes of graft failure (figs. 2.185–2.187). At present, however, no specific MRI findings have been

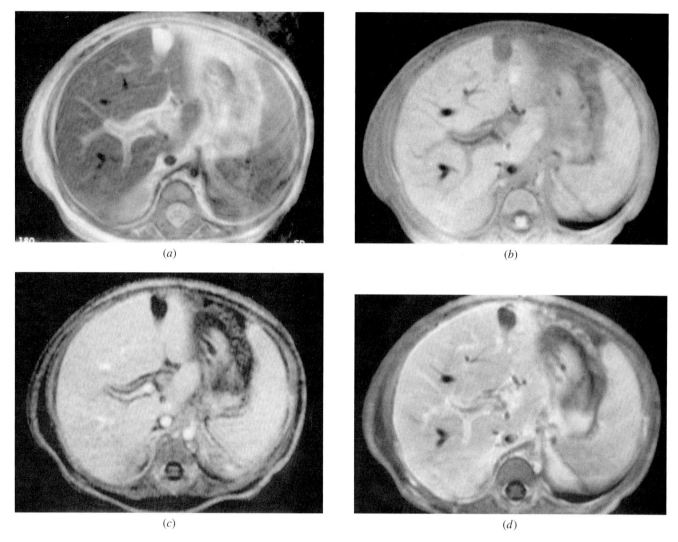

(a)

(b)

(c)

(d)

FIG. 2.182 Periportal inflammation after liver transplant. T2-weighted SE (*a*), T1-weighted SE (*b*), immediate postgadolinium magnetization-prepared gradient-echo (*c*), and T1-weighted interstitial-phase postgadolinium fat-suppressed SE (*d*) images in a 17-month-old patient after liver transplant. There is a moderate amount of periportal inflammatory change, which appears high signal on T2 (*a*) and enhances on interstitial-phase postgadolinium fat-suppressed images (*c*), likely postsurgical changes.

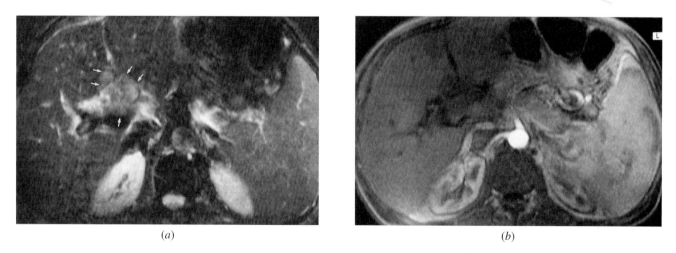

(a)

(b)

FIG. 2.183 Lymphoproliferative disorder. T2-weighted fat-suppressed ETSE (*a*) and immediate postgadolinium SGE (*b*) images. A 3-cm mass is present in the porta hepatis that is moderate in signal on the T2-weighted image (arrows, *a*) and enhances minimally with gadolinium (*b*).

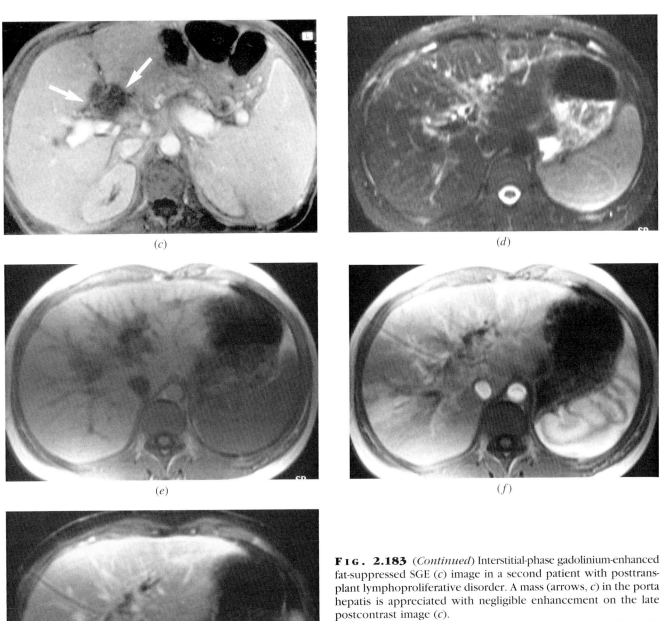

(c)

(d)

(e)

(f)

(g)

FIG. 2.183 (*Continued*) Interstitial-phase gadolinium-enhanced fat-suppressed SGE (*c*) image in a second patient with posttransplant lymphoproliferative disorder. A mass (arrows, *c*) in the porta hepatis is appreciated with negligible enhancement on the late postcontrast image (*c*).

T2-weighted fat-suppressed SS-ETSE (*d*), SGE (*e*), and immediate (*f*) and 90-s fat-suppressed (*g*) postgadolinium SGE images in a third patient. The central portion of the liver shows an abnormal area that is masslike and exhibits high signal intensity on T2-weighted images (*d*), low signal intensity on T1-weighted images (*e*), and moderate enhancement on early-phase images (*f*) and appears homogeneously enhanced on late-phase images (*g*). Histopathology was consistent with lymphoproliferative disorder. Air is present in the biliary tree secondary to the presence of a percutaneous biliary drain.

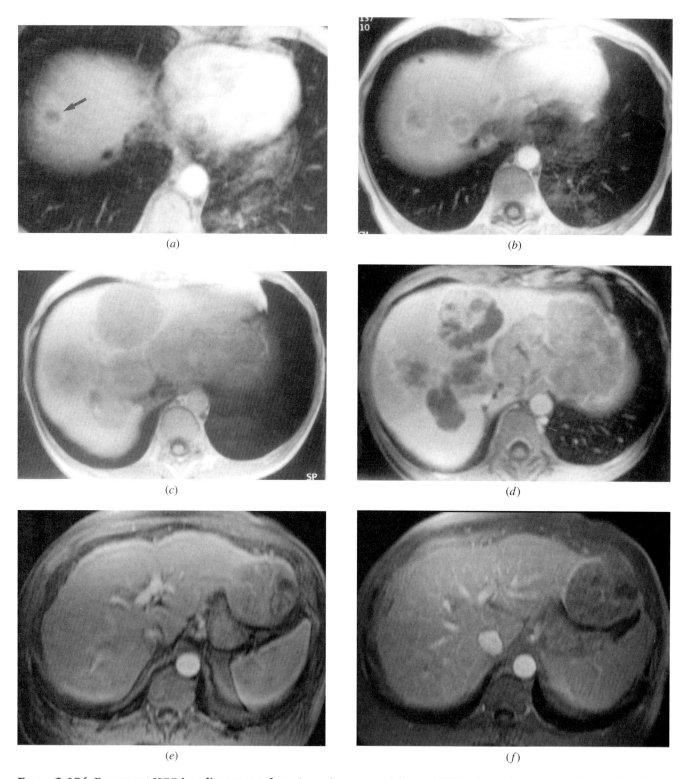

(a)

(b)

(c)

(d)

(e)

(f)

FIG. 2.184 Recurrent HCC in a liver transplant. Immediate postgadolinium SGE (*a*) image in a patient who has developed HCC within a transplanted liver. Multiple small masses involve the dome of the right lobe of the liver that demonstrate ring enhancement on the immediate postgadolinium image (arrow, *a*). Three months later the lesions have increased in size and number, as shown on the immediate postgadolinium SGE image (*b*). One year later, SGE (*c*), and 90-s postgadolinium fat-suppressed SGE (*d*) images demonstrate massive increase in size and number of HCCs. This represents metastases to a liver transplant in a patient who had HCC in her native liver.

T1-weighted fat-suppressed 3D-gradient echo images immediate (*e*), and 90-second (*f*) in a second with HCC imaged **at 3.0T** after liver transplantation. Metastatic foci of HCC are apparent.

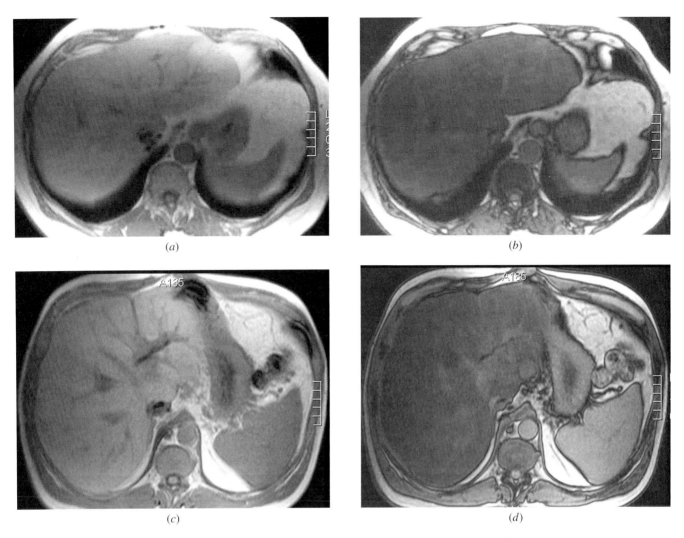

F I G . 2.185 Fatty liver after transplantation. SGE (*a*, *c*) and out-of-phase SGE (*b*, *d*) images in two different patients after liver transplantation that demonstrate signal loss from in-phase T1-weighted images (*a*, *c*) to out-of-phase images (*b*, *d*) compatible with fatty liver.

identified to establish or quantify transplant rejection or hepatocellular function. In the future, hepatocyte-specific contrast agents or MR spectroscopy may play a role in this determination.

DIFFUSE LIVER PARENCHYMAL DISEASE

Chronic Liver Diseases

Autoimmune Diseases

Autoimmune liver disorders are inflammatory liver diseases characterized histologically by a pronounced mononuclear cell infiltrate in the portal tracts and serologically by the presence of non-organ and liver-specific autoantibodies and increased levels of immunoglobulin G (IgG) in the absence of a known etiology

[288]. Primary sclerosing cholangitis (PSC), autoimmune hepatitis (AIH), and primary biliary cirrhosis (PBC) are chronic liver diseases postulated to have an autoimmune basis for their pathogenesis [289].

Primary sclerosing cholangitis (PSC) is a chronic liver disease of unknown etiology. A number of factors have been proposed that might incite injury and cause recurrent damage to the bile ducts. These entities include bacteria, virus, toxins, vascular damage, or genetic abnormalities of immunoregulation. PSC is more common in males and has a high association with inflammatory bowel disease [290]. Also, patients with PSC have a higher risk of developing cholangiocarcinoma than the general population because of chronic biliary inflammatory changes [291].

The morphologic changes of PSC on pathologic evaluation consist of a lymphocytic infiltrate with fibrosing cholangitis of intra- and extrahepatic bile ducts and

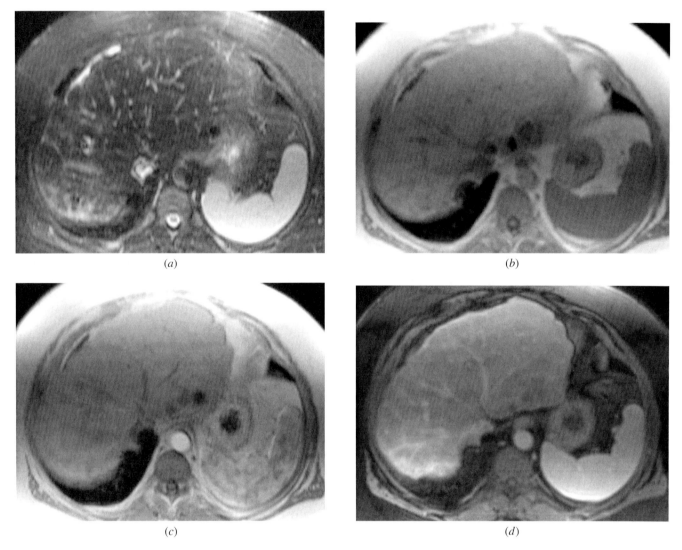

(a)   (b)

(c)   (d)

F I G . 2.186 Fibrosis after liver transplant. T2-weighted SS-ETSE (*a*), SGE (*b*), and immediate (*c*) and 90-s fat-suppressed (*d*) postgadolinium SGE images show strands of fibrosis in a posttransplant liver well shown on late-phase image (*d*).

progressive obliteration of their lumens. Between areas of scarring and progressive stricture, bile ducts become ectatic, presumably the result of downstream obstruction. Such a pattern of multifocal strictures and dilatations produces the well-recognized cholangiographic pattern of "beaded" bile ducts. The disease culminates in cirrhosis.

A prior study [292] described the MR findings of PSC and the association of imaging features with clinical severity by use of the Mayo End-Stage Liver Disease (MELD) and Child–Turcotte–Pugh scales. The association between macronodular morphology, biliary obstruction, and peripheral wedge-shaped atrophy was the most suggestive of PSC, and it was noticed in 23% (12/52) of patients. MR findings of liver cirrhosis were described in 87% of the patients. More than half of the patients had nodules ≥3 cm in the maximum diameter,

and the number of nodules ranged from 1 to 5 in 57% of patients. The majority of nodules enhanced comparably to liver parenchyma. A distinctive feature is that up to 70% of these nodules were located in the central region of the liver. The compression of central ducts by large nodules causes peripheral biliary dilation, and this feature was shown in 29% of patients. The presence of intrahepatic biliary ductal dilatation was described in 85% of the patients, with segmental dilatation, a common finding. Peripheral wedge-shaped areas of parenchymal atrophy were noted in 46% of patients. On MRI, these areas were characterized as high signal on T2-weighted images and low signal on noncontrast T1-weighted images in up to 83%, with atrophic segments occasionally being high signal on T1-weighted images (figs. 2.188 and 2.189). After contrast, the wedge-shaped areas showed minimal enhancement (less than background

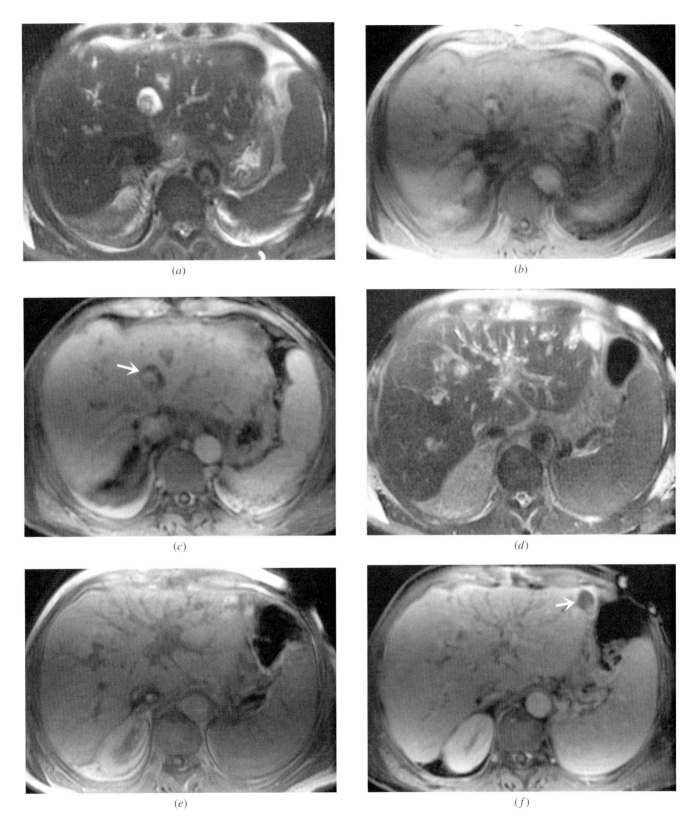

F I G . 2.187 Fungus infection after liver transplant. T2-weighted SS-ETSE (*a, d*), SGE (*b, e*), and 90-s fat-suppressed (*c, f*) postgadolinium SGE images in the same patient at two different tomographic levels. There are two cystic lesions (arrow, *c, f*) in the left hepatic lobe that demonstrate a small focus of internal debris. Note the presence of mild biliary dilatation and ascites.

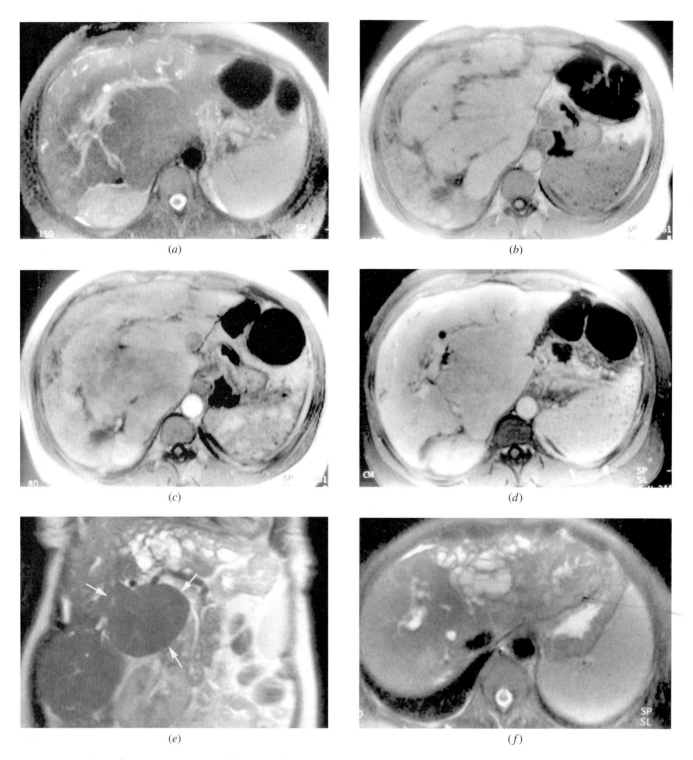

F I G . 2.188 Cirrhosis in primary sclerosing cholangitis. Echo-train STIR (*a*), SGE (*b*), and immediate (*c*) and 90-s fat-suppressed (*d*) postgadolinium SGE images. The liver shows distorted anatomy with heterogeneous signal. The caudate lobe is massively enlarged by large macroregenerative nodules that cause atrophy of the peripheral liver, resulting in signal changes of increased signal on T2 (*a*), decreased signal on T1 (*b*), and early negligible (*c*) and late progressive (*d*) enhancement. There is ductal dilatation in the peripheral liver, due to obstruction from the central hypertrophy. These findings are consistent with cirrhosis due to PSC.

Coronal T2-weighted SS-ETSE (*e*), T2-weighted fat-suppressed SS-ETSE (*f*), and 90-s fat-suppressed (*g, h*) postgadolinium SGE images in a second patient. Note the massive enlargement of the caudate lobe (arrows, *e*), which causes distal obstruction of the biliary tree.

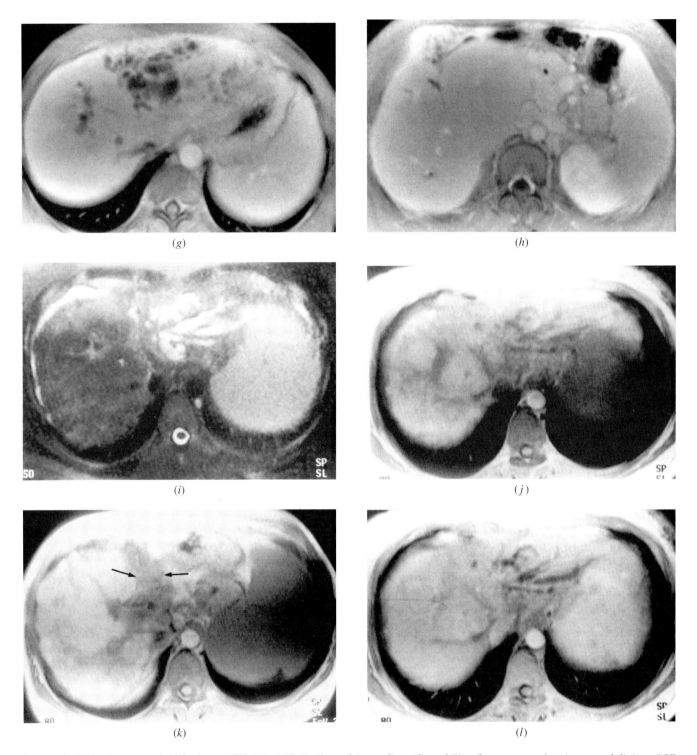

F I G . 2.188 (*Continued*) Echo-train STIR (*i*), SGE (*j*, *k*), and immediate (*l*) and 90-s fat-suppressed (*m*) postgadolinium SGE images in a third patient with PSC. The liver demonstrates a shrunken fibrotic appearance with multiple macroregenerative nodules, which are more widely distributed than in the first 2 patients. Severe lateral segment intrahepatic biliary ductal dilatation is present (*i*) from obstruction by dense fibrous tissue (arrows, *k*).

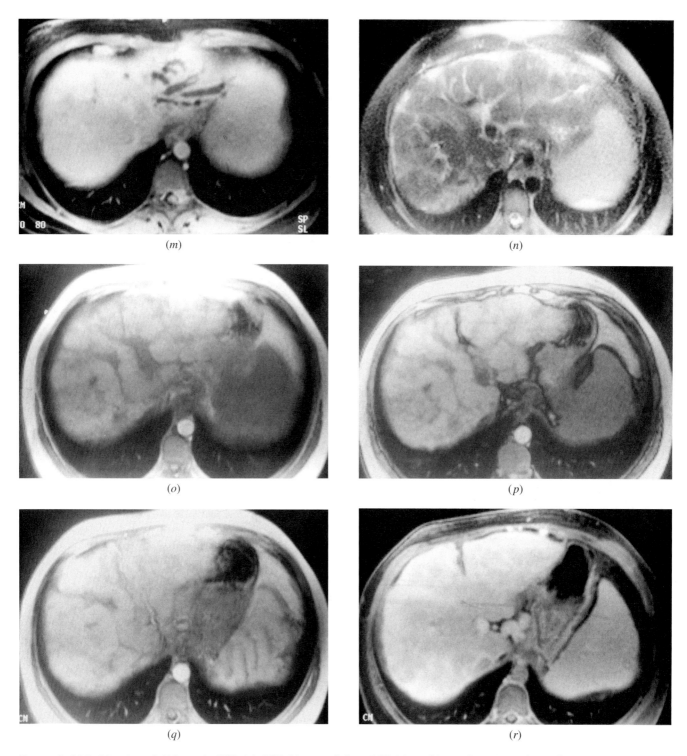

FIG. 2.188 (*Continued*) Echo-train STIR (*n*), SGE (*o*), out-of-phase SGE (*p*), and immediate (*q*) and 90-s fat-suppressed (*r*) post-gadolinium SGE images in a fourth patient with PSC. The liver is heterogeneous in signal on T2-weighted (*n*) and T1-weighted (*o*, *p*) images, with multiple macronodules and fibrotic bands present. This patient does not have the characteristic central macronodular pattern found in PSC.

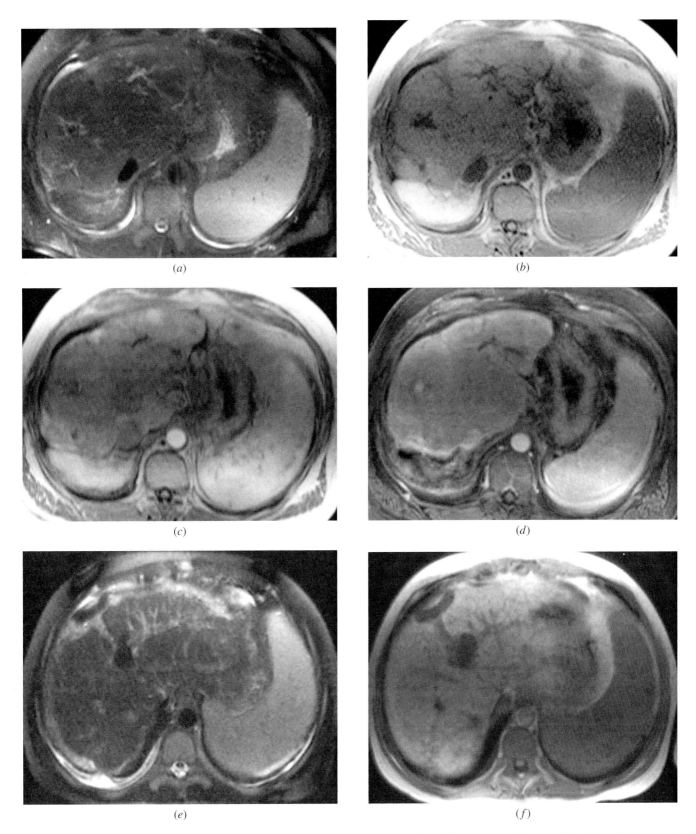

(a)

(b)

(c)

(d)

(e)

(f)

F I G . 2.189 Primary sclerosing cholangitis. T2-weighted fat-suppressed SS-ETSE (*a*), SGE (*b*), immediate (*c*) and 90-second fat-suppressed (*d*) postgadolinium SGE; T2-weighted fat-suppressed SS-ETSE (*e*), SGE (*f*), and immediate (*g*) and 90-second fat-suppressed (*h*) postgadolinium SGE images in two patients with PSC. T2-weighted fat suppressed SS-ETSE fat suppressed (*i, k, n*)

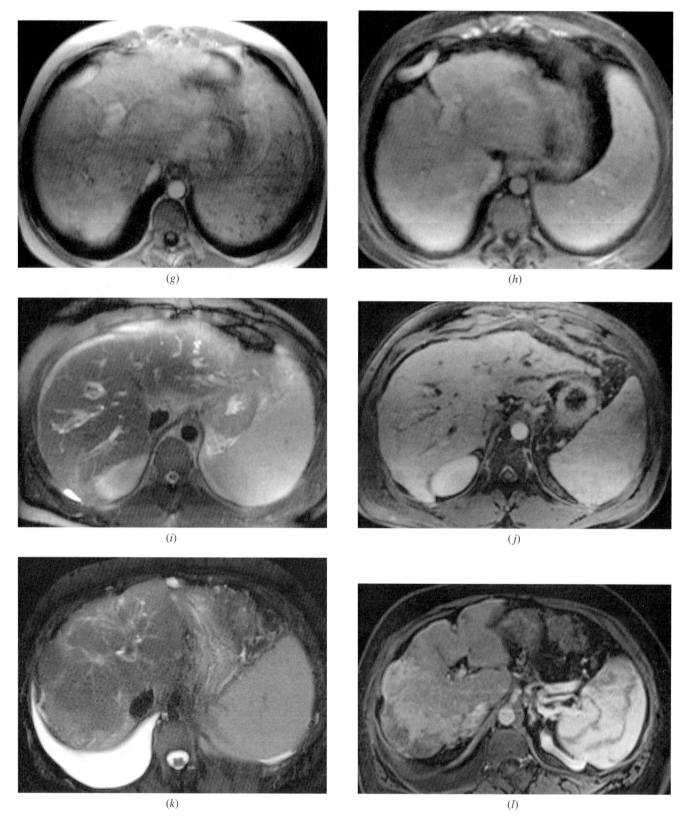

(g)

(h)

(i)

(j)

(k)

(l)

F I G . 2.189 (*Continued*) and T1-weighted fat-supressed 3D-vibe immediate post gadolinium (*l*, *o*) and 90-second post gadolinium (*j*, *m*, *p*) in three different patients imaged **at 3T**. Simlar findings of central regeneration are appreciated.

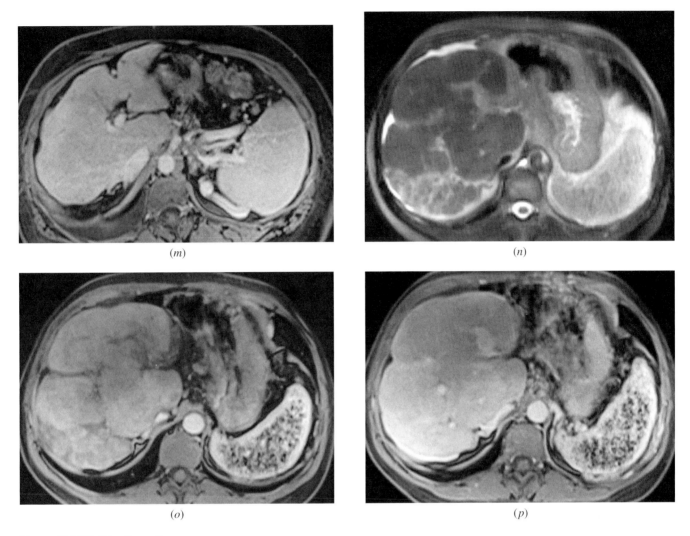

(m)

(n)

(o)

(p)

FIG. 2.189 (*Continued*)

parenchyma) on early-phase images that became more intense on late-phase images in more than half of these patients. The association between the severity of imaging findings and MELD and Child–Turcotte–Pugh were not statistically significant. This suggests that morphologic changes alone may not reflect the extent of hepatic compromise.

Changes of cirrhosis in patients with PSC are associated with extensive fibrotic changes, central macroregenerative nodules, and peripheral atrophy causing architectural distortion. Central macroregenerative nodules may result in true biliary ductal dilatation and peripheral liver atrophy distinct from the beaded biliary ductal changes of PSC. These patterns appear to be both relatively common and distinctive for PSC. Similar findings have been described by others [293–295].

Chronic Budd–Chiari syndrome may present some findings similar to those of PSC. Hypertrophy of the caudate lobe, presence of regenerative nodules and

fibrosis are present in both entities. However, in PSC the regenerative nodules are preferably present in the central portion of the liver parenchyma, commonly causing dilation of bile ducts. A more complete description of Budd–Chiari is in the subsection on liver vascular diseases.

Autoimmune hepatitis (AIH) is a necro-inflammatory chronic liver disease that has an unknown etiology. AIH is characterized serologically by the presence of non-organ and liver-specific autoantibodies and increased levels of transaminases and immunoglobulin G [296]. Histologic features of AIH are not specific and instead are common to other forms of chronic active hepatitis. A dense periportal lymphoplasmacytic inflammatory infiltrate, fibrosis, and lobular necrosis are frequent findings [2]. An overlap between AIH and other chronic liver diseases is reported, most commonly with PSC [297, 298]. The distinction of AIH from other autoimmune liver diseases, namely, PSC and PBC, is particularly important since therapeutic modalities may differ [298, 299].

A prior study [300] reported on the MR appearance of AIH. The great majority of patients were women, with incidence from age 20 and older. Almost all (93%) patients with AIH had a reticular and/or confluent fibrosis shown on MRI. Reticular and/or confluent fibrosis both appear as low signal on short-TE out-of-phase images and show negligible early enhancement with gadolinium and moderate/intense enhancement on delayed images. Four categories were described, based on the thickness of the reticular fibrotic strands and on the liver contour nodularity, as follows: 1) mild when fibrous tissue has a thickness <2 mm and does not cause liver nodularity; 2) moderate when fibrous tissue has a thickness between 2 and 5 mm and causes slight liver nodularity; 3) severe when fibrous tissue has a thickness

>5 mm and causes gross liver nodularity; and 4) confluent fibrosis, which has a localized, masslike configuration. A moderate reticular fibrosis was predominantly observed (44% of patients; 14 of 32) followed by mild fibrosis (34% of patients; 11 of 32). Confluent fibrosis most commonly occurred in *segment* 8 of the liver and was noted along with reticular fibrosis in 18% of patients (6/32) (fig. 2.190). Biliary ductal dilatation was reported in 12.5% of patients with AIH. None of the patients in this study had HCC. AIH was therefore shown to have a prominent pattern of liver fibrosis in the setting of livers with relatively normal contours. At disease onset, AIH is characterized by substantial inflammatory cell infiltration, which should be observed as intense patchy enhancement on hepatic arterial dominant-phase images. All patients in this study were already on treatment for AIH, so the expected appearance of early

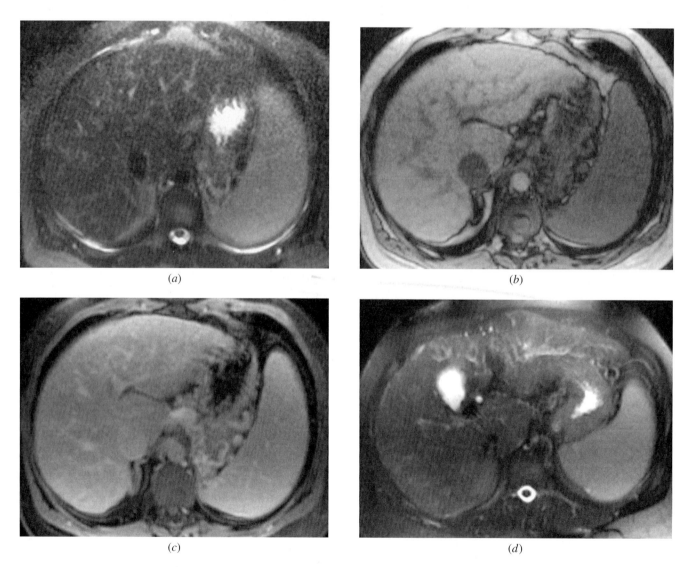

(a)

(b)

(c)

(d)

F I G . 2.190 Autoimmune hepatitis. T2-weighted SS-ETSE (*a*), out-of-phase SGE (*b*), and 90-s fat-suppressed postgadolinium SGE (*c*) images; T2-weighted SS-ETSE (*d*), out-of-phase SGE (*e*), and 90-s fat-suppressed postgadolinium SGE (*f*) images;

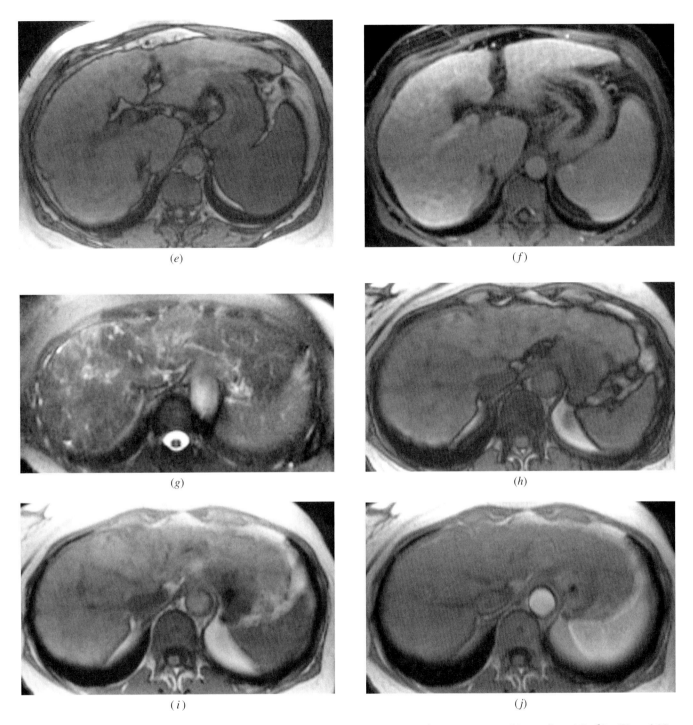

(e) *(f)*

(g) *(h)*

(i) *(j)*

F I G . 2.190 *(Continued)* T2-weighted SS-ETSE (*g*), out-of-phase SGE (*h*), in-phase SGE (*i*), and immediate (*j*), 60-s (*k*) and 90-s (*l*) images in another patient demonstrate diffuse fibrosis that exhibits progressively intense enhancement over time. T2-weighted SS-ETSE fat-suppressed (*m*), SGE (*n*), and immediate (*o*) and 90-s fat-suppressed postgadolinium SGE (*p*) images in a patient with untreated AIH at presentation. Note the early patchy enhancement reflective of acute inflammatory disease. AIH is characterized by a prominent network of fibrosis even early in the course of disease (*d, f*). The hepatic changes are similar to PBC, and both AIH and PBC tend to have less architectural distortion than primary sclerosing cholangitis.

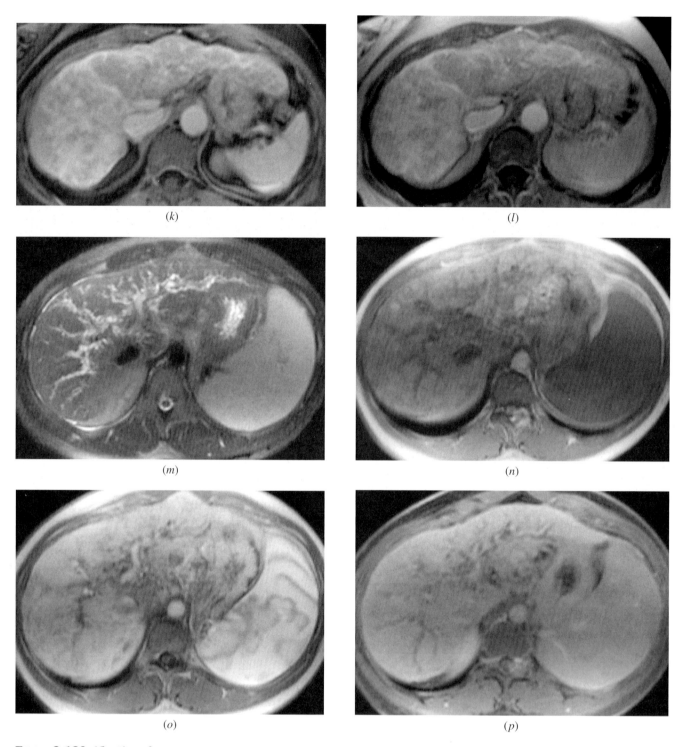

(k)

(l)

(m)

(n)

(o)

(p)

FIG. 2.190 (*Continued*)

intense patchy enhancement of untreated AIH was not observed in any of these patients. The correlation between imaging findings and MELD clinical score was not statistically significant. This again reflects that morphologic findings may not correlate with the severity of liver compromise.

Primary biliary cirrhosis (PBC) is a chronic progressive autoimmune liver disorder that causes the obliteration of the intrahepatic bile ducts, portal inflammation, fibrosis, and cirrhosis [301]. A few imaging studies describe the imaging appearance of PBC. A prior study [302] described the "periportal halo sign" in 43% (9/21)

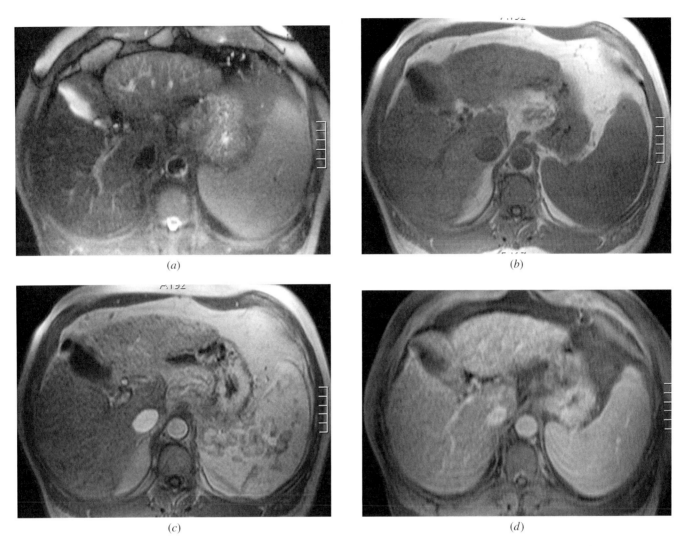

(a)

(b)

(c)

(d)

F I G . 2.191 Primary biliary cirrhosis (PBC). Fat-suppressed T2-weighted SS-ETSE (*a*), SGE (*b*), and immediate (*c*) and 90-s fat-suppressed (*d*) postgadolinium SGE images in a patient with PBC. The liver contains a fine network of fibrosis throughout, and has only mildly distorted morphology.

of patients with PBS, characterized by a hypointense rounded area surrounding the portal vein branches on both T2- and T1-weighted images. The authors attributed this finding to the presence of stellate, periportal hepatocellular parenchyma extension, surrounded by regenerative nodules. This finding was better appreciated on portal venous and interstitial phase. It may be that this appearance reflects a prominent pattern of fibrosis as also observed in AIH (fig. 2.191).

Overlap syndrome represents coexistence of more than one of the autoimmune conditions. MRI features can be helpful to determine the presence of the PSC overlap form. The presence of central regenerative nodules, peripheral atrophy, biliary duct beading, biliary dilation, in patients with laboratory evidence of AIH or PBC should raise suspicion for overlap syndrome (figs. 2.190 and 2.191) [301].

Genetic Diseases

Wilson Disease. Wilson disease is a rare autosomal recessive inherited disorder caused by copper overload in the liver and other organs [2]. The forms of liver disease associated with Wilson disease are highly variable and include fatty change, acute hepatitis, chronic active hepatitis, and cirrhosis [303]. Ultrasound, CT, and MR findings are nonspecific and reflect a full range of hepatic injury including fatty infiltration, acute hepatitis, chronic active hepatitis, and cirrhosis [303]. To date, no characteristic liver imaging finding has been established for Wilson disease (figs. 2.192 and 2.193).

α-1-Antitrypsin Deficiency. α-1-Antitrypsin deficiency is an autosomal recessive inherited disorder characterized by abnormally low serum levels of a major protease inhibitor. Hepatic syndromes are extremely

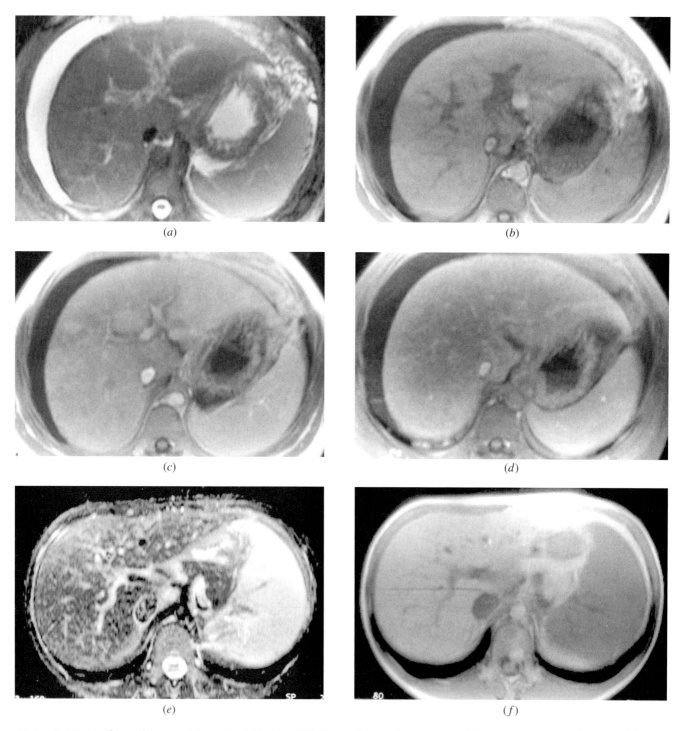

F I G . 2.192 Wilson disease. Echo-train STIR (*a*), SGE (*b*), and immediate (*c*) and 90-s fat-suppressed (*d*) postgadolinium SGE images in a patient with Wilson disease and acute presentation in fulminant liver failure. Early patchy enhancement (*c*) compatible with acute severe hepatitis and late linear stromal enhancement (*d*) are both present, consistent with acute on chronic hepatitis.

Echo-train STIR (*e*), SGE (*f*), out-of-phase SGE (*g*), and immediate (*h*) and 90-s fat-suppressed (*i*) postgadolinium SGE images in a second patient. There are multiple regenerative nodules throughout the liver parenchyma, which are best shown on the out-of-phase image (*g*) because of drop in signal of background fatty liver. Splenomegaly is also present.

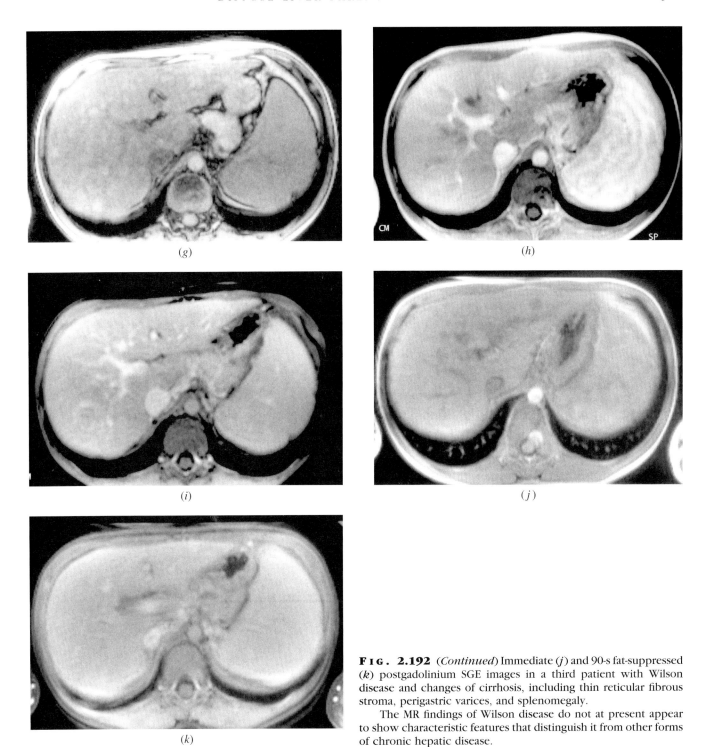

(g)

(h)

(i)

(j)

(k)

FIG. 2.192 (*Continued*) Immediate (*j*) and 90-s fat-suppressed (*k*) postgadolinium SGE images in a third patient with Wilson disease and changes of cirrhosis, including thin reticular fibrous stroma, perigastric varices, and splenomegaly.

The MR findings of Wilson disease do not at present appear to show characteristic features that distinguish it from other forms of chronic hepatic disease.

varied and range from neonatal hepatitis to childhood cirrhosis or cirrhosis late in life when liver fibrosis is advanced [2]. Although no distinctive features of cirrhosis are at present recognized for α-1-antitrypsin deficience. The coexistance of cirrhosis with pulmonary fibrosis should suggest the diagnosis.

Nonalcoholic Fatty Liver Disease. As obesity and type 2 diabetes increase to epidemic proportions, nonalcoholic fatty liver disease (NAFLD) has become the subject of intensified focus and diagnostic refinement. NAFLD has been recognized to be one of the most common causes of chronic liver disease in the U.S. [304]. Emerging evidence cites NAFLD as the most common cause of crytogenic cirrhosis [305]. Cirrhosis related to obesity and NAFLD are risk factors for HCC. The pathologic features of NAFLD are similar to alcohol-induced liver damage and traverse the spectrum of

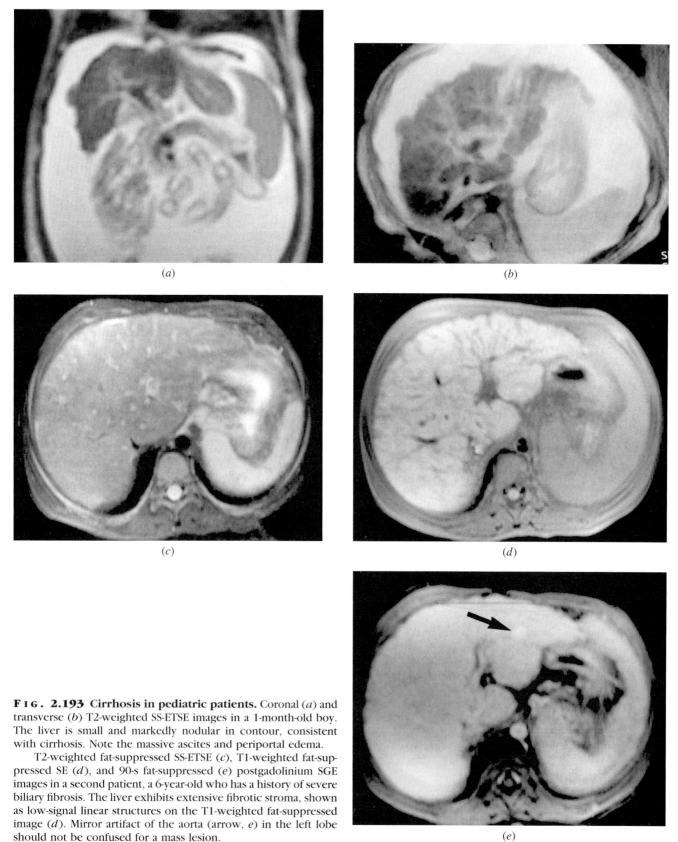

F I G . 2.193 Cirrhosis in pediatric patients. Coronal (*a*) and transverse (*b*) T2-weighted SS-ETSE images in a 1-month-old boy. The liver is small and markedly nodular in contour, consistent with cirrhosis. Note the massive ascites and periportal edema.

T2-weighted fat-suppressed SS-ETSE (*c*), T1-weighted fat-suppressed SE (*d*), and 90-s fat-suppressed (*e*) postgadolinium SGE images in a second patient, a 6-year-old who has a history of severe biliary fibrosis. The liver exhibits extensive fibrotic stroma, shown as low-signal linear structures on the T1-weighted fat-suppressed image (*d*). Mirror artifact of the aorta (arrow, *e*) in the left lobe should not be confused for a mass lesion.

changes, ranging from simple hepatic steatosis (fatty liver) at the most clinically benign, to cirrhosis at the opposite extreme. Nonalcoholic steatohepatitis (NASH) occupies a middle position in the range of NAFLD and represents an intermediate stage of fatty liver damage [306]. NASH is characterized by a constellation of histopathologic features including steatosis, hepatocyte degeneration, inflammation, and fibrosis. A recent study [307] demonstrates a significant correlation between histopathology grades of steatosis and degree of fibrosis in patients with underlying NASH and MRI findings, namely, steatosis and fibrosis. However, no significant correlation was demonstrated between MRI features and Mayo End-stage Liver Disease (MELD) score. It has been estimated that 10–30% of patients with NAFLD (steatosis or NASH) will develop cirrhosis during the ensuing decade [306]. The absence of steatosis in

advanced cirrhosis as a result of NASH is well recognized, and this phenomenon is borne out in MR imaging (fig. 2.194).

From a clinical perspective, there are no laboratory tests that can reliably distinguish steatosis from steatohepatitis or cirrhosis [308]. Although the qualitative and quantitative measurement of hepatic steatosis is accurately assessed by chemical-shift MR imaging [309], there are to date no characteristic imaging findings that point to a specific assessment of NASH [310].

Viral Hepatitis. The term "viral hepatitis" is generally reserved for infection of the liver caused by a small group of hepatotropic viruses. Although agents such as Epstein–Barr virus and cytomegalovirus may produce liver lesions, these are usually a part of a systemic infection in which the liver is only one of several

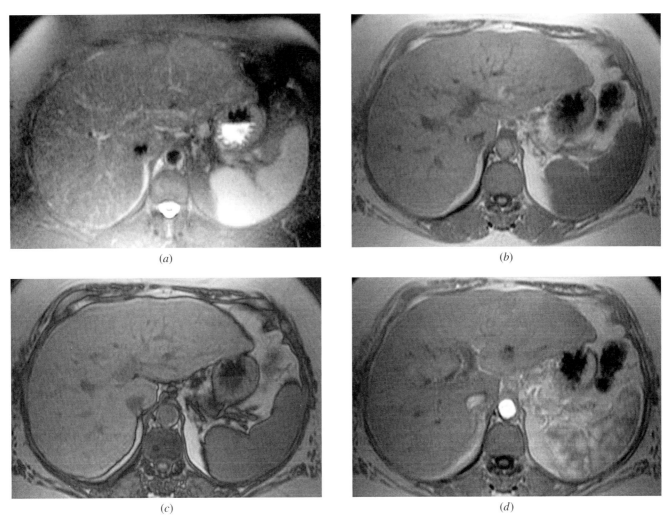

(a)　　　(b)

(c)　　　(d)

F I G . 2.194 Nonalcoholic steatohepatitis. T2-weighted SS-ETSE (*a*), SGE (*b*), out-of-phase SGE (*c*), and immediate (*d*) and 90-s fat-suppressed (*e*) postgadolinium SGE images. The liver is enlarged and shows a higher signal intensity than normal on T1-weighted image (*b*), which converges to the signal intensity of the spleen on out-of-phase image (*c*) suggestive of mild fatty infiltration. On early-phase image, (*d*) there are some patchy areas of enhancement that become homogeneous on late-phase image (*e*), reflecting acute on chronic inflammation. Histopathology was consistent with NASH.

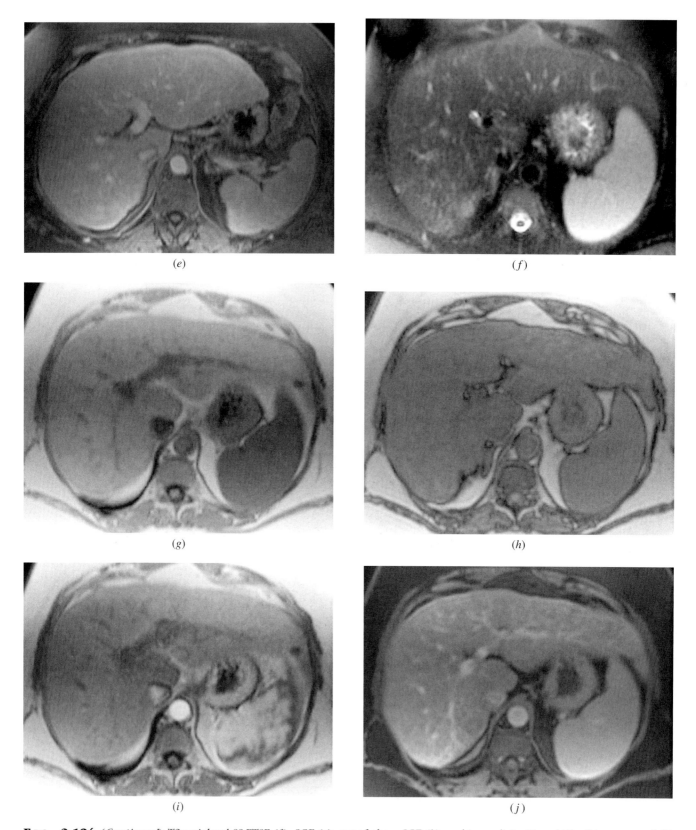

(e)

(f)

(g)

(h)

(i)

(j)

FIG. 2.194 (*Continued*) T2-weighted SS-ETSE (*f*), SGE (*g*), out-of-phase SGE (*h*), and immediate (*i*) and 90-s fat-suppressed (*j*) postgadolinium SGE images in a second patient, who exhibits findings of fatty liver comparing in-phase (*g*) and out-of-phase (*h*) images. Additionally, strands of fibrosis are present, well demonstrated as enhancing reticular structures on late-phase images (*j*). Histopathology was consistent with NASH.

organs or systems involved. Primary viral infection of the liver in the U.S. is caused most commonly by one of three hepatotropic viruses: hepatitis A (HAV), hepatitis B (HBV), and hepatitis C (HCV) [311].

Acute hepatitis is diagnosed by clinical and serologic studies. The major histologic findings in acute viral hepatitis are focal hepatocyte necrosis, inflammatory infiltrates, and evidence of hepatocyte regeneration [2, 3]. Imaging studies are generally not performed unless the clinical picture is complicated. Acute hepatitis may result in heterogeneous hepatic signal intensity, which is most apparent on T2-weighted images and immediate postgadolinium images. Periportal edema may be identified (fig. 2.195).

HBV is a double-stranded DNA virus from the hepadnavirus family that has several genotypes and serotypes capable of causing chronic disease. Two billion people worldwide, or one-third of the world's population, are infected with HBV. Of the 350 million individuals living with chronic HBV, 15-25% risk dying from HBV-related chronic liver disease, including chronic hepatitis, cirrhosis, and hepatocellular carcinoma. In the U.S., 1.25 million people have chronic HBV infection, resulting in more than 5000 deaths each year. Patients with HBV have an increased risk of developing HCC even in the precirrhotic hepatitis phase, when the underlying liver often looks morphologically normal by imaging studies (fig 2.196) [311].

HCV is an RNA virus from the flavivirus family with several known genotypes. The genetic heterogeneity of HCV has important implications for diagnosis, pathogenesis, and treatment. For example, the rapid mutation rate of HCV in opposition to the host immune response renders it a difficult virus to eliminate [311]. HCV infects up to 350 million people worldwide and is currently the leading indication for orthotopic liver transplantation in the U.S. [312]. While up to 50% of individuals clear HCV viremia after acute infection, most people develop persistent infection with chronic hepatitis (fig. 2.197) [312]. Serious sequelae include cirrhosis and hepatocellular carcinoma [313].

Chronic hepatitis may be defined as symptomatic, biochemical, or serologic evidence of continuing inflammation of the liver without improvement for at least 6 months. The microscopic changes of chronic viral hepatitis show chronic inflammation that often extends out from the portal tracts, spilling into the adjacent parenchyma with associated necrosis of hepatocytes. Progressive fibrosis may lead to fully developed cirrhosis [3, 314]. In patients with chronic viral hepatitis, imaging studies are more commonly obtained, usually to detect the presence of cirrhosis or HCC. Focal inflammatory changes or fibrosis may develop in chronic active hepatitis, resulting in diffuse or regional areas of high signal intensity on T2-weighted images and heterogeneous enhancement after contrast on gradient-echo images,

most often appreciated as linear stromal enhancement on late fat-suppressed images (figs. 2.198 and 2.199) [315, 316]. On T2-weighted images, chronic active hepatitis often has periportal high signal intensity, corresponding to inflammation, enlarged lymph nodes, or both (fig. 2.200) [317]. This is a nonspecific finding observed in a number of hepatobiliary and pancreatic diseases [286]. A distinctive feature of HCV chronic liver disease, compared to other chronic diseases, including HBV, is prominent porta hepatis lymph nodes. Nodes measuring 2 cm and larger are common in HCV chronic liver disease.

Radiation-Induced Hepatitis

The liver may be included in radiation portals for a variety of malignancies, metastases in adjacent vertebra, or pancreatic ductal adenocarcinoma. Edema may develop within 6 months of radiation injury. Edema appears as increase signal intensity on T2-weighted images and decreased signal intensity on T1-weighted images (fig. 2.201) [318, 319]. Fat is usually decreased within the radiation portal in patients with fatty liver [320, 321]. This reflects decreased delivery of triglycerides due to diminished portal flow. Increased enhancement is apparent on delayed postgadolinium gradient-echo images in radiation-damaged liver. Increased enhancement is more conspicuous when fat suppression techniques are used (see fig. 2.201). This increased enhancement is related to leaky capillaries in early radiation injury and represents granulation tissue in late injury.

Cirrhosis

A concise definition of cirrhosis is "a diffuse process characterized by fibrosis and a conversion of normal architecture into structurally abnormal nodules" [322]. Cirrhosis is a stage in the evolution of many chronic liver diseases including viral infections, alcohol abuse, hemochromatosis, autoimmune disease, Wilson disease, and primary sclerosing cholangitis. The most common underlying causes in North America include viral hepatitis and alcohol abuse [323].

From a clinicopathologic perspective, cirrhosis is not a static phenomenon but a dynamic process that runs the gamut of inflammation, cell injury and death, fibrosis, and regeneration. Pathologic gross inspection of cirrhotic livers generally shows two types of patterns: 1) micronodular, in which parenchymal nodules are small (<3-mm diameter) and separated by thin fibrous septa, and 2), macronodular in which parenchymal nodules are large (>3mm) and separated by fibrous septa, sometimes reaching proportions of large scars. Because of the underlying pathophysiology of the disease, the conversion from micro- to macronodular cirrhosis is considered to be a general phenomenon. The Copenhagen Study Group for Liver Disease studied 156 cirrhotic patients and observed a conversion ratio

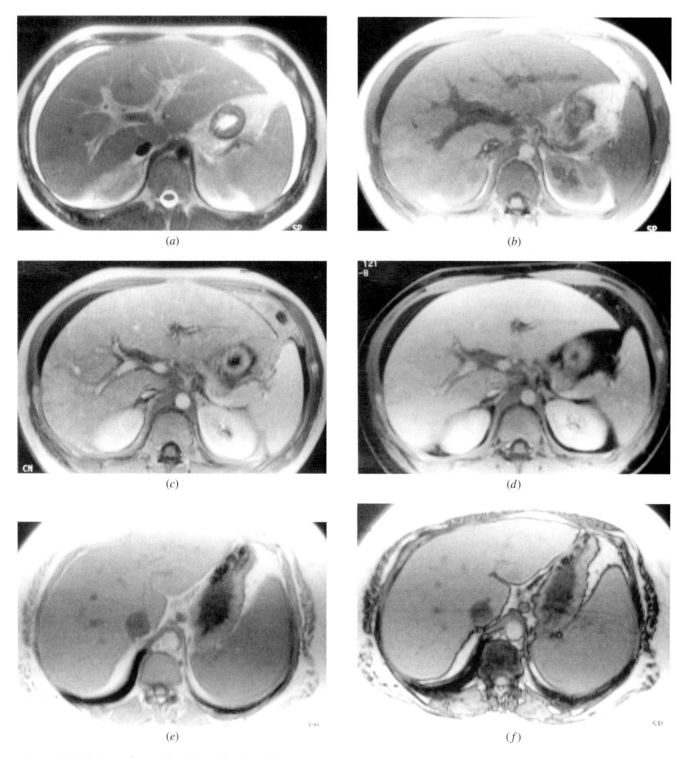

(a)

(b)

(c)

(d)

(e)

(f)

FIG. 2.195 Acute hepatitis. T2-weighted SS-ETSE (*a*), SGE (*b*), immediate (*c*) and 90-s fat-suppressed (*d*) postgadolinium SGE images in a patient with a history of leukemia. The liver is enlarged and demonstrates mild heterogeneous signal on both T2-weighted (*a*) and T1-weighted (*b*) images. On early-phase image (*c*), there is a transient heterogeneous intense patchy enhancement. The liver becomes more uniform in signal intensity on the late images (*d*). Periportal edema is present, which appears as high signal intensity on T2-weighted image (*a*) and does not enhance on postgadolinium images (*c*, *d*). Moderately large volume ascites is shown.

SGE (*e*), out-of-phase SGE (*f*), and immediate (*g*) and 90-s fat-suppressed (*h*) postgadolinium SGE images in a second patient. The liver is unremarkable in signal intensity on T1-weighted image (*e*), with signal intensity of liver and spleen becoming more comparable (converging) on the shorter TE out-of-phase sequence. This appearance of subtle loss of signal of the liver is consistent with mild fat infiltration. There are multiple patchy regions of enhancement after administration of contrast (*g*) throughout the liver consistent with acute on chronic hepatitis.

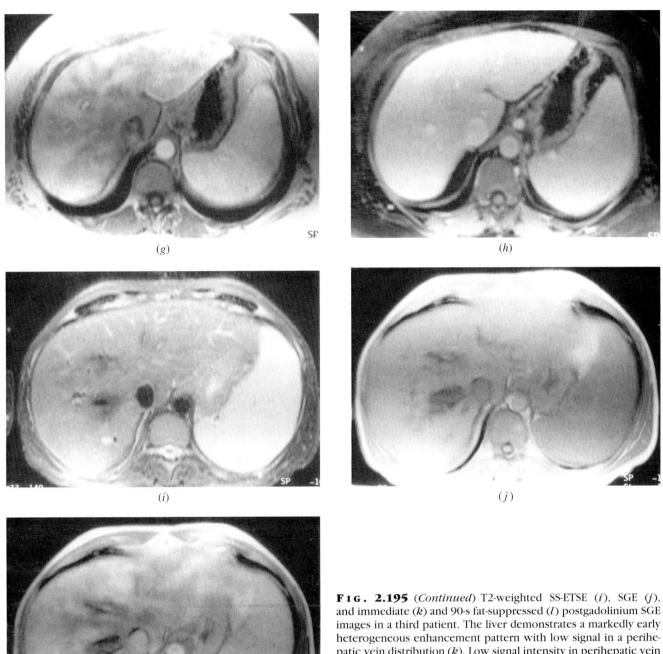

(g)

(h)

(i)

(j)

(k)

FIG. 2.195 (*Continued*) T2-weighted SS-ETSE (*i*), SGE (*j*), and immediate (*k*) and 90-s fat-suppressed (*l*) postgadolinium SGE images in a third patient. The liver demonstrates a markedly early heterogeneous enhancement pattern with low signal in a perihepatic vein distribution (*k*). Low signal intensity in perihepatic vein distribution is also appreciated on the T2-weighted image (*i*).

Coronal T2-weighted SS-ETSE (*m*), SGE (*n*), and immediate (*o*) and 90-s fat-suppressed (*p*) SGE images in a fourth patient. The liver is enlarged and exhibits heterogeneous enhancement on early-phase images (*o*) more evident in the liver periphery. On late-phase images (*p*) the liver demonstrates more homogeneous enhancement.

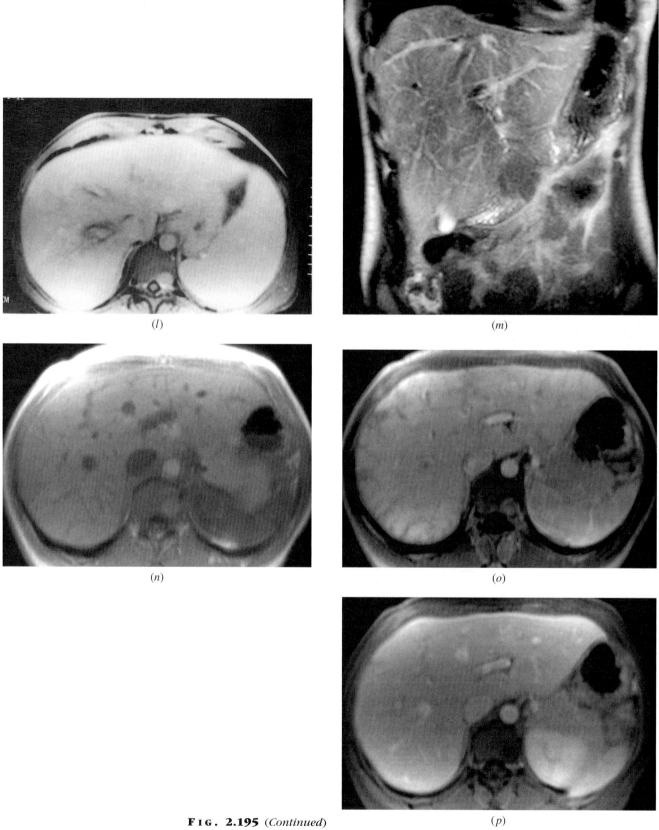

(l)

(m)

(n)

(o)

(p)

FIG. 2.195 (*Continued*)

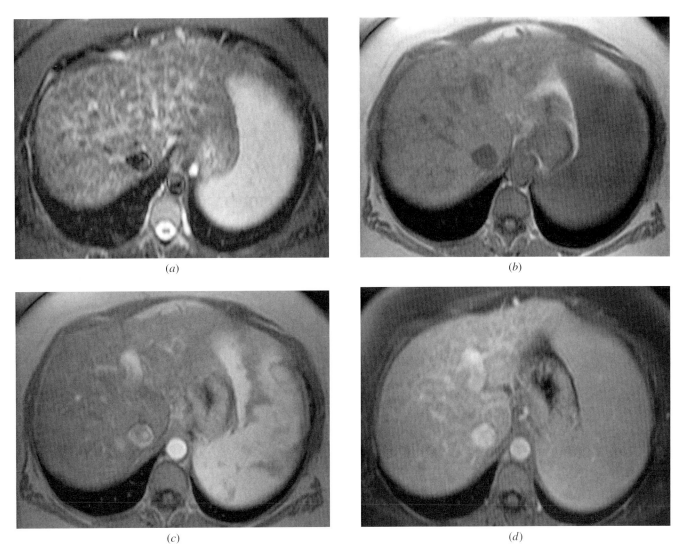

F I G . 2.196 Hepatitis B. T2-weighted fat-suppressed SS-ETSE (*a*), SGE (*b*), and immediate (*c*) and 90-s fat-suppressed (*d*) SGE images in a patient with hepatitis B. In this patient with longstanding disease, the liver is mildly reduced in size and has an irregular contour, with extensive fibrosis on late-phase images (*d*).

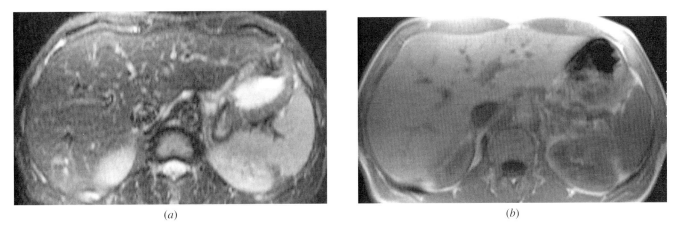

F I G . 2.197 Hepatitis C. T2-weighted SS-ETSE (*a*), SGE (*b*), and immediate (*c*) and 90-s fat-suppressed (*d*) images; T2-weighted

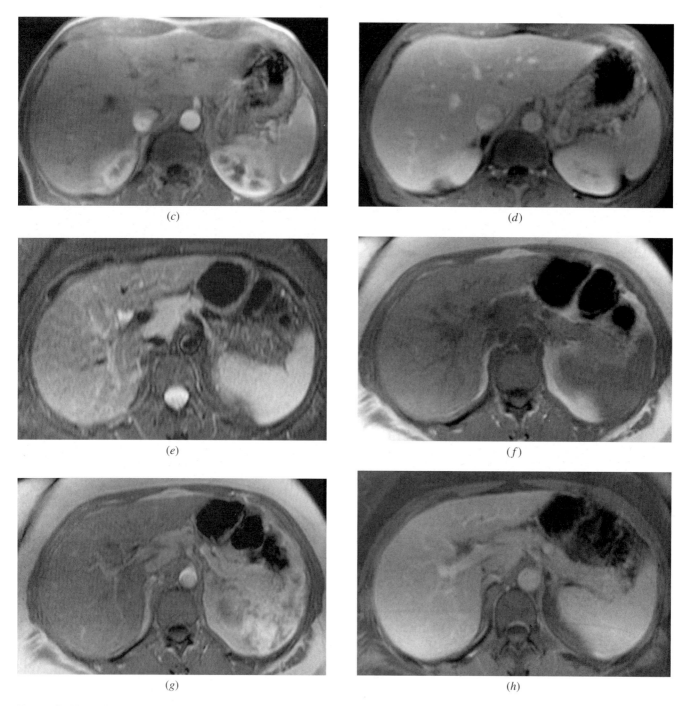

(c)

(d)

(e)

(f)

(g)

(h)

F I G . 2.197 (*Continued*) SS-ETSE (*e*), SGE (*f*), and immediate (*g*) and 90-s fat-suppressed (*h*) images; and T2-weighted SS-ETSE (*i*), out of phase SGE (*j*), and immediate (*k*) and 90-s fat-suppressed (*l*) images in three patients with hepatitis C in different stages. Prominent porta hepatis lymph nodes are usually present (*e*).

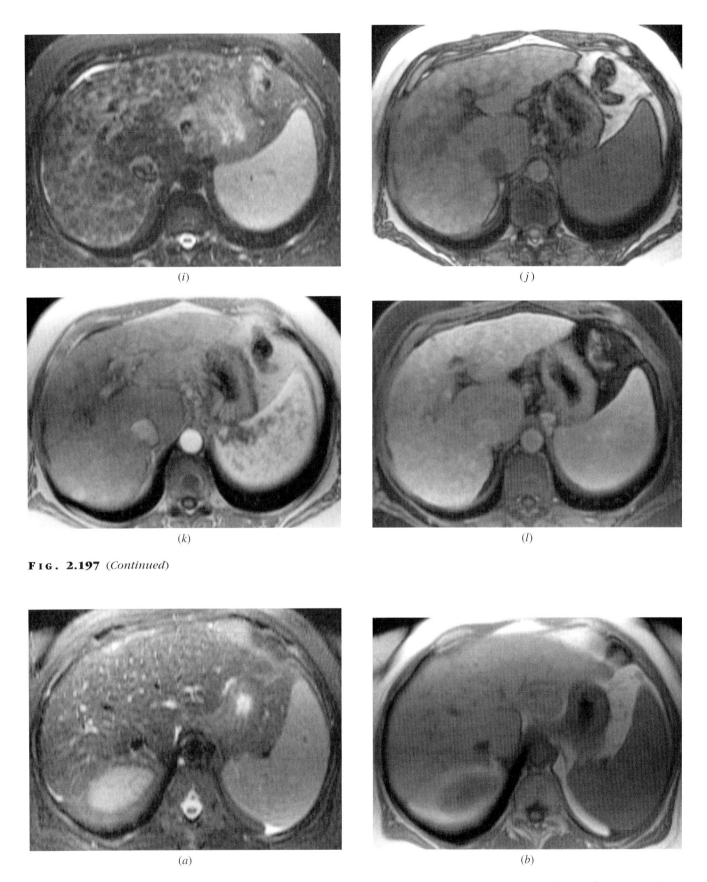

(i)

(j)

(k)

(l)

FIG. 2.197 *(Continued)*

(a)

(b)

FIG. 2.198 Acute on chronic hepatitis. T2-weighted fat-suppressed SS-ETSE (*a, e*), SGE (*b, f, j*), and immediate (*c, g, i, k, m, n*), 45-s (*l*), and 90-s fat-suppressed (*d, h*) SGE images in five different patients. Although these patients demonstrate different stages

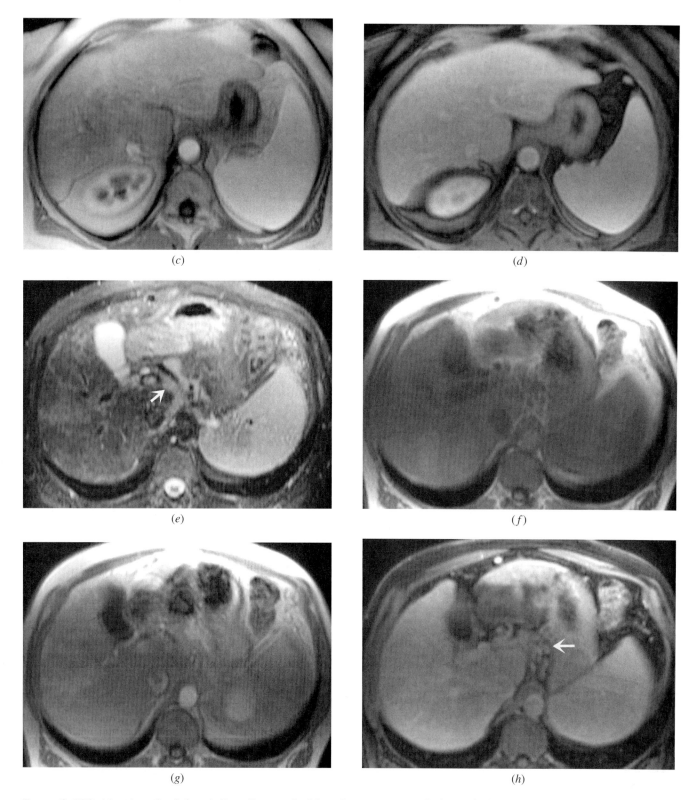

(c)

(d)

(e)

(f)

(g)

(h)

FIG. 2.198 (*Continued*) of chronic liver disease, all of them have a common finding, which is the heterogeneous enhancement on early-phase images (*c, g, k, m, n*) that becomes homogeneous on 45-s image (*l*) and remains homogeneous on late-phase images (*d, h*). This finding is compatible with acute on chronic hepatitis. Note that other signs of chronic liver disease are also appreciated in these patients such as lymphadenopathy (arrow, *e*), varices (arrow, *h*), ascites (*i*), and Gamna–Gandy bodies in the spleen (*m*).

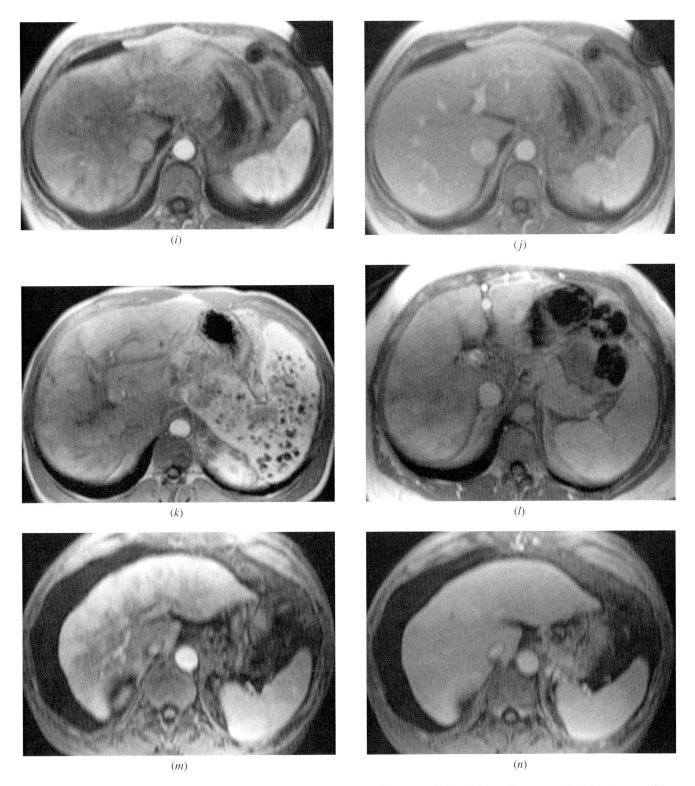

FIG. 2.198 (*Continued*) T1-weighted fat-suppressed 3D-gradient echo (*o*)- and 90-s (*p*)-immediate postgadolinium images show heterogeneous hepatic enhancement on early phase (*m*) that becomer homogeneous on late phase (*n*), features compatible with acute on chronic hepatitis.

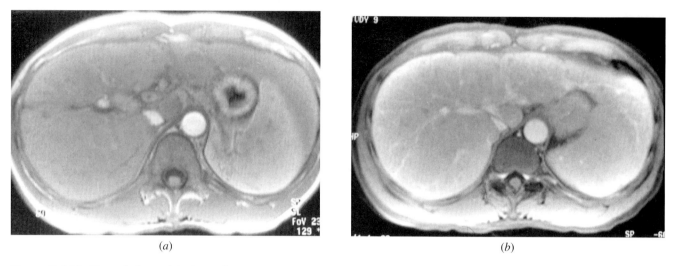

(a)   (b)

FIG. 2.199 Chronic hepatitis. Immediate (*a*) and 90-s fat-suppressed (*b*) postgadolinium SGE images show delayed enhancement of liver fibrous tissue on late-phase image (*b*) consistent with fibrosis.

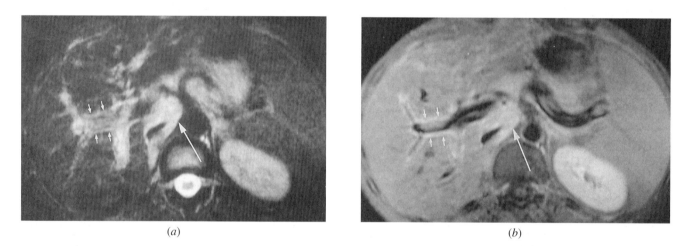

(a)   (b)

FIG. 2.200 Viral hepatitis. T2-weighted fat-suppressed SE (*a*) and 90-s fat-suppressed postgadolinium SE (*b*) images in a patient with HIV infection and positive serology for hepatitis B and C. On the fat-suppressed T2-weighted sequence (*a*), porta hepatis and para-aortic lymph nodes (long arrow, *a*) are clearly shown as high-signal-intensity masses in lower-signal-intensity background. High signal within the liver in a periportal distribution is also present (small arrows, *a*). This periportal abnormality identified on the T2-weighted image is shown to be enhancing tissue (small arrows, *b*) on the gadolinium-enhanced T1-weighted fat-suppressed image (*b*). Gadolinium enhancement distinguishes periportal inflammatory or neoplastic tissue from edema, the latter would appear signal void after contrast. Enhancement of adenopathy (long arrow, *b*) is also appreciated.

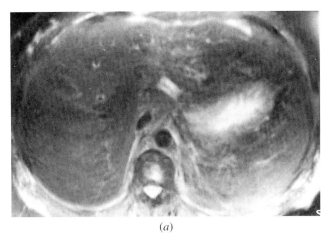

(*a*)

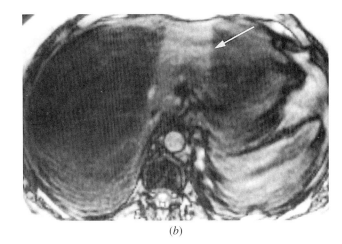

(*b*)

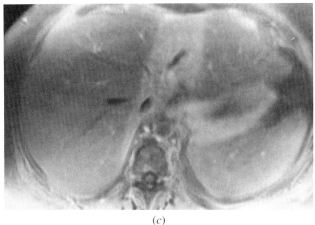

(*c*)

F I G . 2.201 Radiation injury. T2-weighted fat-suppressed SE (*a*), out-of-phase SGE (*b*), and 90-s fat-suppressed postgadolinium SE (*c*) images in a patient who had undergone radiation therapy for a vertebral body metastasis. The out-of-phase image (*b*) shows low-signal-intensity fatty replaced liver with a central, vertically oriented band of higher-signal-intensity nonfatty liver (arrow, *b*). Similar findings are apparent on the fat-suppressed T2-weighted image (*a*), with subtle higher signal intensity of the central band of nonfatty liver. The gadolinium-enhanced T1-weighted fat-suppressed image (*c*) demonstrates increased enhancement of the radiation-damaged liver, which may reflect radiation-induced vasculitis, in conjunction with lower signal of fatty liver due to fat-suppression effects.

of micronodular to macronodular cirrhosis of 90% in 10 years [314]. Cirrhotic nodules may be characterized based on histologic features into three majors categories, namely, 1) regenerative, representing a benign proliferation of hepatocytes surrounded by fibrous septa; 2) dysplastic, representing regenerative nodules with cellular atypia, an intermediate step in the pathogenesis of HCC; and 3) malignant or HCC [93].

By MR imaging, a variety of morphologic changes are common findings. Atrophy of the right lobe and the medial segment of the left lobe is common in cirrhotic livers. Relative sparing of the caudate lobe and lateral segment of the left lobe is often present. In fact, these segments may undergo hypertrophy. The combination of scarring, atrophy, and parenchymal regenerative activity may involve any segment of the liver and occasionally may result in a bizarre hepatic contour that can simulate tumor mass (fig. 2.202). Often the hypertrophic region of the liver possesses imaging and enhancement features comparable to those of normal liver, thus facilitating a correct diagnosis. Morphologic changes of the liver are seen less frequently in early compensated cirrhosis, impairing diagnosis by imaging. In cirrhotic livers, enlargement of the hilar periportal space was

observed in 98% of patients who had atrophy of the medial segment of the left lobe, whereas this finding was seen in only 11% of patients with normal livers [324, 325]. Expansion of the major interlobar fissure may be seen in the late stage of disease, causing extrahepatic fat to fill the space between the left medial and lateral segments [326].

With advanced cirrhosis, morphologic liver changes become more evident. There may be marked atrophy of the right lobe and medial segment of the left lobe and hypertrophy of the caudate lobe and left lateral segment. The combination of these four findings is responsible for the enlargement of the pericholecystic space (gallbladder fossa), which is subsequently filled with fat, known as the "expanded gallbladder fossa sign." This imaging finding is highly suggestive of cirrhosis [324]. Moreover, with progression of the disease, the liver surface shows irregularities and the liver morphology exhibits distortion, both due to the presence of regenerative nodules and confluent or diffuse parenchymal fibrosis [300, 327].

The most consistent morphologic feature of cirrhosis is the demonstration of focal or diffuse fibrous tissue that appears on MRI as a reticular network of linear

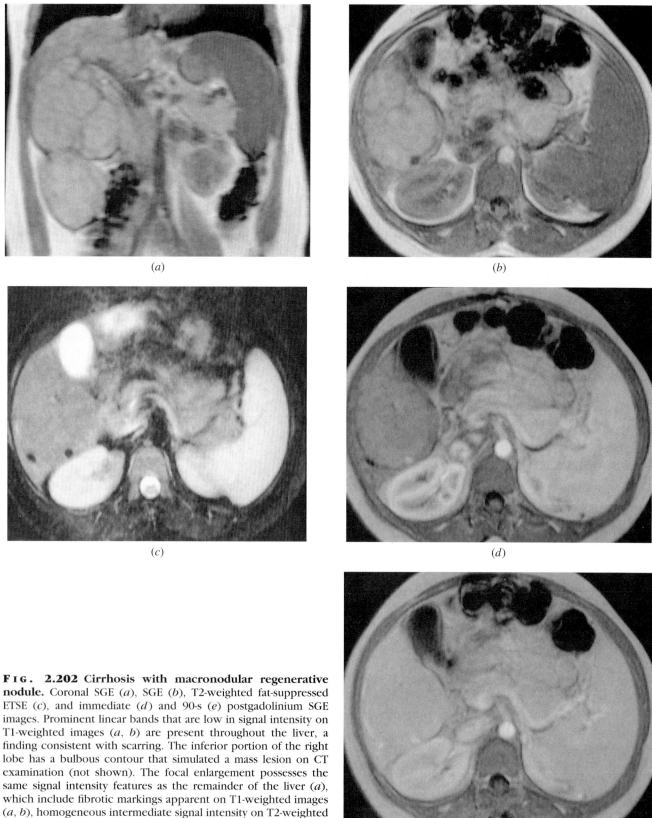

(a)

(b)

(c)

(d)

(e)

F I G . 2.202 Cirrhosis with macronodular regenerative nodule. Coronal SGE (*a*), SGE (*b*), T2-weighted fat-suppressed ETSE (*c*), and immediate (*d*) and 90-s (*e*) postgadolinium SGE images. Prominent linear bands that are low in signal intensity on T1-weighted images (*a, b*) are present throughout the liver, a finding consistent with scarring. The inferior portion of the right lobe has a bulbous contour that simulated a mass lesion on CT examination (not shown). The focal enlargement possesses the same signal intensity features as the remainder of the liver (*a*), which include fibrotic markings apparent on T1-weighted images (*a, b*), homogeneous intermediate signal intensity on T2-weighted images (*c*), early diminished enhancement of scar tissue (*d*), and more uniform enhancement on interstitial-phase images (*e*).

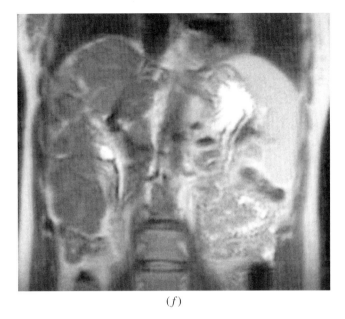

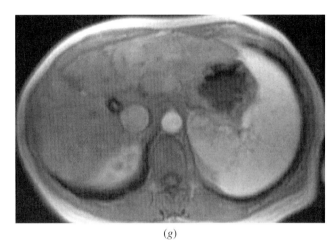

(*f*)   (*g*)

F I G . 2.202 (*Continued*) Coronal T2-weighted SS-ETSE (*f*) and transverse 45-s postgadolinium SGE (*g*) images in a second patient show similar findings.

stroma of varying thickness [328]. On T1-weighted images fibrous tissue is low signal; on T2-weighted images fibrous tissue varies from high signal to low signal, depending on chronicity, with acute fibrous tissue having a higher fluid content and therefore higher signal. On hepatic arterial dominant-phase images, fibrous tissue enhances negligibly and demonstrates late enhancement on hepatic venous phase images (fig. 2.203). Fibrous tissue is most consistently shown on short-TE T1-weighted gradient-echo images and well shown on TE = 2 ms out-of-phase imaging at 1.5 T, appearing as low-signal reticular tissue. Fibrosis is also well shown as late-enhancing stroma on 2-min postgadolinium fat-suppressed gradient-echo images (figs. 2.204 and 2.205) [329].

Many livers in the setting of chronic hepatitis or cirrhosis may contain regions that are high signal intensity on T2-weighted images and low signal intensity on T1-weighted images and enhance moderately intensely on arterial dominant-phase images, secondary to hepatocellular damage, inflammation, or arteriovenous shunts; which are most consistently, or only, shown on hepatic arterial dominant-phase images [330–332]. Acute on chronic liver inflammation is shown as regions of transient increased enhancement on immediate postgadolinium images [329, 332]. Many abnormal regions of enhancement are small with irregular or ill-defined margins. In these cases, distinction from tumor is not problematic. Occasionally, patchy areas of enhancement are large, and they generally fade to near isointensity by 1 min. Rarely, patchy areas of increased enhancement may show variable enhancement on later

postcontrast images. Under these circumstances, distinction from diffuse HCC may be problematic. In the setting of diffuse HCC, an important distinguishing feature is the association with tumor thrombus. Bland thrombus is rare with acute on chronic hepatitis, and enhancing thrombus never occurs. Serum α-fetoprotein level may support the diagnosis, because serum α-fetoprotein is typically very elevated with diffuse HCC and only slightly elevated in patients with acute on chronic hepatitis [333].

Tiny peribiliary cysts may occur in cirrhotic livers. These cysts typically measure 5 mm or less in size [334–336].

In cirrhotic livers, parenchymal nodules are created by the regenerative activity of hepatocytes and the network of fibrosis. The formation of regenerative nodules (RNs) results in gross distortion of hepatic architecture. Micronodular cirrhosis, common in alcoholic liver disease and hemochromatosis, displays RNs ≤3 mm, sheathed by thin fibrous septa. In patients with virus-induced cirrhosis (mainly hepatitis B), the regenerative nodules are 3–15 mm with thick fibrous septa; this pattern is classified as macronodular cirrhosis. Although some diseases are classically associated with one pattern or another, most cirrhotic livers are mixed [337, 338]. MRI demonstrates RNs with greater conspicuity than any other imaging modality. The majority of RNs are isointense on T2- and T1-weighted images. Occasionally, RNs may appear low in signal intensity on T2-weighted images relative to high-signal-intensity inflammatory fibrous septa or damaged liver (figs. 2.206–2.208) [180, 181, 185]. Approximately 16 % (11/68)

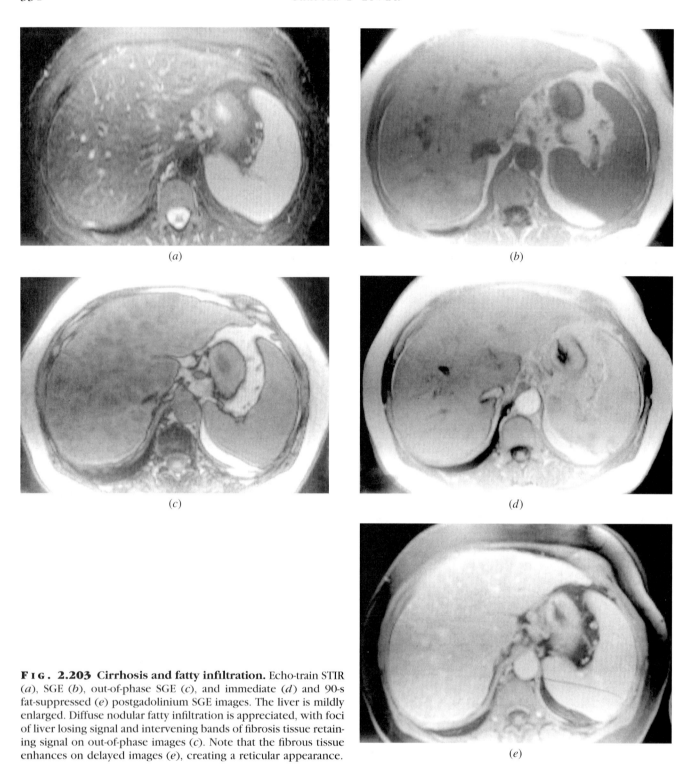

FIG. 2.203 Cirrhosis and fatty infiltration. Echo-train STIR (*a*), SGE (*b*), out-of-phase SGE (*c*), and immediate (*d*) and 90-s fat-suppressed (*e*) postgadolinium SGE images. The liver is mildly enlarged. Diffuse nodular fatty infiltration is appreciated, with foci of liver losing signal and intervening bands of fibrosis tissue retaining signal on out-of-phase images (*c*). Note that the fibrous tissue enhances on delayed images (*e*), creating a reticular appearance.

of RNs are hyperintense on T1-weighted images. The cause for this hyperintensity on T1 is unclear, unrelated to lipid, but possibly reflects high protein content. Because RNs have a portal venous blood supply with minimal contribution from hepatic arteries [339], RNs enhance minimally on hepatic arterial dominant-phase images.

Approximately 25% of RNs accumulate more iron than the surrounding hepatic parenchyma. This feature facilitates the identification of RNs as low signal on T2-weighted and T2*-weighted gradient-echo images and low signal on postgadolinium SGE images because surrounding hepatic parenchyma enhances to a greater degree than iron-containing nodules (fig. 2.209) [339,

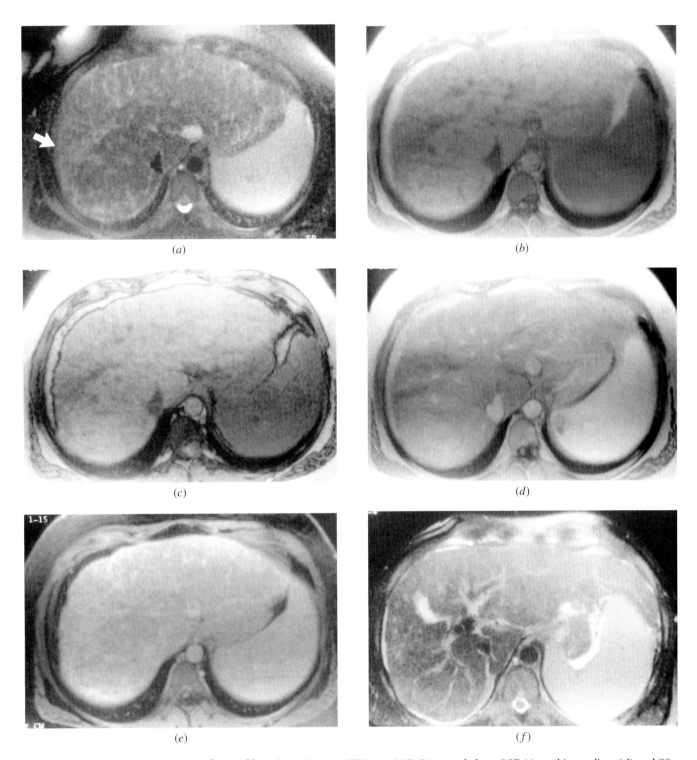

F I G . 2.204 Cirrhosis with confluent fibrosis. Echo-train STIR (*a*), SGE (*b*), out-of-phase SGE (*c*), and immediate (*d*) and 90-s fat-suppressed (*e*) postgadolinium SGE images. There is a linear pattern of fibrosis throughout the liver, with a focal region of confluent fibrosis (arrow, *a*) that is mildly high in signal on T2 (*a*) and mildly low in signal on T1-weighted image (*b*) and demonstrates negligible enhancement on early postcontrast image (*d*) and mild enhancement on late image (*e*). Note that the fine pattern of fibrosis present throughout the liver is particularly well shown on the short TE out-of-phase image (*c*) as low-signal linear structures (*c*) and on late postgadolinium as linear enhancing structures (*e*).

T2-weighted fat-suppressed SS-ETSE (*f*), SGE (*g*), out-of-phase SGE (*h*), and immediate (*i*) and 90-s fat-suppressed postgadolinium SGE (*j*) images in a second patient. The liver is small and nodular in contour and demonstrates a reticular heterogeneous

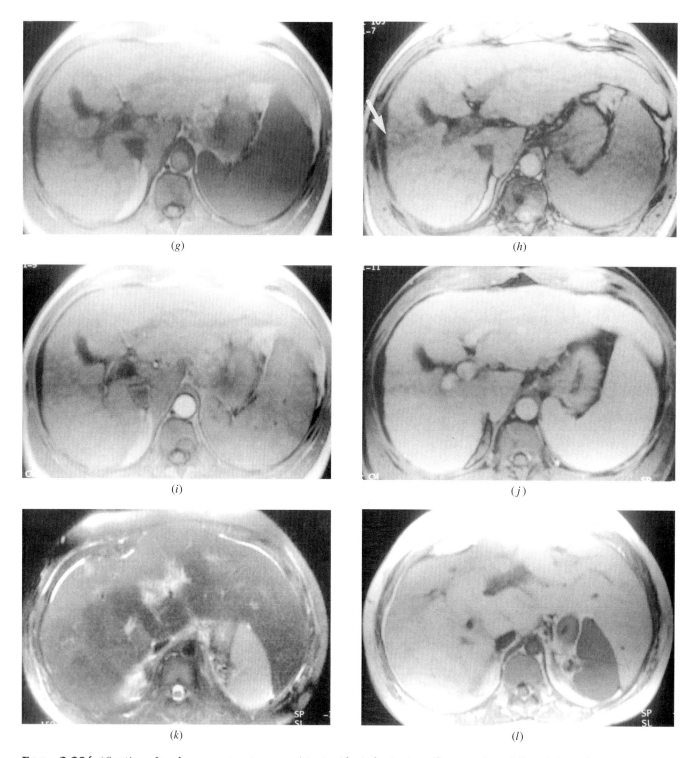

(g)

(h)

(i)

(j)

(k)

(l)

FIG. 2.204 (*Continued*) enhancement pattern consistent with cirrhosis. A confluent region of fibrosis is evident in segment 8 peripherally (arrow, *h*). No focal lesion is identified within the liver. Note the presence of splenomegaly.

T2-weighted fat-suppressed SS-ETSE (*k*), SGE (*l*), out-of-phase (*m*), and immediate (*n*) and 90-s fat-suppressed (*o*) postgadolinium SGE images in a third patient. The liver is enlarged, with the left lobe extending lateral to the spleen. On the out-of-phase image (*m*),

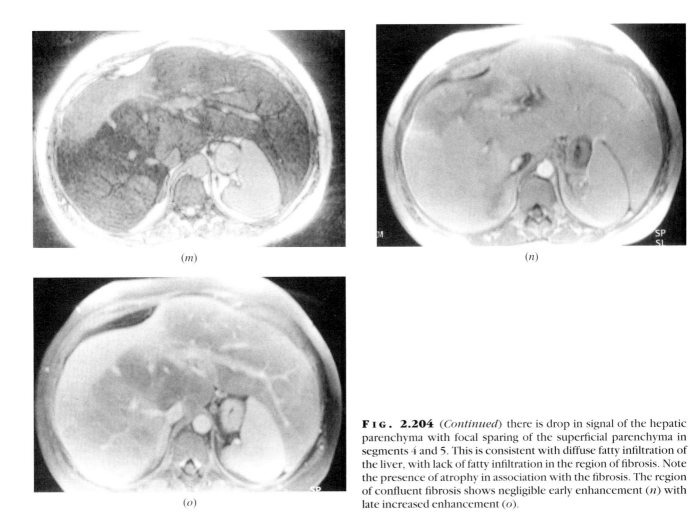

(m)

(n)

(o)

FIG. 2.204 (*Continued*) there is drop in signal of the hepatic parenchyma with focal sparing of the superficial parenchyma in segments 4 and 5. This is consistent with diffuse fatty infiltration of the liver, with lack of fatty infiltration in the region of fibrosis. Note the presence of atrophy in association with the fibrosis. The region of confluent fibrosis shows negligible early enhancement (*n*) with late increased enhancement (*o*).

(a)

(b)

FIG. 2.205 Cirrhosis with extensive and confluent fibrosis. Echo-train STIR (*a*), SGE (*b*), and immediate (*c*), and 90-s fat-suppressed (*d*) postgadolinium SGE and echo-train STIR (*e*), SGE (*f*), out-of-phase SGE (*g*), and immediate (*h*), and 90-s fat-suppressed (*i*) postgadolinium SGE images in two different patients with cirrhosis. In both cases, the liver is diminutive in size and demonstrates

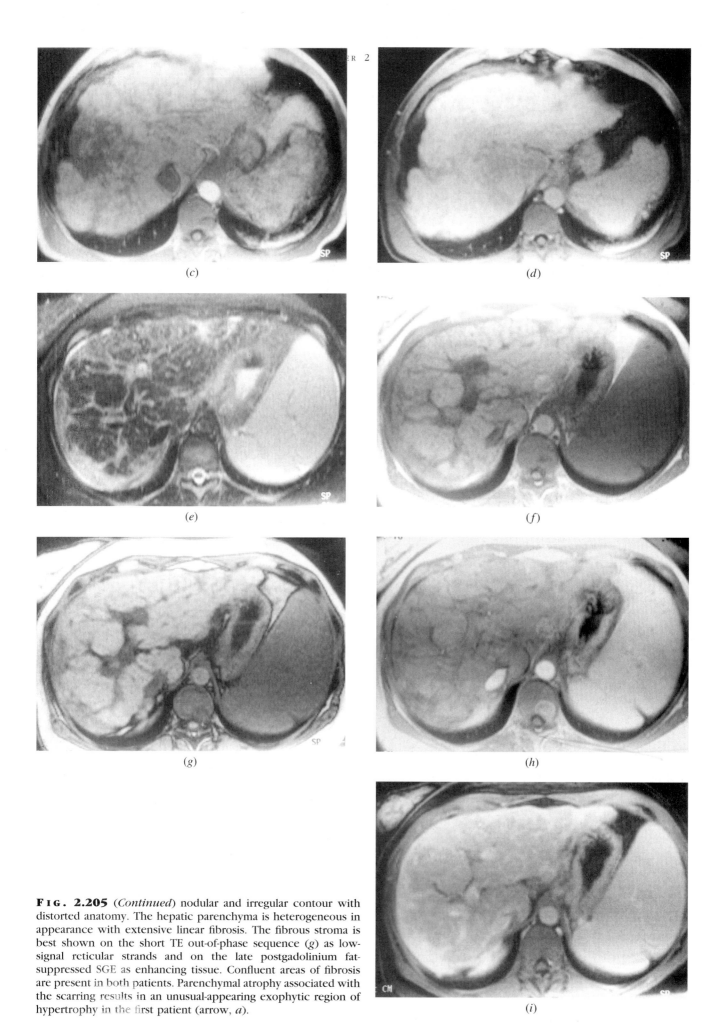

(c)

(d)

(e)

(f)

(g)

(h)

FIG. 2.205 (*Continued*) nodular and irregular contour with distorted anatomy. The hepatic parenchyma is heterogeneous in appearance with extensive linear fibrosis. The fibrous stroma is best shown on the short TE out-of-phase sequence (*g*) as low-signal reticular strands and on the late postgadolinium fat-suppressed SGE as enhancing tissue. Confluent areas of fibrosis are present in both patients. Parenchymal atrophy associated with the scarring results in an unusual-appearing exophytic region of hypertrophy in the first patient (arrow, *a*).

(i)

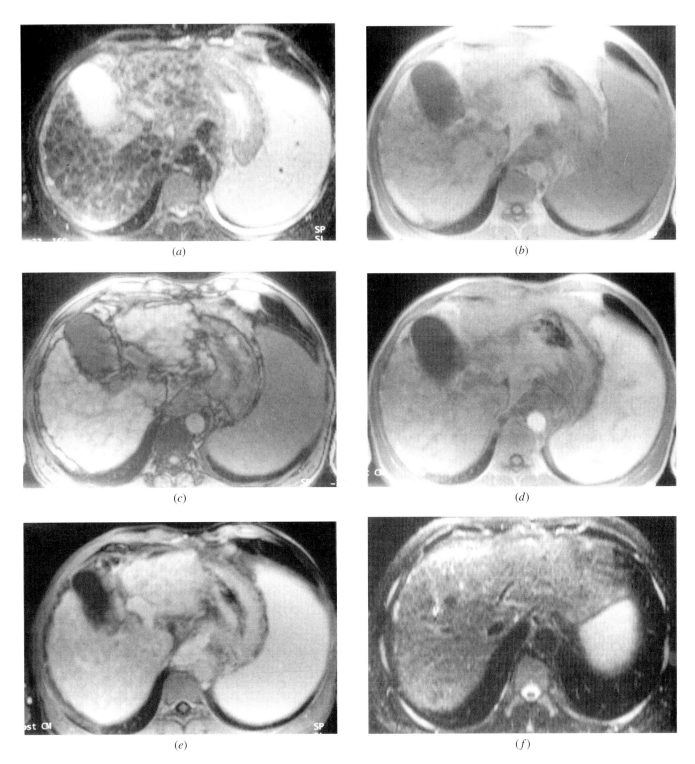

F I G . 2.206 Cirrhosis with regenerative nodules. Echo-train STIR (*a*), SGE (*b*), out-of-phase SGE (*c*), and immediate (*d*), and 90-s fat-suppressed (*e*) postgadolinium SGE images. The liver is small with an extensive nodular pattern. A reticular pattern of fibrosis is present, which is well shown on out-of-phase images (*c*) as low-signal-intensity linear tissue and demonstrates negligible enhancement on immediate postgadolinium images (*d*) with progressive enhancement on late images (*e*). Multiple regenerative nodules appear as rounded <1-cm masses well shown as high-signal lesions on out-of-phase images (*c*). Ascites, splenomegaly, and para-esophageal varices are present.

Echo-train STIR (*f*), SGE (*g*), out-of-phase SGE (*h*), and 45-s (*i*) and 90-s fat-suppressed (*j*) postgadolinium SGE images in a second patient. There are multiple scattered rounded foci throughout the liver that show decreased signal on T2 (*f*) and increased

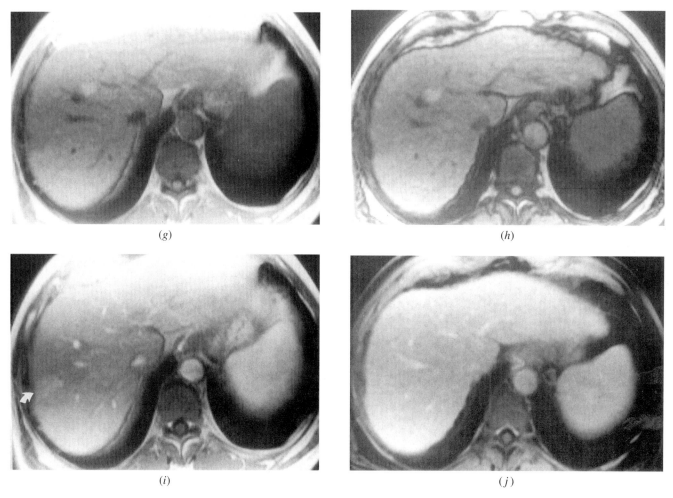

(g)   (h)

(i)   (j)

FIG. 2.206 (*Continued*) signal on noncontrast T1-weighted (*g*) and out-of-phase (*h*) images. Lesions are not apparent on early (*i*) or late (*j*) postgadolinium images, consistent with regenerative or mildly dysplastic nodules. Note also the fine reticular pattern on postgadolinium images (*i, j*) with progressive enhancement, consistent with fibrotic change associated with cirrhosis. A small transiently enhancing focus (curved arrow, *i*) is present in segment 8, which reflects a focal hyperperfusion abnormality.

340]. Although it is suggested that the presence of iron within RNs is a risk factor for HCC [341], this association is not yet well established.

Central large regenerative nodules may be most characteristic of cirrhosis due to PSC. In these cases, regions of atrophic, cirrhotic liver and obstructed bile ducts may be compressed at the periphery of massively expanded regenerative nodules.

The prevalence of RNs in Budd–Chiari syndrome is not known, but it is suggested that they may be observed in up to 25% of patients. In the setting of chronic Budd–Chiari syndrome, RNs may show atypical MR features, namely, high signal on T2- and T1-weighted images and moderate enhancement on arterial dominant phase. It is hypothesized that the hypervascularization of the RNs in this disorder reflects enlargement of hepatic arteries and an abnormality of portal flow [342–344].

Dysplastic nodules (DNs) are defined as neoplastic, clonal lesions that represent an intermediate step in the pathway of carcinogenesis of hepatocytes in cirrhotic livers [93, 338]. They are considered as premalignant nodules and are found in 15–25% of cirrhotic livers [345]. Studies have documented the development of HCC within a DN in as short as a 4-month period [346, 347]. On gross pathologic examination, DNs are usually larger than RNs, but the entities may be impossible to distinguish both pathologically and by MRI [165].

DNs are diagnosed histologically as low or high grade according to the current classification system for nodular hepatocellular lesions by the International Working Party [93]. Low- and high-grade DNs represent parts of a spectrum involving microscopic architectural changes and cytologic atypia [338].

On MR imaging, DNs are most commonly recognized as isointense or hypointense on T2-weighted

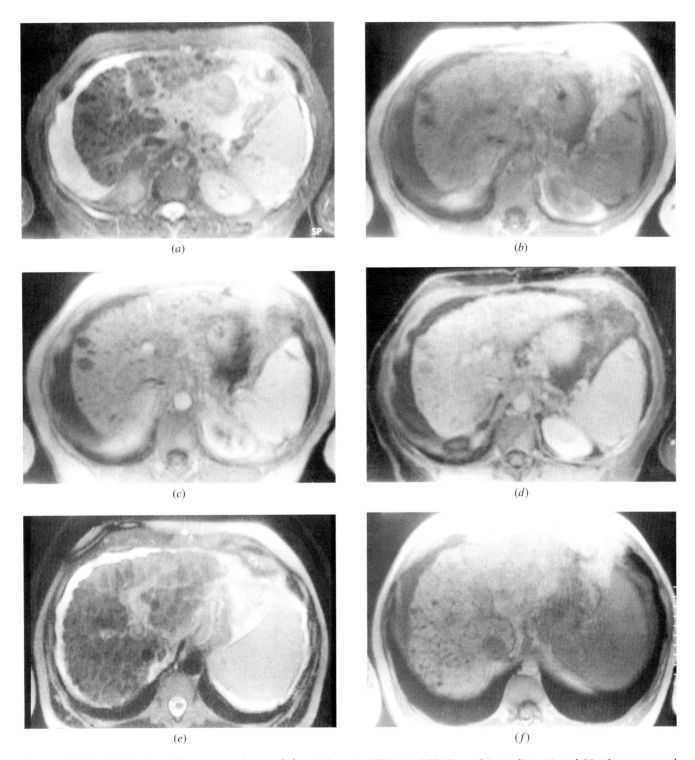

(a)

(b)

(c)

(d)

(e)

(f)

F I G . 2.207 Cirrhosis with regenerative nodules. Echo-train STIR (*a*), SGE (*b*), and immediate (*c*) and 90-s fat-suppressed (*d*) postgadolinium SGE and echo-train STIR (*e*), SGE (*f*), out-of-phase SGE (*g*), and immediate (*h, i*) and 90-s fat-suppressed (*j*) postgadolinium SGE images in two different patients. The livers are diminutive in size and show irregular nodular contours

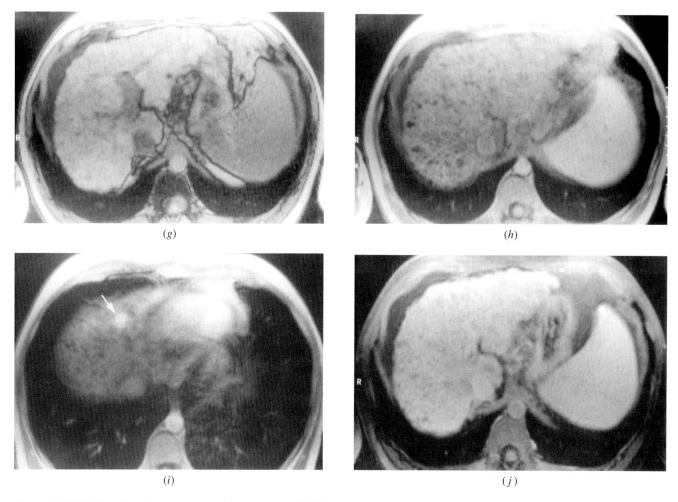

(g)

(h)

(i)

(j)

F I G . 2.207 (*Continued*) consistent with cirrhosis. Multiple varying-sized siderotic nodules are appreciated throughout the hepatic parenchyma that demonstrate low signal on both T2-weighted (*a, e*) and T1-weighted (*b, f*) images and negligible enhancement early (*h*) and late (*j*) after gadolinium administration, compatible with regenerative nodules. In the second patient, an intensely enhancing 1-cm nodule is also shown on early-phase image (arrow, *i*), which fades on late image (not shown) in the dome of the liver, consistent with a high grade dysplastic nodule.

images and hyperintense on T1-weighted images [185, 187, 348]. Like RNs, DNs may also contain iron, which then results in low signal intensity on both T2- and T1-weighted images. Unlike RNs, DNs have been found to contain isolated arteries unaccompanied by bile ducts [338]. Correlations exist between extent of enhancement on arterial dominant images and the grade of DNs. Increase in arterial blood supply and decrease of portal blood supply of hepatic nodules is closely related to the process of malignant transformation to HCC [349, 350]. On MR imaging, low-grade DNs show negligible enhancement or enhancement similar to the background parenchyma (i.e., isointense) on arterial dominant phase (figs. 2.210–2.212), and high-grade DNs may demonstrate enhancement ranging from mild to intense on arterial dominant-phase images (figs. 2.213 and 2.214). There is an overlap in the extent of vascularity and

consequently of imaging findings between high-grade DNs and small HCCs [201, 349]. An ancillary feature of high-grade DNs is the tendency to fade toward background signal of the liver in the interstitial phase of enhancement, whereas small HCCs are more likely to exhibit lesion washout with late capsule enhancement. The signal intensity on T2-weighted images, the degree of lesional enhancement on interstitial-phase images, the interval growth, and the presence of large HCC may help in the distinction of high-grade DNs and small HCCs. Our current practice is to describe lesions that measure less than 1 cm with the imaging features of high DN as DN, recognizing the fact that many of these small lesions resolve on their own, likely reflecting a complex interplay between host and lesion pathophysiology.

Foci of small HCC that develop in a high-grade DN appear as a high-signal-intensity focus within a

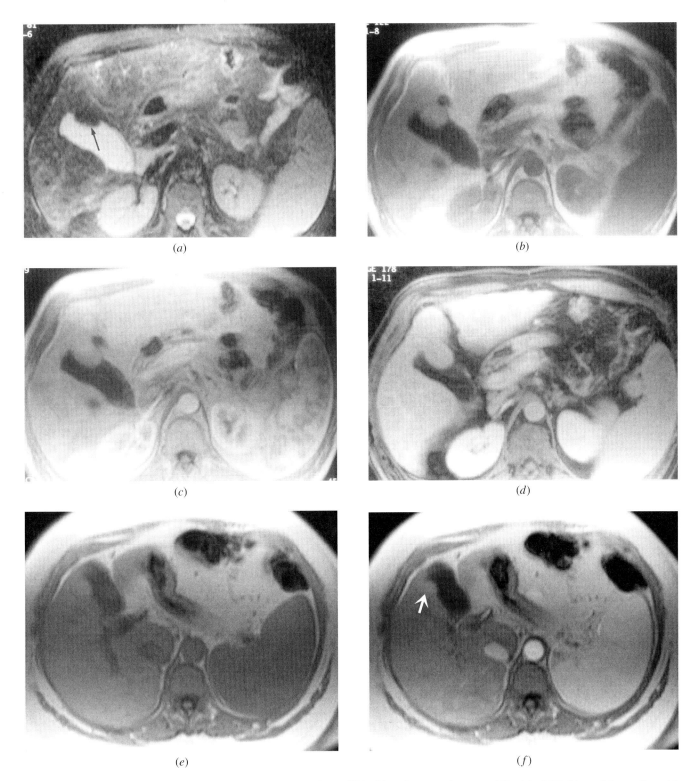

(a)

(b)

(c)

(d)

(e)

(f)

F I G . 2.208 Regenerative nodule extending into the gallbladder fossa. Echo-train STIR (*a*), SGE (*b*), and immediate (*c*) and 90-s fat-suppressed (*d*) postgadolinium SGE images. The liver demonstrates mild diffuse heterogeneous signal on all sequences. There is a hepatic nodule (arrow, *a*) that arises from the tip of segment 4 and indents the anterior wall of the gallbladder, which demonstrates near isointensity with liver on all sequences compatible with a regenerative nodule.

SGE (*e*) and immediate (*f*) images in a second patient that demonstrate a regenerative nodule compressing the posterior wall of the gallbladder (arrow, *f*). It is not uncommon that regenerative nodules bulge into the gallbladder fossa, presumably reflecting that this location experiences less tissue resistance facilitating growth of these nodules as they expand into the gallbladder fossa.

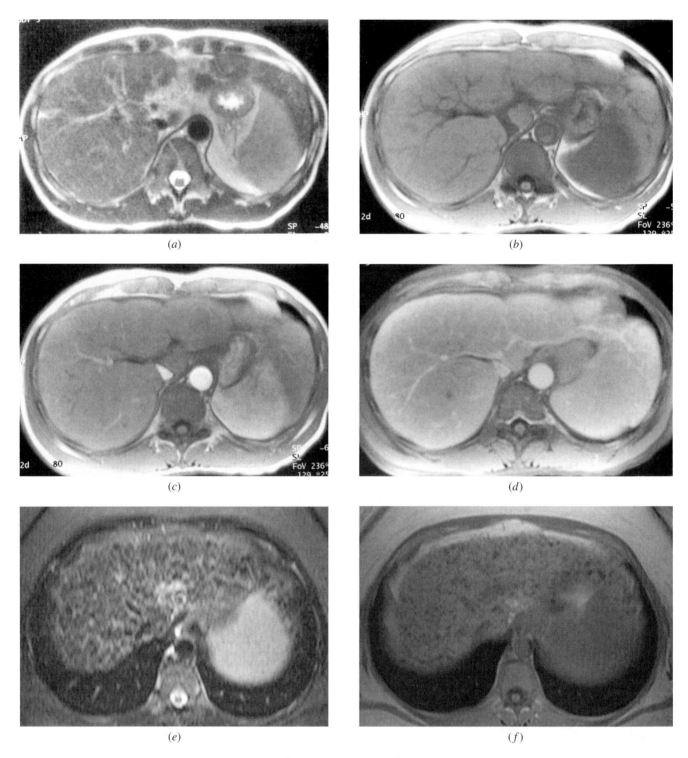

(a)

(b)

(c)

(d)

(e)

(f)

F I G . 2.209 Iron-containing regenerative nodules. T2-weighted ETSE (*a*), SGE (*b*), and immediate (*c*) and 90-s fat-suppressed (*d*) postgadolinium SGE images. There are multiple tiny lesions scattered throughout the liver that demonstrate mild hypointensity to background liver on T2-weighted (*a*) and T1-weighted (*b*) images and negligible enhancement after contrast administration (*c*), consistent with regenerative nodules. Lesions are best seen on the postgadolinium images. Note the fine reticular linear pattern of enhancement on the late image (*d*).

T2-weighted fat-suppressed SS-ETSE (*e*), SGE (*f*), out-of-phase SGE (*g*), and immediate (*h*) and 90-s fat-suppressed (*i*) postgadolinium SGE images (*j*) and SGE (*j*) and immediate (*k*) and 90-s fat-suppressed (*l*) postgadolinium SGE images in two different patients with regenerative nodules. Findings similar to those in the previous case are shown.

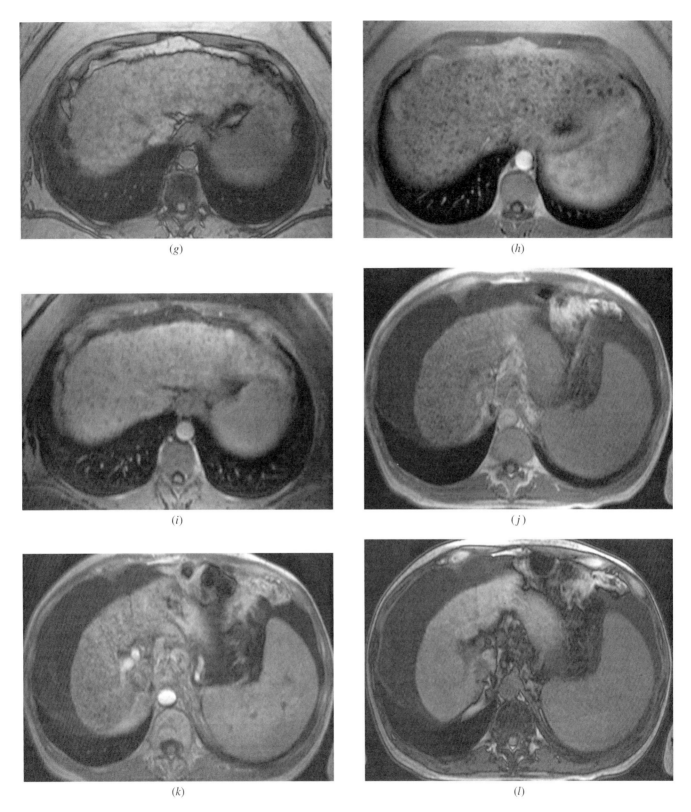

(g)

(h)

(i)

(j)

(k)

(l)

F I G . 2.209 (*Continued*)

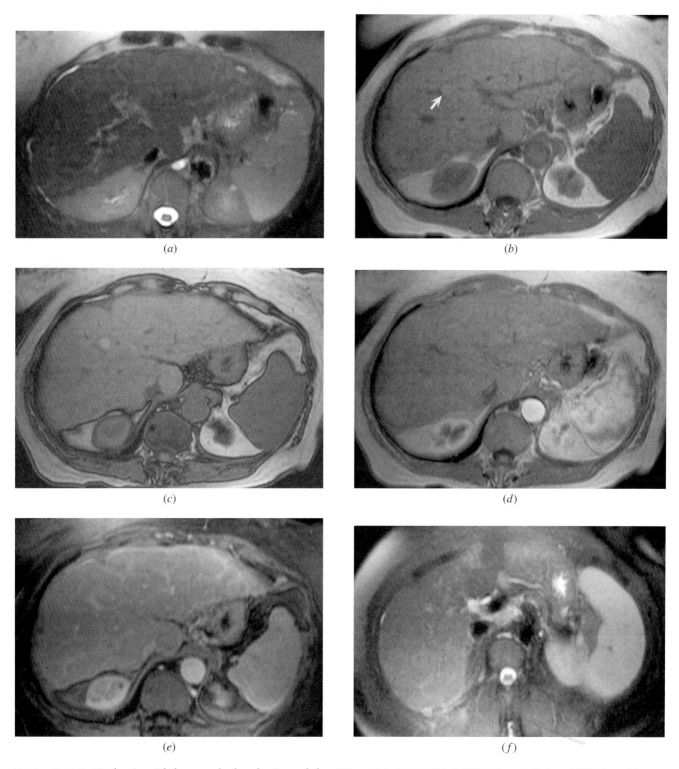

(a)   (b)

(c)   (d)

(e)   (f)

F I G . 2.210 Cirrhosis with low-grade dysplastic nodules. T2-weighted SS-ETSE (*a*), SGE (*b*), out-of-phase SGE (*c*), and immediate (*d*) and 90-s fat-suppressed (*e*) postgadolinium SGE images. There is a nodule in segment 8 of the liver that is isointense on
T2 (*a*) and moderately high signal intensity on T1 (arrow, *b*), does not drop in signal intensity on out-of-phase image (*c*), and shows
negligible enhancement on early-phase postgadolinium image (*d*) and remains isointense to the background parenchyma on late-
phase image (*e*), consistent with a low-grade dysplastic nodule.

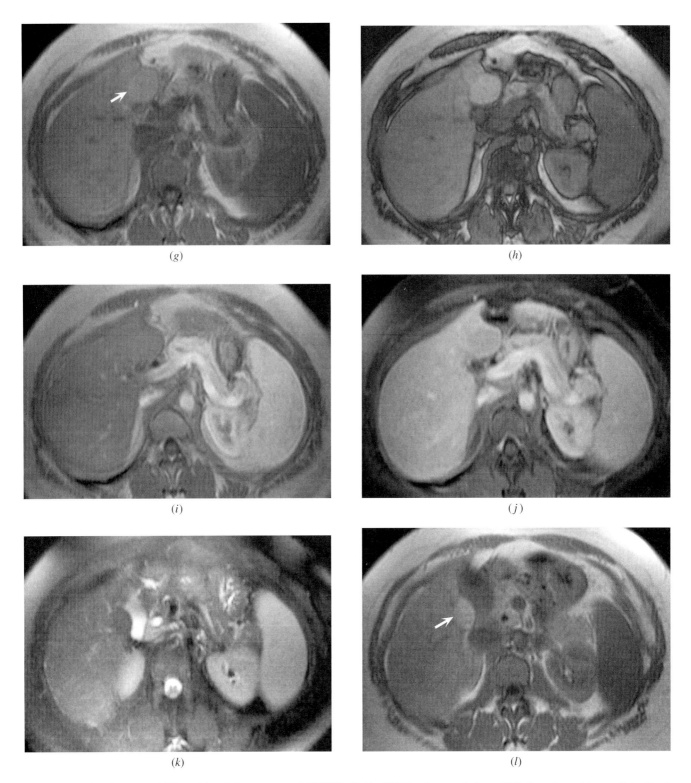

F I G . 2.210 (*Continued*) T2-weighted fat-suppressed SS-ETSE (*f, k*), SGE (*g, l*), out-of-phase SGE (*h, m*), and immediate (*i, n*) and 90-s fat-suppressed (*j, o*) postgadolinium SGE images in a second patient at two different tomographic levels. Nodules are present at both levels (arrow, *g, l*), demonstrating mildly decreased signal intensity on T2 (*f, k*), moderately high signal intensity on T1 (*g, l*), no signal drop on out-of-phase (*h, m*), and enhancement comparable to background parenchyma on early (*i, n*)- and late (*j, o*)-phase images.

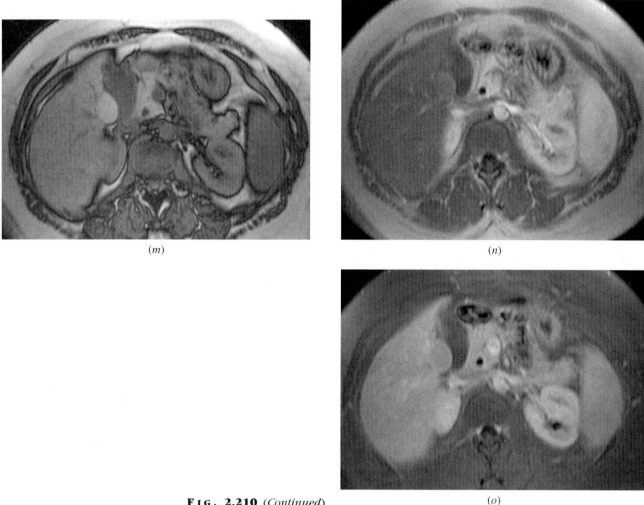

(m)

(n)

(o)

FIG. 2.210 (Continued)

low-signal-intensity nodule on T2-weighted images—a nodule within a nodule. This reflects the development of a high-T2-signal malignancy within a low-T2-signal dysplastic nodule. On T1-weighted images, the high-grade DN exhibits low signal and the foci of small HCC may appear isointense with the liver parenchyma. (fig. 2.215) [351–353].

Portal hypertension results from obstruction at presinusoidal (e.g., portal vein), sinusoidal (e.g., cirrhosis), postsinusoidal (e.g., hepatic vein), or multiple levels [354]. The most common cause of portal hypertension is cirrhosis. Portal hypertension causes or exacerbates complications of cirrhosis such as variceal bleeding, ascites, and splenomegaly. Portosystemic shunts may be identified with 2D time-of-flight techniques or gadolinium-enhanced SGE sequences. Gadolinium-enhanced 3D GE imaging, alone or with fat suppression, is a particularly effective technique. Direction of flow may be determined by using 2D phase-contrast techniques,

or directional information may be derived by observing time-of-flight effects in the main portal vein and correlating it with time-of-flight effects in the aorta and inferior vena cava (IVC). The latter technique is best performed by acquiring superior and inferior multislice slabs, the bottom and top respectively, of the two slabs obtained at the level of the porta hepatis.

In the early stages of portal hypertension, the portal venous system dilates but flow is maintained. Later, substantial portosystemic shunting develops, reducing the volume of flow to the liver and decreasing the size of the portal vein. With advanced portal hypertension, portal flow may reverse and become hepatofugal. Thrombosis of the portal veins may develop, with development of collaterals referred to as cavernous transformation (figs. 2.216 and 2.217).

Mesenteric, omental, and retroperitoneal edema occur commonly in patients with cirrhosis, because of portal hypertension (figs. 2.218–2.220). The appearance

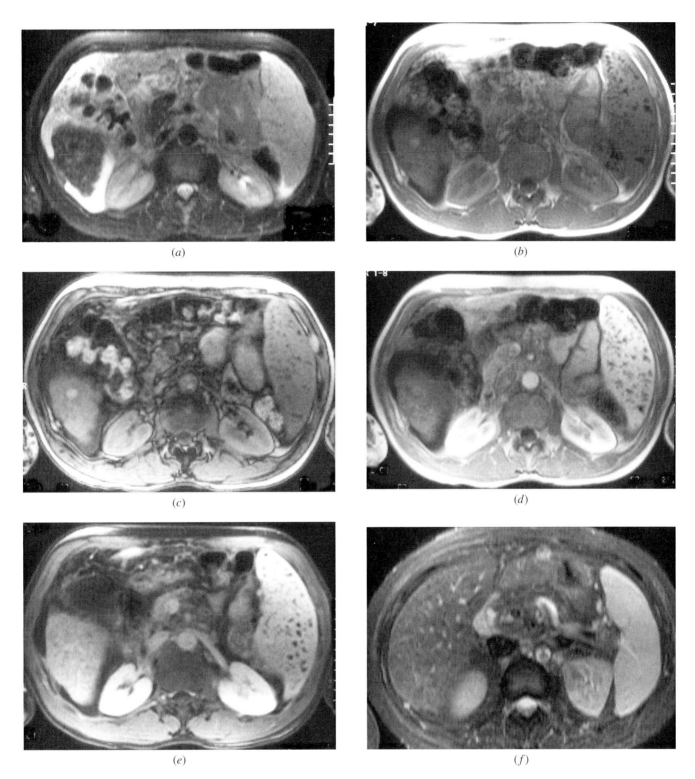

F I G . 2.211 Cirrhosis with low-grade dysplastic nodules. T2-weighted fat-suppressed SS-ETSE (*a*), SGE (*b*), out-of-phase SGE (*c*), and immediate (*d*) and 90-s fat-suppressed (*e*) postgadolinium SGE images. A nodule is present in segment 5 of the liver, which is low signal intensity on T2 (*a*) and high signal intensity on T1 (*b*), does not drop in signal intensity on out-of-phase image (*c*), and enhances to the same extent as background parenchyma on early (*d*)- and late (*e*)-phase images compatible with a low-grade dysplastic nodule.

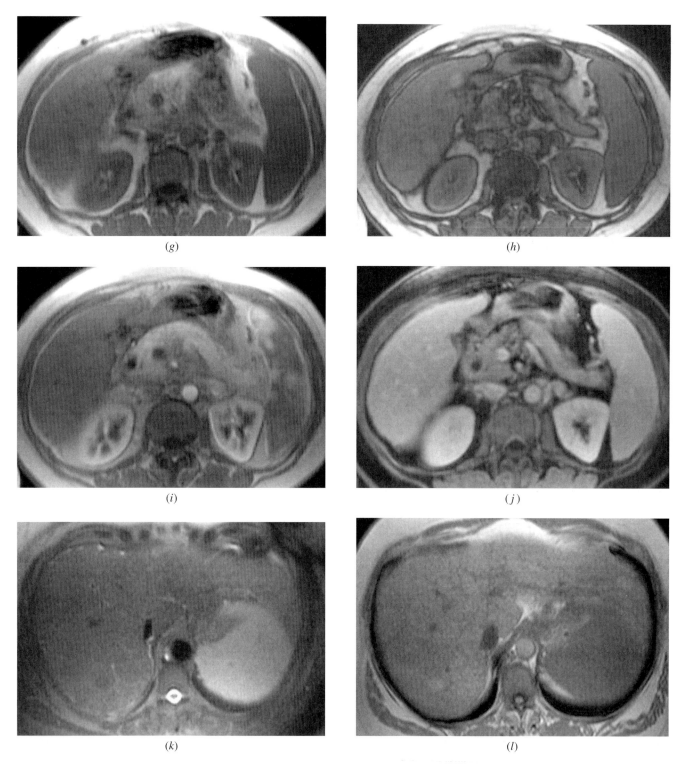

(g) *(h)*

(i) *(j)*

(k) *(l)*

F ɪ ɢ . 2.211 (*Continued*) T2-weighted fat-suppressed SS-ETSE (*f, k*), SGE (*g, l*), out-of-phase SGE (*h, m*), and immediate (*i, n*) and 90-s fat-suppressed (*j, o*) postgadolinium SGE images in a second and third patient with low-grade dysplastic nodules. In both cases, the low-grade dysplastic nodules are most evident on T1 (*g, l*) and out-of-phase (*h, m*) images. On the other sequences, the low-grade dysplastic nodules have signal intensity similar to background parenchyma.

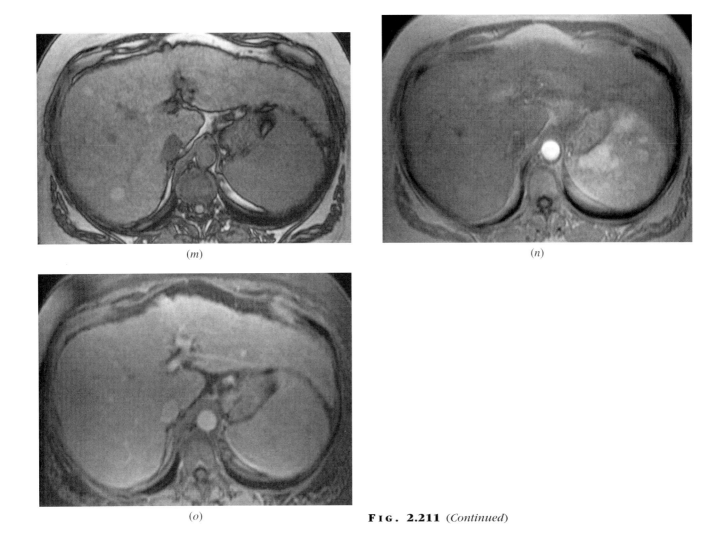

(m)

(n)

(o)   **F I G . 2.211** (*Continued*)

of mesenteric edema varies from a mild infiltrative haze to a substantial masslike sheath that engulfs the mesenteric vessels [322, 355]. Gastrointestinal wall thickening is seen in as many as 25% of patients with end-stage cirrhosis, also secondary to portal hypertension. Many of these patients do not have specific bowel symptoms [322].

Portal varices arise from increased portal pressure, and portal blood is shunted into systemic veins, bypassing hepatic parenchyma. Nutrients absorbed from the gastrointestinal (GI) tract are metabolized less effectively, and hepatic function decreases. Toxic metabolites such as ammonia accumulate in the blood and result in clinical manifestations such as hepatic encephalopathy. Diminished portal flow to the liver parenchyma is a major factor in the production of liver atrophy and prevention of regeneration [356], and portosystemic shunting may play a role in the development of hepatic atrophy in advanced cirrhosis. Major sites of portosys-

temic collateralization include gastroesophageal junction, paraumbilical veins (figs. 2.221 and 2.222), retroperitoneal regions, perigastric, splenorenal, omentum, peritoneum, and hemorrhoidal veins [337]. Esophageal varices are a serious complication because they may rupture and produce life-threatening hemorrhage (fig. 2.223). Flow-sensitive gradient-echo or gadolinium-enhanced gradient-echo images effectively demonstrate varices as high-signal tubular structures (fig. 2.224) [357]. Varices are particularly conspicuous with fat suppression and gadolinium enhancement on gradient-echo images as the competing high signal intensity of fat is removed. Gadolinium-enhanced water excitation gradient echo is another approach to demonstrate varices, as the excitation pulse possesses time-of-flight effects that accentuate the high signal in vessels produced by gadolinium enhancement. These sequences are more sensitive than contrast angiography, endoscopy, or contrast-enhanced CT imaging for detecting varices [358].

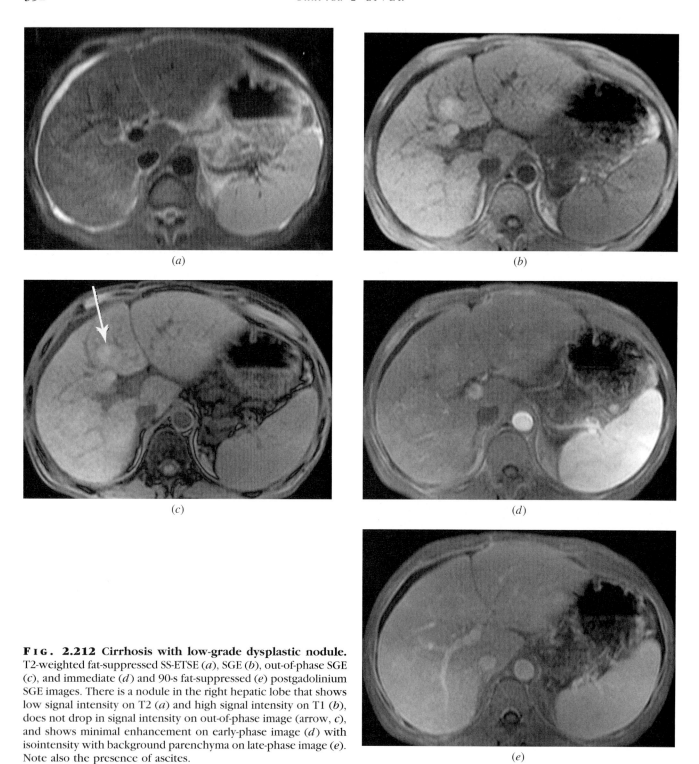

FIG. 2.212 Cirrhosis with low-grade dysplastic nodule. T2-weighted fat-suppressed SS-ETSE (*a*), SGE (*b*), out-of-phase SGE (*c*), and immediate (*d*) and 90-s fat-suppressed (*e*) postgadolinium SGE images. There is a nodule in the right hepatic lobe that shows low signal intensity on T2 (*a*) and high signal intensity on T1 (*b*), does not drop in signal intensity on out-of-phase image (arrow, *c*), and shows minimal enhancement on early-phase image (*d*) with isointensity with background parenchyma on late-phase image (*e*). Note also the presence of ascites.

Porta Hepatis Lymphadenopathy

Porta hepatis lymphadenopathy is a common finding in benign and malignant liver disease. Porta hepatis lymphadenopathy is almost invariably present in chronic liver disease [359]. The detection of malignant porta hepatis lymph nodes is crucial in decision making for management of patients with malignant disease. The most effective approach for the detection of lymph nodes is the combined use of a fat-suppressed T2-weighted sequence and interstitial-phase gadolinium-enhanced T1-weighted fat-suppressed imaging. On the T2 sequence, lymph

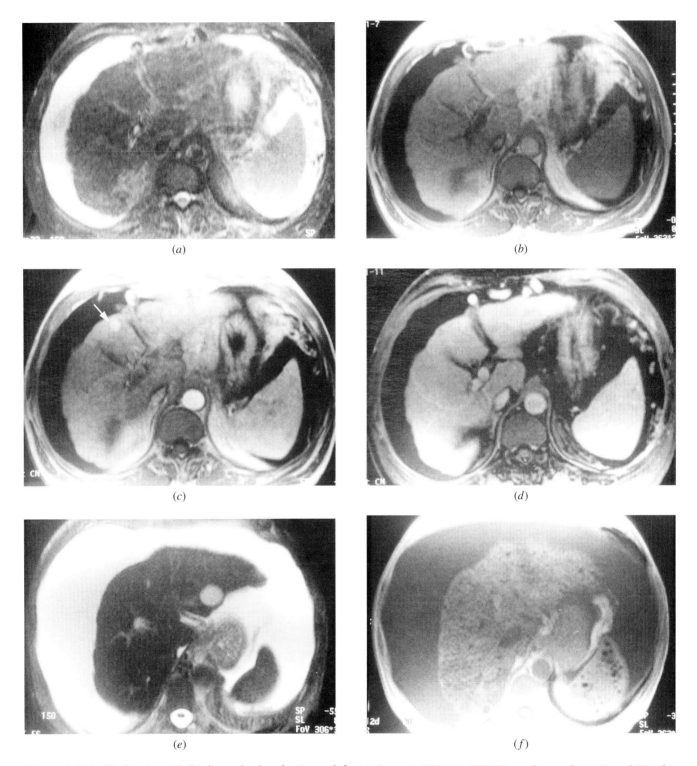

F I G . 2.213 Cirrhosis with high-grade dysplastic nodules. Echo-train STIR (*a*), SGE (*b*), and immediate (*c*) and 90-s fat-suppressed (*d*) postgadolinium SGE images. The liver is small and nodular, compatible with cirrhosis. There is a 1-cm lesion (arrow, *c*) in segment 4 that is not evident on T2 (*a*)- or T1 (*b*)-weighted images but displays intense enhancement on the immediate postgadolinium image (*c*) and fades to isointensity on the late image (*d*), consistent with a high-grade dysplastic nodule. Note also the presence of ascites and collateral vessels.

T2-weighted fat-suppressed SS-ETSE (*e*), SGE (*f*), and immediate (*g*, *h*) and 90-s fat-suppressed (*i*) postgadolinium SGE images in a second patient. The liver is very small, nodular, and irregular in contour, consistent with cirrhosis. Multiple nodules are identified in the liver that demonstrate isointense to mildly high signal intensity on T2 (*e*), low signal intensity on T1 (*f*), and intense enhancement immediately after administration of contrast (*g*, *h*), with persistent enhancement on late images (*i*), compatible with high-grade dysplastic nodules. Note the hemangiomas in the left lobe of the liver, Gamna–Gandy bodies in the spleen and large-volume ascites.

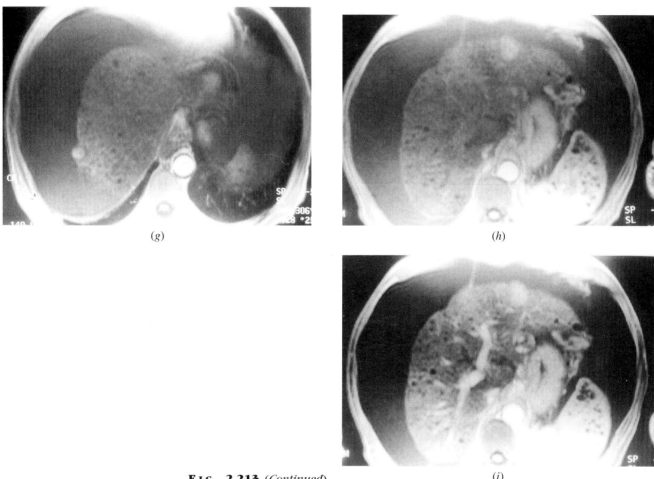

(g)

(h)

FIG. 2.213 (Continued)

(i)

nodes are moderately high signal and both liver and background fat are relatively low signal, rendering excellent conspicuity. Definition of the rounded contour of lymph nodes is optimal with the gadolinium-enhanced T1-weighted fat-suppressed technique and thereby distinguishes rounded lymph nodes from ill-defined inflammatory tissue, which is also high signal on T2 (fig. 2.225).

Iron Overload

Primary (Idiopathic Hemochromatosis)

Genetic Hemochromatosis. Genetic hemochromatosis (GH) is a common genetic disorder among the Caucasian population in the United States [360]. GH results from excessive gastrointestinal absorption and deposition of iron in tissues such as liver, heart, pancreas, anterior pituitary, joints. and skin. Early in the disease process, iron accumulation is restricted to the liver (fig. 2.226) [361]. Pathologic features of hemochromatosis in the liver include iron deposition as hemosiderin pigment granules in hepatocytes. Iron is a direct hepatotoxin. Fibrous septa develop slowly, leading to

micronodular cirrhosis. Kupffer cell (RES) uptake of hemosiderin pigment is not marked. Over time, iron deposition progresses to involve other organs, primarily the pancreas and heart (fig. 2.227). Serologic abnormalities and mild symptoms may occur earlier in life, but the clinical signs and symptoms do not appear until the fifth or sixth decade of life [360]. Disease detection at an early stage, with institution of phlebotomy therapy, may result in a normal life expectancy [362]. Untreated, it results in end-organ damage, which may include cirrhosis and HCC; HCC often is the cause of death [360, 363, 364].

A diagnostic feature of idiopathic hemochromatosis is that signal intensity of the spleen is not substantially decreased on T2-weighted or T2*-weighted images. This finding is due to accumulation of iron within the parenchyma of the liver and pancreas and lack of selective uptake by the RES in the spleen. The presence of iron deposition in the pancreas correlates with irreversible changes of cirrhosis in the liver.

Some patients who present with HCC have previously unsuspected GH (fig. 2.228) [365]. Because tumor

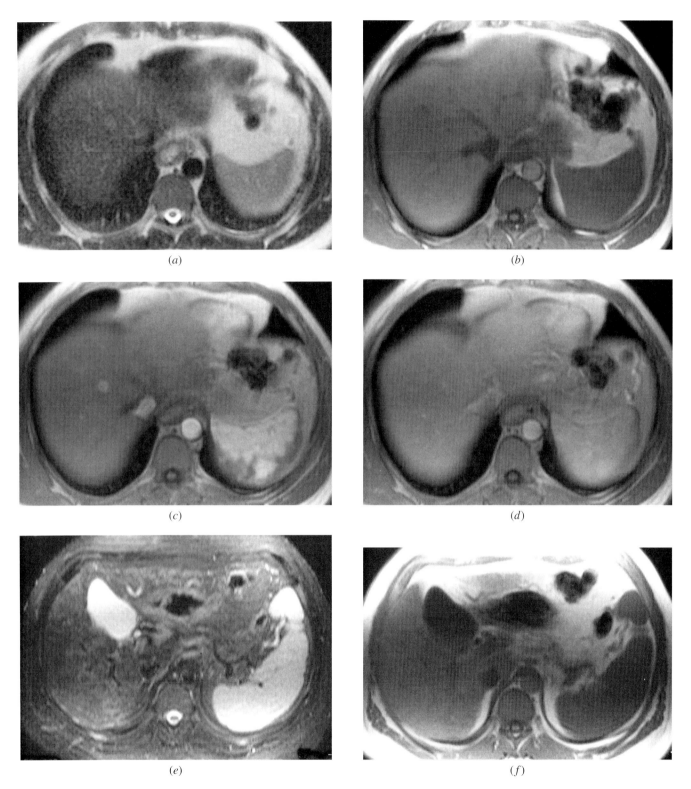

(a)

(b)

(c)

(d)

(e)

(f)

F I G . 2.214 Cirrhosis with high-grade dysplastic nodule. T2-weighted SS-ETSE (*a*), SGE (*b*), and immediate (*c*) and 45-s (*d*) postgadolinium SGE images in a cirrhotic patient. A high-grade dysplastic nodule is appreciated at the junction between segments 8 and 5, which demonstrates mildly high signal intensity on T2 (*a*), isointensity on T1 (*b*), and intense homogeneous enhancement on early-phase image (arrow, *c*) that fades on 45-s image (*d*).

T2-weighted fat-suppressed SS-ETSE (*e*), SGE (*f*), and immediate (*g*) and 90-s fat-suppressed (*h*) postgadolinium SGE images and

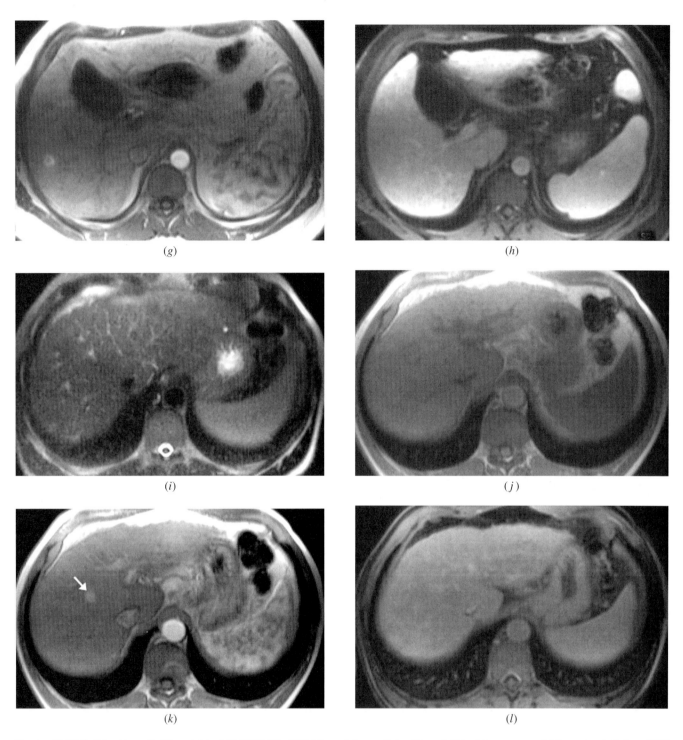

F I G . 2.214 (*Continued*) T2-weighted SS-ETSE (*i*), SGE (*j*), and immediate (*k*) and 90-s fat-suppressed (*l*) postgadolinium SGE images in a second and third cirrhotic patient with a high-grade dysplastic nodule. The nodule shows mildly high signal intensity on T2-weighted image (*e*), mildly low signal intensity on T1-weighted image (*f*), and intense enhancement on early-phase image (*g*) that fades on late-phase image (*h*). The same findings are observed in the third patient (arrow, *k*).

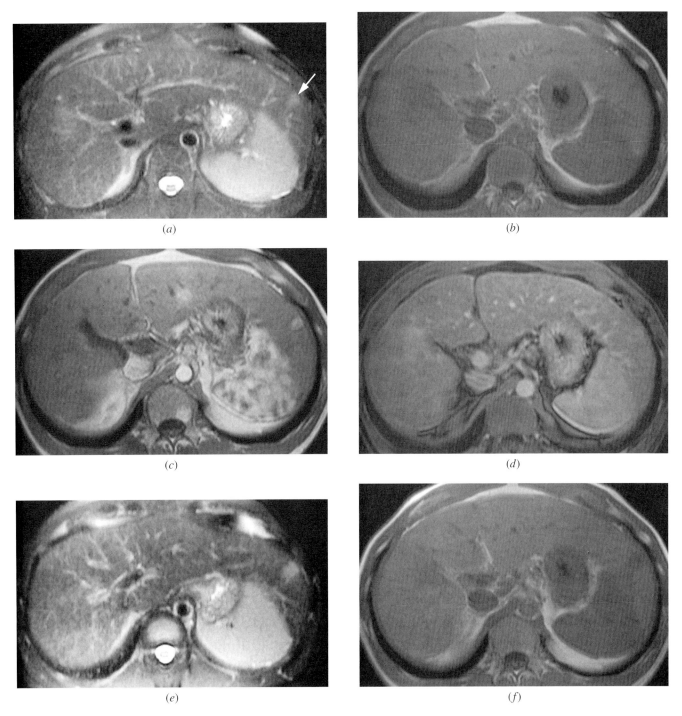

FIG. 2.215 Development of HCC from high-grade dysplastic nodule and nodule-in-nodule appearance of early HCC.
Fat-suppressed T2-weighted SS-ETSE (*a*), SGE (*b*), and immediate (*c*) and 90-s fat-suppressed (*d*) postgadolinium SGE images. A lesion is seen in the left lobe that shows slightly high signal intensity on T2-weighted image (*a*) and slightly low signal intensity on T1-weighted image (*b*) and demonstrates moderate enhancement on early-phase image (*c*) that fades to background parenchyma on late-phase image (*d*), compatible with a high-grade dysplastic nodule. Fat-suppressed T2-weighted SS-ETSE (*e*), SGE (*f*), and

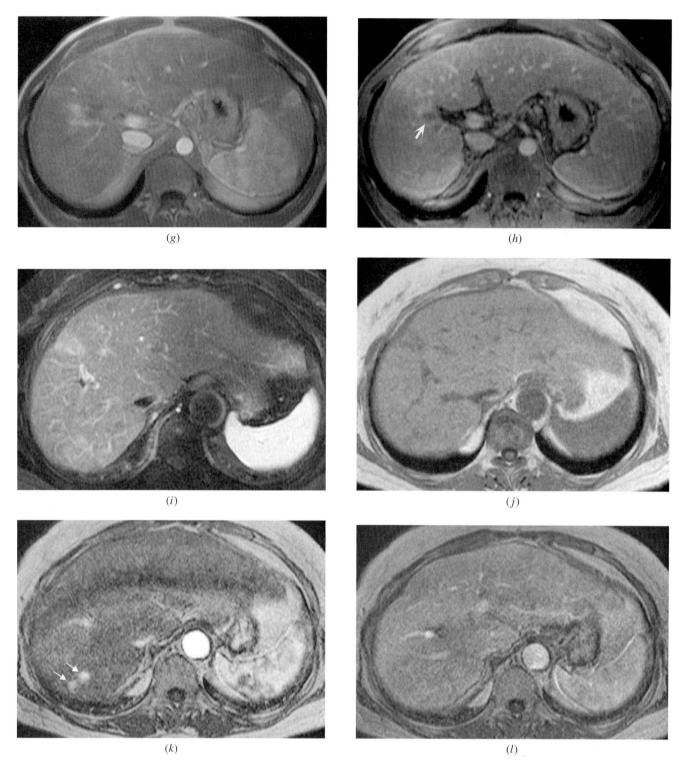

FIG. 2.215 (*Continued*) immediate (*g*) and 90-s fat-suppressed (*h*) postgadolinium SGE images in a 6-month follow-up examination show an intense enhancement on early-phase image (*g*) that washes out with capsule enhancement on late-phase image (arrow, *h*), consistent with HCC. T2-weighted fat-suppressed SE (*i*), T1-weighted SGE (*j*), and T1-weighted immediate (*k*) and 90-s post gadolinium (*l*) images in a second patient. T2-weighted (*i*) and T1-weighted (*j*) images show two areas in the right hepatic lobe that exhibit high and low signal intensity, respectively. After contrast, one of the areas demonstrates two foci (arrows, *k*) of intense enhancement that fades on late-phase images (*l*), consistent with small HCCs within a dysplastic nodule. (Courtesy of Masayuki Kanematsu, M.D., Gifu University, Japan.)

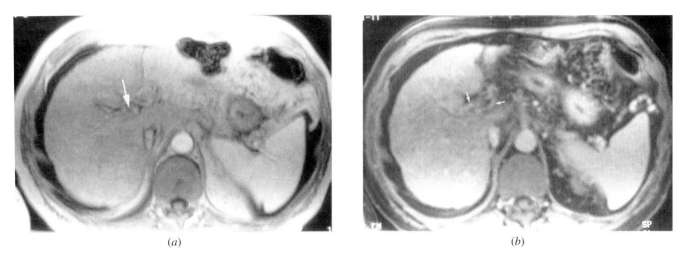

(a)   (b)

F I G . 2.216 Cavernous transformation of the portal vein. Immediate (*a*) and 90-s fat-suppressed (*b*) postgadolinium SGE images in a patient who has a history of cirrhosis. Thrombus (arrow, *a*) is present in a diminutive portal vein, and multiple small serpiginous collateral vessels (arrows, *b*) are identified in the porta hepatis, consistent with cavernous transformation. Note also ascites and splenomegaly.

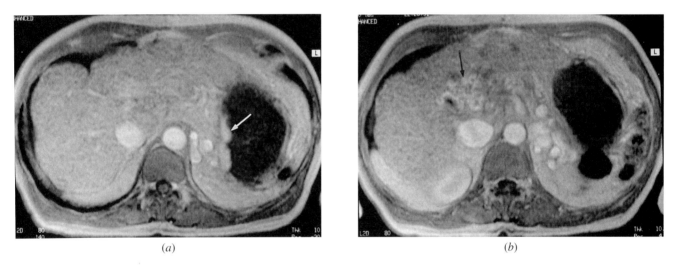

(a)   (b)

F I G . 2.217 Gastric varices and cavernous transformation of the portal vein. Transverse 45-s postgadolinium SGE images (*a, b*) demonstrate a cirrhotic liver with irregular contour and multiple low-signal-intensity <5-mm regenerative nodules. Prominent varices are present along the lesser curvature, which are well shown on portal-phase postgadolinium images. Multiple small serpiginous enhancing structures are present in the porta hepatis (arrow, *b*) that reflect cavernous transformation of the portal vein. A prominent varix is present along the lesser curvature (arrow, *a*). Signal-void small-volume ascites is also present (*a, b*).

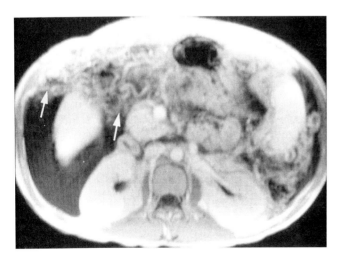

F I G . 2.218 Intraperitoneal and omental varices. Transverse 1-min postgadolinium SGE image demonstrates a tangle of small-caliber varices in the right intraperitoneal space with involvement of the omentum (arrows) and in a perisplenic location.

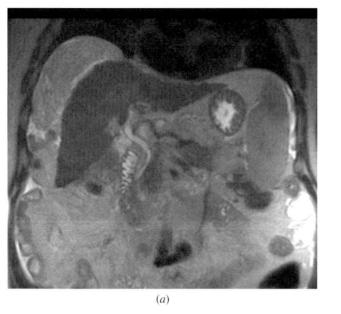

(a)

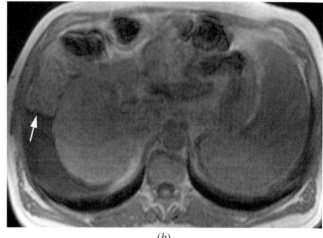

(b)

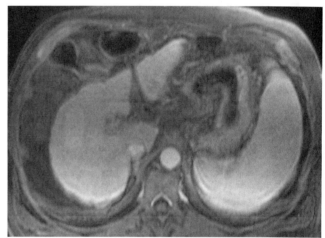

(c)

FIG. 2.219 Omental hypertrophy. Coronal T2-weighted SS-ETSE (*a*), transverse SGE (*b*) and 90-s fat-suppressed (*c*) postgadolinium SGE images in a cirrhotic patient that show substantial omental hypertrophy well shown on coronal image (arrows, *a*). Note that the majority of the omentum suppresses on the fat-suppressed image (*c*).

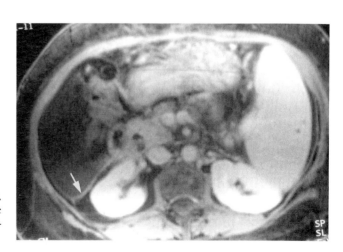

FIG. 2.220 Cirrhosis and peritoneal enhancement. Interstitial-phase gadolinium-enhanced fat-suppressed SGE image demonstrates mild linear peritoneal enhancement (arrow) consistent with microvarices in the peritoneal lining.

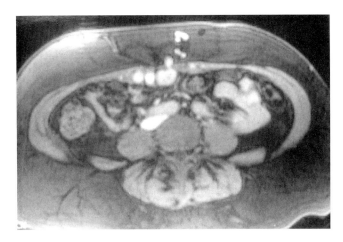

FIG. 2.221 Cirrhosis, paraumbilical varices (caput medusa). Transverse 90-s postgadolinium SGE image demonstrates large varices along the right paramedian peritoneum. Multiple subcutaneous paraumbilical varices are present, which are rendered very conspicuous because of removal of the competing high signal of fat.

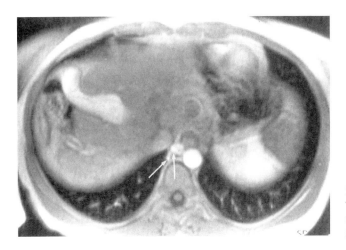

FIG. 2.222 Cirrhosis, varices, recanalized umbilical vein. Transverse 45-s postgadolinium SGE image demonstrates recanalization of a very large umbilical vein. Note that small paraesophageal varices (arrows) are also present.

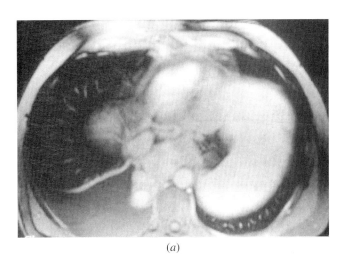

(a)

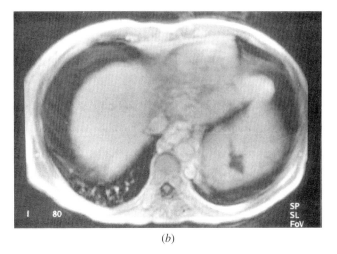

(b)

FIG. 2.223 Cirrhosis, paraesophageal varices. Transverse 45-s postgadolinium SGE images (a, b) in two patients demonstrate large paraesophageal varices.

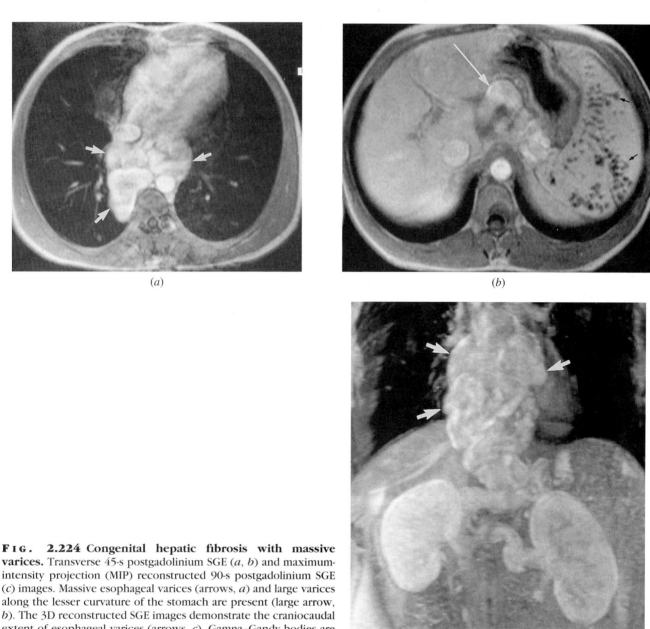

FIG. 2.224 Congenital hepatic fibrosis with massive varices. Transverse 45-s postgadolinium SGE (*a, b*) and maximum-intensity projection (MIP) reconstructed 90-s postgadolinium SGE (*c*) images. Massive esophageal varices (arrows, *a*) and large varices along the lesser curvature of the stomach are present (large arrow, *b*). The 3D reconstructed SGE images demonstrate the craniocaudal extent of esophageal varices (arrows, *c*). Gamna–Gandy bodies are present in the spleen (small arrows, *b*).

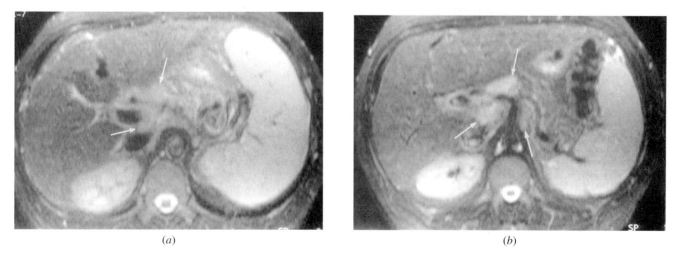

FIG. 2.225 Porta hepatis lymph nodes. Echo-train STIR (*a, b*) and 90-s fat-suppressed postgadolinium SGE (*c, d*) images;

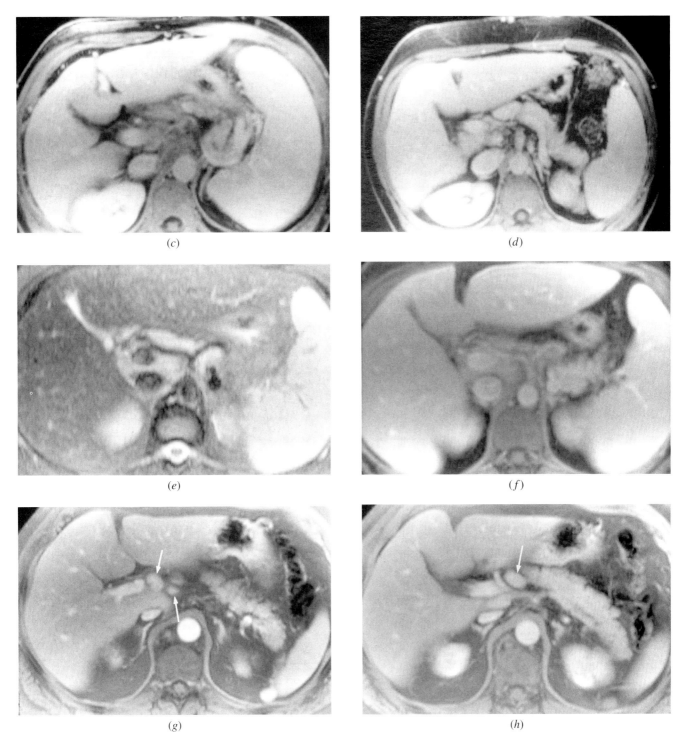

F I G . 2.225 (*Continued*) echo train-STIR (*e*) and 90-s fat-suppressed postgadolinium SGE (*f*) images; and 90-s fat-suppressed postgadolinium SGE images (*g, h*) in three patients with porta hepatis lymph nodes (arrows, *a, b, g, h*). The lymph nodes in the porta hepatis are best detected by the combination of identification of high-signal tissue on T2-weighted fat-suppressed images (*a, b, e*) and demonstration that the high-signal tissue has definable convex margins on interstitial-phase gadolinium-enhanced fat-suppressed SGE images (*c, d, f, g, h*). All of these patients have chronic hepatitis or cirrhosis. Enlarged porta hepatis lymph nodes are common in patients with chronic liver disease, especially secondary to hepatitis C infection.

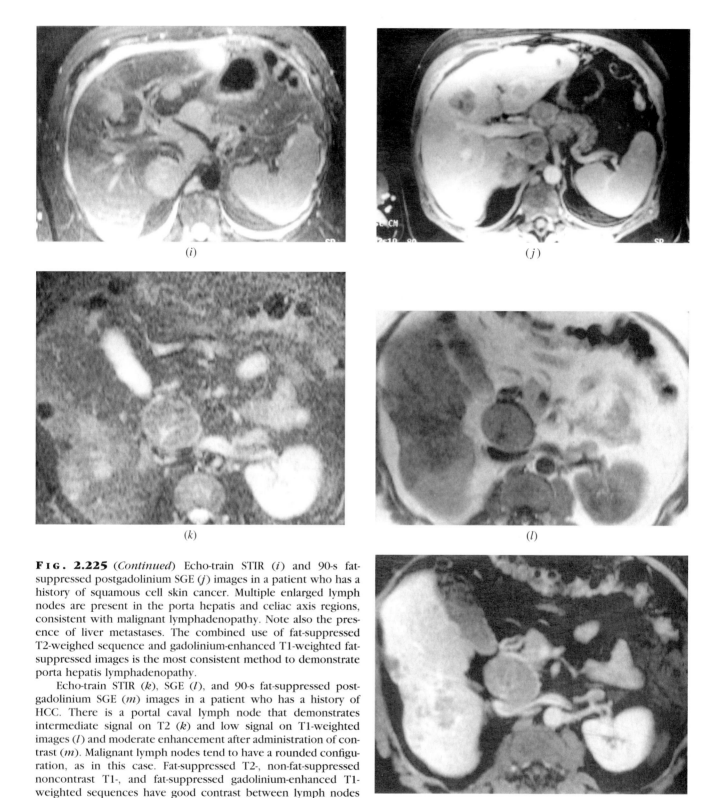

FIG. 2.225 (*Continued*) Echo-train STIR (*i*) and 90-s fat-suppressed postgadolinium SGE (*j*) images in a patient who has a history of squamous cell skin cancer. Multiple enlarged lymph nodes are present in the porta hepatis and celiac axis regions, consistent with malignant lymphadenopathy. Note also the presence of liver metastases. The combined use of fat-suppressed T2-weighed sequence and gadolinium-enhanced T1-weighted fat-suppressed images is the most consistent method to demonstrate porta hepatis lymphadenopathy.

Echo-train STIR (*k*), SGE (*l*), and 90-s fat-suppressed post-gadolinium SGE (*m*) images in a patient who has a history of HCC. There is a portal caval lymph node that demonstrates intermediate signal on T2 (*k*) and low signal on T1-weighted images (*l*) and moderate enhancement after administration of contrast (*m*). Malignant lymph nodes tend to have a rounded configuration, as in this case. Fat-suppressed T2-, non-fat-suppressed noncontrast T1-, and fat-suppressed gadolinium-enhanced T1-weighted sequences have good contrast between lymph nodes and background tissue.

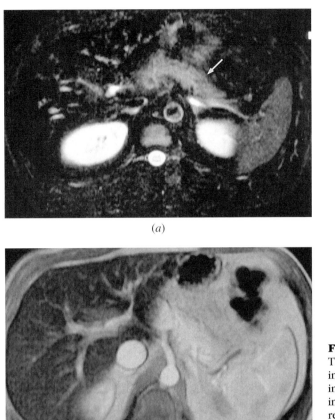

(a)

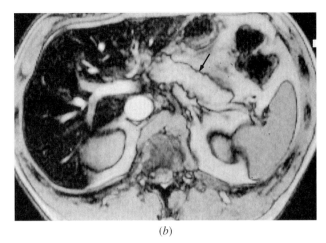

(b)

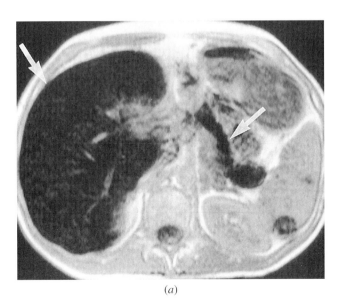

(c)

F I G . 2.226 Idiopathic hemochromatosis, early disease.
T2-weighted fat-suppressed ETSE (*a*), out-of-phase SGE (*b*), and immediate postgadolinium SGE (*c*) images. The liver is low in signal intensity on noncontrast T2-weighted (*a*) and T1-weighted (*b*) images, consistent with substantial iron deposition. The spleen is relatively normal in signal intensity on these sequences, reflecting that iron is not in the RES but in the hepatocytes. The pancreas (arrow, *a*, *b*) is normal in signal intensity on noncontrast images and enhances normally with gadolinium. Iron deposition limited to the liver is consistent with early precirrhotic disease.

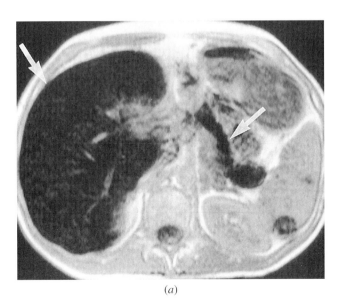

(a)

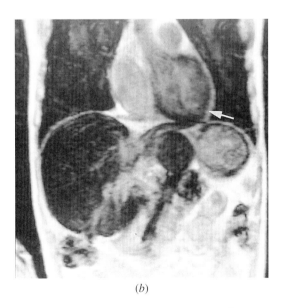

(b)

F I G . 2.227 Idiopathic hemochromatosis, advanced disease. Transverse (*a*) and coronal (*b*) SGE and coronal 45-s postgadolinium SGE (*c*) images. The precontrast T1-weighted image (*a*) demonstrates signal-void liver and pancreas (arrows, *a*). The coronal SGE image (*b*) also demonstrates low-signal-intensity left ventricular myocardium (arrow, *b*). On the 45-s postgadolinium image (*c*), multiple enhanced varices are shown (arrows, *c*), which reflects portal hypertension secondary to cirrhosis.

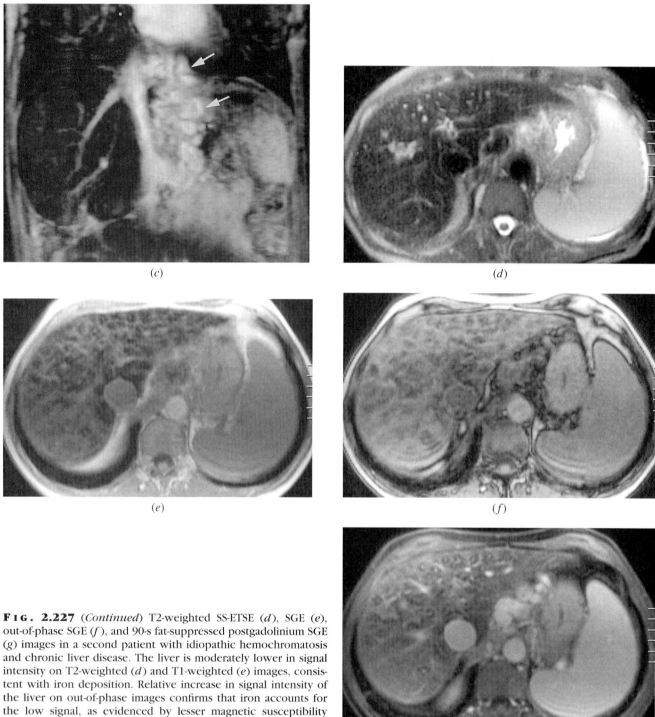

(c)

(d)

(e)

(f)

FIG. 2.227 (*Continued*) T2-weighted SS-ETSE (*d*), SGE (*e*), out-of-phase SGE (*f*), and 90-s fat-suppressed postgadolinium SGE (*g*) images in a second patient with idiopathic hemochromatosis and chronic liver disease. The liver is moderately lower in signal intensity on T2-weighted (*d*) and T1-weighted (*e*) images, consistent with iron deposition. Relative increase in signal intensity of the liver on out-of-phase images confirms that iron accounts for the low signal, as evidenced by lesser magnetic susceptibility effects on shorter TE sequences. Late-phase images (*g*) show enhancement of fibrous tissue consistent with a chronic liver disease.

(g)

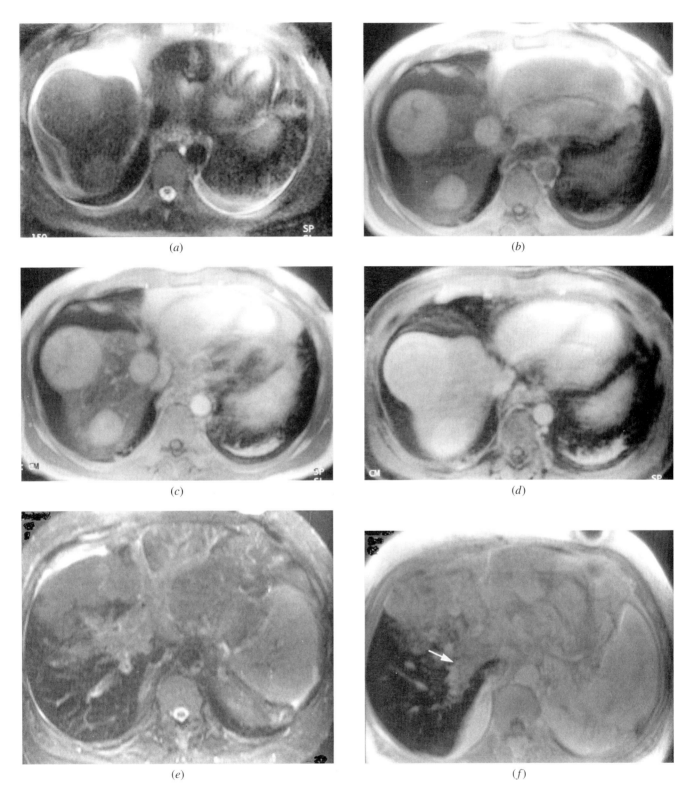

F i g . 2.228 Multifocal HCCs superimposed on idiopathic hemochromatosis. Fat-suppressed T2-weighted SS-ETSE (*a*), SGE (*b*), and immediate (*c*) and 90-s fat-suppressed (*d*) postgadolinium SGE images. There are three HCC nodules that show slight increased signal on T2-weighted (*a*) and T1-weighted (*b*) images and mildly increased enhancement immediately after gadolinium administration (*c*) and fade slightly over time (*d*). The liver is small and irregular in contour and demonstrates diffuse marked decreased signal intensity on T2-weighted (*a*) and T1-weighted (*b*) images, even after contrast, consistent with hepatocellular iron deposition in idiopathic hemochromatosis. Note also ascites.

Echo-train STIR (*e*) and immediate (*f*) and 90-s fat-suppressed (*g*) postgadolinium SGE images in a second patient with idiopathic

(g)

FIG. 2.228 (*Continued*) hemochromatosis. There is a very large HCC involving the entire left lobe and segments 5 and 8 of the right lobe that demonstrates heterogeneous and moderately increased signal on T2-weighted images and heterogeneous gadolinium enhancement. The entire portal venous system is expanded and enhances after gadolinium administration (arrow, *f*), consistent with tumor thrombus. Marked decreased signal intensity of liver parenchyma reflects the iron deposition in idiopathic hemochromatosis.

cells do not contain excess iron [366, 367] they are well shown as high-signal-intensity masses relative to iron-overloaded liver on T2-weighted images. In a patient with hemochromatosis, nonsiderotic nodules that are not hemangiomas or cysts are highly suspicious for HCC [364], because regenerative nodules in these patients contain iron. Dysplastic nodules in patients with increased hepatic iron may contain a different concentration of iron than surrounding hepatic parenchyma.

Secondary Hemochromatosis

Transfusional Iron Overload. Transfusional iron overload is the most common form of excess iron deposition in North America. Fibrosis is usually mild despite even heavy iron stores, and cirrhosis is rare. Iron deposition in the RES results in low signal intensity of the spleen, liver, and bone marrow on MR images, best shown on T2- or T2*-weighted images.

Iron overload from multiple transfusions may be distinguished from genetic hemochromatosis in that large amounts of iron accumulate primarily within the RES of the liver (Kupffer cells) and spleen (monocytes/macrophages) in transfusional overload, with relative sparing of the functional cells within the parenchyma. Evaluation by MRI of pancreatic and splenic signal intensity allows this distinction. Signal intensity of the spleen is usually normal with genetic hemochromatosis, whereas signal intensity of the pancreas is normal with most cases of transfusional overload. In massive iron overload (e.g., >100 units) direct tissue deposition may occur in other cells and tissues, notably the pancreas (fig. 2.229) [361, 365].

Regional variation in iron deposition in the liver parenchyma may occur, such as diffuse heterogeneous (fig. 2.230) or homogeneous iron deposition with focal sparing (fig. 2.231) and focal iron deposition. MR fea-

tures are highly associated with the degree of iron overload in the liver [368–370]. In mild forms of transfusional overload, signal loss is appreciated only on T2- and T2*-weighted images, and signal intensity on T1-weighted images appears relatively normal (fig. 2.232). In moderate to severe forms of iron deposition, the T2-shortening effect of iron results in low signal on T1-weighted images as well (fig. 2.233). If liver and spleen are gray on in-phase SGE (TE = 4.2 ms), we consider iron deposition moderate, and if liver and spleen are near signal void, iron deposition is severe [361, 365].

Hemolytic Anemia. Hepatic signal intensity in patients with hemolytic anemia varies, based on the rate of reincorporation of iron into the bone marrow, the rate of absorption of oral iron, and the transfusional history. Patients with thalassemia vera have increased absorption of oral iron and, in the absence of blood transfusions, will develop erythrogenic hemochromatosis primarily affecting the liver [371]. The appearance is generally indistinguishable from idiopathic hemochromatosis (fig. 2.234). Patients with heterozygous forms of hemolytic anemias may not have low enough red blood cell counts or hemoglobin levels to necessitate transfusion, and may therefore develop this pattern of iron overload. The majority of patients with hemolytic anemias have received blood transfusions and therefore also develop coexisting transfusional iron overload (fig. 2.235).

Patients with sickle cell anemia have rapid turnover of hepatic iron and will have normal hepatic signal intensity unless they have undergone recent blood transfusions [371]. Renal cortical signal intensity may be decreased because of filtration and tubular absorption of free hemoglobin, the severity of which is not dependent on transfusional history (see chapter 9, *Kidneys*)

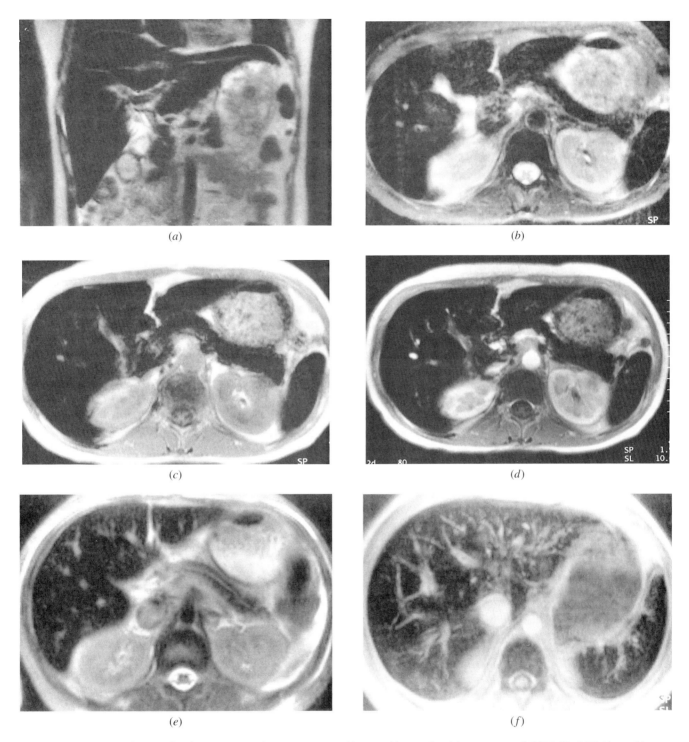

(a)

(b)

(c)

(d)

(e)

(f)

F I G . 2.229 Transfusional siderosis, massive. Coronal SS-ETSE (*a*), T2-weighted fat-suppressed ETSE (*b*), SGE (*c*), and immediate postgadolinium SGE (*d*) images. Massive iron deposition is present in the liver, spleen, and pancreas (*a–c*), demonstrated by
signal-void liver, spleen, and pancreas. Magnetic susceptibility causes a "blooming" appearance surrounding the pancreas (*c*). These
organs remain signal void after gadolinium administration (*d*).

T2-weighted SS-ETSE (*e*) and 1-min postgadolinium SGE (*f*) images in a second patient with massive iron deposition demonstrate
dark liver, spleen, and pancreas on T2-weighted (*e*) and postgadolinium T1-weighted (*f*) images.

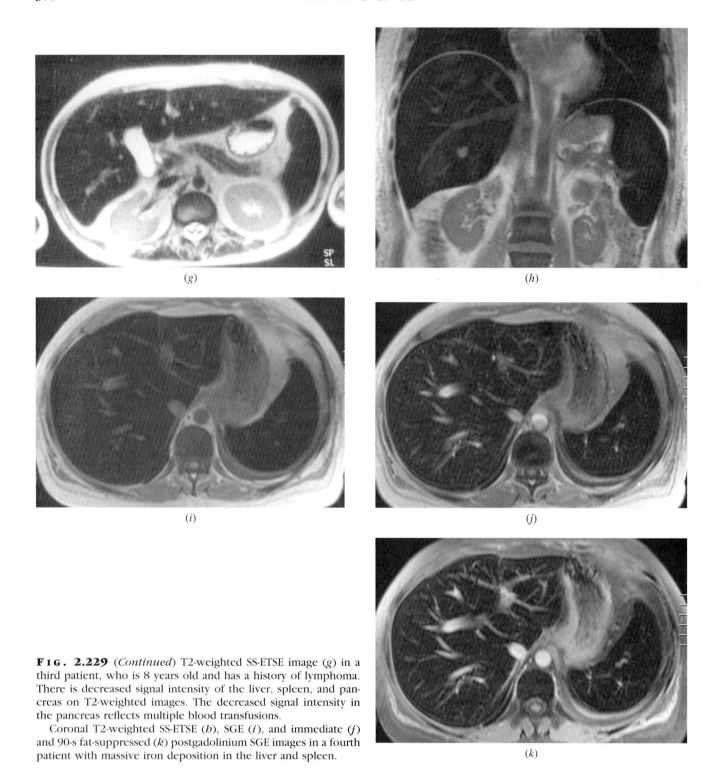

(g) (h)

(i) (j)

(k)

FIG. 2.229 (*Continued*) T2-weighted SS-ETSE image (g) in a third patient, who is 8 years old and has a history of lymphoma. There is decreased signal intensity of the liver, spleen, and pancreas on T2-weighted images. The decreased signal intensity in the pancreas reflects multiple blood transfusions.

Coronal T2-weighted SS-ETSE (h), SGE (i), and immediate (j) and 90-s fat-suppressed (k) postgadolinium SGE images in a fourth patient with massive iron deposition in the liver and spleen.

[361]. Iron overload in the liver and renal cortex is typically seen in patients with paroxysmal nocturnal hemoglobinuria [365].

Cirrhosis. Hepatocellular iron is commonly mildly increased in patients with cirrhosis, particularly those with cirrhosis secondary to ethanol abuse. Anemia, pancreatic insufficiency, and/ or decrease in the synthesis of transferrin probably all contribute to the excess iron deposition [372]. The degree of signal loss of the liver is not as great as that seen with idiopathic hemochromatosis or transfusional siderosis.

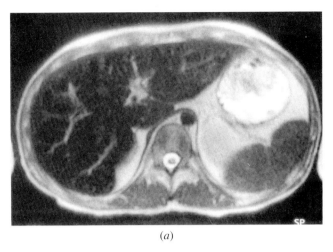

(a)

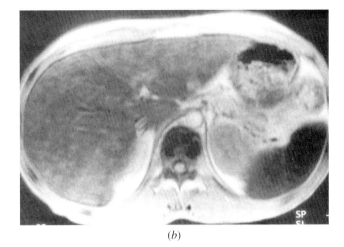

(b)

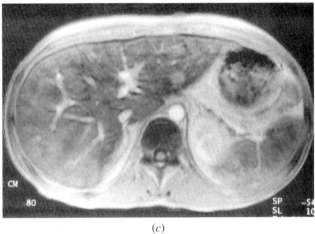

(c)

F I G . 2.230 Transfusional siderosis, heterogeneous iron deposition. T2-weighted SS-ETSE (a), SGE (b), and immediate postgadolinium SGE (c) images in a patient who has a history of acute leukemia. The liver and spleen are low signal intensity on T2-weighted (a) and T1-weighted (b) images, consistent with iron deposition. On pre- and postcontrast T1-weighted images, there is a heterogeneous appearance consistent with heterogeneous distribution of iron deposition, in the setting of transfusional siderosis.

Coexisting Fat and Iron Deposition

Fat and iron deposition may occur concurrently within the liver. Coexisting fat and iron deposition may be demonstrated by using several gradient-echo MR sequences with differing in-phase (TE = 4.2 ms) and out-of-phase (TE = 2.1 ms) echo times. In the presence of iron, signal intensity of the liver will decrease steadily as echo time increases because of T2* effects. At out-of-phase echo time both higher than and lower than the echo time for in-phase images, a disproportionate drop of liver signal intensity will occur relative to spleen because of fat-water phase cancellation. The combined observations that liver and spleen are nearly signal void on T2-weighted images, reflecting iron deposition, and that liver drops in signal intensity relative to spleen, comparing out-of- phase to in-phase SGE images, reflecting fat deposition, are also diagnostic for coexistent iron and fat deposition (fig. 2.236).

Fatty Liver

Fatty liver or steatosis is defined as accumulation of triglycerides within hepatocytes. It constitutes one of the most common abnormalities in liver surgical or autopsy specimens. The causes of hepatic steatosis include alcohol abuse, diabetes mellitus, obesity, malnutrition, and exposure to toxins [388]. Fatty degeneration may present as diffuse, uniform, or patchy and focal or with spared foci of normal liver. At times, focal fatty infiltration or geographic regions of normal liver within fatty liver (fat sparing) may mimic the appearance of mass lesions.

Fatty liver may interfere with the detection of focal liver masses on CT images or sonography [373]. However, out-of-phase gradient-echo (TE = 2.1 ms) imaging is a highly accurate MRI technique to examine for fatty liver and to distinguish focal fat from neoplastic masses (figs. 2.237 and 2.238) [374, 375]. Fat in substantial amount has high signal intensity on in-phase T1-weighted images because of its short T1. Comparing out-of-phase (TE = 2.1 ms) to in-phase (TE = 4.2 ms) gradient-echo images, the presence of fatty metamorphosis results in signal loss. This signal loss on out-of-phase images is progressively more evident in moderate and severe fatty infiltration [309]. The spleen is generally used as the organ of reference for signal loss. As fat content approaches 50% of the voxel element in the

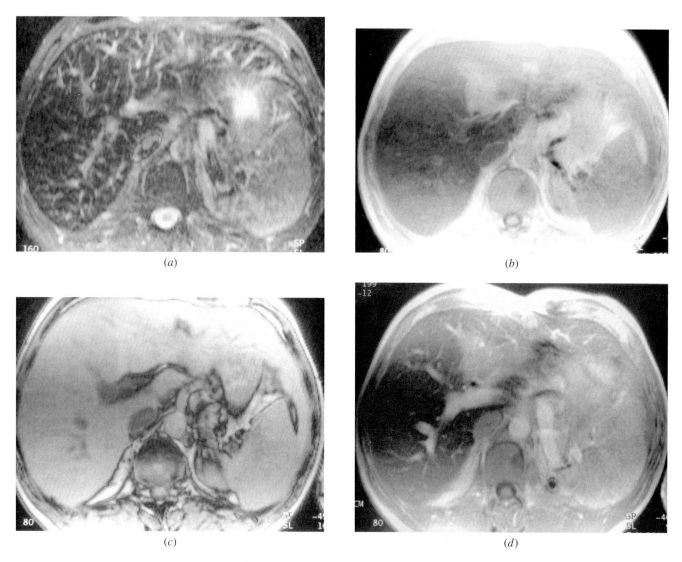

FIG. 2.231 Transfusional siderosis with focal sparing. Echo train-STIR (*a*), SGE (*b*), out-of-phase SGE (*c*), and immediate postgadolinium SGE (*d*) images. The liver is enlarged and demonstrates decreased signal reflecting iron deposition. There is a region in segment 4 with increased signal intensity on the T1-weighted image (*b*). On the short TE out-of-phase image (*c*), the susceptibility artifact from iron diminishes, resulting in a decrease in the signal intensity difference between iron-deposited and normal liver. This is virtually the opposite effect from that seen in focal normal liver in the setting of fat infiltration. Normal vessels are appreciated extending through the focal normal liver on the postgadolinium image (*d*).

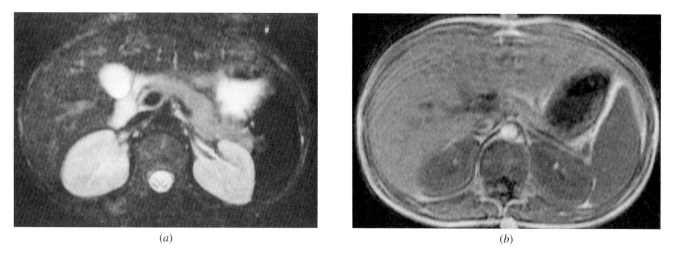

FIG. 2.232 Transfusional siderosis, mild. T2-weighted fat-suppressed ETSE (*a*) and SGE (*b*) images. On the T2-weighted image (*a*), the liver and spleen are low in signal intensity and the pancreas is normal in signal intensity. Signal intensity of the liver, spleen, and pancreas appear normal on the T1-weighted image (*b*). Iron deposition in the liver and spleen that results in signal loss appreciable only on T2-weighted images, and not on T1-weighted images, is compatible with mild transfusional siderosis.

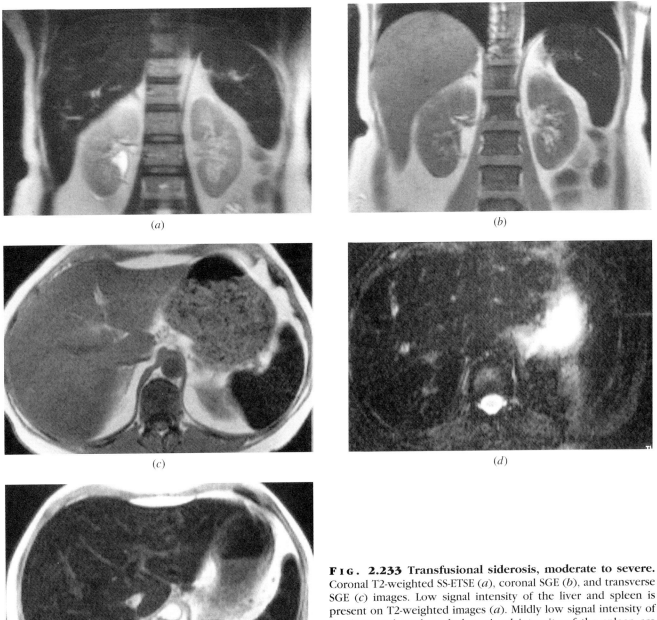

(a)

(b)

(c)

(d)

(e)

FIG. 2.233 Transfusional siderosis, moderate to severe. Coronal T2-weighted SS-ETSE (*a*), coronal SGE (*b*), and transverse SGE (*c*) images. Low signal intensity of the liver and spleen is present on T2-weighted images (*a*). Mildly low signal intensity of the liver and moderately low signal intensity of the spleen are observed on T1-weighted images (*b, c*), consistent with moderate iron deposition.

T2-weighted fat-suppressed ETSE (*d*) and SGE (*e*) images in a second patient demonstrate very low signal intensity of the liver and spleen on T2-weighted (*d*) and T1-weighted (*e*) images consistent with severe iron deposition.

liver, the liver appears blacker relative to the spleen on out-of-phase (TE = 2.1 ms) compared to in-phase (TE = 4.2 ms) sequence. For lesser amounts of fat (<15%) the signal of liver on out-of-phase sequence appears near equivalent to the signal of spleen.

Diffuse liver steatosis can be categorized by MRI based on the degree of fatty infiltration as follows: I, severe; II, moderate; III, mild; and IV, minimal. Severe steatosis demonstrates a very dramatic loss of signal on out-of-phase images compared to in-phase images; moderate steatosis shows that liver signal intensity drops below the signal of the spleen on out-of-phase images but not as intense as severe steatosis; mild steatosis exhibits equivalent signal intensity of liver and spleen on short TE out-of-phase images; and minimal steatosis is a subjective classification that we have begun

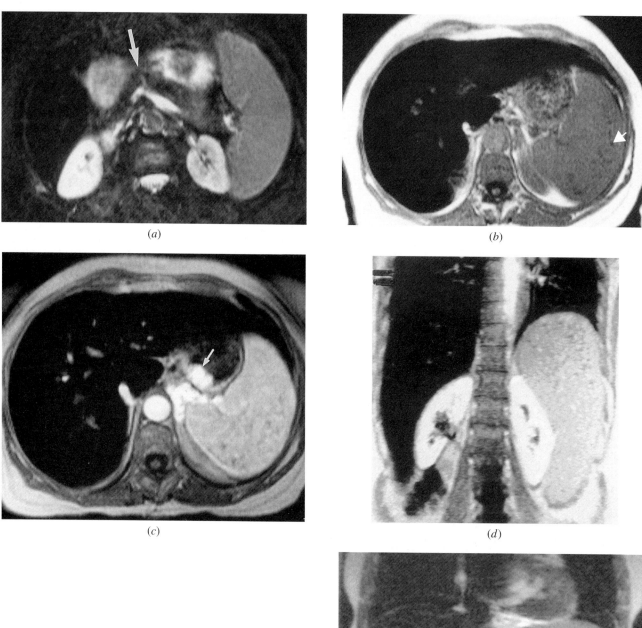

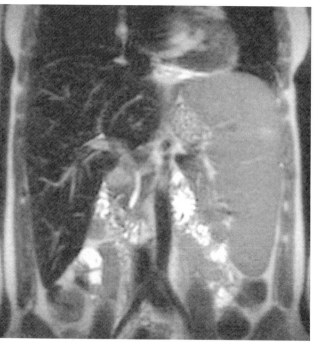

FIG. 2.234 Heterozygous thalassemia. T2-weighted fat-suppressed ETSE (*a*), SGE (*b*), and 45-s (*c*) and coronal 90-s (*d*) postgadolinium SGE images. The liver demonstrates severe iron deposition and is signal void on T2 (*a*)- and T1 (*b*)-weighted images. The spleen is greatly enlarged and shows negligible iron deposition but does contain Gamna–Gandy bodies (arrow, *b*). The pancreas is modestly low in signal intensity (arrow, *a*). Varices along the lesser curvature and within the gastric wall (arrow, *c*) are clearly shown on the 45-s postgadolinium images. Splenomegaly (*d*), Gamma–Gandy bodies, and varices are secondary to portal hypertension. The pattern of iron deposition reflects increased intestinal absorption without transfusional siderosis, which is a common appearance for heterozygous hemolytic anemias because these patients often do not require blood transfusions.

Coronal SS-ETSE (*e*), SGE (*f*), and immediate post gadolinium SGE (*g*) images in a second patient with history of heterozygous thalassemia. The liver is signal void on both T2-weighted (*a*) and

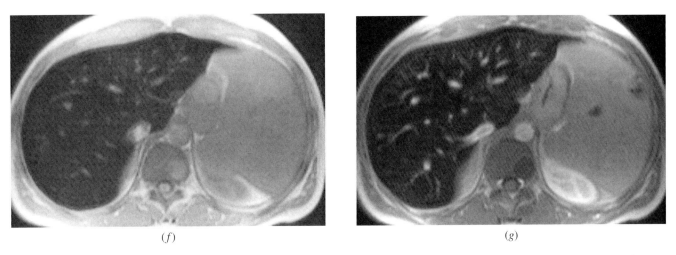

(f)

(g)

FIG. 2.234 (*Continued*) T1-weighted (*f*) images, reflecting iron deposition. The spleen is enlarged and normal in signal intensity, reflecting that the patient has not required blood transfusion. Note the presence of two lesions in the spleen consistent with hemangiomas.

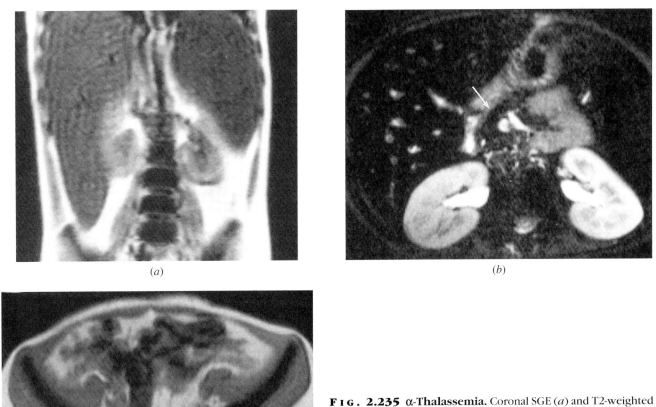

(a)

(b)

(c)

FIG. 2.235 α-Thalassemia. Coronal SGE (*a*) and T2-weighted fat-suppressed ETSE (*b*) images. Enlargement of the liver and spleen is apparent on T1-weighted image (*a*). These organs are also lower in signal intensity than psoas muscle on T1-weighted (*a*) and T2-weighted (*b*) images, consistent with severe iron deposition in the RES. Vertebral bodies are nearly signal void, which also reflects RES iron deposition. The pancreas is nearly signal void (arrow, *b*), reflecting coexistent iron deposition into tissues. SGE image (*c*) through the pelvis shows nearly signal-void pelvic bones secondary to iron deposition in the RES.

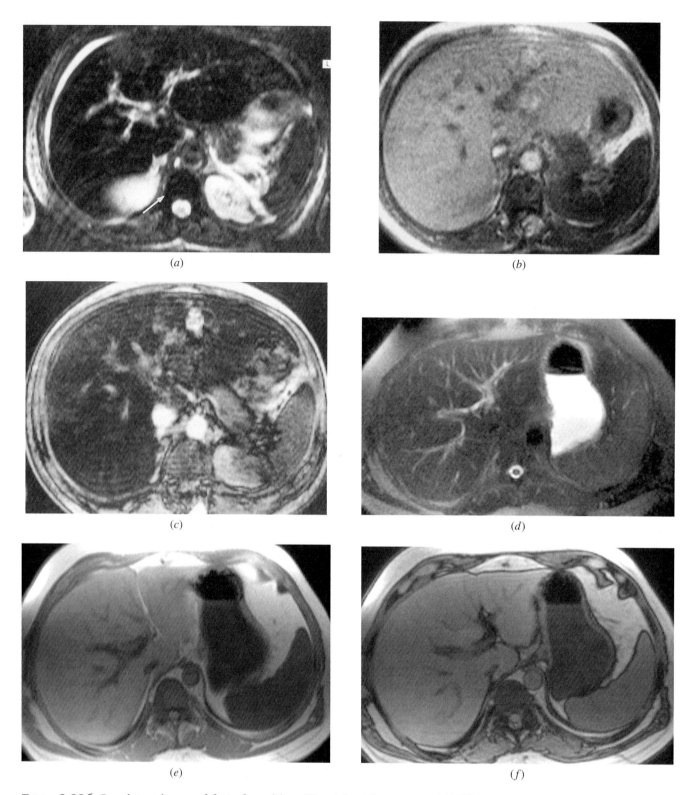

F I G . 2.236 Coexistent iron and fatty deposition. T2-weighted fat-suppressed SS-ETSE (*a*), SGE (*b*), and out-of-phase SGE (*c*) images. On T2-weighted images (*a*), the liver, spleen, and bone marrow (arrow, *a*) are nearly signal void, which is consistent with coexistent iron deposition. On T1-weighted images (*b*), liver and spleen have a normal signal intensity pattern, with the liver higher in signal intensity than the spleen. On the shorter echo-time out-of-phase image (*c*), the liver drops in signal intensity below that of spleen, which is consistent with fatty infiltration. Ascites is well shown as high-signal intensity fluid along the liver margin on the T2-weighted image (*a*).

Echo train STIR (*d*), in-phase SGE (*e*), and out-of-phase SGE (*f*) images in a second patient demonstrate iron deposition and mild fatty infiltration in the liver. Iron deposition is shown by the low signal on T2-weighted image (*d*), and fat is shown by the loss of liver-spleen contrast on the shorter-TE out-of-phase sequence (*f*). Iron alone would result in an increase in liver-spleen contrast on the shorter-TE sequence.

These cases illustrate the effect of iron on T2-weighted images. It is essential to be aware that T1-weighted gradient-echo sequences demonstrate both out-of-phase effects, which cycle with in-phase and out-of-phase times, and susceptibility effects, which increase with increase in TE.

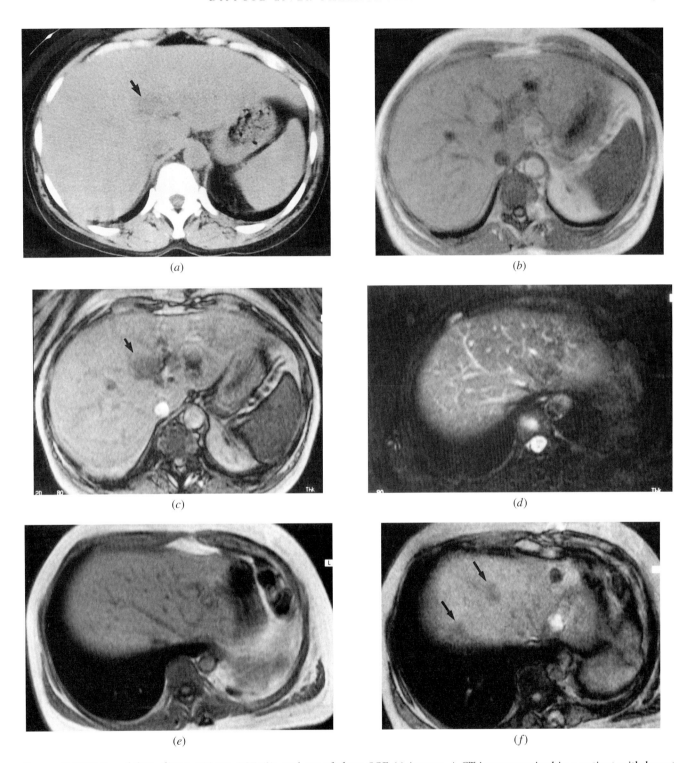

F I G .   2.237   Focal fatty liver. CT (*a*), SGE (*b*), and out-of-phase SGE (*c*) images. A CT image acquired in a patient with breast cancer demonstrates a low-density lesion in the medial segment (arrow, *a*). The in-phase T1-weighted image (*b*) shows no lesion in this location, whereas on the out-of-phase image (*c*), signal drop occurs in the central region of the medial segment (arrow, *c*), which is diagnostic for focal fatty infiltration when combined with the information that enhancement was isointense on the hepatic arterial dominant-phase images.

T2-weighted fat-suppressed ETSE (*d*), SGE (*e*), and out-of-phase SGE (*f*) images in a second patient. Previous ultrasound study in this young boy with acute myelogeneous leukemia demonstrated two liver lesions. No liver lesions are apparent on the in-phase T1-weighted image (*e*). On the out-of-phase image (*f*), two focal low-signal rounded masses are apparent (arrows, *f*). The T2-weighted image (*d*) does not reveal any lesion. No tumor blush was apparent on immediate postgadolinium images (not shown). The identification of lesions only on out-of-phase SGE images is diagnostic for fatty infiltration.

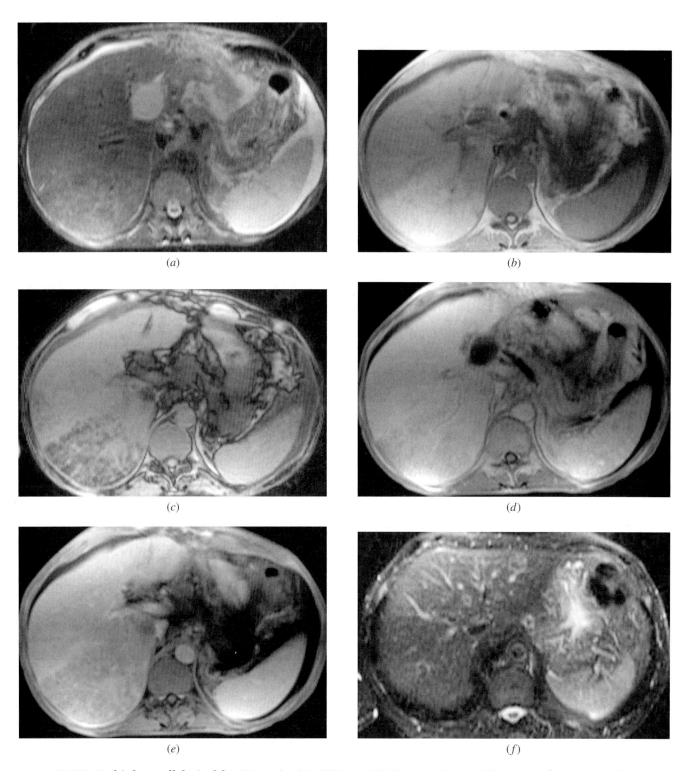

(a) (b) (c) (d) (e) (f)

FIG. 2.238 Multiple small foci of fat. T2-weighted SS-ETSE (*a*), SGE (*b*), out-of-phase SGE (*c*), and 45-s (*d*) and 90-s fat-suppressed (*e*) post gadolinium SGE images. There are multiple small focal fat areas in the right hepatic parenchyma that drop in signal on out-of-phase images (*a*) compared with in-phase images (*b*). Although there is slight hepatic heterogeneity on other sequences, there is no evidence of abnormal enhancement of these foci alone, supporting that this appearance is that of multiple foci of fat deposition.

T2-weighted SS-ETSE (*f*), SGE (*g*), out-of-phase SGE (*h*), and immediate (*i*) and 90-s fat-suppressed (*j*) postgadolinium SGE images in a second patient that show multiple small foci of fat scattered throughout the hepatic parenchyma. The lesions lose signal on the out-of-phase images (*h*) and do not show differing enhancement from background liver.

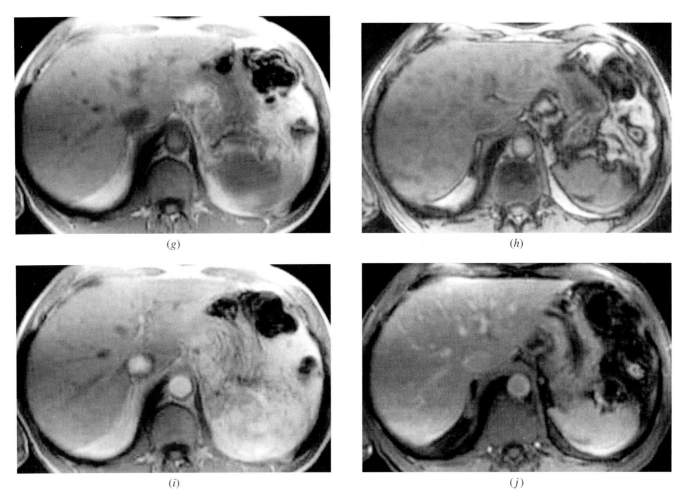

(g)

(h)

(i)

(j)

F I G . 2.238 (*Continued*)

to employ when the signal of liver and spleen converge on shorter TE out-of-phase compared to longer TE in-phase, that is, liver still brighter than spleen but the difference is less than on the in-phase sequence. At the present time, detection of minimal fat has not been substantiated (figs. 2.239–2.242).

FNH and metastases are the most common focal lesions associated with fatty liver. MRI is particularly effective in evaluating patients with fatty liver for the presence of focal lesions. Non-fat-suppressed T1-weighted images and fat-suppressed T2-weighted images maximize the contrast between the liver and lesions. On non-fat-suppressed T1-weighted images, the liver may be higher in signal intensity than normal liver, maximizing the contrast with low-signal-intensity masses, whereas on fat-suppressed T2-weighted images fatty liver is lower in signal intensity than normal liver, maximizing the contrast with moderately high-signal-intensity masses.

An area that is isointense or hyperintense to surrounding background parenchyma on in-phase images and loses signal homogeneously on out-of-phase images is highly diagnostic for focal fatty infiltration. The lack of surrounding mass effect, the presence of vessels, and the morphology of focal fat most often permit distinction from fat within tumors, such as HCC, adenoma, angiomyolipoma, or lipoma [309]. Focal fat usually has angular, wedge-shaped margins that are usually relatively well defined. Masses that contain fat usually have a rounded configuration. Common locations for focal fat are adjacent to the ligamentum teres, the central tip of segment 4, and, less commonly, along the gallbladder [376, 377]. Although the pathogenesis for focal fat is not well established, it is suggested that variations in blood supply may occur [378–380]. An important ancillary observation is that uncomplicated fatty deposition within the liver enhances with gadolinium usually indistinguishably from normal liver on all sequences. Almost invariably masses that contain fat enhance differently than background liver.

Hemorrhage, melanin, copper, and protein may be associated with nonfatty masses with high signal inten-

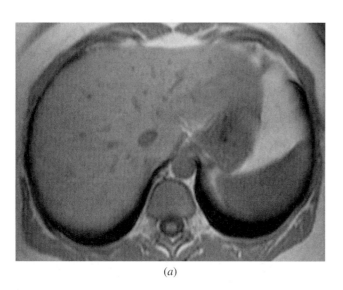

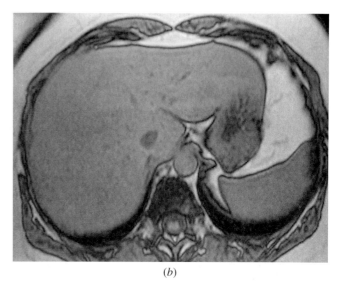

(a)   (b)

FIG. 2.239 Minimal fatty infiltration. In-phase (a) and out-of-phase (b) SGE images. The liver appears unremarkable on the T1-weighted image (a). On out-of-phase image (b), the signal intensity of the liver converges toward the signal intensity of the spleen. Note that although the signal intensity of liver drops on out-of-phase image it remains higher than the signal intensity of the spleen, which may represent minimal fatty infiltration.

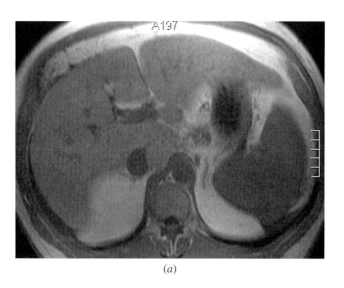

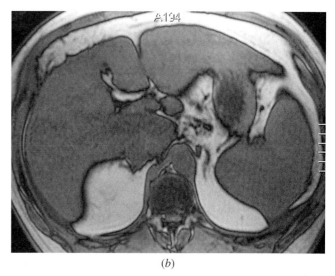

(a)   (b)

FIG. 2.240 Mild fatty infiltration. In-phase (a) and out-of-phase (b) SGE images. The liver appears unremarkable on T1-weighted images (a) and exhibits a drop in signal intensity on out-of-phase image (b), with convergence of the signal intensity of the liver and spleen to comparable signal intensities. Note that the liver has not dropped lower in signal than the spleen, establishing that fatty infiltration is mild.

sity on T1-weighted images. Out-of-phase images distinguish between these tumors and lipid-containing masses or focal fatty infiltration. Although some well-differentiated HCCs contain lipid, most HCCs with high signal intensity on T1-weighted images do not. HCCs that contain lipid tend to be more well-defined masses than focal fatty infiltration. Moreover, HCCs are often encapsulated and are most commonly not homogeneously fatty. They usually contain some elements with high signal intensity on fat-suppressed T2-weighted images. Of all focal hepatic lesions, hepatic adenoma may most closely resemble focal fatty infiltration, as these tumors may have relatively uniform fat content. Demonstration of a capillary blush on arterial dominant images that fades on interstitial-phase postgadolinium images establishes the diagnosis of adenoma. Although angiomyolipoma and lipoma may be composed of fat, they do not drop in signal intensity on out-of-phase images; however, these lesions will demonstrate a phase-cancellation artifact along their margins with

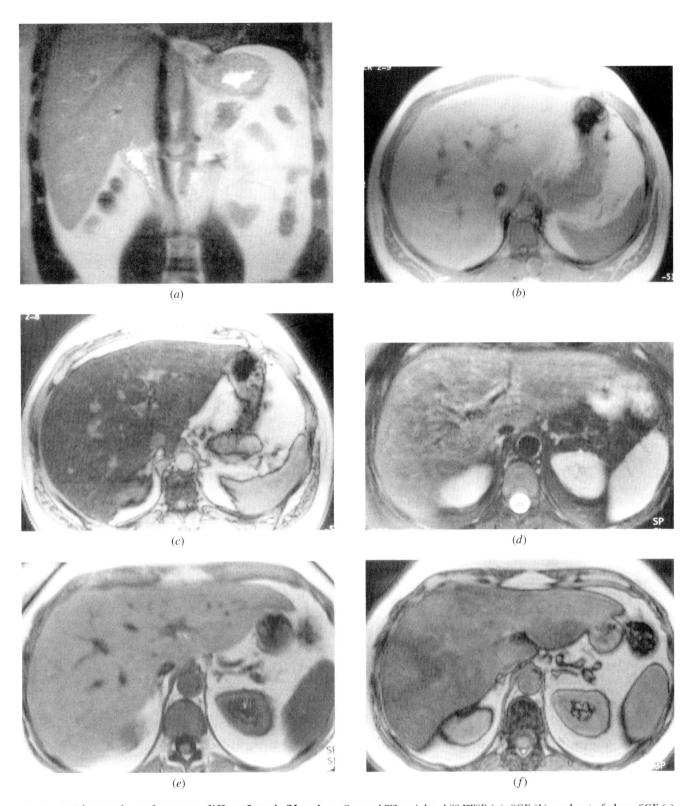

FIG. 2.241 Moderately severe diffuse fatty infiltration. Coronal T2-weighted SS-ETSE (*a*), SGE (*b*), and out-of-phase SGE (*c*) images. The liver is high in signal on T2-weighted image (*a*), which reflects the fact that fat, including fatty liver, is high signal on long echo-train sequences. A useful internal comparison is the psoas muscle: normal liver should be of comparable signal. Note in this patient that the liver is considerably higher in signal than psoas. In-phase (*b*) and out-of-phase (*c*) images confirm moderately severe fatty infiltration.

T2-weighted fat-suppressed ETSE (*d*), SGE (*e*), out-of-phase SGE (*f*), and immediate postgadolinium SGE (*g*) images in a second patient. The liver demonstrates moderately severe heterogeneous drop in signal intensity on out-of-phase image (*f*) with respect to in-phase (*e*) image, consistent with severe diffuse patchy fatty infiltration. Note that enhancement of fatty liver (*g*) is generally

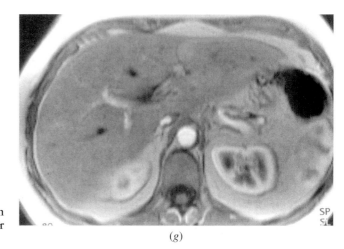

FIG. 2.241 (*Continued*) indistinguishable from normal when an in-phase echo time nonfat-suppressed sequence is used for gadolinium-enhanced imaging.

(g)

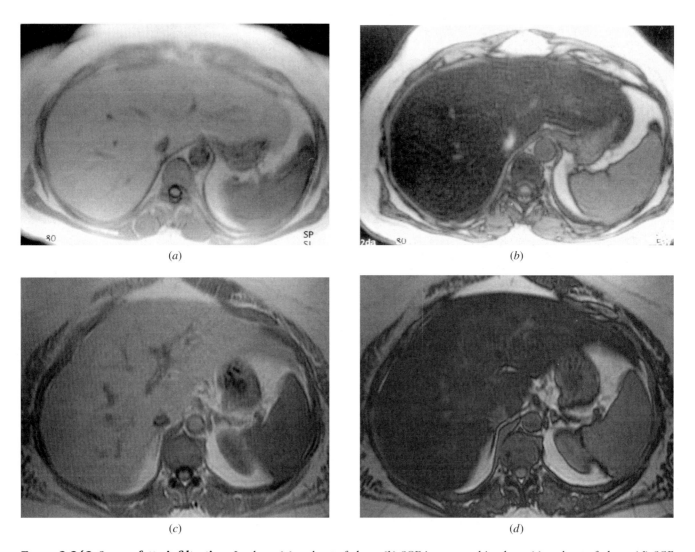

(a)

(b)

(c)

(d)

FIG. 2.242 Severe fatty infiltration. In-phase (*a*) and out-of-phase (*b*) SGE images and in-phase (*c*) and out-of-phase (*d*) SGE images in two different patients both with enlarged liver and marked fatty infiltration.

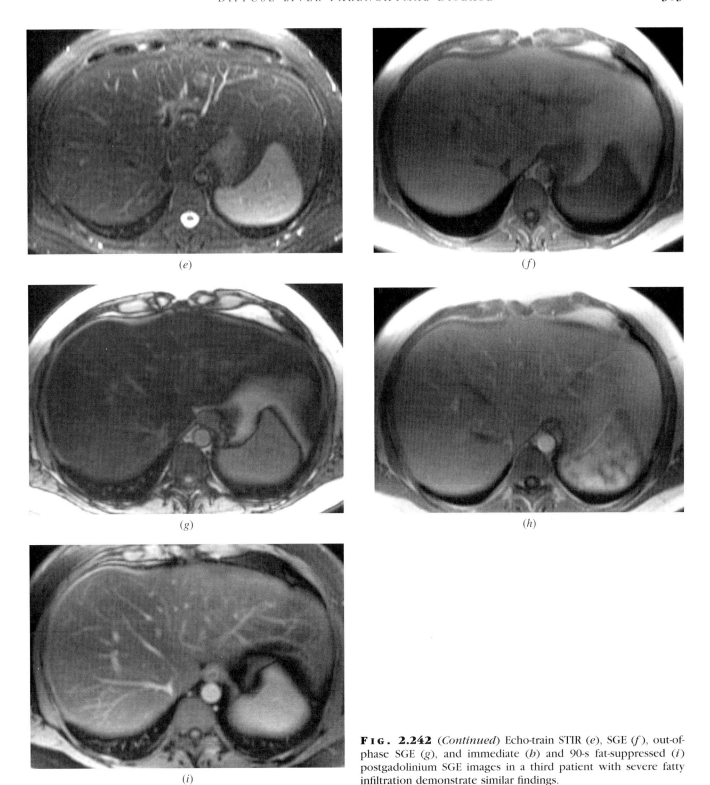

(e)

(f)

(g)

(h)

(i)

F I G . 2.242 (*Continued*) Echo-train STIR (*e*), SGE (*f*), out-of-phase SGE (*g*), and immediate (*h*) and 90-s fat-suppressed (*i*) postgadolinium SGE images in a third patient with severe fatty infiltration demonstrate similar findings.

liver. The extent of fat within those tumors is higher than in severe liver steatosis. Because of this difference, it is possible to distinguish between these tumors and fatty liver. Also, angiomyolipoma and lipoma visibly lose signal when fat-suppressed techniques are

employed because of the very high fat content, which is most apparent with fatty liver.

Focal normal liver in the setting of diffuse fatty infiltration (focal sparing) appears as a focus of high signal intensity in a background of diminished-signal liver on out-of-phase images (figs. 2.243 and 2.244). Arterioportal shunting, occlusion or compression of the portal vein, and decreased portal perfusion causing decreased delivery of lipid are the pathogenetic causes postulated for focal sparing [378–380]. The central tip of segment 4, surrounding gallbladder fossa and adjacent to falciform ligament, most commonly has anomalous vascular supply and, consequently, is more likely to have lesser fat deposition than the rest of the liver [376, 377]. Metastases in the setting of fatty liver may demonstrate peritumoral fat sparing due to vascular compression of this circumferential liver [309, 377, 381, 382].

Mucopolysaccharidoses

The mucopolysaccharidoses are a group of inherited disorders caused by incomplete degradation and storage of acid mucopolysaccharides (glycosaminoglycans). The clinical manifestations result from the accumulation of mucopolysaccharides in somatic and visceral tissues. Mucopolysaccharides are major components of the extracellular substance of connective tissue. Widespread accumulation of mucopolysaccharides along with involvement of many organ systems is observed in this condition. Hepatosplenomegaly, skeletal deformities,

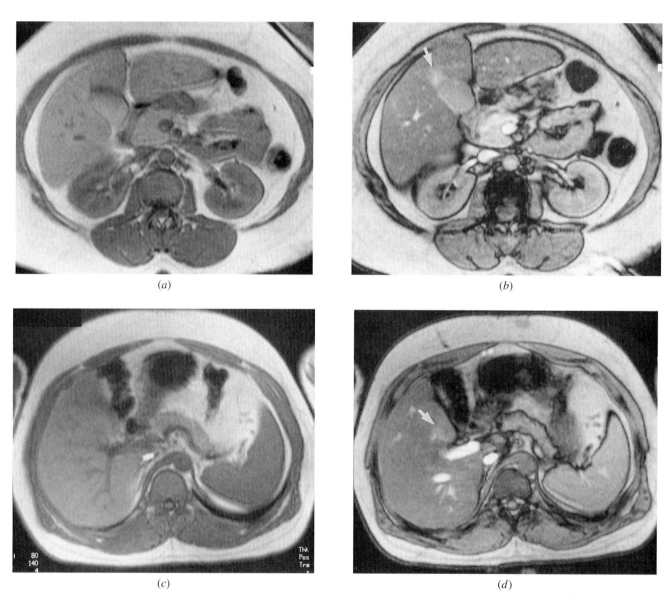

(a)

(b)

(c)

(d)

F I G . 2.243 Fatty infiltration with focal sparing. SGE (*a*) and out-of-phase SGE (*b*) images. Homogeneous signal of the liver is present on the T1-weighted image (*a*). On the out-of-phase image (*b*), the liver drops in signal, with a focus of higher signal adjacent to the gallbladder (arrow, *b*) representing focal normal liver.

SGE (*c*) and out-of-phase SGE (*d*) images in a second patient. The liver is normal in signal intensity on the in-phase image (*c*). On the out-of-phase image (*d*), the liver drops in signal intensity relative to the spleen, with focal sparing present in the tip of segment 4 (arrow, *d*).

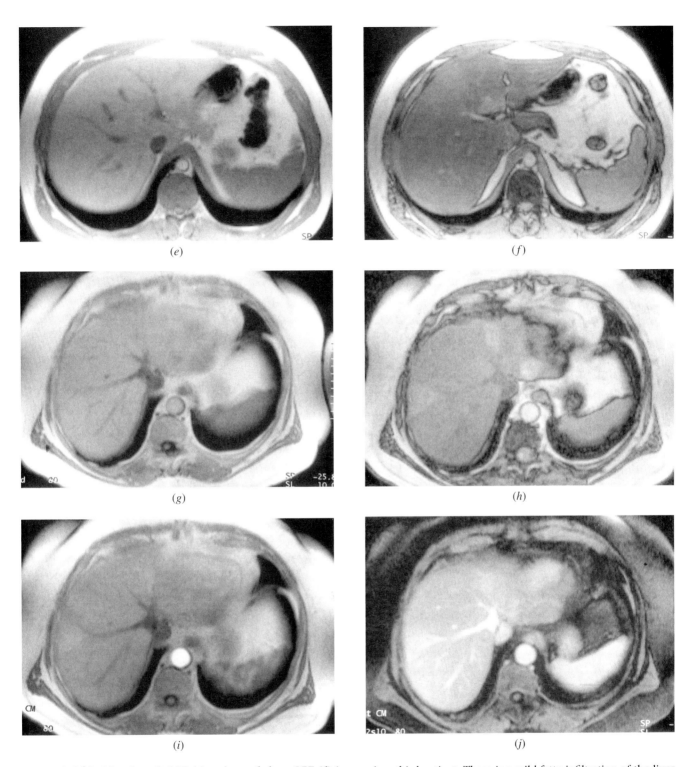

(e)

(f)

(g)

(h)

(i)

(j)

F I G . 2.243 (*Continued*) SGE (*e*) and out-of-phase SGE (*f*) images in a third patient. There is a mild fatty infiltration of the liver with focal sparing of the tip of segment 4 (*f*).

SGE (*g*), out-of-phase SGE (*h*), immediate postgadolinium SGE (*i*), and 90-s postgadolinium fat-suppressed SGE (*j*) images in a fourth patient. Wedge-shaped regions of focal normal liver in a fatty deposited liver are present. Note that on 90-s postgadolinium image (*j*) these same regions are identified as higher signal. This reflects a fat suppression effect of the fatty liver, rather than a gadolinium-enhanced effect of the regions of normal liver.

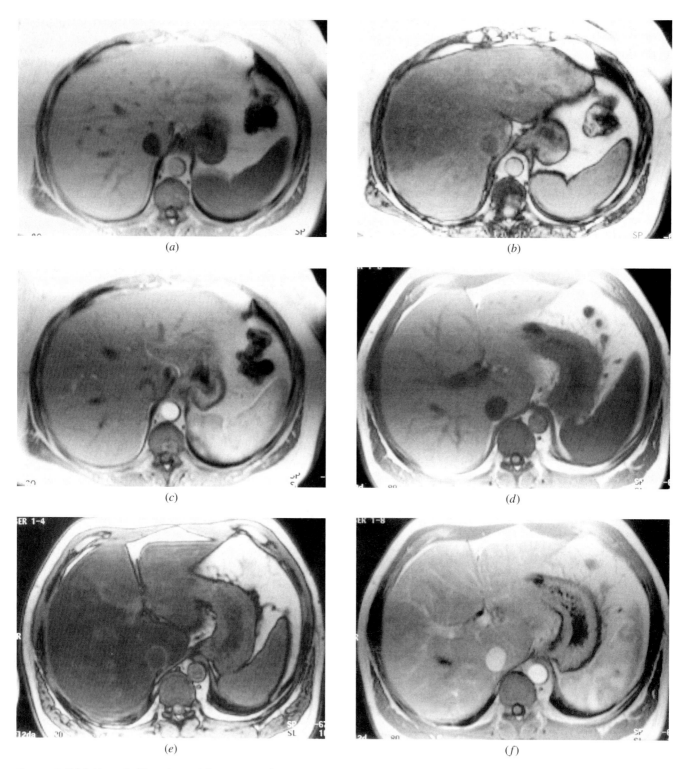

F I G . 2.244 Fatty infiltration with segmental variation in fat content. SGE (*a*), out-of-phase SGE (*b*), and immediate post-gadolinium SGE (*c*) images. On the out-of-phase (*b*) image, there is trisegmental signal loss with relative sparing of the posterior segment of the right lobe. Signal intensity on postgadolinium images (*c*) is unremarkable for the entire liver.

SGE (*d*), out-of-phase SGE (*e*), immediate post-gadolinium SGE (*f*), and 90-s postgadolinium fat-suppressed SGE (*g*) images in a second patient. There is slightly less fatty infiltration of the left lobe compared to the right, reflected by relatively lesser drop in signal on the out-of-phase image (*e*). After contrast, the liver enhances homogeneously.

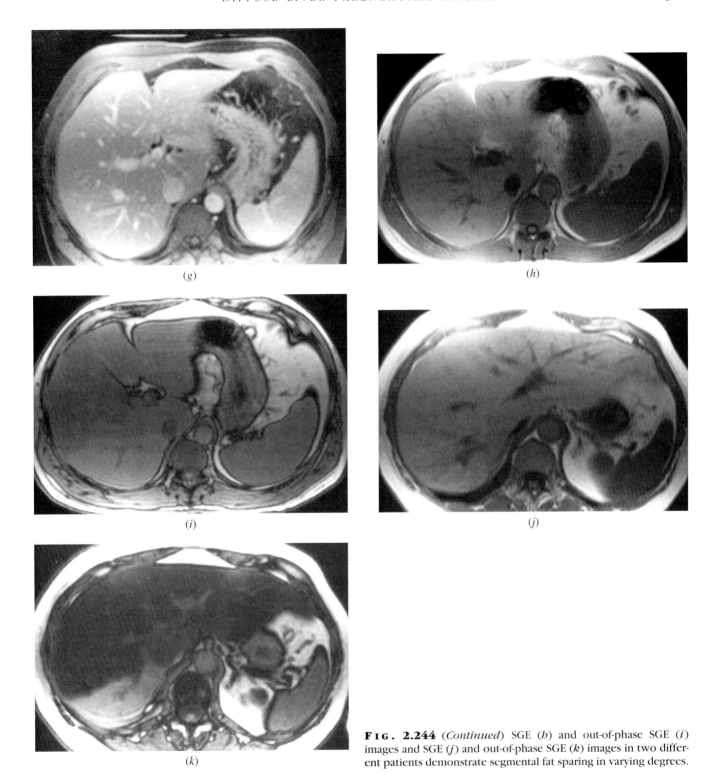

FIG. 2.244 (*Continued*) SGE (*h*) and out-of-phase SGE (*i*) images and SGE (*j*) and out-of-phase SGE (*k*) images in two different patients demonstrate segmental fat sparing in varying degrees.

valvular lesions, subendothelial deposits, particularly within the walls of coronary arteries, and CNS abnormalities are common. On MR images, hepatomegaly is commonly observed (fig. 2.245). Specific MR imaging features are yet to be elucidated. Pathologic macroscopic examination may show extensive fibrosis or cir-

rhosis [2]. A report involving postmortem examination of six cases of mucopolysaccharidoses revealed diffuse liver fibrosis in all cases [383]. Microscopic examination shows swollen hepatocyte and Kupffer cell cytoplasm, filled with abnormal storage material [2]. The degree of disability and overall prognosis in each of the muco-

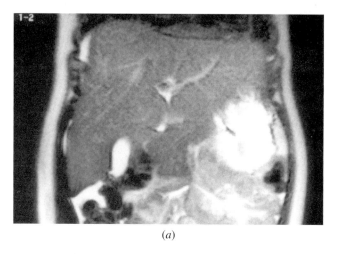
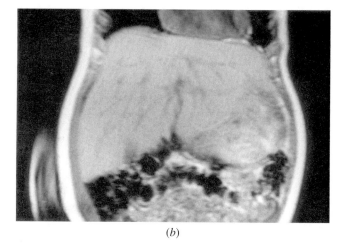

(a)

(b)

FIG. 2.245 Storage disease. Coronal T2-weighted SS-ETSE (*a*) and SGE (*b*) images in a patient who has a history of mucopoly-saccharidosis. Note enlargement of the liver well demonstrated on coronal images.

polysacharidoses are determined by the extent of physical and mental involvement [384].

Arteriovenous Fistulas

Abnormal arterial-venous communications or fistulas may occur in the liver secondary to injury, tumor, or congenital disease. Arteriovenous fistula is a well-known complication of percutaneous liver biopsy [385]. Clinically significant or symptomatic hepatic vascular fistulae are uncommon but are usually caused by trauma, including iatrogenic trauma [386]. Fistulas are well shown with gadolinium-enhanced techniques, either as a 2D or a 3D GRE or MRA technique. MRI features of posttraumatic arterial-vascular communications include dilation of afferent and efferent vessels, transient hepatic parenchymal blush in a watershed distribution, and early opacification of efferent vessels (fig. 2.246) [387]. A critical observation to establish the diagnosis is that the nidus of the shunt follows the enhancement characteristics of comparable intrahepatic vessels (i.e., they often retain contrast); whereas focal hepatic masses with the exception of hemangiomas, follow a different pattern, and often fade more quickly or washout.

Congenital vascular fistulas are rare. One of the more common conditions is hereditary hemorrhagic telangiectasia (Rendu–Osler–Weber syndrome). The disease is characterized by telangiectasias (skin, mucous membranes), arteriovenous fistulas in the liver (30% of cases) lungs. and CNS, and aneurysms [2, 3]. Visceral involvement has been documented in the GI tract, spleen, kidneys, and genital tract. On imaging, the liver may be filled with numerous variably sized abnormal arterial-venous communications. Lesions may appear as multiple well-defined enhancing masses that parallel the enhancement of vessels. A combination of vascularized lesions and thrombosed lesions may be observed, reflecting either the natural history of the condition or treatment approaches such as embolization (fig. 2.247).

Portal Venous Obstruction/Thrombosis

Thrombosis of the portal vein is generally associated with the presence of a hypercoaguable state, vascular injury, or stasis [2]. Obstruction of the portal vein may be insidious and well tolerated or may be an acute, potentially life-threatening event. Most cases fall between these two extremes. Blockage of the portal vein may be extrahepatic or intrahepatic. Common causes of extrahepatic portal vein obstruction include 1) massive hilar lymphadenopathy due to metastatic abdominal cancer; 2) phlebitis resulting from peritoneal sepsis (e.g., appendicitis); 3) propagation of splenic vein or superior mesenteric vein thrombosis secondary to pancreatitis; and 4) postsurgical thrombosis following abdominal procedures. Cirrhosis is the most common intrahepatic cause of portal venous obstruction. Intravascular invasion by primary or secondary malignancy in the liver may occur [388].

On imaging, portal vein thrombosis may be demonstrated by using black-blood techniques (e.g., spin-echo techniques with superior and inferior saturation pulses) and bright-blood techniques (e.g., time-of-flight gradient echo or gadolinium-enhanced gradient echo). A combination of both approaches is often useful to increase diagnostic confidence. Portal veins may be occluded by tumor thrombus, bland thrombus, or extrinsic compression. MRI usually is able to distinguish between these entities. Tumor and bland thrombus may

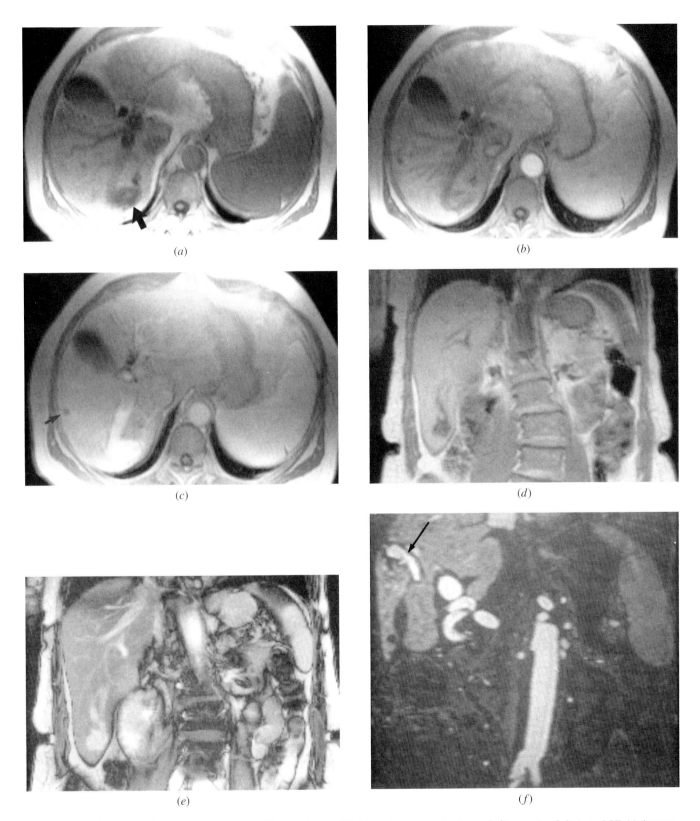

(a)

(b)

(c)

(d)

(e)

(f)

FIG. 2.246 Acquired arterio-venous malformation. SGE (*a*) and immediate (*b*) and 45-s postgadolinium SGE (*c*) images. There is a 2-cm rounded structure (arrow, *a*) in the posterior segment of the right lobe, with a prominent posterior branch of the right portal vein entering the lesion. After contrast administration, there is early minimal enhancement (*b*) and 45-s intense enhancement (*c*) of this lesion in continuity with the portal vein (*c*). Note also the tiny hepatic cyst or biliary hamartoma (arrow, *c*), nodular contour of the liver, and splenomegaly.

Coronal SGE (*d*) and gadolinium-enhanced refocused gradient-echo (*e*) images in a second patient. There is a lesion in the inferior aspect of the right lobe that demonstrates large paired vessels leading into and away from it. This lesion shows decreased signal on the precontrast image (*d*) and intense enhancement after gadolinium administration (*e*), consistent with arterio-venous malformation.

Coronal 3D gradient-echo 2-mm source image (*f*), MIP reconstruction of the 2-mm 3D gradient-echo sections (*g*), and transverse 90-s fat-suppressed SGE image (*h*) in a third patient. The 2D source image (*f*) demonstrates the connection between right hepatic

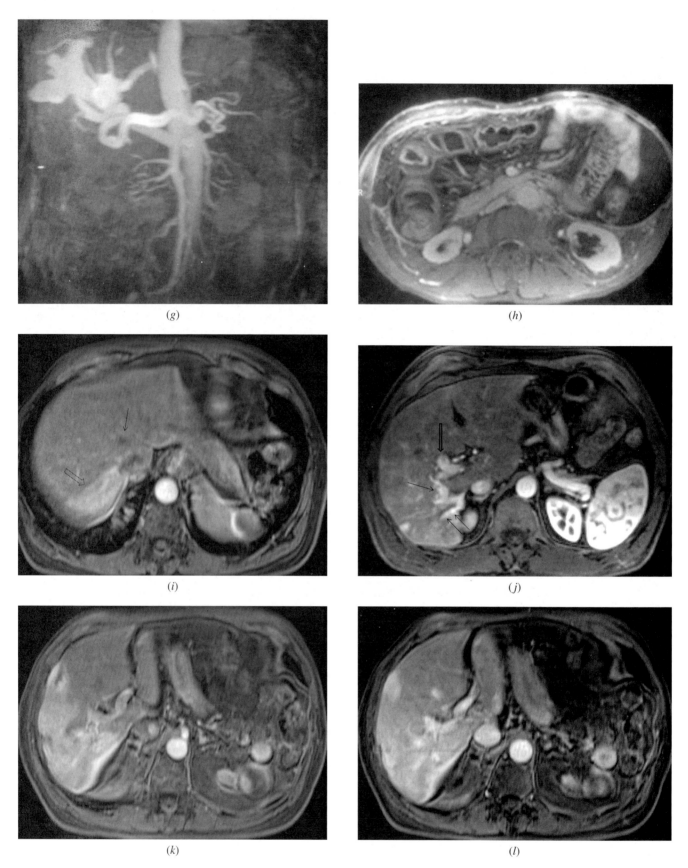

(g)

(h)

(i)

(j)

(k)

(l)

FIG. 2.246 (*Continued*) artery and right portal vein (arrow, *f*) and the MIP reconstruction image (*g*) displays the full length of the dilated right hepatic artery and portal vein. On the interstitial-phase gadolinium-enhanced fat-suppressed SGE image (*h*) there is submucosal edema of the colon with prominent serosal and mucosal enhancement reflecting congestion in the portal venous circulation secondary to the fistula.

T1-weighted fat-suppressed 3D gradient-echo immediate (*i, j, k*) and 45-s (*l*) postgadolinium images in a patient with posttraumatic vascular shunts. The superior tomographic section demonstrates early opacification of the right hepatic vein (thick arrow, *i*). Note that the middle hepatic vein (thin arrow, *i*) is not opacified. A tomographic section through the mid-liver shows dilatation of the right portal vein (thick arrow, *j*). The level of communication is also apparent (thin arrow, *j*).

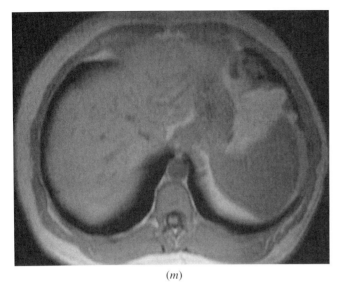

(m)

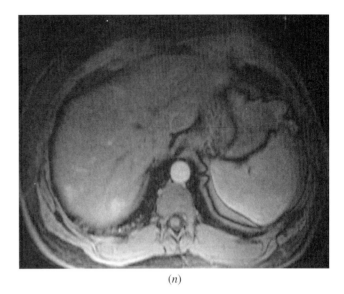

(n)

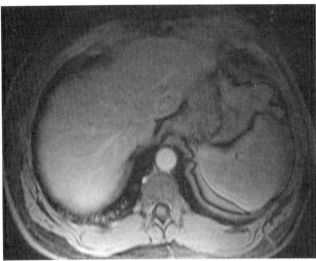

(o)

FIG. 2.246 (*Continued*) On the more inferior tomographic section (*k*), early intense geographic enhancement is noted in the right lobe. On the 45-s postgadolinium images (*l*), the region of increased enhancement has faded to background liver. The three features of traumatic arteriovenous shunts are: i) dilation of afferent vessel, ii) transient early increased parenchymal enhancement in a watershed distribution, and iii) early opacification of efferent vessel. The nidus of the malformation or shunt follows the opacification and enhancement pattern of comparable vessels, which distinguishes them from focal liver lesions. Note that on the late-phase images the transiently enhanced parenchyma tends to be isointense to background parenchyma.

T1-weighted fat-suppressed 3D gradient-echo (*m*), and immediate (*n*) and 90-s (*o*) fat-suppressed 3D gradient-echo image obtained **at 3T** demonstrating focal areas of intense enhancement on early phase (*n*) compatible with focal arteriovenous shunt. Note on the late phase (*o*) the shunt tends to be isointense as background parenchyma. This entity is distinguished from post-traumatic av shunt because there is no dilation of afferent or efferent vessels, or early appearance of contrast in draining veins.

be distinguished from each other by the observation that tumor thrombus is higher in signal intensity on T2-weighted images, has soft tissue signal intensity on time-of-flight gradient-echo images, and enhances with gadolinium (fig. 2.248). Bland thrombus is low in signal intensity on T2-weighted and time-of-flight gradient-echo images and does not enhance with gadolinium (figs. 2.249–2.251). Tumor thrombus is most often observed with hepatocellular carcinoma, most commonly in the diffuse type, although it may also occur with metastases. Bland thrombus may be observed in the setting of cirrhosis and various inflammatory/infectious processes involving organs in the portal circulation, with pancreatitis being the most common. Increased enhancement of the vein wall is appreciated in the setting of infected bland thrombus.

Extrinsic compression of portal veins is most commonly caused by malignant tumors, but may also occur with benign tumors such as hemangiomas. Cholangiocarcinoma, in particular, has a propensity to cause extrinsic compression and obstruction of portal veins. Lobar or segmental portal vein obstruction caused by tumor may result in discrete wedge-shaped regions of high signal intensity on T2-weighted images and enhancement on immediate postgadolinium gradient-echo images [374, 389–393]. Increased signal intensity on T2-weighted images may reflect some degree of hepatocellular injury. Decreased blood supply results in decreased size of hepatocytes, which increases the proportion of liver volume occupied by the vascular and interstitial spaces. Collateral periportal veins may maintain portal perfusion when the main portal vein

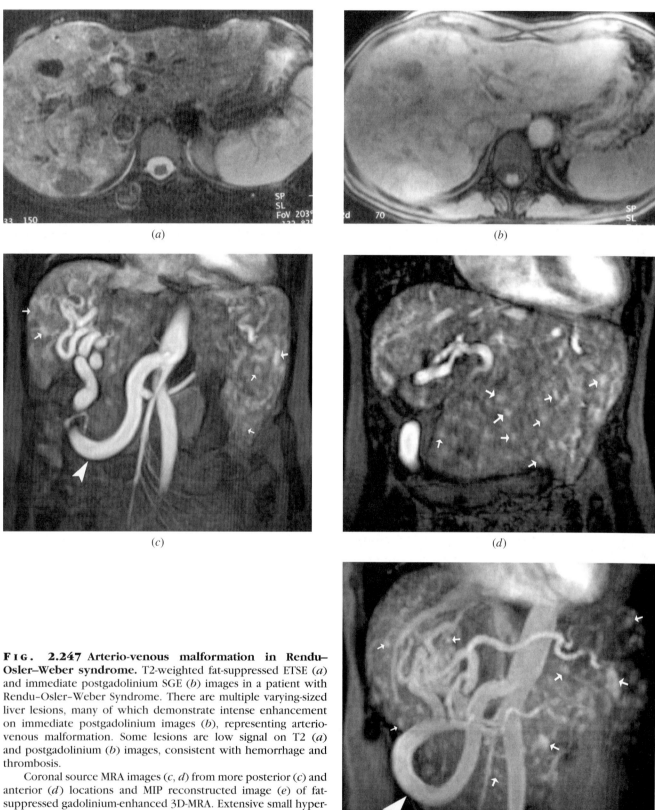

FIG. 2.247 Arterio-venous malformation in Rendu–Osler–Weber syndrome. T2-weighted fat-suppressed ETSE (*a*) and immediate postgadolinium SGE (*b*) images in a patient with Rendu–Osler–Weber Syndrome. There are multiple varying-sized liver lesions, many of which demonstrate intense enhancement on immediate postgadolinium images (*b*), representing arterio-venous malformation. Some lesions are low signal on T2 (*a*) and postgadolinium (*b*) images, consistent with hemorrhage and thrombosis.

Coronal source MRA images (*c, d*) from more posterior (*c*) and anterior (*d*) locations and MIP reconstructed image (*e*) of fat-suppressed gadolinium-enhanced 3D-MRA. Extensive small hypervascular arterio-venous malformations (small arrows, *c, d, e*) are present throughout the liver. Note massive dilatation of the hepatic artery (arrowhead, *c, e*) due to the tremendous blood flow to the liver (Courtesy of Bharat Aggarwal, M.D., Diwan Chand Satya Pal Aggarwal Imaging Research Center, New Delhi, India).

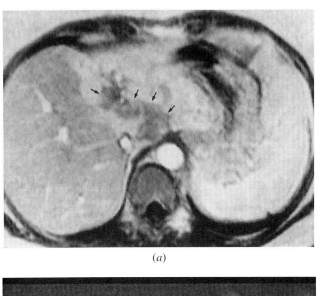

(a)

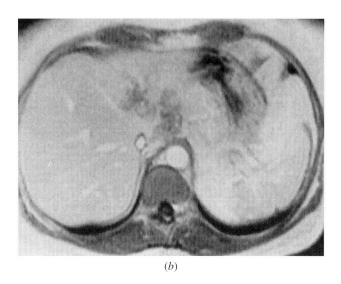

(b)

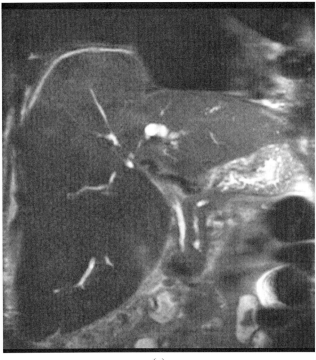

(c)

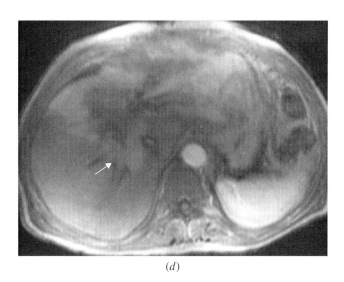

(d)

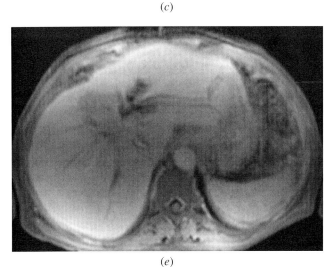

(e)

F I G . 2.248 Portal vein thrombosis, secondary to tumor.
Immediate postgadolinium SGE (*a*) and 90-s postgadolinium SGE
(*b*) images. A liver metastasis is present in the caudate lobe and
the lateral segment associated with heterogeneously enhancing
thrombus extending into the left portal vein (arrows, *a*). On the
immediate postgadolinium image (*a*), there is increased enhancement of the left lobe, which fades by 90 s (*b*).

Coronal T2-weighted SS-ETSE (*c*) and immediate (*d*) and 90-s
fat-suppressed (*e*) postgadolinium SGE images in a second patient
who has HCC. There is a mass in the bifurcation of the portal vein
that shows mild high signal intensity on T2-weighted images (*c*),
low signal intensity on T1-weighted images (not shown), and
negligible enhancement but with perilesional enhancement on
early-phase image (*d*) and becomes homogeneously enhanced on
late-phase image (*e*). Thrombus is present in the main portal vein
extending from the main left branch, which demonstrates low
signal intensity on T2-weighted images and enhances after contrast administration (arrow, *d*), compatible with tumor thrombus.

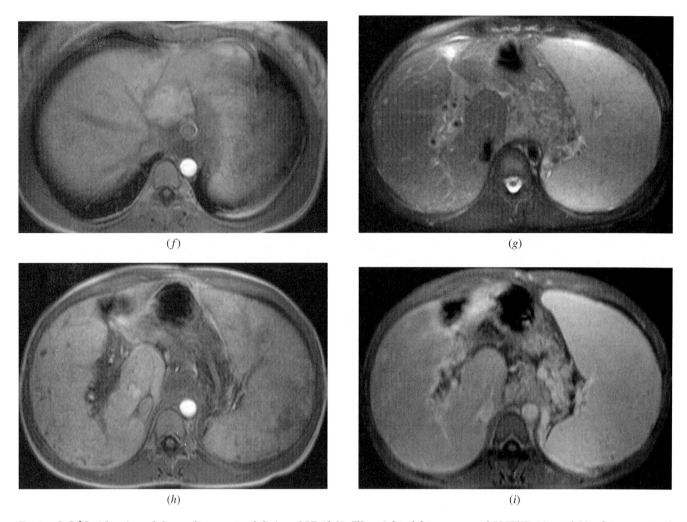

FIG. 2.248 (*Continued*) Immediate postgadolinium SGE (*f, h*), T2-weighted fat-suppressed SS-ETSE (*g*), and 90-s fat-suppressed postgadolinium SGE (*i*) images in a patient with a HCC. There is a mass in the left hepatic lobe that shows faint enhancement on early-phase postgadolinium image (*f*). The left, right, and main portal veins are expanded and appear low signal intensity on T2-weighted images (*g*) and early-phase images (*h*) with mild progressive enhancement on late-phase images (*i*) consistent with tumor thrombus.

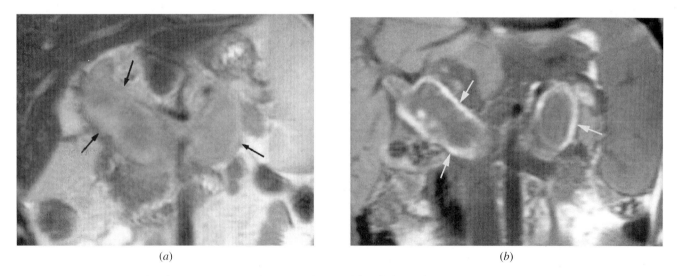

FIG. 2.249 Portal and splenic vein thrombosis—subacute blood thrombus. Coronal T2-weighted SS-ETSE (*a*), coronal SGE (*b*), T2-weighted fat-suppressed SS-ETSE (*c*), SGE (*d*), fat-suppressed SGE (*e*), and 90-s fat-suppressed (*f, g, h*) postgadolinium SGE images in a 21-yr-old man who has a history of spontaneous retroperitoneal hematoma associated with portal and splenic vein thrombosis. There is marked dilatation of the splenic vein, portal vein, and proximal superior mesenteric vein, which contains

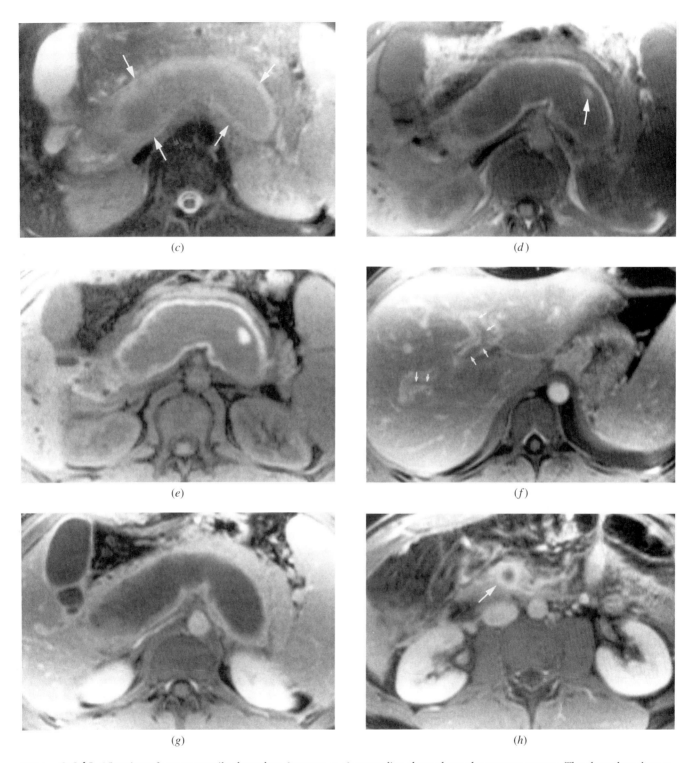

(c)   (d)

(e)   (f)

(g)   (h)

F I G . 2.249 (*Continued*) an expansile thrombus (arrows, *a–c*) extending throughout the venous system. The thrombus demonstrates an increased signal intensity rim on T1-weighted images (*b, d, e*) and a small focus of increased signal intensity (arrow, *d*) within the thrombus, consistent with blood products at different stages of breakdown. Fat-suppressed postgadolinium images (*f, g*) demonstrate no evidence of enhancement within the thrombus. Thrombus is present in normal-caliber intrahepatic portal vein branches (arrows, *f*). Substantially increased enhancement of tissues surrounding the thrombosed SMV (arrow, *h*) suggests an underlying inflammatory process.

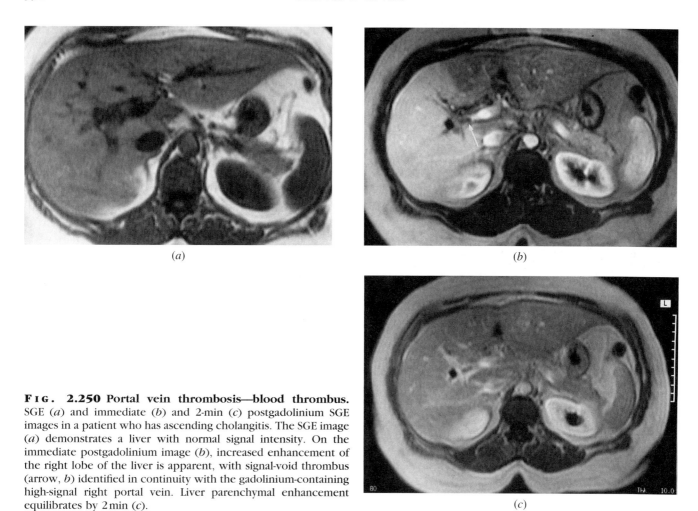

(a)

(b)

(c)

F I G . 2.250 Portal vein thrombosis—blood thrombus. SGE (*a*) and immediate (*b*) and 2-min (*c*) postgadolinium SGE images in a patient who has ascending cholangitis. The SGE image (*a*) demonstrates a liver with normal signal intensity. On the immediate postgadolinium image (*b*), increased enhancement of the right lobe of the liver is apparent, with signal-void thrombus (arrow, *b*) identified in continuity with the gadolinium-containing high-signal right portal vein. Liver parenchymal enhancement equilibrates by 2 min (*c*).

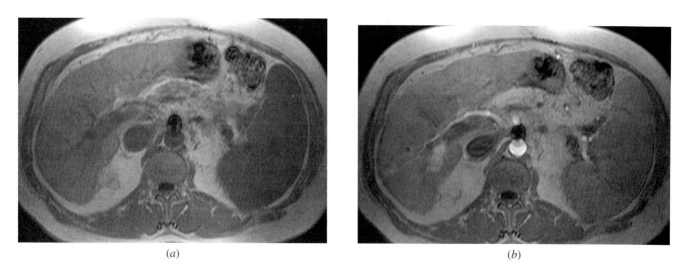

(a)

(b)

F I G . 2.251 Portal vein thrombosis—bland thrombus. SGE (*a*) and immediate (*b*) and 90-s fat-suppressed (*c*) postgadolinium SGE images. There is a bland thrombus in the right branch of the portal vein that is best visualized on the late-phase image as

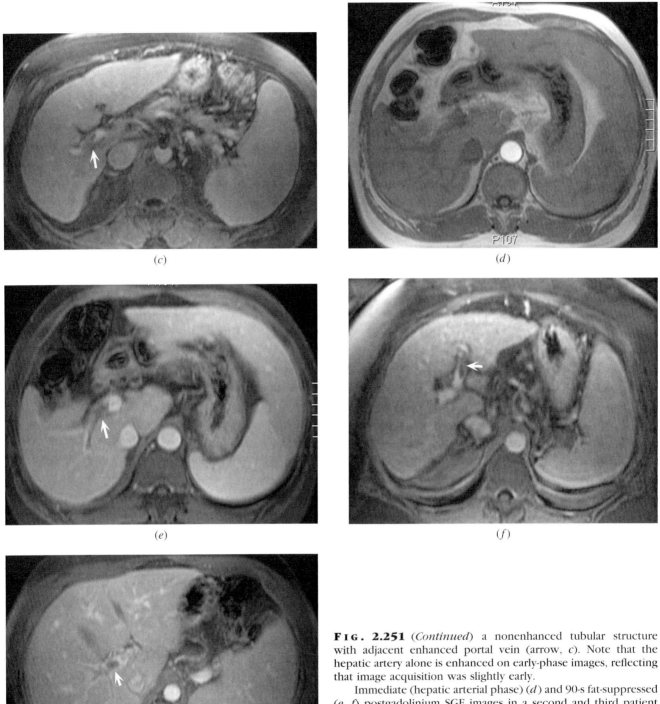

(c)

(d)

(e)

(f)

(g)

F I G . 2.251 (*Continued*) a nonenhanced tubular structure with adjacent enhanced portal vein (arrow, *c*). Note that the hepatic artery alone is enhanced on early-phase images, reflecting that image acquisition was slightly early.

Immediate (hepatic arterial phase) (*d*) and 90-s fat-suppressed (*e, f*) postgadolinium SGE images in a second and third patient with bland thrombus in the main branches of the portal vein (arrow, *e, f*).

Ninety-second fat-suppressed postgadolinium SGE image (*g*) in a fourth patient with bland thrombus within the right portal vein. Note enhancement along the outer margins of the thrombus consistent with flow around the thrombus (arrow, *g*).

is thrombosed. In time, this network of collateral venous channels dilates and the thrombosed portal vein retracts, producing cavernous transformation [394, 395]. Obstruction of segmental portal vein may also cause hepatic atrophy, with compensatory hypertrophy of other segments [374, 389].

After administration of intravenous gadolinium, transient increased enhancement of hepatic parenchyma may be apparent in areas with decreased portal perfusion during the hepatic arterial dominant phase of enhancement (see figs. 2.248 and 2.250) [396]. Exact correlation between perfusion defects on CTAP and regions of transient high signal intensity on immediate postgadolinium gradient-echo images has been reported in eight patients (fig. 2.252) [396]. These findings showed that regions with absent or diminished portal venous supply received increased hepatic arterial supply. This paradoxical increased enhancement of hepatic parenchyma distal to an obstructed portal vein branch largely reflects increased hepatic arterial supply due to an autoregulatory mechanism. Segments with obstructed portal venous supply and increased hepatic arterial supply will display early intense enhancement after contrast administration. Gadolinium delivered in the first pass is more concentrated in hepatic arteries than in portal veins and is delivered earlier by hepatic arteries than by portal veins. On later images, concentration of gadolinium in hepatic arteries and portal veins equilibrates, which explains the transient nature of the increased enhancement. In general, portal venous compromise appears as transient increased enhancement in a segmental distribution of involved liver.

Hepatic Venous Thrombosis

Budd–Chiari

Budd–Chiari syndrome is a disorder with numerous causes resulting from obstruction to hepatic venous outflow. Although originally described for acute, usually fatal, thrombotic occlusion of the major hepatic veins or inferior vena cava, the definition of Budd–Chiari syndrome has been broadened to include subacute and chronic occlusive syndromes.

Obstruction of venous outflow from the liver results in portal hypertension, ascites, and progressive hepatic failure. Budd–Chiari syndrome is more common in women, and an underlying thrombotic tendency is present in up to one-half of patients. Causes include polycythemia vera, pregnancy, postpartum state, and intraabdominal cancer, especially HCC [397]. Pathologically, acute changes after hepatic vein thrombosis show dilatation of veins and congestion of sinusoids. As disease advances, sinusoids become collagenized and hepatocytes become atrophic, with loss of parenchyma [2, 3].

Usually, hepatic venous outflow is not completely eliminated because a variety of accessory hepatic veins may drain above or below the site of obstruction. In some cases, obstruction may be segmental or subsegmental. Although the disease most commonly involves major hepatic veins, demonstration of patent central hepatic veins may be observed as small or intermediate-sized veins may be occluded in isolation [398]. In the chronic setting, regions with completely obstructed hepatic venous outflow will develop shunting of blood from hepatic arteries to portal veins, producing reversed portal venous flow [392, 399–401]. The involved liver parenchyma is thereby deprived of portal vein supply. Hepatic regeneration, hypertrophy, and atrophy depend in part on the degree of portal perfusion [356]. Budd–Chiari syndrome most often results in atrophy of peripheral liver, which experiences severe venous obstruction, and hypertrophy of the caudate lobe and central liver, which are relatively spared.

Absence of hepatic veins may be demonstrated by techniques in which flowing blood is signal void or by techniques in which flowing blood is high in signal intensity such as time-of-flight techniques or portal-phase gadolinium-enhanced gradient echo sequences. Generally, a combination of both approaches results in the highest diagnostic accuracy. However, the bright blood technique is the most accurate and usually suffices.

On immediate postgadolinium MR images, the peripheral atrophic liver in Budd–Chiari syndrome may enhance to a greater or lesser extent than normal or hypertrophied liver, which provides insight into the chronicity of the disease process. One study reported that dynamic enhancement patterns differed for acute, subacute, and chronic Budd-Chiari, with combinations of enhancement patterns present when acute is superimposed on subacute disease [402]. In acute-onset Budd–Chiari syndrome the peripheral liver enhances less than central liver, presumably because of acute increased tissue pressure with resultant diminished blood supply from both hepatic arterial and portal venous systems in the peripheral liver. This is associated with moderately high signal on T2-weighted images and low signal on T1-weighted images, reflecting associated edema. After contrast, the liver demonstrates a dramatic appearance of increased central enhancement compared to decreased enhancement of peripheral liver that persists on late images (figs. 2.253 and 2.254) [403].

In subacute Budd–Chiari syndrome, reversal of flow in portal veins and development of small intra- and extrahepatic venovenous collaterals occurs, features not present in other chronic liver diseases. Many of the collaterals are capsule based. Signal of the peripheral liver is mildly increased on T2-weighted images and mildly decreased on T1-weighted images, similar to

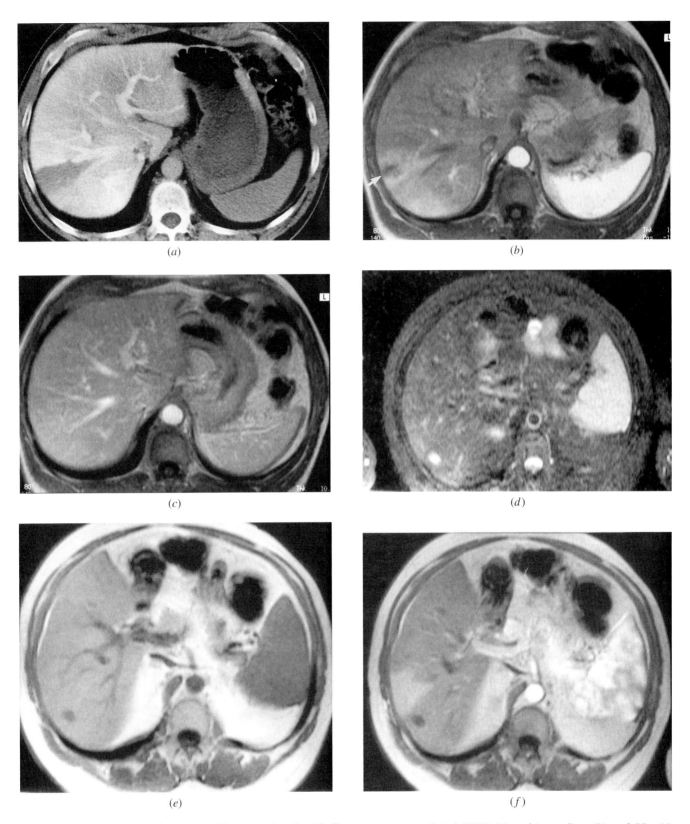

FIG. 2.252 Perfusional abnormality associated with liver metastases. Spiral CTAP (*a*) and immediate (*b*) and 90-s (*c*) postgadolinium SGE images. The CTAP image (*a*) demonstrates a wedge-shaped perfusion defect in the right lobe of the liver. On the immediate postgadolinium SGE image (*b*), wedge-shaped increased enhancement is present surrounding a peripheral 2-cm liver metastasis (arrow, *b*). By 90 s after gadolinium (*c*), both the perfusion defect and the metastases have equilibrated with liver. (Reproduced with permission from Semelka RC, Schlund JF, Molina PL, Willms AG, Kahlenberg M, Mauro MA, Weeks SM, Cance WG. Malignant liver lesions: comparison of spiral CT arterial portography and MR imaging for diagnostic accuracy, cost, and effect on patient management. *J Magn Reson Imaging* 1: 39–43, 1996).

Echo-train STIR (*d*), SGE (*e*), and immediate postgadolinium SGE (*f*) images in a second patient show a perfusional abnormality of transient increased enhancement seen on the immediate postgadolinium image (*f*) in a patient who has a history of colon cancer. Note the small cyst adjacent to the abnormal area. Perfusional abnormalities of transient increased enhancement are not uncommon in patients with colon cancer liver metastases. Many are related to metastases, but in some the cause is not clear, as in this case.

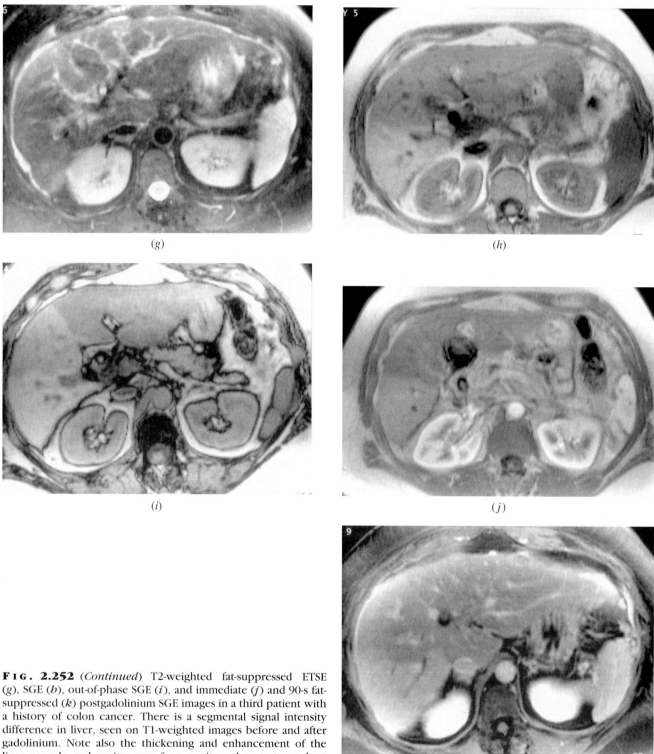

(g)

(h)

(i)

(j)

FIG. 2.252 (*Continued*) T2-weighted fat-suppressed ETSE (*g*), SGE (*h*), out-of-phase SGE (*i*), and immediate (*j*) and 90-s fat-suppressed (*k*) postgadolinium SGE images in a third patient with a history of colon cancer. There is a segmental signal intensity difference in liver, seen on T1-weighted images before and after gadolinium. Note also the thickening and enhancement of the liver capsule and peritoneum from peritoneal metastases, best seen on interstitial-phase fat-suppressed T1-weighted images (*k*).

(k)

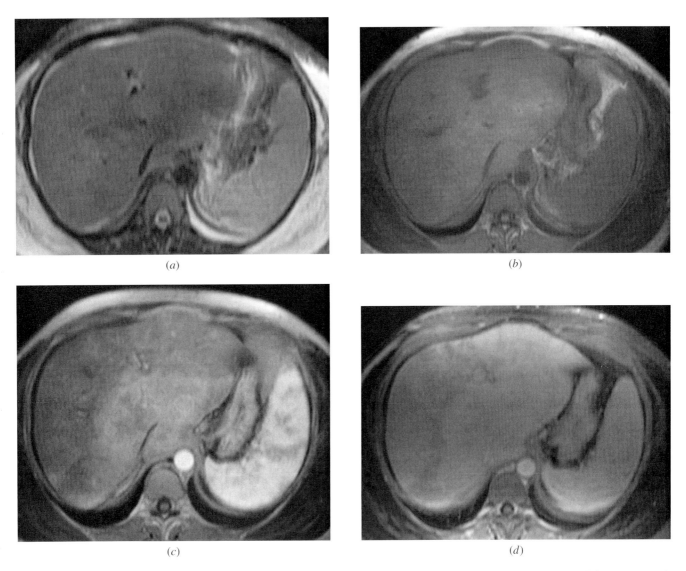

(a)   (b)   (c)   (d)

F I G . 2.253 Acute Budd–Chiari syndrome. T2-weighted ETSE (*a*), SGE (*b*), immediate (*c*), and 90-s postgadolinium SGE (*d*) images. The T2-weighted image (*a*) shows normal signal intensity of the caudate lobe and central liver and mild heterogeneous higher signal intensity of the peripheral liver. On the precontrast T1-weighted image (*b*), the caudate lobe and central portion of the liver are normal in signal intensity, whereas the peripheral liver is low in signal intensity. On the immediate postgadolinium image (*c*), the caudate lobe and central liver enhance heterogeneously and intensely, whereas peripheral liver shows lower enhancement. On late phase (*c*) liver appears more homogeneous than early phase but still shows increased enhancement in central areas.

acute Budd–Chiari syndrome. On dynamic gadolinium-enhanced MR images the enhancement of subacute disease differs substantially from the acute syndrome. Mildly increased and heterogeneous enhancement is apparent in the peripheral liver relative to central liver on hepatic arterial dominant-phase images that, over time, becomes more homogeneous with the remainder of the liver. Caudate lobe hypertrophy is mild to moderate, and collateral vessels are not prominent in the subacute setting (fig. 2.255).

In chronic Budd–Chiari syndrome, hepatic edema is not a prominent feature and fibrosis develops. Fibrosis results in decreased signal of peripheral liver on T2- and

T1-weighted images. Enhancement differences between peripheral and central liver on serial postgadolinium images become more subtle. Venous thrombosis, appreciated in acute and subacute disease, is usually not observed in chronic disease. Massive caudate lobe hypertrophy, massive enlarged bridging intrahepatic collaterals, extrahepatic collaterals, and regenerative nodules are all features observed in chronic Budd–Chiari syndrome.

Curvilinear intrahepatic collaterals and capsule-based collaterals are characteristic of chronic Budd–Chiari syndrome (fig. 2.256). Varices are usually prominent in chronic Budd–Chiari syndrome and are well shown on

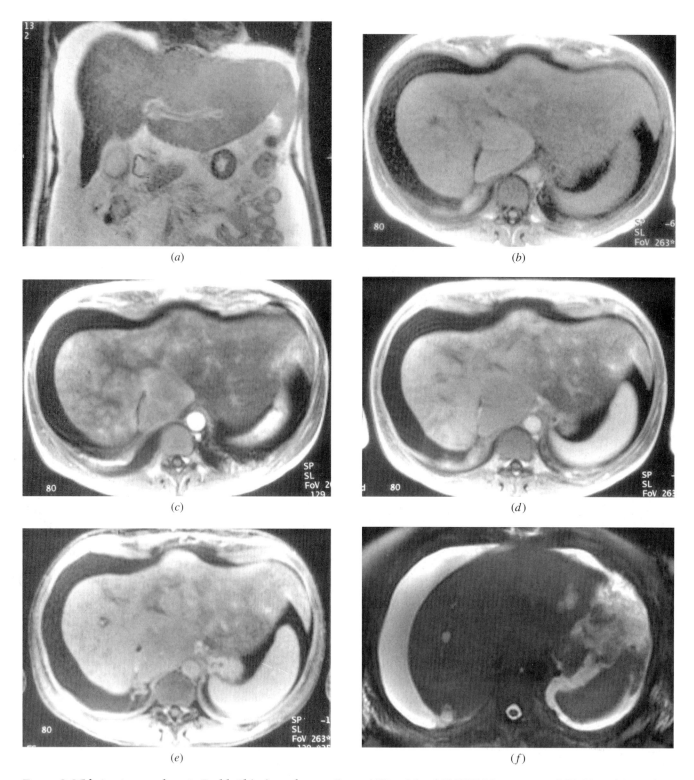

FIG. 2.254 Acute on subacute Budd–Chiari syndrome. Coronal T2-weighted SS-ETSE (*a*), transverse SGE (*b*), and immediate (*c*), 45-s (*d*), and 90-s fat-suppressed (*e*) postgadolinium SGE images. The coronal T2-weighted image (*a*) shows high signal of the lateral segment relative to the right lobe. On the T1-weighted image (*b*), moderately diminished signal is identified in the enlarged lateral segment of the left lobe, with mild diminished signal of the right lobe. The enlarged caudate lobe possesses more normal signal intensity. The immediate postgadolinium image (*c*) reveals markedly diminished enhancement of the lateral segment, consistent with acute changes of Budd–Chiari, and mildly heterogeneous and increase signal of the right lobe, consistent with subacute changes of Budd–Chiari. The caudate lobe has a mild heterogeneity with signal intensity intermediate between the acutely affected lateral segment and subacutely affected right lobe. Enhancement abnormalities diminish but persist on late postcontrast images (*e*).

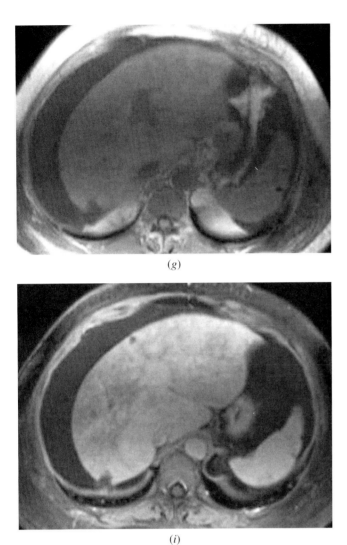
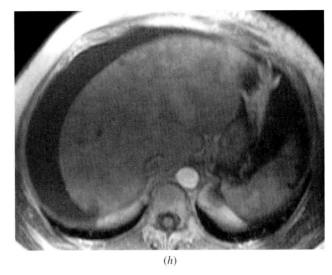

(g)

(h)

(i)

F I G. 2.254 (*Continued*) T2-weighted fat-suppressed SS-ETSE (*f*), SGE (*g*), and immediate (*h*) and 90-s fat-suppressed (*i*) postgadolinium SGE images in a second patient. T2-weighted (*f*) and T1-weighted (*g*) images of the liver demonstrate homogeneous signal intensity. On early-phase images (*h*), a patchy, diffuse faint liver enhancement is appreciated with no dominant segment. However, on late-phase image (*i*) the central portion of the liver becomes homogeneously enhanced while the periphery of the liver maintains the heterogeneous enhancement with a lower signal intensity than central liver.

interstitial-phase fat-suppressed images. Extensive portosystemic varices, as observed in other chronic liver diseases, are also present.

The development of nodular regenerative hyperplasia in the chronic setting is the result of hepatic ischemia caused by hepatic venous obstruction [404, 405]. The nodules are usually round, multiple, range from 0.5 to 4 cm, and cause distortion of the hepatic contour [406–408]. Most commonly, these nodules demonstrate isointensity or low signal intensity on T2-weighted images, and high signal intensity on T1-weighted images similar to macroregenerative nodules (see fig. 2.256). However, these nodules may be moderately hypervascular and tend to possess moderately intense enhancement on immediate postgadolinium gradient-echo images [343, 406, 407, 409]. The high signal intensity of the nodules on the precontrast T1-weighted images likely reflects the presence of protein.

Occasionally, large (>1 cm) regenerative nodules contain a central scar, resembling FNH. It has been postulated that the increased arterial hepatic perfusion in Budd–Chiari syndrome may be responsible for the development of this FNH-like lesion. The scar is characterized by high signal intensity on T2-weighted images, low signal intensity on T1-weighted images, and enhancement on late-phase images, as is typical for FNH [408, 410].

The relationship between Budd–Chiari syndrome and HCC is still controversial. Patients with the diagnosis of HCC may develop acute or subacute Budd–Chiari syndrome because of tumor invasion of major hepatic veins. The involvement of major hepatic veins by HCC has been reported in 6–23% of cases [411]. Few studies suggest that patients with chronic Budd–Chiari syndrome are at increased risk for the development of HCC [343], and there is little evidence to support

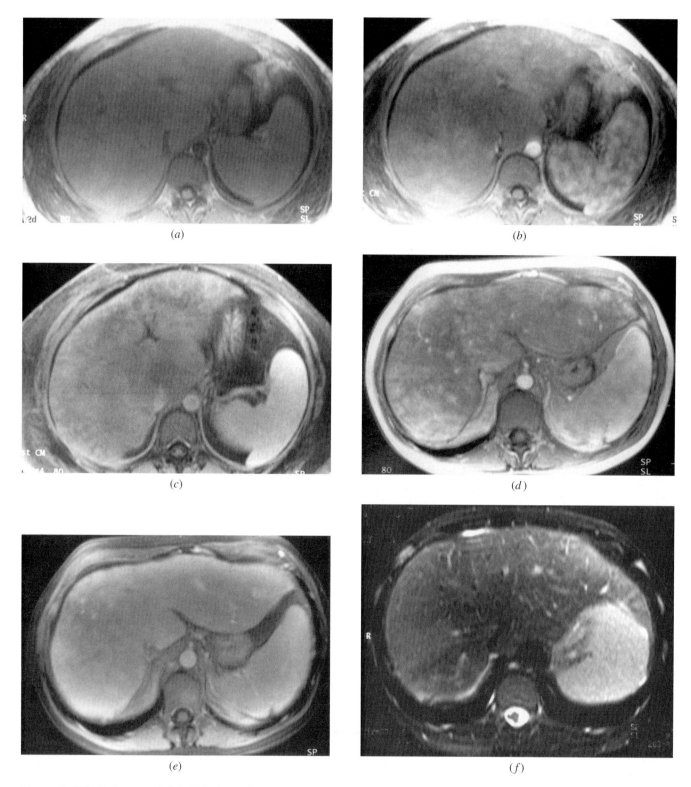

(a)

(b)

(c)

(d)

(e)

(f)

F IG . 2.255 Subacute Budd–Chiari syndrome. SGE (*a*) and immediate (*b*) and 90-s fat-suppressed (*c*) postgadolinium SGE images. Peripheral liver is diminished in signal on T1-weighted image (*a*) and demonstrates a diffuse, heterogeneous mildly increased enhancement on early-phase image (*b*) that persists on later image (*c*), consistent with hepatic vascular compensation to venous thrombosis as observed in subacute Budd–Chiari syndrome (Reproduced with permission from Noone TC, Semelka RC, Siegelman ES, Balci NC, Hussain SM, Kim PN, Mitchell DG. Budd-Chiari Syndrome: spectrum of appearances of acute, subacute, and chronic disease with magnetic resonance imaging. *J Magn Reson Imaging* 11: 44–50, 2000).

Immediate (*d*) and 90-s fat-suppressed (*e*) postgadolinium SGE images in a second patient. The liver is enlarged with an irregular contour. There is mild hypertrophy of the caudate lobe. After administration of contrast (*d*), the liver enhances in a diffusely heterogeneous pattern and becomes more homogeneous on the later image (*e*).

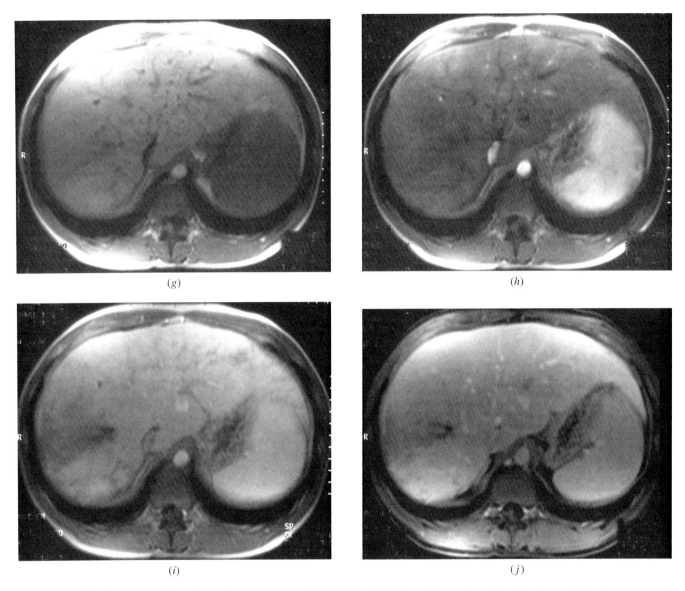

FIG. 2.255 (*Continued*) T2-weighted fat-suppressed SS-ETSE (*f*), SGE (*g*), and immediate (*h*), 45-s (*i*), and 90-s fat-suppressed (*j*) postgadolinium SGE images in a third patient. The liver is enlarged and shows mild hypertrophy of the caudate lobe. On T2-weighted image (*f*), a triangular shaped segmental area is seen in the right hepatic lobe that shows a higher signal intensity than the remainder of the hepatic parenchyma. On T1-weighted image (*g*), this segmental area demonstrates low signal intensity. On early-phase image (*h*), the liver exhibits a dominant peripheral patchy enhancement that becomes homogeneous on late-phase image (*j*). Note that the segmental area observed on precontrast images (*f*, *g*) shows faint enhancement on early-phase images (*h*) that washes out on 45-s (*i*) and late-phase (*j*) images, consistent with ischemic changes.

malignant transformation of the regenerative nodules [406, 407].

Hepatic Vein Thrombosis

Hepatic vein thrombosis affecting minor vessels may occur in the setting of malignant disease and is especially common in HCC. Tumor thrombosis demonstrates gadolinium enhancement, whereas bland thrombus does not enhance. As with the Budd–Chiari syndrome, the degree of enhancement of liver parenchyma that has thrombosed hepatic veins depends on the stage of the thrombosis. In acute thrombosis, involved parenchyma enhances less than surrounding liver in early-phase images [396]. In chronic thrombosis, enhancement is more variable and may be increased.

Hepatic Arterial Obstruction

Hepatic arterial obstruction is much less common than either portal vein or hepatic vein obstruction. Hepatic arterial obstruction is most commonly seen in the setting of liver transplantation. In patients without transplants,

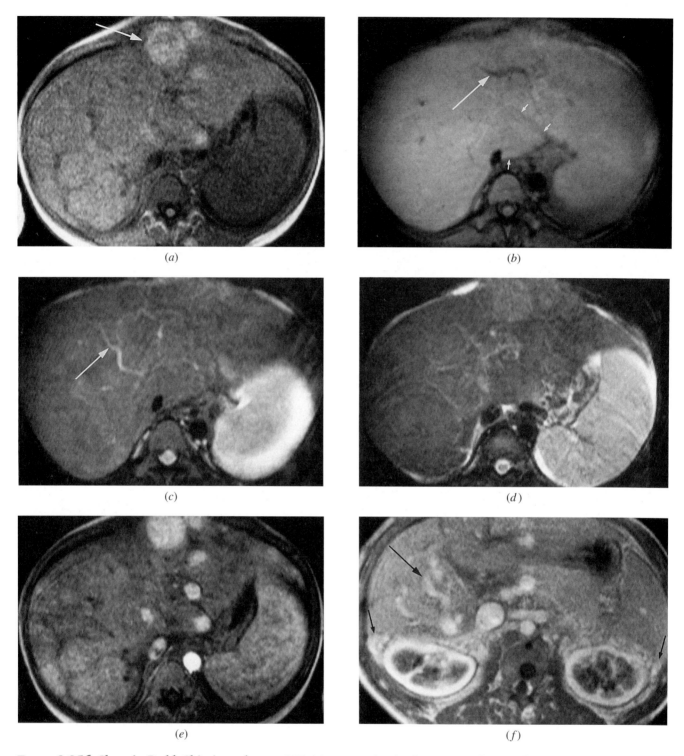

(a)   *(b)*

(c)   *(d)*

(e)   *(f)*

F I G . 2.256 Chronic Budd–Chiari syndrome. SGE (*a*), proton-density fat-suppressed spin-echo (*b*), T2-weighted fat-suppressed ETSE (*c, d*), and immediate postgadolinium SGE (*e*) images. On T1-weighted images (*a*), multiple well-defined high-signal-intensity mass lesions representing regenerative nodules are identified, the largest measuring 3.5 cm in diameter (arrow, *a*). The proton-density image at the expected level of the hepatic veins (*b*) demonstrates absence of hepatic veins, with intrahepatic curvilinear venous collaterals in their stead (arrow, *b*). Enlargement of the caudate lobe is shown (small arrows, *b*). The T2-weighted image (*c*) taken from a slightly higher tomographic section demonstrates curvilinear intrahepatic collaterals (arrow, *c*) with absence of hepatic veins. The immediate postgadolinium image (*e*) acquired at the same tomographic level as the precontrast images (*a, d*) shows enhancement of the regenerative nodules, with multiple enhancing nodules apparent that were not visualized on precontrast images. Slight heterogeneity of hepatic enhancement is present. The enhancement pattern is distinctly different from that of acute Budd–Chiari syndrome.

Immediate postgadolinium SGE image (*f*) in a second patient with chronic Budd–Chiari syndrome. Extensive abdominal collaterals are present (arrows, *f*), including curvilinear intrahepatic collaterals (long arrow, *f*).

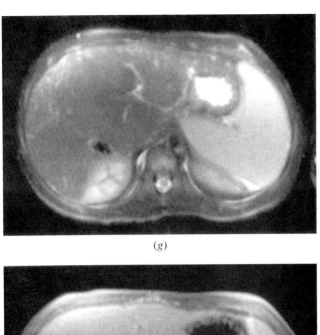

(g)

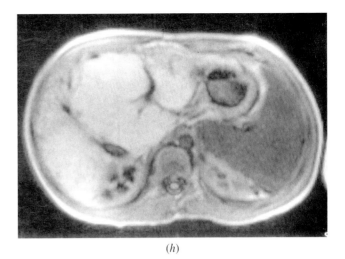

(h)

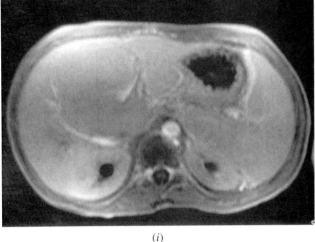

(i)

FIG. 2.256 (*Continued*) T2-weighted fat-suppressed SS-ETSE (*g*), magnetization-prepared gradient-echo (*h*), and immediate postgadolinium magnetization-prepared gradient-echo (*i*) images in an 8-year-old boy. Massive enlargement of the caudate lobe is present, with relative atrophy and peripheral nodularity of the peripheral liver consistent with chronic Budd–Chiari syndrome.

embolic occlusion is the most common cause of hepatic arterial compromise. Diminished enhancement of involved hepatic parenchyma is apparent on early post-contrast images (fig. 2.257). Hepatic arterial occlusion tends to be small, irregularly shaped, and not segmental in appearance. Larger occlusions result in peripheral wedge- or fan-shaped defects with an unusual serrated margin. An unusual feature is that T2- signal may be low, reflecting a lower fluid content.

Preeclampsia and Eclampsia

Hepatic disease is common in preeclampsia and may result in hemolytic anemia, elevated liver function tests, and low platelets (HELLP syndrome), which may cause peripheral vascular occlusions of the liver or hepatic hematoma [412]. Microscopically, sinusoids contain fibrin deposits with hemorrhage into the subendothelial space. Blood may dissect through portal connective tissue to form lakes of hemorrhage. MR images show

peripheral wedge-shaped defects surrounded by regions of increased enhancement on postgadolinium images and heterogeneous high signal intensity on T2-weighted images from edema and, in more severe disease, infarction (figs. 2.258 and 2.259). This pattern reflects central infarction surrounded by a penumbra of ischemic hepatic parenchyma. Hematoma appears as a peripheral fluid collection with signal intensity depending on the age of the blood products, usually deoxyhemoglobin or intracellular methemoglobin reflecting the acute or subacute nature of the disease process.

Congestive Heart Failure

Patients with congestive heart failure may present with hepatomegaly and hepatic enzyme elevations. On early dynamic contrast-enhanced MR images, the liver may enhance in a mosaic fashion with a reticulated pattern of low-signal-intensity linear markings. By 1 min post-contrast, the liver becomes more homogeneous. The

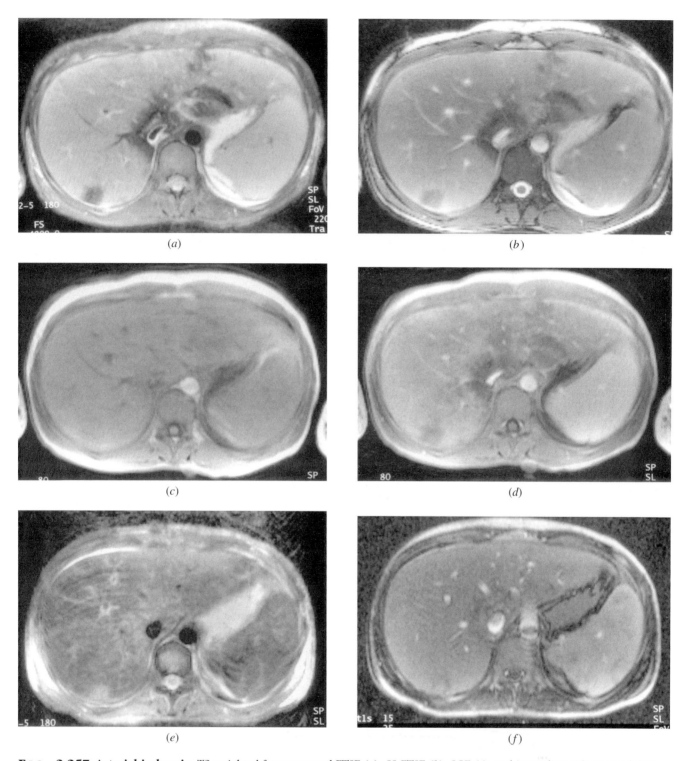

(a)

(b)

(c)

(d)

(e)

(f)

FIG. 2.257 Arterial ischemia. T2-weighted fat-suppressed ETSE (*a*), SS ETSE (*b*), SGE (*c*), and immediate (*d*) postgadolinium SGE images. The liver is enlarged with diffuse increased signal intensity on T2-weighted images (*a*), consistent with edema. There is a 2-cm focus in the right hepatic lobe and a irregular hepatic central region that demonstrate decreased signal intensity on both T2-weighted (*a*) and T1-weighted (*b*) images, most pronounced on T2, and negligible enhancement on early (*d*) postgadolinium images. These features are consistent with arterial ischemia.

T2-weighted fat-suppressed ETSE (*e*) and immediate postgadolinium magnetization-prepared gradient-echo (*f*) images in the same patient 15 days later show a slight increased signal intensity involving the focus in the right lobe and central liver on the T2-weighted image associated with diffuse low signal of the liver secondary to intervening blood transfusion. Note that the previously ischemic areas in the right lobe and central liver demonstrate enhancement on early-phase images (*f*). These findings are consistent with improved perfusion of ischemic regions, which matched the clinical picture.

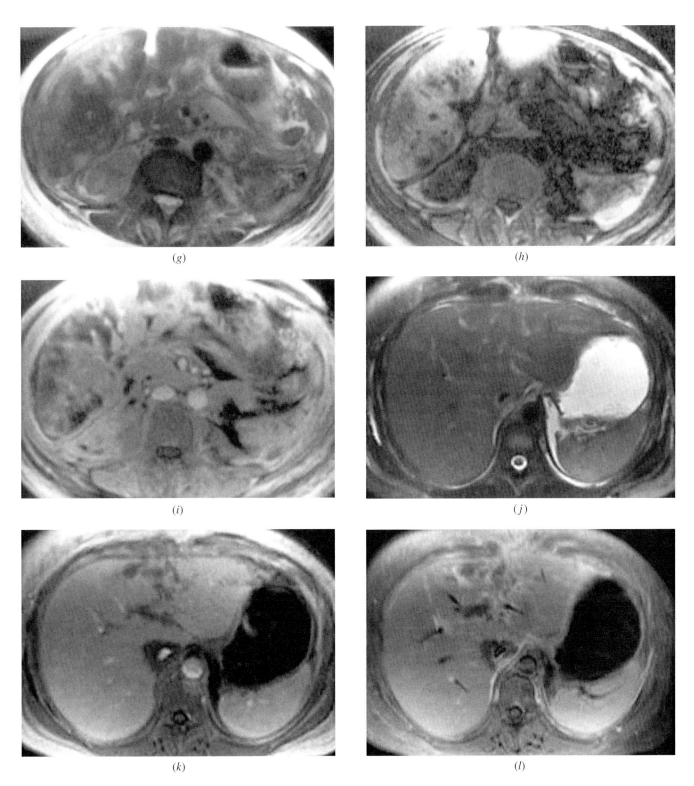

(g)

(h)

(i)

(j)

(k)

(l)

F I G . 2.257 (*Continued*) T2-weighted fat-suppressed SS-ETSE (*g*), SGE (*h*), and 90-s fat-suppressed postgadolinium SGE (*i*) images in a second patient demonstrate irregular peripheral regions in the right lobe inferiorly that are high signal on T2 (*g*) and low signal on T1 (*h*) and show negligible enhancement on late images (*i*), consistent with ischemic or infarcted regions caused by small branch arterial occlusion.

T2-weighted SS-ETSE (*j*) and 45-s (*k*) and 90-s fat-suppressed (*l*) postgadolinium SGE images in a third patient who is status post transplant. Irregular linear areas in the left hepatic lobe are present on early-phase images (*k*) that show peripheral enhancement on late-phase images (*l*) consistent with late enhancement of the ischemic rim. Air is present within bile ducts because of the presence of a biliary stent. Note the presence of air within vessels on the late-phase image (*l*).

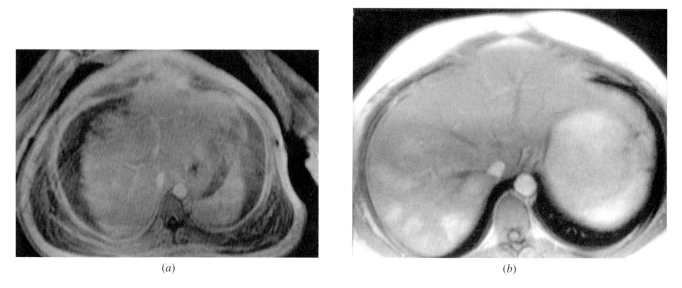

(a)   *(b)*

FIG. 2.258 HELLP syndrome. Transverse 45-s postgadolinium SGE image (*a*) demonstrates an abnormal serrated margin of the liver and massive ascites. Liver changes reflect ischemic injury.

Immediate postgadolinium image (*b*) in a second patient with HELLP syndrome shows an early patchy enhancement of the liver.

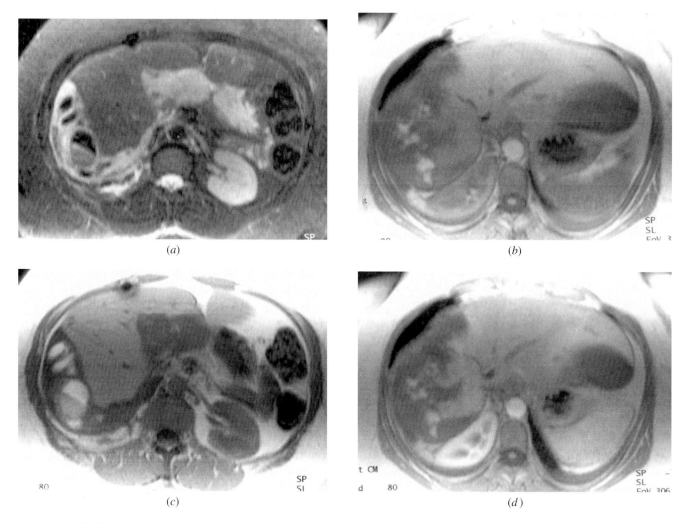

(a)   *(b)*

(c)   *(d)*

FIG. 2.259 Spontaneous intrahepatic hemorrhage. Echo train-STIR (*a*), SGE (*b, c*), immediate postgadolinium SGE (*d, e*),

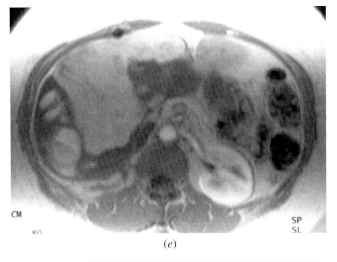

(e)

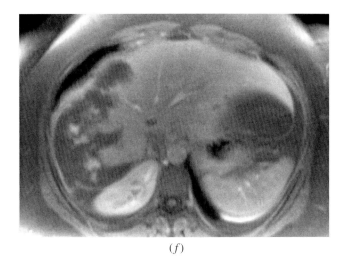

(f)

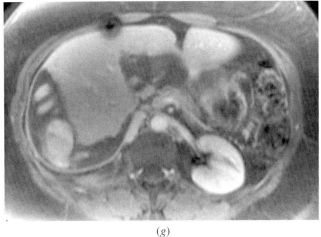

(g)

F I G . 2.259 (*Continued*) and 90-s postgadolinium fat-suppressed SGE (*f, g*) images in a 34-yr-old woman who has a history of spontaneous intrahepatic hematoma. There is a large complex subcapsular collection that demonstrates mixed signal intensity consistent with blood of different ages. Spontaneous intrahepatic hematoma occurs most commonly in patients who are on anticoagulant therapy. Hepatic adenomas are the most common cause in women of child-bearing age who are not on anticoagulation therapy and are taking birth control pills. Note the jagged peripheral margin of the liver (*b, d, f*), which is an appearance also observed in spontaneous hepatic hemorrhage in the HELLP syndrome.

suprahepatic IVC is frequently enlarged with enlargement of the hepatic veins. Contrast injected in a brachial vein may appear earlier in the hepatic veins and suprahepatic IVC than in the portal veins and infrahepatic IVC, reflecting reflux of contrast from the heart (fig. 2.260).

Portal Venous Air

Portal venous air, a serious condition associated with bowel ischemia, appears as signal-void foci within distal branches of the portal vein in the nondependent portion of the liver (typically the left lobe) on all imaging sequences. Magnetic susceptibility artifact may also be identified. Air is best demonstrated with a combination of high-resolution T2-weighted echo-train spin-echo and postgadolinium T1-weighted images in which air will be signal void on both sets of images. The air is most clearly shown on the postcontrast T1-weighted images (fig. 2.261). The T2-weighted images confirm the fact that the tubular structures that are dark on T1-

weighted images are also dark on T2, reflecting signal-void air rather than high-signal fluid.

Air in the Biliary Tree

Air in the biliary tree is usually a relatively benign condition. Air in the biliary tree is less peripheral than air in the portal veins, and is more clearly observed as branching tubular structures conforming to the biliary tree. Air is most commonly observed in the left biliary ducts, reflecting the patient's supine position in the bore of the magnet. Air in the biliary tree is signal void on all MR sequences (fig. 2.262).

Diffuse Hyperperfusion Abnormality

This is a new term that reflects a descriptive, vascular dynamic process that affects the hepatic parenchyma. This entity is characterized by large regions of transient increased enhancement in the liver parenchyma in the hepatic arterial dominant phase that fades to isointensity

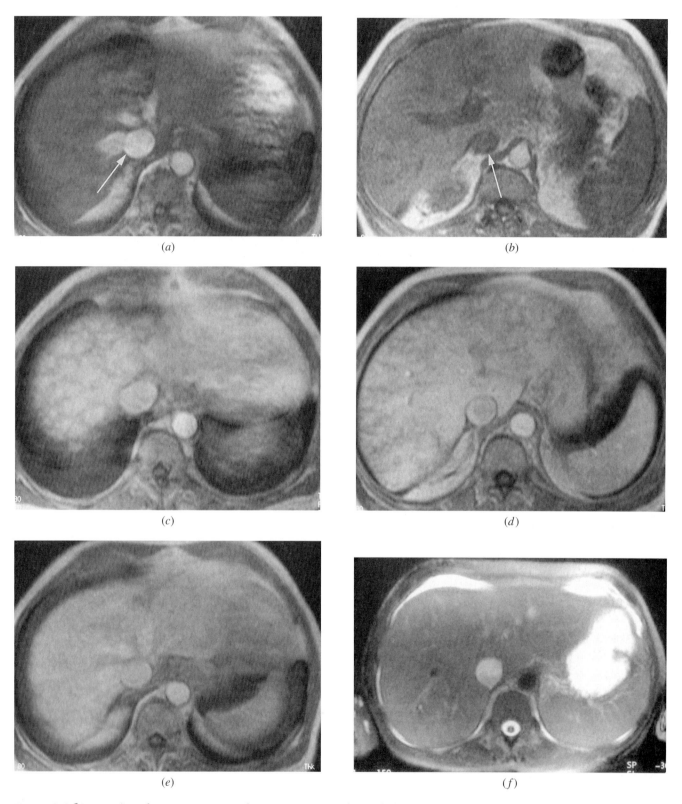

(a)

(b)

(c)

(d)

(e)

(f)

F I G . 2.260 Mosaic enhancement secondary to congestive heart failure. Immediate (*a, b*), 45-s postgadolinium (*c, d*), and 90-s postgadolinium SGE (*e*) images. The immediate postgadolinium images (*a, b*) demonstrate the presence of gadolinium in the superior IVC early in the arterial phase of enhancement with no enhancement of the abdominal organs, because of the low cardiac output state of the patient. Reflux of gadolinium into the dilated suprahepatic IVC and hepatic veins is present (arrow, *a*), with no contrast present in the infrahepatic IVC (arrow, *b*). On the 45-s postgadolinium images (*c, d*), a mosaic enhancement pattern is present throughout the liver, reflecting hepatic congestion. This mosaic enhancement resolves on the 90-s postgadolinium image (*e*).

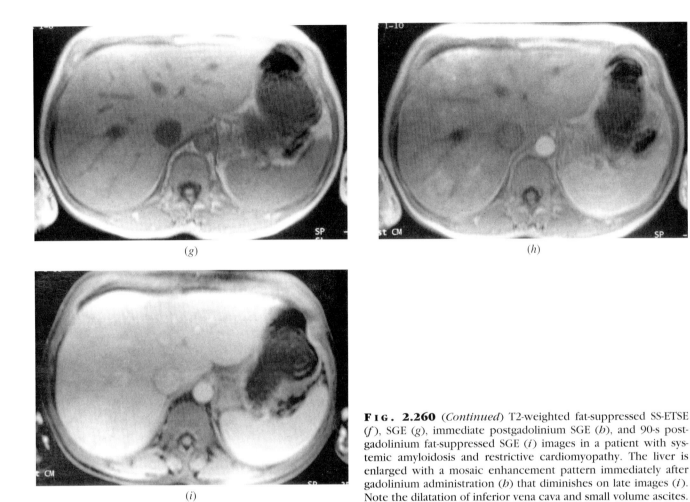

(g)

(h)

(i)

FIG. 2.260 (*Continued*) T2-weighted fat-suppressed SS-ETSE (*f*), SGE (*g*), immediate postgadolinium SGE (*h*), and 90-s postgadolinium fat-suppressed SGE (*i*) images in a patient with systemic amyloidosis and restrictive cardiomyopathy. The liver is enlarged with a mosaic enhancement pattern immediately after gadolinium administration (*h*) that diminishes on late images (*i*). Note the dilatation of inferior vena cava and small volume ascites.

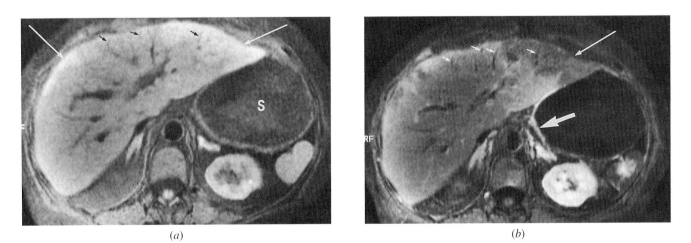

(a)

(b)

FIG. 2.261 Portal venous air. T1-weighted fat-suppressed SE (*a*) and 90-s postgadolinium fat-suppressed SE (*b*) images. On the precontrast T1-weighted fat-suppressed image (*a*), subtle, linear, signal-void, short, vertically oriented markings are present (small arrows, *a*). Regions of peripheral hepatic high signal intensity are present, reflecting hemorrhage (long arrows, *a*). The stomach (S) is dilated. On the gadolinium-enhanced T1-weighted fat-suppressed spin-echo image (*b*), the vertically oriented peripheral collections of portal venous air are more clearly defined (small arrows, *b*). Regions that were hyperintense on the precontrast image are shown to have diminished enhancement (long arrow, *b*). The dilated stomach shows increased mural enhancement (large arrow, *b*) consistent with ischemic changes. Portal venous air is signal void and poorly seen on T2-weighted images (not shown); fluid would be high in signal intensity and well shown on T2-weighted images.

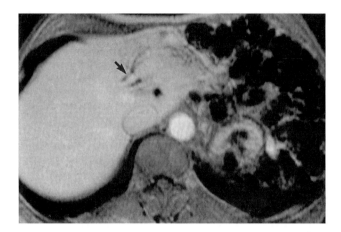

FIG. 2.262 Biliary tree air. Transverse 90-s postgadolinium SGE image in a patient with a choledochojejunostomy shows signal-void, tubular structures with an arborized pattern (arrow). This biliary tree air is more central in location than the portal venous air. The T2-weighted image (not shown) demonstrates signal-void, poorly shown bile ducts consistent with air-containing rather than fluid-containing ducts.

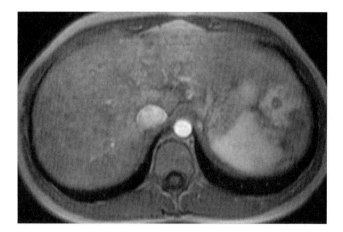

FIG. 2.263 Diffuse hyperperfusion abnormality. Immediate post-gadolinium 3D-gradient echo images demostrates diffuse heterogeneous increased enhancement, that rapidly fades to homogeneous signal on the early hepatic venous phase images (not shown). This appearance is most commonly seen in patients with acute on chronic hepatitis, but may result from a number of conditions. If no underlying explanation is present, then this enhancement is attributed to regional variations in the realtive contributions of hepatic arterial and portal venous supply to the liver. This circumstance may be incidental and not of clinical significance, and it may also be seen in combination with early homogeneous enhacement of the spleen.

rapidly, by the early hepatic venous phase. There are generally no associated signal intensity changes on noncontrast T1- or T2-weighted images. When findings of increased fluid content are apparent on noncontrast T1- or T2-weighted images (i.e., mild low signal on T1, mild high signal on T2) it implies that there is likely associated hepatocellular injury or edema. In its simplest form, diffuse hyperperfusion abnormality represents an imbalance between the normal vascular delivery patterns of blood flow to the liver by hepatic arteries and portal veins, where there is increased hepatic arterial supply. Perhaps the most common entity to result in this vascular phenomenon is acute on chronic hepatitis. A variety of processes, however, can result in this appearance. In patients with no apparent underlying hepatic disease or systemic process, it may reflect anomalous increased hepatic arterial supply (fig. 2.263). A variety of disease entities in addition to acute on chronic hepatitis (fig. 2.264) that can result in this feature are acute hepatitis, generalized systemic disease with generalized vascular effects, ascending cholangitis, drug toxicity, and acute liver transplant rejection, to name some of the more common. As mentioned above, as the disease process affecting the liver becomes more severe, signal intensity changes on T1- and T2-weighted images, and later postgadolinium images may become apparent (fig. 2.246).

Focal Hyperperfusion Abnormality

Focal hyperperfusion abnormalities (FHA) are small regions of transient increased enhancement on hepatic arterial dominant-phase images. These are generally not visible on noncontrast T1- and T2-weighted images. This entity is a new nomenclature for findings that have been previously termed transient hepatic arterial defects (THAD) or transient hepatic signal intensity differences (THID). Frequently these lesions correspond to vascular phenomenon such as arteriovenous shunting but likely can also result from a number of other vascular or inflammatory processes. The morphology of focal hyperperfusion abnormalities frequently allows differentiation from other entities such as dysplastic nodules. Nodules should have a round morphology, whereas FHA frequently appears more oblong or lozenge-shaped, with the more linear configuration rendering this entity more easy to correctly characterize (fig. 2.264).

Inflammatory Parenchymal Disease

Sarcoidosis

Sarcoidosis, a systemic inflammatory granulomatous disease of unknown etiology, is one of the most common causes of hepatic noncaseating granulomas. The liver follows lymph nodes and lung in the frequency of involvement, and the liver is involved histologically in 60–90% of patients [415]. The majority of patients show minimal evidence of clinical or biochemical hepatic

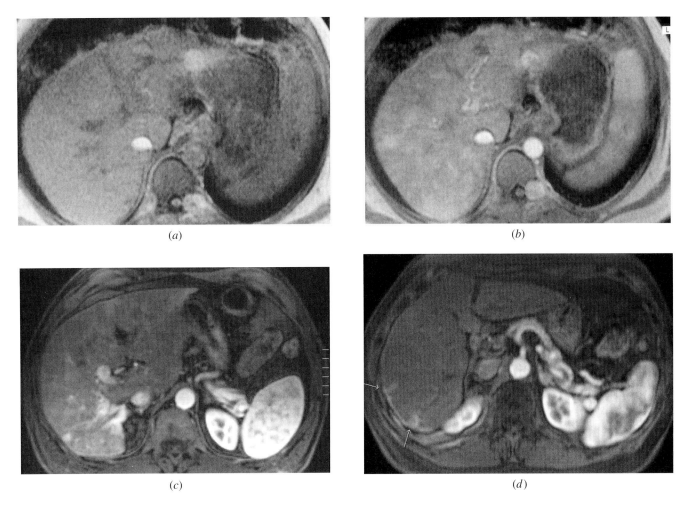

(*a*)   (*b*)

(*c*)   (*d*)

F I G . 2.264 Diffuse Hyperperfusion and Focal Hyperperfusion Abnormalities in the Cirrhotic Liver. SGE (*a*), immediate post-gadolinium SGE (*b*) in 1 patient, and immediate post-gadolinium 3D-gradient echo (*c, d*) images in two other patients with cirrhosis. Diffuse hyperperfusion abnormality may occur secondary to a number of vascular phenomena, but in the cirrhotic liver the most common cause is acute on chronic hepatitis. Note the patchy appearance of increased enhancement throughout the hepatic parenchyma, that is generally apparent only on immediate post-gadolinium images and may not be visible on precontrast or later postcontrast images. In two other patients, small, oval shaped foci of increased enhancement are appreciated on immediate post-gadolinium images (*c, d*, arrows on *d*), which were only apparent on immediate postcontrast images. These represent focal hyperperfusion abnormalities. This entity is also not uncommon in the cirrhotic liver, and the most common underlying mechanism is small intrahepatic arteriovenous shunts. Focal hyperperfusion abnormalities must be distinguished from hepatic nodules, and their non-spherical shape (often lozenge-shaped) and often ill-defined margins usually define their vascular nature.

dysfunction. Granulomas are characterized pathologically by compact aggregates of plump epithelioid cells, sometimes with multinucleated giant cells, surrounded by a cuff of lymphocytes and macrophages. Focal involvement of the liver and spleen in sarcoidosis with noncaseating granulomas is well demonstrated on MR images. Sarcoid granulomas are small (approximately 1 cm in diameter), rounded lesions low in signal intensity on T2- and T1-weighted images that enhance in a diminished, delayed fashion on gadolinium-enhanced gradient-echo images (fig. 2.265) [416, 417]. The diminished enhancement reflects the hypovascular nature of the granuloma. Occasionally, the spleen may be lower in signal intensity than liver on T2-weighted images [416]. Concomitant retroperitoneal lymph nodes are

often present, exhibiting a distinctive, feathery, moderately high signal on T2-weighted images.

Inflammatory Myofibroblastic Tumor (Inflammatory Pseudotumor)

Inflammatory myofibroblastic tumor, formerly termed inflammatory pseudotumor, is an uncommon lesion that rarely presents in the liver [418]. Pathologic macroscopic evaluation may disclose a tumorlike, firm mass within the liver parenchyma or a soft tissue mass encasing the hilar area. Microscopic inspection shows a mixed inflammatory infiltrate consisting of plasma cells, macrophages, chronic inflammatory cells, and histiocytes. Special studies show polyclonality of the inflammatory infiltrate, pointing to the benign nature of the lesion

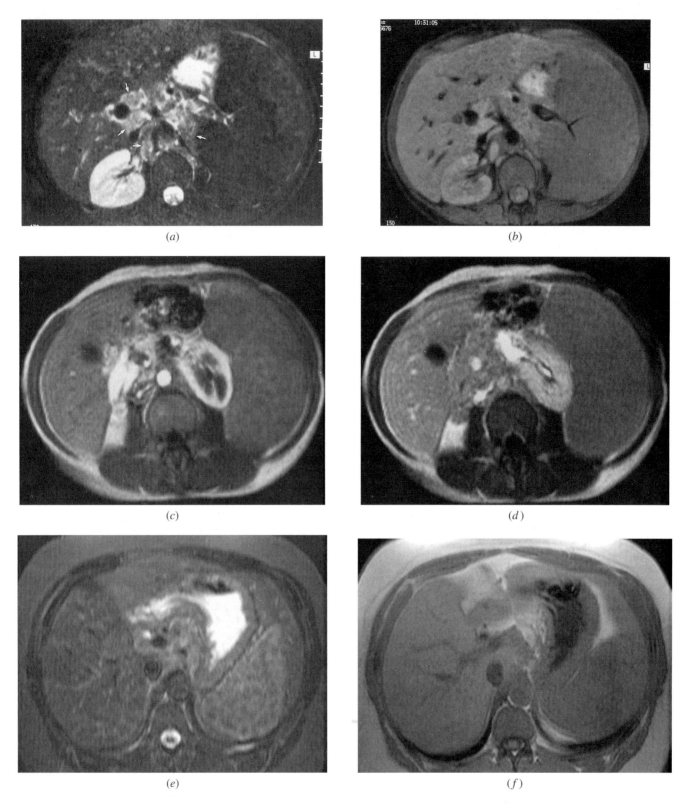

(a)

(b)

(c)

(d)

(e)

(f)

F I G . 2.265 Hepatosplenic sarcoidosis. T2-weighted fat-suppressed SE (*a*), T1-weighted fat-suppressed SE (*b*), and immediate (*c*) and 5-min (*d*) postgadolinium SGE images. The spleen is massively enlarged and contains multiple <1-cm nodules that are moderately low signal intensity on T2-weighted (*a*) and T1-weighted (*b*) images and demonstrate negligible enhancement on early-phase images (*c*) with gradual enhancement over time (*d*). Extensive retroperitoneal, celiac, and periportal lymphadenopathy is also present (*a*, *b*), which has a speckled appearance on the T2-weighted image (arrows, *a*). A speckled signal on T2 has been described for lymph nodes affected by sarcoidosis.

T2-weighted fat-suppressed SS-ETSE (*e*), SGE (*f*), and immediate (*g*) and 90-s fat-suppressed (*h*) postgadolinium SGE images in a second patient with sarcoidosis. The liver shows a patchy enhancement on early-phase image (*g*) that equilibrates on late-phase

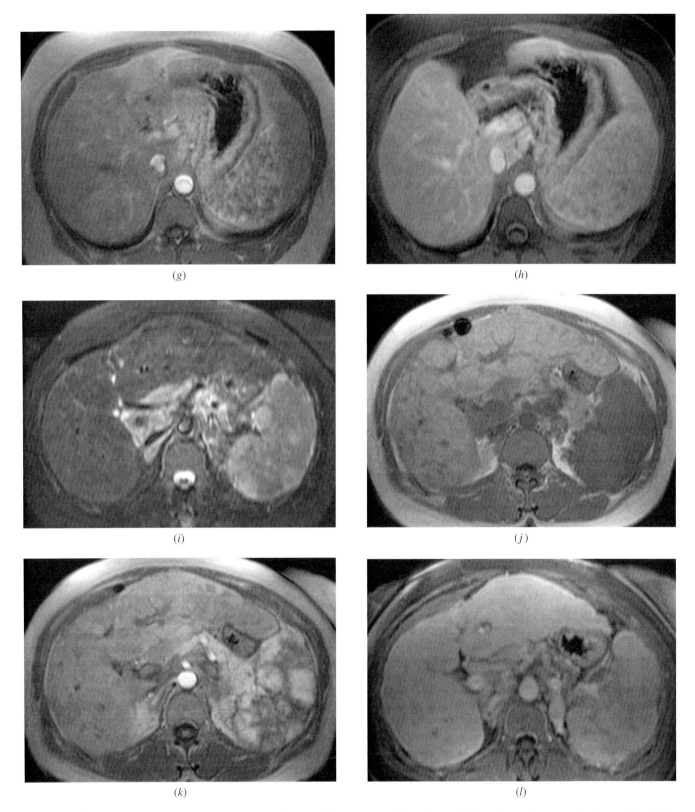

(g)

(h)

(i)

(j)

(k)

(l)

F I G . 2.265 (*Continued*) image (*h*), rendering the liver homogeneously enhanced. The spleen shows multiple small nodules that demonstrate low signal intensity on both T2-weighted (*e*) and T1-weighted (*f*) images, negligible enhancement on early-phase image (*g*), and progressive enhancement on late-phase image (*h*).

T2-weighted fat-suppressed SS-ETSE (*i*), SGE (*j*), and immediate (*k*) and 90-s fat-suppressed (*l*) postgadolinium SGE images in a third patient with sarcoidosis. Multiple nodules are seen in both liver and spleen. The liver nodules appear isointense on T2-weighted (*i*) and T1-weighted (*j*) images and enhance in a fashion similar to background parenchyma. Note that the hepatic architecture is distorted because of the nodules. The spleen nodules are high signal intensity on T2-weighted image (*i*), isointense on T1-weighted image (*j*), and intensely enhanced on early-phase image (*k*), fading on late-phase image (*l*). Lymphadenopathy is best seen on T2-weighted fat-suppressed image (*i*).

[419]. Prominent fibrosis is a characteristic feature. Areas of necrosis and obliteration of blood vessels may occasionally be noted.

Inflammatory myofibroblastic tumor may be associated with systemic symptoms, including fever, weight loss, malaise, and right upper quadrant pain [420]. Although the disease often responds to steroid administration and the prognosis is usually good, fatal outcome has been reported [421]. Inflammatory myofibroblastic tumors are not malignant neoplasms; however, if they occur at the hilum, effects of the lesion can be devastating. Hilar myofibroblastic tumor may encase the portal vein, hepatic artery, and bile duct [418]. Inflammatory infiltrate in the walls and lumen of the portal vein may cause an occlusive phlebitis that extends beyond margins of tumor [418].

On imaging, hepatic myofibroblastic tumor can present as an ill-defined, tumorlike lesion within the parenchyma or as a periportal soft tissue mass involving the hilum [422]. In the former pattern, lesions are usually solitary, but in 20% of cases they are multiple. Masses range from 1 to 20 cm but are generally less than 2 cm in diameter [420].

MRI features of inflammatory myofibroblastic tumor may vary according to the presence of necrosis and fibrosis within the lesion. Tumorlike lesions may demonstrate mild high signal on T2-weighted images, low signal or isointensity on T1-weighted images, and a moderate or intense enhancement on early-phase images that fades away on late-phase images. Soft tissue infiltration along the periportal region may possess MRI features similar to the tumorlike pattern on T2- and T1-weighted precontrast images but tends to demonstrate a lesser degree of enhancement on early-phase images, namely. mild or negligible enhancement (fig. 2.266) [422, 423]. The lesions may regress after treatment or spontaneously and then appear as areas of fibrosis, which in the chronic setting are mildly low signal on T2- and T1-weighted images and exhibit negligible enhancement. Similar to other causes of scarring, the margins of chronic inflammatory myofibroblastic tumors are irregular and angular [422].

Because inflammatory myofibroblastic tumor is a rare entity, lesions are often mistaken for hepatic malignancy. When a mass or tumorlike pattern is present, HCC and abscess should be considered in the differential diagnosis. In addition, the soft tissue infiltration pattern requires distinction from lymphoma and cholangiocarcinoma (see fig. 2.266) [422]. Final diagnosis is based on histologic analysis.

Infectious Parenchymal Disease

Abscesses

Pyogenic Abscess. Pyogenic abscesses are the most frequent form of focal hepatic infections resulting from an infectious process of bacterial origin. Pathologically, pyogenic liver abscesses may occur as solitary or multiple lesions ranging from millimeters to massive lesions. Microscopically, in early stages, lesions are ill defined with intense acute inflammation, purulent debris, and devastation of hepatic parenchyma and stroma. In later stages, the abscesses become circumscribed, surrounded by a shell of granulation tissue consisting of abundant, newly formed blood vessels, fibroblasts, and chronic inflammation. End stages show complete fibrous encapsulation.

Infectious agents reach the liver through hepatic artery, portal vein, biliary tract, and direct extension from contiguous organs [424]. Abscesses may occur in the context of recent surgery, Crohn disease, appendicitis, diverticulitis, and blunt or penetrating injuries [424, 425]. Portal vein thrombosis is frequently associated with bacterial abscesses. The infected bland thrombus is characterized by low signal intensity on T2- and T1-weighted images and time of flight gradient-echo images. The thrombus does not enhance after contrast; however, the vein wall shows a moderate/intense enhancement after contrast administration, best seen on late-phase fat-suppressed images caused by the inflammatory reaction (fig. 2.267).

Characteristic MRI findings of pyogenic abscesses are high signal intensity on T2-weighted images and low signal intensity on T1-weighted images and show moderate enhancement of stroma on immediate postgadolinium images with persistent enhancement on interstitial phase images and no enhancement of additional stroma or progressive fill in of the lesion over time [426]. Pyogenic abscesses also possess markedly thick walls and internal septations, which enhance moderately to intensely on early-phase images and demonstrate persistent enhancement on late-phase images that often appears more intensely enhanced (figs. 2.268–2.270) [424, 427]. Abscesses typically have a moderate perilesional enhancement with indistinct outer margins on immediate postgadolinium images because of a surrounding rim of granulation tissues and a hyperemic inflammatory response in adjacent liver (figs. 2.271 and 2.272) [426]. The perilesional enhancement rapidly diminishes, and is often nearly resolved by 1 min after injection. Layering of debris and gas within the abscess cavity, mainly after biliary drainage, is also commonly appreciated. Gas is identified as signal void on both T2- and T1-weighted images and debris as a low signal on T2- and high signal on T1-weighted images, since debris is usually composed of protein [426, 428].

The higher sensitivity of MRI to gadolinium chelates than of CT imaging to iodinated agents renders dynamic gadolinium-enhanced MRI a useful technique for patients in whom a distinction between simple cysts and multiple abscesses cannot be made on the basis of

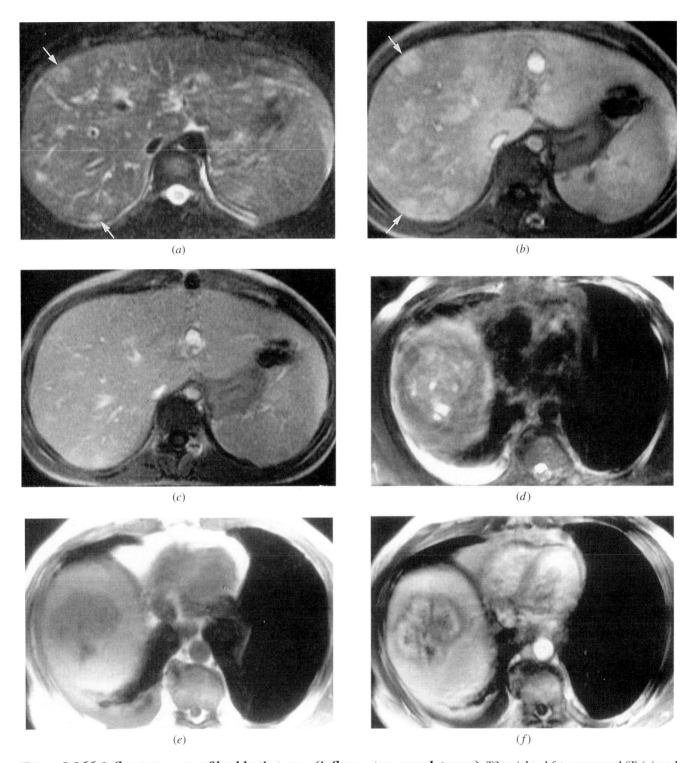

F I G . 2.266 Inflammatory myofibroblastic tumor (inflammatory pseudotumor). T2-weighted fat-suppressed SE (*a*) and immediate (*b*) and 90-s (*c*) postgadolinium SGE images. No definite lesions are apparent on the precontrast T1-weighted image (not shown). Occasional, mildly hyperintense ill-defined lesions are present on the T2-weighted image (arrows, *a*). Multiple small, irregular enhancing foci are demonstrated throughout the liver on early-phase image (arrows, *b*) that fade to isointensity on late-phase image (*c*).

T2-weighted fat-suppressed SS-ETSE (*d*), SGE (*e*), and immediate (*f*) and 90-s fat-suppressed (*g*) postgadolinium SGE images in a second patient. A 6-cm mass lesion is present in the dome of the liver, which is minimally high in signal intensity on T2-weighted image (*d*) and moderately low in signal intensity on T1-weighted image(*e*), enhances in an intense diffuse heterogeneous fashion on early-phase image (*f*), and fades on later images (*g*). The appearance resembles HCC; however, the liver is not cirrhotic. The patient also presented with fever and malaise, which are symptoms often observed with inflammatory pseudotumor.

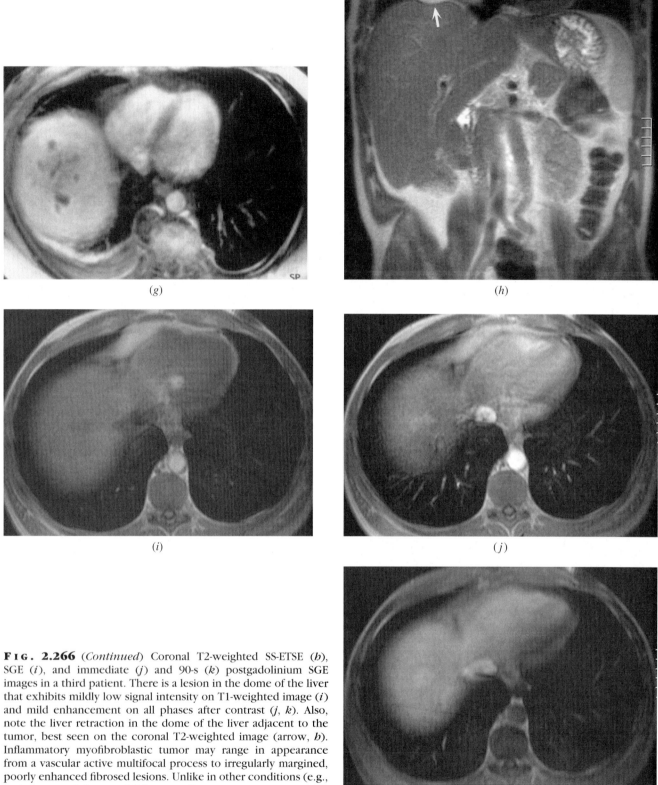

(g)

(h)

(i)

(j)

(k)

FIG. 2.266 (*Continued*) Coronal T2-weighted SS-ETSE (*h*), SGE (*i*), and immediate (*j*) and 90-s (*k*) postgadolinium SGE images in a third patient. There is a lesion in the dome of the liver that exhibits mildly low signal intensity on T1-weighted image (*i*) and mild enhancement on all phases after contrast (*j*, *k*). Also, note the liver retraction in the dome of the liver adjacent to the tumor, best seen on the coronal T2-weighted image (arrow, *h*). Inflammatory myofibroblastic tumor may range in appearance from a vascular active multifocal process to irregularly margined, poorly enhanced fibrosed lesions. Unlike in other conditions (e.g., metastases and abscesses) this range of appearance can occur with no history of treatment of the active disease.

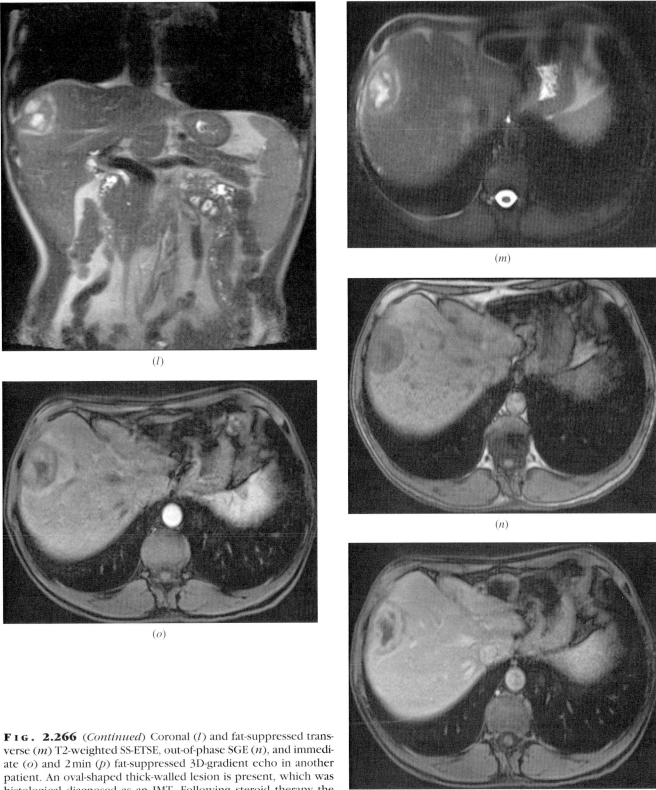

F I G . 2.266 (*Continued*) Coronal (*l*) and fat-suppressed transverse (*m*) T2-weighted SS-ETSE, out-of-phase SGE (*n*), and immediate (*o*) and 2 min (*p*) fat-suppressed 3D-gradient echo in another patient. An oval-shaped thick-walled lesion is present, which was histological diagnosed as an IMT. Following steroid therapy the lesion resolved.

2 LIVER

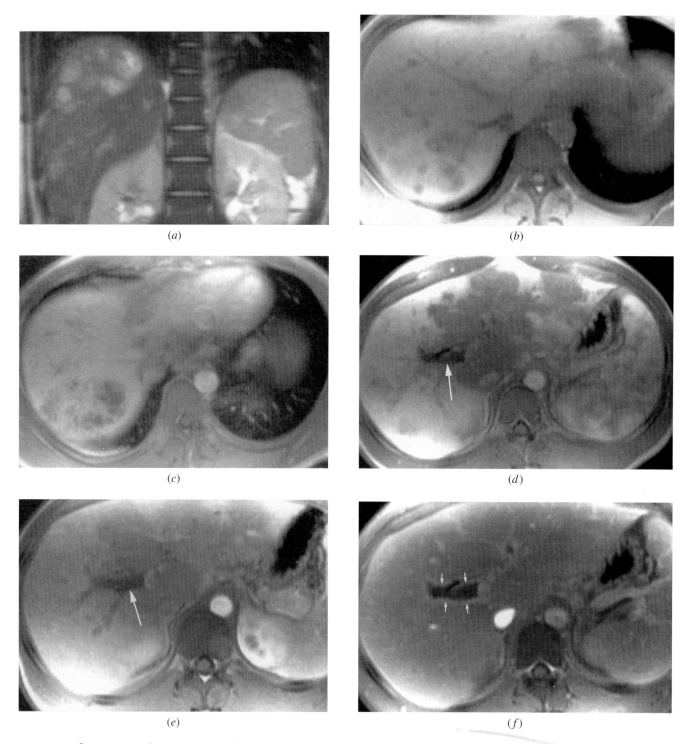

(a)

(b)

(c)

(d)

(e)

(f)

F I G . 2.267 Hepatic abscesses. Coronal T2-weighted SS-ETSE (*a*), transverse SGE (*b*), and immediate (*c, d*), 45-s (*e*), and 90-s fat-suppressed (*f*) postgadolinium SGE images of the abdomen and sagittal T2-weighted SS-ETSE (*g*) and 2.5-min fat-suppressed postgadolinium SGE (*h*) images of the pelvis in a patient with appendicitis and hepatic abscess. There are multiple lesions with a cluster appearance in the right hepatic lobe that demonstrate high signal intensity on T2-weighted image (*a*), low signal intensity on T1-weighted image (*b*), and enhancement of the abscess wall and septations with perilesional enhancement immediately after administration of contrast (*c*). Abnormal enhancement of the liver on the early-phase image (*d*) reflects the presence of portal vein thrombosis, with increased enhancement of the right lobe due to increased hepatic arterial supply. The portal vein is expanded with thrombus (arrow *d, e*) that is low signal on T1-weighted image and does not enhance after administration of contrast, consistent with a bland thrombus. The portal vein wall enhances (small arrows, *f*) on the late-phase images, reflecting that the thrombus is infected. Note on the sagittal images (*g, h*) that the appendix (arrows, *g, h*) is thick walled with increased enhancement, consistent with acute appendicitis.

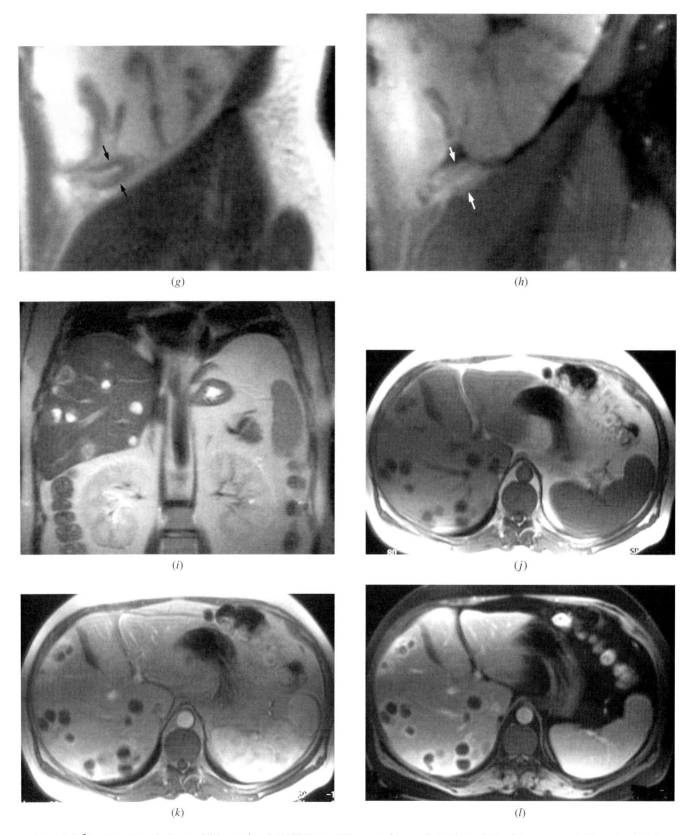

FIG. 2.267 (*Continued*) Coronal T2-weighted SS-ETSE (*i*), SGE (*j*), and immediate (*k*) and 90-s fat-suppressed (*l*) postgadolinium SGE images in a second patient, who has a history of Crohn disease. Multiple abscesses are seen in the right hepatic lobe and demonstrate high signal intensity on T2-weighted image (*i*), low signal intensity on T1-weighted image (*j*), and perilesional enhancement surrounding the whole lesion on early-phase image (*k*) with more intense abscess wall enhancement on late phase image (*l*).

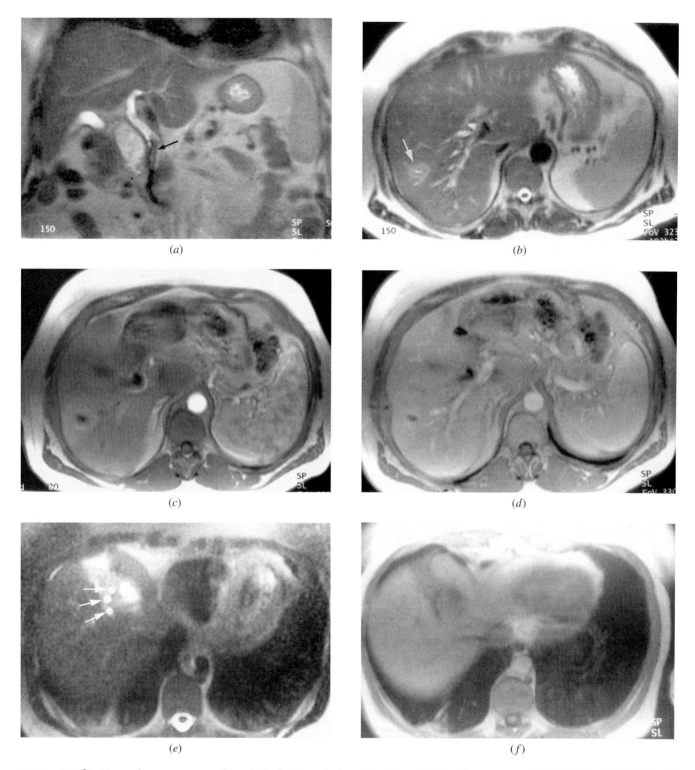

(a)

(b)

(c)

(d)

(e)

(f)

F I G . 2.268 Liver abscesses secondary to infective cholangitis. Coronal (*a*) and transverse (*b*) T2-weighted SS-ETSE and T1-weighted immediate (*c*) and 45-s (*d*) postgadolinium SGE images. There is a lesion in the right hepatic lobe (arrow, *b*) that demonstrates increased signal intensity on T2-weighted image (*b*) and decreased signal on T1-weighted image (not shown). After contrast, the lesion shows a circumferential ill-defined perilesional and capsular enhancement on immediate postgadolinium images (*c*), with fading of the perilesional enhancement but persistent capsular enhancement on 45-s image (*d*). There is no enhancement of internal stroma or fill-in of the lesion with time. Note the biliary stent (arrow, *a*) situated in the common bile duct (*a*).

T2-weighted SS-ETSE (*e*), SGE (*f*), immediate postgadolinium SGE (*g*), and 90-s postgadolinium fat-suppressed SGE (*h*) images in a second patient. There is an irregular region of increased signal on T2-weighted image (*e*) and decreased signal on T1-weighted

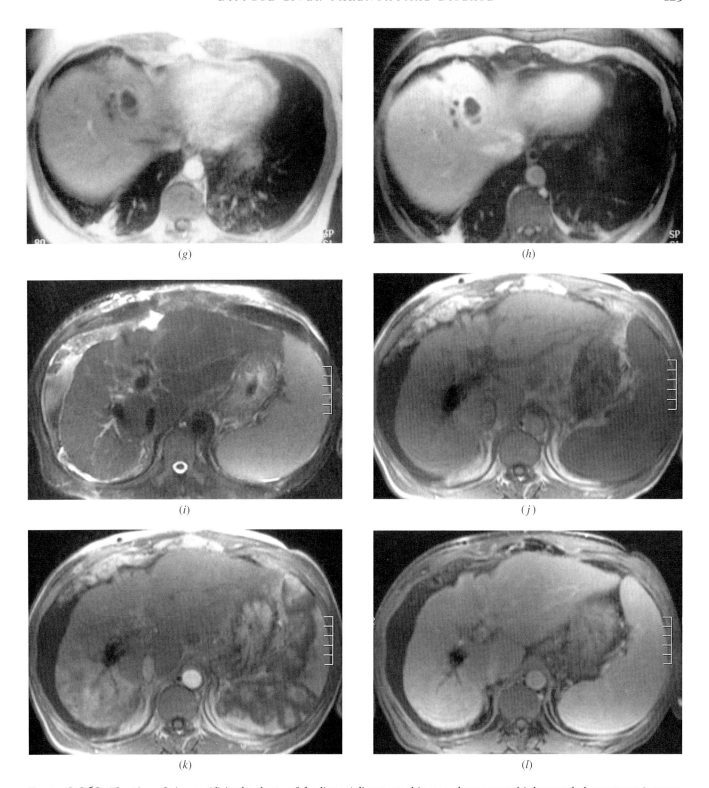

(g)

(h)

(i)

(j)

(k)

(l)

F I G . 2.268 (*Continued*) image (*f*) in the dome of the liver. Adjacent to this area, there are multiple rounded structures (arrows, *e*) that demonstrate increased signal on T2 (*e*) and decreased signal on T1 (*f*), which represent dilated ducts. After gadolinium administration (*g, h*), a cystic mass with a thickened, enhancing wall and internal septations is identified, consistent with an abscess secondary to segmental infective cholangitis.

Fat-suppressed T2-weighted SS-ETSE (*i*), SGE (*j*), and immediate (*k*) and 90-s fat-suppressed (*l*) postgadolinium SGE images in a third patient who has a previous history of cirrhosis and a current history of ascending cholangitis. The right hepatic liver enhances in a heterogeneous fashion on early-phase images (*k*) and becomes homogeneously enhanced on late-phase images (*l*).

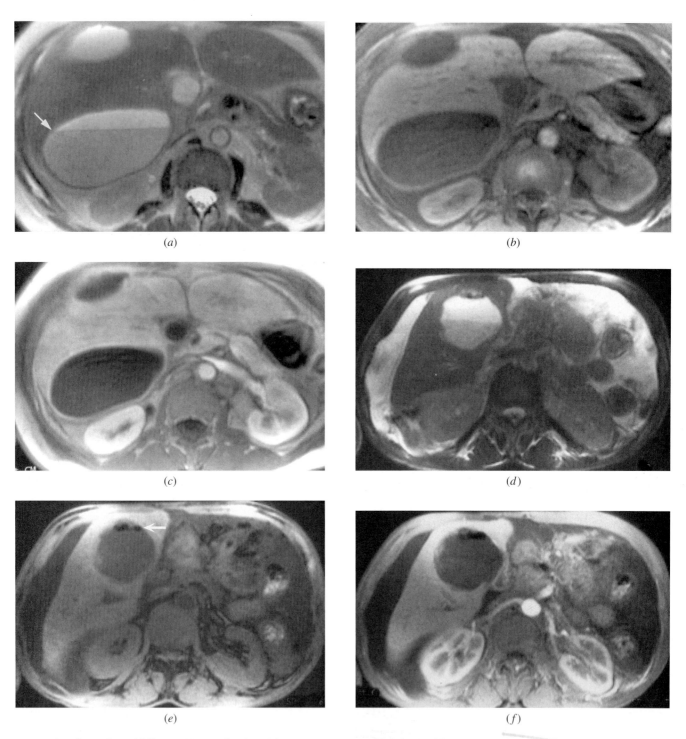

(a)

(b)

(c)

(d)

(e)

(f)

FIG. 2.269 Infected biloma. T2-weighted SS-ETSE (*a*), precontrast fat-suppressed SGE (*b*), and immediate postgadolinium SGE (*c*) images in a 79-year-old woman who has a history of trauma. Large subcapsular fluid collections are observed anterior and posterior to the right hepatic lobe. These collections demonstrate fluid-fluid levels (arrow, *a*) best shown on the breathing-independent single-shot T2-weighted image (*a*) and substantial wall enhancement (*c*) consistent with infection.

T2-weighted fat-suppressed SS-ETSE (*d*), T1-weighted fat-suppressed SGE (*e*), and immediate (*f*) and 90-s fat-suppressed (*g*) postgadolinium SGE images in a second patient, who has a history of trauma. Subcapsular infected biloma with fluid-fluid levels are present, one of which also contains air bubbles (arrow, *e*). Air bubbles appear as signal foci on all sequences.

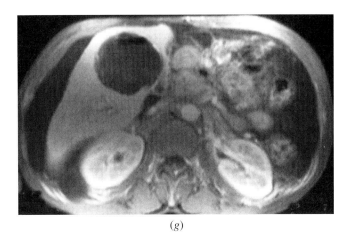

(g)   **FIG. 2.269** *(Continued)*

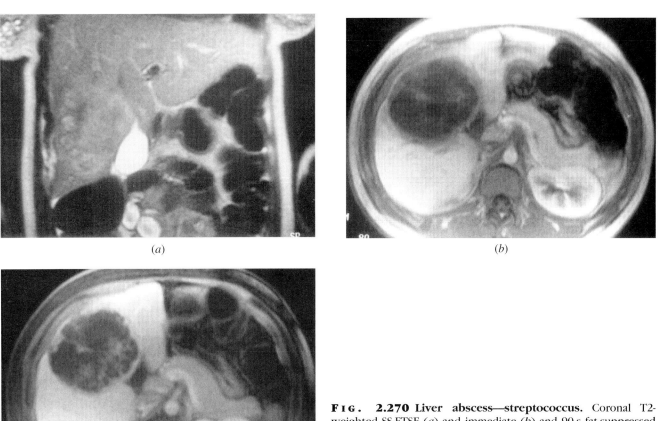

(a)   *(b)*

(c)

FIG. 2.270 Liver abscess—streptococcus. Coronal T2-weighted SS-ETSE (*a*) and immediate (*b*) and 90-s fat-suppressed (*c*) postgadolinium SGE images. A large mass is present in the right lobe of the liver, which is heterogeneous and mildly hyperintense on T2-weighted image (*a*). The mass contains multiple septations that exhibit minimal early enhancement (*b*), with increased intensity on the later image (*c*). No progressive lesion stromal enhancement is present.

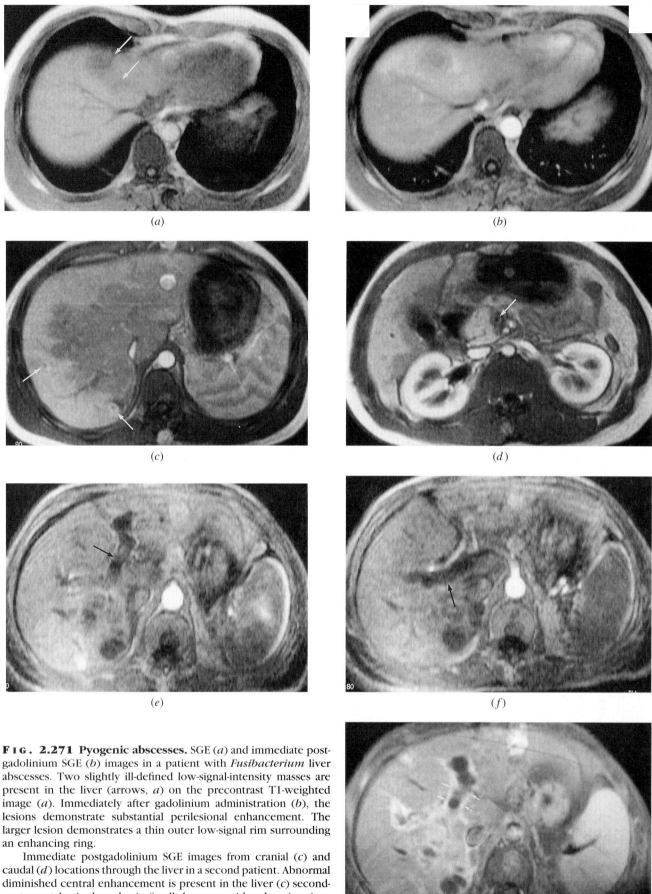

FIG. 2.271 Pyogenic abscesses. SGE (*a*) and immediate post-gadolinium SGE (*b*) images in a patient with *Fusibacterium* liver abscesses. Two slightly ill-defined low-signal-intensity masses are present in the liver (arrows, *a*) on the precontrast T1-weighted image (*a*). Immediately after gadolinium administration (*b*), the lesions demonstrate substantial perilesional enhancement. The larger lesion demonstrates a thin outer low-signal rim surrounding an enhancing ring.

Immediate postgadolinium SGE images from cranial (*c*) and caudal (*d*) locations through the liver in a second patient. Abnormal diminished central enhancement is present in the liver (*c*) secondary to portal vein thrombosis. Small abscesses with enhancing rings (arrows, *c*) are shown in the right hepatic lobe. On the more inferior tomographic image (*d*), thrombus is identified in the SMV with enhancement of the vein wall (arrow, *d*), reflecting infection of the thrombus.

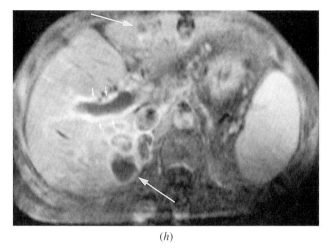

(h)

FIG. 2.271 (*Continued*) Immediate postgadolinium SGE images (*e, f*) and interstitial-phase gadolinium-enhanced T1-weighted fat-suppressed SE images (*g, h*) in a third patient obtained at the level of the left portal vein (*e, g*) and right portal vein (*f, h*). The left (arrow, *e*) and right (arrow, *f*) portal veins are expanded with low-signal thrombus on the immediate postgadolinium images. On the gadolinium-enhanced fat-suppressed images enhancement of the walls of the portal veins is present (small arrows, *g, h*), reflecting the infected nature of the thrombus. The abscesses in the right and left lobes of the liver are well seen on the interstitial-phase images as low-signal-intensity irregular-shaped cystic masses with enhancing rims (long arrows, *g, h*).

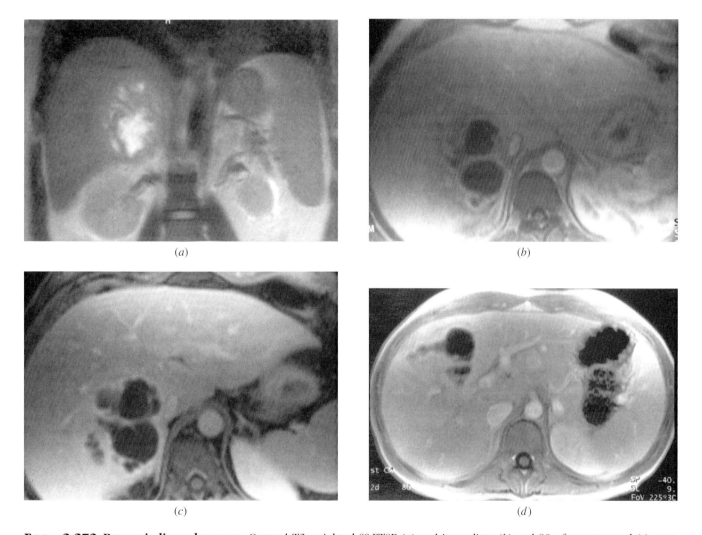

(a)

(b)

(c)

(d)

FIG. 2.272 Pyogenic liver abscesses. Coronal T2-weighted SS-ETSE (*a*) and immediate (*b*) and 90-s fat-suppressed (*c*) postgadolinium SGE images. A large septated lesion is present, which is heterogeneous and high signal intensity on T2-weighted image (*a*) and low signal intensity on T1-weighted images (*b, c*), with intense capsular and internal septa enhancement on early-phase image (*b*) that persists on the late image (*c*). A characteristic feature of abscesses is that the capsule and septa enhance on immediate postgadolinium images and persist in enhancement on 90-s image (*c*), with no progressive internal stromal enhancement. Enhancement of abscess walls frequently becomes more intense on later postcontrast images. Metastases, in distinction, tend to exhibit progressive stromal enhancement.

Transverse 45-s postgadolinium SGE (*d*) image in a second patient demonstrates a lesion with intense mural enhancement consistent with an abscess.

CT imaging. Metastases with large necrotic component may mimic the appearance of hepatic abscesses mainly because both may have prominent rim enhancement [426]. Abscesses exhibit moderately intense enhancement of stroma and internal septations on early-phase postgadolinium images, without progressive enhancement of stroma, whereas necrotic metastases generally show centripetal progression of stromal enhancement. Metastases may also mimic abscesses clinically if they become secondarily infected. The diagnosis of infected metastases should be considered when the lesion wall is thicker than 5 mm and has nodular irregular components and centripetal enhancement is evident.

Nonpyogenic Abscess: Amebic Abscess. Amebic liver abscesses are caused by a protozoan parasite, *Entamoeba histolytica*, and are not uncommon in developing tropical countries [424]. Amebic abscess may arise in patients who live in or have traveled to tropical climates. Amebic abscesses may develop secondary to small ischemic necrotic areas caused by obstruction of small venules by the trophosites and their by-products

[424]. Presenting features include pain, fever, weight loss, nausea and vomiting, diarrhea, and anorexia [429]. Lesions are usually solitary, affect the right lobe more often than the left lobe [424, 428], and are prone to invade the diaphragm with development of pulmonary consolidation and empyema [430]. Lesions are encapsulated and thick walled (5–10 mm) and demonstrate substantial enhancement of the capsule on gadolinium-enhanced images, which permits differentiation from liver cysts (fig. 2.273).

Echinococcal Disease
Echinococcal disease is a worldwide zoonosis produced by two main types of larval forms of equinococcus tapeworms: *E. granulosus* and *E. alveolaris* [431]. *Echinococcus granulosus* is the causative organism for hydatid cysts and is the type of echinococcus indigenous in North America. Pathologically, the typical hydatid cyst is spherical with a fibrous rim. Surrounding liver reaction to the abscess is minimal, with small-volume granulation tissue. The typical imaging feature is in an intrahepatic encapsulated multicystic lesion with daughter cysts arranged peripherally within the larger

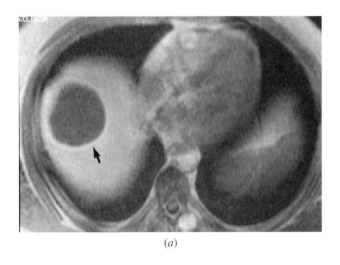
(a)

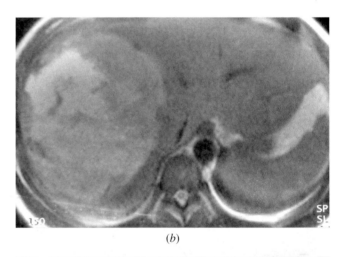
(b)

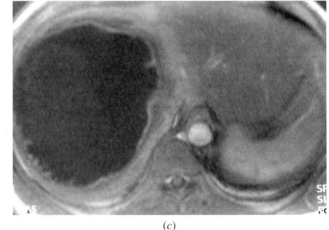
(c)

FIG. 2.273 Amebic abscess. Immediate postgadolinium SGE (*a*) image demonstrates a 7-cm cystic lesion located superiorly in the right lobe of the liver. The amebic abscess has a prominent enhancing wall (arrow, *a*) distinguishing it from a simple cyst.

T2-weighted SS-ETSE (*b*) and immediate postgadolinium magnetization-prepared gradient echo (*c*) images in a second patient. A large cystic lesion is seen in the right hepatic lobe, near the dome of the diaphragm, with a thick irregular wall and perilesional and capsular enhancement after gadolinium administration, consistent with abscess.

cyst. Satellite cysts located exterior to the fibrinous membrane of the main hepatic cyst are not uncommon and have been reported in 16% of hydatid cysts in a series of 185 patients [431]. Lesions are frequently complex, with mixed high signal intensity on T2-weighted images and mixed low signal intensity on T1-weighted images due to the presence of protein-aceous and cellular debris (fig. 2.274).The fibrous capsule and internal septations are well shown on T2-

weighted images and gadolinium-enhanced T1-weighted images. SS-ETSE sequence is particularly effective at showing the architectural detail of cystic lesions. Calcification of the cyst wall and internal calcifications are frequently identified on CT images but may not be distinguishable from the fibrous tissue of the capsule on MR images. Superinfection and cyst rupture, after trauma or spontaneously, are the most frequent com-plications reported with hydatid cysts [428]. The rupture

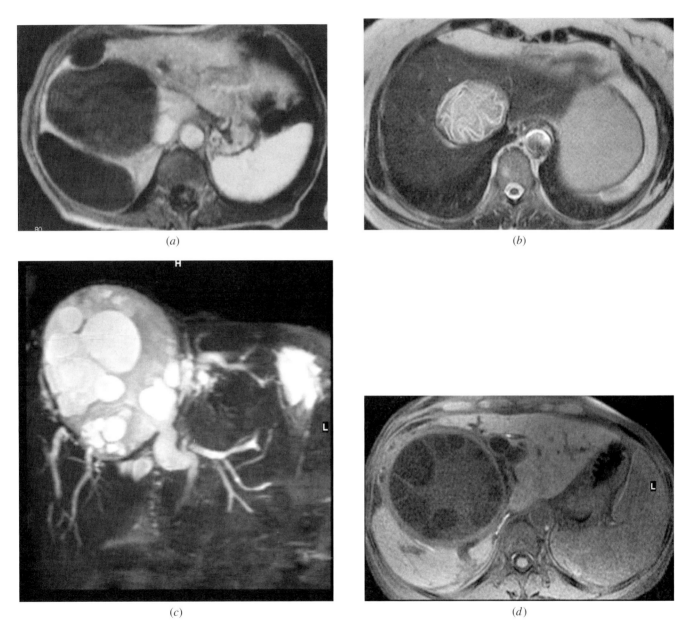

(a)

(b)

(c)

(d)

F I G . 2.274 Hydatid cyst. Immediate postgadolinium SGE image (*a*) exhibits a multicystic lesion in the right hepatic lobe with a dominant cyst centrally and daughter cysts peripherally. There is mild mural enhancement of the hydatid cyst wall.

T2-weighted SS-ETSE image (*b*) in a second patient infected by *E. granulosus*. Note the presence of a cystic lesion with addi-tional small internal cystic lesions (courtesy of N. Cem Balci, M.D.).

Coronal T2-weighted SS-ETSE (*c*) and transverse SGE (*d*) in a third patient show multiple daughter cysts lining the wall of the dominant cystic lesion (courtesy of Bharat Aggarwal, M.D., Diwan Chand Satya Pal Aggarwal Imaging Research Center, New Delhi, India).

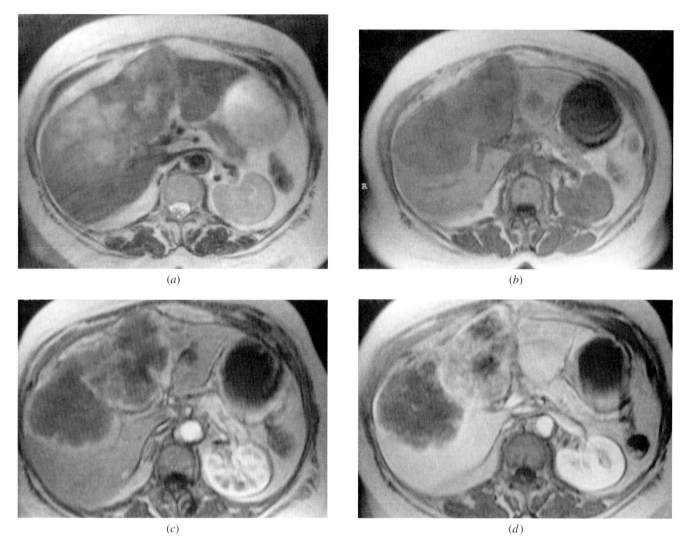

(a)   (b)

(c)   (d)

FIG. 2.275 Hepatic alveolar echinococcosis. T2-weighted ETSE (*a*), SGE (*b*), and immediate (*c*) and 90-s (*d*) postgadolinium SGE images. A large lesion with irregular margins is present in the liver that demonstrates mildly high signal on T2-weighted image (*a*) and low signal on T1-weighted image (*b*), and a peripheral rim of enhancement on early-phase image (*c*) that persists on late images (*d*). There is a substantial solid component within the large infective lesion. The lesions exhibits ill-defined margins. (Courtesy of N. Cem Balci, M.D.)

of a cyst may provoke an intense inflammatory and granulomatous reaction in surrounding tissue.

Echinococcus alveolaris is the causative organism for hepatic alveolar echinococcosis (HAE), a rare parasitic disease in which the fox is the main host of the adult parasite, with dogs and cats being less frequently cited hosts. Pathologically, HAE is characterized grossly by multilocular or confluent cystic, necrotic cavities. A fibrous rim is not present. Balci et al. [431] described the MR appearance of HAE in 13 patients. All lesions were large (mean 9.7 cm), solitary, with mixed cystic/solid components and irregular margins. By MRI, HAE demonstrated heterogeneous signal intensity on T2- and T1-weighted images and negligible lesional enhance-

ment after contrast. A perilesional enhancement was reported in 5 cases (38%) (fig. 2.275).

Calcification is common in HAE and appears as clusters of microcalcifications or large calcified foci. HAE tends to involve extensive regions in the liver in an infiltrative pattern because it does not form membranes or capsules. HAE is more likely to involve the porta hepatitis, causing stenoses of portal veins, intrahepatic bile ducts, and hepatic veins, which commonly result in portal hypertension. The differential diagnosis of HAE includes various infiltrative lesions of the liver, such as HCCs and metastases. The typical pattern of enhancement of HCC and liver metastases, systemic features of infection, and geographic occurrence of the disease may help in the differentiation. HAE can be differentiated from hydatid disease, because the latter process shows well-defined cyst walls and regular contours.

Mycobacterial Infection

Mycobacterium tuberculosis. Hepatic tuberculosis is the most frequent form of infectious hepatic granulomas [428]. The most common pathway for *Mycobacterium tuberculosis* bacilli to reach the liver is through the bloodstream [424]. Although abdominal tuberculosis preferentially affects lymph nodes and the ileocecal junction [424], the liver is also commonly involved. The incidence of hepatic tuberculosis is increasing, reflecting, in part, an increase in numbers of patients who are immunocompromised, such as patients with HIV infection.

Focal hepatic lesions are typically small and multiple with an appearance similar to that of fungal lesions (see next section). Infection has a propensity to involve the portal triads and spread in a superficial infiltrating fashion. This can be visualized as periportal high signal intensity on T2-weighted fat-suppressed images and moderate/intense enhancement on late-phase fat-suppressed postgadolinium images. Associated porta hepatis nodes are common.

Mycobacterium avium intracellulare (MAI). Nontuberculous mycobacterial hepatic infection is common and represents the most frequent hepatic infection in AIDS [432]. MAI infection is found in 50% of livers of patients dying with AIDS [433]. Microscopically, hepatic MAI lesions may show a spectrum of appearances ranging from loose aggregates of histiocytes to tight, well-formed granulomas. CT findings reported to be suggestive of disseminated MAI infection include enlarged mesenteric and/or retroperitoneal lymph nodes, hepatosplenomegaly, and diffuse jejunal wall thickening (fig. 2.276) [434]. Low-density centers of involved lymph nodes are considered a characteristic feature on CT images. Similar findings may be appreciated on MR images.

Fungal Infection

Hepatosplenic or visceral candidiasis is a form of invasive fungal infection that has emerged as a serious complication of the immunocompromised state, especially in AIDS patients, patients on medical therapy for acute myelogeneous leukemia (AML), and patients with bone marrow transplantation [435–437]. Prolonged duration of neutropenia is thought to be the most important risk factor for hepatosplenic candidiasis [437]. The most common infecting organism is *Candida albicans*, but other fungi may be found. Acute hepatosplenic candidiasis involves the liver and spleen, with

renal involvement occurring in less than 50% of patients. Disseminated *C. albicans* infects the liver in a high proportion of cases, leading to development of multifocal microabscesses or granulomas. Although definitive diagnosis requires microbiologic or histologic evidence of infection, the absence of organisms on liver biopsy tissue or negative culture findings in the presence of clinical suspicion does not rule out the diagnosis. Moreover, patient survival depends on early diagnosis. Therefore, cross-sectional imaging is necessary for diagnosis [438]. Liver lesions are frequently smaller than 1 cm and subcapsular in location. The small size and peripheral nature of these lesions make them difficult to detect with CT imaging or standard spin-echo MR sequences. MRI employing T2-weighted fat suppression and dynamic gadolinium-enhanced gradient-echo images have been shown to be more sensitive for the detection of hepatosplenic candidiasis than contrast-enhanced CT imaging [438, 439].

T2-weighted fat-suppressed spin-echo sequences are effective at demonstrating these lesions, because of the high conspicuity of this sequence for small lesions and the absence of chemical shift artifact that may mask small peripheral lesions. STIR images also show these lesions well because of the fat-nulling effect of this sequence [440]. Patients with AML undergo multiple blood transfusions, so the liver and spleen are low in signal intensity on T2-weighted and T1-weighted images [440, 441].

Because acute lesions of fungal disease are abscesses, they are high in signal intensity on T2-weighted images. They also may be seen on gadolinium-enhanced T1-weighted images as signal-void foci with no appreciable abscess wall enhancement (figs. 2.277 and 2.278). It has been observed that patients with hepatosplenic candidiasis who are immunocompetent possess abscesses that demonstrate mural enhancement. The absence of abscess wall enhancement may reflect the patient's neutropenic state. Overall sensitivity of MRI is 100%, and specificity is 96% [438].

After institution of antifungal antibiotics, successful response may be demonstrated. Central high signal develops within lesions on T2-weighted and T1-weighted images that enhances with gadolinium, representing granuloma formation. In addition, a distinctive dark perilesional ring is observed on all sequences, representing collections of iron-laden macrophages throughout granulation tissue at the periphery of lesions (fig. 2.279) [442]. This represents the subacute treated phase, which may be consistent with a good prognostic finding, reflecting the patient's ability to mount an immune response.

MRI also demonstrates chronic healed lesions that have responded to antifungal therapy [439]. Chronic healed lesions are irregularly shaped, isointense and

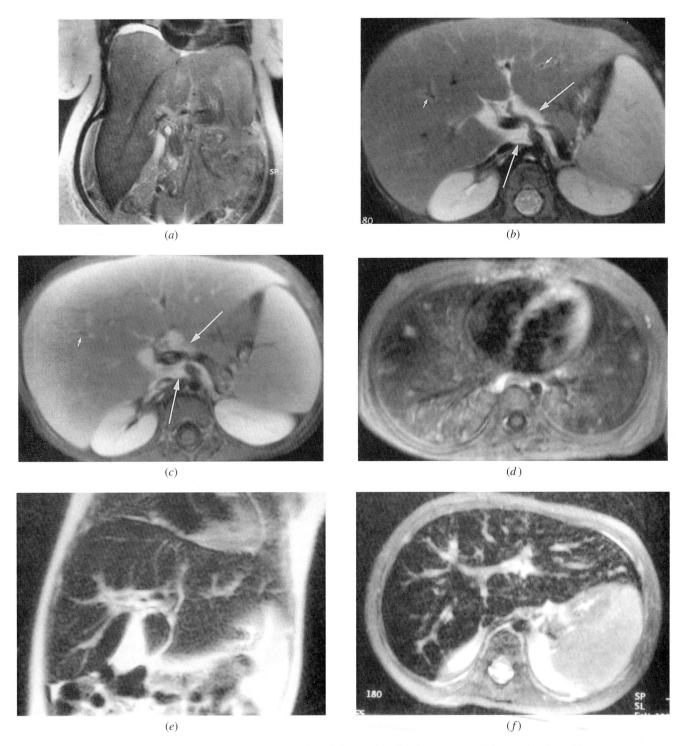

(a)

(b)

(c)

(d)

(e)

(f)

FIG. 2.276 *Mycobacterium avium intracellulare* (MAI) hepatic infection. Coronal T2-weighted SS-ETSE (*a*), transverse T2-weighted fat-suppressed ETSE (*b*), and interstitial-phase gadolinium-enhanced T1-weighted fat-suppressed SE (*c*) images. The coronal image (*a*) demonstrates hepatomegaly. On the fat-suppressed T2-weighted image (*b*), high-signal-intensity soft tissue is present in the porta hepatis (long arrows, *b*) that extends along periportal tracks (short arrows, *b*). After gadolinium administration (*c*), enhancing porta hepatis tissue is clearly shown on the fat-suppressed image (long arrows, *c*), and enhancement is also noted of the periportal tissue (short arrow, *c*). Periportal distribution is a common pattern of involvement with MAI. Gadolinium-enhanced, gated T2-weighted fat-suppressed SE image (*d*) of the lungs demonstrates a ground glass appearance with irregularly marginated 1-cm enhancing nodules consistent with MAI lung infection.

Coronal T2-weighted SS-ETSE (*e*), T2-weighted fat-suppressed SS-ETSE (*f*), immediate postgadolinium SGE (*g*), and 90-s postgadolinium fat-suppressed SGE (*h*) images in a second patient, who has a history of hereditary blood dyscrasia and currently has MAI infection, demonstrate tissue in the porta hepatis and periportal tracks that is high signal on T2 (*e, f*) and enhances on late gadolinium-enhanced fat-suppressed T1-weighted images (arrows, *h*). Note also the iron deposition in the liver from transfusional siderosis.

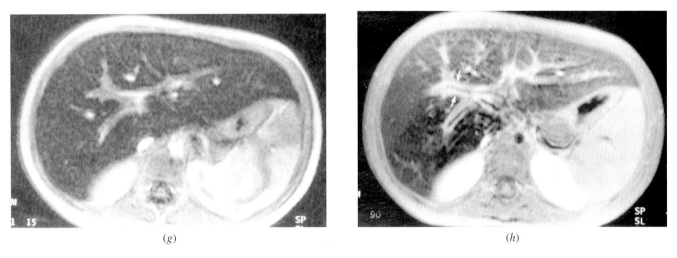

F I G . 2.276 (*Continued*)

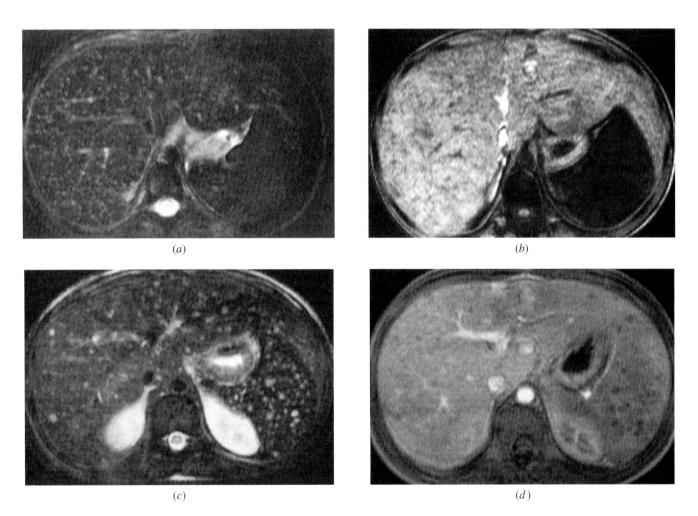

F I G . 2.277 Acute hepatosplenic candidiasis. T2-weighted fat-suppressed ETSE (*a, c*) and immediate postgadolinium SGE (*b, d*) images in two patients. On the T2-weighted images (*a, c*), multiple well-defined <1-cm high-signal-intensity foci are scattered throughout the hepatic parenchyma, with a smaller number of similar lesions apparent in the spleen. On the immediate postgadolinium image (*b, d*), the liver lesions are near signal void and do not show ring or perilesional enhancement.

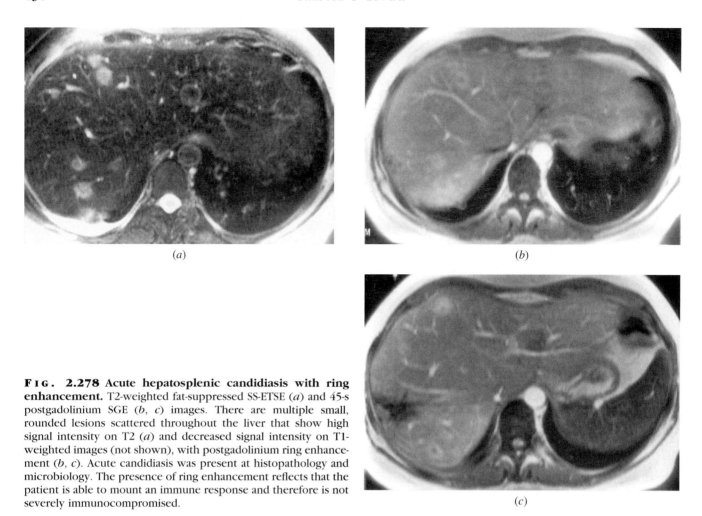

(a)

(b)

(c)

F I G . 2.278 Acute hepatosplenic candidiasis with ring enhancement. T2-weighted fat-suppressed SS-ETSE (*a*) and 45-s postgadolinium SGE (*b*, *c*) images. There are multiple small, rounded lesions scattered throughout the liver that show high signal intensity on T2 (*a*) and decreased signal intensity on T1-weighted images (not shown), with postgadolinium ring enhancement (*b*, *c*). Acute candidiasis was present at histopathology and microbiology. The presence of ring enhancement reflects that the patient is able to mount an immune response and therefore is not severely immunocompromised.

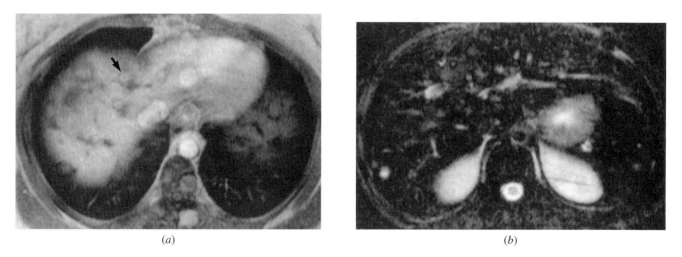

(a)

(b)

F I G . 2.279 Subacute hepatosplenic candidiasis. Immediate postgadolinium SGE image (*a*) demonstrates multiple lesions with a concentric ring pattern with an outer irregular signal-void rim, inner high-signal ring, and central low-signal dot (arrow, *a*).
    T2-weighted fat-suppressed SE (*b*), SGE (*c*), and immediate postgadolinium SGE (*d*) images in a second patient. Multiple concentric ring lesions are evident that are best shown on precontrast and immediate postgadolinium SGE images (*c*, *d*). The outer

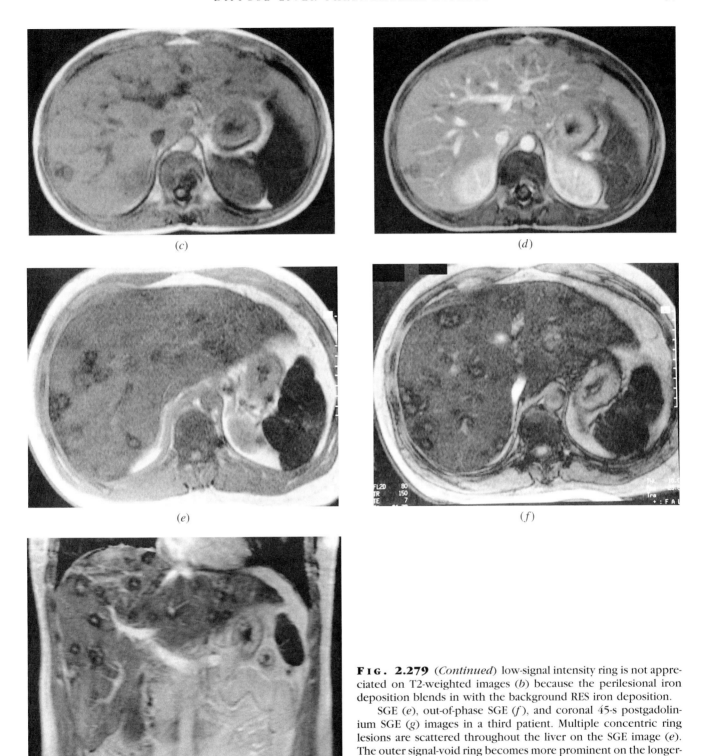

(c)

(d)

(e)

(f)

(g)

F I G . 2.279 (*Continued*) low-signal intensity ring is not appreciated on T2-weighted images (*b*) because the perilesional iron deposition blends in with the background RES iron deposition.

SGE (*e*), out-of-phase SGE (*f*), and coronal 45-s postgadolinium SGE (*g*) images in a third patient. Multiple concentric ring lesions are scattered throughout the liver on the SGE image (*e*). The outer signal-void ring becomes more prominent on the longer-TE out-of-phase image (*f*), because of a magnetic susceptibility artifact from iron. Lesion appearance is largely unchanged on the postgadolinium image (*g*).

poorly shown on T2-weighted images, and hypointense on T1-weighted images and demonstrate negligible enhancement after contrast (fig. 2.280). The lesions are most conspicuous as low-signal intensity defects with angular margins on immediate postgadolinium SGE images. Capsular retraction may also be observed adjacent to the lesions. This constellation of imaging features is consistent with chronic scar formation.

TRAUMA

Liver hematoma, liver laceration, perihepatic hematoma, and hemoperitoneum may be consequences of abdominal trauma and are all well demonstrated on MR images. Liver hematoma can exhibit any morphology; liver laceration is identified as a linear, intraparenchymal defect (figs. 2.281–2.283); perihepatic hematoma is characterized by a fluid collection between parenchyma

and capsule (subcapsular); and hemoperitoneum is seen as free peritoneal fluid. MR features of these entities vary according to the paramagnetic effects of various products of hemoglobin such as oxygen saturation, iron, and protein content [443–448]. The sequence used and the magnetic field strength also play a role in MR findings [447, 449]. Five stages that reflect the age of hemorrhage are described, based on the breakdown products of hemoglobin and the resulting signal

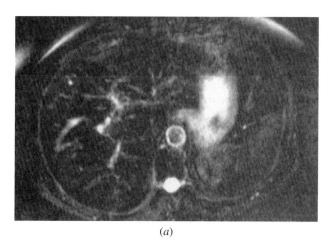
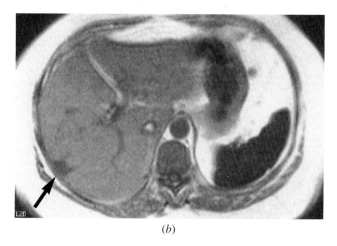

(a)   (b)

FIG. 2.280 Chronic healed candidiasis. T2-weighted fat-suppressed SE (a) and SGE (b) images. On T2-weighted image (a) the area of fibrosis has signal intensity similar to background liver and is not definable. On T1-weighted image (arrow, b), an irregular, polygonal low-signal lesion is present in the right lobe of the liver.

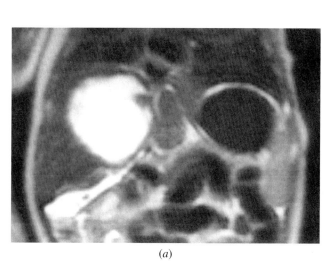
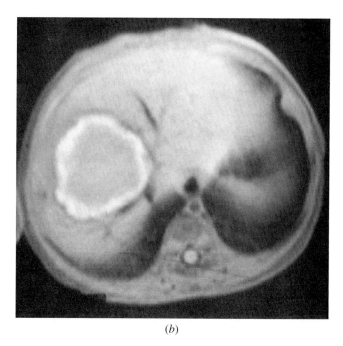

(a)   (b)

FIG. 2.281 Liver hematoma. Coronal T2-weighted SS-ETSE (a) and T1-weighted fat-suppressed SE (b) images in an 8-week-old girl who has a history of malpositioned umbilical venous catheter and subsequent liver hematoma. There is a fluid collection in the right lobe of the liver that is hyperintense on T2-weighted images (a) and isointense centrally with a hyperintense peripheral ring on the fat-suppressed T1-weighted image (b), consistent with hematoma. The appearance on the T1-weighted image, with the high-signal peripheral ring, is diagnostic for a hematoma.

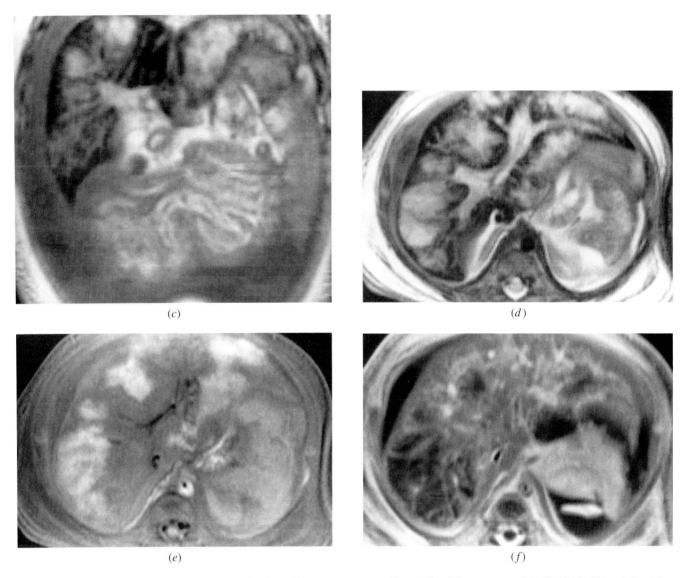

F I G . 2.281 (*Continued*) Coronal T2-weighted SS-ETSE (*c*), transverse T2-weighted fat-suppressed SS-ETSE (*d*), T1-weighted fat-suppressed SE (*e*), and T1-weighted interstitial phase fat-suppressed postgadolinium SE (*f*) images in a newborn patient with disseminated intravascular coagulation. There are abnormal patchy areas throughout the hepatic parenchyma that exhibit high signal intensity on T2-weighted images (*c, d*) and T1-weighted image (*e*) consistent with late subacute blood (extracellular methemoglobin). After contrast, these areas demonstrate negligible enhancement (*f*) compatible with ischemia.

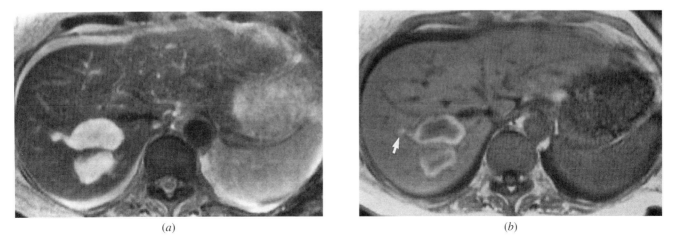

F I G . 2.282 Hepatic hemorrhage after trauma. T2-weighted fat-suppressed ETSE (*a*), SGE (*b*), and 45-s postgadolinium SGE (*c*) images. There are two hematomas in the liver parenchyma that demonstrate heterogeneous moderate high signal on T2-weighted

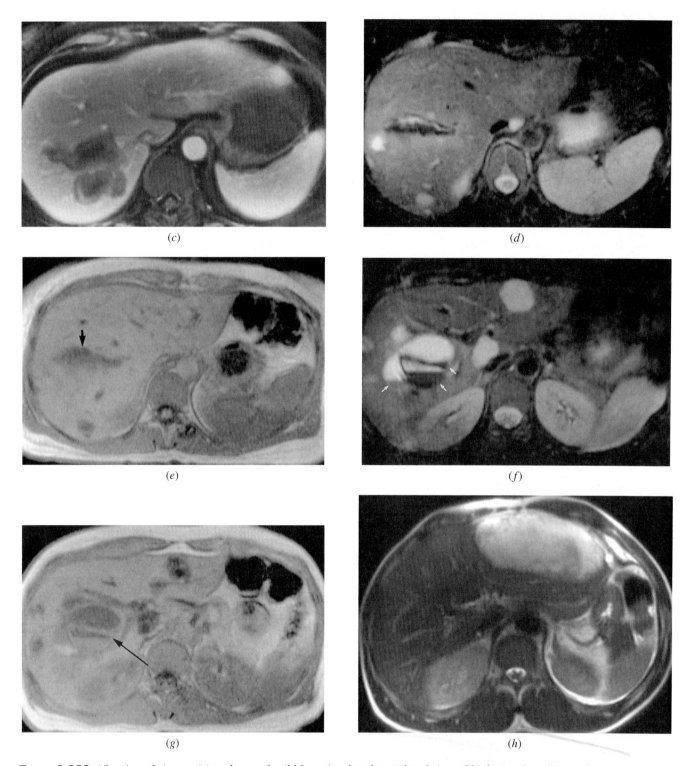

F I G . 2.282 (*Continued*) image (*a*) and central mild low signal and peripheral ring of high signal on T1-weighted precontrast image (*b*), which is diagnostic for subacute hematomas. These lesions do not enhance after gadolinium administration (*c*), but note that the methemoglobin ring remains hyperintense. A high-signal-intensity laceration tract is also noted (arrow, *b*).

T2-weighted fat-suppressed ETSE images (*d, f*) and T1-weighted noncontrast SGE (*e, g*) images acquired in a second patient from two tomographic levels (*d–g*). An acute liver laceration is present (arrow, *e*) through the right lobe of the liver, which contains fluid that is bright and dark (oxyhemoglobin) and dark and dark (deoxyhemoglobin) on T2- and T1-weighted images, respectively. Hemorrhage has extended into two liver cysts that contain a combination of hyperacute blood products including oxyhemoglobin (thin arrow, *g*) and deoxyhemoglobin (dark on T2- and isointense on T1-weighted images; short arrows, *f*).

T2-weighted SS-ETSE (*h*), SGE (*i*), and immediate postgadolinium SGE (*j*) images in a patient after liver trauma. A hematoma is seen in the left hepatic lobe that demonstrates high signal intensity on T2-weighted image (*h*) and low signal intensity on

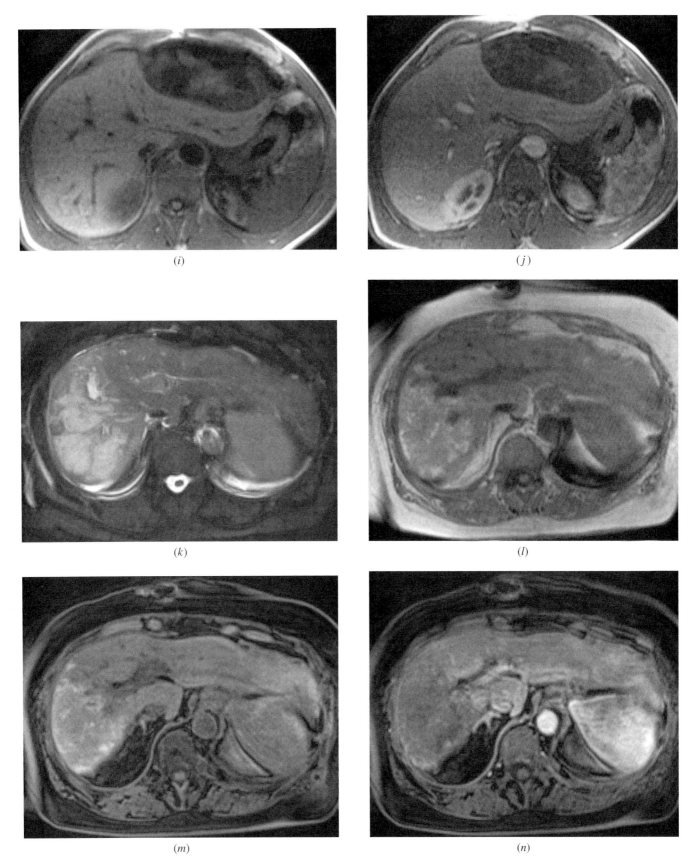

F I G . 2.282 (*Continued*) T1-weighted image with some areas of increased signal within the lesion (*i*). After administration of contrast (*j*), peripheral thin enhancement is appreciated surrounding the lesion. This lesion was compatible with hyperacute hematoma.

T2-weighted fat-suppressed ETSE (*k*), T1 in-phase (*l*), T1-fat-suppressed SGE (*m*), and 45-s postgadolinium fat suppressed SGE (*n*) images. There is area of heterogeneous persistent high signal intensity seen on the right lobe in all sequences, with no enhancement after contrast, compatible with subacute hematoma.

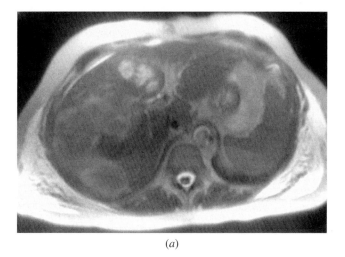

(a)

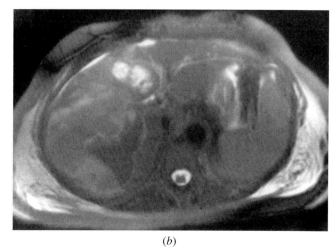

(b)

FIG. 2.283 Intrahepatic hemorrhage after surgery. T2-weighted SS-ETSE (a), T2-weighted fat-suppressed SS-ETSE (b), and single-shot magnetization-prepared gradient-echo (c) images in a patient after laparoscopic cholecystectomy who has a history of end-stage renal disease. There is a large area in the right hepatic lobe extending into the subcapsular space, which demonstrates heterogeneous increased signal intensity on both T2 (a, b)- and T1 (c)-weighted images consistent with late subacute hematoma. Note the peripheral rim of high signal on the T1-weighted image (c). Subcutaneous edema is more readily appreciated on the fat-suppressed T2-weighted image (b) than on the nonsuppressed image (a) because of removal of the competing high signal of fat on these long echo-train sequences.

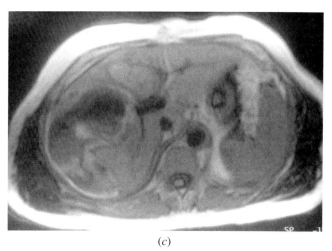

(c)

Table 2.2 Stages of hemorrhage

STAGE	TIME AFTER TRAUMA	HEMOGLOBIN PRODUCTS	T2-W*	T1-W*
Hyperacute	4 to 6 hours	Oxyhemoglobin	High SI	Iso or low SI
Acute	7 to 72 hours	Deoxyhemoglobin	Very low SI	Iso or low SI
Early subacute	4 to 7 days	Intracellular methemoglobin	Very low SI	High SI or high signal in the periphery and isointensity on the central area
Late subacute	1 to 4 weeks	Extracellular methemoglobin	High SI	High SI
Chronic	months to years	Ferritin and hemosiderin	Low SI	Iso SI

*Signal intensity on T2- and T1-weighted images.

intensity on T2- and T1-weighted precontrast images, as follows: hyperacute, acute, early subacute, late subacute, and chronic. In the hyperacute stage, oxyhemoglobin is present, which does not have paramagnetic properties and appears as simple fluid on T2- or T1-weighted images. In the acute stage, deoxyhemoglobin produces a strong effect on T2-weighted images (near signal void), which is a very distinctive finding. In the early subacute stage, intracellular methemoglobin still has a strong effect on T2-weighted images (near signal void) but also has an effect on T1-weighed images (high

signal intensity). In the late subacute stage, extracellular methemoglobin has a pronounced effect on T1-weighted images causing high signal intensity and appears high signal on T2-weighted images. In the chronic stage, hemorrhage is low signal intensity on T2-weighted and T1-weighted images due to hemosiderin and ferritin effects that usually accumulate peripherally located in the region of injury [444, 445, 450–452] (Table 2.2).

Active bleeding can be shown as progressive accumulation of high-signal gadolinium on serial postgadolinium images in a fluid-containing space [451].

REFERENCES

1. Couinaud C. *Le Foie; Etudes Anatomiques et Chirurgicales.* Paris, Masson, 1957.

2. MacSween RNM, Anthony PP, Scheuer PJ, Burt AD, Portamann BC, eds. *Pathology of the Liver.* 3th ed. London, Churchill Livingstone. 1994.

3. Ramalho M, Heredia V, Tsurusaki M, Altun E, Semelka RC. Qualitative and quantitative comparison of 3.0 T and 1.5 T MRI for the liver with chronic liver disease. *J Magn Reson Imaging* 29:869–879, 2009.

4. Goncalves Neto JA, Altun E, Elazzazi M, Chaney M, Vaidean G, Semelka RC. Enhancement of abdominal organs on hepatic arterial phaset: quantitative comparison between 1.5 T and 3.0 T MRI. *Magn Reson Imaging* 2009; Jul 2 (Epub ahead of print).

5. Semelka RC, Heimberger TK. Contrast agents for MR imaging of the liver. *Radiology* 218: 227–238, 2001.

6. Heredia V, Altun E, Ramalho M, Semelka RC. Magnetic resonance imaging of the liver: a review. *Exp Opin Med Diagnostics* 1: 1–11, 2007.

7. Goncalves Neto JA, Altun E, Vaidean G, et al. Early contrast enhancement of the liver: exact description of subphases using MRI. *Magn Reson Imaging* 27:976–987, 2009.

8. Whitney WS, Herfkens RJ, Jeffrey RB, McDonnell CH, Li KC, van Dalsem WJ, Low RN, Francis IR, Dabatin JF, Glazer GM. Dynamic breath-hold multiplanar spoiled gradient recolled MR imaging with gadolinium enhancement for differentiating hepatic hemangiomas from malignancies at 1.5T. *Radiology* 189: 863–870, 1993.

9. Lim KO, Stark DD, Leese PT, Pfefferbaum A, Rocklage SM, Quay SC. Hepatobiliary MR imaging: first human experience with MnDPDP. *Radiology* 178: 79–82, 1991.

10. Hamm B, Vogl TJ, Branding G, Schnell B, Taupitz M, Wolf KJ, Lissner J. Focal liver lesions: MR imaging with Mn-DPDP-initial clinical results in 40 patients. *Radiology* 182: 167–174, 1992.

11. Schuhmann-Giampieri G, Schmitt-Willich H, Press WR, Negishi C, Weinmann HJ, Speck U. Preclinical evaluation of Gd-EOB-DTPA as a contrast agent in MR imaging of the hepatobiliary system. *Radiology* 183: 59–64, 1992.

12. Kettritz U, Schlund JF, Wilbur K, Eisenberg LB, Semelka RA. Comparison of gadolinium chelates with Manganese-DPDP for liver lesion detection and characterization: preliminary results. *Magn Reson Imag* 14 (10): 1185–1190, 1996.

13. Martin DR, Semelka RC, Chung JJ, Balci NC, Wilber K. Sequential use of gadolinium chelate and mangafodipir trisodium for the assessment of focal liver lesions: initial observations. *Magn Reson Imaging* 18: 955–963, 2000.

14. Kim KW, Kim AY, Kim TK, Park SH, Kim HJ, Lee YK, Park MS, Ha HK, Kim PN, Kim JC, Lee MG. Small (< or = 2 cm) hepatic lesions in colorectal cancer patients: detection and characterization on mangafodipir trisodium-enhanced MRI. *AJR Am J Roentgenol* 182: 1233–1240, 2004.

15. Caudana R, Morana G, Pirovano GP, Nicoli N, Portuese A, Spinazzi A, Di Rito R, Pistolesi GF. Focal malignant hepatic lesions: MR imaging enhanced with gadolinium benzoxypropionictetra-acetate (BOPTA)- preliminary results of phase II clinical application. *Radiology* 199: 513–520, 1996.

16. Hamm B, Staks T, Muhler A, Bollow M, Taupitz M, Frenzel T, Wolf KJ, Weinmann HJ, Lange L. Phase I clinical evaluation of Gd-EOB-DTPA as a hepatobiliary MR contrast agent: safety, pharmacokinetics, and MR imaging. *Radiology* 195: 785–792, 1995.

17. Vogl TJ, Kummel S, Hammerstingl R, Schellenbeck M, Schumacher G, Balzer T, Schwarz W, Muller PK, Bechstein WO, Mack MG, Sollner O, Felix R. Liver tumors: comparison of MR imaging with Gd-EOB-DTPA and Gd-DTPA. *Radiology* 200: 59–67, 1996.

18. Reimer P, Rummeny EJ, Shamsi K, Balzer T, Daldrup HE, Tombach B, Hesse T, Berns T, Peters PE. Phase II clinical evaluation of Gd-EOB-DTPA: dose, safety aspects, and pulse sequence. *Radiology* 199: 177–183, 1996.

19. Reimer P, Rummeny EJ, Daldrup HE, Hesse T, Balzer T, Tombach B, Peters PE. Enhancement characteristics of liver metastases, hepatocellular carcinomas, and hemangiomas with Gd-EOB-DTPA: preliminary results with dynamic MR imaging. *Eur Radiol* 7: 275–280, 1997.

20. Petersein J, Spinazzi A, Giovagnoni A et al. Focal liver lesions: evaluation of the efficacy of gadobenate dimeglumine in MR imaging—a multicenter phase III clinical study. *Radiology* 215: 727–736, 2000.

21. Grazioli L, Morana G, Federle MP et al. Focal nodular hyperplasia: morphologic and functional information from MR imaging with gadobenate dimeglumine. *Radiology* 221: 731–739, 2001.

22. Hagspiel KD, Neidl KF, Eichenberger AC, Weder W, Marincek B. Detection of liver metastases: comparison of superparamagnetic iron oxide-enhanced and unenhanced MR imaging at 1.5 T with dynamic CT, intraoperative US, and percutaneous US. *Radiology* 196: 471–478, 1995.

23. Ros PR, Freeny PC, Marms SE et al. Hepatic MR imaging with ferumoxides: a multicenter clinical trial of the safety and efficacy in the detection of focal hepatic lesions. *Radiology* 196: 481–488, 1995.

24. Yamamoto H, Yamashita Y, Yoshimatsu S, Baba Y, Hatanaka Y, Murakami R, Nishiharu T, Takahashi M, Higashida Y, Moribe N. Hepatocellular carcinoma in cirrhotic livers: detection with unenhanced and iron oxide-enhanced MR imaging. *Radiology* 195: 106–112, 1995.

25. Kumano S, Murakami T, Kim T, Hori M, Okada A, Sugiura T, Noguchi Y, Kawata S, Tomoda K, Nakamura H. Using superparamagnetic iron oxide-enhanced MRI to differentiate metastatic hepatic tumors and nonsolid benign lesions. *AJR Am J Roentgenol* 18: 1335–1339, 2003.

26. Montet X, Lazeyras F, Howarth N, Mentha G, Rubbia-Brandt L, Becker CD, Vallee JP, Terrier F. Specificity of SPIO particles for characterization of liver hemangiomas using MRI. *Abdom Imaging* 29: 60–70, 2004.

27. Mori K, Scheidler J, Helmberger T, Holzknecht N, Schauer R, Schirren CA, Bittmann I, Dugas M, Reiser M. Detection of malignant hepatic lesions before orthotopic liver transplantation: accuracy of ferumoxides-enhanced MR imaging. *AJR Am J Roentgenol* 179: 1045–1051, 2002.

28. Ward J, Guthrie JA, Wilson D, Arnold P, Lodge JP, Toogood GJ, Wyatt JI, Robinson PJ. Colorectal hepatic metastases: detection with SPIO-enhanced breath-hold MR imaging—comparison of optimized sequences. *Radiology* 228: 709–718, 2003.

29. Strotzer M, Gmeinwieser J, Schmidt J, Fellner C, Seitz J, Albrich H, Zirngibl H, Feuerbach S. Diagnosis of liver metastases from colorectal adenocarcinoma. Comparison of spiral-CTAP combined with intravenous contrast-enhanced spiral-CT and SPIO-enhanced MR combined with plain MR imaging. *Acta Radiol* 38: 986–992, 1997.

30. Vogl TJ, Schwarz W, Blume S, Pietsch M, Shamsi K, Franz M, Lobeck H, Balzer T, del Tredici K, Neuhaus P, Felix R, Hammerstingl RM. Preoperative evaluation of malignant liver tumors: comparison of unenhanced and SPIO (Resovist)-enhanced MR imaging with biphasic CTAP and intraoperative US. *Eur Radiol* 13: 262–272, 2003.

31. Ward J, Naik KS, Guthrie JA, Wilson D, Robinson PJ. Hepatic lesion detection: comparison of MR imaging after the administration of superparamagnetic iron oxide with dual-phase CT by using alternative-free response receiver operating characteristic analysis. *Radiology* 210: 459–466, 1999.

32. Reimer P, Jahnke N, Fiebich M, Schima W, Deckers F, Marx C, Holzknecht N, Saini S. Hepatic lesion detection and characterization: value of nonenhanced MR imaging, superparamagnetic iron oxide-enhanced MR imaging, and spiral CT-ROC analysis. *Radiology* 217: 152–158, 2000.

33. Hori M, Murakami T, Kim T, Tsuda K, Takahashi S, Okada A, Takamura M, Nakamura H. Detection of hypervascular hepatocellular carcinoma: comparison of SPIO-enhanced MRI with dynamic helical CT. *J Comput Assist Tomogr* 26: 701–710, 2002.

34. Kang BK, Lim JH, Kim SH, Choi D, Lim HK, Lee WJ, Lee SJ. Preoperative depiction of hepatocellular carcinoma: ferumoxides-enhanced MR imaging versus triple-phase helical CT. *Radiology* 226: 79–85, 2003.

35. Semelka RC, Lee JK, Worawattanakul S, Noone TC, Patt RH, Asher SM. Sequential use of ferumoxide particles and gadolinium chelate for the evaluation of focal liver lesions on MRI. *J Magn Reson Imaging* 8: 670–674, 1998.

36. Saini S, Edelman RR, Sharma P, Li W, Mayo-Smith W, Slater GJ, Eisenberg PJ, Hahn PF. Blood-pool MR contrast material for detection and characterization of focal hepatic lesions: initial clinical experience with ultrasmall superparamagnetic iron oxide (AMI-227). *AJR Am J Roentgenol* 164: 1147–1152, 1995.

37. Weissleder R, Lee AS, Fischman AJ, Reimer P, Shen T, Wilkinson R, Callahan RJ, Brady TJ. Polyclonal human immunoglobulin G labeled with polymeric iron oxide: antibody MR imaging. *Radiology* 181: 245–249, 1991.

38. Vogl TJ, Hammerstingl R, Schwarz W et al. Superparamagnetic iron oxide-enhanced versus gadolinium-enhanced MR imaging for differential diagnosis of focal liver lesions. *Radiology* 198: 881–887, 1996.

39. del Frate C, Bazzocchi M, Mortele KJ, Zuiani C, Londero V, Como G, Zanardi R, Ros PR. Detection of liver metastases: comparison of gadobenate dimeglumine-enhanced and ferumoxides-enhanced MR imaging examinations. *Radiology* 225: 766–772, 2002.

40. Kim SK, Kim SH, Lee WJ, Kim H, Seo JW, Choi D, Lim HK, Lee SJ, Lim JH. Preoperative detection of hepatocellular carcinoma: ferumoxides-enhanced versus mangafodipir trisodium-enhanced MR imaging. *AJR Am J Roentgenol* 179: 741–750, 2002.

41. Kim MJ, Kim JH, Chung JJ, Park MS, Lim JS, Oh YT. Focal hepatic lesions: detection and characterization with combination gadolinium- and superparamagnetic iron oxide-enhanced MR imaging. *Radiology* 2003 228: 719–726, 2003.

42. Kim YK, Kim CS, Lee YH, Kwak HS, Lee JM. Comparison of superparamagnetic iron oxide-enhanced and gadobenate dimeglumine-enhanced dynamic MRI for detection of small hepatocellular carcinomas. *AJR Am J Roentgenol* 182: 1217–1223, 2004.

43. Sherlock S and Dooley J. Anatomy and function. In: Sherlock S. and Dooley J. *Diseases of the Liver and Biliary System.* 10th ed. London, Blackwell Science. 1997. p. 4–5.

44. *Ackerman's Surgical Pathology.* 8th ed. St Louis, Mosby. 1995. p. 898–899.

45. Barnes PA, Thomas JL, Bernardino ME. Pitfalls in the diagnosis of hepatic cysts by computed tomography. *Radiology* 141: 129–133, 1981.

46. Semelka RC, Shoenut JP, Greenberg HM, Mickflickier AB. The liver. In: Semelka RC, Shoenut JP, eds. *MRI of the Abdomen with CT Correlation.* New York, Raven Press, 1993. p. 13–41.

47. Vilgrain V, Silbermann O, Benhamou JP, Nahum H. MR imaging in intracystic hemorrhage of simple hepatic cysts. *Abdom Imaging* 18: 164–167, 1993.

48. Kadoya M, Matsui O, Nakanuma Y, Yoshikawa J, Arai K, Takashima T, Amano M, Kimura M. Ciliated hepatic foregut cyst: radiologic features. *Radiology* 175: 475–477, 1990.

49. Shoenut JP, Semelka RC, Levi C, Greenberg H. Ciliated hepatic foregut cysts: US, CT, and contrast-enhanced MR imaging. *Abdom Imaging* 19: 150–152, 1994.

50. Mosetti MA, Leonardou P, Motohara T, Kanematsu M, Armao D, Semelka RC. Autosomal dominant polycystic kidney disease: MR imaging evaluation using current techniques. *J Magn Reson Imaging* 18(2): 210–215, 2003.

51. Itai Y, Ebihara R, Eguchi N, Saida Y, Kurosaki Y, Minami M, Araki T. Hepatobiliary cysts in patients with autosomal dominant polycystic kidney disease: prevalence and CT findings. *AJR Am J Roentgenol* 164: 339–342, 1995.

52. Semelka RC, Hussain SM, Marcos HB, Woosley JT. Biliary hamartomas: solitary and multiple lesions shown on current MR techniques including gadolinium enhancement. *J Magn Reson Imaging* 10: 196–201, 1999.

53. Powers C, Ros PR, Stoupis C, Johnson WK, Segel KH. Primary liver neoplasms: MR imaging with pathologic correlation. *Radiographics* 14: 459–482, 1994.

54. Choi BI, Lim JH, Han MC, Lee DH, Kim SH, Kim YI, Kim CW. Biliary cystadenoma and cystadenocarcinoma: CT and sonographic findings. *Radiology* 171: 57–61, 1989.

55. Kokubo T, Itai Y, Ohtomo K, Itoh K, Kawauchi N, Minami M. Mucin-hypersecreting intrahepatic biliary neoplasms. *Radiology* 168: 609–614, 1988.

56. Palacios E, Shannon M, Solomon C, Guzman M. Biliary cystadenoma: ultrasound, CT, and MRI. *Gastrointest Radiol* 15: 313–316, 1990.

57. Buetow PC, Buck JL, Pantongrag-Brown L, Ros PR, Devaney K, Goodman ZD, Cruess DF. Biliary cystadenoma and cystadenocarcinoma: clinical-imaging-pathologic correlation with emphasis on the importance of ovarian stroma. *Radiology* 196: 805–810, 1995.

58. Semelka RC. Metastatic liver tumor: circumferential versus wedge-shaped perilesional enhancement and quantitative image and pathologic correlation. *Radiology* 219: 298–300, 2001. (comment)

59. Aytaç S, Fitoz S, Akyar S, Atasoy Ç, Erekul S. Focal intrahepatic extramedullary hematopoiesis: color Doppler US and CT findings. *Abdom Imaging* 24: 366–368, 1999.

60. Navarro M, Crespo C, Perez L, Martinez C, Galant J, Gonzalez I. Massive intrahepatic extramedullary hematopoiesis in myelofibrosis. *Abdom Imaging* 25: 184–186, 2000.

61. Nonomura A, Mizukami Y, Cadoya M. Angiomyolipoma of the liver: a collective review. *J Gastroenterol.* 29(1): 95–105, 1994.

62. Worawattanakul S, Kelekis NL, Semelka RC, Woosley JT. Hepatic angiomyolipoma with minimal fat content: MR demonstration. *Magn Reson Imaging* 14: 687–689, 1996.

63. Morton KM, Bluemke DA, Hruban RH, Soyer P, Fishman EK. CT and MR imaging of benign hepatic and biliary tumors. *Radiographics* 19: 431–451, 1999.

64. Craig J, Peters R, Edmondson H. Tumors of the liver and intrahepatic bile ducts. In Hartman H, Sobin L. eds. *Atlas of Tumor Pathology.* 2nd ed. Washington, DC: Armed Forces Institute of Pathology, 1989.

65. Karhunen PJ. Benign hepatic tumours and tumour like conditions in men. *J Clin Pathol* 39: 183–188, 1986.

66. Mitsuodo K, Watanabe Y, Saga T et al. Nonenhanced hepatic cavernous hemangioma with multiple calcifications: CT and pathologic correlation. *Abdom Imaging* 20: 459–461, 1995.

67. Li KC, Glazer GM, Quint LE, Francis IR, Aisen AM, Ensminger WD, Bookstein FL. Distinction of hepatic cavernous hemangioma from hepatic metastases with MR imaging. *Radiology* 169: 409–415, 1988.

68. Lombardo DM, Baker ME, Spritzer CE, Blinder R, Meyers W, Herfkens RJ. Hepatic hemangiomas vs. metastases: MR differentiation at 1.5 T. *AJR Am J Roentgenol* 155: 55–59, 1990.

69. Semelka RC, Shoenut JP, Kroeker MA, Greenberg HM, Simm FC, Minuk GY, Kroeker RM, Micflikier AB. Focal liver disease: comparison of dynamic contrast-enhanced CT and T2-weighted fat-suppressed, FLASH, and dynamic gadolinium-enhanced MR imaging at 1.5 T. *Radiology* 184: 687–694, 1992.

70. Schmiedl U, Kolbel G, Hess CF, Klose U, Kurtz B. Dynamic sequential MR imaging of focal liver lesions: initial experience in 22 patients at 1.5 T. *J Comput Assist Tomogr* 14: 600–607, 1990.

71. Quinn SF and Benjamin GG. Hepatic cavernous hemangiomas: simple diagnostic sign with dynamic bolus CT. *Radiology* 182: 545–548, 1992.

72. Low RN. MRI of the liver using gadolinium chelates. *Magn Reson Imaging Clin N Am.* 9(4): 717–743, 2001.

73. Semelka RC, Brown ED, Ascher SM, Patt RH, Bagley AS, Li W, Edelman RR, Shoenut JP, Brown JJ. Hepatic hemangiomas: a multi-institutional study of appearance on T2-weighted and serial gadolinium-enhanced gradient-echo MR images. *Radiology* 192: 401–406, 1994.

74. Choi BI, Han MC, Park JH, Kim SH, Han MH, Kim CW. Giant cavernous hemangioma of the liver: CT and MR imaging in 10 cases. *AJR Am J Roentgenol* 152: 1221–1226, 1989.

75. Danet IM, Semelka RC, Braga L, Armao D, Woosley JT. Giant hemangioma of the liver: MR imaging characteristics in 24 patients. *Magn Reson Imaging* 21: 95–101, 2003.

76. Semelka RC and Sofka CM. Hepatic hemangiomas. *Magn Reson Imaging Clin N Am* 5(2): 241–253, 1997.

77. Jeong MG, Yu JS, Kim KW. Hepatic cavernous hemangioma: Temporal peritumoral enhancement during multiphase dynamic MR imaging. *Radiology* 216: 692–697, 2000.

78. Wanless IR, Albrecht S, Bilbao J, Frei JV, Heathcote EJ, Roberts EA, Chiasson D. Multiple focal nodular hyperplasia of the liver associated with vascular malformations of various organs and neoplasia of the brain: a new syndrome. *Mod Pathol* 2: 456–462, 1989.

79. Noone TC, Semelka RC, Balci NC, Graham ML. Common occurrence of benign liver lesions in patients with newly diagnosed breast cancer investigated by MRI for suspected liver metastases. *J Magn Reson Imaging* 10: 165–169, 1999.

80. McFarland EG, Mayo-Smith WW, Saini S, Hahn PF, Goldberg MA, Lee MJ. Hepatic hemangiomas and malignant tumors: improved differentiation with heavily T2-weighted conventional spin-echo MR imaging. *Radiology* 193: 43–47, 1994.

81. Hamm B, Thoeni RF, Gould RG, Bernardino ME, Luning M, Saini S, Mahfouz AE, Taupitz M, Wolf KJ. Focal liver lesions: characterization with nonenhanced and dynamic contrast material-enhanced MR imaging. *Radiology* 190: 417–423, 1994.

82. Burdeny DA, Semelka RC, Kelekis NL, Kettritz U, Woosley JT, Cance WG, Lee JKT. Chemotherapy treated liver metastases mimicking hemangiomas on MR images. *Abdom Imag* 24: 378–382, 1999.

83. Dodd GD 3rd, Baron RL, Oliver JH 3rd, Federle MP. Spectrum of imaging findings of the liver in end-stage cirrhosis: Part II, focal abnormalities. *AJR Am J Roentgenol* 173: 1185–1192, 1999.

84. Mastropasqua M, Kanematsu M, Leonardou P, Braga L, Woosley JT, Semelka RC. Cavernous hemangiomas in patients with chronic liver disease: MR imaging findings. *Magn Reson Imaging* 22: 15–18, 2004.

85. Brancatelli G, Federle MP, Blachar A, Grazioli L. Hemangioma in the cirrhotic liver: diagnosis and natural history. *Radiology* 219(1): 69–74, 2001.

86. Siegel MJ. MR imaging of pediatric abdominal neoplasms. *Magn Reson Imaging Clin N Am* 8: 837–851, 2000.

87. Klatskin G, Conn HO. Neoplasms of the liver and intrahepatic bile ducts. *Histopathology of the Liver.* New York, Oxford University Press, 1993. chapter 25, p. 368–370.

88. Buetow PC, Rao P, Marshall H. Imaging of pediatric liver tumors. *Magn Reson Imaging Clin N Am* 5(2): 397–413, 1997.

89. Carneiro RC, Fordham LA, Semelka RC. MR imaging of the pediatric liver. *Magn Reson Imaging Clin N Am* 10(1): 137–164, 2002.

90. Gonzalez A, Canga F, Cardenas F, Castellano G, Garcia H, Cuenca B et al. An unusual case of hepatic adenoma in a male. *J Clin Gastroenterol* 19(2): 179–181, 1994.

91. Kerlin P, Davis GL, McGill DB, Weiland LH, Adson MA, Sheedy PFD. Hepatic adenoma and focal nodular hyperplasia: clinical, pathologic, and radiologic features. *Gastroenterology* 84: 994–1002, 1983.

92. Shortell CK and Schwartz SI. Hepatic adenoma and focal nodular hyperplasia. *Surg Gynecol Obstet* 173: 426–431, 1991.

93. International Working Party: Terminology of nodular hepatocellular lesions. International Working Party. *Hepatology* 22: 983–993, 1995.

94. Meissner K. Hemorrhage caused by ruptured liver cell adenoma following long-term oral contraceptives: a case report. *Hepato-gastroenterology* 45(19): 224–225, 1998.

95. Foster JH, Berman MM. The malignant transformation of liver cell adenomas. *Arch Surg* 129(7): 712–717, 1994.

96. Paulson EK, McClellan JS, Washington K, Spritzer CE, Meyers WC, Baker ME. Hepatic adenoma: MR characteristics and correlation with pathologic findings. *AJR Am J Roentgenol* 163: 113–116, 1994.

97. Arrive L, Flejou JF, Vilgrain V, Belghiti J, Najmark D, Zins M, Menu Y, Tubiana JM, Nahum H. Hepatic adenoma: MR findings in 51 pathologically proved lesions. *Radiology* 193: 507–512, 1994.

98. Psatha EA, Semelka RC, Armao D, Woosley JT, Firat Z, Schneider G. Hepatocellular adenomas in men: MRI findings in four patients. *J Magn Reson Imaging* 22: 258–264, 2005.

99. Hamm B, Vogl TJ, Branding G, Schnell B, Taupitz M, Wolf KJ, Lissner J. Focal liver lesions: MR imaging with Mn-DPDP-initial clinical results in 40 patients. *Radiology* 182: 167–174, 1992.

100. Coffin CM, Diche T, Mahfouz A, Alexandre M, Caseiro-Alves F, Rahmouni A, Vasile N, Mathieu D. Benign and malignant hepatocellular tumors: evaluation of tumoral enhancement after mangafodipir trisodium injection on MR imaging. *Eur Radiol* 19(3): 444–449, 1999.

101. Flejou JF, Barge J, Menu Y et al. Liver adenomatosis: an entity distinct from liver adenoma? *Gastroenterology* 83: 1132–1138, 1985.

102. Grazioli L, Federle MP, Ichikawa T, Balzano E, Nalesnik M, Madariaga J. Liver adenomatosis: clinical, histopathologic, and imaging findings in 15 patients. *Radiology* 216: 395–402, 2000.

103. Bader TR, Braga L, Semelka RC. Exophytic benign tumors of the liver: appearance on MRI. *Magn Reson Imaging* 19: 623–628, 2001.

104. Balci NC, Sirvanci M, Duran C, Akinci A. Hepatic adenomatosis: MRI demonstration with the use of superparamagnetic iron oxide. *Clin Imaging* 26: 35–38, 2002.

105. DeLeve LD. Vascular liver diseases. *Curr Gastroenterol Rep* 5(1): 63–70, 2003.

106. Scheuer PJ, Schachter LA, Mathur S, Burroughs AK, Rolles K. Peliosis hepatitis after liver transplantation. *J Clin Pathol* 43(12): 1036–1037, 1990.

107. Verswijvel G, Janssens F, Colla P, Mampaey S, Verhelst H, Van Eycken P et al. Peliosis hepatis presenting as a multifocal hepatic pseudotumor: MR findings in two cases. *Eur Radiol* 13 *Suppl* 4: L40–L44, 2003.

108. Steinke K, Terraciano L, Wiesner W. Unusual cross-sectional imaging findings in hepatic peliosis. *Eur Radiol* 13(8): 1916–9, 2003.

109. Gouya H, Vignaux O, Legmann P, de Pigneux G, Bonnin A. Peliosis hepatis: triphasic helical CT and dynamic MRI findings. *Abdom Imaging* 26(5): 507–509, 2001.

110. Yekeler E, Dursun M, Tunaci A, Cevikbas U, Rozanes I. Diagnosing of peliosis hepatis by magnetic resonance imaging. *J Hepatol* 41(2): 351, 2004.

111. Ferrozzi F, Tognini G, Zuccoli G, Cademartiri F, Pavone P. Peliosis hepatis with pseudotumoral and hemorrhagic evolution: CT and MR findings. *Abdom Imaging* 26(2): 197–199, 2001.

112. Wanless IR, Mawdsley C, Adams R. On the pathogenesis of focal nodular hyperplasia of the liver. *Hepatology* 5(6): 1194–1200, 1985.

113. Mathieu D, Vilgrain V, Mahfouz AE, Anglade MC, Vullierme MP, Denys A. Benign liver tumor. *Magn Reson Imaging Clin N Am* 5(2): 255–288, 1997.

114. Mortelé KJ, Praet M, Vlierberghe HV, Kunnen M, Ros PR. CT and MR imaging findings in focal nodular hyperplasia of the liver: radiologic- Pathologic correlation. *AJR Am J Roentgenol* 175: 687–692, 2000.

115. Attal P, Vilgrain V, Brancatelli G, Paradis V, Terris B, Belghiti J, Taouli B, Menu Y. Telangiectatic focal nodular hyperplasia: US, CT, and MR imaging findings with histopathologic correlation in 13 cases. *Radiology* 228: 465–472, 2003.

116. Ferlicot S, Kobeiter H, Tran Van Nhieu J, Cherqui D, Dhumeaux D, Mathieu D, Zafrani ES. MRI of atypical focal nodular hyperplasia of the liver: Radiology-pathology correlation. *AJR Am J Roentgenol* 182: 1227–1231, 2004.

117. Lee MJ, Saini S, Hamm B, Taupitz M, Hahn PF, Seneterre E, Ferrucci JT. Focal nodular hyperplasia of the liver: MR findings in 35 proved cases. *AJR Am J Roentgenol* 156: 317–320, 1991.

118. Vilgrain V, Flejou JF, Arrive L, Belghiti J, Najmark D, Menu Y, Zins M, Vullierme MP, Nahum H. Focal nodular hyperplasia of the liver: MR imaging and pathologic correlation in 37 patients. *Radiology* 184: 699–703, 1992.

119. Schiebler ML, Kressel HY, Saul SH, Yeager BA, Axel L, Gefter WB. MR imaging of focal nodular hyperplasia of the liver. *J Comput Assist Tomogr* 11: 651–654, 1987.

120. Haggar AM, Bree RL. Hepatic focal nodular hyperplasia: MR imaging at 1.0 and 1.5T. *J Magn Reson Imaging* 2: 85–88, 1992.

121. Mahfouz AE, Hamm B, Taupitz M, Wolf KJ. Hypervascular liver lesions: differentiation of focal nodular hyperplasia from malignant tumors with dynamic gadolinium-enhanced MR imaging. *Radiology* 186: 133–138, 1993.

122. Eisenberg LB, Warshauer DM, Woosley JT, Cance WG, Bunzendahl H, Semelka RC. CT and MRI of hepatic focal nodular hyperplasia with peripheral steatosis. *J Comput Assist Tomogr* 19: 498–500, 1995.

123. Hamm B, Vogl TJ, Branding G, Schnell B, Taupitz M, Wolf KJ, Lissner J. Focal liver lesions: MR imaging with Mn-DPDP-initial clinical results in 40 patients. *Radiology* 182: 167–174, 1992.

124. Vogl TJ, Hamm B, Schnell B, McMahon C, Branding G, Lissner J, Wolf KJ. Mn-DPDP enhancement patterns of hepatocellular lesions on MR images. *J Magn Reson Imaging* 3: 51–58, 1993.

125. Grazioli L, Morana G, Federle MP et al. Focal nodular hyperplasia: morphologic and functional information from MR imaging with gadobenate dimeglumine. *Radiology* 221: 731–739, 2001.

126. Rummeny EJ, Wernecke K, Saini S, Vassallo P, Wiesmann W, Oestmann JW, Kivelitz D, Reers B, Reiser MF, Peters PE. Comparison between high-field-strength MR imaging and CT for screening of hepatic metastases: a receiver operating characteristic analysis. *Radiology* 182: 879–886, 1992.

127. Nelson RC, Chezmar JL, Sugarbaker PH, Murray DR, Bernardino ME. Preoperative localization of focal liver lesions to specific liver segments: utility of CT during arterial portography. *Radiology* 176: 89–94, 1990.

128. Sugarbaker PH and Kemeny N. Management of metastatic cancer to the liver. *Adv Surg* 22: 1–56, 1989.

129. Hughes KS, Rosenstein RB, Songhorabodi S, Adson MA, Ilstrup DM, Fortner JG, Maclean BJ, Foster JH, Daly JM, Fitzherbert D et al. Resection of the liver for colorectal carcinoma metastases: a multi-institutional study of long-term survivors. *Dis Colon Rectum* 31: 1–4, 1988.

130. Semelka RC, Hricak H, Bis KG, Werthmuller WC, Higgins CB. Liver lesion detection: comparison between excitation-spoiling fat suppression and regular spin-echo at 1.5T. *Abdom Imaging* 18: 56–60, 1993.

131. De Lange EE, Mugler JP III, Bosworth JE, DeAngelis GA, Gay SB, Hurt NS, Berr SS, Rosenblatt JM, Merickel LW, Harris EK. MR imaging of the liver: breath-hold T1-weighted MP-GRE compared with conventional T2-weighted SE imaging-lesion detection, localization, and characterization. *Radiology* 190: 727–736, 1994.

132. Larson RE, Semelka RC, Bagley AS, Molina PL, Brown ED, Lee JK. Hypervascular malignant liver lesions: comparison of various MR imaging pulse sequences and dynamic CT. *Radiology* 192: 393–399, 1994.

133. Semelka RC, Shoenut JP, Ascher SM, Kroeker MA, Greenberg HM, Yaffe CS, Micflikier AB. Solitary hepatic metastasis: comparison of dynamic contrast-enhanced CT and MR imaging with fat-suppressed T2-weighted, breath-hold T1-weighted FLASH, and dynamic gadolinium-enhanced FLASH sequences. *J Magn Reson Imaging* 4: 319–323, 1994.

134. Stark DD, Wittenberg J, Butch RJ, Ferrucci JT Jr. Hepatic metastases: randomized, controlled comparison of detection with MR imaging and CT. *Radiology* 165: 399–406, 1987.

135. Zeman RK, Dritschilo A, Silverman PM, Clark LR, Garra BS, Thomas DS, Ahlgren JD, Smith FP, Korec SM, Nauta RJ et al. Dynamic CT vs. 0.5T MR imaging in the detection of surgically proven hepatic metastases. *J Comput Assist Tomogr* 13: 637–644, 1989.

136. Balci NC, Semelka RC, Altun E. Fundamentals of MR imaging techniques applied to the abdomen and pelvis. *Applied Radiology* 35: 30–35, 2006.

137. Semelka RC, Worawattanakul S, Kelekis NL, John G, Woosley JT, Graham M, Cance WG. Liver lesion detection and characterization. Comparison of single-phase spiral CT and current MR techniques. *J Magn Reson Imaging* 7(6): 1040–1047, 1997.

138. Semelka RC, Martin DR, Balci Cem, Lance T. Focal liver lesions: comparison of dual phase CT and multisequence multiplanar MR imaging including dynamic gadolinium enhancement. *J Magn Reson Imaging* 13: 397–401, 2001.

139. Semelka RC, Unal B, Altun E. MRI and treatment response. *Imaging Economics* 2006 October Issue.

140. Semelka RC, Cance WG, Marcos HB, Mauro MA. Liver metastases: comparison of current MR techniques and spiral CT during arterial portography for detection in 20 surgically staged cases. *Radiology* 213: 86–91, 1999.

141. Danet IM, Semelka RC, Leonardou P, Braga L, Vaidean G, Woosley JT, Kanematsu M. Spectrum of MRI appearances of untreated metastases of the liver. *AJR Am J Roentgenol* 181(3): 809–817, 2003.

142. Braga L, Semelka RC, Pietrobon R, Martin D, de Barros N, Guller U. Does hypervascularity of liver metastases as detected on MRI predict disease progression in breast cancer patients? *AJR Am J Roentgenol* 182(5): 1207–1213, 2004

143. Larson RE, Semelka RC, Bagley AS, Molina PL, Brown ED, Lee JK. Hypervascular malignant liver lesions: comparison of various MR imaging pulse sequences and dynamic CT. *Radiology* 192: 393–399, 1994.

144. Semelka RC, Cumming MJ, Shoenut JP, Magro CM, Yaffe CS, Kroeker MA, Greenberg HM. Islet cell tumors: comparison of dynamic contrast-enhanced CT and MR imaging with dynamic gadolinium enhancement and fat suppression. *Radiology* 186: 799–802, 1993.

145. Mahfouz AE, Hamm B, Wolf KJ. Peripheral washout: a sign of malignancy on dynamic gadolinium-enhanced MR images of focal liver lesions. *Radiology* 190: 49–52, 1994.

146. Silva AC, Evans JM, McCullough AE, Jatoi MA, Vargas HE, Hara AK. MR imaging of hypervascular liver masses: a review of current techniques. *Radiographics* 29: 385–402, 2009.

147. Outwater E, Tomaszewski JE, Daly JM, Kressel HY. Hepatic colorectal metastases: correlation of MR imaging and pathologic appearance. *Radiology* 180(2): 327–32, 1991.

148. Muramatsu Y, Nawano S, Takayasu K, Moriyama N, Yamada T, Yamasaki S, Hirohashi S. Early hepatocellular carcinoma: MR imaging. *Radiology* 181: 209–213, 1991.

149. Gabata T, Matsui O, Kadoya M, Yoshikawa J, Ueda K, Kawamori Y et al. Delayed MR imaging of the liver: correlation of delayed enhancement of hepatic tumors and pathologic appearance. *Abdom Imaging* 23(3): 309–13, 1998.

150. Larson RE, Semelka RC. Magnetic resonance imaging of the liver. *Top Magn Reson Imaging* 7(2): 71–81, 1995.

151. Semelka RC, Hussain SM, Marcos HB, Woosley JT. Perilesional enhancement of hepatic metastases: correlation between MR imaging and histopathologic findings: initial observations. *Radiology* 215: 89–94, 2000.

152. Danet IM, Semelka RC, Nagase LL, Woosely JT, Leonardou P, Armao D. Liver metastases from pancreatic adenocarcinoma: MR imaging characteristics. *J Magn Reson Imaging.* 18(2): 181–188, 2003.

153. Terayama N, Matsui O, Ueda K, Kobayashi S, Sanada J, Gabata T, et al. Peritumoral rim enhancement of liver metastasis: hemodynamics observed on single-level dynamic CT during hepatic arteriography and histopathologic correlation. *J Comput Assist Tomogr* 26(6): 975–980, 2002.

154. Semelka RC, Bagley AS, Brown ED, Kroeker MA. Malignant lesions of the liver identified on T1- but not T2-weighted MR images at 1.5 T. *J Magn Reson Imaging* 4: 315–318, 1994.

155. Pedro MS, Semelka RC, Braga L. MR imaging of hepatic metastases. *Magn Reson Imaging Clin N Am.* 10(1): 15–29, 2002.

156. Outwater E, Tomaszewski JE, Daly JM, Kressel HY. Hepatic colorectal metastases: correlation of MR imaging and pathologic appearance. *Radiology* 180: 327–332, 1991.

157. Braga L, Semelka RC, Danet IM, Venkataraman S, Woosley JT. Liver metastases from unknown primary site: demonstration on MR images. *Magn Reson Imaging.* 21(8): 871–877, 2003.

158. Bader TR, Semelka RC, Chiu VC, Armao DM, Woosley JT. MRI of carcinoid tumors: spectrum of appearances in the gastrointestinal tract and liver. *J Magn Reson Imaging* 14(3): 261–269, 2001.

159. Soyer P, Riopel M, Bluemke DA, Scherrer A. Hepatic metastases from leiomyosarcoma: MR features with histopathologic correlation. *Abdom Imaging* 22(1): 67–71, 1997.

160. Jones EC, Chezmar JL, Nelson RC, Bernardino ME. The frequency and significance of small (less than or equal to 15 mm) hepatic lesions detected by CT. *AJR Am J Roentgenol* 158: 535–539, 1992.

161. Bruneton JN, Raffaelli C, Maestro C, Padovani B. Benign liver lesions: implications of detection in cancer patients. *Eur Radiol* 5: 387–390, 1995.

162. Mathieu D, Vilgrain V, Mahfouz AE, Anglade MC, Vullierme MP, Denys A. Benign liver tumor. *Magn Reson Imaging Clin N Am* 5(2): 255–288, 1997.

163. Trump DL, Fahnestock R, Cloutier CT, Dickman MD. Anaerobic liver abscess and intrahepatic metastases- a case report and review of the literature. *Cancer* 41(2): 682–686, 1978.

164. Eckel F, Lersch C, Huber W, Weiss W, Berger H, Schulte-Frohlinde E. Multimicrobial sepsis including clostridium perfringens after chemoembolization of a single liver metastases from common bile duct cancer. *Digestion* 62: 208–212, 2000.

165. Taouli B, Losada M, Holland A, Krinsky G. Magnetic resonance imaging of hepatocellular carcinoma. *Gastroenterology* 127(5 *Suppl* 1): S144–S152, 2004.

166. Fung J, Marsh W. The quandary over liver transplantation for hepatocellular carcinoma: the greater sin? *Liver Transpl* 8(9): 775–777, 2002.

167. El-Serag HB, Mason AC. Rising incidence of hepatocellular carcinoma in the United States. *N Engl J Med* 340(10): 745–750, 1999.

168. Yuen MF, Cheng CC, Lauder IJ, Lam SK, Ooi CG, Lai CL. Early detection of hepatocellular carcinoma increases the chance of treatment: Hong Kong experience. *Hepatology* 31(2): 330–335, 2000.

169. Hytiroglou P. Morphological changes of early human hepatocarcinogenesis. *Semin Liver Dis* 24(1): 65–75, 2004.

170. Ahn J, Flamm SL. Hepatocellular carcinoma. *Dis Mon* 50(10): 556–573, 2004.

171. Kerr M. Increase of liver cancer rate outpaces all other cancers. *Internal Medicine News*, 2005. p.72

172. Mastropasqua, M, Braga L, Kanematsu M, Vaidean G, Shrestha R, Polytimi L, Firat Z, Woosley JT, Semelka RC. Hepatic nodules in liver transplantation candidates: MR imaging and underlying hepatic disease. *Magn Reson Imaging* 23: 557–562, 2005.

173. Ahn J, Flamm SL. Hepatocellular carcinoma. *Dis Mon* 50(10): 556–573, 2004.

174. Miller WJ, Baron RL, Dodd GD III, Federle MP. Malignancies in patients with cirrhosis: CT sensitivity and specificity in 200 consecutive transplant patients. *Radiology* 193: 645–650, 1994.

175. Oi H, Murakami T, Kim T, Matsushita M, Kishimoto H, Nakamura H. Dynamic MR imaging and early-phase helical CT for detecting small intrahepatic metastases of hepatocellular carcinoma. *AJR Am J Roentgen* 166: 369–374, 1996.

176. Yamashita Y, Mitsuzaki K, Yi T, Ogata I, Nishiharu T, Urata J, Takahashi M. Small heptacellular carcinoma in patients with chronic liver damage: prospective comparison of detection with dynamic MR imaging and helical CT of the whole liver. *Radiology* 200: 79–84, 1996.

177. Yu JS, Kim KW, Lee JT, Yoo HS. MR imaging during arterial portography for assessment of hepatocellular carcinoma: comparison with CT during arterial portography. *AJR Am J Roentgenol* 170: 1501–1506, 1998.

178. Lim JH, Kim CK, Lee WJ, Park CK, Koh KC, Paik SW, Joh JW. Detection of hepatocellular carcinomas and dysplastic nodules in cirrhotic livers: accuracy of helical CT in transplant patients. *AJR Am J Roentgenol* 175(3): 693–698, 2000.

179. Valls C, Cos M, Figueras J, Andia E, Ramos E, Sanchez A, Serrano T, Torras J. Pretransplantation diagnosis and staging of hepatocellular carcinoma in patients with cirrhosis: value of dual-phase helical CT. *AJR Am J Roentgenol* 182(4): 1011–1007, 2004.

180. Ebara M, Watanabe S, Kita K, Yoshikawa M, Sugiura N, Ohto M, Kondo F, Kondo Y. MR imaging of small hepatocellular carcinoma: effect of intratumoral copper content on signal intensity. *Radiology* 180: 617–621, 1991.

181. Yamashita Y, Fan ZM, Yamamoto H, Matsukawa T, Yoshimatsu S, Miyazaki T, Sumi M, Harada M, Takahashi M. Spin-echo and dynamic gadolinium-enhanced FLASH MR imaging of hepatocellular carcinoma: correlation with histopathologic findings. *J Magn Reson Imaging* 4: 83–90, 1994.

182. Yasemin M K-B, Braga L, Birchard KR, Gerber D, Firat Z, Woosley JT, Shrestha R, Semelka R. Hepatocellular carcinoma missed on gadolinium enhanced MR imaging, discovered in liver explants: retrospective evaluation. *J Magn Reson Imaging* 23: 210–205, 2006.

183. Kelekis NL, Semelka RC, Worawattanakul S, de Lange EE, Ascher SM, Ahn IO, Reinhold C, Remer EM, Brown JJ, Bis KG, Woosley JT, Mitchell DG. Hepatocellular carcinoma in North America: a

multiinstitutional study of appearance on T1-weighted, T2-weighted, and serial gadolinium-enhanced gradient-echo images. *AJR Am J Roentgenol* 170: 1005–1013, 1998.

184. Hirai K, Aoki Y, Majima Y, Abe H, Nakashima O, Kojiro M, Tanikawa K. Magnetic resonance imaging of small hepatocellular carcinoma. *Am J Gastroenterol* 86: 205–209, 1991.

185. Kadoya M, Matsui O, Takashima T, Nonomura A. Hepatocellular carcinoma: correlation of MR imaging and histopathologic findings. *Radiology* 183: 819–825, 1992.

186. Muramatsu Y, Nawano S, Takayasu K, Moriyama N, Yamada T, Yamasaki S, Hirohashi S. Early hepatocellular carcinoma: MR imaging. *Radiology* 181: 209–213, 1991.

187. Earls JP, Theise ND, Weinreb JC, DeCorato DR, Krinsky GA, Rofsky NM, et al. Dysplastic nodules and hepatocellular carcinoma: thin-section MR imaging of explanted cirrhotic livers with pathologic correlation. *Radiology* 201(1): 207–214, 1996.

188. Ebara M, Fukuda H, Kojima Y, Morimoto N, Yoshikawa M, Sugiura N, Satoh T, Kondo F, Yukawa M, Matsumoto T, Saisho H. Small hepatocellular carcinoma: relationship of signal intensity to histopathologic findings and metal content of the tumor and surrounding hepatic parenchyma. *Radiology* 210(1): 81–88, 1999.

189. Kelekis NL, Semelka RC, Woosley JT. Malignant lesions of the liver with high signal intensity on T1-weighted MR images. *J Magn Reson Imaging* 6: 291–294, 1996.

190. Jeong YY, Mitchell DG, Kamishima T. Small (<20 mm) enhancing hepatic nodules seen on arterial phase MR imaging of the cirrhotic liver: clinical implications. *AJR Am J Roentgenol* 178(6): 1327–1334, 2002.

191. Shimizu A, Ito K, Koike S, Fujita T, Shimizu K, Matsunaga N. Cirrhosis or chronic hepatitis: evaluation of small (< or = 2-cm) early-enhancing hepatic lesions with serial contrast-enhanced dynamic MR imaging. *Radiology* 226(2): 550–555, 2003.

192. Peterson MS, Baron RL, Murakami T. Hepatic malignancies: usefulness of acquisition of multiple arterial and portal venous phase images at dynamic gadolinium-enhanced MR imaging. *Radiology* 201: 337–345, 1996.

193. Rummeny E, Weissleder R, Stark DD, Saini S, Compton CC, Bennett W, Hahn PF, Wittenberg J, Malt RA, Ferrucci JT. Primary liver tumors: diagnosis by MR imaging. *AJR Am J Roentgenol* 152: 63–72, 1989.

194. Matsui O, Kadoya M, Kameyama T, Yoshikawa J, Arai K, Gabata T, Takashima T, Nakanuma Y, Terada T, Ida M. Adenomatous hyperplastic nodules in the cirrhotic liver: differentiation from hepatocellular carcinoma with MR imaging. *Radiology* 173: 123–126, 1989.

195. Rosenthal RE, Davis PL. MR imaging of hepatocellular carcinoma at 1.5 tesla. *Gastrointest Radiol* 17: 49–52, 1992.

196. Itoh K, Nishimura K, Togashi K, Fujisawa I, Noma S, Minami S, Sagoh T, Nakano Y, Itoh H, Mori K et al. Hepatocellular carcinoma: MR imaging. *Radiology* 164: 21–25, 1987.

197. Mahfouz AE, Hamm B, Wolf KJ. Dynamic gadopentetate dimeglumine-enhanced MR imaging of hepatocellular carcinoma. *Eur Radiol* 3: 453–458, 1993.

198. Yoshida H, Itai Y, Ohtomo K, Kokubo T, Minami M, Yashiro N. Small hepatocellular carcinoma and cavernous hemangioma: differentiation with dynamic FLASH MR imaging with Gd-DTPA. *Radiology* 171: 339–342, 1989.

199. Yamamoto T, Ikebe T, Mikami S, Shuto T, Hirohashi K, Kinoshita H, Sakurai M. Immunohistochemistry and angiography in adenomatous hyperplasia and small hepatocellular carcinoma. *Pathol Int* 46: 364–371, 1996.

200. Yamamoto T, Hirohashi K, Kaneda K, Ikebe T, Mikami S, Uenishi T, Kanazawa A, Takemura S, Shuto T, Tanaka H, Kubo S, Sakurai M, Kinoshita H. Relationship of the microvascular type to the tumor size, arterialization and dedifferentiation of human hepatocellular carcinoma. *Jpn J Cancer Res* 92: 1207–1213, 2001.

201. Mikami S, Kubo S, Hirohashi K, Shuto T, Kinoshita H, Nakamura K, Yamada R. Computed tomography during arteriography and arterial portography in small hepatocellular carcinoma and dysplastic nodule: a prospective study. *Jpn J Cancer Res* 91: 859–863, 2000.

202. Kanematsu M, Semelka RC, Leonardou P, Mastropasqua M, Armao D, Vaidean G et al. Angiogenesis in hepatocellular nodules: correlation of MR imaging and vascular endothelial growth factor. *J Magn Reson Imaging* 2004;20(3): 426–434.

203. Hussain SM, Semelka RC, Mitchell DG. MR imaging of hepatocellular carcinoma. *Magn Reson Imaging Clin N Am* 10(1): 31–52, 2002.

204. Kadoya M, Matsui O, Takashima T, Nonomura A. Hepatocellular carcinoma: correlation of MR imaging and histopathologic findings. *Radiology* 183(3): 819–825, 1992.

205. Kierans AS, Leonardou P, Hayashi P, Elazazzi M, Shaikh F, Semelka RC. MR imaging findings of rapidly progressive hepatocellular carcinoma (submitted).

206. McKenzie CA, Lim D, Ransil BJ, Morrin M, Pedrosa I, Yeh EN, Sodickson DK, Rofsky NM. Shortening MR image acquisition for volumetric interpolated breath-hold examination with a recently developed parallel imaging reconstruction technique: clinical feasibility. *Radiology* 230: 589–594, 2004.

207. Kanematsu M, Semelka RC, Leonardou P, Mastropasqua M, Lee JK. Hepatocellular carcinoma of diffuse type: MR imaging findings and clinical manifestations. *Magn Reson Imaging* 18(2): 189–195, 2003.

208. Okuda K, Noguchi T, Kubo Y, Shimokawa Y, Kojiro M, Nakashima T. A clinical and pathological study of diffuse type hepatocellular carcinoma. *Liver* 1(4): 280–289, 1981.

209. Craig JR, Peters RL, Edmondson HA, Omata M. Fibrolamellar carcinoma of the liver: a tumor of adolescents and young adults with distinctive clinico-pathologic features. *Cancer* 46: 372–379, 1980.

210. Corrigan K and Semelka RC. Dynamic contrast-enhanced MR imaging of fibrolamellar hepatocellular carcinoma. *Abdom Imaging* 20: 122–125, 1995.

211. Ichikawa T, Federle MP, Grazioli L, Madariaga J, Nalesnik M, Marsh W. Fibrolamellar hepatocellular carcinoma: imaging and pathologic findings in 31 recent cases. *Radiology* 213(2): 352–361, 1999.

212. Scheimberg IB, Pollock DJ, Collins PW, Doran HM, Newland AC, van der Walt JD. Pathology of the liver in leukemia and lymphoma. A study of 110 autopsies. *Histopathology* 26: 311–322, 1995.

213. Kelekis NL, Semelka RC, Siegelman ES, Ascher SM, Outwater EK, Woosley TJ, Reinhold C, Mitchell DG. Focal hepatic lymphoma: MR demonstration using current techniques including gadolinium enhancement. *J Magn Reson Imaging* 15(6): 625–636, 1997.

214. Kelekis NL, Warshauer DM, Semelka RC, Sallah AS. Nodular liver involvement in light chains multiple myeloma: appearance on US and MRI. *Clin Imaging* 21: 207–209, 1997.

215. Anthony PP. Primary carcinoma of the liver: a study of 282 cases in Ugandan Africans. *J Pathol* 110(1):37–48, 1973.

216. Hamrick-Turner J, Abbitt PL, Ros PR. Intrahepatic cholangiocarcinoma: MR appearance. *AJR Am J Roentgenol* 158:77–79, 1992.

217. Low RN, Sigeti JS, Francis IR, Weinman D, Bower B, Shimakawa A, Foo TK. Evaluation of malignant biliary obstruction: efficacy of fast multiplanar spoiled gradient-recalled MR imaging vs. spin-echo MR imaging, CT, and cholangiography. *AJR Am J Roentgenol* 162:315–323, 1994.

218. Buetow PC, Buck JL, Ros PR, Goodman ZD. Malignant vascular tumors of the liver: radiologic-pathologic correlation. *Radiographics* 14:153–166, 1994.

219. Koyama T, Fletcher JG, Johnson CD, Kuo MS, Notohara K, Burgart LJ. Primary hepatic angiosarcoma: findings at CT and MR imaging. *Radiology* 222(3): 667–673, 2002.

220. Worawattanakul S, Semelka RC, Kelekis NL, Woosley JT. Angiosarcoma of the liver: MR imaging pre- and post-chemotherapy. *Magn Reson Imaging* 15(5): 613–617, 1997.

221. Leonardou P, Semelka RC, Kanematsu M, Braga L, Woosley JT. Primary malignant mesothelioma of the liver: MR imaging findings. *Magn Reson Imaging* 21(9): 1091–1093, 2003.

222. Moran CA, Ishak KG, Goodman ZD. Solitary fibrous tumor of the liver: a clinicopathologic and immunohistochemical study of nine cases. *Ann Diagn Pathol* 2(1): 19–24, 1998.

223. Dean PJ, Haggitt RC, O'Hara CJ. Malignant epithelioid hemangioendothelioma of the liver in young women. Relationship to oral contraceptive use. *Am J Surg Pathol* 9(10): 695–704, 1985.

224. Leonardou P, Semelka RC, Mastropasqua M, Kanematsu M, Woosley JT. Epithelioid hemangioendothelioma of the liver. MR imaging findings. *Magn Reson Imaging* 20(8): 631–633, 2002

225. Buetow PC, Rao P, Marshall H. Imaging of pediatric liver tumors. *Magn Reson Imaging Clin N Am* 5(2): 397–413, 1997.

226. Helmberger TK, Ros PR, Mergo PJ, Tomczak R, Reiser MF. Pediatric liver neoplasms: a radiologic-pathologic correlation. *Eur Radiol* 9(7): 1339–1347, 1999.

227. Ros PR, Olmsted WW, Dachman AH, Goodman ZD, Ishak KG, Hartman DS. Undifferentiated (embryonal) sarcoma of the liver: radiologic-pathologic correlation. *Radiology* 161(1): 141–145, 1986.

228. Buetow PC, Buck JL, Pantongrag-Brown L, Marshall WH, Ros PR, Levine MS, Goodman ZD. Undifferentiated (embryonal) sarcoma of the liver: pathologic basis of imaging findings in 28 cases. *Radiology* 203(3): 779–783, 1997.

229. Carneiro RC, Fordham LA, Semelka RC. MR imaging of the pediatric liver. *Magn Reson Imaging Clin N Am* 10(1): 137–164, 2002.

230. Psatha EA, Semelka RC, Fordham L, Firat Z, Woosley JT. Undifferentiated (embryonal) sarcoma of the liver (USL): MRI findings including dynamic gadolinium enhancement. *Magn Reson Imaging* 22(6): 897–900, 2004.

231. Arrive L, Hricak H, Goldberg HI, Thoeni RF, Margulis AR. MR appearance of the liver after partial hepatectomy. *AJR Am J Roentgenol* 152: 1215–1220, 1989.

232. Bartolozzi C, Lencioni R, Caramella D, Falaschi F, Cioni R, DiCoscio G. Hepatocellular carcinoma: CT and MR features after transcatheter arterial embolization and percutaneous ethanol injection. *Radiology* 191: 123–128, 1994.

233. Bartolozzi C, Lencioni R, Caramella D, Mazzeo S, Ciancia EM. Treatment of hepatocellular carcinoma with percutaneous ethanol injection: evaluation with contrast-enhanced MR imaging. *AJR Am J Roentgenol* 162: 827–831, 1994.

234. Giovagnoni A, Paci E, Terilli F, Cellerino R, Piga A. Quantitative MR imaging data in the evaluation of hepatic metastases during systemic chemotherapy. *J Magn Reson Imaging* 5: 27–32, 1995.

235. Lee MJ, Mueller PR, Dawson SL, Gazelle SG, Hahn PF, Goldberg MA, Boland GW. Percutaneous ethanol injection for the treatment of hepatic tumors: indications, mechanism of action, technique, and efficacy. *AJR Am J Roentgenol* 164: 215–220, 1995.

236. Nagel HS and Bernardino ME. Contrast-enhanced MR imaging of hepatic lesions treated with percutaneous ethanol ablation therapy. *Radiology* 189: 265–270, 1993.

237. Sironi S, De Cobelli F, Livraghi T, Villa G, Zanello A, Taccagni G, Del Maschio AL. Small hepatocellular carcinoma treated with percutaneous ethanol injection: unenhanced and gadolinium-enhanced MR imaging follow-up. *Radiology* 192: 407–412, 1994.

238. Shirkhoda A and Baird S. Morphologic changes of the liver following chemotherapy for metastatic breast carcinoma: CT findings. *Abdom Imaging* 19: 39–42, 1994.

239. Soyer P, Bluemke DA, Zeitoun G, Marmuse JP, Levesque MLC. Detection of recurrent hepatic metastases after partial hepatectomy: value of CT combined with arterial portography. *AJR Am J Roentgenol* 162: 1327–1330, 1994.

240. Young ST, Paulson EK, Washington K, Gulliver DJ, Vredenburgh JJ, Baker ME: CT of the liver in patients with metastatic breast carcinoma treated by chemotherapy: findings simulating cirrhosis. *AJR Am J Roentgenol* 163: 1385–1388, 1994.

241. Harned RK, II, Chezmar JL, Nelson RC. Recurrent tumor after resection of hepatic metastases from colorectal carcinoma: location and time of discovery as determined by CT. *AJR Am J Roentgenol* 163: 93–97, 1994.

242. Lang EK, Brown CL Jr. Colorectal metastases to the liver: selective chemoembolization. *Radiology* 189: 417–422, 1993.

243. Scwickert HC, Stiskal M, Roberts TPL, van Dijke CF, Mann J, Muehler A, Shames DM, Demsar F, Disston A, Brasch RC. Contrast-enhanced MR imaging assessment of tumor capillary permeability: effect of irradiation on delivery of chemotherapy. *Radiology* 198: 893–898, 1996.

244. Matsumoto R, Selig AM, Colucci VM, Jolesz FA. MR monitoring during cryotherapy in the liver: predictability of histologic outcome. *J Magn Reson Imaging* 3: 770–776, 1993.

245. Matsumoto R, Oshio K, Jolesz FA. Monitoring of laser and freezing-induced ablation in the liver with T1-weighted MR imaging. *J Magn Reson Imaging* 2: 555–562, 1992.

246. Vogl TJ, Muller PK, Hammerstingl R et al. Malignant liver tumors treated with MR imaging-guided laser-induced thermotherapy: technique and prospective results. *Radiology* 196: 257–265, 1995.

247. Kuszyk BS, Choti MA, Urban BA, Chambers TP, Bluemke DA, Sitzmann JV, Fishman EK. Hepatic tumors treated by cryosurgery: normal CT appearance. *AJR Am J Roentgenol* 166: 363–368, 1996.

248. McLoughlin RF, Saliken JF, McKinnon G, Wiseman D, Temple W. CT of the liver after cryotherapy of hepatic metastases: imaging findings. *AJR Am J Roentgenol* 165: 329–332, 1995.

249. Braga L, Guller U, Semelka, RC. Pre-, peri-, and post-treatment imaging of the liver. *Radiol Clin N Am* 43(5): 915–927, 2005.

250. Braga L, Semelka RC, Pedro MS, de Barros N. Post-treatment malignant liver lesions. MR imaging. *Magn Reson Imaging Clin N Am*. 10(1): 53–73, 2002.

251. Marn CS, Andrews JC, Francis IR, Hollett MD, Walker SC, Ensminger WD. Hepatic parenchymal changes after intraarterial Y-90 therapy: CT findings. *Radiology* 187: 125–128, 1993.

252. Bilimoria MM, Lauwers GY, Doherty DA, Nagorney DM, Belghiti J, Do KA et al. Underlying liver disease, not tumor factors, predicts long-term survival after resection of hepatocellular carcinoma. *Arch Surg* 136(5): 528–535, 2001.

253. Harmon KE, Ryan JA, Jr., Biehl TR, Lee FT. Benefits and safety of hepatic resection for colorectal metastases. *Am J Surg* 177(5): 402–404, 1999.

254. Holbrook RF, Koo K, Ryan JA. Resection of malignant primary liver tumors. *Am J Surg* 171(5): 453–455, 1996.

255. Goshima S, Kanematsu M, Matsuo M, Kondo H, Kako N, Yokoyama R et al. Malignant hepatic tumor detection with ferumoxide-enhanced magnetic resonance imaging: is chemical-shift-selective fat suppression necessary for fast spin-echo sequence? *J Magn Reson Imaging* 20(1): 75–82, 2004.

256. Haran EF, Maretzek AF, Goldberg I, Horowitz A, Degani H. Tamoxifen enhances cell death in implanted MCF7 breast cancer by inhibiting endothelium growth. *Cancer Res.* 54: 5511–5514, 1994.

257. Semelka RC, Worawattanakul S, Mauro M, Bernard SA, Cance WG. Malignant hepatic tumors: changes on MRI after hepatic arterial chemoembolization—preliminary findings. *J Magn Reson Imaging* 8(1): 48–56, 1998.

258. Kierans AS, Elazzazi M, Braga L, Leonardou P, Gerber D, Burke C, Qureshi W, Kanematsu M, Semelka RC. Thermo-ablative focal treatments for malignant liver lesions: 10-year experience of MRI appearances of treatment response. AJR, 2009 (in press).

259. Dromain C, de Baere T, Elias D, Kuoch V, Ducreux M, Boige V et al. Hepatic tumors treated with percutaneous radio-frequency ablation: CT and MR imaging follow-up. *Radiology* 223(1): 255–262, 2002.

260. Goldberg SN, Charboneau JW, Dodd GD 3rd, Dupuy DE, Gervais DA, Gillams AR et al. International Working Group on Image-Guided Tumor Ablation. Image-guided tumor ablation: proposal for standardization of terms and reporting criteria. *Radiology* 228(2): 335–345, 2003.

261. Choi D, Lim HK, Kim MJ, Lee SH, Kim SH, Lee WJ, et al. Recurrent hepatocellular carcinoma: percutaneous radiofrequency ablation after hepatectomy. *Radiology* 230(1): 135–141, 2004.

262. Limanond P, Zimmerman P, Raman SS, Kadell BM, Lu DS. Interpretation of CT and MRI after radiofrequency ablation of hepatic malignancies. *AJR Am J Roentgenol.* 181(6): 1635–1640, 2003.

263. Kuszyk BS, Boitnott JK, Choti MA, Bluemke DA, Sheth S, Magee CA, et al. Local tumor recurrence following hepatic cryoablation: radiologic-histopathologic correlation in a rabbit model. *Radiology* 217(2): 477–486, 2000.

264. Lim HK, Choi D, Lee WJ, Kim SH, Lee SJ, Jang HJ et al. Hepatocellular carcinoma treated with percutaneous radio-frequency ablation: evaluation with follow-up multiphase helical CT. *Radiology* 221(2): 447–454, 2001.

265. Goldberg SN, Gazelle GS, Compton CC, Mueller PR, Tanabe KK. Treatment of intrahepatic malignancy with radiofrequency ablation: radiologic-pathologic correlation. *Cancer* 88(11): 2452–2463, 2000.

266. Chopra S, Dodd GD 3rd, Chanin MP, Chintapalli KN. Radiofrequency ablation of hepatic tumors adjacent to the gallbladder: feasibility and safety. *AJR Am J Roentgenol* 180(3): 697–701, 2003.

267. Joseph FB, Baumgarten DA, Bernardino ME. Hepatocellular carcinoma: CT appearance after percutaneous ethanol ablation therapy. Work in progress. *Radiology* 186(2): 553–556, 1993.

268. Mitsuzaki K, Yamashita Y, Nishiharu T, Sumi S, Matsukawa T, Takahashi M, et al. CT appearance of hepatic tumors after microwave coagulation therapy. *AJR Am J Roentgenol* 171(5): 1397–1403, 1998.

269. Schlund JF, Semelka RC, Kettritz U, Weeks SM, Kahlenberg M, Cance WG. Correlation of perfusion abnormalities on CTAP and immediate postintravenous gadolinium-enhanced gradient echo MRI. *Abdom Imaging* 21(1): 49–52, 1996.

270. Centers for Disease Control, National Center of Health Statistics (NCHS) Vital Statistics System (1998).

271. Bassignani M, Fulcher AS, Szucs RA, Chong WK, Prasad UR, Marcos A. Use of imaging for living donor liver transplantation. *Radiographics* 21: 39–52, 2001.

272. Weisner R, Demetris A, Belle S et al. Acute hepatic allograft rejection: incidence risk factor and impact on outcome. *Hepatology* 28: 638–645,1998.

273. Demetris AJ, Lasky S, Van Thiel DH, Starzl TE, Dekker A. Pathology of hepatic transplantation: a review of 62 adult allograft recipients immunosuppressed with a cyclosporine/steroid regimen. *Am J Pathol* 118: 151–161, 1985.

274. Wozney P, Zajko AB, Bron KM, Point S, Starzl TE. Vascular complications after liver transplantation: a 5-year experience. *AJR Am J Roentgenol* 147: 657–663, 1986.

275. Glockner JF, Forauer AR, Solomon H, Varma CR, Perman WH. Three-dimensional gadolinium-enhanced MR angiography of vascular complications after liver transplantation. *AJR Am J Roentgenol* 174: 1447–1452, 2000.

276. Ito K, Siegelman ES, Stolpen AH, Mitchell DG. MR imaging of complications after liver transplantation. *AJR Am J Roentgenol* 175: 1145–1149, 2000.

277. Stange BJ, Glanemann M, Nuessler NC, Settmacher U, Steinmuller T, Neuhaus P. Hepatic artery thrombosis after adult liver transplantation. *Liver Transpl* 9(6): 612–620, 2003.

278. Stafford-Johnson DB, Hamilton BH, Dong Q, Cho KJ, Turcotte JG, Fontana RJ et al. Vascular complications of liver transplantation: evaluation with gadolinium-enhanced MR angiography. *Radiology* 207(1): 153–160, 1998.

279. Kim BS, Kim TK, Jung DJ, Kim JH, Bae IY, Sung KB, Kim PN, Ha HK, Lee SG, Lee MG. Vascular complications after living related liver transplantation: evaluation with gadolinium-enhanced three-dimensional MR angiography. *AJR Am J Roentgenol* 181: 467–474, 2003.

280. Zajko AB, Bennett MJ, Campbell WL, Koneru B. Mucocele of the cystic duct remnant in eight liver transplant recipients: findings at cholangiography, CT, and US. *Radiology* 177: 691–693, 1990.

281. Lang P, Schnarkowski P, Grampp S, van Dijke C, Gindele A, Steffen R, Neuhaus P, Felix R. Liver transplantation: significance of the periportal collar on MRI. *J Comput Assist Tomogr* 19: 580–585, 1995.

282. Marincek B, Barbier PA, Becker CD, Mettler D, Ruchti C. CT appearance of impaired lymphatic drainage in liver transplants. *AJR Am J Roentgenol* 147: 519–523, 1986.

283. Pickhardt PJ and Siegel MJ. Posttransplantation lymphoproliferative disorders of the abdomen: CT evaluation in 51 patients. *Radiology* 213: 73–78, 1999.

284. Strouse PJ, Platt JF, Francis IR, Bree RL. Tumorous intrahepatic lymphoproliferative disorder in transplanted livers. *AJR Am J Roentgenol* 167: 1159–1162, 1996.

285. Nalesnik MA. The diverse pathology of post-transplant lymphoproliferative disorders: the importance of a standardized approach. *Transpl Infect Dis* 3: 88–96, 2001

286. Matsui O, Kadoya M, Takashima T, Kameyama T, Yoshikawa J, Tamura S. Intrahepatic periportal abnormal intensity on MR images: an indication of various hepatobiliary diseases. *Radiology* 171: 335–338, 1989.

287. Ferris JV, Baron RL, Marsh JW Jr, Oliver JH 3rd, Carr BI, Dodd GD 3rd. Recurrent hepatocellular carcinoma after liver transplantation: spectrum of CT findings and recurrence patterns. *Radiology* 198: 233–238, 1996.

288. Mieli-Vergani G, Vergani D. Autoimmune liver disease. *Indian J Pediatr* 69(1): 93–98, 2002.

289. Feld JJ, Heathcote EJ. Epidemiology of autoimmune liver disease. *J Gastroenterol Hepatol* 18(10): 1118–1128, 2003.

290. Lee YM, Kaplan MM. Primary sclerosing cholangitis. *N Engl J Med* 332(14): 924–933, 1999.

291. Burak K, Angulo P, Pasha TM, Egan K, Petz J, Lindor KD. Incidence and risk factors for cholangiocarcinoma in primary sclerosing cholangitis. *Am J Gastroenterol* 99(3): 523–526, 2004.

292. Bader TR, Beavers KL, Semelka RC. MR imaging features of primary sclerosing cholangitis: patterns of cirrhosis in relationship to clinical severity of disease. *Radiology* 226(3): 675–685, 2003.

293. Dodd GD 3rd, Baron RL, Oliver JH 3rd, Federle MP. End-stage primary sclerosing cholangitis: CT findings of hepatic morphology in 36 patients. *Radiology* 211(2): 357–362, 1999.

294. Ito K, Mitchell DG, Outwater EK, Blasbalg R. Primary sclerosing cholangitis: MR imaging features. *AJR Am J Roentgenol* 172(6): 1527–1533, 1999.

295. Revelon G, Rashid A, Kawamoto S, Bluemke DA. Primary sclerosing cholangitis: MR imaging findings with pathologic correlation. *AJR Am J Roentgenol* 173(4): 1037–1042, 1999.

296. Vergani D, Alvarez F, Bianchi FB, Cancado EL, Mackay IR, Manns MP et al. Liver autoimmune serology: a consensus statement from the committee for autoimmune serology of the International Autoimmune Hepatitis Group. *J Hepatol* 41(4): 677–683, 2004.

297. Ben-Ari Z, Czaja AJ. Autoimmune hepatitis and its variant syndromes. *Gut* 49(4): 589–594, 2001.

298. Krawitt EL. Autoimmune hepatitis. *N Engl J Med* 354(1): 54–66, 2006.

299. Autoimmune Hepatitis Group Report: review of criteria for diagnosis of autoimmune hepatitis. *J Hepatol* 31(5): 929–938, 1999.

300. Bilaj F, Hyslop WB, Rivero H, Firat Z, Vaidean G, Shrestha R, Woosley JT, Semelka R. MRI findings in autoimmune hepatitis: correlation with clinical staging. *Radiology* 236(3): 896–902, 2005.

301. Hyslop WB, Kierans AS, Leonardou P, Fritchie K, Darling J, Elazzazi M, Semelka RC. Overlap syndrome of autoimmune chronic liver diseases: MR imaging findings. JMRI, 2007 (in press).

302. Wenzel JS, Donohoe A, Ford KL 3rd, Glastad K, Watkins D, Molmenti E. Primary biliary cirrhosis: MR imaging findings and description of MR imaging periportal halo sign. *AJR Am J Roentgenol* 176(4): 885–9, 2001.

303. Akhan O, Akpinar E, Oto A, Koroglu M, Ozmen MN, Akata D, et al. Unusual imaging findings in Wilson's disease. *Eur Radiol* 12 *Suppl* 3: S66–9, 2002.

304. Marrero JA, Fontana RJ, Su GL, Conjeevaram HS, Emick DM, Lok AS. NAFLD may be a common underlying liver disease in patients with hepatocellular carcinoma in the United States. *Hepatology* 36(6): 1349–54, 2002.

305. Ratziu V, Bonyhay L, Di Martino V, Charlotte F, Cavallaro L, Sayegh-Tainturier MH, et al. Survival, liver failure, and hepatocellular carcinoma in obesity-related cryptogenic cirrhosis. *Hepatology* 35(6): 1485–93, 2002.

306. Clark JM, Diehl AM. Nonalcoholic fatty liver disease: an underrecognized cause of cryptogenic cirrhosis. *JAMA* 289(22): 3000–4, 2003.

307. Elias J Jr, Altun E, Zacks S, Armao D, Woosley JT, Semelka RC. MRI findings in nonalcoholic steatohepatitis: Correlation with histopathology and clinical staging. *Magn Reson Imaging* 27: 976–987, 2009.

308. Clouston AD, Powell EE. Nonalcoholic fatty liver disease: is all the fat bad? *Intern Med J* 34(4): 187–91, 2004.

309. Venkataraman S, Braga L, Semelka RC. Imaging the fatty liver. *Magn Reson Imaging Clin N Am* 10(1): 93–103, 2002.

310. Saadeh S, Younossi ZM, Remer EM, Gramlich T, Ong JP, Hurley M, et al. The utility of radiological imaging in nonalcoholic fatty liver disease. *Gastroenterology* 123(3): 745–50, 2002.

311. Hochman JA, Balistreri WF. Chronic viral hepatitis: always be current! *Pediatr Rev* 24(12): 399–410, 2003.

312. Feld JJ, Liang TJ. HCV persistence: cure is still a four letter word. *Hepatology* 41: 23–5, 2005

313. Alter MJ, Kruszon-Moran D, Nainan OV, McQuillan GM, Gao F, Moyer LA, Kaslow RA, Margolis HS. The prevalence of hepatitis C virus infection in the United States, 1988 through 1994. *N Engl J Med*. 341(8): 556–62, 1999.

314. Fauerholdt L, Schlichting P, Christensen E, Poulsen H, Tygstrup N, Juhl E. Conversion of micronodular cirrhosis into macronodular cirrhosis. *Hepatology* 3: 928–931, 1983.

315. Itai Y, Ohtomo K, Kokubo T, Minami M, Yoshida H. CT and MR imaging of postnecrotic liver scars. *J Comput Assist Tomogr* 12: 971–975, 1988.

316. Stark DD, Goldberg HI, Moss AA, Bass NM: Chronic liver disease: Evaluation by magnetic resonance. *Radiology* 150: 149–151, 1984.

317. Zhang XM, Mitchell DG, Shi H, Holland GA, Parker L, Herrine SK, et al. Chronic hepatitis C activity: correlation with lymphadenopathy on MR imaging. *AJR Am J Roentgenol* 179(2): 417–22, 2002.

318. Unger EC, Lee JK, Weyman PJ. CT and MR imaging of radiation hepatitis. *J Comput Assist Tomogr* 11: 264–268, 1987.

319. Yankelevitz DF, Knapp PH, Henschke CI, Nisce L, Yi Y, Cahill P. MR appearance of radiation hepatitis. *Clin Imaging* 16: 89–92, 1992.

320. Cutillo DP, Swayne LC, Fasciano MG, Schwartz JR. Absence of fatty replacement in radiation damaged liver: CT demonstration. *J Comput Assist Tomogr* 13: 259–261, 1989.

321. Garra BS, Shawker TH, Chang R, Kaplan K, White RD. The ultrasound appearance of radiation-induced hepatic injury. Correlation with computed tomography and magnetic resonance imaging. *J Ultrasound Med* 7: 605–609, 1988.

322. Anthony PP, Ishak KG, Nayak NC, Poulsen HE, Scheuer PJ, Sobin LH. The morphology of cirrhosis. The morphology of cirrhosis. Recommendations on definition, nomenclature, and classification by a working group sponsored by the World Health Organization. *J Clin Pathol* 31: 395–414, 1978.

323. Gore RM. Diffuse liver disease. In: Gore RM, Levine NS, Laufer I, eds. *Textbook of Gastrointestinal Radiology.* Philadelphia, Saunders, 1994. p.1968–2017.

324. Ito K, Mitchell DG, Gabata T, Hussain SM. Expanded gallbladder fossa: simple MR imaging sign of cirrhosis. *Radiology* 211: 723–726, 1999.

325. Ito K, Mitchell DG, Gabata T. Enlargement of hilar periportal space: a sign of early cirrhosis at MR imaging. *J Magn Reson Imaging* 11(2): 136–40, 2000.

326. Lafortune M, Matricardi L, Denys A, Favret M, Dery R, Pomier-Layrargues G. Segment 4 (the quadrate lobe): a barometer of cirrhotic liver disease at US. *Radiology* 206(1): 157–60, 1998.

327. Ito K, Mitchell DG, Siegelman ES. Cirrhosis: MR imaging features. *Magn Reson Imaging Clin N Am* 10(1): 75–92, 2002.

328. Mitchell DG, Lovett KE, Hann HW, Ehrlich S, Palazzo J, Rubin R. Cirrhosis: Multiobserver analysis of hepatic MR imaging findings in a heterogeneous population. *J Magn Reson Imaging* 3: 313–321, 1993.

329. Semelka RC, Chung JJ, Hussain SM, Marcos HB, Woosley JT. Chronic hepatitis: correlation of early patchy and late linear enhancement patters on gadolinium-enhanced MR images with histopathology-initial experience. *J Magn Reson Imaging* 13: 385–391, 2001.

330. Marti-Bonmati L, Talens A, del Olmo J, de Val A, Serra MA, Rodrigo JM, Ferrandez A, Torres V, Rayon M, Vilar JS. Chronic hepatitis and cirrhosis: evaluation by means of MR imaging with histologic correlation. *Radiology* 188: 37–43, 1993.

331. Shimizu A, Ito K, Koike S, Fujita T, Shimizu K, Matsunaga N. Cirrhosis or chronic hepatitis: evaluation of small (< or = 2-cm) early-enhancing hepatic lesions with serial contrast-enhanced dynamic MR imaging. *Radiology* 226(2): 550–555, 2003.

332. Kanematsu M, Danet MI, Leonardou P, Mastropasqua M, Mosetti MA, Braga L, Woosley JT, Semelka RC. Early heterogeneous enhancement of the liver: magnetic resonance imaging findings and clinical significance. *J Magn Reson Imaging* 20(2): 242–249, 2004.

333. *Harrison's Principle of Internal Medicine.* 16th ed. / New York: McGraw-Hill.

334. Baron RL, Campbell WL, Dodd GD. Peribiliary cysts associated with severe liver disease: imaging-pathologic correlation. *AJR Am J Roentgenol* 162: 631–636, 1994.

335. Itai Y, Ebihara R, Tohno E, Tsunoda HS, Kurosaki Y, Saida Y, Doy M. Hepatic peribiliary cysts: multiple tiny cysts within the larger portal tract, hepatic hilum, or both. *Radiology* 191: 107–110, 1994.

336. Terayama N, Matsui O, Hoshiba K, Kadoya M, Yoshikawa J, Gabata T, Takashima T, Terada T, Nakanuma Y, Shinozaki K, et al. Peribiliary cysts in liver cirrhosis: US, CT, and MR findings. *J Comput Assist Tomogr* 19: 419–423, 1995.

337. Anthony PP, Ishak KG, Nayak NC, Poulsen HE, Scheuer PJ, Sobin LH. The morphology of cirrhosis. The morphology of cirrhosis. Recommendations on definition, nomenclature, and classification by a working group sponsored by the World Health Organization. *J Clin Pathol* 31: 395–414, 1978.

338. Hytiroglou P, Theise NH. Differential diagnosis of hepatocellular nodular lesions. *Semin Diag Pathol* 15: 285–299, 1998.

339. Ohtomo K, Itai Y, Ohtomo Y, Shiga J, Iio M. Regenerating nodules of liver cirrhosis: MR imaging with pathologic correlation. *AJR Am J Roentgenol* 154: 505–507, 1990.

340. Terada T, Nakanuma Y. Survey of iron-accumulative macroregenerative nodules in cirrhotic livers. *Hepatology* 10: 851–854, 1989.

341. Ito K, Mitchell DG, Gabata T, Hann HW, Kim PN, Fujita T, Awaya H, Honjo K, Matsunaga N. Hepatocellular carcinoma: association with increased iron deposition in the cirrhotic liver at MR imaging. *Radiology* 212(1): 235–240, 1999.

342. Soyer P, Lacheheb D, Caudron C, Levesque M. MRI of adenomatous hyperplastic nodules of the liver in Budd-Chiari syndrome. *J Comput Assist Tomogr* 17(1): 86–89, 1993.

343. Vilgrain V, Lewin M, Vons C, Denys A, Valla D, Flejou JF, Belghiti J, Menu Y. Hepatic nodules in Budd-Chiari syndrome: imaging features. *Radiology* 210(2): 443–450, 1999.

344. Cazals-Hatem D, Vilgrain V, Genin P, Denninger MH, Durand F, Belghiti J, Valla D, Degott C. Arterial and portal circulation and parenchymal changes in Budd-Chiari syndrome: a study in 17 explanted livers. *Hepatology* 37(3): 510–519, 2003.

345. Theise ND, Schwartz M, Miller C, Thung SN. Macroregenerative nodules and hepatocellular carcinoma in forty-four sequential adult liver explants with cirrhosis. *Hepatology* 16(4): 949–955, 1992.

346. Sakamoto M, Hirohashi S, Shimosato Y. Early stages of multistep hepatocarcinogenesis: adenomatous hyperplasia and early hepatocellular carcinoma. *Hum Pathol* 22(2): 172–178, 1991.

347. Takayama T, Makuuchi M, Hirohashi S, Sakamoto M, Okazaki N, Takayasu K, Kosuge T, Motoo Y, Yamazaki S, Hasegawa H. Malignant transformation of adenomatous hyperplasia to hepatocellular carcinoma. *Lancet* 10;336(8724): 1150–1153, 1990.

348. Kadoya M, Matsui O, Takashima T, Nonomura A. Hepatocellular carcinoma: correlation of MR imaging and histopathologic findings. *Radiology* 183: 819–825, 1992.

349. Roncalli M, Roz E, Coggi G, Di Rocco MG, Bossi P, Minola E, et al. The vascular profile of regenerative and dysplastic nodules of the cirrhotic liver: implications for diagnosis and classification. *Hepatology* 30(5): 1174–8, 1999.

350. Ward J, Guthrie JA, Schott DJ, Atchley J, Wilson D, Davies MH, Wyatt JI, Robinson PJ. Hepatocellular carcinoma in the cirrhotic liver: double-contrast MR imaging for diagnosis. *Radiology* 216: 154–162, 2000.

351. Mitchell DG, Rubin R, Siegelman ES, Burk DL Jr, Rifkin MD. Hepatocellular carcinoma within siderotic regenerative nodules: appearance as a nodule within a nodule on MR images. *Radiology* 178(1): 101–103, 1991.

352. Muramatsu Y, Nawano S, Takayasu K, Moriyama N, Yamada T, Yamasaki S, Hirohashi S. Early hepatocellular carcinoma: MR imaging. *Radiology* 181(1): 209–213, 1991.

353. Sadek AG, Mitchell DG, Siegelman ES, Outwater EK, Matteucci T, Hann HW. Early hepatocellular carcinoma that develops within macroregenerative nodules: growth rate depicted at serial MR imaging. *Radiology* 195(3): 753–756, 1995.

354. Groszmann RJ, Atterbury CE. The pathophysiology of portal hypertension: a basis for classification. *Semin Liver Dis* 2: 177–186, 1982.

355. Chopra S, Dodd GD, Chintapalli KN, Esola CC, Ghiatas AA. Mesenteric, omental, and retroperitoneal edema in cirrhosis: frequency and spectrum of CT findings. *Radiology* 211: 737–742, 1999.

356. Starzl TE, Francavilla A, Halgrimson CG, Francavilla FR, Porter KA, Brown TH, Putnam CW. The origin, hormonal nature, and action of hepatotrophic substances in portal venous blood. *Surg Gynecol Obstet* 137: 179–199, 1973.

357. Matsuo M, Kanematsu M, Kim T, Hori M, Takamura M, Murakami T, Kondo H, Moriyama N, Nakamura H, Hoshi H. Esophageal varices: diagnosis with gadolinium-enhanced MR imaging of the liver for patients with chronic liver damage. *AJR Am J Roentgenol.* 180(2): 461–466, 2003.

358. Finn JP, Edelman RR, Jenkins RL, Lewis WD, Longmaid HE, Kane RA, Stokes KR, Mattle HP, Clouse ME. Liver transplantation: MR angiography with surgical validation. *Radiology* 179: 265–269, 1991.

359. Zhang XM, Mitchell DG, Shi H, Holland GA, Parker L, Herrine SK, Pasqualin D, Rubin R. Chronic hepatitis C activity: correlation with lymphadenopathy on MR imaging. *AJR Am J Roentgenol.* 179(2): 417–422, 2002.

360. Brandhagen DJ, Fairbanks VF, Batts KP, Thebodeau SN. Update on hereditary hemochromatosis and the HFE gene. *Mayo Clin Proc* 74: 917–9121, 1999.

361. Siegelman ES, Mitchell DG, Semelka RC. Abdominal iron deposition: metabolism, MR findings, and clinical importance. *Radiology* 199: 13–22, 1996.

362. Barton JC, McDonnell SM, Adams PC, Brissot P, Powell LW, Edwards CQ, Cook JD, Kowdley KV. Management of hemochromatosis. Hemochromatosis Management Working Group. *Ann Intern Med* 129: 932–939, 1998.

363. McLaren G, Muir W, Kellermeyer R. Iron overload disorders: natural history, pathogenesis, diagnosis and therapy. *Crit Rev Clin Lab Sci* 19: 205–226, 1984.

364. Guyader D, Gandon Y, Sapey T, Turlin B, Mendler MH, Brissot P, Deugnier Y. Magnetic resonance iron-free nodules in genetic hemochromatosis. *Am J Gastroenterol* 94: 1083–1086, 1999.

365. Siegelman ES, Mitchell DG, Rubin R, Hann HW, Kaplan KR, Steiner RM, Rao VM, Schuster SJ, Burk DL, Jr., Rifkin MD. Parenchymal versus reticuloendothelial iron overload in the liver: distinction with MR imaging. *Radiology* 179: 361–366, 1991.

366. Terada T, Kadoya M, Nakanuma Y, Matsui O. Iron-accumulating adenomatous hyperplastic nodule with malignant foci in the cirrhotic liver. Histopathologic, quantitative iron, and magnetic resonance imaging in vitro studies. *Cancer* 65: 1994–2000, 1990.

367. Terada T, Nakanuma Y. Iron-negative foci in siderotic macroregenerative nodules in human cirrhotic liver. A marker of incipient neoplastic lesions. *Arch Pathol Lab Med* 113: 916–920, 1989.

368. Ernst O, Sergent G, Bonvarlet P, Canva-Delcambre V, Paris JC, L'Hermine. Hepatic iron overload: diagnosis and quantification with MR imaging. *AJR Am J Roentgenol.* 168: 1205–8, 1997.

369. Bonkovsky HL, Rubin RB, Cable EE, Davidoff A, Rijcken TH, Stark DD. Hepatic iron concentration: noninvasive estimation by means of MR imaging techniques. *Radiology* 212: 227–34, 1999.

370. Alustiza JM, Artetxe J, Castiella A, Agirre C, Emparanza JI, Otazua P, Garcia-Bengoechea M, Barrio J, Mujica F, Recondo JA; Gipuzkoa Hepatic Iron Concentration by MRI Study Group. MR quantification of hepatic iron concentration. *Radiology* 230: 479–84, 2004.

371. Siegelman ES, Outwater E, Hanau CA, Ballas SK, Steiner RM, Rao VM, Mitchell DG. Abdominal iron distribution in sickle cell disease: MR findings in transfusion and nontransfusion dependent patients. *J Comput Assist Tomogr* 18: 63–67, 1994.

372. Pomerantz S and Siegelman ES. MR imaging of iron depositional disease. *Magn Reson Imaging Clin North Am* 10(1): 105–120, 2002.

373. Yates CK, Streight RA. Focal fatty infiltration of the liver simulating metastatic disease. *Radiology* 159: 83–84, 1986.

374. Mitchell DG. Focal manifestations of diffuse liver disease at MR imaging. *Radiology* 185: 1–11, 1992.

375. Mitchell DG, Kim I, Chang TS, Vinitski S, Consigny PM, Saponaro SA, Ehrlich SM, Rifkin MD, Rubin R. Fatty liver. Chemical shift phase-difference and suppression magnetic resonance imaging techniques in animals, phantoms, and humans. *Invest Radiol* 26: 1041–1052, 1991.

376. Matsui O, Kadoya M, Takahashi S, Yoshikawa J, Gabata T, Takashima T, Kitagawa K. Focal sparing of segment IV in fatty livers shown by sonography and CT: correlation with aberrant gastric venous drainage. *AJR Am J Roentgenol* 164: 1137–1140, 1995.

377. Itai Y. Focal sparing versus a hepatic tumor in fatty liver. *AJR Am J Roentgenol* 172: 242–243, 1999.

378. Arai K, Matsui O, Takashima T, Ida M, Nishida Y. Focal spared areas in fatty liver caused by regional decreased portal flow. *AJR Am J Roentgenol* 151: 300–302, 1988.

379. Arita T, Matsunaga N, Honma Y, Nishikawa E, Nagaoka S. Focally spared area of fatty liver caused by arterioportal shunt. *J Comput Assist Tomogr* 20: 360–362, 1996.

380. Kawamori Y, Matsui O, Takahashi S, Kadoya M, Takashima T, Miyayama S. Focal hepatic fatty infiltration in the posterior edge of the medial segment associated with aberrant gastric venous drainage: CT, US, and MR findings. *J Comput Assist Tomogr.* 20: 356–359, 1996.

381. Grossholz M, Terrier F, Rubbia L, Becker C, Stoupis C, Hadengue A, Mentha G. Focal sparing in the fatty liver as a sign of an adjacent space-occupying lesion. *AJR Am J Roentgenol* 17: 1391–1395, 1998.

382. Chung JJ, Kim MJ, Kim JH, Lee JT, Yoo HS. Fat sparing of surrounding liver from metastasis in patients with fatty liver: MR imaging with histopathologic correlation. *AJR Am J Roentgenol* 180: 1347–50, 2003.

383. Parfrey NA, Hutchins GN. Hepatic fibrosis in the mucopolysaccharises. *Am J Med* 81: 825–829, 1986.

384. Matalan, RH. Metabolic diseases. In: Behrman RE, Kligman RM, Nelson WE, Vaughan III VC, eds. *Textbook of Pediatrics.* 14 ed. Philadelphia, W.B. Saunders, 1992. p. 372–77.

385. Hurwitz LM, Thompson WM. Calcified hepatic arteriovenous fistula found after biopsy of the liver: unusual cause of calcification in the right upper quadrant. *AJR Am J Roentgenol* 79(5): 1293–5, 2002.

386. Sharlock S and Dooley J. *Diseases of the Liver and Biliary System.* p. 1086. 10 edition. Blackwell science. 1997.

387. Semelka RC, Lessa T, Shaikh F, Miller FH, Elazzazi M, Dyson M. MRI findings of intrahepatic vascular shunts. *J Magn Reson Imag* 29: 617–620, 2009.

388. Cotran RS, Cumar V, Robbins SL. *Pathologic Basis of Disease.* P. 872. 5th edition. W.B. Saunders Company Philadelphia, 1994.

389. Itai Y, Ohtomo K, Kokubo T, Okada Y, Yamauchi T, Yoshida H. Segmental intensity differences in the liver on MR images: a sign of intrahepatic portal flow stoppage. *Radiology* 167: 17–19, 1988.

390. Lorigan JG, Charnsangavej C, Carrasco CH, Richli WR, Wallace S. Atrophy with compensatory hypertrophy of the liver in hepatic neoplasms: Radiographic findings. *AJR Am J Roentgenol* 150: 1291–1295, 1988.

391. Carr DH, Hadjis NS, Banks LM, Hemingway AP, Blumgart LH. Computed tomography of hilar cholangiocarcinoma: a new sign. *AJR Am J Roentgenol* 145: 53–56, 1985.

392. Itai Y, Murata S, Kurosaki Y. Straight border sign of the liver: spectrum of CT appearances and causes. *Radiographics* 15: 1089–1102, 1995.

393. Schlund JF, Semelka RC, Kettritz U, Eisenberg LB, Lee JKT. Transient increased segmental hepatic enhancement distal to portal vein obstruction on dynamic gadolinium-enhanced gradient echo MR images. *J Magn Reson Imaging* 5: 375–377, 1995.

394. De Gaetano AM, Lafortune M, Patriquin H, De Franco A, Aubin B, Raradis K. Cavernous transformation of the portal vein: patterns of intrahepatic and splanchnic collateral circulation detected with Doppler sonography. *AJR Am J Roentgenol* 165: 1151–1156, 1995.

395. Nakao N, Miura K, Takahashi H, Miura T, Ashida H, Ishikawa Y, Utsunomiya J. Hepatic perfusion in cavernous transformation of the portal vein: evaluation by using CT angiography. *AJR Am J Roentgenol* 152: 985–986, 1989.

396. Schlund JF, Semelka RC, Kettritz U, Weeks SM, Kahlenberg M, Cance WG. Correlation of perfusion abnormalities on CTAP and immediate postintravenous gadolinium-enhanced gradient echo MRI. *Abdom Imaging* 21: 49–52, 1996.

397. Gilchrist AJ and Hayes PC. Vascular disorders of the liver. In: *Diseases of the Gastrointestinal Tract and Liver.* Shearman DJC, Finlayson NDC, Camilleri M. eds. 3 ed. New York, Churchill Livingstone, 1997. p. 1079–81.

398. Miller WJ, Federle MP, Straub WH, Davis PL. Budd-Chiari syndrome: imaging with pathologic correlation. *Abdom Imaging* 18: 329–335, 1993.

399. Mathieu D, Vasile N, Menu Y, Van Beers B, Lorphelin JM, Pringot J. Budd-Chiari syndrome: dynamic CT. *Radiology* 165: 409–413, 1987.

400. Murata S, Itai Y, Hisashi K, Nakajima K, et al. Effect of temporary occlusion of the hepatic vein on dual blood supply in the liver: evaluation with spiral CT. *Radiology* 195: 351–356, 1995.

401. Pollard JJ, Nebesar RA. Altered hemodynamics in the Budd-Chiari syndrome demonstrated by selective hepatic and selective splenic angiography. *Radiology* 89: 236–243, 1967.

402. Noone TC, Semelka RC, Siegelman ES, Balci NC, Hussain SM, et al. Budd-Chiari syndrome: spectrum of appearances of acute, subacute, and chronic disease with magnetic resonance imaging. *J Magn Reson Imaging* 11: 44–50, 2000.

403. Noone T, Semelka RC, Woosley JT, Pisano ED. Ultrasound and MR findings in acute Budd-Chiari syndrome with histopathologic correlation. *J Comput Assist Tomogr* 20: 819–822, 1996.

404. Castellano G, Canga F, Solis-Herruzo JA, Colina F, Martinez-Montiel MP, Morillas JD. Budd-Chiari syndrome associated with nodular regenerative hyperplasia of the liver. *J Clin Gastroenterol* 11: 698–702, 1989.

405. de Sousa JM, Portmann B, Williams R. Nodular regenerative hyperplasia of the liver and the Budd-Chiari syndrome. Case report, review of the literature and reappraisal of pathogenesis. *J Hepatol* 12: 28–35, 1991.

406. Brancatelli G, Federle MP, Grazioli L, Golfieri R, Lencioni R. Large regenerative nodules in Budd-Chiari syndrome and other vascular disorders of the liver: CT and MR imaging findings with clinicopathologic correlation. *AJR Am J Roentgenol.* 178: 877–83, 2002.

407. Brancatelli G, Federle MP, Grazioli L, Golfieri R, Lencioni R. Benign regenerative nodules in Budd-Chiari syndrome and other vascular disorders of the liver: radiologic-pathologic and clinical correlation. *Radiographics* 22: 847–62, 2002.

408. Maetani Y, Itoh K, Egawa H, Haga H, Sakurai T, Nishida N, Ametani F, Shibata T, Kubo T, Tanaka K, Konishi J. Benign hepatic nodules in Budd-Chiari syndrome: radiologic-pathologic correlation with emphasis on the central scar. *AJR Am J Roentgenol.* 178: 869–75, 2002.

409. Soyer P, Lacheheb D, Caudron C, Levesque M. MRI of adenomatous hyperplastic nodules of the liver in Budd-Chiari syndrome. *J Comput Assist Tomogr* 17: 86–89, 1993.

410. Cazals-Hatem D, Vilgrain V, Genin P, Denninger MH, Durand F, Belghiti J, Valla D, Degott C. Arterial and portal circulation and parenchymal changes in Budd-Chiari syndrome: a study in 17 explanted livers. *Hepatology* 37: 510–9, 2003.

411. Nakashima T, Okuda K, Kojiro M, et al. Pathology of hepatocellular carcinoma in Japan. 232 consecutive cases autopsied in 10 years. *Cancer* 51: 863–877, 1983.

412. Rooholamini SA, Au AH, Hansen GC, Kioumehr F, Dadsetan MR, Chow PP, Kurzel RB, Mikhail G. Imaging of pregnancy-related complications. *Radiographics* 13: 753–770, 1993.

413. Brown JJ, Borrello JA, Raza HS, Balfe DM, Baer AB, Pilgram TK, Atilla S. Dynamic contrast-enhanced MR imaging of the liver: parenchymal enhancement patterns. *Magn Reson Imaging* 13: 1–8, 1995.

414. Kanematsu M, Semelka RC, Matsuo M, Kondo H, Enya M, Goshima S, Moriyama N, Hoshi H. Gadolinium-enhanced MR imaging of the liver: optimizing imaging delay for hepatic arterial and portal venous phases–a prospective randomized study in patients with chronic liver damage. *Radiology* 225(2): 407–15, 2002.

415. Seeff LC, Seeff LB. Pulmonary disorders and the liver. In: *The Liver and Systemic Disease.* Gitlin N, ed. New York, Churchill Livingstone, New York, 1997. p. 29–31.

416. Kessler A, Mitchell DG, Israel HL, Goldberg BB. Hepatic and splenic sarcoidosis: Ultrasound and MR imaging. *Abdom Imaging* 18: 159–163, 1993.

417. Warshauer DM, Semelka RC, Ascher SM. Nodular sarcoidosis of the liver and spleen: appearance on MR images. *J Magn Reson Imaging* 4: 553–557, 1994.

418. Dasgupta D, Guthrie A, McClean P, Davison S, Luntley J, Rajwal S, et al. Liver transplantation for a hilar inflammatory myofibroblastic tumor. *Pediatr Transplant* 8(5): 517–21, 2004.

419. Horiuchi R, Uchida T, Kojima T, Shikata T. Inflammatory pseudotumor of the liver. Clinicopathologic study and review of the literature. *Cancer* 65(7): 1583–90, 1990.

420. Shek TW, Ng IO, Chan KW. Inflammatory pseudotumor of the liver. Report of four cases and review of the literature. *Am J Surg Pathol* 17: 231–238, 1993.

421. Horiuchi R, Uchida T, Kojima T, Shikata T. Inflammatory pseudotumor of the liver. Clinicopathologic study and review of the literature. *Cancer* 65: 1583–1590, 1990.

422. Venkataraman S, Semelka RC, Braga L, Woosley JT. Inflammatory myofibroblastic tumor of the hepato-biliary system: appearances on MRI. *Radiology* 227: 758–763, 2003.

423. Kelekis NL, Warshauer DM, Semelka RC, Eisenberg LB, Woosley JT. Inflammatory pseudotumor of the liver: appearance on contrast enhanced helical CT and dynamic MR images. *J Magn Reson Imaging* 5: 551–553, 1995.

424. Oto A, Akhan O, Ozmen M. Focal inflammatory diseases of the liver. *Eur J Radiol* 32: 61–75, 1999

425. Bertel CK, van Heerden JA, Sheedy PF. Treatment of pyogenic hepatic abscesses. Surgical vs. percutaneous drainage. *Arch Surg* 121: 554–558, 1986.

426. Balci NC, Semelka RC, Noone TC, Siegelman ES, Beeck BO, Brown JJ, Lee MG. Pyogenic hepatic abscesses: MRI findings on T1- and T2-weighted and serial gadolinium-enhanced gradient-echo images. *J Magn Reson Imaging* 9: 285–290, 1999.

427. Mendez RJ, Schiebler ML, Outwater EK, Kressel HY. Hepatic abscesses: MR imaging findings. *Radiology* 190: 431–436, 1994.

428. Balci NC and Sirvanci M. MR imaging of infective liver lesions. *Magn Reson Imaging.* 10 (1): 121–135, 2002.

429. Ralls PW, Henley DS, Colletti PM, Benson R, Raval JK, Radin DR, Boswell WD, Jr., Halls JM. Amebic liver abscess: MR imaging. *Radiology* 165: 801–804, 1987.

430. Balci NC, Tunaci A, Semelka RC, Tunaci M, Özden I, Rezanu IB. Hepatic alveolar echinococcosis: MRI findings. *Magn Reson Imaging* 18: 537–541, 2000.

431. Landay MJ, Setiawan H, Hirsch G, Christensen EE, Conrad MR. Hepatic and thoracic amaebiasis. *AJR Am J Roentgenol.* 135: 449–454, 1980.

432. Lebovics E, Thung SN, Schaffner F. The liver in the acquired immunodeficiency syndrome: a clinical and histologic study. *Hepatology* 5: 293–298, 1995

433. Schneiderman DJ, Arenson DM, Cello JP. Hepatic disease in patients with acquired immune deficiency syndrome (AIDS). *Hepatology* 7: 925–930,1987.

434. Pantongrag-Brown L, Krebs TL, Daly BD, et al. Frequency of abdominal CT findings in AIDS patients with *M. Avium* complex bacteraemia. *Clin Radiol.* 53: 816–819, 1998.

435. Shirkhoda A, Lopez-Berestein G, Holbert JM, Luna MA. Hepatosplenic fungal infection: CT and pathologic evaluation after treatment with liposomal amphotericin B. *Radiology* 159: 349–353, 1986.

436. Lewis JH, Patel HR, Zimmerman HJ. The spectrum of hepatic candidiasis. *Hepatology* 2: 479–487, 1982.

437. Sallah S, Semelka RC, Kelekis N, Worawattanakul S, Sallah W. Diagnosis and monitoring response of treatment of hepatosplenic candidiasis in patients with acute leukemia using magnetic resonance imaging. *Acta Haematol* 100: 77–81, 1998.

438. Semelka RC, Kelekis NL, Sallah S, Worawattanakul S, Ascher SM. Hepatosplenic fungal disease: diagnostic accuracy and spectrum of appearance on MR imaging. *AJR Am J Roentgenol.* 169(5): 1311–6, 1997.

439. Semelka RC, Shoenut JP, Greenberg HM, Bow EJ. Detection of acute and treated lesions of hepatosplenic candidiasis: comparison of dynamic contrast-enhanced CT and MR imaging. *J Magn Reson Imaging* 2: 341–345, 1992.

440. Cho JS, Kim EE, Varma DG, Wallace S. MR imaging of hepatosplenic candidiasis superimposed on hemochromatosis. *J Comput Assist Tomogr* 14: 774–776, 1990.

441. Lamminen AE, Anttila VJ, Bondestam S, Ruutu T, Ruutu PJ. Infectious liver foci in leukemia: comparison of short-inversion-time inversion-recovery, T1-weighted spin-echo, and dynamic gadolinium-enhanced MR imaging. *Radiology* 191: 539–543, 1994.

442. Kelekis NL, Semelka RC, Jeon HJ, Sallah AS, Shea TC, Woosley JT. Dark ring sign: finding in patients with fungal liver lesions and transfusional hemosiderosis undergoing treatment with antifungal antibiotics. *Magn Reson Imaging* 14: 615–618, 1996.

443. Grossman RI, Kemp SS, Ip CY, Fishman JE, Gomori JM, Joseph PM, Asakura T. Importance of oxygenation in the appearance of acute subarachnoid hemorrhage on high field magnetic resonance imaging. *Acta Radiol Suppl* 369: 56–58, 1986.

444. Gomori JM, Grossman RI, Yu-Ip C, Asakura T. NMR relaxation times of blood: dependence on field strength, oxidation state, and cell integrity. *J Comput Assist Tomogr* 11: 684–90, 1987.

445. Grossman RI, Gomori JM, Goldberg HI, Hackney DB, Atlas SW, Kemp SS, Zimmerman RA, Bilaniuk LT. MR imaging of hemorrhagic conditions of the head and neck. *Radiographics* 8: 441–454, 1988.

446. Hayman LA, Taber KH, Ford JJ, Saleem A, Gurgun M, Mohamed S, Bryan RN. Effect of clot formation and retraction on spin-echo MR images of blood: an in vitro study. *AJNR Am J Neuroradiol* 10: 1155–8, 1989.

447. Hayman LA, Taber KH, Ford JJ, Bryan RN. Mechanisms of MR signal alteration by acute intracerebral blood: old concepts and new theories. *AJNR Am J Neuroradiol* 12: 899–907, 1991.

448. Janick PA, Hackney DB, Grossman RI, Asakura T. MR imaging of various oxidation states of intracellular and extracellular hemoglobin. *AJNR Am J Neuroradiol* 12: 891–897, 1991.

449. Bradley WG Jr. MR appearance of hemorrhage in the brain. *Radiology* 189: 15–26, 1994.

450. Balci NC, Semelka RC, Noone TC, Ascher SM. Acute and subacute liver-related hemorrhage. MRI findings. *Magn Reson Imaging* 17(2): 207–211, 1999.

451. Hasegawa S, Eisenberg LB, Semelka RC. Active intrahepatic gadolinium extravasation following TIPS. *Magn Reson Imaging.* 16: 851–855, 1998.

452. Gomori JM, Grossman RI, Hackney DB, Goldberg HI, Zimmerman RA, Bilaniuk LT. Variable appearances of subacute intracranial hematomas on high-field spin-echo MR. *AJR Am J Roentgenol* 150: 171–8, 1988.

CHAPTER

3

GALLBLADDER AND BILIARY SYSTEM

ERSAN ALTUN, TILL BADER, JORGE ELIAS, JR., FAIQ SHAIKH, AND RICHARD C. SEMELKA

INTRODUCTION

Significant technical improvements of MRI hardware and software during recent years have led to the development of new and faster imaging sequences that are capable of demonstrating soft tissue well and visualizing the biliary and pancreatic ductal systems with excellent image quality, sharpness, and resolution previously only provided by endoscopic retrograde cholangiopancreatography (ERCP). In several studies, these MR techniques, termed magnetic resonance cholangiopancreatography (MRCP), have been shown to be comparable to ERCP in the diagnosis of choledocholithiasis, malignant obstruction of the biliary and pancreatic ducts, congenital anomalies, and chronic pancreatitis [1–8]. The advantages of MRCP over other imaging techniques include the following: 1) The examination is noninvasive and requires no anesthesia; 2) the examination is not operator dependent, and high-quality images can be obtained consistently; 3) no administration of intraductal or intravenous contrast agent is necessary; 4) no ionizing radiation is employed; 5)

visualization of ducts proximal to an obstruction is superior to that achieved by ERCP; 6) MRCP can be successfully performed in the presence of biliary-enteric anastomoses (e.g., hepaticojejunostomy, choledochojejunostomy, Billroth II anastomosis); and 7) combination with conventional MR sequences is possible and helpful for the evaluation of duct wall and extraductal disease [9]. A significant advantage of ERCP is that it allows therapeutic interventions at the time of initial diagnosis. Although generally considered a safe procedure, ERCP is associated with morbidity and mortality rates of 8% and 1%, respectively [10]. In addition, unsuccessful cannulation of the common bile duct (CBD) or pancreatic duct occurs in 3–10% of cases [11, 12]. Therefore, in many institutions MRCP has become the primary imaging modality for diagnostic purposes in the biliary system, with ERCP reserved for therapeutic interventions (e.g., sphincterotomy, stone removal, dilatation of strictures, stent placement) [1, 13, 14]. Ultrasound, because of its lower costs, remains the modality of choice for the evaluation of cholecystolithiasis, which accounts for 90% of gallbladder diseases.

Abdominal-Pelvic MRI, Third Edition, edited by Richard C. Semelka. Copyright © 2010 John Wiley & Sons, Inc.

NORMAL ANATOMY

The intrahepatic bile ducts are a component of the intrahepatic portal triad. They follow the course of portal venous branches along their ventral aspect. Subsegmental branches join to form segmental branches that join to form the right and left hepatic biliary ducts, which join to form the common hepatic duct (CHD). The confluence of both hepatic ducts is usually at the level of the porta hepatis, but it can be substantially lower. The gallbladder is situated in the gallbladder fossa, located between the right and left lobes of the liver, between Couinaud segments four and five. Anatomically, the gallbladder is composed of the fundus, body, and neck. The gallbladder is usually oval in shape, measuring approximately 7–10 cm in length and 2–3.5 cm in width, which can vary substantially depending on dietary status. The wall thickness of a normal, well-filled gallbladder does not exceed 3 mm. The gallbladder is connected to the CHD via the cystic duct, which has a mucosal endoluminal fold (called the spiral fold or valve). The confluence of the cystic duct and the CHD is typically located superior to the head of the pancreas to form the common bile duct (CBD). The CBD enters the head of the pancreas and usually joins with the main pancreatic duct (Wirsung) just before it enters the duodenum through the sphincter of Oddi in the major papilla (papilla of Vater).

MRI TECHNIQUE

T2-Weighted Sequences/MRCP

Magnetic resonance cholangiopancreatography (MRCP) is based on the acquisition of heavily T2-weighted images to provide visualization of stationary or slow-moving fluids (e.g., bile) with high signal intensity. Because of the heavy T2 weighting of these sequences, the signal from the pancreatico-biliary system appears hyperintense, whereas the background tissue (e.g., hepatic and pancreatic tissue, peritoneal fat, fast-flowing blood) is either very low signal or signal void, resulting in excellent contrast and depiction of the pancreatico-biliary system. The use of phased-array surface coil imaging, small field of view, and fat suppression techniques has resulted in higher signal-to-noise and contrast-to-noise ratios, allowed the acquisition of thinner sections and measurement of T2 rather than T2* decay, decreased susceptibility artifacts, and diminished sensitivity to motion artifacts and slow blood flow [15–18].

Current MRCP techniques are based on echo-train spin-echo techniques that allow two-dimensional (2D) and three-dimensional (3D) approaches. Multiple 180° pulses with successive echoes (echo train) are acquired

with a separate phase encoding gradient applied before each echo. Each of these detected echoes represents a different line within k-space. Ultrafast single-shot echo-train spin-echo techniques are capable of acquiring images in less than 1 s [19, 20]. After a single 90° excitation pulse, an extremely long echo train of 100–150 refocusing 180° pulses is obtained as a single-shot technique. After acquiring slightly more than half of k-space after the single 90° pulse, the remainder of k-space is filled by extrapolation, because of the intrinsic symmetry of k-space (half-Fourier technique). The extremely long echo train leads to diminution of echo signal intensity as the echo train progresses and, consequently, to decreased signal-to-noise and contrast-to-noise ratios. However, this effect is counteracted by the ultrashort acquisition time (less than 1 s), which "freezes" any physiological motion and avoids misregistration, and by the very low signal intensity from background tissue, which is an effect of the very long TE (600–1000 ms). Overall, this leads to a reduction of noise and an increase in contrast. The half-Fourier single-shot echo-train spin-echo sequences that are currently most widely used are half-Fourier RARE (rapid acquisition with relaxation enhancement) and HASTE (half-Fourier acquisition single-shot turbo spin echo) [21–23]. Acquisition of images with a very long TE renders very little signal from tissue with short TE such as fat and parenchymal organs, which makes the application of fat suppression techniques unnecessary. Fluids with relatively short TE, such as concentrated bile or mucinous fluid, however, will also give very little signal, which may hinder the depiction of small biliary ducts or mucinous lesions. An intermediate TE (80–100 ms) results in images in which all fluid, including concentrated bile and mucinous fluid, is bright and even small ducts are well depicted. The use of fat suppression to diminish the signal from surrounding tissue is advisable and makes maximum-intensity projection (MIP) postprocessing possible. To suppress signal from intestinal fluid, oral application of iron- or manganese-containing contrast agents has been investigated. The diagnostic benefits, however, are questionable [24–26].

MRCP can be performed with thick-section and thin-section sequences. For thick-section images, a thick-collimation single section of 4- to 5-cm thickness is acquired in a right anterior oblique coronal plane, obtained in less than 2 s (figs. 3.1 and 3.2). Several slabs can be acquired in various rotations to view the ducts from different angles. The images resemble conventional ERCP images and are particularly useful to provide an overview of the pancreatico-biliary system and to visualize nondilated ducts. However, thick-section technique is not appropriate to investigate intraductal pathologies because visualization of small intraductal signal-void structures (e.g., calculi) is masked by partial

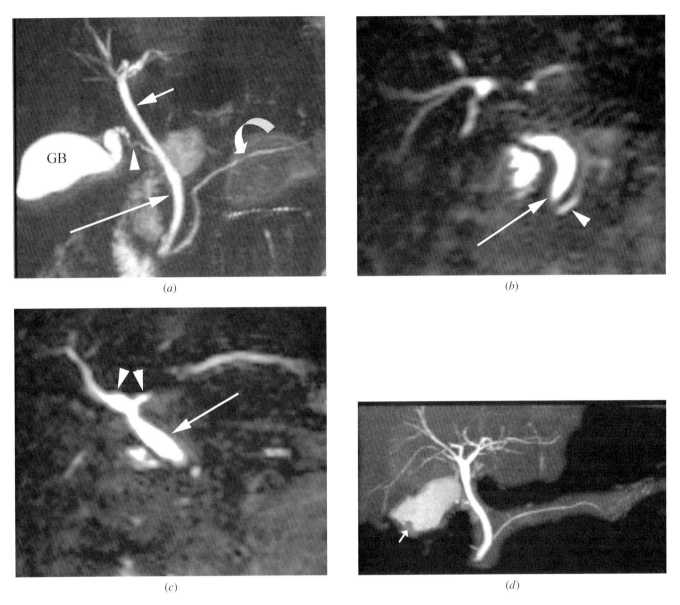

FIG. 3.1 Normal biliary system, MRCP. Thick-slab T2-weighted fat-suppressed single-shot echo-train spin-echo image (*a*) showing a good overview of the normal intra- and extrahepatic biliary system depicting the gallbladder (GB, *a*), the common bile duct (long arrow, *a*), the common hepatic duct (short arrow, *a*), the cystic duct (arrowhead, *a*), and the pancreatic duct (curved arrow, *a*). Thin-slab T2-weighted fat-suppressed single-shot echo-train spin-echo images (*b, c*) in a different patient demonstrate more detail and allow exact evaluation of the lumen and walls of the preampullary section of the common bile duct (long arrow, *b*), the pancreatic duct (short arrow, *b*), the common hepatic duct (long arrow, *c*), and the confluence of the right and left hepatic ducts (arrowheads, *c*). Navigator pulse triggered 30-MRCP in a third patient shows excellent depiction of biliary and pancreatic ducts. A gallstone is present in the gallbladder (arrow, *d*).

volume averaging with intraductal high signal from fluid (e.g., bile). Therefore, the additional acquisition of thin-section images with a thin-collimation multisection sequence is essential. Images in a right anterior oblique plane provide a cholangiographic display capturing the bifurcation of the CHD into right and left hepatic ducts (figs. 3.1 and 3.3). An additional acquisition in the axial plane provides a useful evaluation of the distal CBD and the pancreatic duct. Alternatively, thick-slab images in the coronal and axial planes can be used as localizers to focus the acquisition of thin-collimation images on the middle and distal CBD in the coronal plane. As another alternative, coronal thick-section images can be used to assess the range for axial thin-section images covering the entire biliary and pancreatic ductal system. On these images, a thin-section paracoronal series can be exactly targeted to depict the bifurcation of the CHD and the entire course of the CBD. Slice thickness of

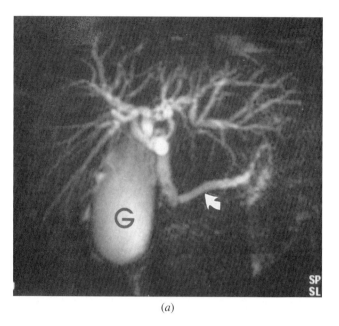

(a)

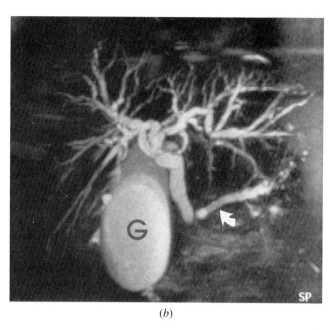

(b)

F I G . 3.2 Thick-section MRCP versus 3D MIP reconstruction image. T2-weighted fat-suppressed thick-section MRCP single-shot echo-train spin-echo (*a*) and 3D MIP reconstruction image (*b*) from a series of thin-section single-shot echo-train spin-echo images. A pancreatic head carcinoma obstructs the preampullary CBD and pancreatic duct. The entire biliary tree and the pancreatic duct (curved arrow, *a*, *b*) are dilated. Note the finer resolution and detail of the 3D MIP image (*b*). G = gallbladder.

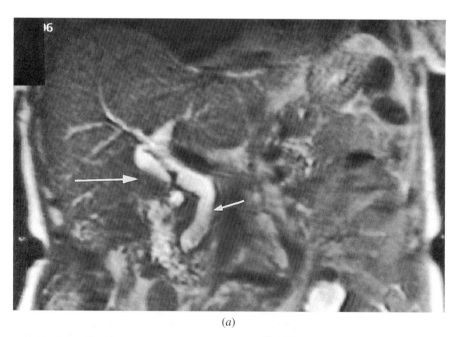

(a)

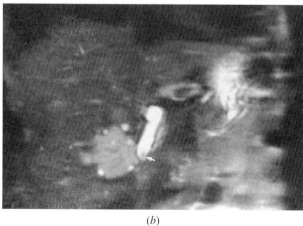

(b)

F I G . 3.3 Thin-section MRCP versus 3D MIP reconstruction image. MRCP 3D MIP reconstruction (*a*) and coronal T2-weighted fat-suppressed thin-section single-shot echo-train spin-echo (*b*) images. On the MIP image (*a*), severe dilation of the CBD (short arrow, *a*) is shown, but no CBD calculus is visualized. Multiple signal-void calculi are demonstrated in the gallbladder (long arrow, *a*). The coronal thin-section image (*b*) reveals a 5-mm preampullary CBD stone (arrow, *b*). Coronal T2-weighted thin-section echo-train

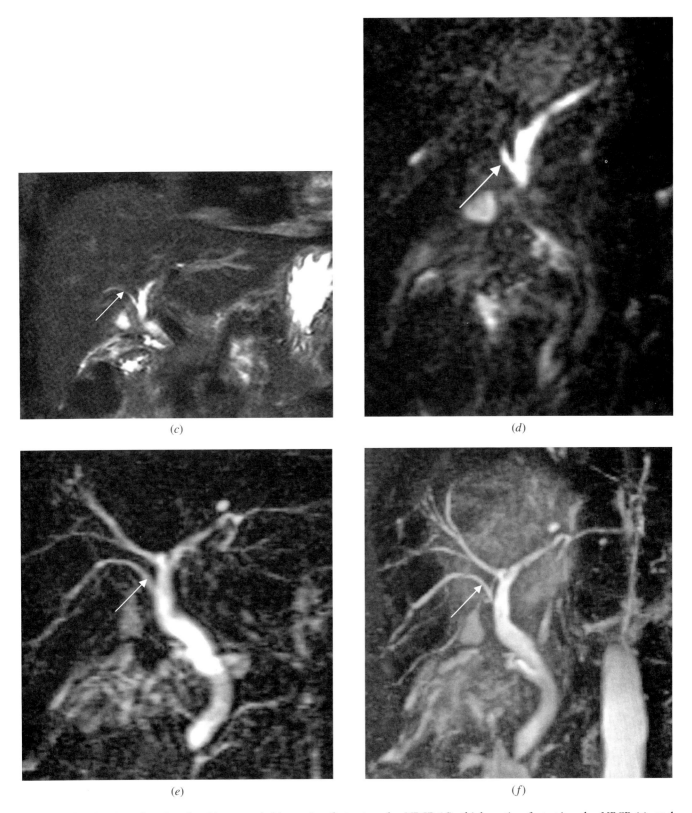

F I G . 3.3 (*Continued*) spin-echo (*c*), coronal thin-section fast spin-echo MRCP (*d*), thick-section fast spin-echo MRCP (*e*), and reconstructed 3D MIP MRCP (*f*) images demonstrate the right accessory bile duct in another patient.

1–3 mm provides sufficient signal to obtain good-quality images and is sufficiently thin to detect small calculi (see figs. 3.1 and 3.3). Thin-collimation images can be obtained as multiple single-section acquisitions with no gap in an interleaved fashion to avoid cross-talk.

Three-dimensional reconstruction can also be performed on the thin-collimation source images, using a maximum-intensity projection (MIP) algorithm that generates images that closely resemble conventional cholangiograms (see figs. 3.1 and 3.3). However, volume averaging effects degrade spatial and contrast resolution, which makes it necessary to use the thin-source images for the evaluation of pathology, in particular for the detection of small stones and subtle mural irregularity.

Single-shot echo-train spin-echo sequences, such as HASTE and RARE techniques, can be applied as breath-hold or breathing-independent sequences. The breathing-independent thick-section approach is the fastest technique and is especially useful in patients who are uncooperative or cannot hold their breath (e.g., infants, the very sick, and old patients). For thin-section acquisitions, misregistrations due to respiratory motion should be avoided and thus breath-hold sequences are generally preferable. A new non-breath-hold respiratory-triggered turbo spin echo (TSE) technique uses navigator pulses to register the movement of the diaphragm in order to compensate for respiratory motion [27, 28]. In this technique the high-resolution data set is acquired over several respiratory cycles. A series of navigator pulses are acquired in order to measure the diaphragm position and thus to detect when the patient has reached the relatively long quiet phase at end expiration. At that point, the sequence switches from navigation to imaging and acquires several lines of k-space using a TSE approach. The respiratory navigator then resumes in order to ensure that the next repetition is also acquired with the diaphragm in roughly the same position. With the use of a volumetric, heavily T2-weighted sequence (TE ~600 ms), 3D Turbo Spin-Echo images are acquired over a period of several minutes, which allows the reconstruction of 3D images and thin 2D images [27, 28].

T1-Weighted Sequences

T1-weighted sequences are useful for the evaluation of duct walls and parenchymal lesions. These can be acquired as T1-weighted gradient-echo sequences in a 2D or a 3D technique, obtained before and after gadolinium administration. Fat suppression techniques are essential as they improve the delineation of enhancing duct walls, inflammatory tissue, small lymph nodes, and tumor infiltration from surrounding fatty tissue [29]. The use of breath-hold T1-weighted gradient-echo sequences

after gadolinium administration also provides information on the blood supply and interstitial space of diseased tissue that facilitates characterization.

In addition to standard nonspecific extracellular gadolinium chelates, T1-shortening intravenous contrast agents that are partly eliminated in bile have been used for the evaluation of the biliary system, including gadobenate dimeglumine (Multihance) and gadoxetic acid (Eovist) [30, 31]. Manganese-based contrast agent Mn-DPDP is also eliminated through the biliary route; however, it is not currently available in the USA. Owing to their lipophilic character, these contrast agents are taken up by hepatocytes and secreted into the biliary ductal system. Gadoxetic acid (Eovist) has a greater fractional elimination by the biliary system than gadobenate dimeglumine (Multihance), and as a result biliary elimination is visualized at 15 min with gadoxetic acid (Eovist) compared to 1 h with gadobenate dimeglumine (Multihance) [31]. On T1-weighted images, this leads to bright signal of contrasted bile in biliary ducts and gallbladder (fig. 3.4). Bright bile images can be generated with 2D or 3D T1-weighted gradient-echo techniques. However, in the presence of high-grade biliary obstruction the bile ducts distal to the obstruction may remain noncontrasted, and in patients with diminished hepatocyte function the biliary system may be poorly opacified. Laceration or injury to the biliary system may be revealed as high-signal fluid leaking beyond the biliary system.

NORMAL APPEARANCE AND VARIANTS

Gallbladder

On T2-weighted sequences, the walls of the gallbladder and bile ducts are of low signal intensity and normal bile shows high signal intensity (fig. 3.5). On T1-weighted images, the wall of the gallbladder is of intermediate signal intensity, comparable to adjacent soft tissue such as liver. Bile within the gallbladder may vary from very low to high signal intensity on T1-weighted images, because of variations in the concentration of water, cholesterol, and bile salts (see fig. 3.5) [32]. Nonconcentrated bile accumulates in the gallbladder and demonstrates low signal intensity on T1-weighted sequences, similar to water. With reabsorption of water and increased cholesterol and bile salt concentration, the T1 relaxation time decreases and the signal from concentrated bile becomes increasingly high with increased concentration (fig. 3.6) [32]. In the presence of concentrated bile (e.g., in prolonged fasting state), a layering effect is often appreciated, with the concentrated hyperintense bile in the dependent portion of the

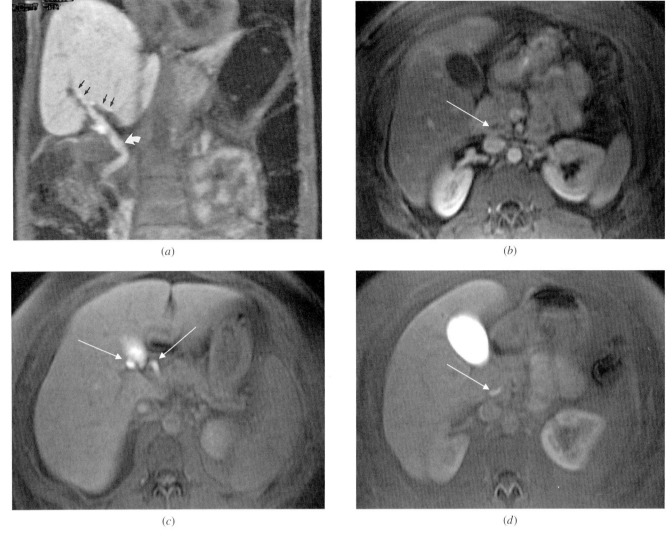

(a)

(b)

(c)

(d)

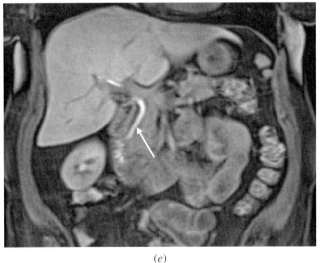

(e)

FIG. 3.4 Contrast-enhanced normal biliary tree. T1-weighted coronal Mn-DPDP-enhanced GE image (*a*) with fat suppression. The normal intrahepatic (small arrows) and extrahepatic (curved arrow) bile ducts demonstrate high signal intensity due to the T1 shortening of Mn-DPDP, which is excreted in the bile. Note also the enhancement of normal liver parenchyma. T1-weighted postgadolinium fat-suppressed 3D-GE images acquired after the administration of gadobenate dimeglumine (Multihance) (*b*–*d*) and gadoxetic acid (Eovist) (*e*). The common bile duct is seen as a hypointense structure on hepatic venous phase 3D-GE image (*b*) after the administration of gadobenate dimeglumine in another patient. The extrahepatic bile ducts (arrows, *c*), the common bile duct (arrow, *d*), and the gallbladder show contrast enhancement on 1-h delayed 3D-GE images (*c, d*) after the administration of gadobenate dimeglumine. The common bile duct (arrow, *e*) also shows enhancement on 15-min delayed coronal 3D-GE image (*e*) after the administration of gadoxetic acid in another patient. Gadobenate dimeglumine and gadoxetic acid have both extracellular and intracellular properties. They are hepatocyte-specific contrast agents (intracellular property) and are taken up by hepatocytes and excreted into the bile ducts. Therefore, they have dual elimination, including biliary and renal. They can be used as routine extracellular gadolinium agents for the acquisition of arterial, venous, and interstitial phase images. Delayed imaging also allows us to obtain additional morphologic and functional information for the liver and biliary system and their pathologies. Note that the liver is enhanced on delayed images (*c*–*e*). The enhancement of the liver is more with gadoxetic acid because of its higher biliary elimination (50%) compared to the biliary elimination of gadobenate dimeglumine (3%).

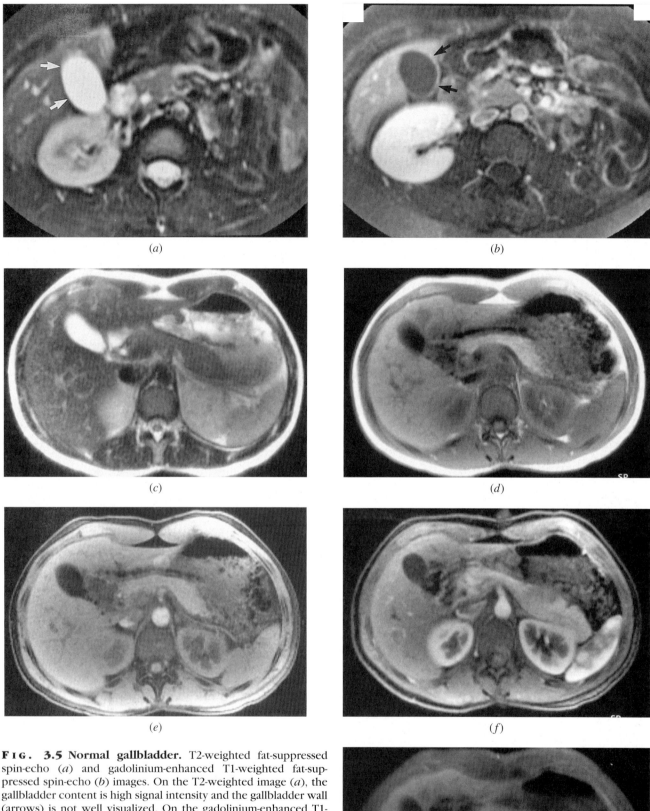

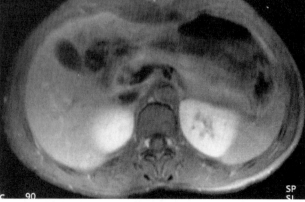

FIG. 3.5 Normal gallbladder. T2-weighted fat-suppressed spin-echo (*a*) and gadolinium-enhanced T1-weighted fat-suppressed spin-echo (*b*) images. On the T2-weighted image (*a*), the gallbladder content is high signal intensity and the gallbladder wall (arrows) is not well visualized. On the gadolinium-enhanced T1-weighted fat-suppressed spin-echo image (*b*), the gallbladder wall (arrows) is well shown as a thin enhancing structure. The gallbladder wall adjacent to the liver is not clearly defined because the enhancement of gallbladder wall and liver are similar.

T2-weighted simple shot echo-train spin-echo (*c*), T1-weighted GE (*d*), fat-suppressed GE (*e*), immediate postgadolinium fat-suppressed GE (*f*), and 2-min postgadolinium fat-suppressed spin-echo (*g*) images in a second patient with normal gallbladder. The bile is high in signal on the T2-weighted image (*c*) and low in signal on the T1-weighted images (*d–g*).The normal gallbladder wall is barely perceptible as a thin line, best shown on the immediate postgadolinium image (*f*).

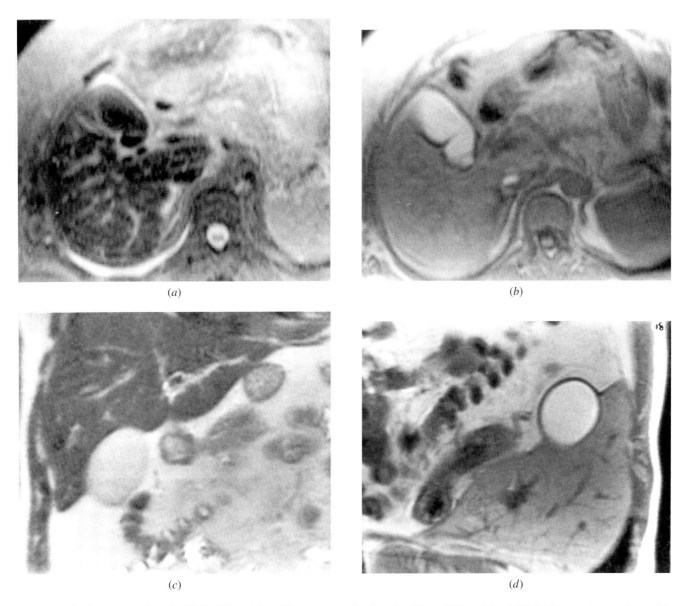

(a)

(b)

(c)

(d)

F I G . 3.6 Abnormal signal of bile. T2-weighted fat-suppressed spin-echo (*a*) and T1-weighted GE (*b*) images in a patient with primary biliary cirrhosis. The bile in the gallbladder is highly concentrated, resulting in low signal on the T2-weighted image (*a*) and high signal on the T1-weightcd image (*b*). A small pleural effusion is present in the right posterior pleural recess showing high signal on the T2-weighted image (*a*).

Coronal T2-weighted single-shot echo-train spin-echo (*c*) and coronal T1-weighted GE (*d*) images in a second patient with concentrated bile in the gallbladder showing moderately high signal on the T2-weighted image (*c*) and high signal on the T1-weighted image (*d*). Note that on the T2-weighted image (*c*), both fluid and fat are higher signal than bile.

gallbladder fundus (fig. 3.7). After intravenous gadolinium administration, the normal gallbladder wall enhances homogeneously comparable to the enhancement of adjacent liver parenchyma (see fig. 3.5). Variations of the gallbladder include phrygian cap configuration, ectopic location (i.e., intrahepatic, retrohepatic, or beneath the left lobe), and septations. Septations are best visualized on single-shot T2-weighted sequences, in which they appear low signal in a background of high-signal fluid.

Bile Ducts

With MRCP sequences, the intrahepatic ducts can be visualized as an arborizing system of high signal intensity that can be followed into the outer third of the liver in over 90% of patients (see fig. 3.1) [33]. Anatomic variants, however, occur relatively frequently and are of clinical importance in laparoscopic cholecystectomy and in living donor liver transplantation because preoperatively unrecognized bile duct variations may result

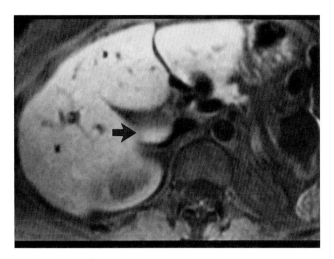

F I G . 3.7 Layering of gallbladder bile. T1-weighted fat-suppressed spin-echo image. Layering of the bile in the gall-bladder is observed with the more concentrated, hyperintense bile (arrow) in the dependent portion of the gallbladder.

in complications [34]. The clinically most important variants are aberrant intrahepatic ducts that may join the common hepatic duct (CHD), common bile duct (CBD), cystic duct, gallbladder, or an anomalous right hepatic duct that joins the CBD, all of which place the patient at increased risk for bile duct injury at endoscopic cholecystectomy (fig 3.3) [35]. A right dorsocaudal intrahepatic branch draining into the left hepatic duct, known as crossover anomaly, is the most frequent bile duct variation. MRCP can play a valuable role in the preoperative evaluation of the biliary tree because of its excellent capability of noninvasively detecting aberrant or accessory ducts [6, 36].

The extrahepatic ducts (CHD, cystic duct, CBD) are consistently well evaluated (fig. 3.8). Occasionally, surgical clips, metallic stents, or pneumobilia may render segments of the ducts signal void. The cystic duct can be visualized in its full extent, including its insertion into the CBD (see fig. 3.1). A number of variations of its insertion are of clinical significance for laparoscopic cholecystectomy because they also have been shown to increase the risk of bile duct injury. Such variants include a low or medial duct insertion, insertion into the right hepatic duct, a long parallel course of the cystic and common hepatic ducts, and a short cystic duct [6, 37].

The CBD empties into the duodenum through the major papilla. This is a small mucosal protrusion into the duodenum resulting from the muscles that surround the distal CBD and ventral pancreatic duct. Its signal intensity is isointense to duodenal wall on T1- and T2-weighted images. Along the superior aspect of the major papilla is the superior papillary fold, which often forms a hood over the papilla that may be quite prominent.

Inferior to the papilla is the longitudinal fold. The shape and size of the major papilla can vary, with reported average diameters of 15 × 7 mm (longitudinal × transverse) [38]. The minor papilla is the orifice of the dorsal pancreatic duct and is located proximal to the major papilla. With MRCP, the major papilla is visualized in 40% of cases [39]. The minor papilla is seen less frequently.

On T1-weighted sequences, the signal of bile in intrahepatic ducts is usually low because of its high water content. In the CBD, however, the signal can be variable, reflecting the concentration of bile, although concentrated bile is observed much less frequently in the CBD compared to the gallbladder. On postgadolinium fat-suppressed images acquired approximately 2 min after gadolinium administration, the bile duct walls are best depicted and show moderate enhancement that may be slightly higher than that of normal liver parenchyma.

Biliary Anastomoses

In the presence of end-to-end anastomosis (e.g., after orthotopic liver transplantation), Roux-en-Y, or other choledochoenteric anastomoses, ERCP is technically very difficult to perform or contraindicated. In such instances, MRCP is the imaging modality of choice and may be particularly useful to exclude strictures (e.g., at the anastomosis) and to demonstrate the morphology and diameter of the bile ducts distal and proximal to the anastomosis (fig. 3.9) [40]. The presence of a biliary-enteric anastomosis can be suspected when small bowel is noted tucked into the porta hepatis (see fig. 3.9).

DISEASES OF THE GALLBLADDER

Nonneoplastic Disease

Gallstone Disease
Predisposing factors for cholelithiasis can be summarized as "female, forty, fat, fair, fertile," preexisting cholestasis, inflammatory bowel disease, and metabolic disorders (e.g., diabetes mellitus, pancreatic disease, hypercholesterolemia, cystic fibrosis). The primary imaging modality for cholecystolithiasis is sonography. However, because of the high prevalence of this disease, gallstones frequently are encountered incidentally and familiarity with their MRI appearance is essential.

MRCP sequences are highly sensitive and accurate in depicting cholecystolithiasis and can outperform ultrasound and computed tomography [2]. Gallstones generally present as intraluminal, signal-void, round or faceted structures on both T1- and T2-weighted images (fig. 3.10). Occasionally, areas of high signal intensity will be present in gallstones on T1- and T2-weighted

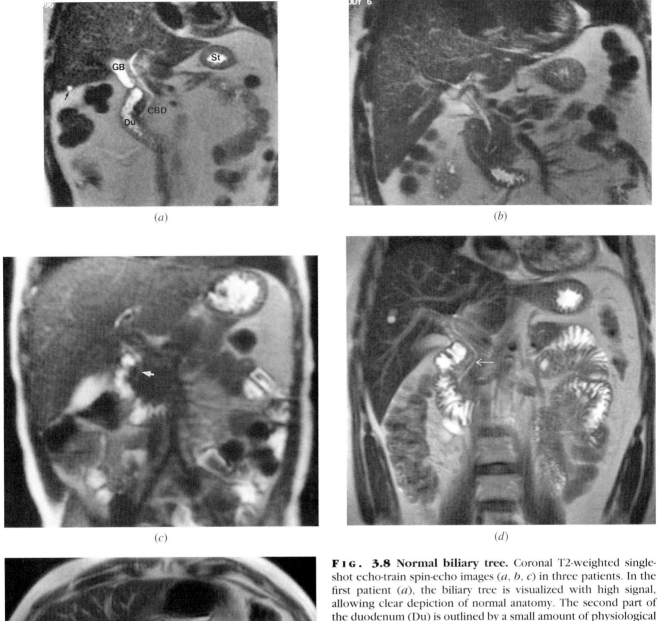

(a)

(b)

(c)

(d)

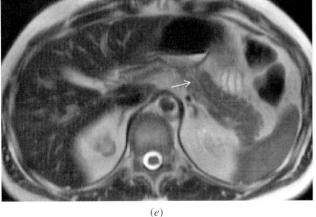

(e)

F I G . 3.8 Normal biliary tree. Coronal T2-weighted single-shot echo-train spin-echo images (*a*, *b*, *c*) in three patients. In the first patient (*a*), the biliary tree is visualized with high signal, allowing clear depiction of normal anatomy. The second part of the duodenum (Du) is outlined by a small amount of physiological fluid in this fasting patient (*a*) (CBD, common bile duct; GB, gallbladder; St, stomach). A small liver cyst (arrow, *a*) is present in the right lobe. In a second adult patient (*b*), the right and left hepatic, common hepatic, and common bile ducts are demonstrated. A short portion of the pancreatic duct is also seen. In a 1-yr-old child (*c*), the CBD (arrow) is well visualized despite the lack of patient cooperation. Coronal (*d*) and transverse (*e*) T2-weighted single-shot echo-train spin-echo images at 3.0 T demonstrate normal common bile duct (arrow, *d*) and pancreatic duct (arrow, *e*) in another patient. Note that valvula conniventes of the small intestine are seen very well, and there are biliary hamartomas in the liver.

sequences, or, less commonly, the stones will appear largely hyperintense on T1-weighted sequences (fig. 3.11) [41, 42]. The exact cause for the increased signal intensity has not yet been established. It has been shown, with spectroscopy and chemical analysis of gallstones, that it is not caused by high lipid content [42]. Therefore, the presence of protein macromolecules or dispersed calcium microparticles, which shorten T1

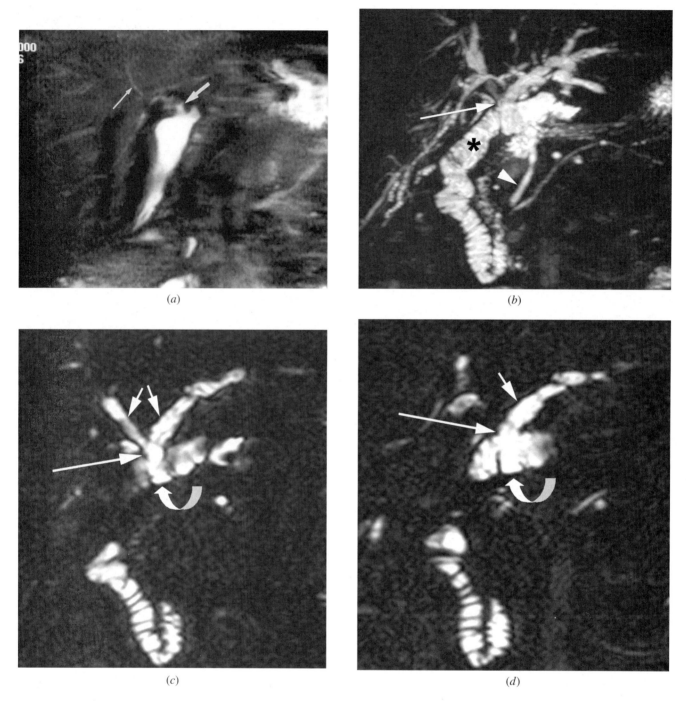

(a)   (b)

(c)   (d)

F I G . 3.9 Biliary anastomosis. Coronal T2-weighted fat-suppressed thin-section MRCP image (*a*) in a patient with hepatico-porto-enterostomy (after Kasai operation) showing the normal anastomosis between a bowel loop and the porta hepatis (arrow). Intrahepatic nondilated bile ducts are also well depicted (thin arrow). Paracoronal T2-weighted fat-suppressed thick-section MRCP image (*b*) and thin-section MRCP images (*c*, *d*) in a different patient with hepaticojejunostomy after liver transplantation. The thick-slab MRCP image (*b*) gives an excellent overview of the anatomic situation. The biliary anastomosis (long arrow, *b–d*) between the common hepatic duct and the jejunal bowel loop (asterisk, *b*; curved arrow, *c*, *d*) shows normal diameter and regular fluid signal. The intrahepatic bile ducts are mildly dilated, and the right and left hepatic ducts (short arrows, *c*, *d*) are well visualized. The remaining original common bile duct (arrowhead, *b*) and the adjacent pancreatic duct are also visualized. T2-weighted coronal

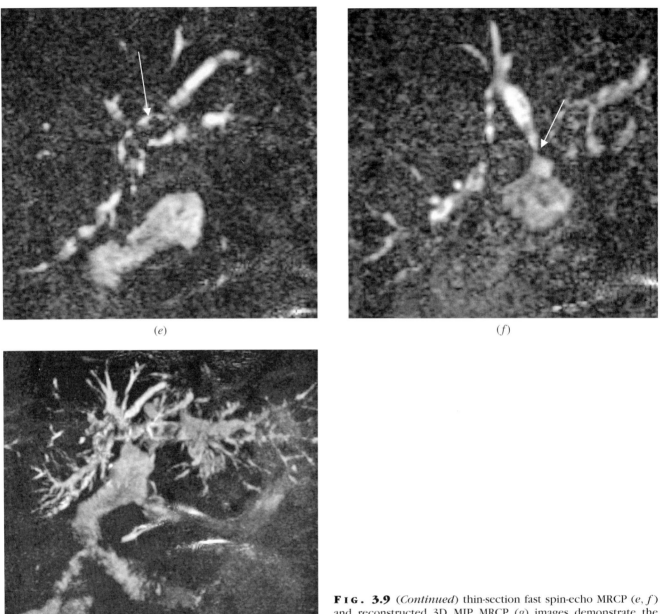

(e)

(f)

(g)

FIG. 3.9 (*Continued*) thin-section fast spin-echo MRCP (*e*, *f*) and reconstructed 3D MIP MRCP (*g*) images demonstrate the common bile duct-jejunum anastomosis in another patient. There is stenosis (arrow, *f*) in the region of anastomosis, and there are stones (arrows, *e*) proximally in the dilated bile ducts.

relaxation times, may be a reasonable explanation [43, 44]. Occasionally, the specific weight of a gallstone is lower than that of bile and the gallstone will float in the nondependent portion of the gallbladder (fig. 3.12). In this case, a gallstone can be differentiated from a gallbladder polyp by the lack of enhancement on T1-weighted postgadolinium images.

Acute Cholecystitis

Acute inflammation of the gallbladder is caused by obstruction of the cystic duct (e.g., by cystic duct stones) in 80–95% of patients. Morphologic criteria to establish the diagnosis have been described in the ultrasound literature. A combination of gallbladder wall thickening (>3 mm), three-layered appearance of the wall, hazy delineation of the gallbladder, localized pain (Murphy's sign), presence of gallstones, gallbladder hydrops, and fluid surrounding the gallbladder indicate a high probability of acute cholecystitis. In the presence of acalculous cholecystitis, or if many of these signs are absent, establishing the correct diagnosis with ultrasound is challenging and findings can be equivocal.

Acute cholecystitis results in increased blood flow and capillary leakage due to inflammatory changes,

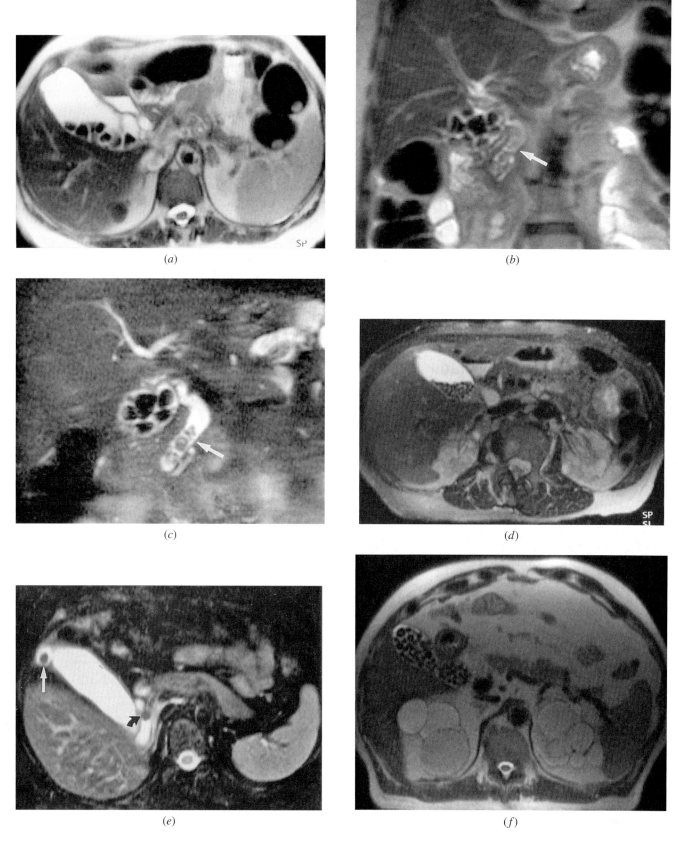

(a)

(b)

(c)

(d)

(e)

(f)

F I G. 3.10 Gallstone disease. T2-weighted 8-mm transverse (*a*) and coronal (*b*) single-shot echo-train spin-echo images and coronal thin-section MRCP single-shot echo-train spin-echo image with fat suppression (*c*). Multiple calculi are demonstrated as round or faceted signal-void structures in the gallbladder (*a, b, c*) and the CBD (arrows, *b* and *c*), outlined by high-signal bile. Note how much better the CBD stones are visualized on the thin-section MRCP image (*c*) compared to the standard 8-mm image (*b*).

Transverse T2-weighted single-shot echo-train spin-echo image (*d*) in a second patient showing multiple tiny signal-void calculi in the dependent portion of the gallbladder.

Transverse T2-weighted fat-suppressed spin-echo image (*e*) in a third patient showing stones in the phrygian cap of the gallblad-der (straight arrow, *e*) and in the cystic duct (curved arrow, *e*). T2-weighted single-shot echo-train spin-echo (*f*), T1-weighted

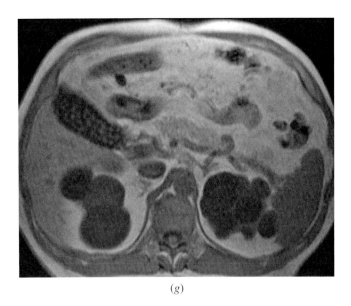
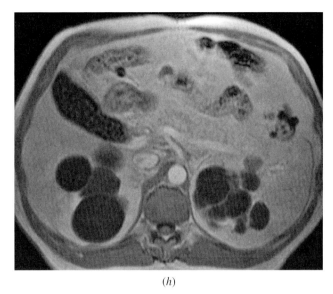

(g)   (h)

F I G .   3.10 (*Continued*) SGE (*g*), and T1-weighted postgadolinium interstitial phase SGE (*h*) images demonstrate multiple hypointense stones in the gallbladder in another patient. Note that there are multiple cysts in the kidneys and this finding is consistent with autosomal dominant polycystic kidney disease.

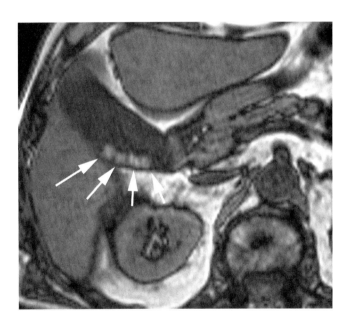

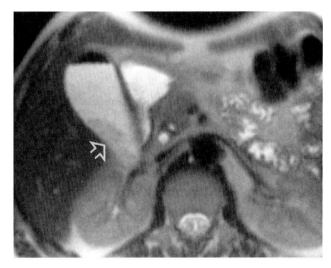

F I G .   3.12 Floating gallstones. Transverse T2-weighted single-shot echo-train spin-echo image demonstrating multiple small, signal-void calculi floating in the nondependent portion of the gallbladder. Concentrated bile (sludge), appears as moderately hypointense material in the dependent portion of the gallbladder (open arrow).

F I G .   3.11 Hyperintense gallstones. T1-weighted opposed-phase GE image showing several small gallstones (arrows) of uniform high signal intensity in the dependent portion of the gallbladder.

which is reflected on MRI by increased enhancement on postgadolinium images. The high sensitivity of MRI for gadolinium enhancement, especially with the use of fat suppression techniques, makes it an effective technique for the diagnosis of acute cholecystitis, demonstrating higher sensitivity and accuracy than ultrasound [45, 46]. The enhancement is most pronounced along the mucosal layer of the gallbladder wall on T1-weighted

immediate postgadolinium images and progresses to involve the entire thickness of the wall on more delayed images (fig. 3.13). The percentage of contrast enhancement of the gallbladder wall has been shown to correlate well with the presence of acute cholecystitis and was more accurate than wall thickness in distinguishing acute from chronic cholecystitis and gallbladder malignancy [46, 47]. An important finding in acute

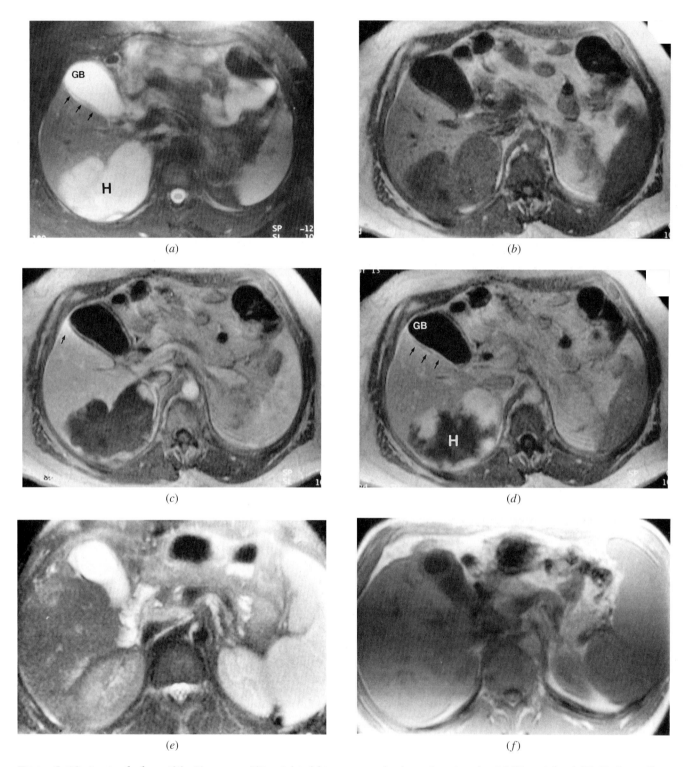

F I G . 3.13 Acute cholecystitis. Transverse T2-weighted fat-suppressed echo-train spin-echo (*a*), T1-weighted GE (*b*), immediate postgadolinium GE (*c*), and 90-s postgadolinium GE (*d*) images. The wall of the gallbladder (GB) is mildly thickened (4 mm) and shows increased signal intensity on the T2-weighted image (arrows, *a*). A giant hemangioma (H) is seen in *segment 6* of the liver. On the immediate postgadolinium image (*c*), increased enhancement of the gallbladder mucosa and transient increased enhancement of liver parenchyma adjacent to the gallbladder is apparent (arrow, *c*). On the 90-s postgadolinium image (*d*), increased enhancement of the entire gallbladder wall (arrows, *d*) is shown. Also note the peripheral nodular enhancement of the hemangioma (H).

T2-weighted fat-suppressed spin-echo (*e*), T1-weighted GE (*f*), immediate postgadolinium GE (*g*), and 2-min postgadolinium fat-suppressed GE (*h*) images in another patient. The gallbladder wall shows increased signal and wall thickening on the T2-weighted

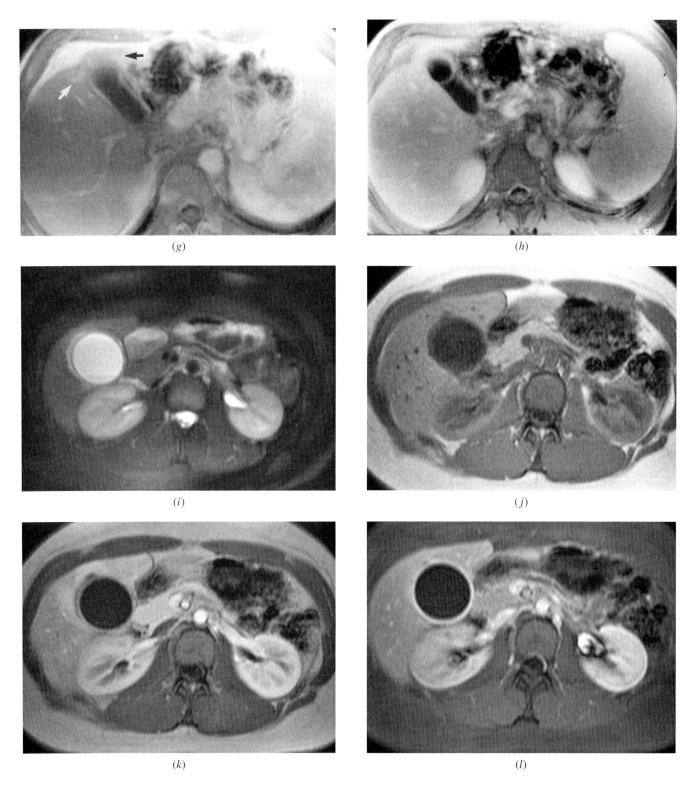

F I G . 3.13 (*Continued*) image (*e*). Increased enhancement of the gallbladder mucosa and transient increased enhancement of adjacent liver parenchyma (arrows, *g*) are seen on the immediate postgadolinium image (*g*). T2-weighted fat-suppressed single-shot echo-train spin-echo (*i*), T1-weighted SGE (*j*), T1-weighted postgadolinium hepatic arterial dominant phase SGE (*k*), and T1-weighted postgadolinium interstitial phase fat-suppressed SGE (*l*) images demonstrate acalculous cholecystitis in another patient. The gallbladder wall is thickened and shows hyperintense signal on T2-weighted image due to edema (*i*). There is transient increased pericholecystic hepatic parenchymal enhancement, which is a highly specific finding associated with acute inflammation, on the hepatic arterial dominant phase (*k*). The gallbladder wall shows intense enhancement on the interstitial phase (*l*). Note that

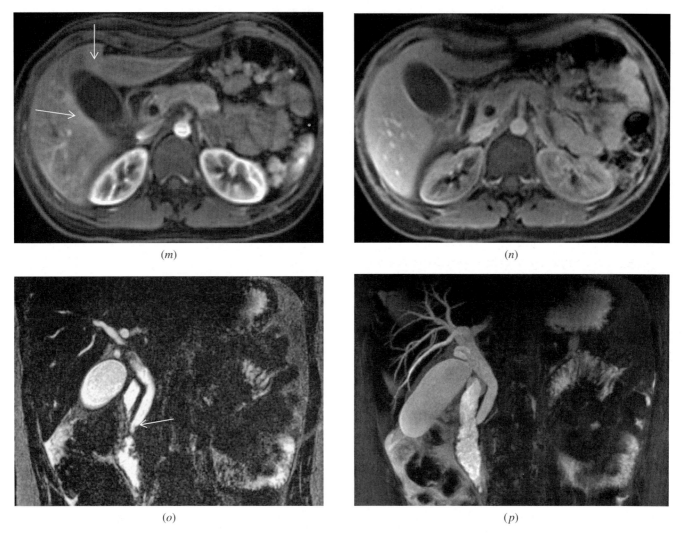

(m)   (n)

(o)   (p)

Fig. 3.13 (*Continued*) the bile shows layering on T2-weighted image (*i*) and the gallbladder is enlarged. T1-weighted postgado-linium fat-suppressed 3D-GE (*m, n*) and T2-weighted thin section fast spin echo MRCP (*o*) and reconstructed 3D MIP MRCP (*p*) images at 3.0 T demonstrate mild acalculous cholecystitis in another patient. There is transient increased pericholecystic hepatic parenchymal enhancement (arrows, *m*) on the hepatic arterial dominant phase (*m*), which fades to isointensity with the remaining liver parenchyma on the hepatic venous phase (*n*). The gallbladder wall shows prominent enhancement on the hepatic venous phase (*n*). MRCP images show the dilated biliary system due to ampullary stenosis secondary to passed stone. Fusiform ending of the common bile duct (arrow, *o*) suggests the presence of ampullary stenosis. Note that the gallbladder is enlarged.

cholecystitis is the transient increased enhancement of adjacent liver tissue on immediate postgadolinium images, which can be observed in approximately 70% of patients (figs. 3.13–3.15) [46, 47]. This reflects a hyperemic inflammatory response to the adjacent acute inflammation in the gallbladder wall. Thus findings that are indicative of acute cholecystitis on postgadolinium T1-weighted images include 1) increased wall enhance-ment, 2) transient increased enhancement of adjacent liver parenchyma on immediate postgadolinium images, and 3) increased thickness of the gallbladder wall [48]. Findings on T2-weighted images that are helpful to establish the diagnosis are 1) presence of gallstones, 2) presence of pericholecystic fluid, 3) presence of intra-

mural edema or abscesses appearing as hyperintense foci in the gallbladder wall, and 4) increased wall thick-ness (see figs. 3.13–3.15) [47]. Periportal high signal intensity may be observed but is a nonspecific finding.

Acute acalculous cholecystitis comprises about 5–15% of all acute cholecystitis cases. It can be caused by depressed motility (e.g., in patients with severe trauma/surgery, burns, shock, anesthesia, diabetes mellitus), by decreased blood flow in the cystic artery due to extrinsic obstruction or embolization, or by bacterial infection (fig. 3.16). MR imaging may be espe-cially useful for the diagnosis of acute acalculous cholecystitis in critically ill patients [46]. Complications of acute cholecystitis including abscess formation and

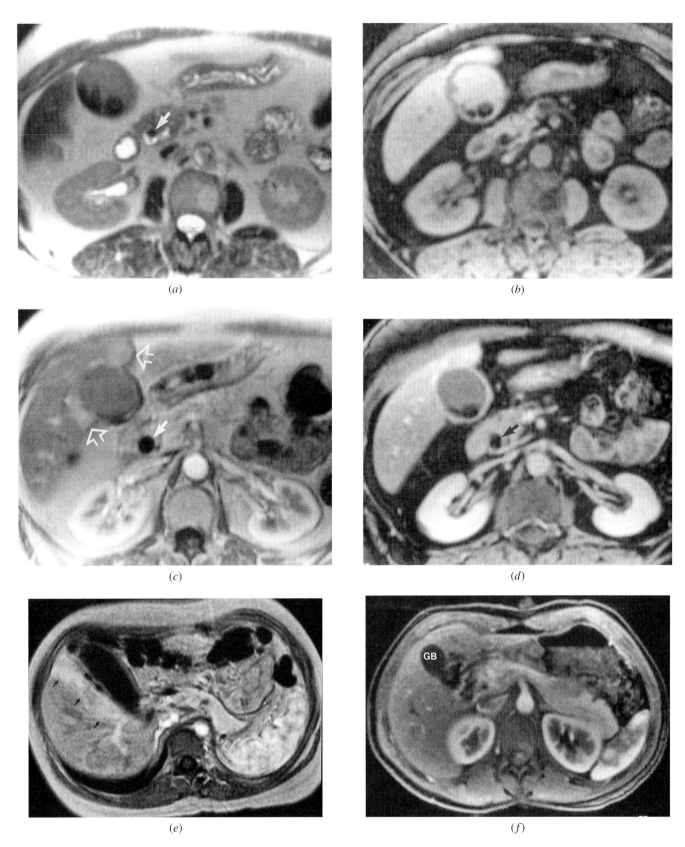

F I G . 3.14 Acute cholecystitis with gallstones. T2-weighted single-shot echo-train spin-echo (*a*),T1-weighted fat-suppressed GE (*b*), immediate postgadolinium GE (*c*), and 2-min postgadolinium fat-suppressed GE (*d*) images. The bile in the gallbladder is highly concentrated, showing low signal on the T2-weighted image (*a*) and high signal on the T1-weighted image (*b*).

Several low-signal gallstones are visualized in the gallbladder and the CBD (arrows, *a*, *c*, *d*). The gallbladder wall is thickened. On the immediate postgadolinium image (*c*), the adjacent liver parenchyma demonstrates transient increased enhancement (open arrows, *c*). Immediate postgadolinium GE image (*e*) in another patient demonstrating transient hyperemic enhancement of the liver (arrows, *e*) adjacent to the gallbladder. Immediate postgadolinium fat-suppressed GE image (*f*) in a normal subject for comparison,

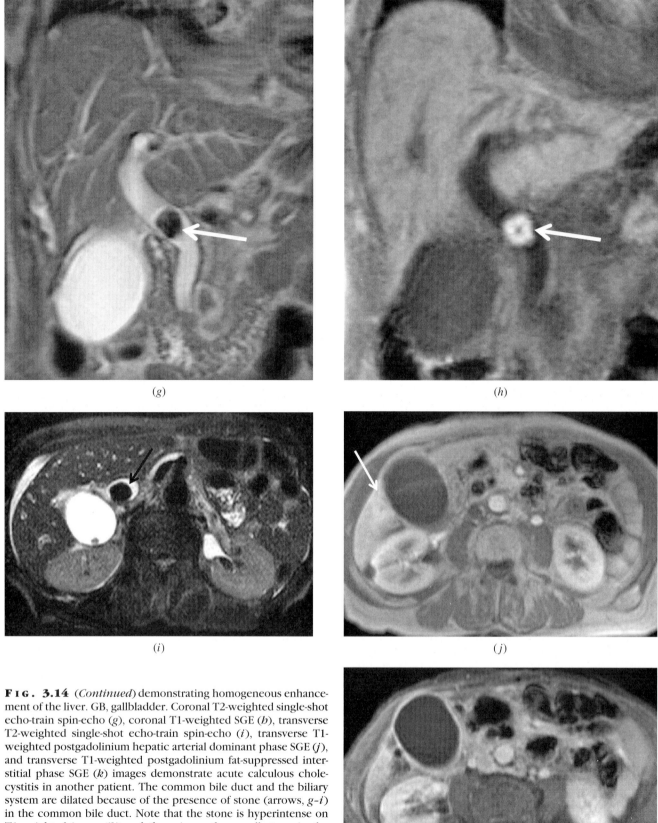

(g)

(h)

(i)

(j)

FIG. 3.14 (*Continued*) demonstrating homogeneous enhancement of the liver. GB, gallbladder. Coronal T2-weighted single-shot echo-train spin-echo (*g*), coronal T1-weighted SGE (*h*), transverse T2-weighted single-shot echo-train spin-echo (*i*), transverse T1-weighted postgadolinium hepatic arterial dominant phase SGE (*j*), and transverse T1-weighted postgadolinium fat-suppressed interstitial phase SGE (*k*) images demonstrate acute calculous cholecystitis in another patient. The common bile duct and the biliary system are dilated because of the presence of stone (arrows, *g–i*) in the common bile duct. Note that the stone is hyperintense on T1-weighted image (*h*) and there is another small stone in the gallbladder. The gallbladder is enlarged. The gallbladder wall is thickened and edematous. There is transient increased pericholecystic hepatic parenchymal enhancement (arrow, *j*) on the hepatic arterial dominant phase. The gallbladder wall shows prominent enhancement on the interstitial phase (*k*). Note the free fluid in the abdomen.

(k)

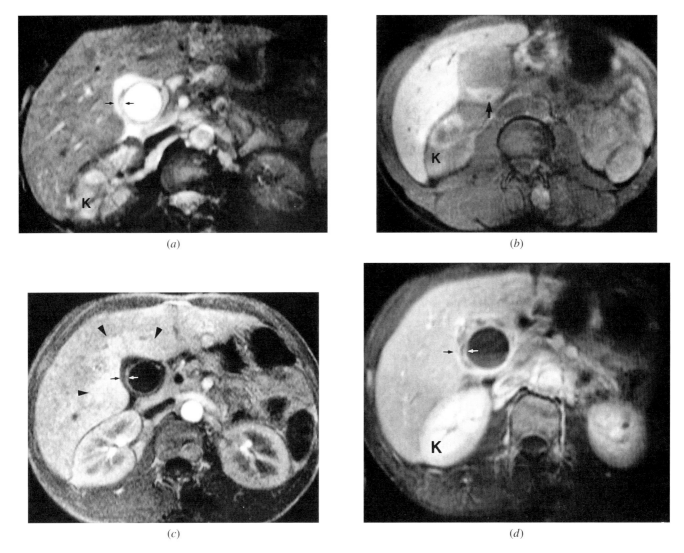

(a) (b)

(c) (d)

F I G . 3.15 Acute on chronic cholecystitis. T2-weighted fat-suppressed echo-train spin-echo (*a*),T1-weighted fat-suppressed spin-echo (*b*), immediate postgadolinium GE (*c*), and 2-min postgadolinium fat-suppressed spin-echo (*d*) images. The gallbladder wall is thickened (arrows, *a, c, d*) with increased mural signal intensity on the T2-weighted image (*a*). On the T1-weighted image (*b*), layering of high-signal concentrated bile in the dependent portion and a small, hypointense, gallbladder stone (arrow, *b*) are shown.

On the immediate postgadolinium image (*c*), moderate enhancement of the gallbladder mucosa and transient increased enhancement of adjacent liver parenchyma (arrowheads, *c*) are consistent with acute cholecystitis. Delayed heterogeneous enhancement of the markedly thickened gallbladder wall, demonstrated on the 2-min postgadolinium image (*d*), is suggestive of chronic inflammatory changes. The low signal intensity of the renal cortex is due to iron deposition in this patient with sickle cell anemia. K, kidney.

perforation can also be evaluated with high accuracy with MRI.

Hemorrhagic Cholecystitis

Hemorrhagic cholecystitis is more prevalent in patients with acalculous cholecystitis than in patients with calculous cholecystitis. Blood breakdown products in the gallbladder wall and lumen can be clearly identified with precontrast MRI sequences. Because of the specific signal intensity characteristics of these blood breakdown products on T1- and T2-weighted sequences, the

age of the hemorrhage may be determined (fig. 3.17). High signal on T1-weighted images is a distinctive feature of this condition, and MRI may be uniquely able to establish the diagnosis of hemorrhagic cholecystitis.

Chronic Cholecystitis

Chronic cholecystitis is more common than acute cholecystitis. However, the clinical findings of acute cholecystitis and chronic cholecystitis may overlap, and MR imaging may be used for the differentiation [46]. Because of the longstanding inflammatory process, a variable

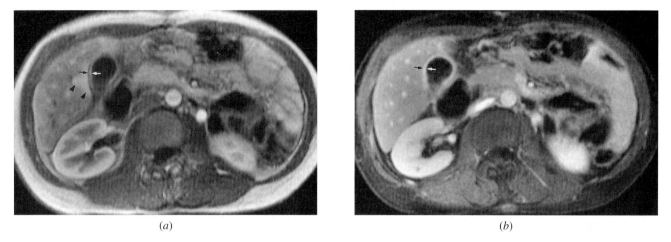

(a)   (b)

FIG. 3.16 Chemoembolization-induced acute cholecystitis. Immediate (*a*) and 90-s (*b*) postgadolinium GE images. Transient pericholecystic enhancement of the liver parenchyma (arrowheads, *a*) is noted on the immediate postgadolinium image (*a*). Homogeneous enhancement is observed after 90 s (*b*). The thickened gallbladder wall (arrows, *a*, *b*) shows progressive enhancement from *a* to *b*.

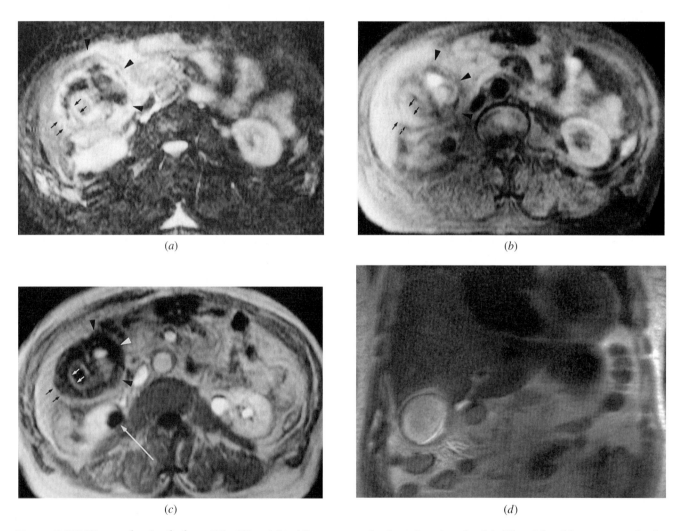

(a)   (b)

(c)   (d)

FIG. 3.17 Hemorrhagic cholecystitis. T2-weighted fat-suppressed echo-train spin-echo (*a*), T1-weighted fat-suppressed spin-echo (*b*), and immediate postgadolinium GE (*c*) images. On the T2-weighted image (*a*), the thickened gallbladder wall (small arrows, *a*) shows areas of high and low signal. A pericholecystic area of predominantly low signal (arrowheads, *a*) is located anteromedially. On the T1-weighted image (*b*), areas of high signal intensity consistent with hemorrhage are noted within the substantially thickened gallbladder wall (small arrows, *b*). The large complex anteromedial area (arrowheads, *b*) is predominantly of high signal, which in combination with the low signal on the T2-weighted image is consistent with intracellular methemoglobin in an area of hemorrhage. The delayed postgadolinium GE image (*c*) shows to better advantage the thick gallbladder wall (small arrows, *c*) and the hemorrhagic pericholecystic fluid collection (arrowheads, *c*). A calculus (long arrow, *c*) is incidentally shown in the right renal collecting system. Coronal T2-weighted single-shot echo-train spin-echo (*d*), transverse T1-weighted fat-suppressed 3D-GE (*e*),

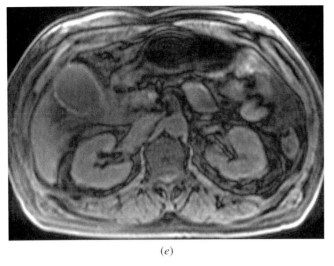

(e)

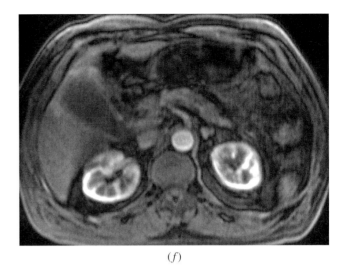

(f)

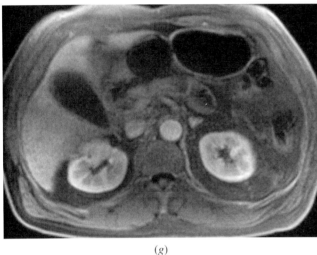

(g)

FIG. 3.17 (*Continued*) transverse T1-weighted postgadolinium arterial phase (*f*), and hepatic venous phase (*g*) fat-suppressed 3D-GE images at 3.0T demonstrate acute hemorrhagic cholecystitis in another patient. The gallbladder is enlarged and its wall is thickened. The wall shows hypointense signal on T2-weighted image (*d*) and hyperintense signal on T1-weighted image (*e*), which is consistent with hemorrhage. There is transient increased pericholecystic hepatic parenchymal enhancement on the arterial phase (*f*), which fades to isointensity with the remaining liver parenchyma on the hepatic venous phase (*g*).

degree of fibrosis occurs, causing wall thickening and shrinkage of the gallbladder. In contrast to acute cholecystitis, mural gadolinium enhancement is mild and most prominent on delayed postgadolinium images. Pericholecystic enhancement is minimal or absent, because of the lesser severity of the inflammatory process (fig. 3.18). The adjacent liver parenchyma usually does not show increased enhancement [46, 49]. A recent report has shown that increased gallbladder wall enhancement and increased transient pericholecystic hepatic enhancement were the most significant differences between acute and chronic cholecystitis [46]. The wall of the gallbladder may calcify, resulting in porcelain gallbladder (fig. 3.19). On MR images, calcifications may appear as signal-void foci. Patients with porcelain gallbladder may be at increased risk for gallbladder carcinoma. Therefore, enhancing nodular tissue arising from the gallbladder wall, best shown on fat-suppressed late postgadolinium images, should raise suspicion of malignant disease in these patients. A uniform wall of less than 4 mm, however, excludes the presence of malignancy (see fig. 3.19).

Xanthogranulomatous Cholecystitis

Xanthogranulomatous cholecystitis (fibroxanthogranulomatous inflammation) is a rare, focal or diffuse, destructive inflammatory disease of the gallbladder that is assumed to be a variant of chronic cholecystitis. The pathogenesis is thought to be occlusion of mucosal outpouchings (Rokitansky–Aschoff sinuses) with subsequent rupture and intramural extravasation of inspissated bile and mucin that causes an inflammatory reaction with multiple intramural xanthogranulomatous nodules. The importance of this disease is that it mimics gallbladder carcinoma both clinically and radiologically [50]. The MRI findings are focal or diffuse gallbladder wall thickening with contrast enhancement. Small intramural abscesses may be demonstrated as foci of high signal on T2-weighted images and low signal on T1-weighted images [51].

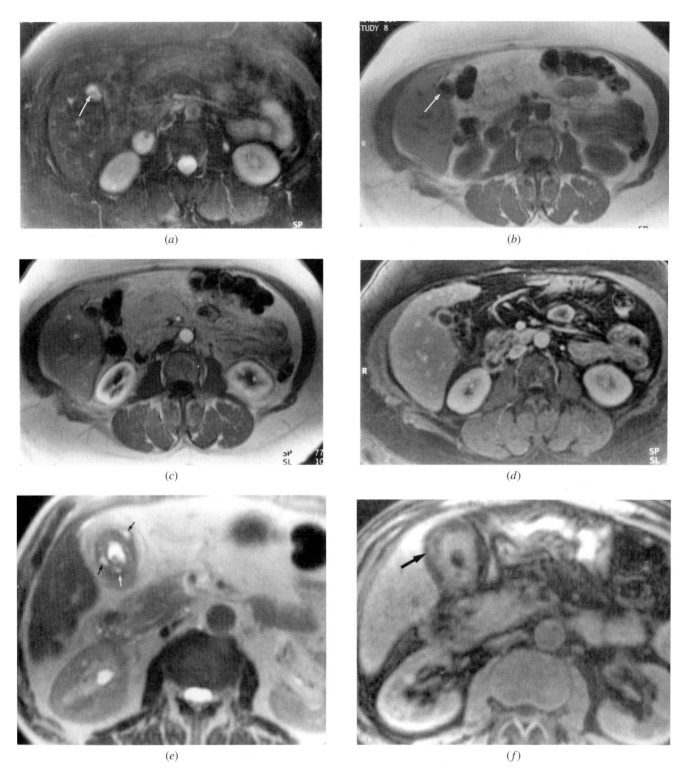

(a)

(b)

(c)

(d)

(e)

(f)

F i g . 3.18 Chronic cholecystitis. T2-weighted fat-suppressed spin-echo (*a*),T1-weighted GE (*b*), immediate postgadolinium GE (*c*), and 90-s postgadolinium fat-suppressed GE (*d*) images. On the T2-weighted image (*a*), the gallbladder is shrunken and irregular in shape, with poorly defined walls and a low-signal gallstone (arrow, *a*). On the precontrast T1-weighted image (*b*), the gallbladder wall is partly hyperintense (arrow, *b*). It enhances mildly on the immediate postgadolinium image (*c*), but no increased enhancement is noted in the adjacent liver parenchyma. On the 90-s postgadolinium fat-suppressed image (*d*), the gallbladder wall shows progressive enhancement.

T2-weighted single-shot echo-train spin-echo (*e*),T1-weighted fat-suppressed GE (*f*), and 2-min postgadolinium fat-suppressed GE (*g*) images in a second patient with chronic cholecystitis. The gallbladder is shrunken and irregular in shape and shows

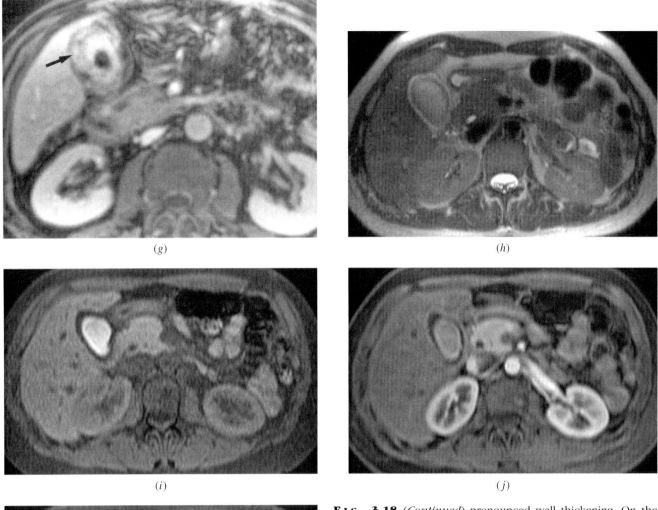

(g)

(h)

(i)

(j)

(k)

F I G . 3.18 (*Continued*) pronounced wall thickening. On the T2-weighted image (*e*), small hyperintense foci (short arrows, *e*) represent intramural fluid collections.

The gallbladder shows enhancement on the 2-min postgadolinium image (*g*). In the pericholecystic space, complex septations (arrows, *f*, *g*) demonstrating enhancement on the postgadolinium image (*g*) are suggestive of fibrous inflammatory tissue. Small low-signal calculi are seen in the gallbladder lumen (*e–g*). T2-weighted single-shot echo-train spin-echo (*h*), T1-weighted fat-suppressed SGE (*i*), T1-weighted fat-suppressed postgadolinium hepatic arterial dominant phase 3D-GE (*j*), and interstitial phase SGE (*k*) images demonstrate chronic cholecystitis in another patient. The gallbladder wall is thickened and shows hyperintense signal on T2-weighted image (*h*) due to edema. The gallbladder wall shows minimal enhancement on the hepatic arterial dominant phase (*j*) and moderate enhancement on the interstitial phase (*k*). The absence of associated transient increased pericholecystic hepatic parenchymal enhancement in combination with other findings suggest the presence of chronic cholecystitis. Note that the bile has high signal on T1-weighted image (*i*).

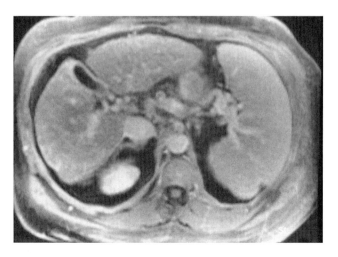

F I G . 3.19 Porcelain gallbladder. Diffuse calcification of the gallbladder wall was seen on a CT examination (not shown). The T1-weighted 2-min postgadolinium fat-suppressed GE image demonstrates uniform enhancement of a smooth 3-mm-thick gallbladder wall, which excludes superimposed malignancy.

Diffuse Gallbladder Wall Thickening

Diffuse gallbladder wall thickening may be present in a number of hepatic, biliary, and pancreatic diseases. Among nontumorous causes are hepatitis, liver cirrhosis, hypoalbuminemia, renal failure, systemic or hepatic venous hypertension, AIDS cholangiopathy, and graft-versus-host disease. Important features to discriminate these conditions from cholecystitis are minimal enhancement of the gallbladder wall and lack of increased enhancement of adjacent structures on postgadolinium images, in particular the lack of transient increased enhancement of adjacent liver parenchyma (fig. 3.20).

Neoplastic Disease

Gallbladder Polyps

Gallbladder polyps are often incidentally identified arising from the gallbladder wall and are either sessile or pedunculated. They comprise a wide spectrum of histologic types; however, the vast majority are benign. Nevertheless, gallbladder polyps pose a dilemma with respect to diagnosis of potential malignancy and determination of proper long-term management. The majority are cholesterol polyps that do not have malignant potential. Approximately 10% of gallbladder polyps, however, are adenomas, which are thought to have malignant potential [52]. However, this determination may be reliably established only by histology. Polyps are typically homogeneously low to intermediate in signal intensity on T1- and T2-weighted MR images. On T1-weighted postgadolinium images, they show moderate homogeneous enhancement that is most pronounced

on delayed images (fig. 3.21). Polyps can be readily distinguished from calculi on the basis of gadolinium enhancement, or by location: While the polyp is located on the nondependent surface of the gallbladder wall, calculi generally layer on the dependent surface or float horizontally within the gallbladder. Polyp size may be used as an indicator for malignant potential: Polyps 1 cm or smaller have minimal risk for malignancy and can be managed by imaging follow-up [53]. Symptomatic lesions, irregular polyps, polyps larger than 1 cm, or interval increase in size are worrisome for malignancy, and cholecystectomy is indicated [54].

Gallbladder Adenomyomatosis

Adenomyomatosis is a relatively common disease with a reported incidence of up to 5% [55]. This disease entity is characterized by hyperplasia of epithelial and muscular elements with mucosal outpouching of epithelium-lined cystic spaces into a thickened muscularis layer. These changes can involve the entire gallbladder or may be focal. The mucosal outpouchings are termed Rokitansky–Aschoff sinuses, and they form small intramural diverticula that are pathognomonic. On MR images, these fluid-filled sinuses appear as small intramural foci of low signal intensity on T1-weighted images and high signal intensity on T2-weighted images [55–57]. After gadolinium administration, early mucosal enhancement and late homogeneous enhancement can be observed (fig. 3.22) [55]. Demonstration of Rokitansky–Aschoff sinuses with a breath-hold or breathing-independent T2-weighted sequence has been shown to be a useful imaging finding to differentiate adenomyomatosis from gallbladder carcinoma [55]. However, this differentiation may be difficult on the basis of imaging.

Gallbladder Carcinoma

Gallbladder carcinoma is the most common biliary malignancy and occurs predominantly in the sixth and seventh decades with a slight female predominance [58]. Porcelain gallbladder has been considered a predisposing factor for gallbladder carcinoma. A recent large series, however, has cast doubt on this supposition [59]: In a review of 10,741 cholecystectomies, 15 specimens were porcelain gallbladder, and none of these 15 had gallbladder carcinoma [59]. Other diseases that are associated with gallbladder carcinoma are cholecystolithiasis, inflammatory bowel disease (predominantly ulcerative colitis), and chronic cholecystitis. However, fewer than 1% of patients with gallstones develop gallbladder carcinoma, and the risk for carcinoma is minimal if the stones are small and asymptomatic. The risk of developing carcinoma is increased if the stones are large and symptomatic, warranting prophylactic cholecystectomy. The most common histologic type of gallbladder carcinoma is adenocarcinoma, with squamous

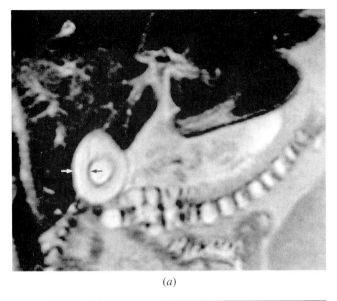

(a)

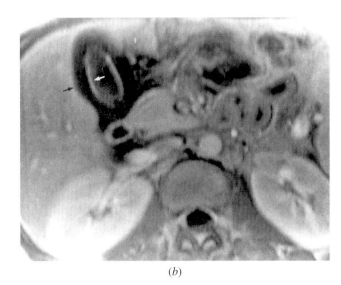

(b)

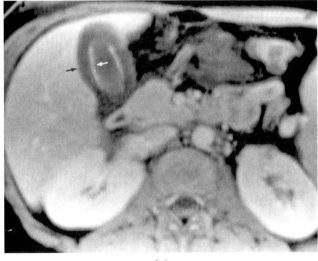

(c)

FIG. 3.20 Gallbladder wall edema. Coronal T2-weighted fat-suppressed single-shot echo-train spin-echo (*a*), T1-weighted immediate postgadolinium GE (*b*), and 2-min postgadolinium fat-suppressed GE (*c*) images. In this patient after bone marrow transplantation, the gallbladder wall is markedly edematous and thickened (arrows, *a–c*). Because of the high fluid content of the wall, the signal intensity is high on the T2-weighted image (*a*) and low on the T1-weighted images (*b*, *c*). The gallbladder mucosa shows moderate early and late enhancement (*b*, *c*). The adjacent liver parenchyma is normal.

cell tumor being far less common [60]. The 5-year survival rate is very poor (approximately 6%), reflecting that up to 75% of tumors are unresectable at initial presentation because of local invasion of adjacent organs.

Findings at MRI that are suggestive of gallbladder carcinoma are 1) a mass either protruding into the gallbladder lumen or replacing the lumen completely; 2) focal or diffuse thickening of the gallbladder wall greater than 1 cm; and 3) soft tissue (tumor) invasion of adjacent organs such as the liver, duodenum, and pancreas, which occurs frequently (fig. 3.23) [58, 61, 62]. On T1-weighted MR images, the tumor is hypo- or isointense compared to adjacent liver. On T2-weighted sequences, it is usually hyperintense relative to the liver and poorly delineated (see fig. 3.23) [62, 63]. The tumor usually

enhances on T1-weighted immediate postgadolinium images in a heterogeneous fashion, which facilitates differentiation from chronic cholecystitis [64]. However, superimposed infection or perforation of gallbladder carcinoma may be indistinguishable from severe acute cholecystitis. Invasion of the tumor into adjacent organs and the presence of lymph node metastases are features of advanced disease and can be best visualized with a combination of a T2-weighted fat-suppressed sequence, T1-weighted immediate postgadolinium gradient echo, and 2-min postgadolinium fat-suppressed gradient-echo sequence (see fig. 3.23) [62]. Preservation of a fat plane between tumor and surrounding structures excludes invasion. Delayed fat-suppressed gadolinium-enhanced images are particularly useful to delineate tumor spread along bile ducts and into the mesenteric fatty tissue.

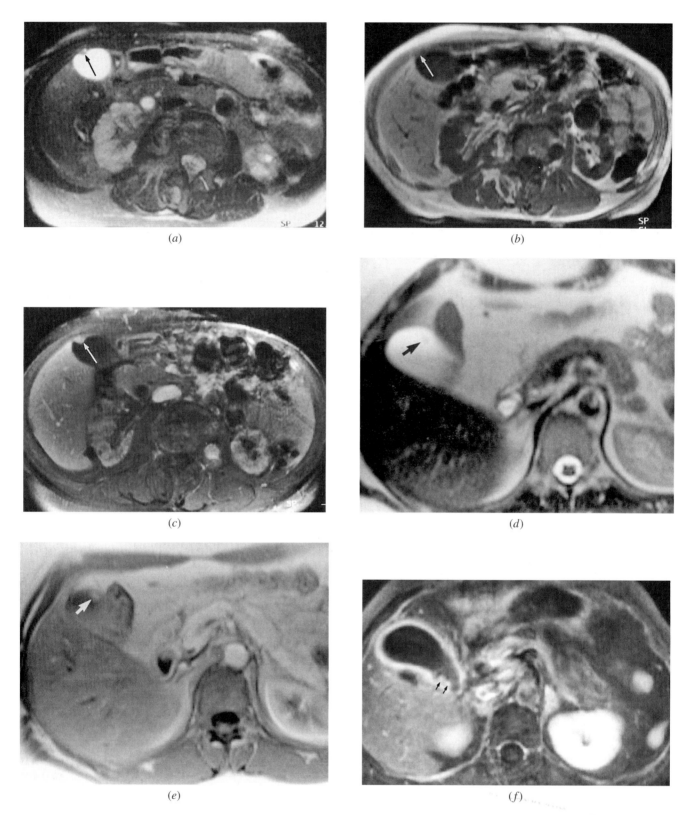

(a)

(b)

(c)

(d)

(e)

(f)

F I G . 3.21 Gallbladder polyps. T2-weighted fat-suppressed single-shot echo-train spin-echo (*a*),T1-weighted GE (*b*), and 2-min postgadolinium fat-suppressed GE (*c*) images. A 1-cm polyp (arrows, *a–c*) is shown on the nondependent surface of the gallbladder. The polyp is intermediate signal on the T2-weighted image (*a*), showing high contrast against bile. The polyp is low signal on the T1-weighted image (*b*) and can barely be seen. Intense uniform enhancement of the polyp is appreciated on the 2-min postgadolinium image (*c*). Enhancement and nondependent location distinguish the polyp from a gallbladder calculus. T2-weighted single-shot echo-train spin-echo (*d*) and T1-weighted 60-s postgadolinium GE (*e*) images in a second patient.

A polyp (arrows, *d, e*) is demonstrated in the nondependent portion of the gallbladder, showing intermediate signal on the T2-weighted image (*d*) and enhancement on the postgadolinium image (*e*). Layering of concentrated bile in the dependent portion of the gallbladder is seen on both sequences (*d, e*).

Transverse interstitial phase gadolinium-enhanced fat-suppressed SE image (*f*) in a third patient, with coexistent acute acalculous cholecystitis, demonstrates two small enhancing polyps (arrows, *f*). Note the intense enhancement of the acutely inflamed and

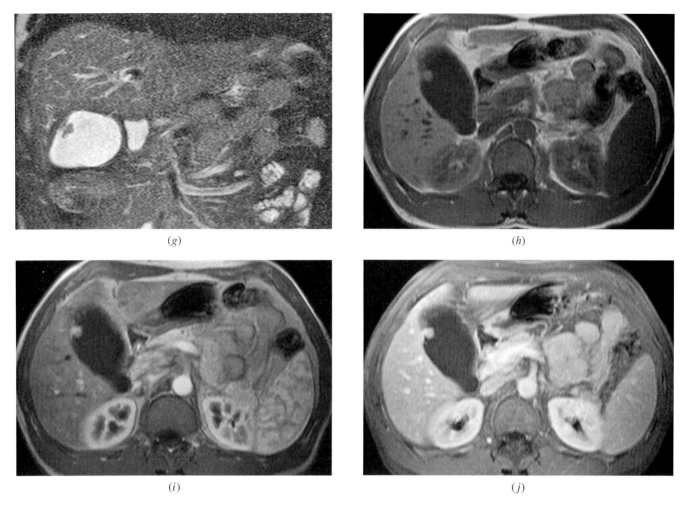

(g)

(h)

(i)

(j)

F I G . 3.21 *(Continued)* thickened gallbladder wall. Coronal T2-weighted echo train spin echo *(g)*, transverse T1-weighted SGE *(h)*, transverse T1-weighted postgadolinium hepatic arterial dominant phase SGE *(i)*, and hepatic venous phase fat-suppressed SGE *(j)* images demonstrate the gallbladder wall polyp, which shows prominent enhancement on postgadolinium images in another patient. The size of the polyp is relatively large, and its contours are irregular. These findings suggest that the lesion has malignant features, and the histopathologic findings are consistent with adenocarcinoma not extending beyond the serosa.

Metastases to the Gallbladder

A number of malignant diseases can metastasize to the gallbladder. Among the most common primary malignancies are breast carcinoma, melanoma, and lymphoma. Breast cancer and melanoma more commonly show focal gallbladder involvement, whereas lymphoma more commonly presents with diffuse mural involvement and thickening (fig. 3.24).

DISEASES OF THE BILE DUCTS

One of the main indications for MRCP and/or conventional MRI of the biliary system is to reveal the cause for biliary obstruction and to characterize the lesion process as benign or malignant. MRCP has become the first-line imaging modality for the diagnostic evaluation of bile ducts including the obstruction. In patients in whom ERCP is difficult to perform or contraindicated (e.g., patients who have undergone liver transplantation or biliary-enteric anastomosis), MRCP is the primary modality to evaluate biliary obstruction [65]. Common causes for benign obstruction are gallstone disease or strictures as a sequel to inflammation or surgery [66]. Malignant causes are pancreatic head tumors, primary biliary tumors, ampullary tumors, and compression from adjacent malignancies. In all cases it is necessary to define the level, grade, and cause of the biliary obstruction. Therefore, demonstration of the lumen and the walls of the bile ducts, as well as the surrounding tissue, is required. This can be achieved with a combination of MRCP and conventional MRI sequences acquired before and after intravenous administration of gadolinium.

The normal maximal diameters of the CBD as visualized with MRCP (measured on coronal source images)

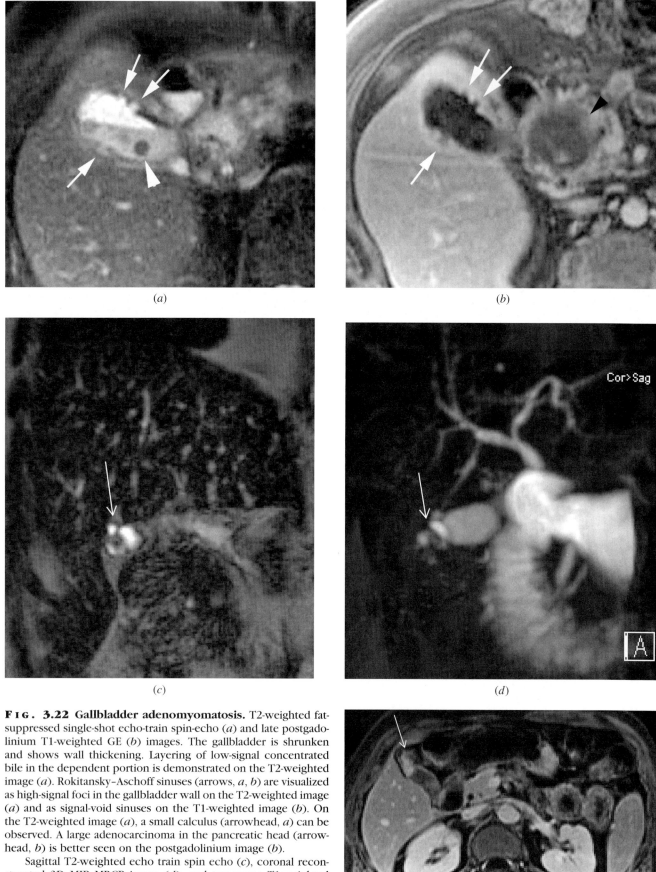

(a)

(b)

(c)

(d)

(e)

F I G . 3.22 Gallbladder adenomyomatosis. T2-weighted fat-suppressed single-shot echo-train spin-echo (*a*) and late postgadolinium T1-weighted GE (*b*) images. The gallbladder is shrunken and shows wall thickening. Layering of low-signal concentrated bile in the dependent portion is demonstrated on the T2-weighted image (*a*). Rokitansky–Aschoff sinuses (arrows, *a*, *b*) are visualized as high-signal foci in the gallbladder wall on the T2-weighted image (*a*) and as signal-void sinuses on the T1-weighted image (*b*). On the T2-weighted image (*a*), a small calculus (arrowhead, *a*) can be observed. A large adenocarcinoma in the pancreatic head (arrowhead, *b*) is better seen on the postgadolinium image (*b*).

Sagittal T2-weighted echo train spin echo (*c*), coronal reconstructed 3D MIP MRCP image (*d*), and transverse T1-weighted postgadolinium fat-suppressed 3D-GE image (*e*) demonstrate adenomyomatosis in another patient. Aschoff–Rokitansky sinuses (arrows, *c*, *d*) are seen as high signal intensity cystic spaces on T2-weighted image (*c*) and MRCP image (*d*). The gallbladder wall shows homogeneously enhancing thickening and unenhanced sinuses on postgadolinium image (*e*).

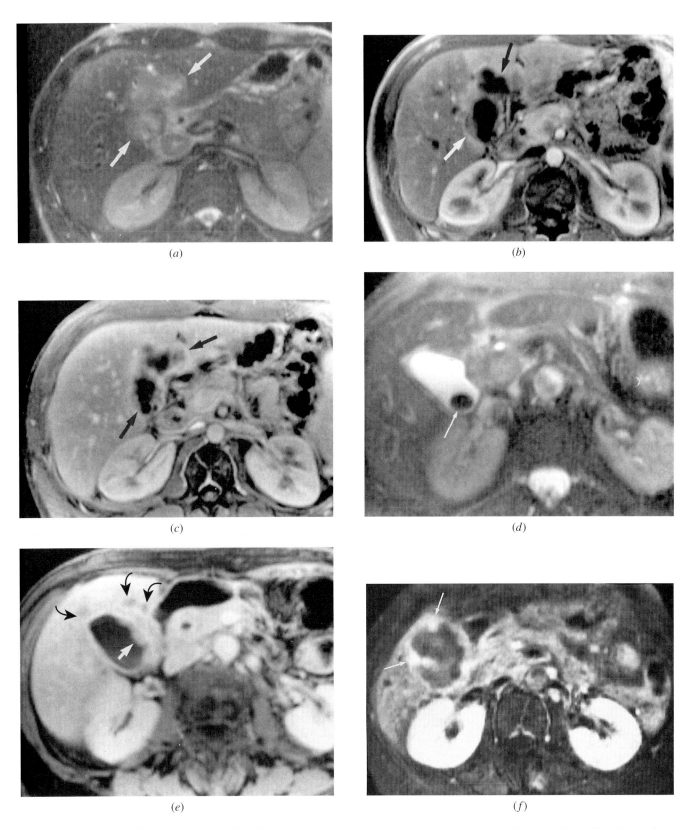

FIG. 3.23 Gallbladder carcinoma. T2-weighted fat-suppressed single-shot echo-train spin-echo (*a*), T1-weighted immediate postgadolinium GE (*b*), and 2-min postgadolinium fat-suppressed GE (*c*) images. The gallbladder (arrows, *a*–*c*) has a masslike appearance and shows an irregular and markedly thickened wall (arrows) that is moderately hyperintense on the T2-weighted image (*a*). Intense, slightly heterogeneous enhancement is demonstrated on the immediate and 2-min postgadolinium images (*b*, *c*), showing poor delineation from liver parenchyma.

T2-weighted fat-suppressed single-shot echo-train spin-echo (*d*) and T1-weighted 2-min postgadolinium fat-suppressed GE (*e*) images in a second patient with adenocarcinoma of the gallbladder. A signal-void stone is shown on the T2-weighted image (*d*). The gallbladder wall demonstrates partial irregular thickening (arrow, *e*), best visualized on the postgadolinium image (*e*). Small hypoenhancing areas in the adjacent liver parenchyma (curved arrows, *e*) are suggestive of metastases to the liver.

Transverse T1-weighted 2-min postgadolinium fat-suppressed GE image (*f*) in a third patient with gallbladder cancer demonstrates irregular nodular thickening of the gallbladder wall (arrows, *f*).

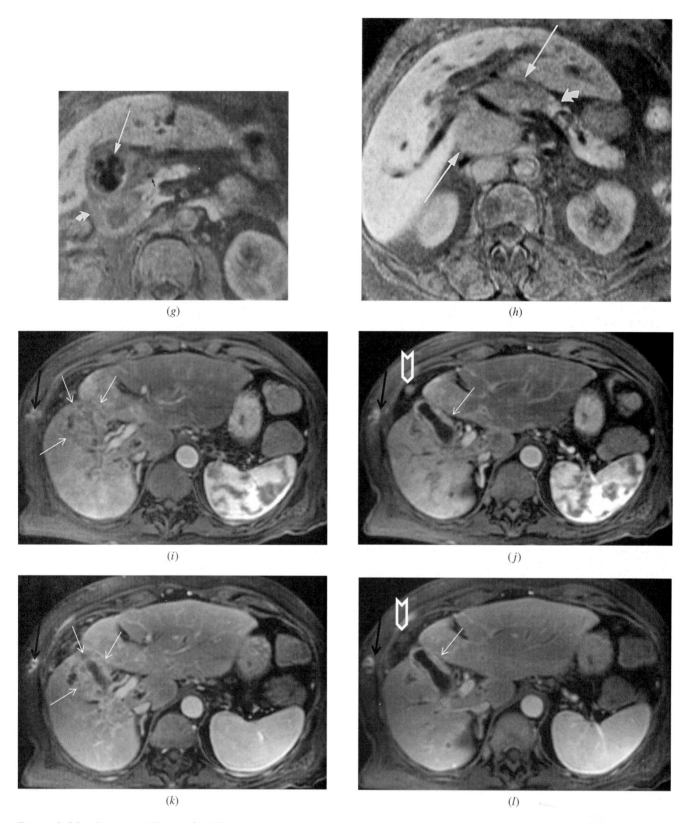

(g)

(h)

(i)

(j)

(k)

(l)

FIG. 3.23 (*Continued*) T1-weighted fat-suppressed spin-echo images (*g, h*) in a fourth patient demonstrating gallbladder cancer, which is intermediate in signal intensity and infiltrates along the duodenal wall (curved arrow, *g*) and head of the pancreas encasing the gastroduodenal artery (short arrow, *g*). Signal-void calculi are present within the gallbladder (long arrow, *g*). On a more superior image at the level of the porta hepatis (*h*), a large tumor (straight arrows, *h*) is demonstrated. Good contrast is observed between intermediate-signal tumor and high-signal pancreas (curved arrow, *h*).

T1-weighted postgadolinium hepatic arterial dominant phase (*i, j*) and hepatic venous phase (*k, l*) fat-suppressed 3D-GE images demonstrate gallbladder carcinoma in another patient. The gallbladder wall is irregularly thickened because of the tumor (white arrows, *j, l*). The adjacent liver parenchyma (white arrows, *i, k*) is heterogeneous because of tumor invasion. Multiple peripherally enhancing liver metastases are detected. Abdominal wall metastasis (black arrows, *i–l*) and peritoneal metastasis (open arrows, *j, l*) are also shown. There is increased differential enhancement in the right hepatic lobe on the hepatic arterial dominant phase (*i, j*) due to right portal vein thrombosis. Increased differential enhancement becomes isointense with the remaining liver parenchyma on the hepatic venous phase (*k, l*).

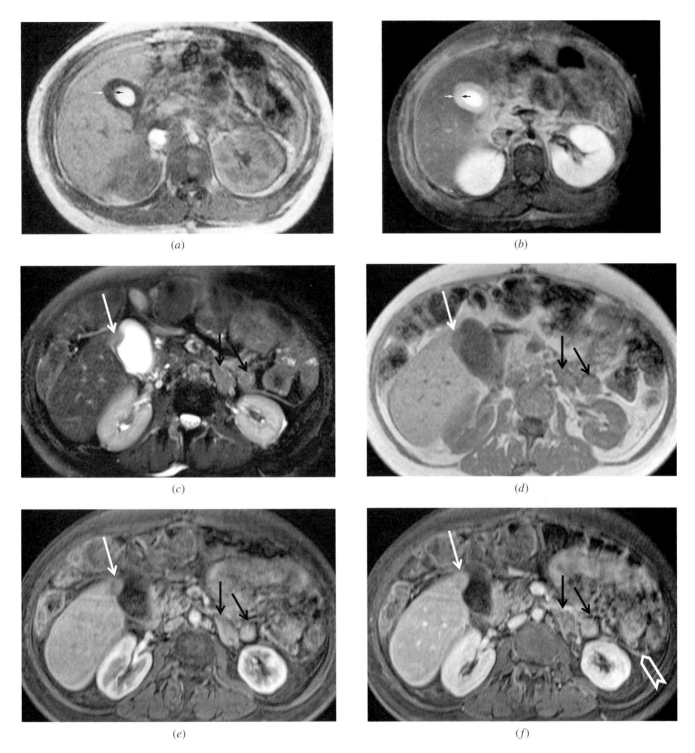

(a)   (b)

(c)   (d)

(e)   (f)

F I G . 3.24 Burkitt lymphoma of the gallbladder. T1-weighted GE (*a*) and 2-min postgadolinium fat-suppressed spin-echo (*b*) images. The gallbladder wall (arrows, *a*, *b*) is diffusely thickened because of infiltration by lymphoma. Note the uniform moderate enhancement of the wall after contrast administration (*b*), which is less than that observed for acute cholecystitis. **Gallbladder metastasis from ovarian cancer.** T2-weighted fat-suppressed single-shot echo-train spin-echo (*c*), T1-weighted SGE (*d*), and T1-weighted postgadolinium fat-suppressed hepatic arterial dominant phase (*e*) and interstitial phase (*f*) 3D-GE images demonstrate the gallbladder wall metastases (white arrows, *c-f*) from ovarian cancer. The tumor shows moderate enhancement on postgadolinium images (*e*, *f*). Note that there are lymph node (black arrows, *c-f*) and peritoneal (open arrow, *f*) metastases.

is considered 7 mm in patients with their gallbladder in place and 10 mm in patients after cholecystectomy. Duct diameter, however, increases slightly with increasing patient age. Normal intrahepatic bile ducts show smooth walls that taper slowly toward the periphery.

Benign Disease

Choledocholithiasis

Calculi in the biliary ducts, although less frequent than in the gallbladder, are the most common cause of extrahepatic obstructive jaundice. With the increase of laparoscopic cholecystectomy over recent years, the interest in preoperative diagnosis of choledocholithiasis has surged, because the presence of bile duct stones renders laparoscopic procedures extremely difficult. Ultrasound and CT imaging are not well suited for the diagnosis of choledocholithiasis because of their relatively low sen-

sitivity and accuracy [67–70]. ERCP is still considered the gold standard technique for the evaluation of the biliary ductal system and allows therapeutic interventions such as sphincterotomy for the release of CBD stones. However, significant complications (e.g., pancreatitis) after sphincterotomy occur in 6–13% of patients, with an overall mortality rate up to 1.5% [71–73]. Even with diagnostic ERCP alone, the rate of major complications or death is 5–8% and the rate of failed ERCP is 5–20% [10, 74, 75].

MRCP is a noninvasive technique that is ideally suited for detecting bile duct stones because of the high contrast of calculi as intraluminal low-signal-intensity or signal-void structures against high-signal-intensity bile (fig. 3.25). A number of studies have shown that MRCP is superior to CT or ultrasound and comparable or superior to ERCP in detecting choledocholithiasis [2, 5, 21, 76, 77]. A study of 366 patients by Topal et al. [78]

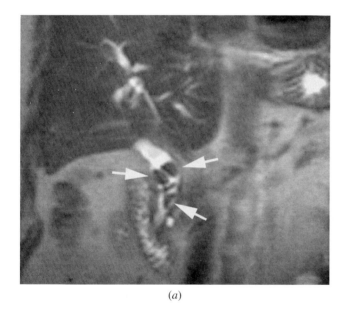

(a)

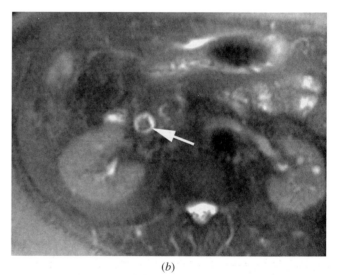

(b)

F I G . 3.25 Choledocholithiasis, MRCP. T2-weighted single-shot echo-train spin-echo images in the coronal (*a*) and transverse plane with fat suppression (*b*) and coronal thin-section MRCP single-shot echo-train spin-echo image with fat suppression (*c*). Multiple faceted low-signal calculi (arrows, *a*, *b*) are shown in the dilated CBD with good contrast against surrounding high-signal bile. On the thin-section MRCP image (*c*), the dilated intrahepatic ducts (short arrows, *c*) and a stone in the CHD (long arrow, *c*) are visualized more clearly. The normal pancreatic duct (curved arrow, *c*) is also well depicted.

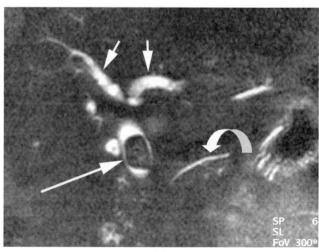

(c)

came to the conclusion that in patients with a predicted probability of CBD stones of more than 5%, MRCP is recommended to confirm or rule out choledocholithiasis. For the detection of intrahepatic stones, MRCP proved to be even more effective than ERCP, with sensitivity and specificity of 97% and 93%, respectively, for MRCP versus 59% and 97%, respectively, for ERCP [79].

At MRI, ductal biliary stones typically have a rounded or oval-shaped configuration with a meniscus of fluid above their proximal edge (fig. 3.26). On thin-section source images, stones consistently appear as signal-void foci and can be detected as small as 2 mm in dilated and nondilated ducts [2]. On thick-section images, however, the detection rate of stones depends on their size. Large or medium-sized stones in normal-caliber ducts are readily detectable as signal-void structures, but small stones that are completely surrounded by fluid may escape detection because of volume averaging effects. Another potential missed diagnosis is an impacted stone in the ampulla, not surrounded by fluid, that may be misinterpreted as a stricture (fig. 3.27). Soto et al. [80] compared the performance of thick-slab, thin-slab, and 3D fast-SE MRCP sequences with ERCP for detecting choledocholithiasis in 49 patients. They found sensitivity and specificity rates exceeding 92% and 92%, respectively, for all sequences. There was 100% agreement between MRCP and ERCP in the detection of ductal dilatation.

Mirizzi's syndrome is a rare condition in which the stone in the cystic duct compresses the common bile duct and causes obstruction. This condition can also be successfully evaluated with MRCP (fig. 3.27).

Pitfalls of MRCP. A common pitfall in the diagnosis of choledocholithiasis is intraductal air bubbles (pneumobilia), which can be differentiated from stones by observing that air-filling defects lie on the nondependent portion of the bile duct against the wall or by recognition of an air-fluid level (fig. 3.28). Blood clots, however, may be indistinguishable from biliary stones (fig. 3.28). Other pitfalls that may mimic calculi include 1) tortuosity of the bile duct that results in the duct traveling in and out of the imaging plane; 2) insertion of the cystic duct into the CBD, which when observed en face on coronal images may appear as a round hypointense focus mimicking a stone; 3) flow artifacts in bile ducts (fig. 3.29); 4) metallic clips; and 5) external compression artifact from the right hepatic or gastroduodenal artery, which may result in a signal void focus (see fig. 3.29) [3, 81, 82]. Careful attention to the exact location of these defects (e.g., air in a nondependent location, continuation of the cystic duct or right hepatic or gastroduodenal arteries on adjacent images, clips in the gallbladder fossa) and interpretation of MRCP MIP reconstruction images in conjunction with thin-section

source images most often permits correct exclusion of these entities as representing stones. Flow of bile that occurs intermittently during biliary contractions is fastest in the center of the ducts and can cause small flow-void artifacts, especially when the flow is perpendicular to the image plane. Acquiring thin-slab MRCP images in two perpendicular planes is most helpful to confirm or exclude the presence of a stone. The intraductal central location of this flow void is another hint to differentiate this artifact from stones because the latter tend to be located in the dependent portion of the ducts (see fig. 3.29).

Another pitfall is complete filling of the biliary system with debris, with the absence of visible high-signal bile within the biliary system. This may mask the fact that the bile ducts are dilated and debris-filled (fig. 3.29) [83].

Ampullary Stenosis

The clinical symptoms of ampullary stenosis include recurrent, intermittent upper abdominal pain, abnormal liver tests, and dilatation of the common bile duct.

Ampullary Fibrosis. The most common cause of benign ampullary stenosis is fibrosis, which occurs most frequently as a sequel to stone passage in the context of choledocholithiasis. The degree of biliary ductal dilatation is usually mild to moderate but can be severe. In the acute phase, swelling and edema of the ampulla may be present, shown as enlarged prominence of the ampulla and increased signal intensity on T2-weighted images. In the chronic stage, fibrosis of the ampulla appears as low signal intensity on T2-weighted images without enlargement of the ampulla. Rarely, these fibrotic changes are proliferative and lead to pronounced enlargement of the ampulla, which may give the impression of an obstructing tumor. T1-weighted immediate postgadolinium images are a useful tool to show normal enhancement of the periampullary pancreatic parenchyma to exclude pancreatic tumor (figs. 3.30 and 3.31). Nevertheless, endoscopic biopsy may sometimes be necessary to establish the correct diagnosis.

Papillary Dysfunction. Functional stenosis of the sphincter of Oddi includes spasm of the sphincter of Oddi and abnormalities of the sequencing or frequency rate of sphincteric contraction waves [84]. This results in delayed drainage of the CBD with clinical symptoms and radiologic signs of biliary obstruction at the level of the papilla. MRI can aid in establishing the diagnosis by ruling out morphologic causes for biliary ductal dilatation (fig. 3.32). To visualize the function of the sphincter of Oddi, serial thick-section MRCP single-shot echo-train spin-echo images ("functional MRCP") can help to show regular relaxation of the sphincter [84, 86].

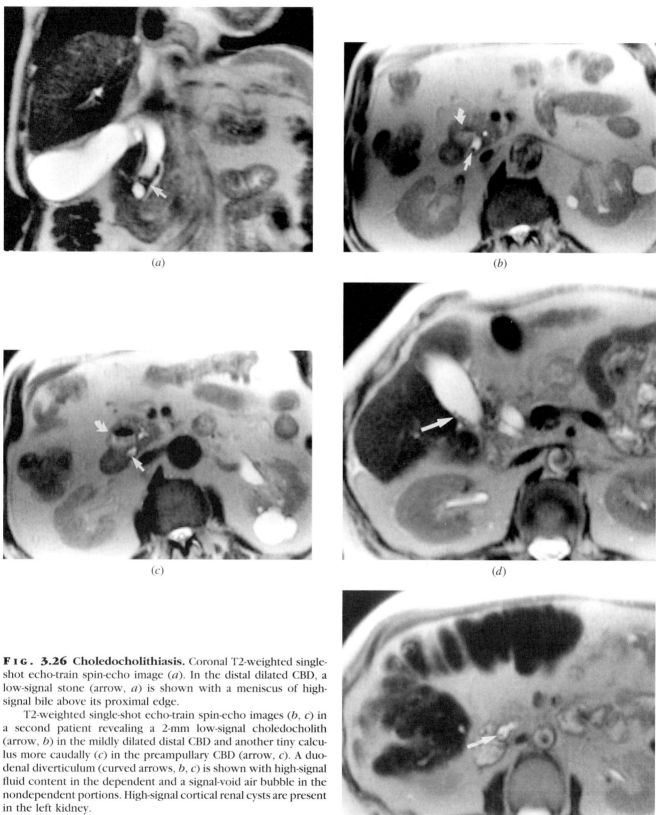

(a)

(b)

(c)

(d)

(e)

FIG. 3.26 Choledocholithiasis. Coronal T2-weighted single-shot echo-train spin-echo image (*a*). In the distal dilated CBD, a low-signal stone (arrow, *a*) is shown with a meniscus of high-signal bile above its proximal edge.

T2-weighted single-shot echo-train spin-echo images (*b*, *c*) in a second patient revealing a 2-mm low-signal choledocholith (arrow, *b*) in the mildly dilated distal CBD and another tiny calculus more caudally (*c*) in the preampullary CBD (arrow, *c*). A duodenal diverticulum (curved arrows, *b*, *c*) is shown with high-signal fluid content in the dependent and a signal-void air bubble in the nondependent portions. High-signal cortical renal cysts are present in the left kidney.

Transverse T2-weighted single-shot echo-train spin-echo images (*d*, *e*) in a third patient demonstrating several low-signal 2-mm calculi in the gallbladder (arrow, *d*) and in the preampullary CBD (arrow, *e*).

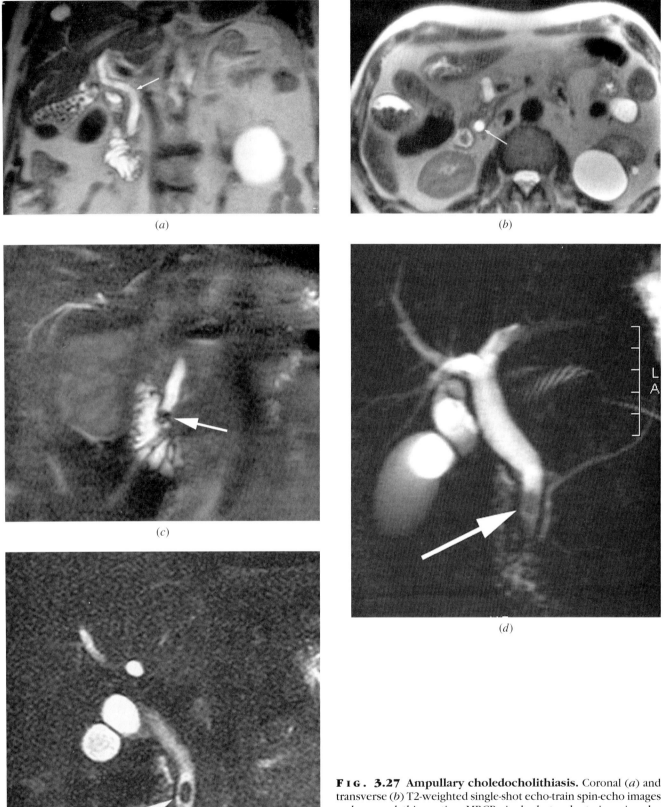

(a)

(b)

(c)

(d)

(e)

FIG. 3.27 Ampullary choledocholithiasis. Coronal (*a*) and transverse (*b*) T2-weighted single-shot echo-train spin-echo images and coronal thin-section MRCP single-shot echo-train spin-echo image with fat suppression (*c*). Multiple small low-signal calculi are demonstrated in the gallbladder (*a*, *b*). The CHD and CBD (arrows, *a*, *b*) are dilated but no intraductal stone is visualized on the 8-mm coronal and transverse images (*a*, *b*). The thin-section MRCP image (*c*) reveals a small choledocholith (arrow, *c*) that is lodged in the ampulla and obstructs the CBD. The duodenum is filled with fluid outlining its folds (*a*, *c*). High-signal cysts are incidentally revealed in the dome of the liver (*a*) and the left kidney (*a*, *b*). Paracoronal thick-section MRCP (*d*), thin-section MRCP (*e*), and axial T2-weighted single-shot echo-train spin-echo

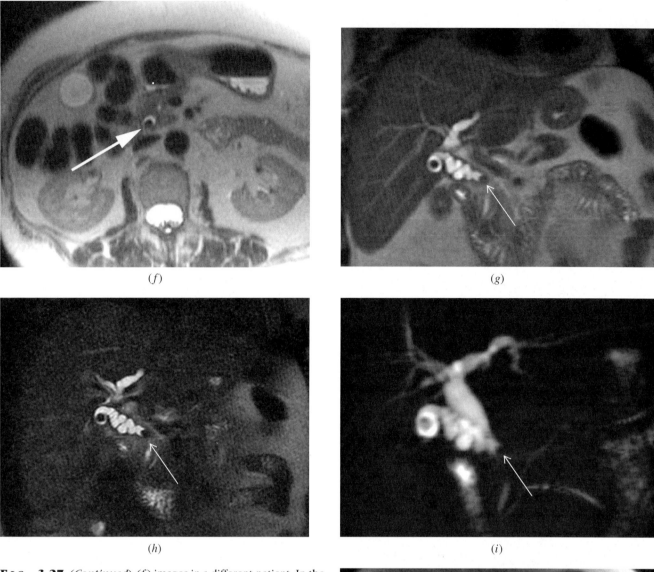

(f)

(g)

(h)

(i)

F IG . 3.27 (*Continued*) (*f*) images in a different patient. In the distal CBD, a low-signal stone (arrow, *d–f*) is shown with a meniscus of high-signal bile above its proximal edge. Note the dilatation of the proximal CBD. The paracoronal thin-section MRCP image (*e*) better visualizes the stone (arrow, *e*) and shows its preampullary position. The axial T2-weighted single-shot echo-train spin-echo image (*f*) shows the stone (arrow, *f*) in the dependent portion of the preampullary CBD and better demonstrates the adjacent organs.

Coronal T2-weighted single-shot echo-train spin-echo (*g*), coronal T2-weighted thin-section echo-train spin-echo (*h*), coronal thick-section fast spin-echo MRCP (*i*), and transverse T2-weighted fat-suppressed single-shot echo-train spin-echo (*j*) images demonstrate Mirizzi's syndrome in another patient with prior cholecystectomy. The common bile duct and proximal biliary ducts are dilated because of the compression of the common bile duct resulting from the presence of a stone (arrows, *g–j*) in the cystic duct. The cystic duct is also dilated, and there is another stone in the stump.

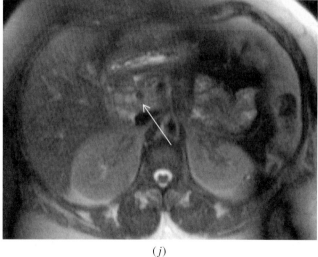

(j)

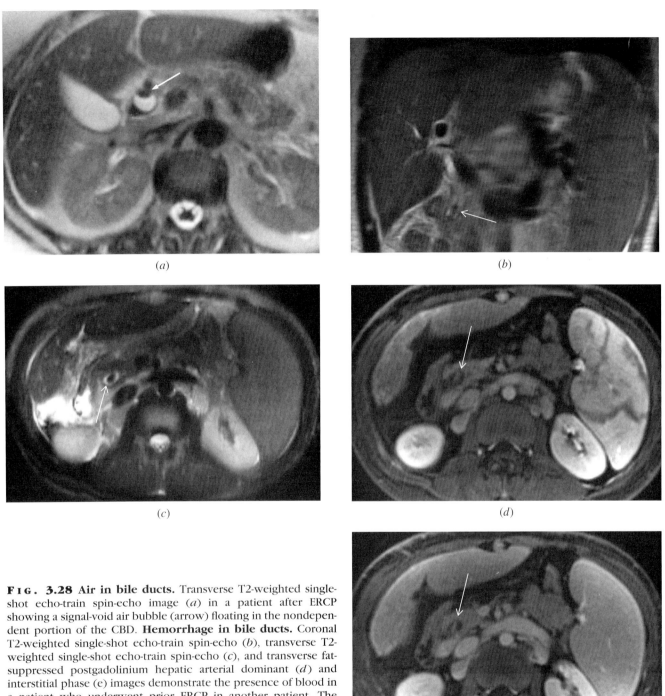

(a)

(b)

(c)

(d)

(e)

F I G . 3.28 Air in bile ducts. Transverse T2-weighted single-shot echo-train spin-echo image (*a*) in a patient after ERCP showing a signal-void air bubble (arrow) floating in the nondependent portion of the CBD. **Hemorrhage in bile ducts.** Coronal T2-weighted single-shot echo-train spin-echo (*b*), transverse T2-weighted single-shot echo-train spin-echo (*c*), and transverse fat-suppressed postgadolinium hepatic arterial dominant (*d*) and interstitial phase (e) images demonstrate the presence of blood in a patient who underwent prior ERCP in another patient. The common bile duct is dilated, and there is a distal intraluminal structure (arrows, *b–e*) which shows low signal on T2-weighted images (*b, c*) and intermediate signal on T1-weighted images (*d, e*). The findings are consistent with blood products. Note the portal hypertension findings.

MRCP performed after intravenous administration of 1 unit of secretin per kilogram of body weight ("pharmacodynamic MRCP") with images acquired every 30–60 s over a period of 10 min is under investigation for its role in papillary dysfunction [87, 88].

Sclerosing Cholangitis

Inflammation and obliterative fibrosis of intrahepatic and extrahepatic bile ducts characterize this disease entity. Progressive periductal fibrosis eventually leads to disappearance of small ducts and strictures of larger

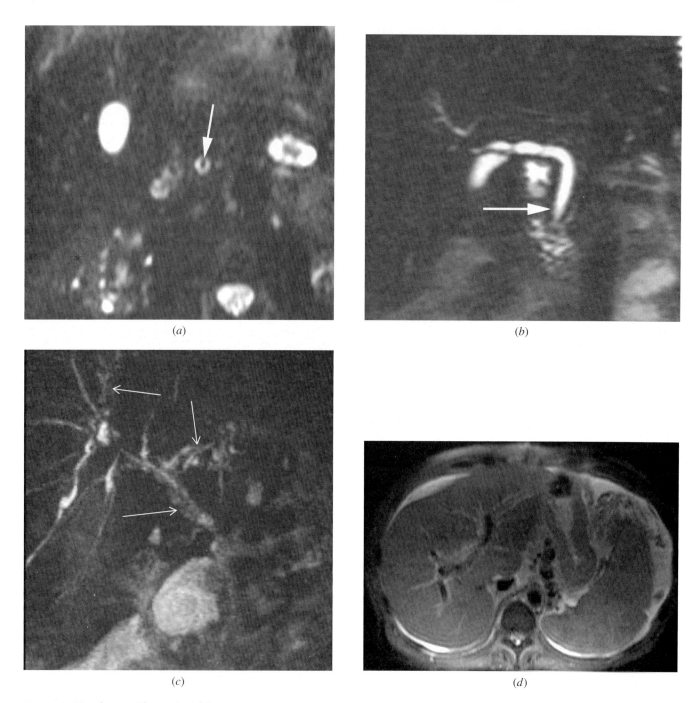

F I G . 3.29 Flow artifact mimicking a stone in an asymptomatic person. The axial thin-slab MRCP image (*a*) shows a small, signal-void round area (arrow, *a*) in the center of the preampullary common bile duct (CBD). The paracoronal thin-slab MRCP image (*b*) demonstrates a normal, fluid-filled CBD (arrow, *b*), excluding the presence of a stone. **Low signal of debris filled ducts masks dilated bile ducts.** Coronal thick-section fast spin-echo (*c*) and transverse T2-weighted fat-suppressed single-shot echo-train spin-echo (*d*) images demonstrate dilated and debris-filled bile ducts developing secondary to an obstruction in another patient who had prior liver transplantation. Dilated and debris-filled CBD and intrahepatic bile ducts show less signal (arrows, *c*). Note the portal hypertension findings and ascites on T2-weighted image (*d*).

ducts. The anatomic changes in the biliary tract and the hepatic histologic changes are nonspecific and can either be secondary to infection or hepatic arterial damage, or "primary" when immune factors are thought to underlie the disease [89].

Primary Sclerosing Cholangitis. Approximately 71% of patients with primary sclerosing cholangitis (PSC) also have inflammatory bowel disease [90]. Approximately 87% of these patients have ulcerative colitis, and 13% have Crohn disease [89]. PSC results in cholestasis with

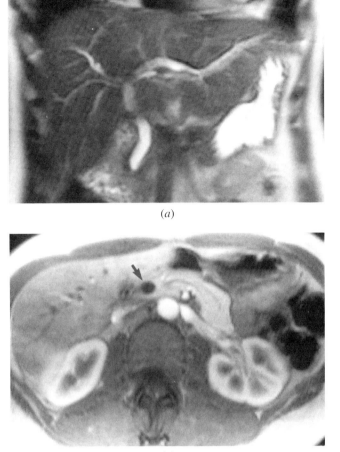

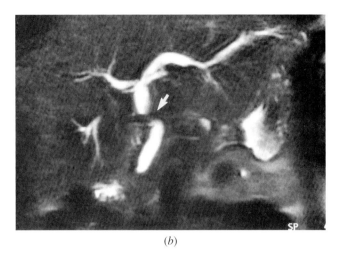

(a)

(b)

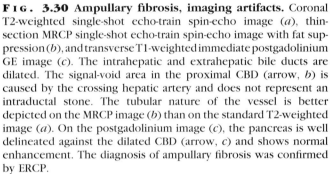

(c)

F I G . 3.30 Ampullary fibrosis, imaging artifacts. Coronal T2-weighted single-shot echo-train spin-echo image (*a*), thin-section MRCP single-shot echo-train spin-echo image with fat suppression (*b*), and transverse T1-weighted immediate postgadolinium GE image (*c*). The intrahepatic and extrahepatic bile ducts are dilated. The signal-void area in the proximal CBD (arrow, *b*) is caused by the crossing hepatic artery and does not represent an intraductal stone. The tubular nature of the vessel is better depicted on the MRCP image (*b*) than on the standard T2-weighted image (*a*). On the postgadolinium image (*c*), the pancreas is well delineated against the dilated CBD (arrow, *c*) and shows normal enhancement. The diagnosis of ampullary fibrosis was confirmed by ERCP.

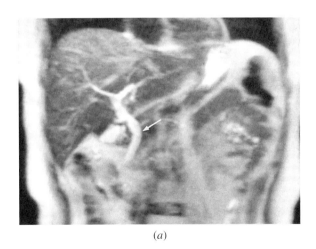

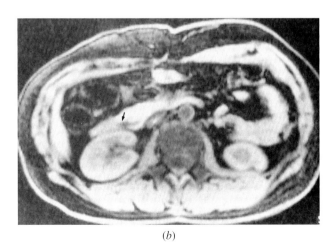

(a)

(b)

F I G . 3.31 Ampullary fibrosis. Coronal T2-weighted thin-section MRCP single-shot echo-train spin-echo image (*a*) shows the entire dilated CBD (arrow, *a*), excluding ductal calculi. Transverse T1-weighted fat-suppressed GE (*b*) and immediate postgadolinium

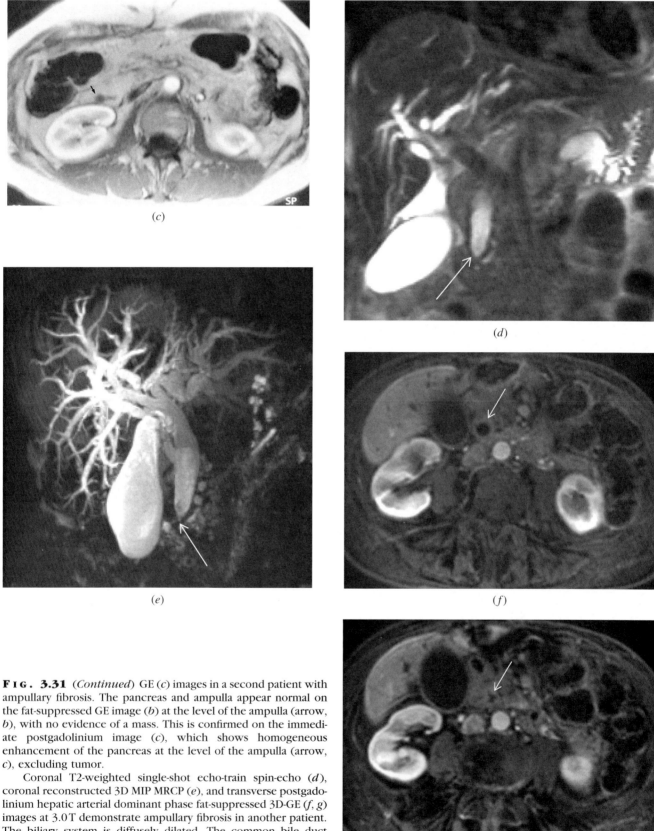

FIG. 3.31 (*Continued*) GE (*c*) images in a second patient with ampullary fibrosis. The pancreas and ampulla appear normal on the fat-suppressed GE image (*b*) at the level of the ampulla (arrow, *b*), with no evidence of a mass. This is confirmed on the immediate postgadolinium image (*c*), which shows homogeneous enhancement of the pancreas at the level of the ampulla (arrow, *c*), excluding tumor.

Coronal T2-weighted single-shot echo-train spin-echo (*d*), coronal reconstructed 3D MIP MRCP (*e*), and transverse postgadolinium hepatic arterial dominant phase fat-suppressed 3D-GE (*f, g*) images at 3.0 T demonstrate ampullary fibrosis in another patient. The biliary system is diffusely dilated. The common bile duct shows fusiform ending, and the distal common bile duct shows minimal enhancement and thickening (arrows, *d–g*). These findings suggest the presence of ampullary fibrosis.

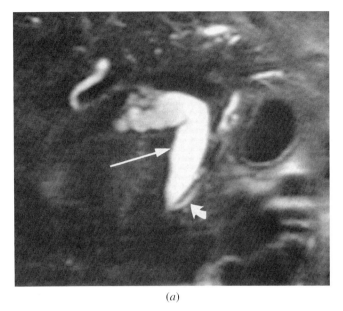

(a)

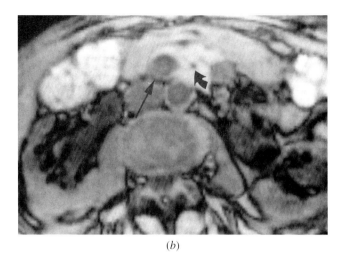

(b)

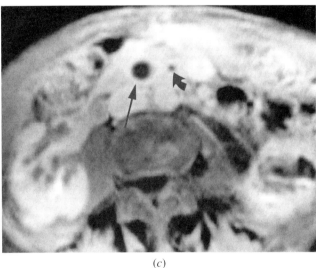

(c)

FIG. 3.32 Papillary dysfunction. Coronal T2-weighted thin-section MRCP single-shot echo-train spin-echo image with fat suppression (a) and transverse T1-weighted fat-suppressed GE (b) and 2-min postgadolinium fat-suppressed GE (c) images. The CBD (straight arrow, a–c) is severely dilated without evidence of an intraductal stone on the thin-section MRCP image (a). The pancreatic duct (curved arrow, a–c) is also mildly dilated. The pancreas and region of the ampulla show no evidence of a tumor on the precontrast (b) and postgadolinium (c) images. Papillary dysfunction was diagnosed on ERCP.

progression to secondary biliary cirrhosis and hepatic failure. Current hypotheses hold immune factors or toxic bacterial products that cross the inflamed colonic mucosa and enter the portal venous bloodstream accountable for PSC by inducing pericholangitic inflammation and fibrosis [90]. The diagnosis of PSC is made using cholangiographic findings supported by histologic results. Clinical features, such as ulcerative colitis or cholestasis, may be supportive but are not diagnostic.

The imaging appearance of PSC is characterized by multifocal, irregular strictures and dilatations of segments of the intra- and extrahepatic biliary tree. The strictures are usually short and annular, alternating with normal or slightly dilated segments, producing a beaded appearance (fig. 3.33). Because of fibrosis of higher-order intrahepatic bile ducts the biliary tree has the appearance of cut-off peripheral ducts, described as

"pruning." The disease may involve intrahepatic ducts, extrahepatic ducts, or both, with the cystic duct usually spared. All of these findings are not pathognomonic for PSC and can be found in secondary forms as well. If the intrahepatic ducts are involved in isolation, differentiation must be made from primary biliary cirrhosis, which can be distinguished clinically from PSC. The conventional imaging modality to establish the diagnosis of PSC is ERCP. However, this method is associated with risks of pancreatitis and perforation and has been shown to result in progression of cholestasis in patients with PSC [74, 91]. MRCP has shown to be an adequate method for the diagnosis and follow-up of PSC [92, 93]. The imaging features that can be depicted in PSC are identical to the findings described for ERCP. In a comparative study with ERCP involving 150 patients, MRCP showed a sensitivity and specificity to depict PSC of

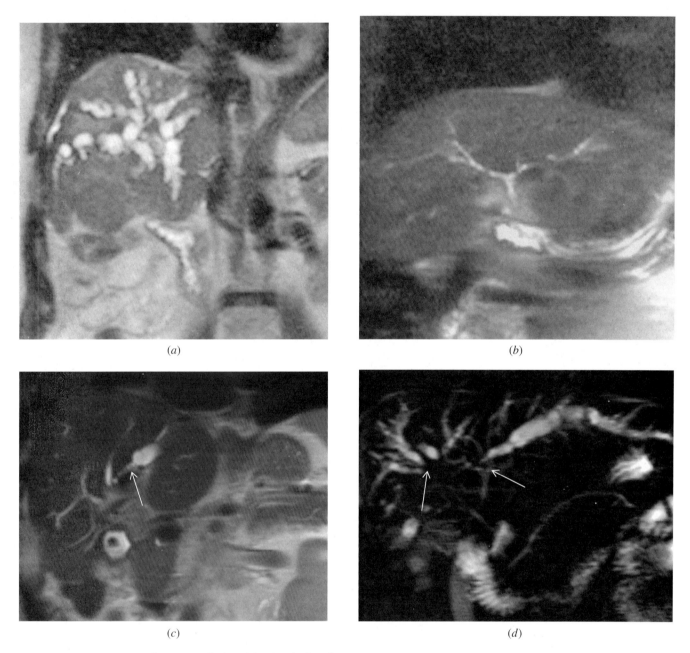

F I G . 3.33 Primary sclerosing cholangitis (PSC), beading. Coronal T2 weighted single-shot echo-train spin-echo images without (*a*) and with (*b*) fat suppression in two different patients (*a*, *b*, respectively). The high-signal intrahepatic bile ducts demonstrate beading caused by short strictures alternating with dilated (*a*) or normal-caliber (*b*) segments. Coronal T2-weighted single-shot echo-train spin-echo (*c*), coronal thick-section fast spin-echo MRCP (*d*), transverse T2-weighted single-shot echo-train spin-echo

88% and 99%, respectively, showing that its diagnostic accuracy is comparable to that of ERCP [93]. Factors that can lead to difficulties in interpreting the MR images and to false-positive and false-negative diagnoses are 1) the presence of liver cirrhosis and 2) PSC limited to the peripheral intrahepatic ducts. Cirrhosis may lead to distortion of the biliary tree that may mimic PSC even on ERCP images. If PSC is limited to the peripheral ductal system, the higher image resolution of ERCP makes this a more sensitive test compared to current MRCP

sequences. However, a limitation of ERCP is that the presence of severe strictures may lead to inadequate opacification of proximal bile ducts and to false-negative diagnoses [93]. MRCP provides visualization of bile ducts proximal to even severe stenoses and demonstrates bile duct stones in these locations, where they often escape detection with ERCP. In fact, visualization of bile ducts is considered easier with MRCP in the presence of severe ductal obstruction, because of the expanded fluid-filled state of the obstructed ducts. In

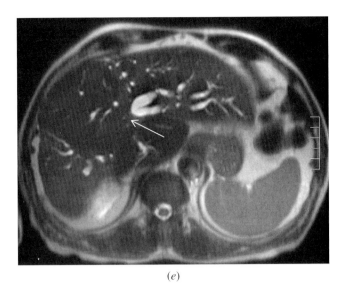
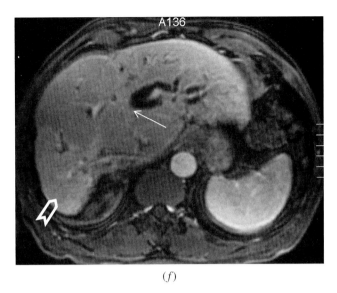

(e)   (f)

FIG. 3.33 (*Continued*) (*e*), and transverse postgadolinium hepatic venous phase fat-suppressed 3D-GE (*f*) images at 3.0 T demonstrate PSC in another patient. Dilated intrahepatic bile ducts in combination with strictures and beading are detected (arrows, *c-f*). Pruning is seen both in the intrahepatic and extrahepatic bile ducts (*d*). Central regeneration and peripheral atrophy are also detected. Note that there is minimal inflammatory patchy enhancement (open arrow, *f*) in the right lobe posterior segment on postgadolinium image (*f*) and the liver is enlarged.

our experience, however, subtle changes of mild PSC can be difficult to detect with current MR techniques.

The use of conventional MR sequences and intravenous gadolinium provides information on the liver parenchyma and bile duct walls, which is valuable for a thorough evaluation [94, 95]. In a study of patients with PSC by Revelon et al. [96], peripheral, wedge-shaped zones of hyperintense signal on T2-weighted images were found in the liver in 72% of patients. These triangular areas ranged from 1 to 5 cm in diameter (fig. 3.34). Periportal edema or inflammation, seen as high signal intensity along the porta hepatis on T2-weighted images, was present in 40% of patients. A study by Ito et al. [97] evaluated the imaging features of PSC on dynamic gadolinium-enhanced MRI. Thickening of bile duct walls and wall enhancement were seen in 50% and 67% of patients, respectively (see fig. 3.34). On pregadolinium T1-weighted images, 23% of patients showed areas of increased signal intensity in the liver that did not represent focal fatty infiltration. On immediate postgadolinium images, 56% of all patients showed areas of increased parenchymal enhancement that were patchy, peripheral, segmental, or a combination of these patterns. These regions remained mildly or markedly hyperintense on delayed-phase images in 90% of patients. Other findings occasionally associated with PSC are atrophy of liver segments, periportal lymphadenopathy, and findings attributable to liver cirrhosis and portal hypertension, such as hypertrophy of the caudate lobe, regenerative nodules, and abdominal varices. In our experience, cirrhosis secondary to PSC often results in large central regenerative nodules that may cause periportal obstruction of bile ducts and, eventually, segmental atrophy of peripheral liver (see fig. 3.34) [94].

PSC is associated with an increased malignant potential, and the most important and common malignant entity that may occur in these patients is cholangiocarcinoma. Cholangiocarcinoma is the second most common cause of death, after liver failure, in patients with PSC, occurring in up to 20% of patients [98]. The diagnosis of superimposed cholangiocarcinoma in patients with PSC is difficult because of the underlying morphologic bile duct changes. The MR appearance of cholangiocarcinoma is described below.

Infectious Cholangitis

Infectious, bacterial, or ascending cholangitis is a clinically defined syndrome caused by complete or partial biliary obstruction with associated ascending infection from the intestine. It encompasses a wide spectrum of clinical manifestations ranging from a mild form to a fulminating form that constitutes a life-threatening surgical emergency. Predisposing conditions are the presence of microorganisms in the bile and the presence of partial or complete biliary obstruction. The typical clinical symptoms that lead to the diagnosis of ascending cholangitis are jaundice, abdominal pain, and sepsis (chills and fever), referred to as Charcot's triad. This triad is present in approximately 70% of patients.

The distribution of inflammatory changes may be diffuse or segmental. The most consistent imaging finding in infectious cholangitis is generalized or segmental

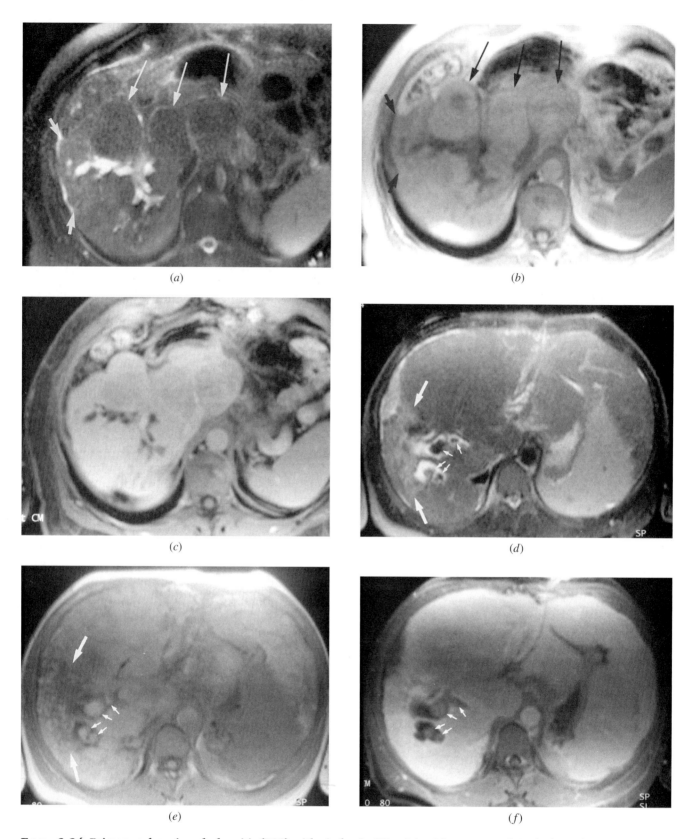

(a)

(b)

(c)

(d)

(e)

(f)

F I G . 3.34 Primary sclerosing cholangitis (PSC) with cirrhosis. T2-weighted fat-suppressed single-shot echo-train spin-echo (*a*), T1-weighted SGE (*b*), and 2-min postgadolinium fat-suppressed SGE (*c*) images. The intrahepatic bile ducts are dilated and demonstrate beading. The liver is nodular and cirrhotic in this patient with late-stage PSC. Three large macroregenerative nodules (long arrows, *a*, *b*) located in the central portion of the liver appear to obstruct the bile ducts centrally. The nodules are slightly hypoenhancing on the 2-min postgadolinium image (*c*). A subsegmental distal area of atrophic liver parenchyma (short arrows, *a*, *b*) appears slightly hyperintense on the T2-weighted image (*a*) and hypointense on the T1-weighted image (*b*). T2-weighted fat-suppressed single-shot echo-train spin-echo (*d*), T1-weighted SGE (*e*), and 2-min postgadolinium fat-suppressed SGE (*f*) images in a second patient. The liver shows multiple large macroregenerative nodules. The bile ducts in the right lobe of the liver are severely dilated and contain several calculi (arrows, *d-f*) that are high signal on the T1-weighted image (*e*). A wedge-shaped peripheral area of liver parenchyma (short arrows, *d-f*) is atrophic, showing high signal on the T2-weighted image (*d*) and low signal on the T1-weighted image (*e*) with late enhancement on the 2-min postgadolinium image (*f*). T1-weighted 2-min postgadolinium

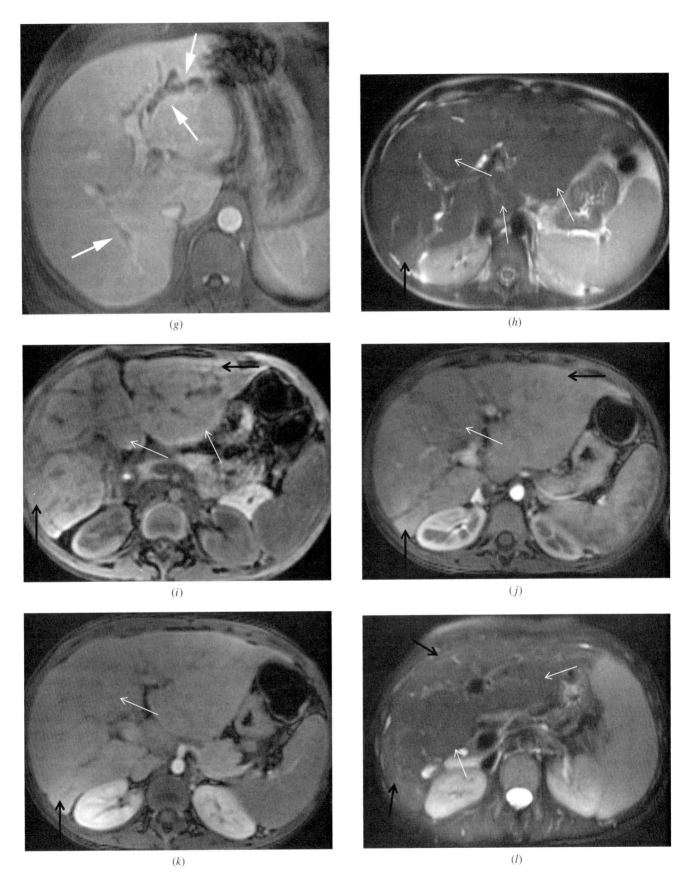

(g)

(h)

(i)

(j)

(k)

(l)

F I G . 3.34 (*Continued*) GE image with fat suppression (g) in a third patient demonstrating a beaded appearance of the intrahepatic bile ducts (arrows, g). The branches of the portal vein are enhanced, facilitating differentiation from low-signal dilated intrahepatic bile ducts. The walls of the bile ducts show increased enhancement. The liver demonstrates nodular enlargement of the left lobe and the caudal lobe.

T2-weighted single-shot echo-train spin-echo (*h*), T1-weighted fat-suppressed 3D-GE (*i*), and T1-weighted postgadolinium fat-suppressed hepatic arterial dominant phase (*j*) and interstitial phase (*k*) 3D-GE images at 3.0 T demonstrate PSC with cirrhosis in another patient. Central regeneration (white arrows, *h–k*) and peripheral atrophy (black arrows, *h–k*) are shown. Dilated bile ducts and periportal edema are also detected in combination with liver contour irregularity and hepatomegaly. T2-weighted fat-suppressed single-shot echo train spin echo (*l*), T1-weighted fat-suppressed 3D-GE (*m*), and T1-weighted postgadolinium fat-suppressed hepatic

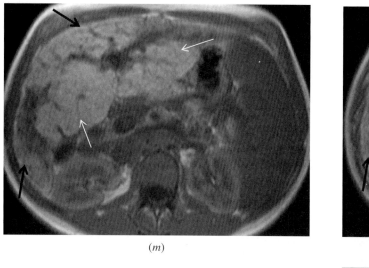

(*m*)

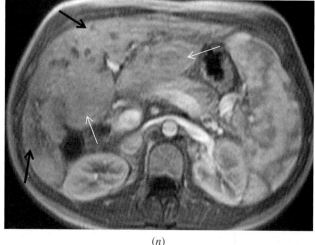

(*n*)

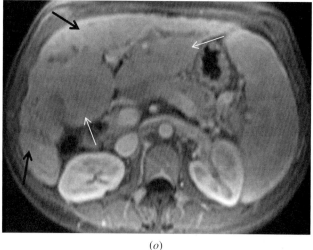

(*o*)

FIG. 3.34 (*Continued*) arterial dominant phase (*n*) and interstitial phase (*o*) 3D-GE images demonstrate PSC with severe cirrhosis and portal hypertension findings in another patient. Central regeneration (white arrows; *l–o*) and peripheral atrophy (black arrows; *l–o*) cause bizarre-shaped cirrhosis in patients with advanced PSC. Note that there are dilated bile ducts, periportal edema, and liver contour irregularity.

biliary dilatation that can be mild or severe but does not correlate well with the severity or stage of the disease [99]. Bile duct walls are commonly mild to moderately thickened and show increased enhancement, which can be best appreciated on T1-weighted fat-suppressed 2-min postgadolinium images (fig. 3.35). Imaging findings on T2-weighted images are streaky increased signal in the periportal area and wedge-shaped hyperintense regions in the liver parenchyma (see fig. 3.35) [100]. On pregadolinium T1-weighted images, these wedge-shaped regions in the liver are usually hypointense but may also show increased signal intensity. On immediate postgadolinium images, increased focal parenchymal enhancement can frequently be observed, consistent with inflammation (see fig. 3.35) [100]. The greater inflammatory nature of infectious cholangitis compared to PSC is reflected by the more common occurrence of regions of increased enhancement on immediate postgadolinium images in the former condition. Liver abscesses may complicate infectious cholangitis and are best visualized on T2-weighted and T1-weighted dynamic postgadolinium images. Thrombosis of the portal vein is not uncommonly associated with infectious cholangitis (fig. 3.36) and aids in the distinction from sclerosing cholangitis, in which this occurrence is uncommon.

A particular form of infectious cholangitis is recurrent pyogenic cholangitis (oriental cholangitis), which is caused by infestation of the biliary tract by *Clonorchis sinensis* or other parasites. This leads to inflammatory infiltration of bile ducts, proliferative fibrosis, periductal abscesses, and calculi (pigment stones). MR imaging findings are disproportionally severe dilatation of the extrahepatic bile ducts proximal and distal to calculi, stricture of bile ducts, thickening of duct walls, and hepatic abscesses [101] (fig. 3.37). Liver segments that contain biliary duct stones frequently undergo atrophy. Absence of a tumor mass helps to differentiate this condition from cholangiocarcinoma. However, cautious interpretation of findings is essential as these patients have an increased incidence of cholangiocarcinoma [101].

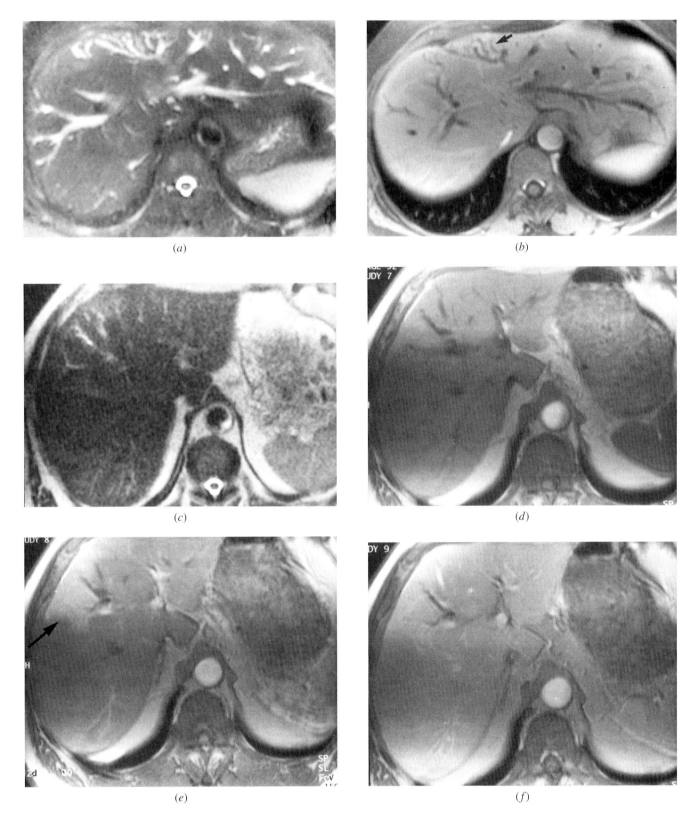

FIG. 3.35 Infectious cholangitis. T2-weighted fat-suppressed single-shot echo-train spin-echo (*a*) and T1-weighted 2-min postgadolinium fat-suppressed GE (*b*) images. The entire intrahepatic biliary tree is severely dilated, visualized as high signal on the T2-weighted image (*a*). On the T1-weighted image (*b*), the low-signal ducts are well differentiated from gadolinium-enhanced vessels. The walls of the bile ducts show increased enhancement that is most pronounced in *segment 4* of the liver (arrow, *b*).

T2-weighted single-shot echo-train spin-echo (*c*), T1-weighted GE (*d*), immediate postgadolinium GE (*e*), and 2-min postgadolinium fat-suppressed GE (*f*) images in a second patient. A peripheral wedge-shaped area of liver parenchyma between *segments 4* and *8* shows moderate biliary ductal dilatation. The liver parenchyma in this area demonstrates increased signal on both the T2 (*c*)- and T1 (*d*)-weighted images, consistent with inspissated bile. Increased enhancement of this area (arrow, *e*) is demonstrated on the postgadolinium images (*e, f*), reflecting local inflammation and hyperemia in the liver parenchyma. The bile duct walls show increased enhancement, best visualized on the 2-min postgadolinium image (*f*).

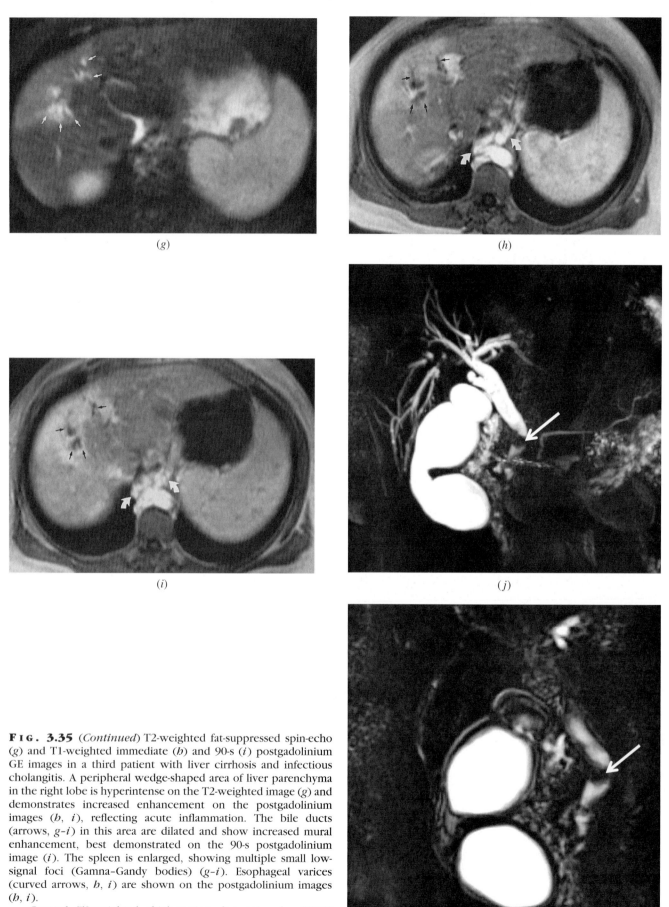

(g)

(h)

(i)

(j)

(k)

FIG. 3.35 (*Continued*) T2-weighted fat-suppressed spin-echo (*g*) and T1-weighted immediate (*h*) and 90-s (*i*) postgadolinium GE images in a third patient with liver cirrhosis and infectious cholangitis. A peripheral wedge-shaped area of liver parenchyma in the right lobe is hyperintense on the T2-weighted image (*g*) and demonstrates increased enhancement on the postgadolinium images (*h, i*), reflecting acute inflammation. The bile ducts (arrows, *g–i*) in this area are dilated and show increased mural enhancement, best demonstrated on the 90-s postgadolinium image (*i*). The spleen is enlarged, showing multiple small low-signal foci (Gamna–Gandy bodies) (*g–i*). Esophageal varices (curved arrows, *h, i*) are shown on the postgadolinium images (*h, i*).

Coronal T2-weighted thick-section fast spin-echo MRCP (*j*), coronal T2-weighted thin-section fast spin-echo MRCP (*k*),

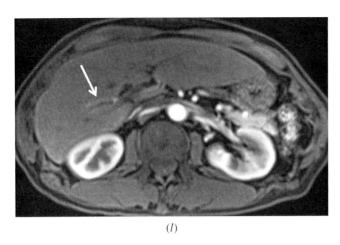
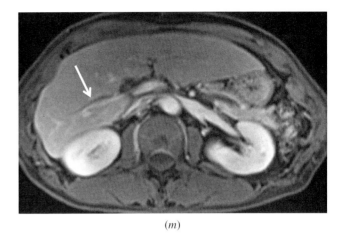

(l)   (m)

FIG. 3.35 (*Continued*) transverse T1-weighted postgadolinium fat-suppressed true late hepatic arterial phase (*l*), and hepatic venous phase (*m*) 3D-GE images demonstrate ascending cholangitis and choledocholithiasis in another patient. The common bile duct and intrahepatic bile ducts are dilated because of the stone (arrows, *j, k*) in the common bile duct. A dilated duct (arrows, *l, m*), which shows increased wall enhancement on postgadolinium images, is shown (*l, m*). These findings are suggestive of ascending cholangitis.

AIDS Cholangiopathy

In HIV-positive patients, involvement of the pancreatico-biliary tract may be an early feature of AIDS (acquired immunodeficiency syndrome) [102]. Inflammation and edema of the biliary mucosa resulting in mucosal thickening and irregularity is the hallmark of AIDS cholangiopathy. This may lead to strictures, dilatations, and pruning resembling sclerosing cholangitis [2, 102]. When the papilla of Vater is involved, ampullary stenosis with common bile duct dilatation may result. The gall-bladder may also be involved and show acalculous cholecystitis with imaging features similar to acute cholecystitis. Furthermore, patients have a predisposition for superimposed infectious cholangitis, often by unusual pathogens (e.g., cytomegalovirus, cryptosporidium, mycobacteria, *Candida albicans*) [102].

Cystic Diseases of Bile Ducts

Congenital biliary cysts comprise choledochal cysts, diverticula originating from extrahepatic ducts, choledochocele, Caroli disease, and segmental cysts, depending on the location of the dilatation of the biliary tract. MRCP with 3D MIP reconstructions can display the anatomic extent and degree of these lesions, diagnose associated findings such as stone disease, and, in combination with gadolinium-enhanced T1-weighted images, evaluate for malignancy [103]. A classification system that groups all types of biliary cystic diseases together has been introduced by Todani et al. [104]: Type I, choledochal cyst; Type II, diverticulum of extra-hepatic ducts; Type III, choledochocele; Type IV, multiple segmental cysts; and Type V, Caroli disease. It is, however, unclear whether they represent variations of the same disease or are separate entities with distinct etiologies. For clinical purposes, however, description of morphology and location is usually adequate.

Choledochal Cyst. The most common cystic dilatations are choledochal cysts (77–87%), which present before the age of 10 in approximately 50% of cases. Choledochal cysts are segmental aneurismal dilatations of the CBD alone or the CBD and CHD (fig. 3.38). The etiology is an anomalous junction of the CBD and the pancreatic duct, proximal to the major papilla, where there is no ductal sphincter. This allows a free reflux of pancreatic enzymes into the biliary system, weakening the walls of the bile ducts. Choledochal cysts are associated with an increased incidence of other biliary anomalies, gallstone disease, pancreatitis, and cholangiocarcinoma. Choledochal cysts may also be coexistent with intrahepatic bile duct cysts (multiple segmental cysts) (fig. 3.39). Cystic expansion of the common bile duct may also be short in length (see fig. 3.39); the etiology of these is at present uncertain.

Choledochocele. Choledochoceles are cystic dilatations of the distal CBD that herniate into the lumen of the duodenum and create a "cobra head" appearance on cholangiographic images (fig. 3.40).

Caroli Disease. Caroli disease is an uncommon form of congenital dilatations of intrahepatic bile ducts with normal extrahepatic ducts. Demonstration that these multiple cystic spaces communicate with the biliary tree is mandatory for the differentiation from cystic disease of the liver and abscesses. This can be

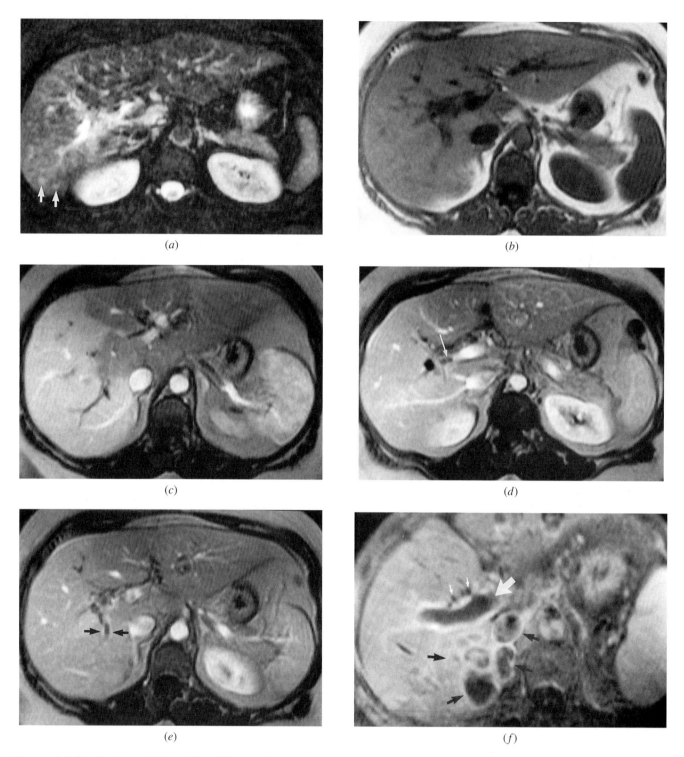

(a)

(b)

(c)

(d)

(e)

(f)

F I G . 3.36 Infectious cholangitis with portal vein thrombosis. T2-weighted fat-suppressed spin-echo (*a*),T1-weighted GE (*b*), immediate postgadolinium GE (*c*), and 1-min postgadolinium GE (*d, e*) images. The right lobe of the liver is hyperintense on both the T2 (*a*)- and T1 (*b*)-weighted images, consistent with edema and inspissated bile. On the T2-weighted image (*a*), small hyperintense areas (arrows, *a*) likely represent foci of infection. The liver parenchyma shows increased enhancement of the right lobe on the postgadolinium GE images (*c, d*) due to thrombosis of the right portal vein (arrow, *d*) and consequent arterial hyperperfusion. The thrombus (arrow, *d*) is best visualized as a near signal-void filling defect of the right portal vein on the 1-min postgadolinium image (*d*). Increased enhancement of bile duct walls is demonstrated on the 1-min postgadolinium GE images (arrows, *e*).

T1-weighted 2-min postgadolinium fat-suppressed GE image (*f*) in a second patient. The portal vein (large white arrow, *f*) is dilated and shows lack of central enhancement with increased enhancement of the vessel walls, consistent with thrombosis. Several liver abscesses (black arrows, *f*) are visualized as round hypointense lesions with enhancing rims. Several bile ducts (small white arrows, *f*) are moderately dilated.

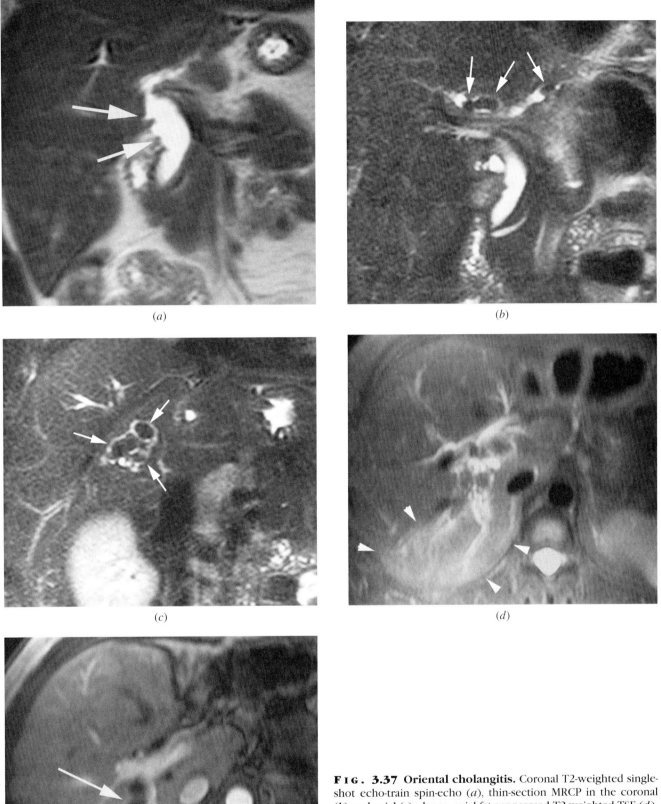

F I G . 3.37 Oriental cholangitis. Coronal T2-weighted single-shot echo-train spin-echo (*a*), thin-section MRCP in the coronal (*b*) and axial (*c*) planes, axial fat-suppressed T2-weighted TSE (*d*), and immediate postgadolinium GE (*e*) images. Disproportionate dilatation of the CBD (arrows, *a*) with slight wall irregularity is noted on the coronal T2-weighted image (*a*). Multiple intrahepatic bile duct stones (arrows, *b*, *c*) are best visualized on the thin-section MRCP images (*b*, *c*). Intrahepatic bile ducts show wall irregularities and strictures (arrow, *e*). The adjacent hepatic parenchyma (arrowheads, *d*, *e*) shows hyperintense signal on the T2-weighted image (*d*) and arterial hyperenhancement (*e*) indicative of inflammation.

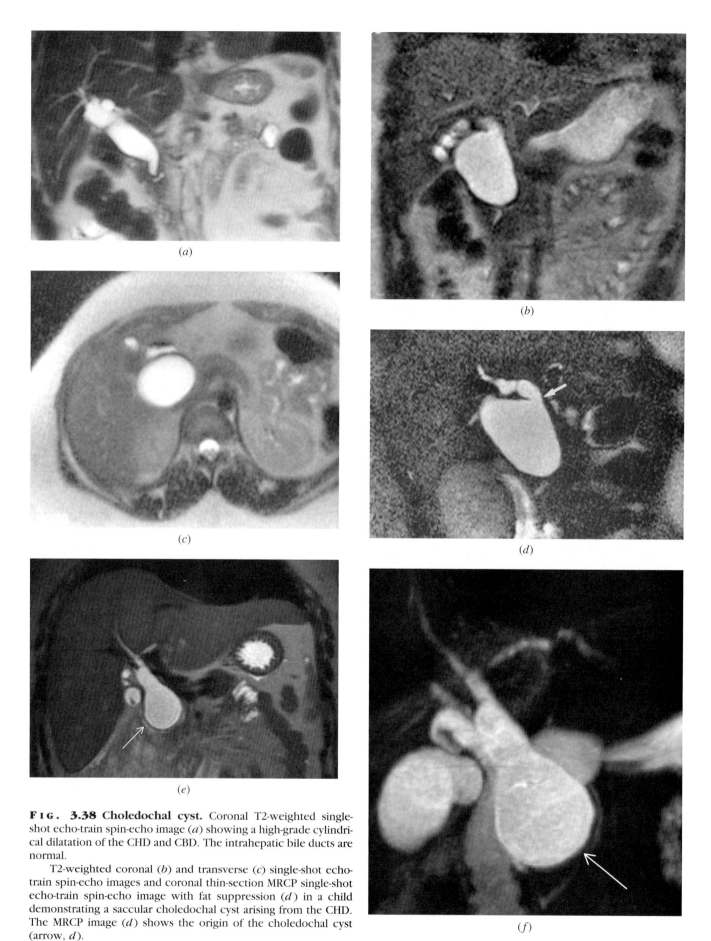

(a)

(b)

(c)

(d)

(e)

(f)

FIG. 3.38 Choledochal cyst. Coronal T2-weighted single-shot echo-train spin-echo image (*a*) showing a high-grade cylindrical dilatation of the CHD and CBD. The intrahepatic bile ducts are normal.

T2-weighted coronal (*b*) and transverse (*c*) single-shot echo-train spin-echo images and coronal thin-section MRCP single-shot echo-train spin-echo image with fat suppression (*d*) in a child demonstrating a saccular choledochal cyst arising from the CHD. The MRCP image (*d*) shows the origin of the choledochal cyst (arrow, *d*).

Coronal T2-weighted single-shot echo-train spin-echo (*e*), coronal thick-section fast spin-echo MRCP (*f*), transverse T1-weighted

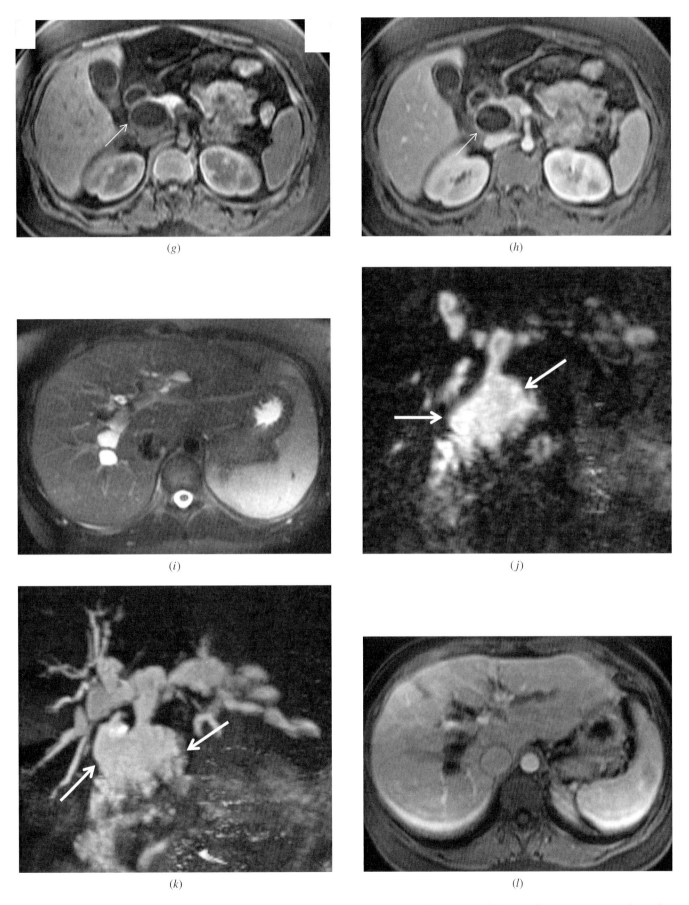

(g)

(h)

(i)

(j)

(k)

(l)

FIG. 3.38 (*Continued*) fat-suppressed 3D-GE (*g*), and transverse T1-weighted postgadolinium hepatic venous phase fat-suppressed 3D-GE (*h*) images demonstrate the choledochal cyst (arrows, *e–h*) in another patient. Transverse T2-weighted single-shot echo-train spin-echo (*i*), coronal thin-section fast spin-echo MRCP (*j*), coronal thick-section fast spin-echo MRCP (*k*), and transverse T1-weighted fat-suppressed postgadolinium hepatic venous phase 3D-GE (*l*) images demonstrate an irregular cyst (arrows, *j*, *k*) arising from the common bile duct in another patient. The proximal bile ducts are dilated. The histopathology of the large cystic lesion was consistent with cystadenoma.

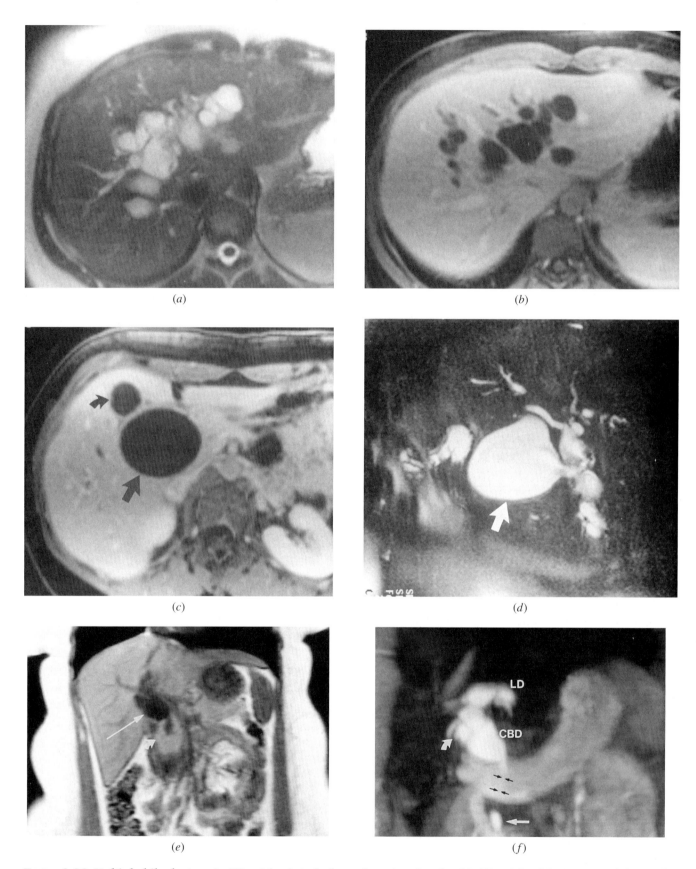

(a)

(b)

(c)

(d)

(e)

(f)

F I G . 3.39 Multiple bile duct cysts. T2-weighted single-shot echo-train spin-echo (*a*), T1-weighted 2-min postgadolinium fat-suppressed GE (*b, c*) images, and coronal T2-weighted thin-section MRCP single-shot echo-train spin-echo image with fat suppression (*d*). Multiple intrahepatic bile duct cysts are demonstrated showing high signal on the T2 (*a*)- and low signal on the T1 (*b*)-weighted images. A large choledochal cyst (straight arrow, *c, d*) is revealed abutting the gallbladder (curved arrow, *c*). The MRCP image (*d*) nicely demonstrates the intra- and extrahepatic extent of biliary cystic disease.

Coronal T1-weighted GE (*e*) and MRCP MIP reconstruction (*f*) images in a second patient. A cystic dilatation of the proximal CBD (long arrow, *e*) above the head of the pancreas (curved arrow, *e*) is appreciated on the GE image (*e*). The left hepatic duct (LD, *f*) shown with high signal on the MRCP MIP image (*f*) also demonstrates fusiform dilatations. Cystic dilatations are also visualized in the cystic duct at its insertion into the CHD (curved arrow, *f*) and of the preampullary CBD (straight arrow, *f*). The mid-CBD (small arrows, *f*) is of normal caliber.

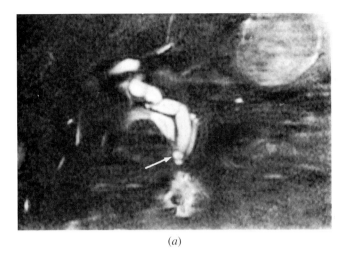

(a)

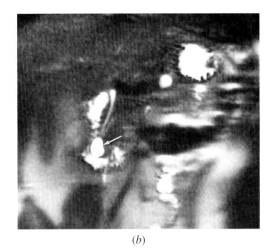

(b)

FIG. 3.40 Choledochocele. Coronal thin-section MRCP single-shot echo-train spin-echo image with fat suppression (*a*). The ampullary section of the CBD shows a small cystic dilatation (arrow, *a*) that protrudes into the lumen of the duodenum. The rest of the CBD is also dilated.

T2-weighted single-shot echo-train spin-echo images in the coronal plane with fat suppression (*b*) and the transverse plane without fat suppression (*c*) in a second patient. The CBD shows a cystic expansion (white arrows, *b*, *c*) of its ampullary section. The transverse image (*c*) demonstrates that the choledochocele (white arrows, *c*) bulges into the duodenum (black arrow, *c*), which contains high-signal intensity intraluminal fluid.

(c)

best demonstrated with thin-section T2- or T1-weighted images, on which Caroli disease presents with rounded cystic dilatations of equivalent signal intensity compared to bile (bright on T2- and low on T1-weighted images) communicating with bile ducts (fig. 3.41) [105].

Mass Lesions

Benign tumors that involve the biliary tract are relatively uncommon. Tumors can be solitary or multiple. Benign mass lesions can result in ductal obstruction and hepatic atrophy, resembling an imaging appearance comparable to malignant disease, as illustrated by a rare benign tumor, giant cell tumor of the bile duct (fig. 3.42).

Papillary Adenoma. Papillary adenomas of the biliary tract are rare benign epithelial tumors that have an increased risk for malignant transformation. Multiple small papillomas scattered throughout the biliary tree are characteristic of biliary papillomatosis. This condition is associated with an irregular pattern of intrahepatic bile duct dilatation due to obstruction by the papillomas. These small tumors are best visualized on 2-min postgadolinium fat-suppressed T1-weighted

gradient-echo images as tiny enhancing mass lesions (fig. 3.43).

Ampullary Adenoma. Neoplasms that arise at the ampulla may have a benign histology. The most common benign ampullary tumor is an ampullary adenoma. The MRI appearance of this rare entity shows a well-defined mass, often polypoid, that shows no evidence of local invasion. Masses are generally small and enhance homogeneously (fig. 3.44).

Postsurgical Biliary Complications

Benign biliary strictures are a sequel of surgical injury (e.g., laparoscopic cholecystectomy, gastric and hepatic resection, biliary-enteric anastomosis, biliary reconstruction after liver transplantation) in 90–95% of cases [106, 107]. The remainder are secondary to penetrating or blunt trauma, inflammation associated with gallstone disease, chronic pancreatitis, ampullary fibrosis, toxic or ischemic lesions of the hepatic artery, or primary infection. The advent of minimally invasive therapeutic procedures, performed by interventional radiology or endoscopy, has greatly increased the need for preoperative diagnosis and

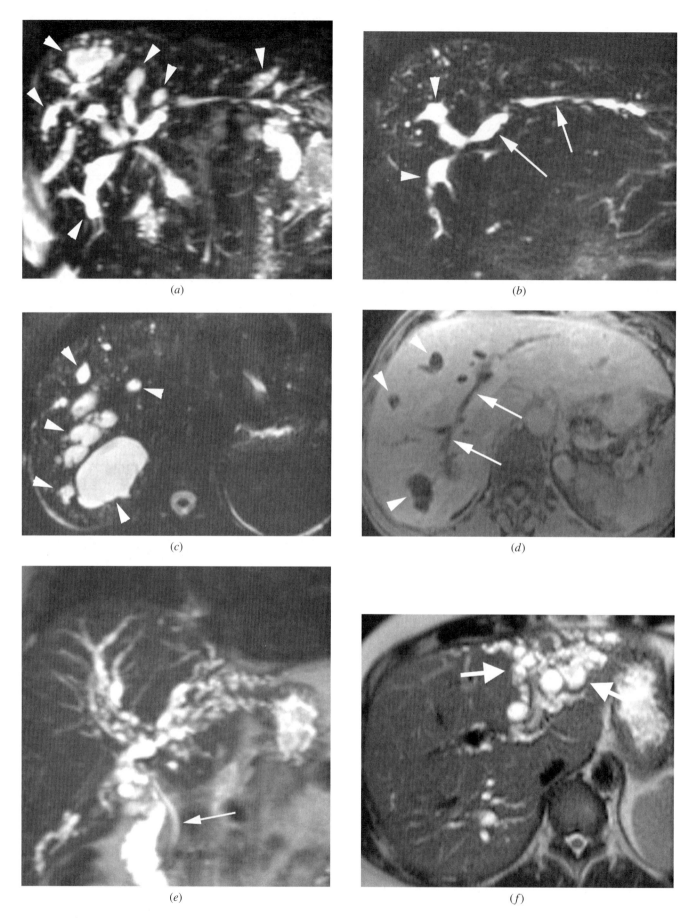

(a)

(b)

(c)

(d)

(e)

(f)

F I G . 3.41 Caroli disease. Paracoronal thick-section MRCP (*a*), paracoronal thin-section MRCP (*b*), axial fat-suppressed T2-weighted single-shot echo-train spin-echo (*c*), and axial 2-min postgadolinium GE (*d*) images. Cystic intrahepatic biliary dilatations (arrowheads, *a–d*) are present in the right and left lobes of the liver. Differentiation from liver cysts is made by demonstration of continuity with mildly dilated bile ducts (arrows, *b*, *d*). Differentiation of bile ducts from portal vein branches is facilitated on the postgadolinium image (*d*), where the latter demonstrate enhancement. MIP reconstruction MRCP (*e*), axial T2-weighted single-shot echo-train spin-echo (*f*), and axial 2-min postgadolinium GE (*g*) images of another patient with Caroli disease (Courtesy of

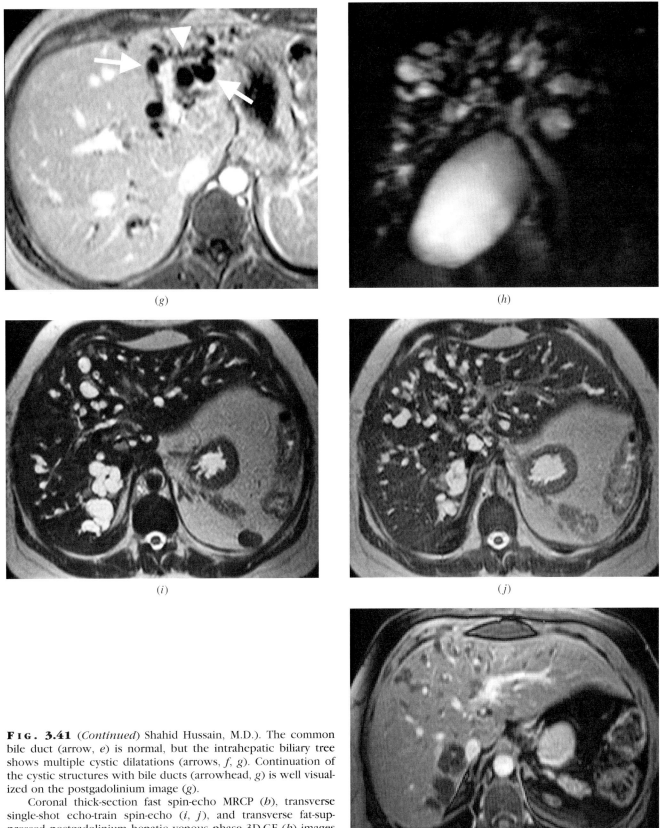

FIG. 3.41 (*Continued*) Shahid Hussain, M.D.). The common bile duct (arrow, *e*) is normal, but the intrahepatic biliary tree shows multiple cystic dilatations (arrows, *f, g*). Continuation of the cystic structures with bile ducts (arrowhead, *g*) is well visualized on the postgadolinium image (*g*).

Coronal thick-section fast spin-echo MRCP (*h*), transverse single-shot echo-train spin-echo (*i, j*), and transverse fat-suppressed postgadolinium hepatic venous phase 3D-GE (*k*) images demonstrate multiple cystic dilatations of intrahepatic bile ducts in another patient (Courtesy of Frank Miller, M.D.). There is no involvement in the extrahepatic ducts. No enhancement is detected in the cystic dilatations. Note that there is no spleen.

(g)

(h)

(i)

(j)

(k)

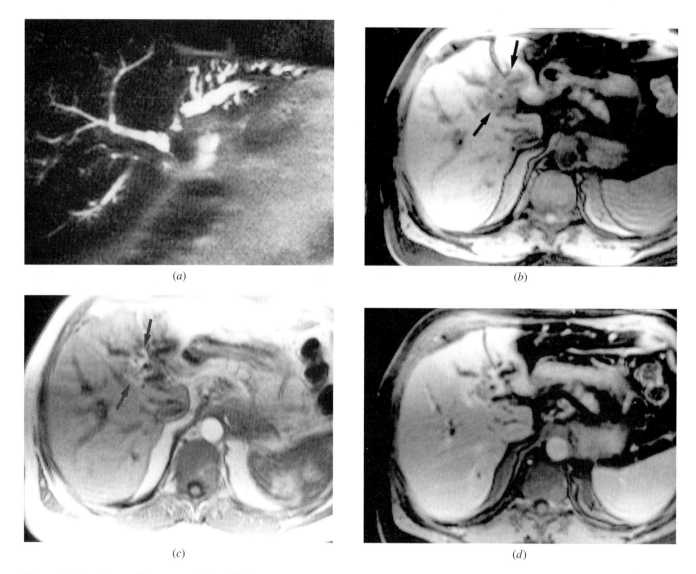

(a)   (b)   (c)   (d)

F I G . 3.42 Giant cell tumor of the bile duct. Coronal thin-section MRCP single-shot echo-train spin-echo image with fat suppression (a), transverse T1-weighted fat-suppressed GE (b), immediate postgadolinium GE (c), and 2-min postgadolinium fat-suppressed GE (d) images. An obstruction at the confluence of the right and left main hepatic ducts is visualized on the MRCP image (a) with dilatation of the right and left intrahepatic biliary system. The tumor (arrows, b) appears moderately low signal intensity on the T1-weighted image (b). The tumor demonstrates increased enhancement (arrows, c) on the immediate postgadolinium image (c), with persistent enhancement on the 2-min postgadolinium image (d). The liver parenchyma distal to the tumor shows delayed increased enhancement (d). The tumor mimics the MRI appearance of Klatskin tumor but was diagnosed as giant cell tumor of the left hepatic duct at histopathology.

imaging in order to plan the optimal therapeutic approach. The major advantage of MRCP is the ability to visualize the biliary tree above and below a high-grade stricture or complete obstruction. The bile ducts distal to a stenosis, however, may be collapsed and nonvisualized on MIP-reconstruction images, leading to overestimation of the stricture. Thin-section source images must be used to evaluate the extent of high-grade stenoses, as even minimal amounts of fluid in collapsed ducts can be depicted on these images.

Other biliary complications of cholecystectomy are retained bile duct stones, biliary leak, and biliary fistula

(fig. 3.45). In a study of such complications by Coakley et al. [108], two readers correctly categorized post-surgical complications in 88% and 76%, respectively. However, high-grade biliary stricture and transsection of bile ducts both presented as abrupt termination of a dilated duct, and, consequently, MRCP failed to distinguish between those entities but grouped them together as occlusion.

In patients with biliary-enteric anastomoses, ERCP can often not be performed. MRCP, however, is very effective in visualizing the anatomy of the anastomosis, strictures of the anastomosis or of intrahepatic ducts,

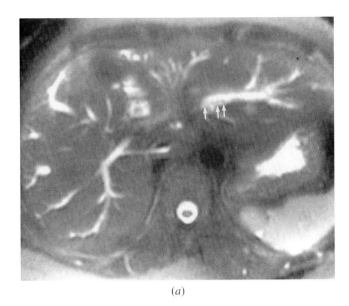 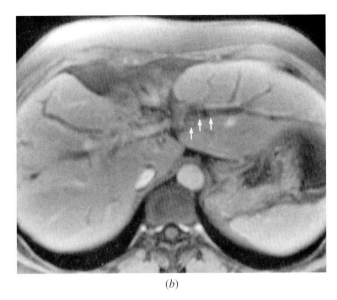

(a)   (b)

F I G . 3.43 Biliary papillomatosis. T2-weighted single-shot echo-train spin-echo (*a*) and T1-weighted 2-min postgadolinium fat-suppressed GE (*b*) images. Several small, biliary intraductal, papillary tumors (arrows, *a*, *b*) are revealed showing enhancement on the postgadolinium image (*b*). The entire biliary tree is moderately dilated because of obstruction by papillomas in the CHD and CBD.

and biliary tract stones proximal to the anastomosis, in up to 100% of patients (see figs. 3.9, 3.43) [2, 109]. Close scrutiny of the thin-section source images is mandatory because the biliary-enteric anastomosis and stones can be obscured on thick-section and MIP-reconstruction images by the high signal intensity of surrounding bile and bowel fluid (fig. 3.46). Metallic surgical clips and pneumobilia can also produce artifacts that should not be mistaken as stones or strictures. Ischemic changes of the biliary system and obstruction secondary to a stricture following liver transplantation operations can also be well evaluated with MRI (fig. 3.46).

Malignant Disease

Cholangiocarcinoma
Cholangiocarcinomas are well-differentiated sclerosing adenocarcinomas in two-thirds of cases; the remainder are anaplastic, squamous cell, or cystadenocarcinomas. The most common predisposing diseases in Western countries are ulcerative colitis and sclerosing cholangitis. In Far Eastern countries, recurrent pyogenic cholangitis (caused by *Clonorchis sinensis* infestation) is the most common cause. Other predisposing factors are Caroli disease, choledochal cysts, α-1-antitrypsin deficiency, and autosomal dominant polycystic kidney disease. Cholangiocarcinoma is typically a malignancy of older patients (>50 yr). Patients usually present with jaundice and weight loss. Three types of cholangiocarcinomas can be differentiated based on anatomic distribution: the peripheral (or intrahepatic) type arising from peripheral bile ducts in the liver, the hilar type (Klatskin

tumor) with its origin at the confluence of the right and left hepatic ducts, and the extrahepatic type arising from the main hepatic ducts, CHD or CBD [110, 111].

The peripheral type constitutes approximately 10% of all cholangiocarcinomas and is the second most common primary liver tumor after hepatocellular carcinoma (HCC). Peripheral cholangiocarcinomas usually present as masslike lesions that do not obstruct the central bile ducts [112]. Therefore, they can obtain a large size and show intrahepatic metastases before they cause clinical symptoms. Their typical MR imaging appearance is a mass lesion that is mildly heterogeneous with moderately low signal intensity on T1-weighted images and mildly to moderately hyperintense signal on T2-weighted images (fig. 3.47) [95]. On immediate postgadolinium images, they usually show mild to moderate enhancement that is usually diffuse heterogeneous in pattern. Progressive enhancement may be observed on late fat-suppressed images, reflecting a high content of fibrous tissue (see fig. 3.47). This feature, if present, may suggest this type of tumor and differentiate it from HCC, which typically shows intense, diffuse heterogeneous enhancement on immediate postgadolinium images and washout on delayed images [113]. Additional features that help differentiate cholangiocarcinomas from HCC are lack of vascular invasion and rare occurrence of cholangiocarcinoma in cirrhotic livers [113]. Peripheral cholangiocarcinoma is also described in Chapter 2, *Liver*.

Klatskin tumors are usually small-volume superficial spreading tumors that result in early biliary obstruction and dilatation of proximal ducts (fig. 3.48). These tumors

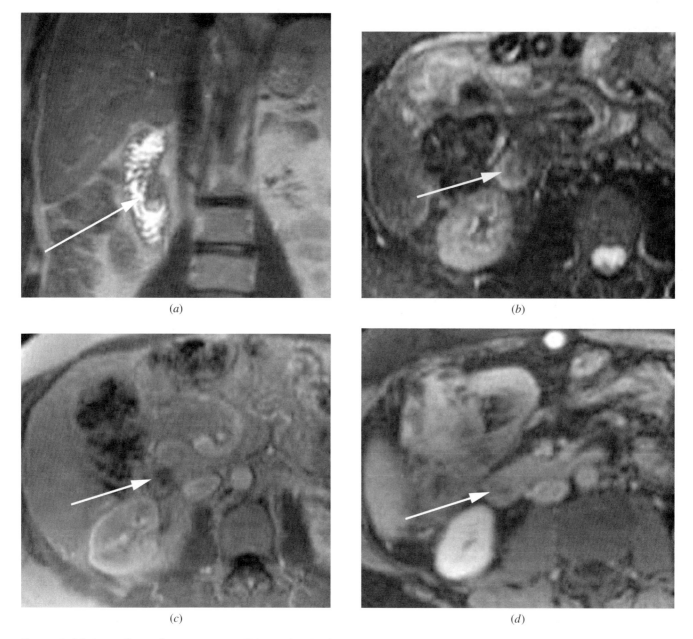

FIG. 3.44 Ampullary adenoma. Coronal T2-weighted echo-train spin-echo (*a*), axial STIR (*b*), axial immediate postgadolinium GE (*c*), and 2-min postgadolinium fat-suppressed GE (*d*) images. A prominent, masslike major papilla (arrows, *a–d*) is observed protruding into the duodenal lumen. Signal intensity and contrast enhancement are equivalent to a normal papilla. No sign of malignancy is observed.

may uncommonly present as masslike lesions similar to peripheral tumors. Most often, they show circumferential growth and spread along bile ducts with poor conspicuity on noncontrast MR images (fig. 3.49). Biliary dilatation can involve one or both lobes of the liver, depending on the location of the tumor. Lobar atrophy of the liver combined with marked biliary dilatation should raise suspicion of cholangiocarcinoma (fig. 3.50), but this feature is not pathognomonic [114].

Extrahepatic cholangiocarcinomas usually grow in a circumferential pattern similar to Klatskin tumors.

They arise in the CBD and result in biliary obstruction in the vast majority of patients. The imaging features of Klatskin tumors and extrahepatic cholangiocarcinomas at MRCP are dilatation of the proximal biliary tree with stricture or abrupt termination at the tumor, typically showing a shoulder sign (fig. 3.51) [115]. Irregularity of the ductal wall is indicative of infiltration and raises a high suspicion of malignancy. Occasionally, tumors can show intraluminal papillary growth presenting as a filling defect on MRCP images. ERCP may on occasion poorly evaluate tumors because of incomplete biliary

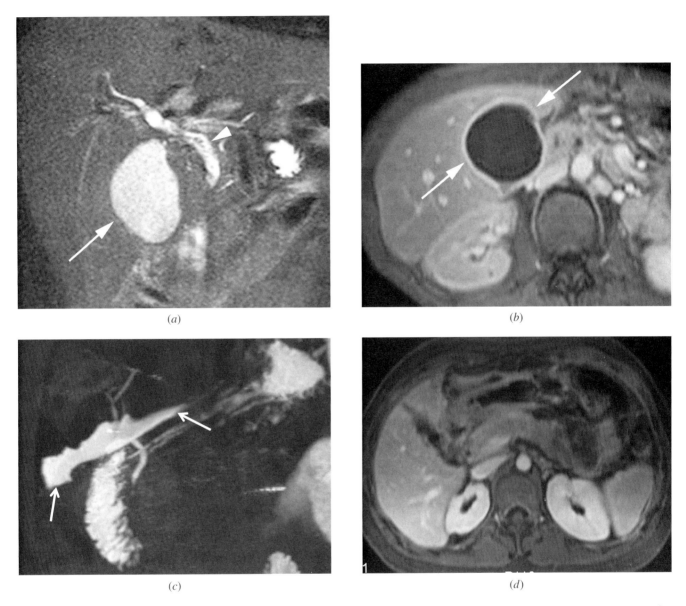

(a)   *(b)*

(c)   *(d)*

F I G . 3.45 Biloma. T2-weighted fat-suppressed single-shot echo-train spin-echo (*a*) and T1-weighted 2-min postgadolinium fat-suppressed GE (*b*) images in a 44-yr-old woman with a history of open cholecystectomy and persistent right upper quadrant pain. A fluid collection (arrows, *a*, *b*) is depicted in the gallbladder bed, resembling a gallbladder. The fluid collection (biloma) has an enhancing wall (arrows, *b*) caused by an inflammatory reaction of the surrounding peritoneum. The common bile duct (arrowhead, *a*) shows inhomogeneous internal signal caused by a T-tube drain.

Coronal T2-weighted reconstructed 3D MIP MRCP image (*c*), transverse T1-weighted postgadolinium interstitial phase 3D-GE (*d*), and T1-weighted postgadolinium 1-h delayed fat-suppressed coronal and transverse 3D-GE (*e*, *f*) images acquired with gadobenate

opacification. An advantage of MRCP in combination with conventional MRI is that it can also visualize the biliary tree proximal to an occlusion, which often is not possible or advisable with ERCP, as well as detecting distant disease such as liver metastases or lymph node involvement.

On T1-weighted MR images with or without fat suppression, cholangiocarcinomas appear mildly to moderately hypointense but may also be isointense relative to liver parenchyma. On T2-weighted images, they are isointense or mildly hyperintense (see Figs. 3.47–3.49) [113]. Thickening of bile duct walls greater than 5 mm is highly suggestive of cholangiocarcinoma [95]. However, this measurement is not sensitive, as at least 50% of tumors show thinner wall diameters [113]. The finding of relatively minor increase of wall thickness (3–4 mm) in association with high-grade biliary obstruction is highly suggestive of cholangiocarcinoma in patients without a history of recent gallbladder surgery. On immediate postgadolinium images, cholangiocarcinomas

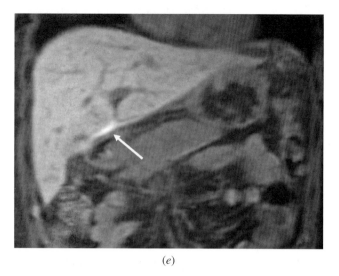

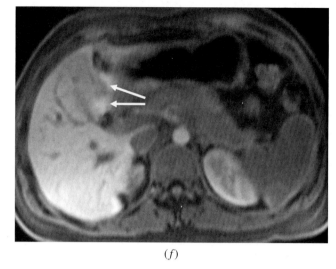

(e)   (f)

F I G . 3.45 (*Continued*) dimeglumine (Multihance) demonstrate the bile leak (arrows, *e, f*) following the cholecystectomy operation in another patient. Free fluid (arrows, *c*) is detected along the inferior surface of the liver and gallbladder fossa. Because gadobenate dimeglumine is taken up by hepatocytes and excreted into the biliary ducts, intrabdominal bile leaks resulting from disruptions of the biliary system can be detected as high-signal intensity fluid (arrows, *e, f*) on delayed images. Note that high-signal-intensity intrabdominal bile cannot be detected on early postgadolinium image (*d*).

are usually hypovascular, showing minimal or moderate enhancement that intensifies on delayed images (see figs. 3.47–3.49) [113]. A combination of early and late fat-suppressed gadolinium-enhanced images is very helpful to identify these tumors. Fat suppression also reduces the signal of fatty tissue in the porta hepatis, which improves the conspicuity of cholangiocarcinomas and facilitates the evaluation of the extent of tumor and infiltration into adjacent tissues and organs.

Findings that indicate that a tumor is unresectable are vascular encasement and direct invasion of liver parenchyma. Large tumor size generally also confers inoperability (see fig. 3.50). Most cholangiocarcinomas are unresectable at the time of initial diagnosis and can be treated only with palliative biliary drainage. Biliary stent placement results in mild inflammation of bile duct walls, which appears as increased gadolinium enhancement with an appearance indistinguishable from superficial spread of cholangiocarcinoma (fig. 3.52). If feasible, it is preferable to image patients suspected of biliary tumor before stent placement to avoid the problem of incorrectly staging the tumor because of inflammatory changes secondary to the presence of the stent. Lymphadenopathy with portocaval and porta hepatis nodes is an associated finding in up to 73% of patients with cholangiocarcinoma (see fig. 3.50). This is best demonstrated with a combination of T2-weighted fat-suppressed and T1-weighted 2-min postgadolinium fat-suppressed images [113]. On these late postgadolinium images, fine tumor strands are frequently observed, and 5-mm or smaller lymph nodes are con-

sistent with tumor extension if three or more of them are clustered in the region of the tumor. In advanced cholangiocarcinoma, intraperitoneal tumor spread may occasionally be found and is also best seen on late postgadolinium fat-suppressed images (fig. 3.53).

Periampullary and Ampullary Carcinoma
Carcinomas arising from the ampulla of Vater, periampullary duodenum, or distal CBD are grouped together and termed periampullary carcinomas. Their presentation is similar to that of pancreatic head ductal adenocarcinoma, including obstruction of both the CBD and pancreatic duct. The prognosis of periampullary carcinoma is significantly better than that of pancreatic carcinoma, with a 5-year survival rate up to 85% [116]. Periampullary carcinomas can cause ampullary obstruction and become clinically symptomatic even when they are only a few millimeters in size. Therefore, signs and symptoms of dilatation of the biliary tree and the pancreatic duct are observed relatively early in the course of these tumors, which likely accounts in part for their better prognosis. MRCP is very effective for the visualization of biliary and pancreatic ductal dilatation and the determination of the level of obstruction [117]. On T1-weighted fat-suppressed images, periampullary carcinomas typically appear as low-signal-intensity masses (fig. 3.54). Obstruction of the pancreatic duct eventually results in chronic pancreatitis. Chronic pancreatitis results in a reduced signal intensity of the pancreas on precontrast T1-weighted images, which diminishes the conspicuity of periampullary carcinomas on this

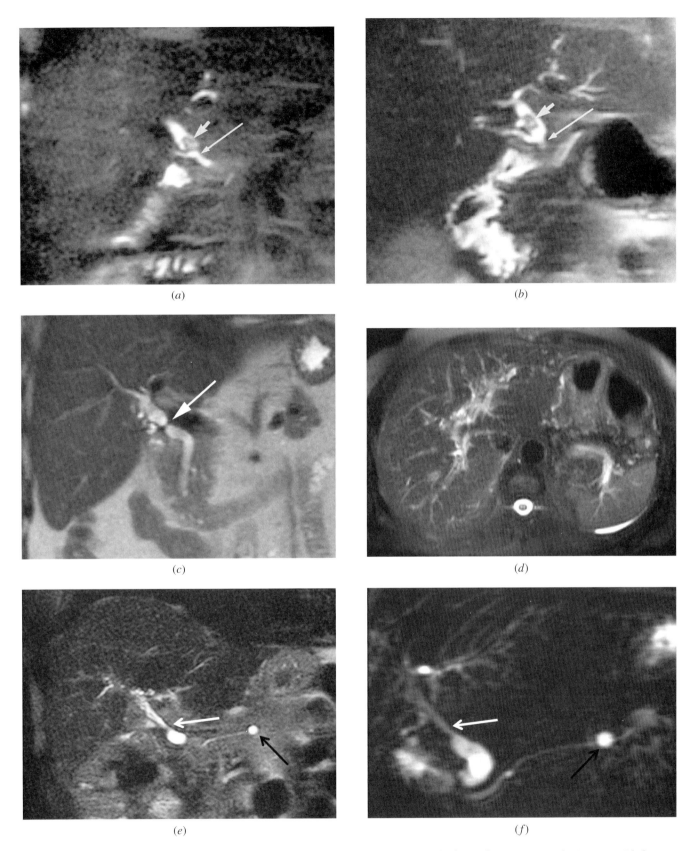

(a)

(b)

(c)

(d)

(e)

(f)

F I G. 3.46 MRCP after liver transplantation. Coronal thin-section MRCP single-shot echo-train spin-echo images with fat suppression (*a*, *b*). Slight narrowing of the anastomosis (long arrows, *a*, *b*) between the graft CBD and the host CBD is observed. A low-signal stone (short arrows, *a*, *b*) is visualized in the dilated graft CBD immediately proximal to the anastomosis. Coronal T2-weighted echo-train spin-echo image in another patient after liver transplantation (*c*). A circumscribed stricture (arrow, *c*) is observed at the anastomosis of the donor and recipient CBD. The proximal bile ducts are slightly dilated.

Transverse T2-weighted fat-suppressed single-shot echo-train spin-echo (*d*), coronal T2-weighted thin-section echo-train spin-echo (*e*), coronal thick-section fast spin-echo MRCP (*f*), and coronal reconstructed 3D MIP MRCP (*g*) images demonstrate ischemic

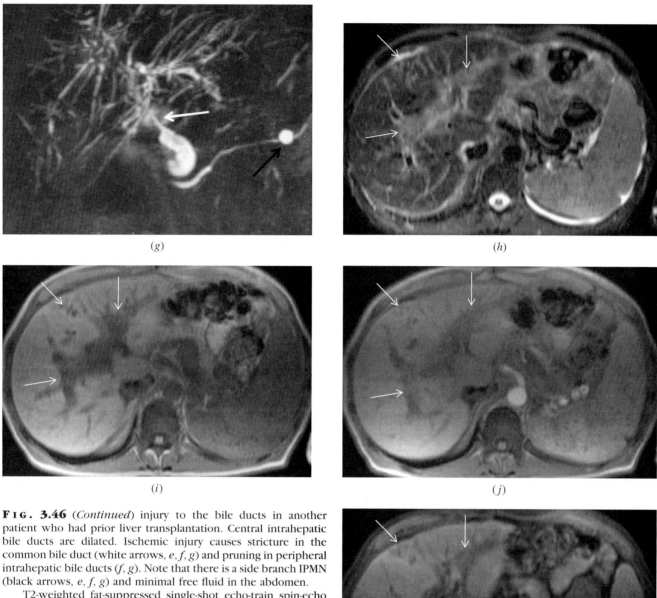

(g)

(h)

(i)

(j)

(k)

FIG. 3.46 (*Continued*) injury to the bile ducts in another patient who had prior liver transplantation. Central intrahepatic bile ducts are dilated. Ischemic injury causes stricture in the common bile duct (white arrows, *e, f, g*) and pruning in peripheral intrahepatic bile ducts (*f, g*). Note that there is a side branch IPMN (black arrows, *e, f, g*) and minimal free fluid in the abdomen.

T2-weighted fat-suppressed single-shot echo-train spin-echo (*h*), T1-weighted SGE (*i*), and T1-weighted postgadolinium late hepatic arterial phase SGE (*j*) and interstitial phase fat-suppressed 3D-GE (*k*) images demonstrate debris-filled dilated bile ducts in a patient who had liver transplantation. Debris-filled ducts (arrows, *h–k*) may have low or intermediate signal on T2-weighted images and this appearance of debris-filled dilated bile ducts and periportal edema mimics infiltrative lesions extending along the portal tracts such as posttransplant lymphoproliferative disorder. Debris filled bile ducts show mild enhancement, which suggests the presence of inflammation as well. Note the portal hypertension findings and ascites.

sequence. On immediate postgadolinium T1-weighted images, pancreatic parenchyma enhances greater than tumor, even in the presence of chronic pancreatitis. Periampullary carcinomas enhance minimally on early postgadolinium images because of their hypovascular character (figs. 3.54, 3.55) [118]. On 2-min postgadolinium fat-suppressed images, delayed enhancement is a typical finding [117]. A thin rim of enhancement is commonly observed along the periphery of these tumors and may also be a relatively specific finding (see

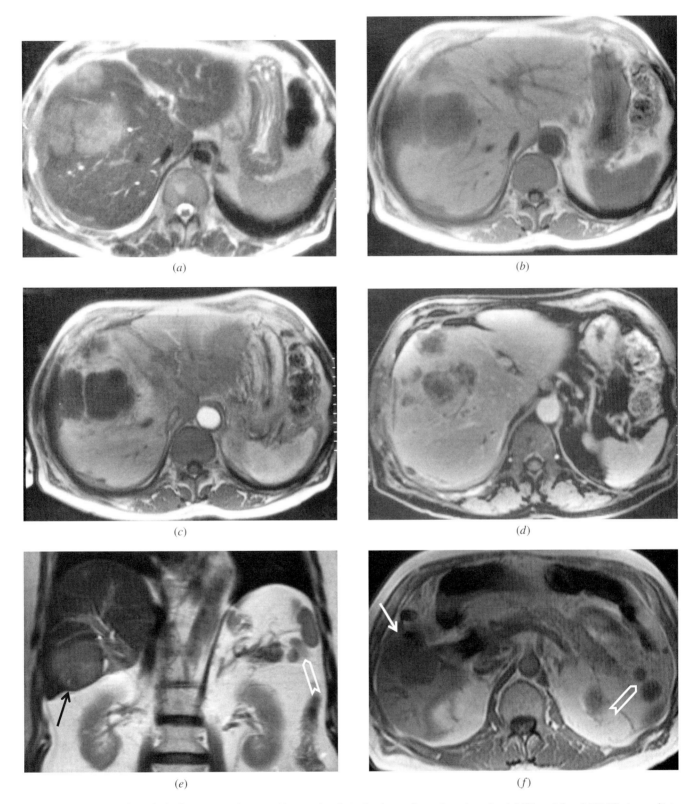

(a)

(b)

(c)

(d)

(e)

(f)

F I G . 3.47 Peripheral cholangiocarcinoma. T2-weighted single-shot echo-train spin-echo (*a*),T1-weighted GE (*b*), immediate postgadolinium GE (*c*), and 2-min postgadolinium fat-suppressed GE (*d*) images. A large tumor with intrahepatic metastases is observed in the right lobe of the liver. The signal is moderately hyperintense on the T2-weighted image (*a*) and hypointense on the T1-weighted image (*b*). On the immediate postgadolinium image (*c*), the tumors are hypoenhancing and demonstrate mild perilesional enhancement. Progressive heterogeneous enhancement of the tumors is observed on the 2-min postgadolinium image (*d*).

Coronal T2-weighted single-shot echo-train spin-echo (*e*), transverse T1-weighted SGE (*f*), transverse T1-weighted postgadolinium hepatic arterial dominant phase (*g*), and hepatic venous phase (*h*) fat-suppressed 3D-GE images at 3.0 T demonstrate a peripheral

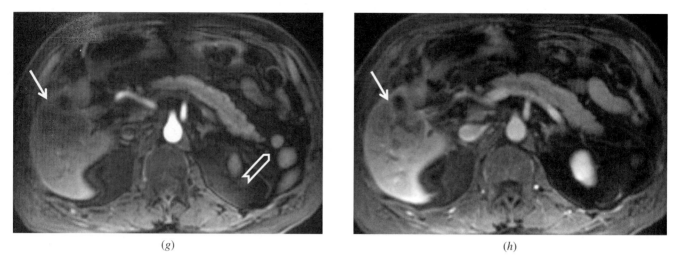

(g)   (h)

F I G . 3.47 (*Continued*) cholangiocarcinoma (solid arrows, *e–h*) in another patient with prior splenectomy and splenosis (open arrows, *e, f, g*). The tumor shows heterogeneous progressive enhancement on postgadolinium images and obstructs the peripheral biliary ducts.

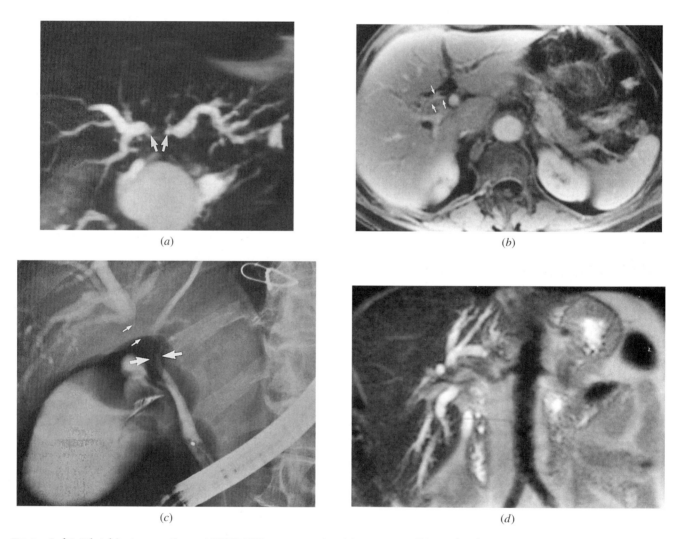

(a)   (b)

(c)   (d)

F I G . 3.48 Klatskin tumor. Coronal MRCP MIP reconstruction (*a*), transverse T1-weighted 2-min postgadolinium fat-suppressed GE (*b*), and ERCP (*c*) images. Obstruction of the right and left main hepatic ducts (arrows, *a*) at the level of the porta hepatis with dilatation of peripheral ducts is visualized on the MRCP image (*a*). A small enhancing tumor (small arrows, *b*), measuring 4 mm in diameter, extends from the CHD into the right main hepatic duct, as shown on the postgadolinium image (*b*). ERCP (*c*) also shows the obstruction (arrows, *c*) at the level of the porta hepatis and the extension of the tumor into the right main hepatic duct (small arrows, *c*). Note the poor visualization of the left biliary ductal system on the ERCP image (*c*) because of underfilling.

Coronal T2-weighted single-shot echo-train spin-echo (*d*), transverse T1-weighted fat-suppressed GE (*e*), and 2-min postgadolinium fat-suppressed GE (*f*) images in a second patient. Dilatation of the right and left intrahepatic biliary tree is observed on the

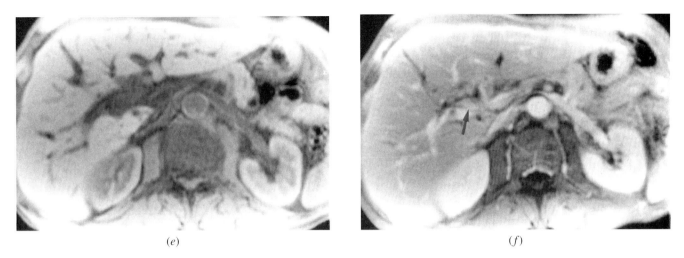

(e)　　　　　　　　　　　　　　　　　　(f)

F I G . 3.48 (*Continued*) T2-weighted image (*d*).The tumor shows poor conspicuity on the precontrast GE image (*e*). On the 2-min postgadolinium image (*f*), the small Klatskin tumor (arrow, *f*) in the porta hepatis demonstrates enhancement and can be well differentiated from surrounding structures.

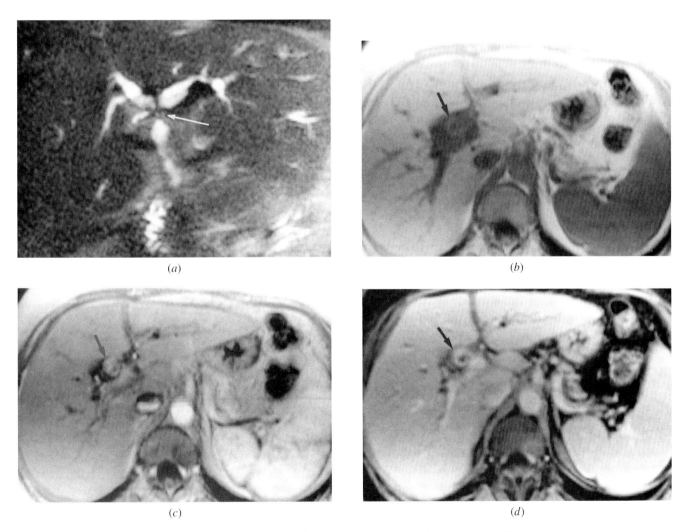

(a)　　　　　　　　　　　　　　　　　　(b)

(c)　　　　　　　　　　　　　　　　　　(d)

F I G . 3.49 Klatskin tumor, circumferential growth. Coronal T2-weighted thin-section MRCP single-shot echo-train spin-echo image with fat suppression (*a*) and transverse T1-weighted GE (*b*), immediate postgadolinium GE (*c*), and 2-min postgadolinium fat-suppressed GE (*d*) images. A short obstruction at the confluence of the right and left main hepatic ducts (arrow, *a*) is revealed on the MRCP image (*a*). It is difficult to delineate the tumor (arrow, *b*) from surrounding structures on the T1-weighted precontrast image (*b*). After gadolinium administration, the tumor shows moderately intense enhancement (arrows, *c, d*) on the immediate (*c*) and late (*d*) postgadolinium images. Note the circumferential growth and small volume of the Klatskin tumor, best visualized on the postgadolinium images (*c, d*).

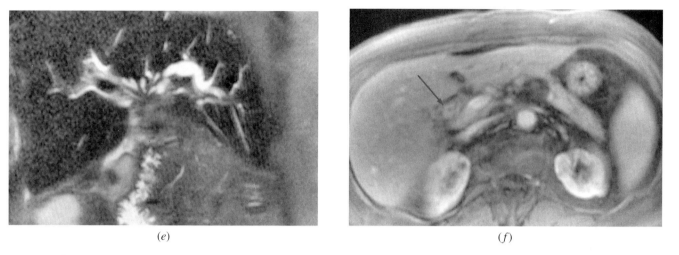

(e)   *(f)*

F I G . 3.49 *(Continued)* Coronal T2-weighted thin-section MRCP single-shot echo-train spin-echo image with fat suppression *(e)* and transverse T1-weighted 2-min postgadolinium fat-suppressed GE image *(f)* in a second patient. The Klatskin tumor obstructs the intrahepatic biliary system at the porta hepatis, demonstrated on the MRCP image *(e)*. The tumor shows circumferential growth in the CHD (arrow, *f*) and increased enhancement on the late postgadolinium image *(f)*.

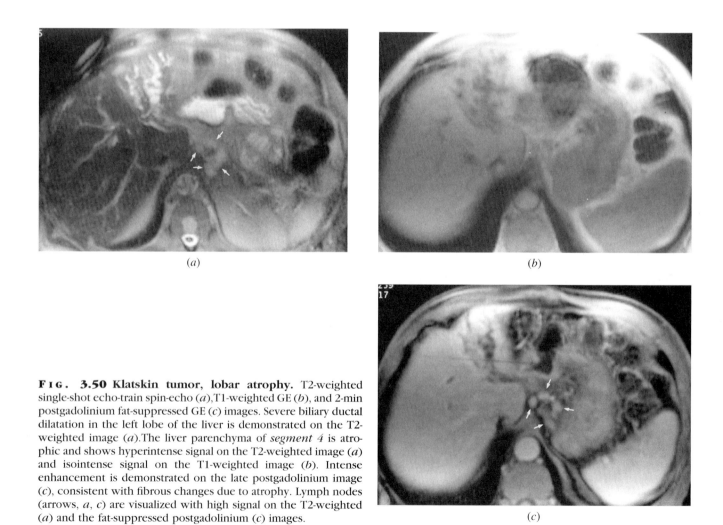

(a)   *(b)*

F I G . 3.50 Klatskin tumor, lobar atrophy. T2-weighted single-shot echo-train spin-echo *(a)*, T1-weighted GE *(b)*, and 2-min postgadolinium fat-suppressed GE *(c)* images. Severe biliary ductal dilatation in the left lobe of the liver is demonstrated on the T2-weighted image *(a)*. The liver parenchyma of *segment 4* is atrophic and shows hyperintense signal on the T2-weighted image *(a)* and isointense signal on the T1-weighted image *(b)*. Intense enhancement is demonstrated on the late postgadolinium image *(c)*, consistent with fibrous changes due to atrophy. Lymph nodes (arrows, *a*, *c*) are visualized with high signal on the T2-weighted *(a)* and the fat-suppressed postgadolinium *(c)* images.

(c)

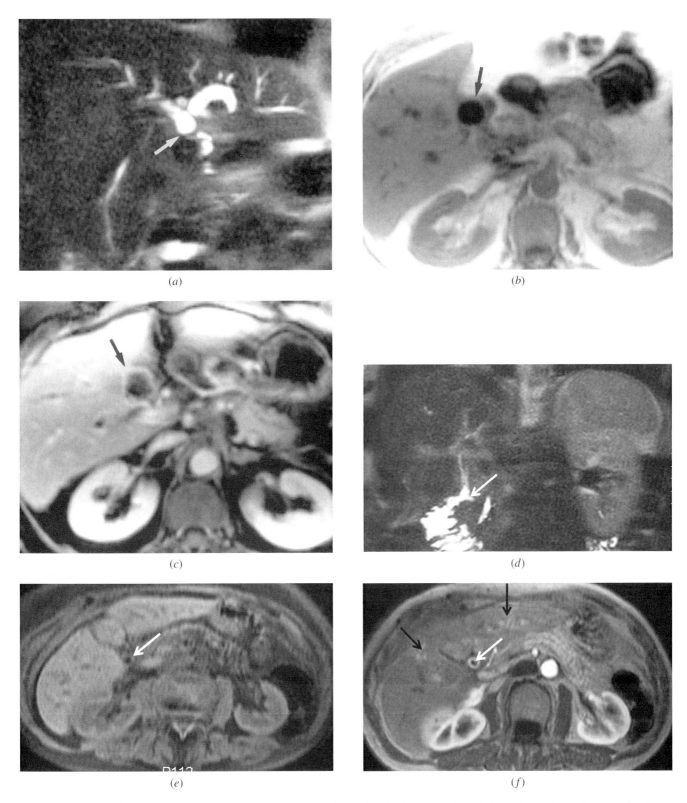

(a)

(b)

(c)

(d)

(e)

(f)

F I G . 3.51 Extrahepatic cholangiocarcinoma. Coronal T2-weighted thin-section MRCP single-shot echo-train spin-echo image with fat suppression (*a*) and transverse T1-weighted GE (*b*) and 2-minute postgadolinium fat-suppressed GE (*c*) images. Obstruction of the proximal CBD (arrow, *a*) is present, showing an abrupt cut-off ("shoulder sign") on the MRCP image (*a*). The intrahepatic biliary tree is markedly dilated (*a*). The extrahepatic cholangiocarcinoma shows circumferential growth along the dilated proximal CBD (arrows, *b*, *c*). On the late postgadolinium image (*c*), the tumor shows intense enhancement (arrow, *c*) and can be differenti-ated from adjacent liver parenchyma.

Coronal T2-weighted thin-section echo-train spin-echo (*d*), transverse T1-weighted fat-suppressed 3D-GE (*e*), transverse T1-weighted postgadolinium hepatic arterial dominant phase SGE (*f*), and hepatic venous phase fat-suppressed 3D-GE (*g*) images

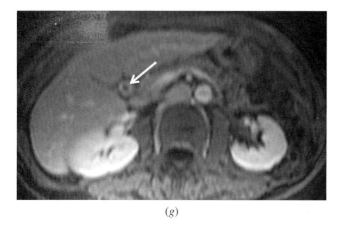

(g)

FIG. 3.51 (*Continued*) demonstrate distal common bile duct cholangiocarcinoma (arrows, *d-g*) in another patient. There is a stent in the common bile duct. There is an abrupt angulation and shoulder sign (arrow, *d*) between the common bile duct and duodenum. The common bile duct wall shows thickening and prominent enhancement (arrows, *e*, *f*, *g*), which may result from the involvement of the tumor and inflammation secondary to the stent placement and infectious cholangitis. Intrahepatic bile ducts show prominent enhancement suggestive of ascending cholangitis (black arrows, *f*).

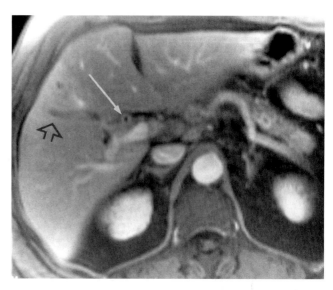

FIG. 3.52 Klatskin tumor and biliary stent. Transverse 2-min postgadolinium fat-suppressed GE image. A biliary stent (white arrow) is present in this patient with Klatskin tumor of the right hepatic duct. The bile duct walls around the stent show intense enhancement that makes differentiation between reactive inflammation caused by the stent placement and tumor spread along the bile duct impossible. *Segment 8* of the liver (open arrow) shows biliary dilatation with increased enhancement of bile duct walls and increased parenchymal enhancement, which may reflect inflammatory changes.

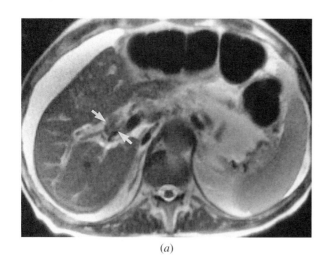

(a)

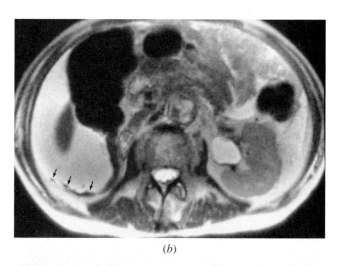

(b)

FIG. 3.53 Cholangiocarcinoma with peritoneal metastases. T2-weighted single-shot echo-train spin-echo (*a*, *b*) and 2-min postgadolinium fat-suppressed GE (*c*) images. In the porta hepatis (*a*), a tumor (arrows, *a*) is shown that is isointense compared to liver. Ascites surrounding the liver is demonstrated with high signal on the T2-weighted (*a*, *b*) and low signal on the T1-weighted (*c*) images. More caudally (*b*, *c*), nodular peritoneal implants (arrows, *b*, *c*) are visualized, demonstrating intense enhancement on the 2-min postgadolinium fat-suppressed image (*c*).

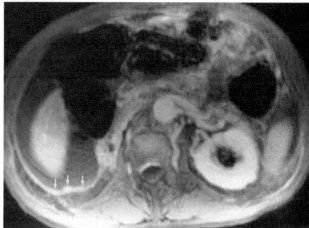

(c)

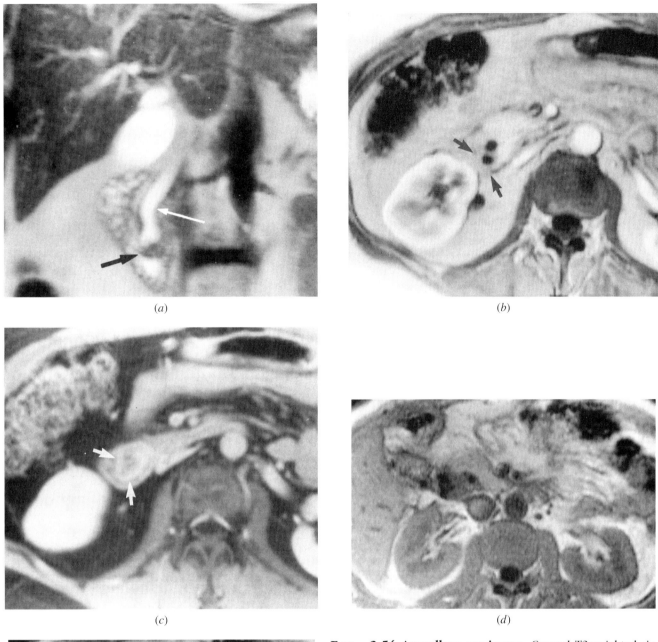

(a)

(b)

(c)

(d)

(e)

FIG. 3.54 Ampullary carcinoma. Coronal T2-weighted single-shot echo-train spin-echo (a), transverse T1-weighted immediate postgadolinium GE (b), and 2-min postgadolinium fat-suppressed GE (c) images. The ampullary carcinoma (black arrow, a) obstructs the CBD (white arrow, a), as visualized on the T2-weighted image (a). On the immediate postgadolinium image (b), the tumor (arrows, b) is hypoenhancing compared to normal pancreas and is well delineated. It surrounds the CBD completely and the pancreatic duct partially, which are both dilated and visualized as signal-void structures. Note the peripheral rim enhancement of the tumor (arrows, c) on the 2-min postgadolinium image (c) on a more inferior section where the tumor protrudes into the duodenum.

T1-weighted GE (d) and immediate postgadolinium GE (e) images in a second patient demonstrating a 2.5-cm ampullary carcinoma of low signal intensity that shows good contrast against high-signal pancreas on the precontrast image (d). The tumor is hypoenhancing compared to pancreatic parenchyma (e), surrounds the distal CBD (straight arrow, e), and protrudes into the duodenum (curved arrow, e).

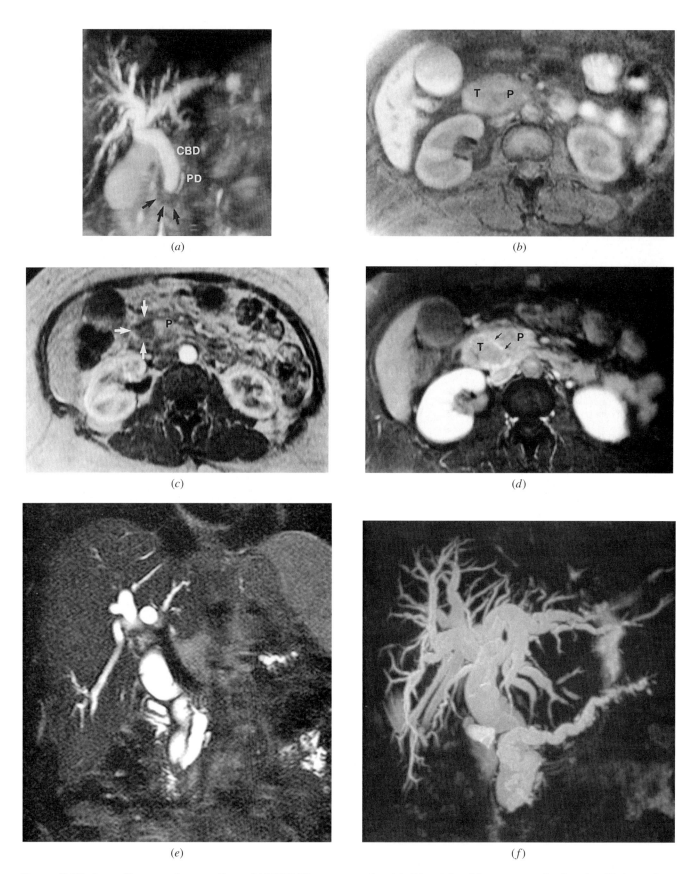

(a)

(b)

(c)

(d)

(e)

(f)

F I G . 3.55 Ampullary carcinoma. Coronal MRCP MIP reconstruction (*a*), T1-weighted fat-suppressed spin-echo (*b*), immediate postgadolinium GE (*c*), and 2-min postgadolinium fat-suppressed spin-echo (*d*) images. On the MRCP image (*a*), an obstructing mass (arrows, *a*) is visualized at the level of the ampulla resulting in severe dilatation of the intra- and extrahepatic biliary system and moderate dilatation of the pancreatic duct. On the precontrast T1-weighted image (*b*), the tumor (T, *b*) cannot be differentiated from the pancreas (P, *b*), which shows abnormal low signal intensity due to pancreatitis. On the immediate postgadolinium image (*c*), the tumor (arrows, *c*) is well visualized, demonstrating decreased enhancement compared to pancreas (P). Note a peripheral rim of enhancement (arrows, *d*) of the tumor on the 2-min postgadolinium image (*d*). CBD, common bile duct; GB, gallbladder; PD, pancreatic duct.

Small ampullary cancer shown on a combination of sequences in a second patient. Source MRCP (*e*), MIP reconstruction 3D-MRCP (*f*), immediate (*g*), and 90-s (*h*) fat-suppressed postgadolinium 3D gradient-echo images. Obstruction at the level of

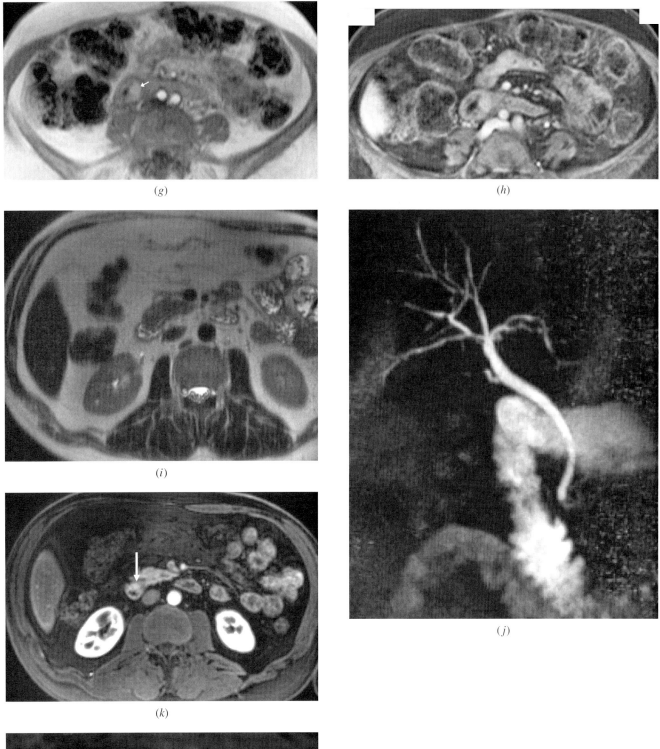

(g)

(h)

(i)

(j)

(k)

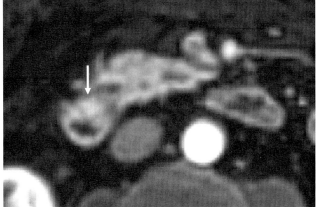

(l)

FIG. 3.55 (*Continued*) the ampulla is identified on MRCP images. A small mass is well shown at the ampulla (arrow, *g*) that was not shown at CT or at initial ERCP and biopsy. Ampullary adenocarcinoma was present in the post-Whipple procedure pathological specimen.

Transverse (*i*) T2-weighted single-shot echo-train spin-echo, coronal reconstructed 3D MIP MRCP image (*j*) and transverse T1-weighted postgadolinium hepatic arterial dominant phase fat-suppressed 3D-GE (*k*, *l*) images at 3.0 T demonstrate a small ampullary neuroendocrine carcinoma (arrow, *k*, *l*) in another patient. The enhancing tumor is under 1 cm in size, and it is detected on postgadolinium image because of higher spatial resolution at 3.0 T. Note that the findings are normal on T2-weighted images and there is no biliary obstruction.

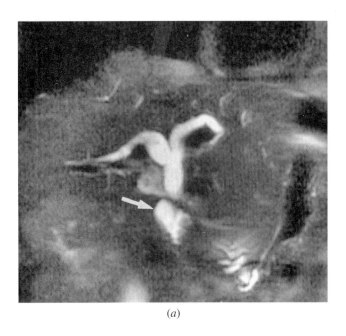

(a)

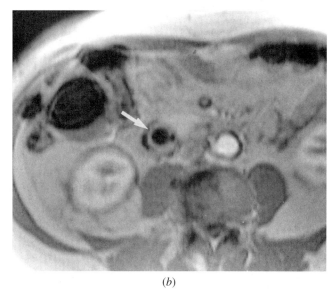

(b)

FIG. 3.56 Ampullary carcinoma superimposed on choledochocele. Coronal T2-weighted thin-section MRCP single-shot echo-train spin-echo image with fat suppression (*a*) and transverse immediate postgadolinium T1-weighted GE (*b*) and 2-min postgadolinium fat-suppressed GE (*c*) images in a patient with a choledochocele. The choledochocele (arrows, *a–c*) is visualized protruding into the duodenal lumen, and biliary obstruction with dilated intra- and extrahepatic ducts is observed on the MRCP image (*a*). The walls of the choledochocele are minimally thickened and show moderately intense enhancement on the 2-min postgadolinium image (*c*). On surgical resection, this was found to represent cholangiocarcinoma in the wall of the choledochocele. This patient had sudden development of jaundice and abdominal pain. Sudden development of these symptoms in the absence of stone disease should raise clinical suspicion of malignancy in patients with underlying cystic disease of the biliary tree.

(c)

figs. 3.54 and 3.55) [6]. Combining MRCP techniques with T1-weighted precontrast fat-suppressed and immediate and 2-min postgadolinium sequences is a very effective approach for the noninvasive evaluation of biliary obstructions [119]. Periampullary carcinomas may arise in the setting of choledochocele, fostered by longstanding chronic inflammation. A sudden change in clinical status or sudden development of jaundice may indicate the presence of cancer even if the tumor volume is small (fig. 3.56).

Metastases to the Bile Ducts and Ampulla

Metastases to the bile ducts or ampulla may occur in rare instances. Breast cancer, melanoma, and lymphoma are the most common malignancies involved. They result in biliary obstruction and resemble the appearance of primary tumors of the bile ducts and ampulla.

REFERENCES

1. Park MS, Kim TK, Kim KW et al. Differentiation of extrahepatic bile duct cholangiocarcinoma from benign stricture: findings at MRCP versus ERCP. *Radiology* 233(1): 234–240, 2004.

2. Fulcher AS, Turner MA, Capps GW et al. Half-Fourier RARE MR cholangiopancreatography: experience in 300 subjects. *Radiology* 207(1): 21–32, 1998.

3. Holzknecht N, Gauger J, Sackmann M et al. Breath-hold MR cholangiography with snapshot techniques: prospective com-

parison with endoscopic retrograde cholangiography. *Radiology* 206(3): 657–664, 1998.

4. Reinhold C, Taourel P, Bret PM et al. Choledocholithiasis: evaluation of MR cholangiography for diagnosis. *Radiology* 209(2): 435–442, 1998.

5. Guibaud L, Bret PM, Reinhold C et al. Bile duct obstruction and choledocholithiasis: diagnosis with MR cholangiography. *Radiology* 197(1): 109–115, 1995.

6. Taourel P, Bret PM, Reinhold C et al. Anatomic variants of the biliary tree: diagnosis with MR cholangiopancreatography. *Radiology* 199(2): 521–527, 1996.

7. Soto JA, Barish MA, Yucel EK et al. Pancreatic duct: MR cholangiopancreatography with a three-dimensional fast spin-echo technique. *Radiology* 196(2): 459–464, 1995.

8. Hirohashi S, Hirohashi R, Uchida H et al. Pancreatitis: evaluation with MR cholangiopancreatography in children. *Radiology* 203(2): 411–415, 1997.

9. Motohara T, Semelka RC, Bader TR. MR cholangiopancreatography. *Radiol Clin North Am* 41(1): 89–96, 2003.

10. Cohen SA, Siegel JH, Kasmin FE. Complications of diagnostic and therapeutic ERCP. *Abdom Imaging* 21(5): 385–394, 1996.

11. Rieger R, Wayand W. Yield of prospective, noninvasive evaluation of the common bile duct combined with selective ERCP/sphincterotomy in 1390 consecutive laparoscopic cholecystectomy patients. *Gastrointest Endosc* 42(1): 6–12, 1995.

12. Soto JA, Yucel EK, Barish MA et al. MR cholangiopancreatography after unsuccessful or incomplete ERCP. *Radiology* 199(1): 91–98, 1996.

13. Fulcher AS, Turner MA. MR cholangiopancreatography. *Radiol Clin North Am* 40(6): 1363–1376, 2002.

14. Park DH, Kim MH, Lee SS et al. Accuracy of magnetic resonance cholangiopancreatography for locating hepatolithiasis and detecting accompanying biliary strictures. *Endoscopy* 36(11): 987–992, 2004.

15. Ichikawa T, Nitatori T, Hachiya J et al. Breath-held MR cholangiopancreatography with half-averaged single shot hybrid rapid acquisition with relaxation enhancement sequence: comparison of fast GRE and SE sequences. *J Comput Assist Tomogr* 20(5): 798–802, 1996.

16. Hundt W, Petsch R, Scheidler J et al. Clinical evaluation of further-developed MRCP sequences in comparison with standard MRCP sequences. *Eur Radiol* 12(7): 1768–1777, 2002.

17. Takehara Y, Ichijo K, Tooyama N et al. Breath-hold MR cholangiopancreatography with a long-echo-train fast spin-echo sequence and a surface coil in chronic pancreatitis. *Radiology* 192(1): 73–78, 1994.

18. Reinhold C, Guibaud L, Genin G et al. MR cholangiopancreatography: comparison between two-dimensional fast spin-echo and three-dimensional gradient-echo pulse sequences. *J Magn Reson Imaging* 5(4): 379–384, 1995.

19. Hennig J, Nauerth A, Friedburg H. RARE imaging: a fast imaging method for clinical MR. *Magn Reson Med* 3(6): 823–833, 1986.

20. Augui J, Vignaux O, Argaud C et al. Liver: T2-weighted MR imaging with breath-hold fast-recovery optimized fast spin-echo compared with breath-hold half-Fourier and non-breath-hold respiratory-triggered fast spin-echo pulse sequences. *Radiology* 223(3): 853–859, 2002.

21. Regan F, Fradin J, Khazan R et al. Choledocholithiasis: evaluation with MR cholangiography. *AJR Am J Roentgenol* 167(6): 1441–1445, 1996.

22. Miyazaki T, Yamashita Y, Tsuchigame T et al. MR cholangiopancreatography using HASTE (half-Fourier acquisition single-shot turbo spin-echo) sequences. *AJR Am J Roentgenol* 166(6): 1297–1303, 1996.

23. Soto JA, Alvarez O, Munera F et al. Diagnosing bile duct stones: comparison of unenhanced helical CT, oral contrast-enhanced CT cholangiography, and MR cholangiography. *AJR Am J Roentgenol* 175(4): 1127–1134, 2000.

24. Riordan RD, Khonsari M, Jeffries J et al. Pineapple juice as a negative oral contrast agent in magnetic resonance cholangiopancreatography: a preliminary evaluation. *Br J Radiol* 77(924): 991–999, 2004.

25. Lorenzen M, Wedegartner U, Fiehler J et al. [Quality rating of MR-cholangiopancreatography with oral application of iron oxide particles]. *Rofo* 175(7): 936–941, 2003.

26. Sugita R, Nomiya T. Disappearance of the common bile duct signal caused by oral negative contrast agent on MR cholangiopancreatography. *J Comput Assist Tomogr* 26(3): 448–450, 2002.

27. Chavhan GB, Babyn PS, Manson D et al. Pediatric MR cholangiopancreatography: principles, technique, and clinical applications. *Radiographics* 28(7): 1951–1962, 2008.

28. Glockner JF. Hepatobiliary MRI: current concepts and controversies. *J Magn Reson Imaging* 25(4): 681–695, 2007.

29. Semelka RC, Shoenut JP, Greenberg HM et al. The liver. In: Semelka RC, Shoenut JP, editors. *MRI of the Abdomen with CT correlation.* New York: Raven Press, 1993, p. 13–41.

30. Hamm B, Staks T, Muhler A et al. Phase I clinical evaluation of Gd-EOB-DTPA as a hepatobiliary MR contrast agent: safety, pharmacokinetics, and MR imaging. *Radiology* 195(3): 785–792, 1995.

31. Dahlstrom N, Persson A, Albiin N et al. Contrast-enhanced magnetic resonance cholangiography with Gd-BOPTA and Gd-EOB-DTPA in healthy subjects. *Acta Radiol* 48(4): 362–368, 2007.

32. Demas BE, Hricak H, Moseley M et al. Gallbladder bile: an experimental study in dogs using MR imaging and proton MR spectroscopy. *Radiology* 157(2): 453–455, 1985.

33. Macaulay SE, Schulte SJ, Sekijima JH et al. Evaluation of a non-breath-hold MR cholangiography technique. *Radiology* 196(1): 227–232, 1995.

34. Limanond P, Raman SS, Ghobrial RM et al. The utility of MRCP in preoperative mapping of biliary anatomy in adult-to-adult living related liver transplant donors. *J Magn Reson Imaging* 19(2): 209–215, 2004.

35. Strasberg SM, Hertl M, Soper NJ. An analysis of the problem of biliary injury during laparoscopic cholecystectomy. *J Am Coll Surg* 180(1): 101–125, 1995.

36. Hirao K, Miyazaki A, Fujimoto T et al. Evaluation of aberrant bile ducts before laparoscopic cholecystectomy: helical CT cholangiography versus MR cholangiography. *AJR Am J Roentgenol* 175(3): 713–720, 2000.

37. Soper NJ, Brunt LM. The case for routine operative cholangiography during laparoscopic cholecystectomy. *Surg Clin North Am* 74(4): 953–959, 1994.

38. Sterling JA. The common channel for bile and pancreatic ducts. *Surg Gynecol Obstet* 98(4): 420–424, 1954.

39. David V, Reinhold C, Hochman M et al. Pitfalls in the interpretation of MR cholangiopancreatography. *AJR Am J Roentgenol* 170(4): 1055–1059, 1998.

40. Fulcher AS, Turner MA, Ham JM. Late biliary complications in right lobe living donor transplantation recipients: imaging findings and therapeutic interventions. *J Comput Assist Tomogr* 26(3): 422–427, 2002.

41. Moeser PM, Julian S, Karstaedt N et al. Unusual presentation of cholelithiasis on T1-weighted MR imaging. *J Comput Assist Tomogr* 12(1): 150–152, 1988.

42. Baron RL, Shuman WP, Lee SP et al. MR appearance of gallstones in vitro at 1.5 T: correlation with chemical composition. *AJR Am J Roentgenol* 153(3): 497–502, 1989.

43. Dell LA, Brown MS, Orrison WW et al. Physiologic intracranial calcification with hyperintensity on MR imaging: case report and experimental model. *AJNR Am J Neuroradiol* 9(6): 1145–1148, 1988.

44. Bangert BA, Modic MT, Ross JS et al. Hyperintense disks on T1-weighted MR images: correlation with calcification. *Radiology* 195(2): 437–443, 1995.

45. Hakansson K, Leander P, Ekberg O et al. MR imaging in clinically suspected acute cholecystitis. A comparison with ultrasonography. *Acta Radiol* 41(4): 322–328, 2000.

46. Altun E, Semelka RC, Elias J, Jr. et al. Acute cholecystitis: MR findings and differentiation from chronic cholecystitis. *Radiology* 244(1): 174–183, 2007.

47. Loud PA, Semelka RC, Kettritz U et al. MRI of acute cholecystitis: comparison with the normal gallbladder and other entities. *Magn Reson Imaging* 14(4): 349–355, 1996.

48. Semelka RC, Shoenut JP, Micflikier AB et al. The gallbladder and biliary tree. In: Semelka RC, Shoenut JP, editors. *MRI of the Abdomen with CT correlation.* New York: Raven Press, 1993, pp. 43–52.

49. Kelekis NL, Semelka RC. MR imaging of the gallbladder. *Top Magn Reson Imaging* 8(5): 312–320, 1996.

50. Chun KA, Ha HK, Yu ES et al. Xanthogranulomatous cholecystitis: CT features with emphasis on differentiation from gallbladder carcinoma. *Radiology* 203(1): 93–97, 1997.

51. Furuta A, Ishibashi T, Takahashi S et al. MR imaging of xanthogranulomatous cholecystitis. *Radiat Med* 14(6): 315–319, 1996.

52. Roa I, Araya JC, Villaseca M et al. Preneoplastic lesions and gallbladder cancer: an estimate of the period required for progression. *Gastroenterology* 111(1): 232–236, 1996.

53. Chijiiwa K, Tanaka M. Polypoid lesion of the gallbladder: indications of carcinoma and outcome after surgery for malignant polypoid lesion. *Int Surg* 79(2): 106–109, 1994.

54. Kubota K, Bandai Y, Noie T et al. How should polypoid lesions of the gallbladder be treated in the era of laparoscopic cholecystectomy? *Surgery* 117(5): 481–487, 1995.

55. Yoshimitsu K, Honda H, Jimi M et al. MR diagnosis of adenomyomatosis of the gallbladder and differentiation from gallbladder carcinoma: importance of showing Rokitansky-Aschoff sinuses. *AJR Am J Roentgenol* 172(6): 1535–1540, 1999.

56. Haradome H, Ichikawa T, Sou H et al. The pearl necklace sign: an imaging sign of adenomyomatosis of the gallbladder at MR cholangiopancreatography. *Radiology* 227(1): 80–88, 2003.

57. Kim MJ, Oh YT, Park YN et al. Gallbladder adenomyomatosis: findings on MRI. *Abdom Imaging* 24(4): 410–413, 1999.

58. Rooholamini SA, Tehrani NS, Razavi MK et al. Imaging of gallbladder carcinoma. *Radiographics* 14(2): 291–306, 1994.

59. Towfigh S, McFadden DW, Cortina GR et al. Porcelain gallbladder is not associated with gallbladder carcinoma. *Am Surg* 67(1): 7–10, 2001.

60. Roa I, Araya JC, Villaseca M et al. Gallbladder cancer in a high risk area: morphological features and spread patterns. *Hepatogastroenterology* 46(27): 1540–1546, 1999.

61. Schwartz LH, Black J, Fong Y et al. Gallbladder carcinoma: findings at MR imaging with MR cholangiopancreatography. *J Comput Assist Tomogr* 26(3): 405–410, 2002.

62. Sagoh T, Itoh K, Togashi K et al. Gallbladder carcinoma: evaluation with MR imaging. *Radiology* 174(1): 131–136, 1990.

63. Rossmann MD, Friedman AC, Radecki PD et al. MR imaging of gallbladder carcinoma. *AJR Am J Roentgenol* 148(1): 143–144, 1987.

64. Demachi H, Matsui O, Hoshiba K et al. Dynamic MRI using a surface coil in chronic cholecystitis and gallbladder carcinoma: radiologic and histopathologic correlation. *J Comput Assist Tomogr* 21(4): 643–651, 1997.

65. Czako L, Takacs T, Morvay Z et al. Diagnostic role of secretin-enhanced MRCP in patients with unsuccessful ERCP. *World J Gastroenterol* 10(20): 3034–3038, 2004.

66. Khalid TR, Casillas VJ, Montalvo BM et al. Using MR cholangiopancreatography to evaluate iatrogenic bile duct injury. *AJR Am J Roentgenol* 177(6): 1347–1352, 2001.

67. Pasanen P, Partanen K, Pikkarainen P et al. Ultrasonography, CT, and ERCP in the diagnosis of choledochal stones. *Acta Radiol* 33(1): 53–56, 1992.

68. O'Connor HJ, Hamilton I, Ellis WR et al. Ultrasound detection of choledocholithiasis: prospective comparison with ERCP in the postcholecystectomy patient. *Gastrointest Radiol* 11(2): 161–164, 1986.

69. Cronan JJ. US diagnosis of choledocholithiasis: a reappraisal. *Radiology* 161(1): 133–134, 1986.

70. Stott MA, Farrands PA, Guyer PB et al. Ultrasound of the common bile duct in patients undergoing cholecystectomy. *J Clin Ultrasound* 19(2): 73–76, 1991.

71. Cotton PB, Lehman G, Vennes J et al. Endoscopic sphincterotomy complications and their management: an attempt at consensus. *Gastrointest Endosc* 37(3): 383–393, 1991.

72. Halme L, Doepel M, von Numers H et al. Complications of diagnostic and therapeutic ERCP. *Ann Chir Gynaecol* 88(2): 127–131, 1999.

73. Mehta SN, Pavone E, Barkun AN. Outpatient therapeutic ERCP: a series of 262 consecutive cases. *Gastrointest Endosc* 44(4): 443–449, 1996.

74. Duncan HD, Hodgkinson L, Deakin M et al. The safety of diagnostic and therapeutic ERCP as a daycase procedure with a selective admission policy. *Eur J Gastroenterol Hepatol* 9(9): 905–908, 1997.

75. Loperfido S, Angelini G, Benedetti G et al. Major early complications from diagnostic and therapeutic ERCP: a prospective multicenter study. *Gastrointest Endosc* 48(1): 1–10, 1998.

76. NIH. State-of-the-science statement on endoscopic retrograde cholangiopancreatography (ERCP) for diagnosis and therapy. *NIH Consens State Sci Statements* 19(1): 1–26, 2002.

77. Tang Y, Yamashita Y, Arakawa A et al. Pancreaticobiliary ductal system: value of half-Fourier rapid acquisition with relaxation enhancement MR cholangiopancreatography for postoperative evaluation. *Radiology* 215(1): 81–88, 2000.

78. Topal B, Van de Moortel M, Fieuws S et al. The value of magnetic resonance cholangiopancreatography in predicting common bile duct stones in patients with gallstone disease. *Br J Surg* 90(1): 42–47, 2003.

79. Kim TK, Kim BS, Kim JH et al. Diagnosis of intrahepatic stones: superiority of MR cholangiopancreatography over endoscopic retrograde cholangiopancreatography. *AJR Am J Roentgenol* 179(2): 429–434, 2002.

80. Soto JA, Barish MA, Alvarez O et al. Detection of choledocholithiasis with MR cholangiography: comparison of three-dimensional fast spin-echo and single- and multisection half-Fourier rapid acquisition with relaxation enhancement sequences. *Radiology* 215(3): 737–745, 2000.

81. Sugita R, Sugimura E, Itoh M et al. Pseudolesion of the bile duct caused by flow effect: a diagnostic pitfall of MR cholangiopancreatography. *AJR Am J Roentgenol* 180(2): 467–471, 2003.

82. Irie H, Honda H, Kuroiwa T et al. Pitfalls in MR cholangiopancreatographic interpretation. *Radiographics* 21(1): 23–37, 2001.

83. Shaikh F, Elazzazi M, Ryan A, Semelka RC. Debris-filled biliary system: a difficult diagnosis on MRI and MRCP. *Magn Reson Imaging* 2009, Submitted.

84. Takehara Y. Fast MR imaging for evaluating the pancreaticobiliary system. *Eur J Radiol* 29(3): 211–232, 1999.

85. Kim JH, Kim MJ, Park SI et al. Using kinematic MR cholangiopancreatography to evaluate biliary dilatation. *AJR Am J Roentgenol* 178(4): 909–914, 2002.

86. Mariani A, Curioni S, Zanello A et al. Secretin MRCP and endoscopic pancreatic manometry in the evaluation of sphincter of Oddi function: a comparative pilot study in patients with idiopathic recurrent pancreatitis. *Gastrointest Endosc* 58(6): 847–852, 2003.

87. Hosoki T, Hasuike Y, Takeda Y et al. Visualization of pancreati-cobiliary reflux in anomalous pancreaticobiliary junction by secretin-stimulated dynamic magnetic resonance cholangiopan-creatography. *Acta Radiol* 45(4): 375–382, 2004.

88. Matos C, Metens T, Deviere J et al. Pancreatic duct: morphologic and functional evaluation with dynamic MR pancreatography after secretin stimulation. *Radiology* 203(2): 435–441, 1997.

89. Sherlock S. Pathogenesis of sclerosing cholangitis: the role of nonimmune factors. *Semin Liver Dis* 11(1): 5–10, 1991.

90. Textor HJ, Flacke S, Pauleit D et al. Three-dimensional magnetic resonance cholangiopancreatography with respiratory triggering in the diagnosis of primary sclerosing cholangitis: comparison with endoscopic retrograde cholangiography. *Endoscopy* 34(12): 984–990, 2002.

91. Beuers U, Spengler U, Sackmann M et al. Deterioration of cho-lestasis after endoscopic retrograde cholangiography in advanced primary sclerosing cholangitis. *J Hepatol* 15(1-2): 140–143, 1992.

92. Ernst O, Asselah T, Sergent G et al. MR cholangiography in primary sclerosing cholangitis. *AJR Am J Roentgenol* 171(4): 1027–1030, 1998.

93. Fulcher AS, Turner MA, Franklin KJ et al. Primary sclerosing cholangitis: evaluation with MR cholangiography—a case-control study. *Radiology* 215(1): 71–80, 2000.

94. Bader TR, Beavers KL, Semelka RC. MR imaging features of primary sclerosing cholangitis: patterns of cirrhosis in relationship to clinical severity of disease. *Radiology* 226(3): 675–685, 2003.

95. Semelka RC, Shoenut JP, Kroeker MA et al. Bile duct disease: prospective comparison of ERCP, CT, and fat suppression MRI. *Gastrointest Radiol* 17(4): 347–352, 1992.

96. Revelon G, Rashid A, Kawamoto S et al. Primary sclerosing cholangitis: MR imaging findings with pathologic correlation. *AJR Am J Roentgenol* 173(4): 1037–1042, 1999.

97. Ito K, Mitchell DG, Outwater EK et al. Primary sclerosing chol-angitis: MR imaging features. *AJR Am J Roentgenol* 172(6): 1527–1533, 1999.

98. LaRusso NF, Wiesner RH, Ludwig J et al. Current concepts. Primary sclerosing cholangitis. *N Engl J Med* 310(14): 899–903, 1984.

99. Balthazar EJ, Birnbaum BA, Naidich M. Acute cholangitis: CT evaluation. *J Comput Assist Tomogr* 17(2): 283–289, 1993.

100. Bader TR, Braga L, Beavers KL et al. MR imaging findings of infectious cholangitis. *Magn Reson Imaging* 19(6): 781–788, 2001.

101. Kim MJ, Cha SW, Mitchell DG et al. MR imaging findings in recurrent pyogenic cholangitis. *AJR Am J Roentgenol* 173(6): 1545–1549, 1999.

102. Miller FH, Gore RM, Nemcek AA, Jr. et al. Pancreaticobiliary manifestations of AIDS. *AJR Am J Roentgenol* 166(6): 1269–1274, 1996.

103. Matos C, Nicaise N, Deviere J et al. Choledochal cysts: compari-son of findings at MR cholangiopancreatography and endoscopic retrograde cholangiopancreatography in eight patients. *Radiology* 209(2): 443–448, 1998.

104. Todani T, Watanabe Y, Narusue M et al. Congenital bile duct cysts: classification, operative procedures, and review of thirty-seven cases including cancer arising from choledochal cyst. *Am J Surg* 134(2): 263–269, 1977.

105. Pavone P, Laghi A, Catalano C et al. Caroli's disease: evaluation with MR cholangiopancreatography (MRCP). *Abdom Imaging* 21(2): 117–119, 1996.

106. Lillemoe KD, Pitt HA, Cameron JL. Current management of benign bile duct strictures. *Adv Surg* 25: 119–174, 1992.

107. Laghi A, Pavone P, Catalano C et al. MR cholangiography of late biliary complications after liver transplantation. *AJR Am J Roentgenol* 172(6): 1541–1546, 1999.

108. Coakley FV, Schwartz LH, Blumgart LH et al. Complex postcho-lecystectomy biliary disorders: preliminary experience with evaluation by means of breath-hold MR cholangiography. *Radiology* 209(1): 141–146, 1998.

109. Pavone P, Laghi A, Catalano C et al. MR cholangiography in the examination of patients with biliary-enteric anastomoses. *AJR Am J Roentgenol* 169(3): 807–811, 1997.

110. Soyer P, Bluemke DA, Reichle R et al. Imaging of intrahepatic cholangiocarcinoma. 1. Peripheral cholangiocarcinoma. *AJR Am J Roentgenol* 165(6): 1427–1431, 1995.

111. Soyer P, Bluemke DA, Reichle R et al. Imaging of intrahepatic cholangiocarcinoma. 2. Hilar cholangiocarcinoma. *AJR Am J Roentgenol* 165(6): 1433–1436, 1995.

112. Hamrick-Turner J, Abbitt PL, Ros PR. Intrahepatic cholangiocar-cinoma: MR appearance. *AJR Am J Roentgenol* 158(1): 77–79, 1992.

113. Worawattanakul S, Semelka RC, Noone TC et al. Cholangiocarcinoma: spectrum of appearances on MR images using current techniques. *Magn Reson Imaging* 16(9): 993–1003, 1998.

114. Soyer P. Capsular retraction of the liver in malignant tumor of the biliary tract MRI findings. *Clin Imaging* 18(4): 255–257, 1994.

115. Fulcher AS, Turner MA. HASTE MR cholangiography in the evaluation of hilar cholangiocarcinoma. *AJR Am J Roentgenol* 169(6): 1501–1505, 1997.

116. Yamaguchi K, Enjoji M. Carcinoma of the ampulla of Vater. A clinicopathologic study and pathologic staging of 109 cases of carcinoma and 5 cases of adenoma. *Cancer* 59(3): 506–515, 1987.

117. Irie H, Honda H, Shinozaki K et al. MR imaging of ampullary carcinomas. *J Comput Assist Tomogr* 26(5): 711–717, 2002.

118. Semelka RC, Kelekis NL, John G et al. Ampullary carcinoma: demonstration by current MR techniques. *J Magn Reson Imaging* 7(1): 153–156, 1997.

119. Pavone P, Laghi A, Passariello R. MR cholangiopancreatography in malignant biliary obstruction. *Semin Ultrasound CT MR* 20(5): 317–323, 1999.

PANCREAS

ERSAN ALTUN, JORGE ELIAS, JR., DIANE ARMAO,
BUSAKORN VACHIRANUBHAP, AND RICHARD C. SEMELKA

When health is absent, wisdom cannot reveal itself, art cannot manifest, strength cannot fight, wealth becomes useless, and intelligence cannot be applied.
> Herophilus, Greek anatomist, credited
> with the discovery of the pancreas, meaning
> "all flesh," in 336 B.C.

NORMAL ANATOMY

The pancreas is a soft, fleshy, lobulated gland retroperitoneally located against the posterior body wall. The anatomic divisions of the pancreas include the head, uncinate process, neck, body, and tail. The broad head is embraced by the curve of the duodenum. An extension of the head, the uncinate process hooks behind the superior mesenteric artery and vein. The border between the head and body is a slightly narrowed region, the neck. On the posterior aspect of the neck is a shallow groove marking the passage of the superior mesenteric vein and the beginning of the portal vein. The body is oriented in an oblique fashion extending to the right of midline, and the tail is located in the region of the splenic hilum. The anatomic relationship

of the head of the pancreas includes the second portion of the duodenum laterally, the gastroduodenal artery anteriorly, the inferior vena cava posterolaterally, the third portion of the duodenum posteroinferiorly, and the superior mesenteric vessels medially.

The splenic vein lies along the posterior surface of the body and tail of the pancreas. This constant relationship is an important landmark for the identification of the pancreatic body. The left adrenal gland is seated posterior to the splenic vein. The tail of the pancreas often drapes over the left kidney and terminates in the splenic hilum. The tail may be folded anteriorly over the body of the pancreas. The stomach lies anterior to the pancreas and is separated from it by parietal peritoneum and the lesser sac. The transverse mesocolon forms the inferior boundary of the lesser sac and is formed by the fusion of leaves of the parietal peritoneum, which covers the anterior surface of the pancreas. The lesser sac and transverse mesocolon are common pathways for the tracking and accumulation of fluid in acute pancreatitis.

In elderly patients, fatty replacement of the pancreas occurs frequently as a normal degenerative process

Abdominal-Pelvic MRI, Third Edition, edited by Richard C. Semelka. Copyright © 2010 John Wiley & Sons, Inc.

and results in a feathery, lobulated appearance on imaging. The posterior aspect of the pancreas does not have a serosal covering, which accounts for the extensive dissemination of fluid in pancreatitis and the early spread of pancreatic ductal cancer into retroperitoneal fat.

The pancreatic duct measures 1–2 mm in diameter in normal subjects. Although considerable variation in the size of the head occurs, the normal pancreatic head is 2–2.5 cm in diameter, with the remainder of the gland approximately 1–2 cm thick. The main pancreatic duct extends from the tail of the pancreas through the head and empties via the sphincter of Oddi into the second part of the duodenum at the major papilla. The main duct is termed the duct of Wirsung. A smaller accessory duct, the duct of Santorini, is frequently present, extends from the body of the pancreas through the neck, and enters separately into the duodenum in a more proximal location at the minor papilla.

The pancreas is a mixed exocrine and endocrine gland. The main mass of pancreatic microstructure is exocrine in nature, composed of acinar cells, which store and release digestive enzymes. Embedded in acinar tissue are small, scattered islets of Langerhans composed of endocrine cells, which synthesize hormones. The major hormones released by the pancreas are insulin and glucagon.

MRI TECHNIQUE

New MRI techniques that limit artifacts in the abdomen have increased the role of MRI in detection and characterization of pancreatic disease. Breath-hold T1 weighted gradient-echo sequences obtained either as 2D or 3D gradient echo, fat suppression techniques, and dynamic administration of gadolinium chelate have resulted in image quality of the pancreas sufficient to detect and characterize focal pancreatic mass lesions smaller than 1 cm in diameter, and to evaluate diffuse pancreatic disease [1–4]. The use of high spatial resolution MR imaging at 3.0 T improves the detection of small focal lesions particularly.

MR cholangiopancreatography (MRCP) permits good demonstration of the biliary and pancreatic ducts to assess ductal obstruction, dilatation, and abnormal duct pathways [5–7]. The combination of tissue-imaging sequences and MRCP provides comprehensive information to evaluate the full range of pancreatic disease.

MRI of the pancreas is optimal at high field (1.5 T or 3.0 T) because of a good signal-to-noise (S/N) ratio, which facilitates breath-hold imaging, and increased fat-water frequency shift, which facilitates chemically selective excitation-spoiling fat suppression or water

excitation. T1-weighted chemically selective fat suppression and T1-weighted breath-hold gradient echo are effective techniques for imaging pancreatic parenchyma. The highest image quality of the pancreas is achieved with imaging at 3.0 T [8]. The combination of higher signal to noise ratio, greater spectral separation, and increased sensitivity to gadolinium results in the acquisition of images with high quality, and high spatial and temporal resolution. Particularly, the image quality of postgadolinium sequences is superb at 3.0 T. This allows for improved detection and characterization of very small lesions [8]. The normal pancreas is high in signal intensity on T1-weighted fat-suppressed images because of the presence of aqueous protein in the acini of the pancreas [1]. Normal pancreas is well shown with this technique (fig. 4.1) [9, 10]. In elderly patients, the signal intensity of the pancreas may diminish and be lower than that of liver [2]. This may reflect changes of fibrosis secondary to the aging process.

Our standard MR protocol includes T1-weighted fat-suppressed gradient-echo and postgadolinium imaging in the capillary phase (immediate postcontrast, hepatic arterial dominant phase) and interstitial phase (1–10 min postcontrast) [4]. There may be advantages in performing postgadolinium gradient-echo imaging as a 3D gradient-echo technique for the following reasons: a) thinner sections can be obtained (3 mm vs. 5 mm for 2D-SGE) and b) the absence of mirror artifact from the aorta, which is problematic on 2D-SGE. T2-weighted echo-train spin-echo sequences such as T2-weighted half-Fourier acquisition snapshot turbo spin-echo (HASTE) provide a sharp anatomic display of the common bile duct (CBD) on coronal plane images and of the pancreatic duct on transverse plane images. MRCP images can be acquired oriented in the plane of the pancreatic duct, in an oblique coronal projection, to delineate longer segments of the pancreatic duct in continuity [11]. T2-weighted fat-suppressed images are useful for demonstrating liver metastases and islet cell tumors. T2-weighted images also provide information on the complexity of the fluid in pancreatic pseudocysts, which may reflect the presence of complications such as necrotic debris or infection. Regarding gadolinium enhancement, the pancreas demonstrates a uniform capillary blush on immediate postcontrast images, which renders it markedly higher in signal intensity than liver, neighboring bowel, and adjacent fat (fig. 4.2) [4]. By 1 min after contrast the pancreas shows approximately isointense signal with fat on non-fat-suppressed T1-weighted SGE, and moderately higher signal than background fat on fat-suppressed SGE or 3D-GE sequences (see fig. 4.1). Pancreatic head is readily distinguished from duodenum or adjacent bowel on immediate post-gadolinium images

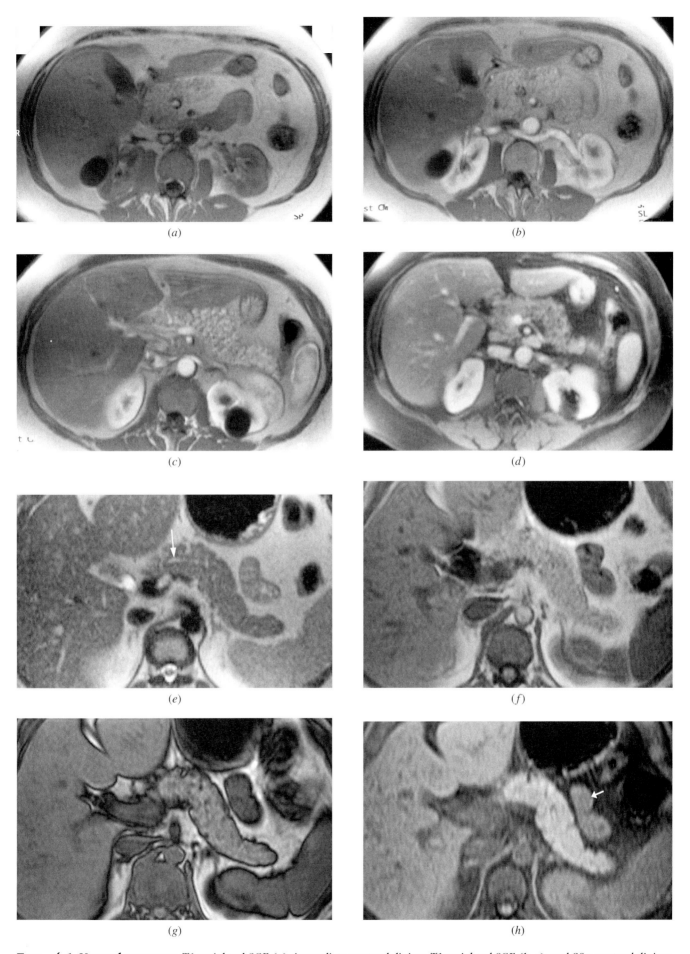

F I G . 4.1 Normal pancreas. T1-weighted SGE (*a*), immediate postgadolinium T1-weighted SGE (*b, c*), and 90-s postgadolinium fat-suppressed SGE (*d*) images. The pancreas has a marbled appearance, which is a normal finding associated with aging.

T2-weighted SS-ETSE (*e*), in-phase (*f*) and out-of-phase (*g*) T1-weighted gradient-echo, fat-suppressed T1-weighted gradient-echo (*h*),

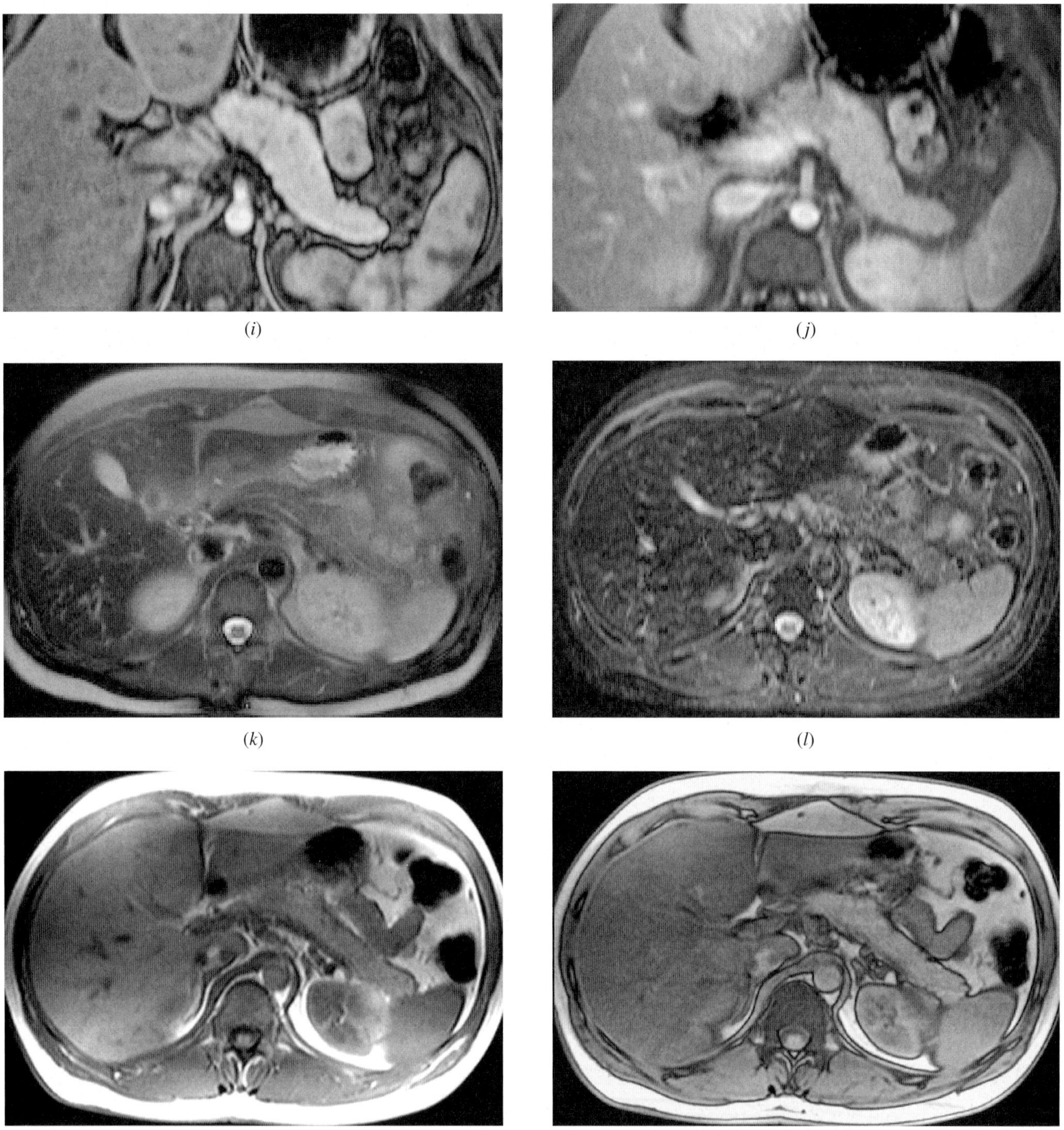

(*i*) (*j*)

(*k*) (*l*)

(*m*) (*n*)

FIG. 4.1 (*Continued*) and immediate (*i*) and interstitial-phase (*j*) postgadolinium fat-suppressed T1-weighted gradient-echo images of pancreatic body and tail in a second patient. The normal pancreas is high in signal intensity on T1-weighted fat-suppressed image (*h*) because of the presence of aqueous protein in the acini of the pancreas. A uniform capillary blush is apparent on the immediate postgadolinium image (*i*). Small bowel is moderate in signal intensity on T1-weighted fat-suppressed image (arrow, *h*), which is clearly different from the homogeneous or marbled high signal intensity of the pancreas. The normal-caliber pancreatic duct is well shown (arrow, *e*) on T2-weighted image.

T2-weighted single-shot echo-train spin-echo (*k*), T2-weighted short-tau inversion recovery (*l*), T1-weighted in-phase (*m*) and out-of-phase (*n*) SGE, T1-weighted fat-suppressed SGE (*o*), and T1-weighted postgadolinium hepatic arterial dominant phase (*p*) and

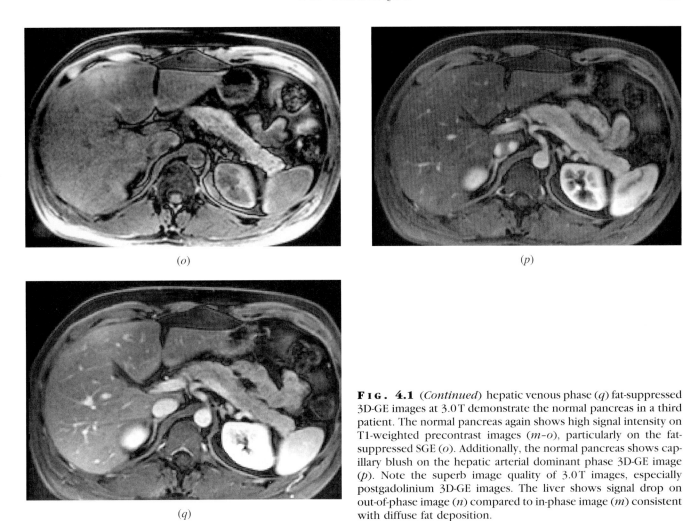

(o)

(p)

(q)

F IG. 4.1 (*Continued*) hepatic venous phase (*q*) fat-suppressed 3D-GE images at 3.0 T demonstrate the normal pancreas in a third patient. The normal pancreas again shows high signal intensity on T1-weighted precontrast images (*m–o*), particularly on the fat-suppressed SGE (*o*). Additionally, the normal pancreas shows capillary blush on the hepatic arterial dominant phase 3D-GE image (*p*). Note the superb image quality of 3.0 T images, especially postgadolinium 3D-GE images. The liver shows signal drop on out-of-phase image (*n*) compared to in-phase image (*m*) consistent with diffuse fat deposition.

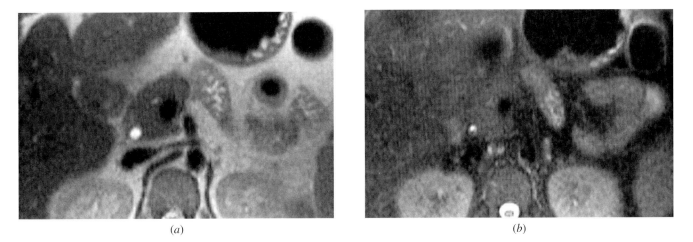

(a)

(b)

F IG. 4.2 Normal head of the pancreas. T2-weighted SS-ETSE (*a*), fat-suppressed T2-weighted SS-ETSE (*b*), fat-suppressed

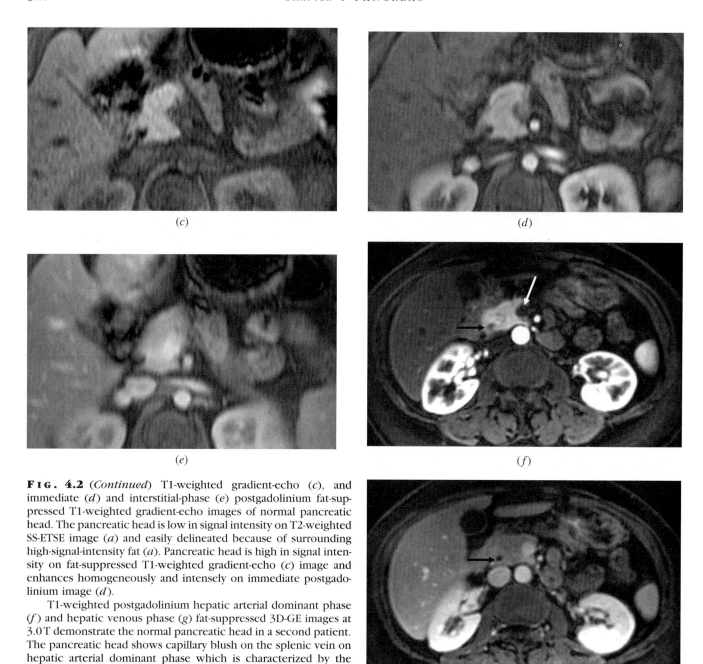

FIG. 4.2 (*Continued*) T1-weighted gradient-echo (*c*), and immediate (*d*) and interstitial-phase (*e*) postgadolinium fat-suppressed T1-weighted gradient-echo images of normal pancreatic head. The pancreatic head is low in signal intensity on T2-weighted SS-ETSE image (*a*) and easily delineated because of surrounding high-signal-intensity fat (*a*). Pancreatic head is high in signal intensity on fat-suppressed T1-weighted gradient-echo (*c*) image and enhances homogeneously and intensely on immediate postgadolinium image (*d*).

T1-weighted postgadolinium hepatic arterial dominant phase (*f*) and hepatic venous phase (*g*) fat-suppressed 3D-GE images at 3.0 T demonstrate the normal pancreatic head in a second patient. The pancreatic head shows capillary blush on the splenic vein on hepatic arterial dominant phase which is characterized by the presence of contrast in the portal and splenic vein but not in the superior mesenteric vein (white arrow, *f*). Additionally, the normal common bile duct (black arrow, *f*, *g*) is very well seen on both images.

because the pancreas enhances substantially greater than bowel (see fig. 4.1 and fig. 4.2). MRI combining T1, T2, early and late postgadolinium images, MRCP, and MRA generates comprehensive information on the pancreas [12].

Recognition of the characteristic high signal intensity of normal pancreas on precontrast T1-weighted fat-suppressed and immediate postgadolinium images is useful in circumstances of abnormalities of position. After left nephrectomy, the tail of the pancreas falls into the renal fossa, which can simulate recurrent disease on CT examination. Normal pancreas can be readily distinguished by its high signal intensity (fig. 4.3).

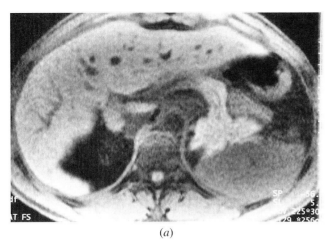

(a)

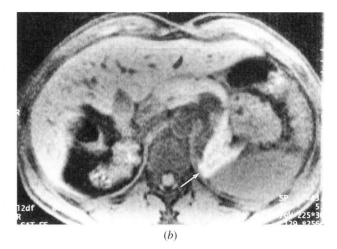

(b)

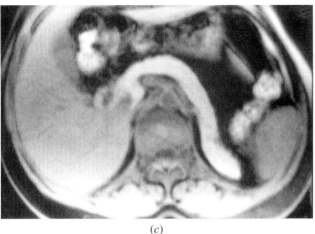

(c)

F I G . 4.3 Pancreatic tail seated in the left renal fossa after left nephrectomy. T1-weighted fat-suppressed SGE images (*a, b*) demonstrate normal high-signal-intensity pancreas situated in the left renal fossa (arrow, *b*).

T1-weighted fat-suppressed SGE image (*c*) in a second patient who underwent a bilateral nephrectomy shows the pancreatic tail seated posteriorly, filling the space in the renal fossa.

DEVELOPMENTAL ANOMALIES

Pancreas Divisum

Pancreas divisum is the most clinically important and common major anatomic variant. Although a misleading term, pancreas divisum is, by definition, a superficially normal-appearing pancreas in which no communication has developed between the duct of the dorsally derived pancreas and the duct of the embryonic ventral pancreas, which normally forms most of the main pancreatic duct [13]. The result of this congenital abnormality is that portions of the pancreas have separate ductal systems: A very short ventral duct of Wirsung drains only the lower portion of the head, whereas the dorsal duct of Santorini drains the tail, body, neck and upper aspect of the head. The incidence of this anomaly varies between 1.3 to 6.7% of the population [14]. One study described 108 patients who underwent both endoscopic retrograde cholangiopancreatography (ERCP) and MRCP and reported exact correlation between these modalities for the detection and exclusion of pancreas divisum [6]. On MRCP images, separate entries of the ducts of Santorini

and Wirsung into the duodenum are consistently demonstrated because of the good conspicuity of the linear high-signal-intensity tubular structures (fig. 4.4). Variations in pancreas divisum are also shown, which include the dominant dorsal duct syndrome (see fig. 4.4).

Pancreas divisum has been reported to be a predisposing factor in recurrent pancreatitis [15, 16]. It is postulated that in some subjects the disproportion between the small caliber of the minor papilla and the large amount of secretion from the dorsal part of the gland leads to a relative outflow obstruction from the dorsal pancreas, resulting in pain or pancreatitis [17]. Compared with patients with pancreatitis and normal duct anatomy, the pancreas in pancreas divisum may appear normal in signal intensity on T1-weighted fat-suppressed images and immediate postgadolinium gradient echo-images because the attacks of recurrent pancreatitis tend to be less severe and changes of chronic pancreatitis may not develop.

Annular Pancreas

Annular pancreas is an uncommon congenital anomaly in which glandular pancreatic tissue, in continuity with

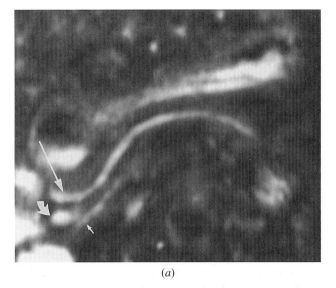

(a)

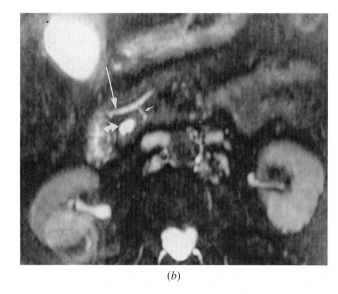

(b)

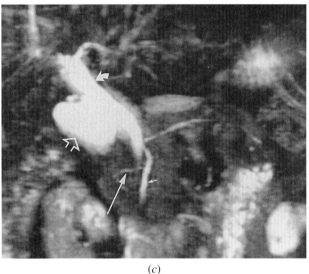

(c)

FIG. 4.4 Pancreas divisum. MRCP image (*a*) formatted in an oblique transverse plane demonstrates separate entry of the ducts of Santorini (long arrow, *a*) and Wirsung (short arrow, *a*) into the duodenum with no communication between the ductal systems. MRCP image (*b*) in a second patient with dominant dorsal duct syndrome shows a large duct of Santorini (long arrow, *b*) and a small communication with a diminutive duct of Wirsung (short arrow, *b*). The common bile duct (curved arrow, *a*, *b*) is identified between the ducts of Santorini and Wirsung. Oblique coronal MRCP (*c*) in a patient with normal ductal anatomy shows a small duct of Santorini (long arrow, *c*) and a larger duct of Wirsung (short arrow, *c*). The common bile duct (curved arrow, *c*) and gallbladder (open arrow, *c*) are also shown. MR pancreatography has the advantage of being a noninvasive diagnostic method for pancreas divisum. (Courtesy of Caroline Reinhold, M.D., Dept. of Radiology, McGill University.)

the head of the pancreas, encircles the duodenum. In most cases, the annular portion surrounds the second part of the duodenum. Patients may present with duodenal obstruction. On MR images, pancreatic tissue is identified encasing the duodenum. Noncontrast T1-weighted fat-suppressed and/or immediate postgadolinium gradient-echo images are particularly effective at demonstrating this entity because of the high signal intensity of pancreatic tissue, which is readily distinguished from the lower signal intensity of adjacent tissue and duodenum (fig. 4.5) [18].

Congenital Absence of the Dorsal Pancreatic Anlage

Congenital absence of the dorsal pancreatic anlage is a very rare anomaly. This abnormality predisposes to recurrent attacks of pancreatitis with eventual exocrine and endocrine pancreatic failure [13]. The head of the pancreas terminates with a rounded contour (fig. 4.6), unlike surgical or posttraumatic absence of the distal pancreas, which has more squared-off or irregular terminations.

Uneven Fatty Infiltration of the Pancreas

Variation in fat content between the posterior head of pancreas and the anterior head through tail of pancreas may be observed. The underlying mechanism likely reflects the differing embryological origin of these portions of the pancreas. The importance of recognizing this condition is that it may simulate a mass lesion (fig. 4.6). MRI is superior to CT in correctly diagnosing this entity.

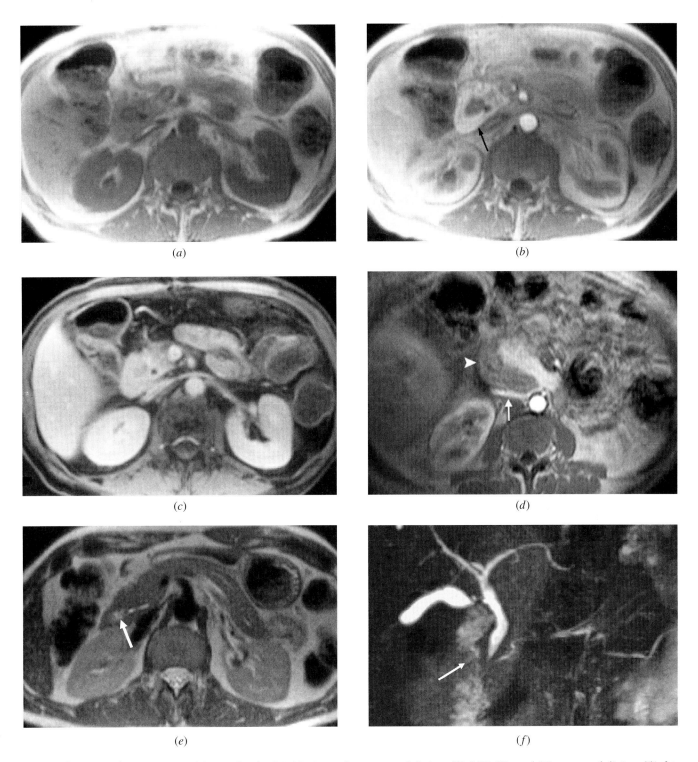

FIG. 4.5 Annular pancreas. T1-weighted SGE (*a*), immediate postgadolinium T1 SGE (*b*), and 90-s postgadolinium T1 fat-suppressed SGE (*c*) images. Normal pancreatic parenchyma (arrow, *b*) surrounds the second portion of the duodenum, diagnostic for annular pancreas. This is best shown on noncontrast T1-weighted fat-suppressed and immediate postgadolinium (*b*) images.

Immediate postgadolinium T1-weighted gradient-echo image (*d*) in a second patient demonstrates that the pancreatic head partially encircles the duodenum (arrowhead, *d*), suggestive of a variant of annular pancreas (arrow, *d*).

T2-weighted single-shot echo-train spin-echo (*e*), reconstructed MRCP image (*f*), T1-weighted fat-suppressed SGE (*g*), and T1-weighted postgadolinium hepatic arterial dominant phase SGE (*h*) images demonstrate an annular pancreas in another patient.

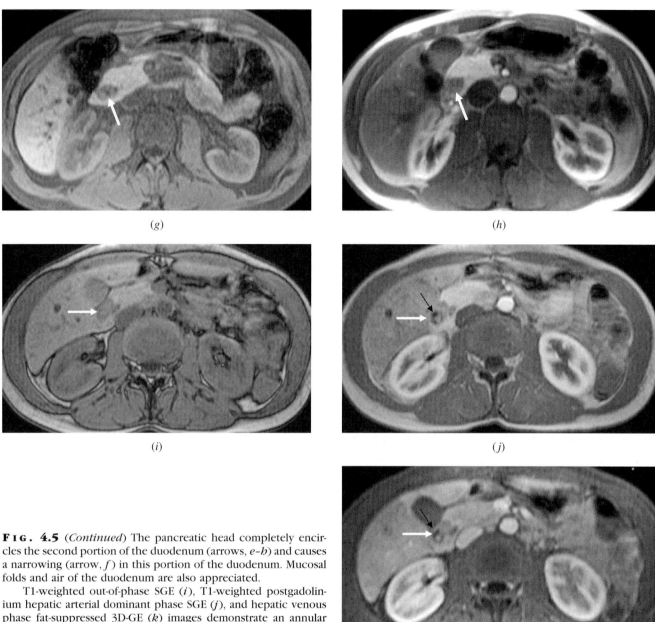

(g)

(h)

(i)

(j)

(k)

FIG. 4.5 (*Continued*) The pancreatic head completely encircles the second portion of the duodenum (arrows, *e–h*) and causes a narrowing (arrow, *f*) in this portion of the duodenum. Mucosal folds and air of the duodenum are also appreciated.

T1-weighted out-of-phase SGE (*i*), T1-weighted postgadolinium hepatic arterial dominant phase SGE (*j*), and hepatic venous phase fat-suppressed 3D-GE (*k*) images demonstrate an annular pancreas in another patient. The pancreatic head incompletely encircles the second portion of the duodenum (white arrows, *i–k*). Note the air in the second portion of the duodenum (black arrows, *j*, *k*).

Short Pancreas in the Polysplenia Syndrome

Polysplenia syndrome is a congenital syndrome characterized by multiple, misplaced small spleens characteristic in the right upper quadrant and isomerism (bilateral left-sidedness) [19]. In a study involving adults with polysplenia syndrome discovered incidentally, four of eight patients evaluated with CT showed a short pancreas. The short pancreas may also have an abnormal orientation (fig. 4.7). A possible explanation for the anomaly is disturbance in the blood supply to the pancreas-spleen region during embryonal life [20].

GENETIC DISEASE

Cystic Fibrosis

Cystic fibrosis is the most common lethal genetic disease affecting Caucasians, with an incidence of 1 in 2000 live births. It is an autosomal recessive multisystem disease with an abnormality of the long arm of chromosome 7, and homozygotes express the disease fully. The disease is characterized by a dysfunction of the secretory process of all exocrine glands and reduced mucociliar transport, which results in mucous plugging of the exocrine glands. The diagnosis is made during childhood when the

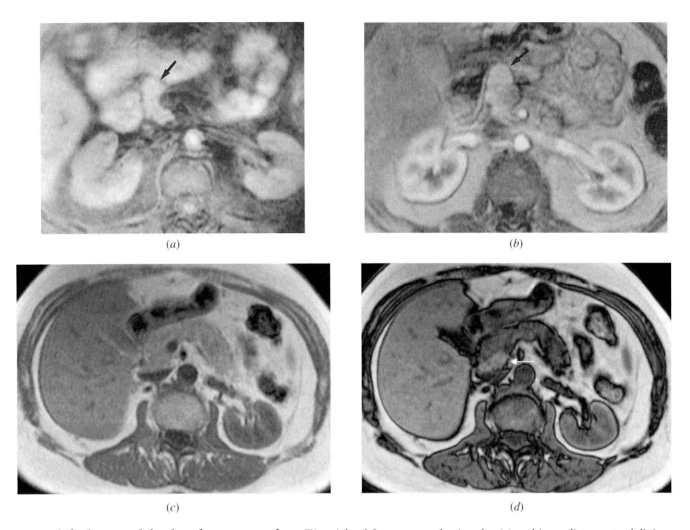

F I G . 4.6 Absence of the dorsal pancreas anlage. T1-weighted fat-suppressed spin-echo (*a*) and immediate postgadolinium T1-weighted SGE (*b*) images. A normal-appearing head of the pancreas is apparent. The pancreas terminates with a rounded contour (arrow, *a*, *b*) at the level of the pancreatic neck.

Uneven fatty infiltration of the pancreas. T1-weighted in-phase (*c*) and out-of-phase (*d*) SGE images demonstrate fatty infiltration of the pancreas with sparing of the posterior portion of the pancreatic head. The anterior portion of the pancreatic head and the pancreatic body shows signal drop on out-of-phase image (*d*), which is consistent with fatty infiltration. The posterior portion of the pancreatic head (arrow, d) does not show signal drop on out-of-phase image (*d*). This can be mistaken for a pancreatic head mass on CT, but the combination of standard and fat attenuated MR images clearly demonstrate that this appearance is due to varying fat content between anatomic regions of the pancreas.

patient has clinical manifestations of recurrent broncho-pulmonary infections leading to chronic lung disease, malabsorption secondary to pancreatic insufficiency, and an increased sweat sodium concentration. MRI has proven to be an effective modality in demonstrating pancreas changes in patients with cystic fibrosis [21–23]. It is superior to ultrasound in showing fatty infiltration and avoids ionizing radiation used in computed tomography. The disadvantage of MRI is that it does not show small calcifications, which are encountered in a small percentage of patients with cystic fibrosis.

Pathologic examination of the pancreas in patients who have survived until early adulthood shows a spectrum of changes involving atrophy and fibrosis of the exocrine pancreas with varying degrees of fatty replace-ment. Three basic imaging patterns of pancreatic abnor-malities have been described: pancreatic enlargement with complete fatty replacement with or without loss of the lobulated contour, atrophic pancreas with partial fatty replacement (fig. 4.8), and diffuse atrophy of the pancreas without fatty replacement [21–23]. Pancreatic enlargement with complete fatty replacement is the most common pattern observed in cystic fibrosis [23]. Fatty replacement is high in signal intensity on T1-weighted images and demonstrates loss of signal intensity on T1-weighted fat-suppressed images (see fig. 4.8). These findings correlate with the pathologic description of mature adipose tissue and isolated foci of Langerhans cell islets in the pancreas of patients with cystic fibrosis.

Another manifestation of cystic fibrosis is pancreatic cysts secondary to duct obstruction by secretion. Pancreatic cystosis is a rare manifestation characterized by large cysts. MRCP is valuable in demonstrating pancreatic duct abnormalities (narrowing, dilatation, stricture, beading).

Primary Hemochromatosis

Primary hemochromatosis is an autosomal recessive heritable disease in which there is excessive accumula-

tion of body iron, most of which is deposited in the parenchyma of various organs. The liver, pancreas, and heart are primarily affected. Iron deposition results in a loss of signal intensity that is more pronounced on T2 or T2*-weighted sequences, but in severe deposition a loss of signal intensity is also apparent on T1-weighted images (fig. 4.9). Iron deposition in primary hemochromatosis is most substantial in the liver. Deposition of iron in the pancreas tends to occur late in the course of disease after liver damage is irreversible [24, 25].

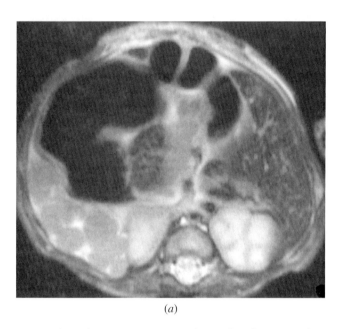
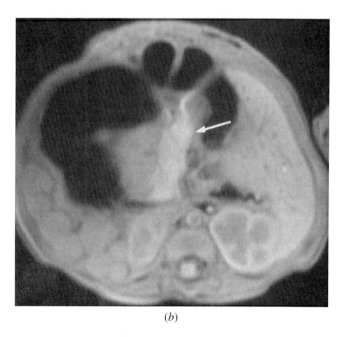

(a)   (b)

F I G . 4.7 Short pancreas in the polysplenia syndrome. T2-weighted fat-suppressed SS-ETSE (a) and T1-weighted fat-suppressed spin-echo (b) images in a 9-wk-old boy with polysplenia syndrome. The pancreas has an abnormal anterior-posterior orientation and appears short (arrow, b), but the parenchyma signal intensity is normal. The most common pancreatic finding in polysplenia syndrome is short pancreas. Note situs inversus and multiple small spleens.

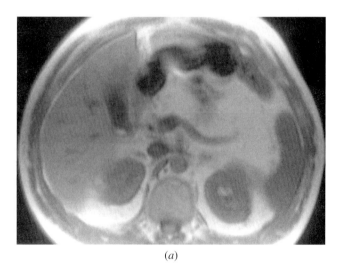
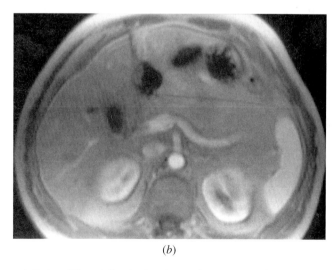

(a)   (b)

F I G . 4.8 Cystic fibrosis. T1-weighted SGE (a), immediate postgadolinium T1-weighted SGE (b), and 90-s postgadolinium T1-weighted fat-suppressed SGE (c) images in a patient with cystic fibrosis. The pancreas is markedly enlarged and hyperintense on

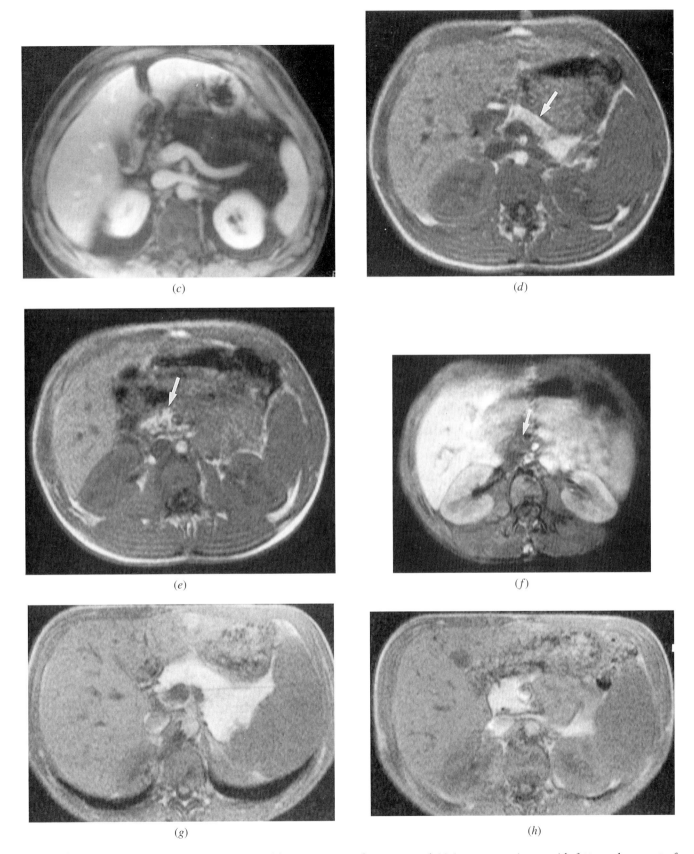

F I G . 4.8 (*Continued*) T1-weighted image and hypointense on fat-suppressed (*c*) images, consistent with fatty replacement of the pancreatic parenchyma by adipose tissue. The complete fatty replacement of the pancreas is the most common manifestation of cystic fibrosis. T1-weighted SGE (*d*, *e*) and T1-weighted fat-suppressed spin-echo (*f*) images in a second patient. The pancreas is atrophic and demonstrates fatty replacement. T1-weighted SGE (*g*, *h*), T1-weighted fat-suppressed spin-echo (*i*, *j*), and gated

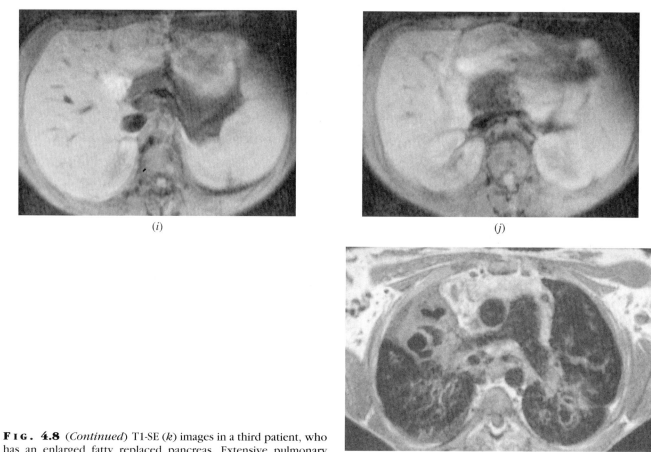

F I G . 4.8 (*Continued*) T1-SE (*k*) images in a third patient, who has an enlarged fatty replaced pancreas. Extensive pulmonary fibrosis is present (*k*).

(*i*)

(*j*)

(*k*)

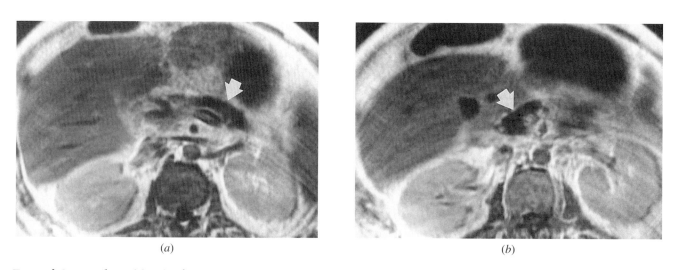

(*a*)

(*b*)

F I G . 4.9 Iron deposition in the pancreas from primary hemochromatosis. T1-weighted SGE (*a*, *b*) images. The pancreas (arrow, *a*, *b*) is signal void on T1-weighted images because of the susceptibility effect of iron. The liver is a transplanted liver and

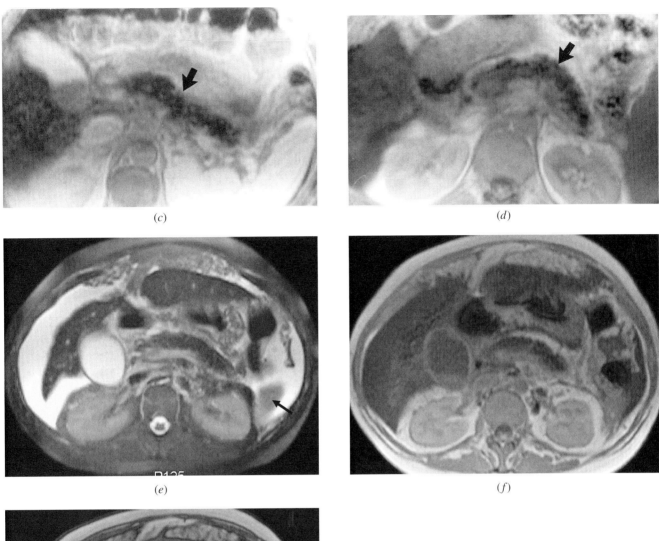

(c)

(d)

(e)

(f)

(g)

F I G . 4.9 (*Continued*) therefore has not sustained iron deposition. Transverse 1-min postgadolinium SGE image (*c*) in a second patient with primary hemochromatosis. Both the pancreas (arrow, *c*) and liver show decreased signal intensity. Gallstones are also present. T1-weighted SGE (*d*) image in a third patient with primary hemochromatosis shows a low-signal pancreas (arrow, *d*). T2-weighted single-shot echo-train spin-echo (*e*) and T1-weighted in-phase (*f*) and out-of-phase (*g*) SGE images demonstrate the deposition of iron in the liver and pancreas but not in the spleen in another patient. The diagnosis, therefore, is consistent with primary hemochromatosis. The liver and pancreas show decreased signal on T2-weighted and T1-weighted in-phase images. The liver and pancreas show signal increase on out-of-phase image compared to in-phase image because of shorter TE. The spleen (arrow, *e*) shows normal signal on all images. Note that the liver is cirrhotic, and there are ascites and omental hypertrophy.

von Hippel–Lindau Syndrome

Von Hippel–Lindau syndrome is an autosomal dominant condition with variable penetration. This condition is characterized by tumors in the cerebellum and retina. Patients may have cysts of the liver and kidney, with a strong propensity to develop renal cell carcinoma. Patients with von Hippel–Lindau syndrome may develop pancreatic cysts, islet cell tumors, or microcystic cystadenoma. In one series, cysts were the most common pancreatic lesions and were present in 19 of 52 patients in whom no other pancreatic lesions were present (fig. 4.10) [26].

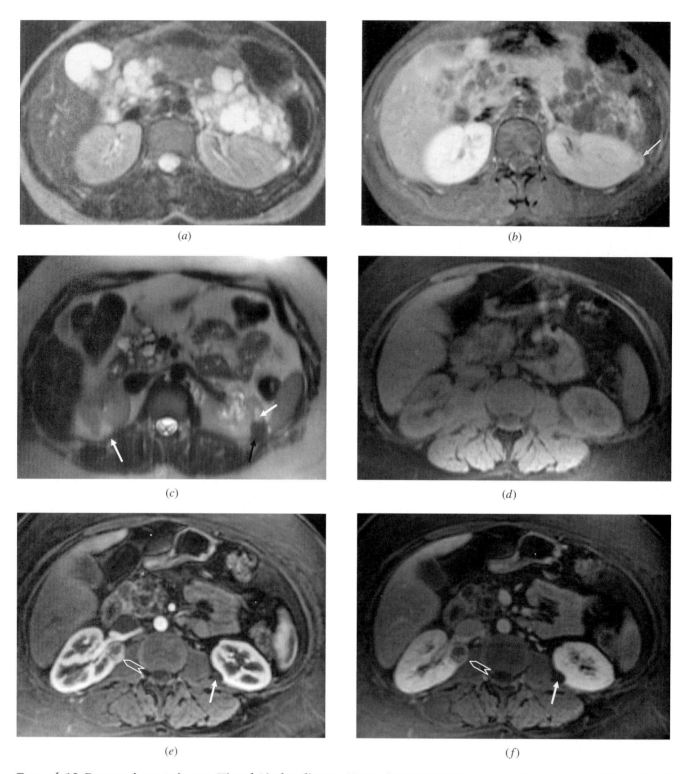

(a)

(b)

(c)

(d)

(e)

(f)

FIG. 4.10 Pancreatic cysts in von Hippel–Lindau disease. T2-weighted SS-ETSE (*a*) and gadolinium-enhanced T1-weighted fat-suppressed spin-echo (*b*) images. Multiple pancreatic cysts are scattered throughout the pancreas, which are high in signal intensity on T2-weighted images (*a*) and low in signal intensity on gadolinium-enhanced images (*b*). Thick septations are present between many of the clustered cysts. A small renal cancer is identified in the left kidney (arrow, *b*).

T2-weighted single-shot echo-train spin-echo (*c*), T1-weighted fat-suppressed SGE (*d*), T1-weighted postgadolinium true late hepatic arterial phase (*e*), and hepatic venous phase (*f*) fat-suppressed 3D-GE images at 3.0T demonstrate multiple cysts located in the pancreatic head and bilateral kidneys in another patient with von Hippel–Lindau disease. Thick septations located between pancreatic cysts show enhancement. T2-weighted image shows simple cysts in both kidneys (white arrows, *c*) and a hemorrhagic cyst (black arrow, *c*) in the left kidney. Additionally, there is an enhancing lesion (open arrow, *e*, *f*) in the right kidney suggestive of renal cell carcinoma.

NEOPLASMS

Pancreatic mass lesions can be detected and successfully characterized with a pattern recognition approach using T1, T2, and immediate and late postgadolinium images. Table 4.1 summarizes a pattern recognition approach for the most common pancreatic tumors.

SOLID NEOPLASMS

Benign Solid Neoplasms

Lipoma

Lipoma is the most common benign solid tumor that affects the pancreas. Rounded morphology and larger

Table 4.1 Pattern Recognition: Focal Pancreatic Lesions

	T1	T2	EARLY Gd	LATE Gd	OTHER FEATURES
Ductal Adeno Ca (small)	ø	Δ	ø	ø–≠	Usually no background chronic pancreatitis, so tumor is well seen on precontrast T1.
Ductal Adeno Ca (large)	ø–Δ	Δ–≠	ø	ø	Usually background chronic pancreatitis; tumor is not well seen on precontrast T1.
					Focal mass with definable margins shown on early post Gd images is the most common imaging characteristic.
Islet Cell Tumors Insulinoma	ø	≠	≠, homogeneous and benign	Δ–≠	Tumors are usually <1 cm.
Gastrinoma	ø	≠	≠, ring	Δ–≠	Tumors are usually located in the region of the pancreatic head.
					Approximately 50% have metastases at initial diagnosis.
					Liver metastases tend to be uniform population of numerous smooth ring enhancing tumors shown on immediate postgadolinium images that exhibit peripheral washout on delayed images.
Somastostatinoma, Glucagonoma, Untyped	ø	≠	≠, diffuse heterogeneous	Δ heterogeneous	Tumors are usually large at initial diagnosis, with the majority having liver metastases. Liver metastases are numerous and vary in size with irregular ring enhancement.
VIPoma	ø	≠	≠	Δ	Primary tumor is usually small at initial diagnosis with few varying size liver metastases with irregular ring enhancement.
Serous Cystadenoma	ø	≠≠	Δ–≠	Δ	Small cysts best seen on single-shot T2 sequences.
					Septations usually thin and regular but may measure up to 4 mm in thickness with regular thickness.
					Septations may enhance moderately on immediate post-Gd images of larger tumors with thicker septations, and these tumors may possess a central scar that shows delayed enhancement.
Mucinous Cystadenoma	ø	≠≠	Δ–≠	Δ	Cysts >2 cm.
					Septations are uniform in thickness, and there is no evidence of irregular tumor tissue or nodule.
Macrocystic Cystadenocarcinoma	ø	≠	Δ–≠	Δ–≠	Cysts vary in signal and >2 cm,
					Septations are irregular in thickness with irregular-shaped tumor tissue and tumor nodule.
					Tumor may be very locally aggressive and may have liver metastases.
					Liver metastases may be high signal on T1 weighted images because of presence of mucin.

size distinguish this tumor from prominent fat within the interstices of the pancreas. The diagnosis is readily made with non-fat-suppressed and fat-attenuating techniques (fig. 4.11).

Malignant Solid Neoplasms

Adenocarcinoma

Adenocarcinoma of the pancreas refers to carcinoma arising in the exocrine portion of the gland. Pancreatic ductal adenocarcinoma accounts for 95% of malignant tumors of the pancreas. Pancreatic adenocarcinoma is the fourth most common cause of cancer death in the United States [27]. The lesion is more common in males and blacks [28]. The age range for tumor occurrence is the fourth through the eighth decade, with tumor incidence peaking in the eighth decade [29]. The tumor has a poor prognosis, with a 5-year survival of 5% [28].

Approximately 60–70% of pancreatic adenocarcinomas occur in the head (figs. 4.12–4.22), 15% in the body (figs. 4.23 and 4.24), 5% in the tail (fig. 4.25), and 10–20% with diffuse involvement (fig. 4.26) [30]. Tumors in the head of the pancreas are in a strategic position to encroach on the common bile duct, major papilla, and duodenum. They tend to present smaller in size than tumors in the body or tail because of the development of jaundice secondary to obstruction of the common bile duct. Painless jaundice is the classical presenting feature of carcinomas within the pancreatic head.

In general, the diagnosis of pancreatic adenocarcinoma is made when the tumor is relatively large (about 5 cm) and has extended beyond the pancreas (85% of cases). Carcinoma involving the body and tail of the pancreas grows insidiously and often has already metastasized widely at the time of diagnosis [31]. The most common sites of metastases, in order of decreasing frequency, are liver, regional lymph nodes, peritoneum, and lungs [30]. The rich lymphatic supply and lack of a capsule account for the early spread of cancer to regional lymph nodes. The nodal groups involved include parapancreatic, paraaortic, paracaval, paraportal, and celiac. Calcification is a rare constituent of the mass itself, although adenocarcinoma may occur in a pancreas containing calcification.

Pancreatic cancer arising in the head of the pancreas may cause obstruction of the CBD and pancreatic duct [32]. This appearance on MRCP studies results in the "double duct sign," which was originally described on ERCP (see fig. 4.15). A characteristic imaging appearance of pancreatic carcinoma consists of enlargement of the head of the pancreas with dilatation of the pancreatic and common bile duct and atrophy of the body and tail of the pancreas. However, enlargement of the head of the pancreas with obstruction of both ducts is not a feature unique to pancreatic cancer, as this same

appearance may be appreciated, although less commonly, in patients with focal pancreatitis. One study evaluated the accuracy of MRI emphasizing T1-weighted 3D-GE sequences, for differentiating pancreatic carcinoma from chronic pancreatitis. The results showed a sensitivity of 93% and specificity of 75% [33]. The most discriminative finding for pancreatic carcinoma was relative demarcation of the mass compared to background pancreas in contrast to chronic pancreatitis on post-Gd 3D-GE sequences (fig. 4.15) [33]. Additional features included that chronic pancreatitis demonstrated progressively more intense enhancement on serial post gadolinium images than that of pancreatic cancer, and that destruction of pancreatic architecture was present with cancer and often absent with chronic pancreatitis [33].Other features that assist in the diagnosis of pancreatic cancer include the presence of lymphadenopathy, encasement of the celiac axis or superior mesenteric artery, and liver metastases (figs. 4.27 and 4.28) [30, 34]. On tomographic images, vascular encasement is observed as a loss of the fat plane around vessels [35]. Liver metastases are the only absolute indication of malignancy, as lymphadenopathy and vascular encasement may rarely occur in inflammatory disease. Because liver metastases are not common at initial presentation, the most useful imaging feature for the diagnosis of pancreatic cancer is the demonstration of a focal hypovascular mass within pancreatic parenchyma. Detection of carcinoma is best performed by immediate postgadolinium T1-weighted gradient-echo images (see fig. 4.12) [1, 4, 36–38]. Pancreatic tissue is well delineated from tumors, and tumor margins are clearly shown with this sequence in all regions of the pancreas. Small tumors or tumors of the pancreatic tail are also well demonstrated on noncontrast T1-weighted fat-suppressed images. Larger tumors in the pancreatic head are revealed less consistently with noncontrast T1weighted fat-suppressed images, as explained below. Conventional spin-echo images are generally limited in the detection of pancreatic cancer [39]. Tumors are usually minimally hypointense relative to pancreas on T2-weighted images and are therefore difficult to visualize. One study evaluated MRI, including noncontrast T1-weighted fat-suppressed spin echo and immediate postgadolinium gradient echo, for the detection or exclusion of pancreatic cancer in 16 patients with findings indeterminate for cancer on spiral CT imaging [37]. Immediate postgadolinium gradient echo was found to be the most sensitive approach to detect pancreatic cancer, particularly in the head of the pancreas. Both immediate postgadolinium gradient-echo and noncontrast T1-weighted fat-suppressed imaging performed well at excluding cancer, and both were significantly superior to spiral CT imaging (see figs. 4.13 and 4.17). These findings are similar to those reported by Gabata et al. [36], who

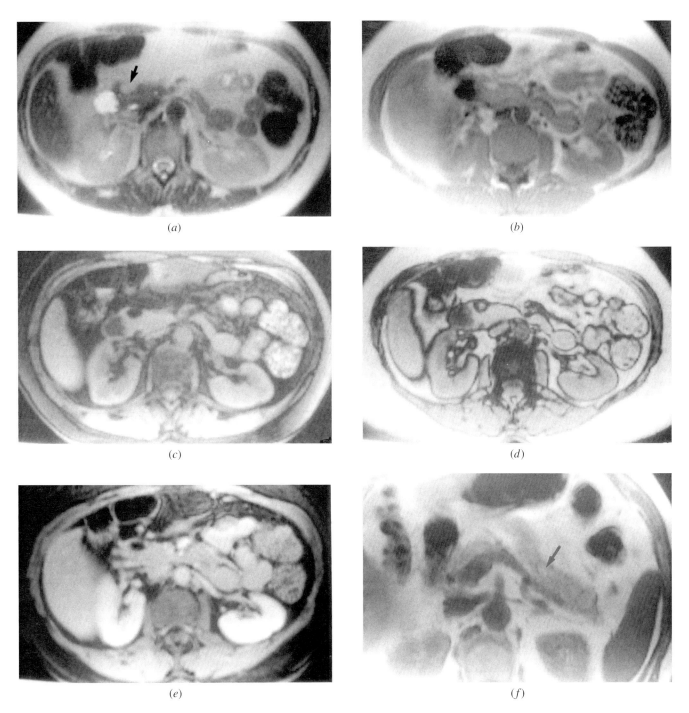

FIG. 4.11 Pancreatic lipoma. T2-weighted SS-ETSE (*a*), T1-weighted SGE (*b*), T1-weighted fat-suppressed SGE (*c*), T1-weighted out-of-phase SGE (*d*), and 90-s postgadolinium T1-weighted fat-suppressed SGE (*e*) images. There is a small lesion in the anterior aspect of the head of the pancreas (arrow, *a*), which appears isointense with adjacent intraperitoneal fat on T1 (*b*)- and T2 (*a*)-weighted images, with drop in signal intensity on fat-suppressed images (*c, e*). A phase-cancellation artifact surrounds the lesion on the T1 out-of-phase image (*d*).These findings are diagnostic for a pancreatic lipoma.

compared these MR techniques to dynamic contrast-enhanced CT imaging.

Because of their abundant fibrous stroma and relatively sparse vascularity, pancreatic cancers enhance to a lesser extent than surrounding normal pancreatic tissue on early postcontrast images [36]. It is therefore critical to exploit this difference in vascularity in contrast-enhanced studies by imaging in the dynamic capillary phase of enhancement (see figs. 4.12, 4.13, and 4.17) [36, 37]. Thin section thickness is also helpful, but

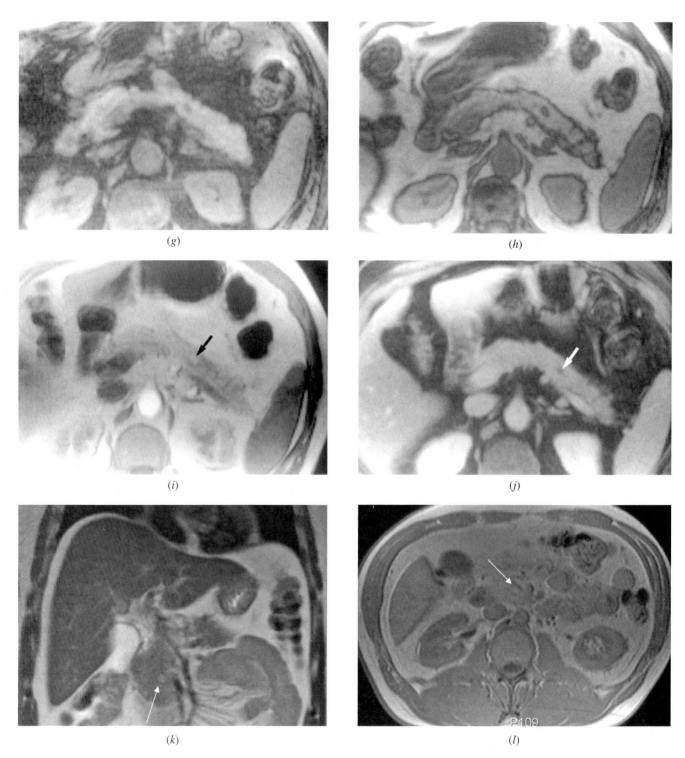

(g)

(h)

(i)

(j)

(k)

(l)

FIG. 4.11 (*Continued*) T1-weighted SGE (*f*), T1-weighted fat-suppressed SGE (*g*), T1-weighted out-of-phase SGE (*h*), immediate postgadolinium T1-weighted SGE (*i*), and 90-s postgadolinium fat-suppressed SGE (*j*) images in a second patient with a small lipoma (arrow, *f*) in the pancreatic body/tail. An important reason to correctly identify a lesion as a lipoma is not to misinterpret high signal on immediate postgadolinium nonsuppressed images as consistent with enhancement (arrow, *i*), nor to misinterpret low signal on interstitial-phase gadolinium-enhanced fat-suppressed images as consistent with washout (arrow, *j*).

Coronal T2-weighted single-shot echo-train spin-echo (*k*), transverse T1-weighted in-phase (*l*) and out-of-phase (*m*) SGE, and transverse T1-weighted postgadolinium hepatic arterial dominant phase (*n*) and hepatic venous phase (*o*) fat-suppressed 3D-GE

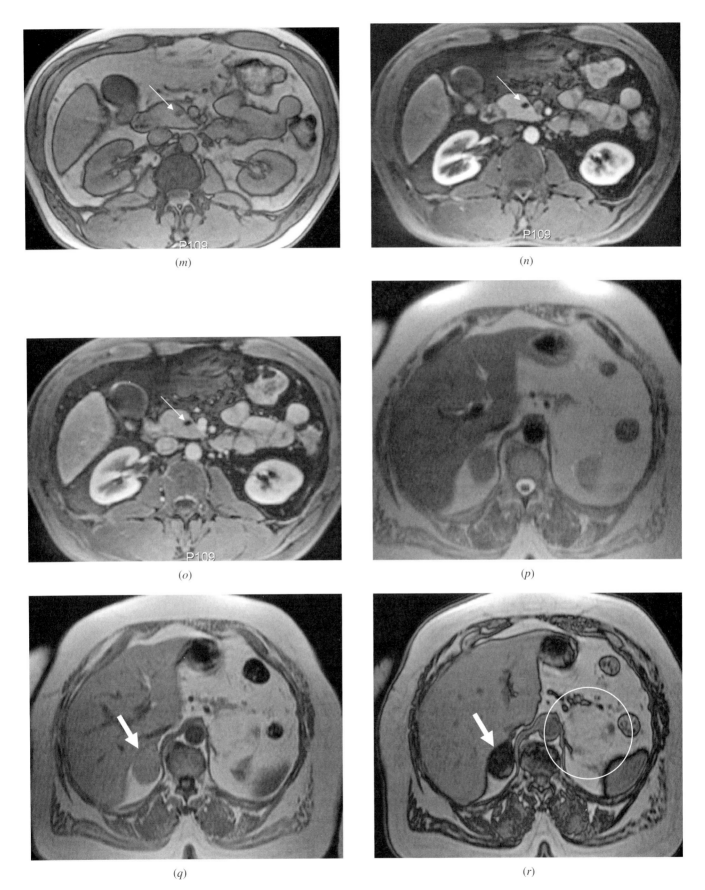

(m)

(n)

(o)

(p)

(q)

(r)

FIG. 4.11 (*Continued*) images at 3.0 T demonstrate a small pancreatic lipoma (arrows, *k–o*) in the pancreatic head of another patient, showing similar and characteristic findings.

T2-weighted single-shot echo-train spin-echo (*p*), T1-weighted in-phase (*q*) and out-of-phase (*r*) SGE, T1-weighted fat-suppressed SGE (*s*), and T1-weighted postgadolinium hepatic venous phase fat-suppressed 3D-GE (*t*) images demonstrate a large pancreatic lipoma

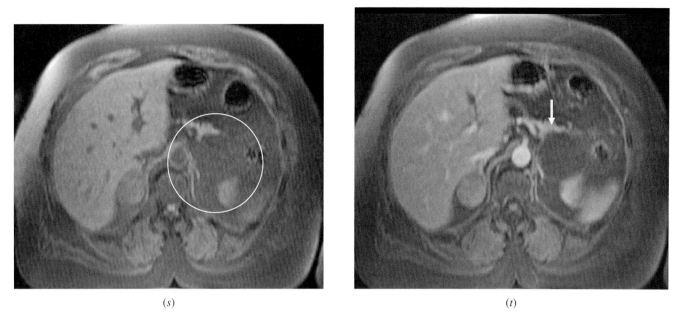

(s)   (t)

FIG. 4.11 (*Continued*) originating from the tail region and a right adrenal adenoma. The large pancreatic lipoma (circle, *r*, *s*) shows phase cancellation artifact on out-of-phase SGE image (*r*) and suppression on fat-suppressed SGE image (*s*). The pancreatic tail shows beaking (arrow, *t*) and the capsule of lipoma shows enhancement on postgadolinium image (*t*). The right adrenal adenoma (arrows, *q*, *r*) shows prominent signal drop on out-of-phase SGE (*r*) compared to in-phase SGE (*q*) and homogenous enhancement on post-gadolinium image (*t*). While the lipoma consisting of 100% fat demonstrates signal loss on fat-suppressed images, the adenoma shows signal loss on out-of-phase image due to its water and fat components.

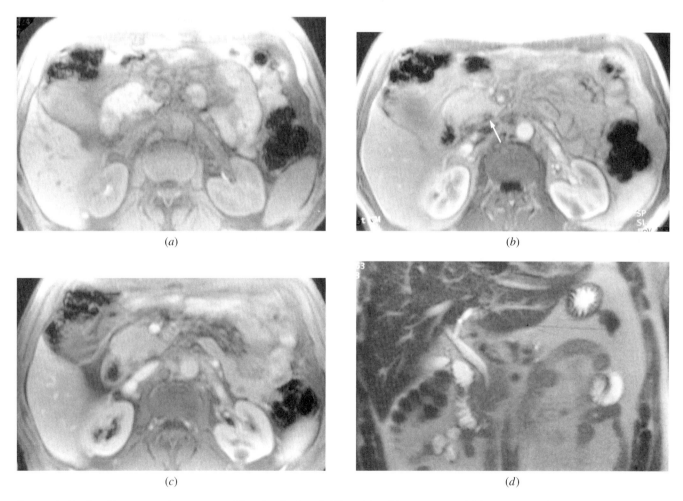

(a)   (b)

(c)   (d)

FIG. 4.12 Small pancreatic cancer arising in the head. T1-weighted fat-suppressed SGE (*a*), immediate postgadolinium T1-weighted SGE (*b*), and 90-s postgadolinium fat-suppressed SGE (*c*) images. A 6-mm tumor (arrow, *b*) is present in the uncinate process of the pancreas, which does not result in ductal obstruction because of its small size and location. Note that the mass is most clearly shown on the immediate postgadolinium image (*b*) as a small hypoenhancing lesion. Coronal (*d*) and transverse (*e*)

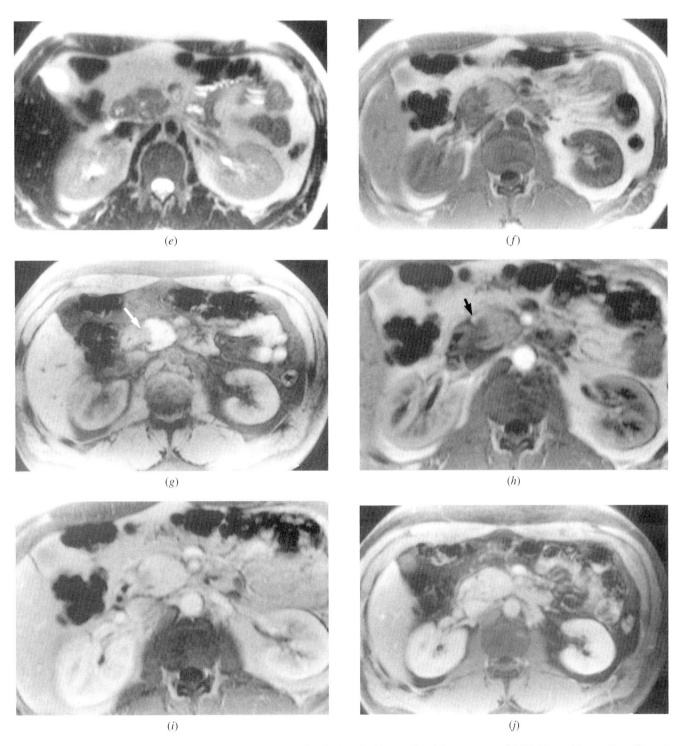

F I G . 4.12 (*Continued*) T2-weighted SS-ETSE, T1-weighted SGE (*f*), T1-weighted fat-suppressed SGE (*g*), and immediate (*h*) and 45-s (*i*) postgadolinium T1-weighted SGE and 90-s postgadolinium fat-suppressed SGE (*j*) images in a second patient with moderately differentiated adenocarcinoma. There is a 1.5-cm mass arising in the lateral aspect of the pancreatic head, which invades the duodenal wall and causes biliary ductal dilatation. On the T2-weighted images (*d, e*), CBD obstruction is well shown, but the tumor itself is almost imperceptible. The tumor (arrow, *g*) is most clearly appreciated on the noncontrast T1-weighted fat-suppressed SGE image (*g*) and the immediate postgadolinium SGE image (*h*). Progressive tumor enhancement and pancreatic parenchyma wash-out over time (*i, j*) diminishes the tumor-pancreas contrast, which is most problematic with small tumors. The gastroduodenal artery (arrow, *h*) is well shown on the immediate postgadolinium image as an enhancing structure. The tumor is shown to abut this vessel. Approximately one-quarter of all pancreas head cancers exhibit some degree of duodenal wall invasion.

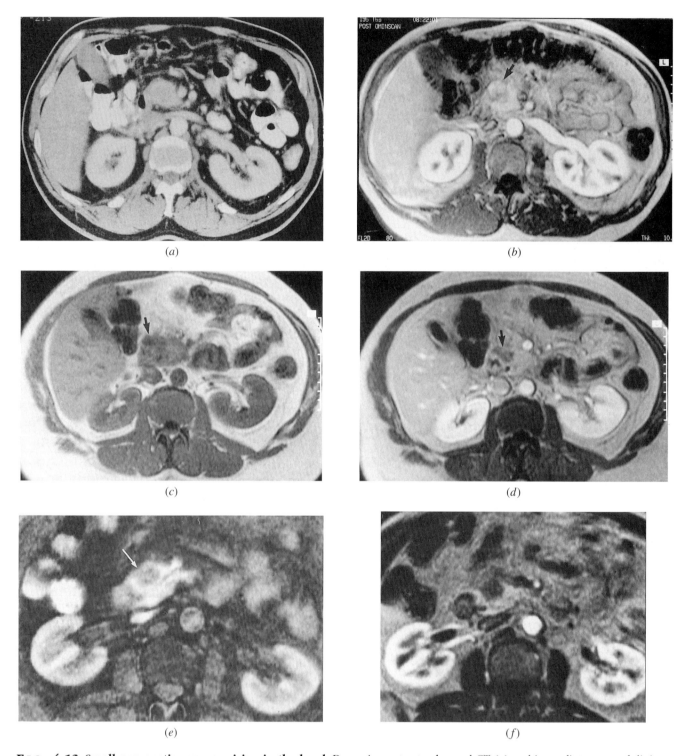

F I G . 4.13 Small pancreatic cancer arising in the head. Dynamic contrast-enhanced CT (*a*) and immediate postgadolinium T1-weighted SGE (*b*) images. The non-organ-deforming cancer is not apparent on the CT image (*a*). On the immediate postgadolinium image (*b*), a heterogeneous low-signal-intensity tumor (arrow, *b*) is identified in the head of the pancreas, clearly demarcated from uniform-enhancing pancreatic tissue.

T1-weighted SGE (*c*) and 45-s postgadolinium T1-weighted SGE (*d*) images in a second patient. A 2-cm pancreatic cancer is present that is minimally lower in signal intensity than pancreas on the precontrast image (*c*) and enhances substantially less than pancreas on the early postgadolinium image (arrow, *d*). T1-weighted fat-suppressed spin-echo (*e*), immediate postgadolinium T1-weighted SGE (*f*), and interstitial-phase gadolinium-enhanced T1-weighted fat-suppressed spin-echo (*g*) images in a third patient.

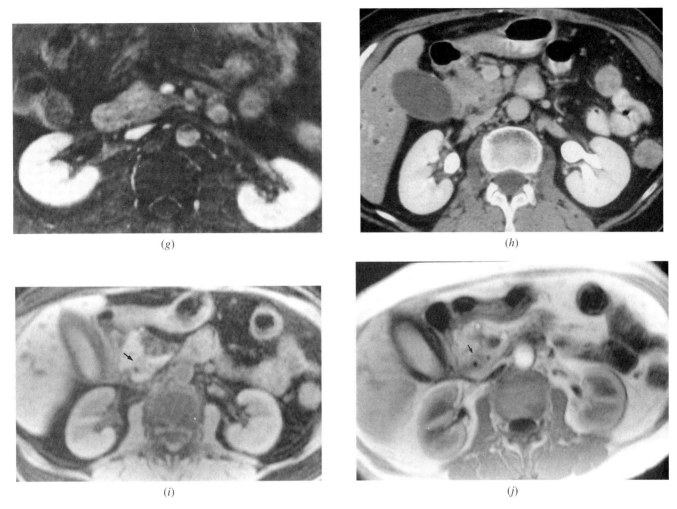

(g)

(h)

(i)

(j)

FIG. 4.13 (*Continued*) A small non-organ-deforming cancer is present in the head of the pancreas (arrow, *e*). The tumor does not obstruct the main pancreatic duct, so background pancreas remains high in signal intensity on T1-weighted fat-suppressed images (*e*). The immediate postgadolinium T1-weighted SGE image (*f*) demonstrates normal capillary enhancement of the pancreas with minimal enhancement of the cancer. The interstitial-phase gadolinium-enhanced T1-weighted fat-suppressed image (*g*) demonstrates minimally higher signal intensity of the tumor compared to the background pancreas, reflecting a greater accumulation of gadolinium by the tumor and obscuring the cancer.

Spiral CT (*h*), T1-weighted fat-suppressed SGE (*i*), and immediate postgadolinium T1-weighted SGE (*j*) images in a fourth patient. The pancreatic cancer is not visualized on the spiral CT image (*h*). On the T1-weighted fat-suppressed image, the tumor is low in signal intensity (arrow, *i*) relative to background pancreas. On the immediate postgadolinium image (*j*), the tumor (arrow, *j*) enhances less than background pancreas.

8-mm-thick sections may be sufficiently thin to detect even small (<1 cm) cancers because of the high contrast resolution on 2D-SGE images. An adequate signal-to-noise ratio may be achieved with section thickness of 5 mm by using a phased-array surface coil. On newer MR systems, 3D-GE is a good technique to detect small pancreatic cancers with 3 mm section thickness (see figs. 4.17 and 4.18). Although pancreatic cancers are lower in signal intensity than pancreas on immediate postgadolinium (capillary phase) images, the appearance of cancers on ≥1-min postgadolinium (interstitial phase) images is variable [36]. The enhancement of cancer relative to pancreas on interstitial phase images reflects the volume of extracellular space and venous drainage of cancers compared to pancreatic tissue. In general, large pancreatic tumors tend to remain low in signal intensity on later images (see figs. 4.23 and 4.25), whereas smaller tumors may range from hypointense to hyperintense.

Pancreatic cancers appear as low-signal-intensity masses on noncontrast T1-weighted fat-suppressed images and are clearly separated from normal pancreatic tissue, which is high in signal intensity [4, 36, 37]. Pancreatic tissue distal to pancreatic cancer is often lower in signal intensity than normal pancreatic tissue [36, 37]. This finding may be explained by

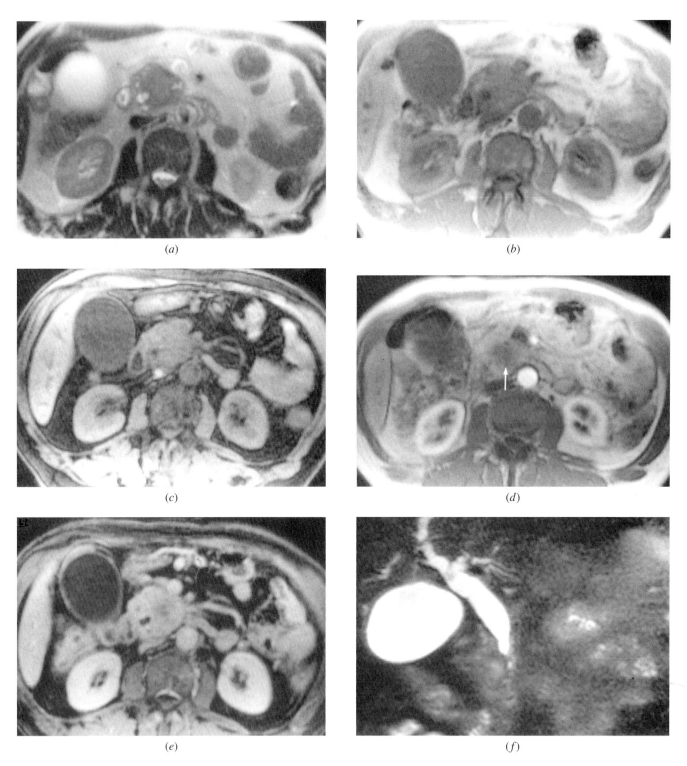

(a)   (b)

(c)   (d)

(e)   (f)

F ig . 4.14 Pancreatic cancer arising in the head. T2-weighted echo-train spin-echo (*a*), T1-weighted SGE (*b*), T1-weighted fat-suppressed SGE (*c*), immediate postgadolinium T1-weighted SGE (*d*), and 90-s postgadolinium fat-suppressed SGE (*e*) images. There is a 4-cm tumor arising in the pancreatic head, which appears hypointense on T1 (*b, c*)- and T2 (*a*)-weighted images. On immediate postgadolinium images (*c*), the tumor exhibits diminished enhancement compared to normal adjacent pancreatic paren-chyma, with demarcation of the tumor edges (arrow, *d*) with background pancreas.

MRCP (*f*), immediate postgadolinium T1-weighted SGE (*g*), and 90-s postgadolinium fat-suppressed SGE (*h*) images in a second patient with poorly differentiated pancreatic adenocarcinoma. The pancreatic cancer appears as a hypoenhancing mass (arrow, *g*)

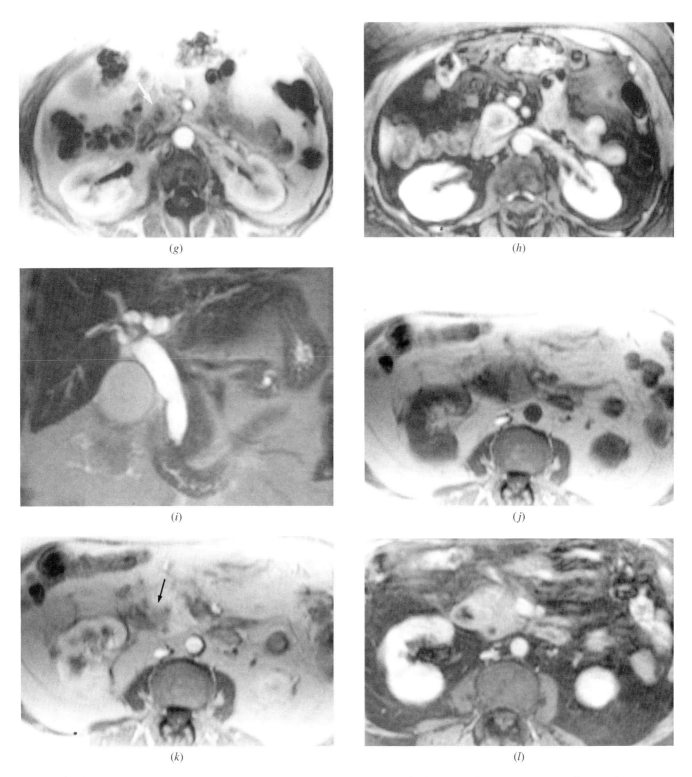

(g)

(h)

(i)

(j)

(k)

(l)

F I G . 4.14 (*Continued*) on the immediate postgadolinium image (*g*) with demarcated margins. Relationship to the superior mesenteric vessels, which are spared, is well shown on the interstitial phase gadolinium-enhanced fat-suppressed image (*h*). Coronal T2-weighted echo-train spin-echo (*i*), T1-weighted SGE (*j*), immediate postgadolinium T1-weighted SGE (*k*), and 90-s postgadolinium fat-suppressed SGE (*l*) images. A 2-cm moderately differentiated adenocarcinoma of the pancreatic head is present (arrow, *k*), which is most clearly depicted on the immediate postgadolinium image (*k*). On the interstitial-phase gadolinium-enhanced fat-suppressed image (*l*), the tumor has decreased in conspicuity because of progressive tumor enhancement and pancreatic parenchymal wash-out. Invasion of the medial duodenal wall is shown by contiguous extension of tumor to the wall.

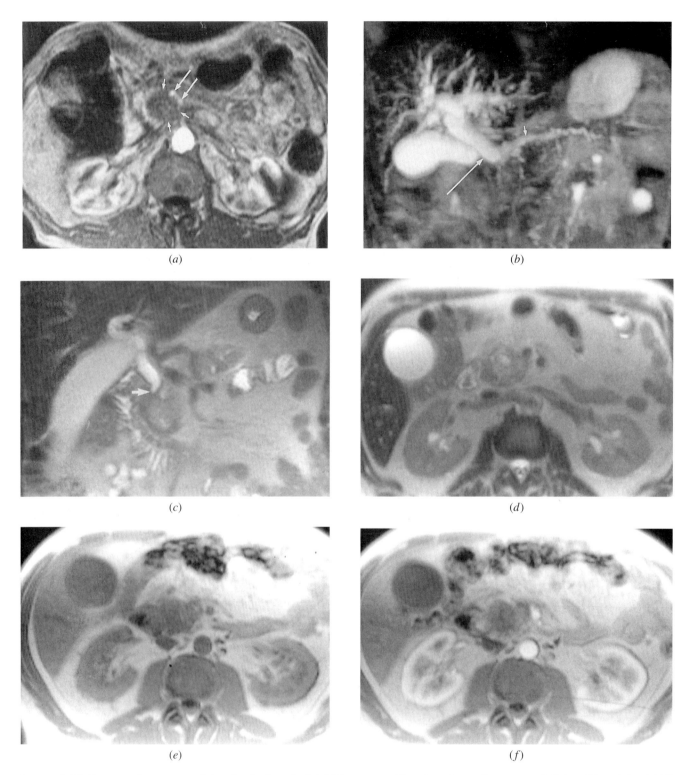

(a)

(b)

(c)

(d)

(e)

(f)

FIG. 4.15 Pancreatic cancer arising in the head with biliary tree dilatation. Immediate postgadolinium T1-weighted SGE (*a*) and non-breath-hold 3D MIP MRCP (*b*) images. A 3.5-cm cancer arises from the head of the pancreas. On the immediate post-contrast image (*a*), the tumor is well shown as a low-signal intensity mass (small arrows, *a*) that is closely applied to the superior mesenteric vein and superior mesenteric artery (long arrows, *a*). The MRCP image (*b*) demonstrates obstruction of the CBD (long arrow, *b*) and pancreatic duct (small arrow, *b*) creating the "double duct" sign.

Coronal (*c*) and transverse (*d*) T2-weighted SS-ETSE, T1-weighted SGE (*e*), immediate (*f*) and 45-s (*g*) postgadolinium T1-weighted SGE, and transverse (*h*) and coronal (*i*) interstitial-phase gadolinium-enhanced fat-suppressed SGE images in a second

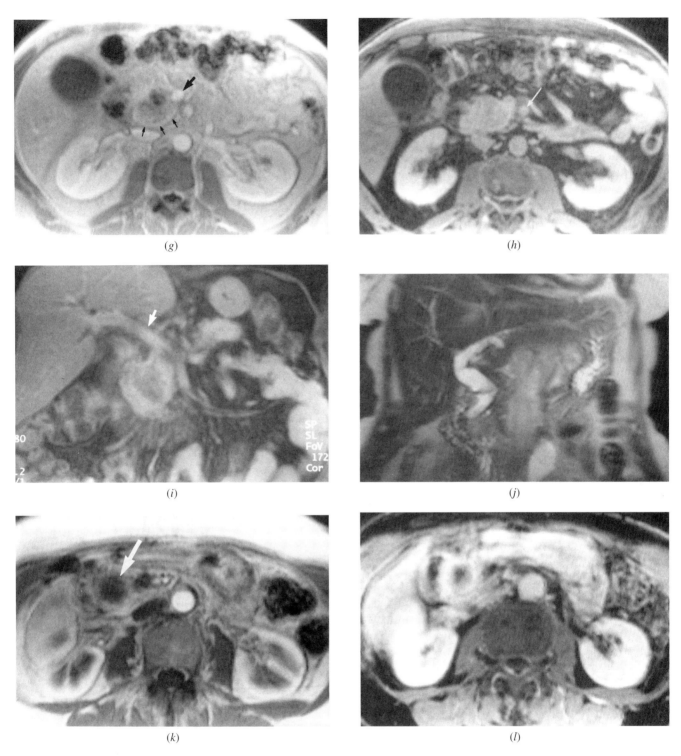

(g)

(h)

(i)

(j)

(k)

(l)

FIG. 4.15 (*Continued*) patient with a poorly differentiated pancreatic adenocarcinoma arising in the head. Obstruction of the CBD (arrow, *c*) by the pancreatic head cancer is clearly shown on the coronal image (*c*). The pancreatic mass is mildly heterogeneous and hyperintense on T2-weighted (*c, d*) images, with minimal enhancement on early postcontrast images (*f*) and progressive enhancement on later images (*h*). The tumor partially encases the superior mesenteric vein (arrow, *h*), and a definable margin with a thin rim of adjacent pancreas (small arrows, *g*) is appreciated. Duskiness of the fat around the superior mesenteric artery (arrow, *h*) is shown on the interstitial-phase gadolinium-enhanced fat-suppressed image (*h*). The coronal gadolinium-enhanced fat-suppressed image shows a patent portal vein (arrow, *i*) and its relationship with the cancer. Coronal T2-weighted SS-ETSE (*j*), immediate post-gadolinium T1-weighted SGE (*k*), and 90-s postgadolinium fat-suppressed SGE (*l*) images in a third patient with pancreatic cancer. Obstruction of the CBD is present. A hypoenhancing tumor (arrow, *k*) with definable margins with adjacent pancreas is clearly shown on the immediate postgadolinium image (*k*), which has central necrotic areas and causes biliary tree dilatation.

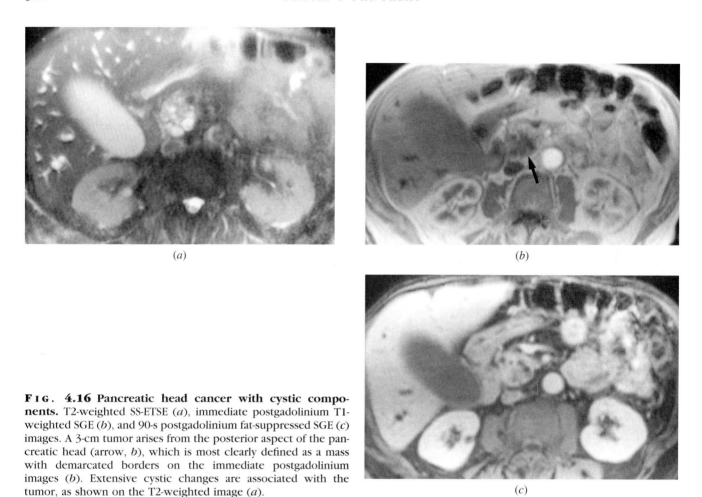

FIG. 4.16 Pancreatic head cancer with cystic components. T2-weighted SS-ETSE (*a*), immediate postgadolinium T1-weighted SGE (*b*), and 90-s postgadolinium fat-suppressed SGE (*c*) images. A 3-cm tumor arises from the posterior aspect of the pancreatic head (arrow, *b*), which is most clearly defined as a mass with demarcated borders on the immediate postgadolinium images (*b*). Extensive cystic changes are associated with the tumor, as shown on the T2-weighted image (*a*).

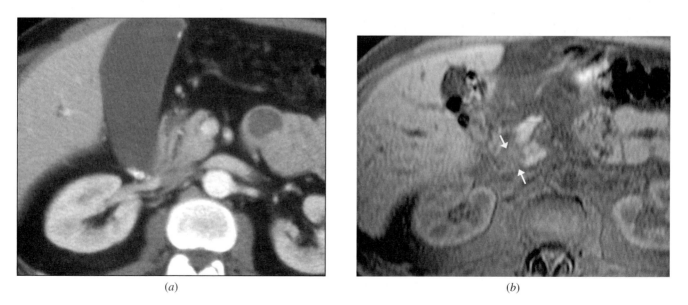

FIG. 4.17 Small pancreatic cancer arising in the head. Dynamic contrast-enhanced CT (*a*), fat-suppressed T1-weighted gradient-echo (*b*), immediate postgadolinium fat-suppressed T1-weighted 3D gradient-echo (*c*), and coronal reformat of

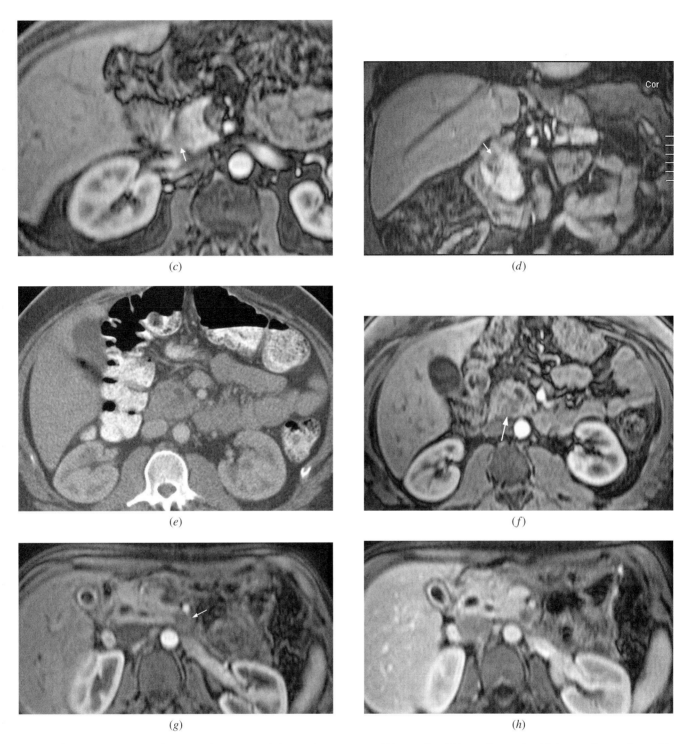

(c)

(d)

(e)

(f)

(g)

(h)

F I G . 4.17 (*Continued*) the immediate postgadolinium fat-suppressed T1-weighted 3D gradient-echo (*d*) images in a patient with small pancreatic cancer. A small cancer is present in the pancreatic head (arrows, *c*, *d*), which is most clearly defined as a mass with demarcated borders on fat-suppressed T1-weighted images (arrows, *b*). The small, non-organ-deforming tumor is not apparent on CT image. The tumor appears as a hypoenhancing mass (arrow, *c*) on the immediate postgadolinium image (*c*) with demarcated margins. Dynamic contrast-enhanced CT (*e*) and immediate postgadolinium fat-suppressed T1-weighted 3D gradient-echo (*f*) images in a second patient. A small cancer seen on the immediate postgadolinium image (arrow, *f*), is not appreciated on CT image.

Immediate and interstitial postgadolinium fat-suppressed T1-weighted gradient-echo images (*g*, *h*) in a third patient demonstrate a small hypoenhancing mass arising from the tip of the uncinate process. This mass is seen well only on the immediate postgadolinium 3D gradient-echo image (arrow, *g*).

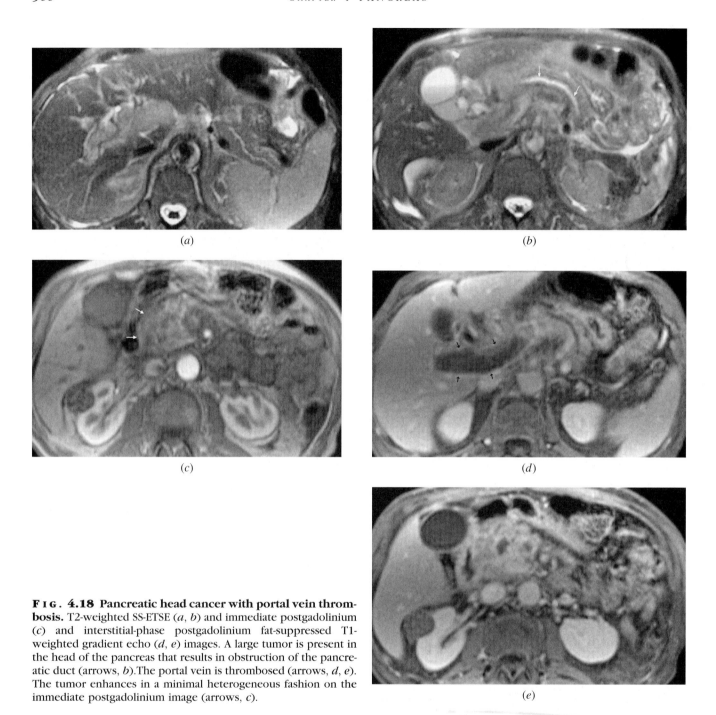

(a)

(b)

(c)

(d)

(e)

FIG. 4.18 **Pancreatic head cancer with portal vein thrombosis.** T2-weighted SS-ETSE (*a*, *b*) and immediate postgadolinium (*c*) and interstitial-phase postgadolinium fat-suppressed T1-weighted gradient echo (*d*, *e*) images. A large tumor is present in the head of the pancreas that results in obstruction of the pancreatic duct (arrows, *b*).The portal vein is thrombosed (arrows, *d*, *e*). The tumor enhances in a minimal heterogeneous fashion on the immediate postgadolinium image (arrows, *c*).

tumor-associated pancreatitis occurring distal to the tumor because of obstruction of the main pancreatic duct. With chronic inflammation of the pancreas, there is progressive fibrosis and glandular atrophy and the proteinaceous fluid of the gland diminishes [36, 40]. In these cases, depiction of cancer is poor on noncontrast T1-weighted fat-suppressed images [36, 37]. However, immediate postgadolinium gradient-echo images are able to define the size and extent of cancers that obstruct the pancreatic duct [36, 37]. Demonstration of a rim of

increased enhancement representing surrounding pancreas is commonly observed in pancreatic cancer, particularly that arising in the head. This is an important imaging feature, which helps to establish the focal nature of the disease process (see fig. 4.15). These tumors appear as low-signal-intensity mass lesions in a background of slightly greater-enhancing chronically inflamed pancreas. Tumors are usually large when they cause changes of surrounding chronic pancreatitis, and in this setting diagnosis is not problematic. In carcino-

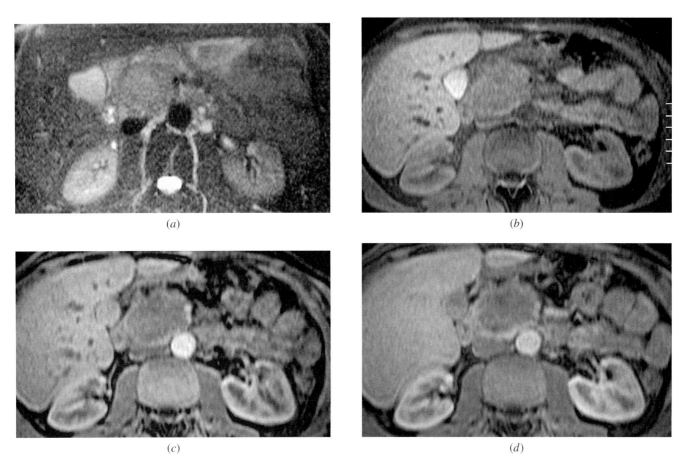

(a) (b)

(c) (d)

F I G . 4.19 Large pancreatic cancer arising in the head. Fat-suppressed T2-weighted SS-ETSE (*a*), fat-suppressed T1-weighted gradient-echo (*b*), and immediate (*c*) and interstitial-phase (*d*) postgadolinium fat-suppressed T1-weighted gradient-echo images in a patient with pancreatic cancer. A 5-cm mass is present in the pancreatic head. It is mildly hypointense relative to pancreas and demonstrates diminished enhancement on immediate and late postgadolinium T1-weighted images (*c, d*).

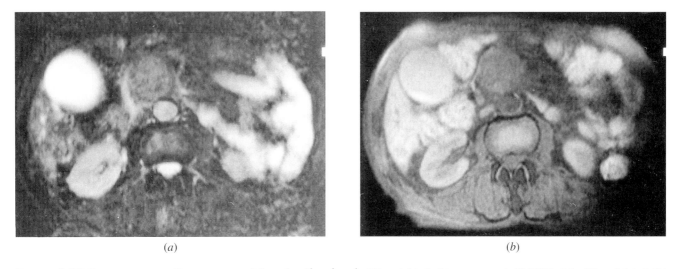

(a) (b)

F I G . 4.20 Large pancreatic cancer arising in the head. T2-weighted fat-suppressed SS-ETSE (*a*), T1-weighted fat-suppressed spin-echo (*b*), immediate postgadolinium T1-weighted SGE (*c*), and interstitial-phase gadolinium-enhanced T1-weighted

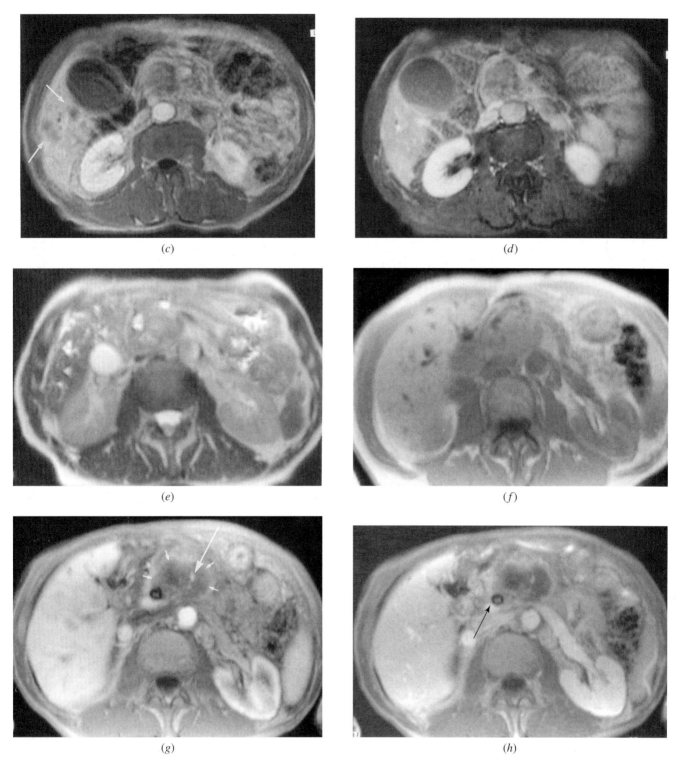

(c) *(d)*

(e) *(f)*

(g) *(h)*

FIG. 4.20 (*Continued*) fat-suppressed spin-echo (*d*) images. A large 5-cm cancer is present in the head of the pancreas that is low in signal intensity on T1-weighted images (*b*) and low in signal intensity on T2-weighted images (*a*) and enhances minimally on early (*c*) and late (*d*) postgadolinium images. This represents the typical appearance of a large pancreatic ductal cancer. Liver metastases are present and are most clearly defined on immediate postgadolinium images as focal low-signal intensity masses with irregular rim enhancement (arrows, *c*). The liver is the most common site for metastatic lesions from primary pancreatic cancer.

T2-weighted SS-ETSE (*e*), T1-weighted SGE (*f*), immediate postgadolinium T1-weighted SGE (*g*), and 90-s postgadolinium fat-suppressed T1-weighted SGE (*h*) images in a second patient. There is a 5.5-cm adenocarcinoma (small arrows, *g*) arising in the pancreatic head, which encases the superior mesenteric artery (long arrow, *g*). The superior mesenteric vein is thrombosed and not visualized. There is a stent in the CBD that causes susceptibility artifact (arrow, *h*).

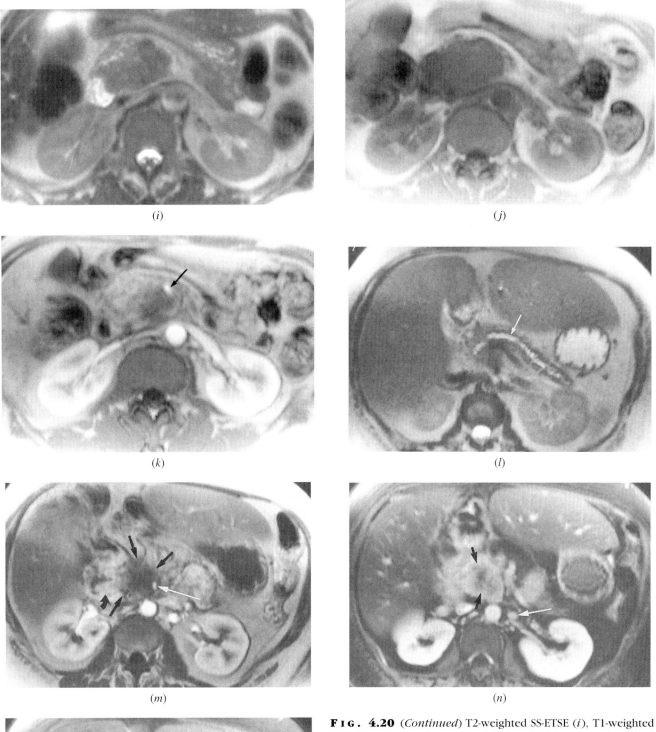

(i)

(j)

(k)

(l)

(m)

(n)

(o)

FIG. 4.20 (*Continued*) T2-weighted SS-ETSE (*i*), T1-weighted SGE (*j*), and immediate postgadolinium SGE (*k*) images in a third patient. A 6 × 5-cm cancer arises in the head and uncinate process of the pancreas, with an appearance comparable to the prior examples. Note encasement of the SMA (arrow, *k*).

T2-weighted single-shot SS-ETSE (*l*), immediate postgadolinium T1-weighted SGE (*m*), and 2-min postgadolinium fat-suppressed T1-weighted SGE (*n, o*) images in a fourth patient. A large 4-cm tumor is present in the head of the pancreas that results in obstruction of the pancreatic duct (arrow, *l, m*). The tumor is markedly low in signal intensity on the immediate postgadolinium image (short arrows, *m*), and encasement of the SMA is shown (thin arrow, *m*). Adjacent duodenum is thick walled, which is consistent with invasion (curved arrow, *m*). The tumor shows diminished central enhancement on the interstitial-phase fat-suppressed T1-weighted SGE image (arrows, *n*). Small periaortic lymph nodes are identified (long arrow, *n*). Tumor extension into the porta hepatis is present (large arrow, *o*).

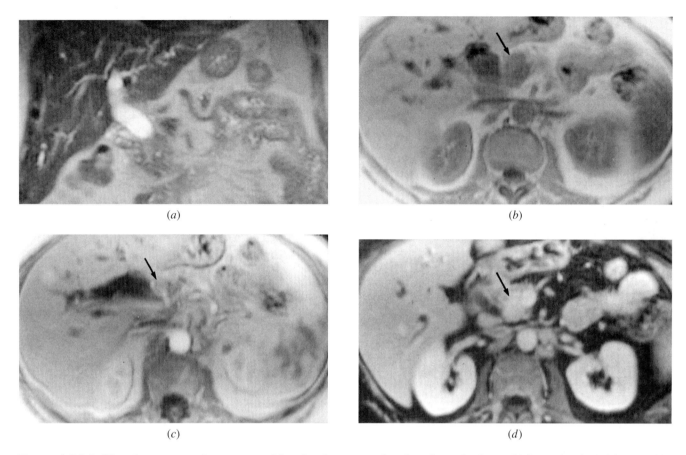

(a)

(b)

(c)

(d)

F I G . 4.21 Infiltrative pancreatic cancer arising in the upper head and neck. Coronal T2-weighted SS-ETSE (*a*), T1-weighted SGE (*b*), immediate postgadolinium T1-weighted SGE (*c*), and 90-s postgadolinium fat-suppressed SGE (*d*) images. A 3-cm poorly differentiated infiltrative adenocarcinoma is present in the pancreatic head, which causes high-grade obstruction of the CBD. The tumor is ill defined on all imaging sequences (arrow, *b*, *c*) and demonstrates late increased enhancement (arrow, *d*).These are features of an infiltrative desmoplastic neoplasm.

mas involving the tail, uninvolved pancreatic parenchyma proximal to the tumor usually is uninvolved and high in signal intensity on T1-weighted fat-suppressed images (see fig. 4.25). This differs from the circumstance of carcinoma within the pancreatic head and reflects the fact that chronic pancreatitis occurs distal to tumor that causes obstruction of the main pancreatic duct. An additional imaging feature, which assists in the distinction between carcinoma and chronic pancreatitis, is effacement of the fine, lobular contours of the gland by carcinoma. In contrast, in the setting of chronic pancreatitis, although there may be focal enlargement of the gland, the internal pancreatic architecture is generally preserved and retains the lobular, marbled or feathery appearance on MRI. On immediate postgadolinium images, pancreatic carcinoma has diminished signal intensity without well-defined internal structure, but with a mild heterogeneous morphology, whereas with chronic pancreatitis, although enhancement is diminished, the architectural pattern is often preserved.

In general, pancreatic carcinoma usually appears as a focal mass that is readily detected and characterized on immediate postgadolinium images. In these instances, the tumor is relatively well demarcated from adjacent uninvolved pancreas, which shows greater enhancement [41]. Pancreatic cancer may occasionally be poorly marginated [41]. In this setting, tumors will be ill defined without clear margination with adjacent pancreas and little or no definition of a mass [41]. These poorly-marginated tumors may have decreased enhancement on immediate postgadolinium images and may show slightly increased enhancement on 2-min postgadolinium fat suppressed gradient-echo images. This appearance is commonly observed in pancreatic cancer that has been treated with chemotherapy and radiation therapy (see below) but may also, uncommonly, be seen at initial presentation (see fig. 4.26). One study has showed that poorly-marginated appearance of pancreatic ductal carcinoma on MRI most commonly possessed moderate- to well-differentiated histopathology

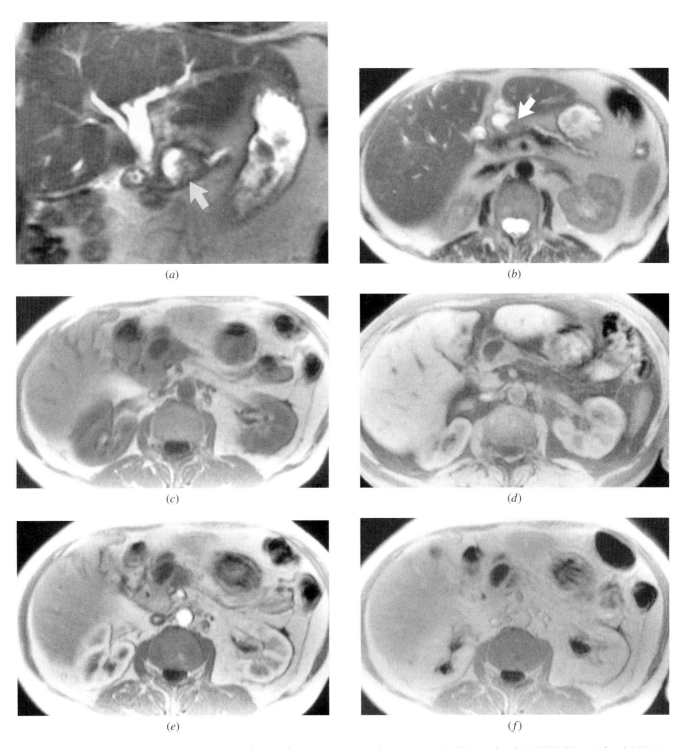

F I G . 4.22 Pancreatic cancer arising in the neck. Coronal (*a*) and transverse (*b*) T2-weighted SS-ETSE, T1-weighted SGE (*c*), T1-weighted fat-suppressed SGE (*d*), and immediate (*e*) and 45-s (*f*) postgadolinium T1-weighted SGE images in a patient with a pancreatic adenocarcinoma arising in the neck of the pancreas. There is a heterogeneous mass in the pancreatic neck (arrow, *a*, *b*), which contains a cystic component. The body and tail of the pancreas are atrophic with dilatation of the main pancreatic duct. The biliary tree is markedly dilated (*a*). Note diminished enhancement of the solid component of the mass (*e*, *f*).

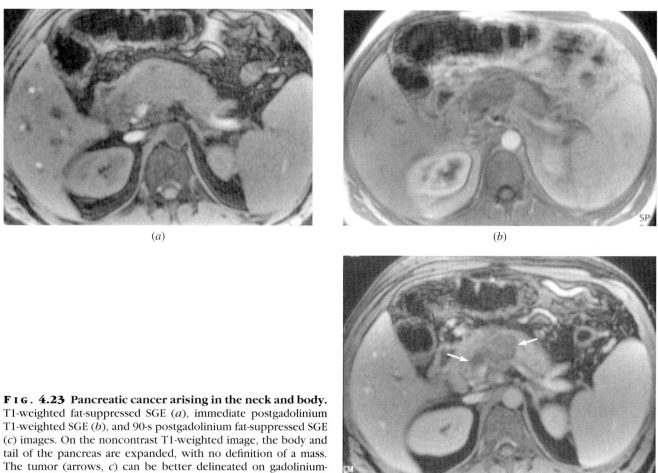

FIG. 4.23 Pancreatic cancer arising in the neck and body.
T1-weighted fat-suppressed SGE (*a*), immediate postgadolinium
T1-weighted SGE (*b*), and 90-s postgadolinium fat-suppressed SGE
(*c*) images. On the noncontrast T1-weighted image, the body and
tail of the pancreas are expanded, with no definition of a mass.
The tumor (arrows, *c*) can be better delineated on gadolinium-
enhanced images (*b*, *c*) because of lesser enhancement of the
tumor in relation to the pancreatic parenchyma.

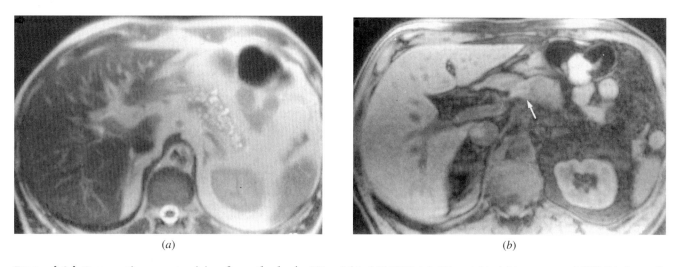

FIG. 4.24 Pancreatic cancer arising from the body. T2-weighted SS-ETSE (*a*), T1-weighted fat-suppressed SGE (*b*), immediate postgadolinium T1-weighted SGE (*c*), and 90-s postgadolinium fat-suppressed SGE (*d*) images. There is a 3-cm tumor arising in

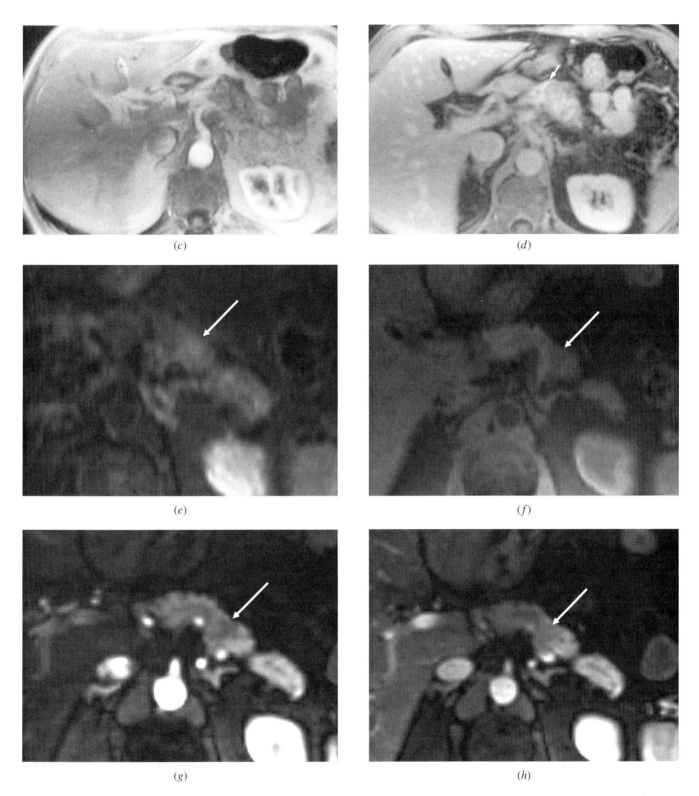

F I G. 4.24 (*Continued*) the midpancreatic body. A sharp transition is apparent between proximal normal pancreas and tumor (arrow, *b*), which causes distal chronic pancreatitis on T1-weighted fat-suppressed images (*b*) and postcontrast images (*c*, *d*). A claw sign is appreciated (arrow, *d*), reflecting that the mass arises from the pancreas. Dilated ectatic pancreatic duct side branches are present in the distal body and tail, which enhances less than the normal parenchyma.

T2-weighted short-tau inversion recovery (STIR) (*e*), T1-weighted fat-suppressed SGE (*f*), T1-weighted postgadolinium hepatic arterial dominant phase (*g*) and hepatic venous phase (*h*) fat-suppressed 3D-GE images at 3.0 T demonstrate a very small lesion (arrows; *e*–*h*) showing mildly high signal on T2-weighted image (*e*), moderately low signal on T1-weighted SGE (*f*), and initial low signal with progressive enhancement on postgadolinium images (*g*, *h*) in another patient. The diagnosis was pancreatic adenocarcinoma histopathologically.

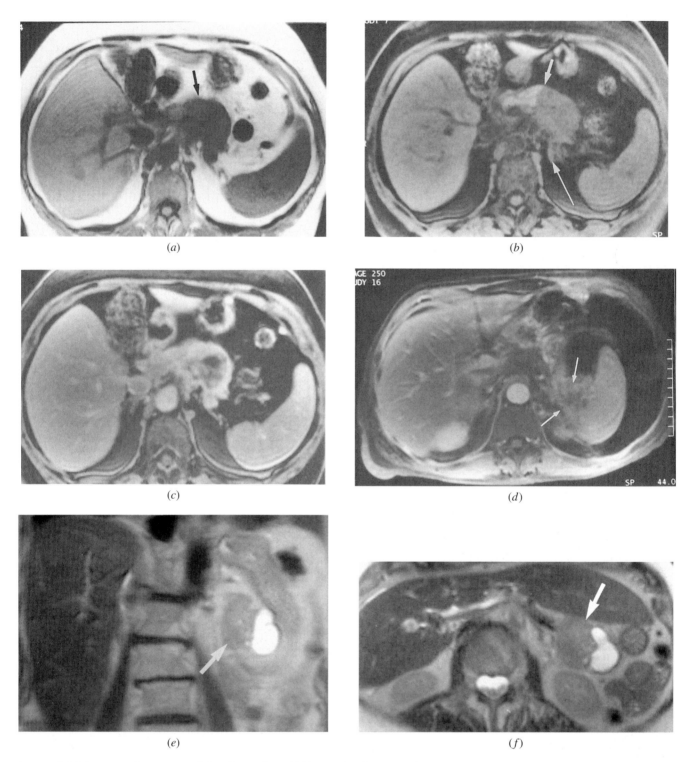

F I G . 4.25 Pancreatic cancer arising from the tail. T1-weighted SGE (*a*), fat-suppressed T1-weighted SGE (*b*), and interstitial-phase gadolinium-enhanced T1-weighted SGE (*c*) images. A large pancreatic tail cancer is present that has encased the splenic vein. The tumor is low in signal intensity on the T1-weighted image (arrow, *a*). Demarcation of tumor from uninvolved pancreas (short arrow, *b*) is clearly shown on the precontrast T1-weighted fat-suppressed image (*b*). The left adrenal is involved (long arrow, *b*). Heterogeneous enhancement with central low signal intensity is apparent on the interstitial-phase image (*c*).

Interstitial-phase gadolinium-enhanced T1-weighted SGE image (*d*) in a second patient demonstrates a pancreatic tail cancer (arrows, *d*) that invades the splenic hilum.

Coronal (*e*) and transverse (*f*) T2-weighted SS-ETSE, T1-weighted SGE (*g*), T1-weighted fat-suppressed SGE (*h*), immediate postgadolinium T1-weighted SGE (*i*), and 90-s postgadolinium fat-suppressed SGE (*j*) images in a third patient. A 5-cm cancer

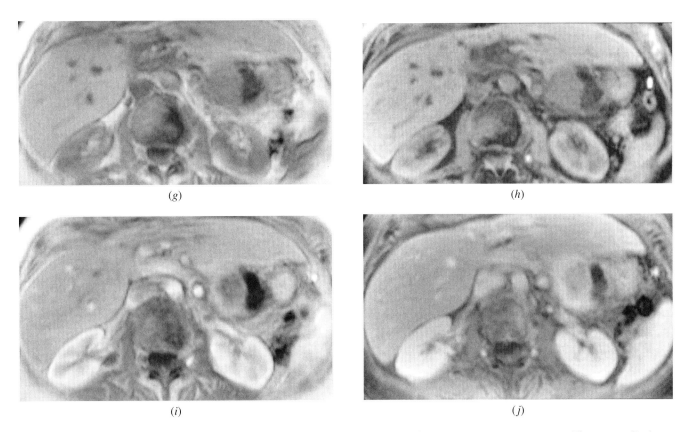

FIG. 4.25 (*Continued*) (arrow, *e*, *f*) arises from the tail of the pancreas and contains a cystic component. The tumor displaces the lesser gastric curvature laterally, best appreciated on the coronal image (*e*).

compared to focally-defined cancers which had more poorly differentiated histology [41]. Features that may aid in the distinction from chronic pancreatitis are the relatively short history of clinical findings (e.g., pain, jaundice), and the high-grade biliary and/or pancreatic ductal obstruction despite apparently small-volume disease.

Regarding tumor staging, local extension of cancer and lymphovascular involvement may be evaluated on nonsuppressed T1-weighted images [42, 43]. Low-signal-intensity tumor is well shown in a background of high-signal-intensity fat. Gadolinium-enhanced fat-suppressed gradient-echo images, acquired in the interstitial phase of enhancement (1–10 min postcontrast), demonstrate intermediate-signal-intensity tumor tissue extension into low-signal-intensity-suppressed fat (figs. 4.29 and 4.30). In comparison, noncontrast T1-weighted fat-suppressed images generally show minimal signal intensity difference between tumor, which is low in signal intensity, and suppressed background fat [36]. When tumor involves the body or tail of the pancreas, invasion of adjacent organs, such as the left adrenal gland, is well shown on a combination of sequences including nonsuppressed T1-weighted

images and interstitial-phase gadolinium-enhanced fat-suppressed T1-weighted images (see figs. 4.29 and 4.30).

Vascular encasement by tumor is best shown with thin-section 3D gradient-echo images, which can be analyzed both as source images in the transverse plane and reformatted images in the coronal plane. Coronal plane reformatted images are of value to determine the relationship between tumor and the portal vein as it enters the porta hepatis and tumor and the superior mesenteric vein along the medial margin of the head of pancreas. Immediate postgadolinium gradient echo-images are useful for evaluating arterial patency and immediate and 45-s postgadolinium gradient-echo images for evaluating venous patency (see fig. 4.27).

When comparing approaches by CT and MRI, interstitial-phase gadolinium-enhanced fat-suppressed sequence is an effective technique to delineate peritoneal metastases and is superior to CT [44, 45]. MR does not perform well at local staging if this technique is not employed [46]. Peritoneal metastases appear moderately high signal in a dark background of suppressed fat and are very conspicuous even if peritoneal disease is of thin volume and relatively linear (fig. 4.31). Demonstration of focal thickening or nodules increases the likelihood

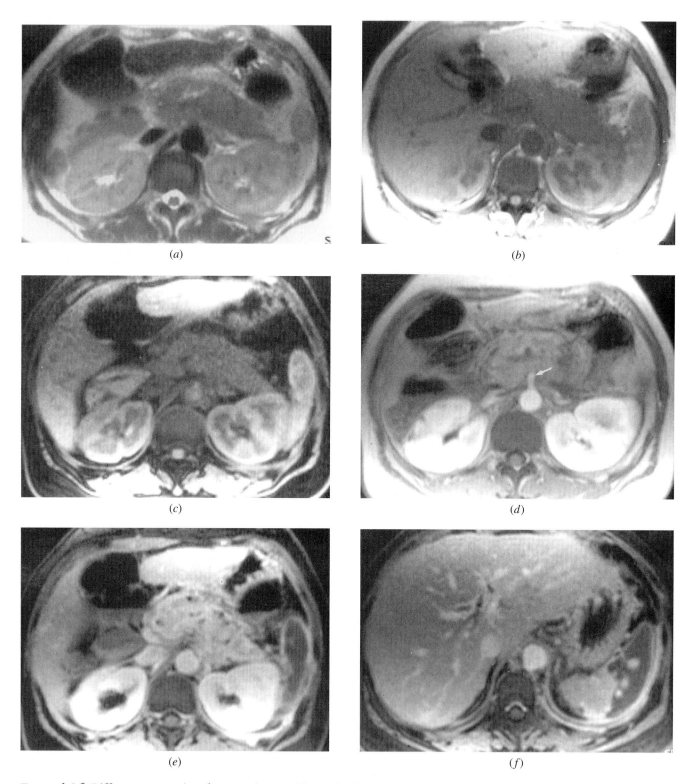

(a)   *(b)*

(c)   *(d)*

(e)   *(f)*

FIG. 4.26 Diffuse pancreatic adenocarcinoma. T2-weighted echo-train spin-echo (*a*), T1-weighted SGE (*b*), T1-weighted fat-suppressed SGE (*c*), immediate postgadolinium T1-weighted SGE (*d*), and 90-s postgadolinium fat-suppressed SGE (*e, f*) images. The pancreas is diffusely enlarged and hypointense on T2 (*a*) and T1 (*b*)-weighted images, with diminished and heterogeneous enhancement on early (*d*) and late (*e*) gadolinium-enhanced images. The tumor encases the superior mesenteric artery (arrow, *d*) and occludes the superior mesenteric vein and splenic vein. Extensive infarction of the spleen (*f*) reflects the vascular occlusion of splenic vessels.

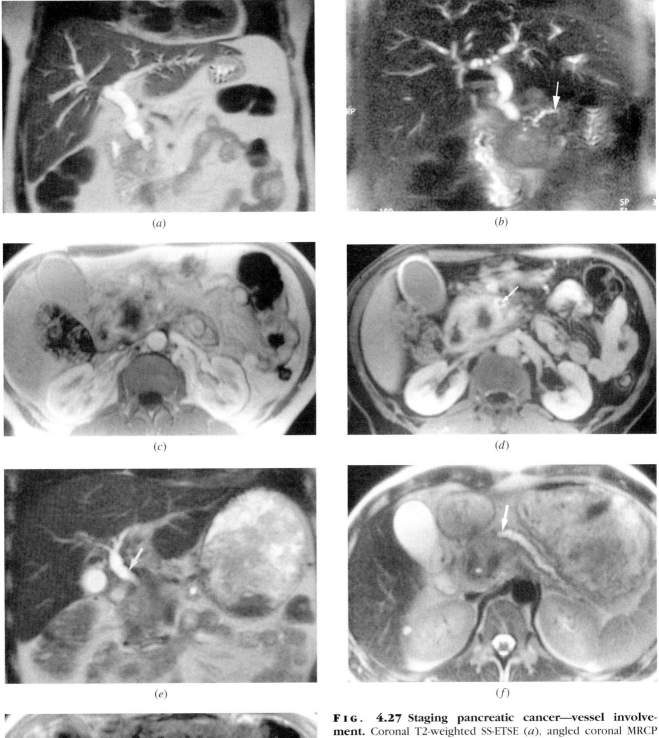

(a)

(b)

(c)

(d)

(e)

(f)

(g)

FIG. 4.27 Staging pancreatic cancer—vessel involvement. Coronal T2-weighted SS-ETSE (*a*), angled coronal MRCP (*b*), immediate postgadolinium T1-weighted SGE (*c*), and 90-s postgadolinium fat-suppressed SGE (*d*) images. A 5-cm tumor arises from the pancreatic head and obstructs the CBD and pancreatic duct (arrow, *b*), which is well shown on the MRCP image (*b*). The interstitial-phase gadolinium-enhanced image (*d*) shows a nonocclusive thrombus in the superior mesenteric vein (arrow, *d*) and tumor stranding around both superior mesenteric vessels.

Coronal (*e*) and transverse (*f*) T2-weighted SS-ETSE and immediate postgadolinium T1-weighted SGE (*g*) images in a second patient with pancreatic head adenocarcinoma. Note atrophy of the pancreatic body and tail with dilatation of main pancreatic duct. Ductal dilatations of the CBD (arrow, *e*) and pancreatic duct (arrow, *f*) are best shown on single shot T2-weighted images (including MRCP). The tumor is best shown on immediate postgadolinium images (*g*). Encased superior mesenteric artery is shown (arrow, *g*).

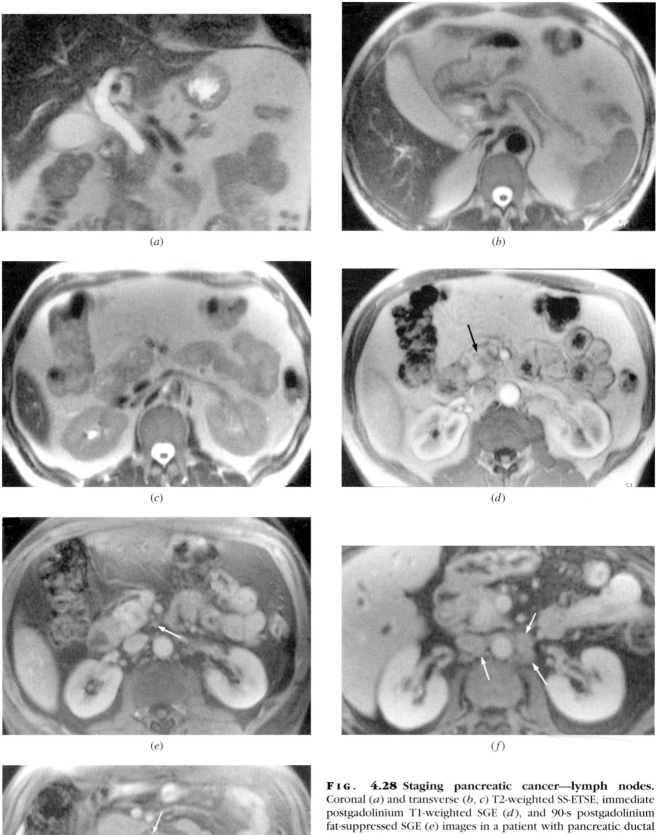

(a)

(b)

(c)

(d)

(e)

(f)

(g)

FIG. 4.28 Staging pancreatic cancer—lymph nodes.
Coronal (*a*) and transverse (*b*, *c*) T2-weighted SS-ETSE, immediate postgadolinium T1-weighted SGE (*d*), and 90-s postgadolinium fat-suppressed SGE (*e*) images in a patient with pancreatic ductal adenocarcinoma (arrow, *d*) arising from the head. The CBD is markedly dilated (*a*), with mild dilatation of the pancreatic duct (*b*). Tumors are generally not well seen on T2 (*c*). Optimal tumor demonstration is on immediate postgadolinium images (*d*). Small regional nodes (arrow, *e*) are best seen on interstitial-phase gadolinium-enhanced fat-suppressed SGE images (*e*).

Interstitial-phase gadolinium-enhanced fat-suppressed SGE images (*f*, *g*) in two other patients demonstrate malignant retroperitoneal lymph nodes (arrows, *f*, *g*). In the latter patient (*g*), the lymph nodes have low-signal centers consistent with central necrosis.

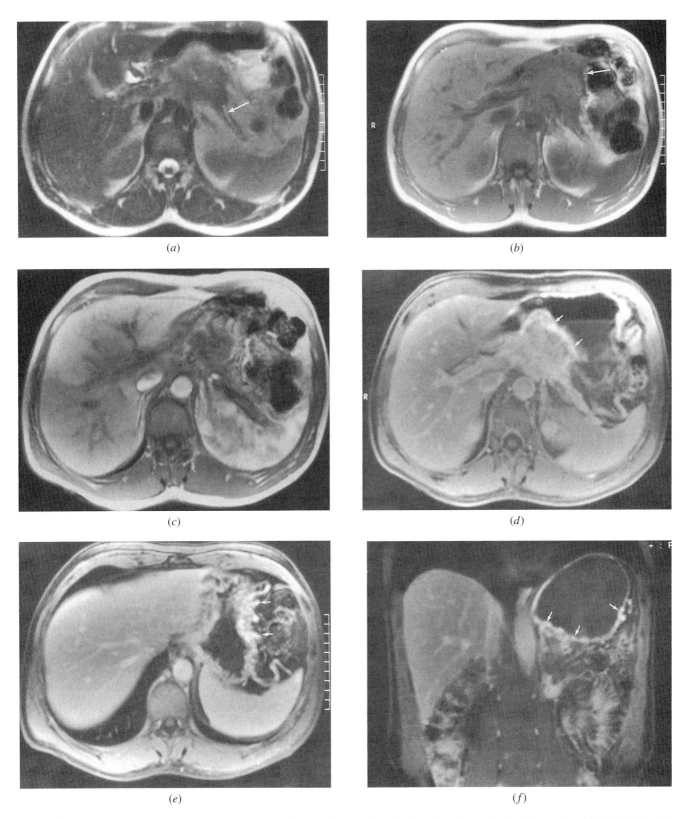

F I G . 4.29 Staging pancreatic cancer—stomach invasion and splenic vein thrombosis. T2-weighted SS-ETSE (*a*), T1-weighted SGE (*b*), immediate postgadolinium T1-weighted SGE (*c*), interstitial-phase gadolinium-enhanced T1-weighted fat-suppressed SGE (*d, e*), and coronal interstitial-phase gadolinium-enhanced T1-weighted fat-suppressed SGE (*f*) images. A large cancer is present arising from the body of the pancreas (arrow, *b*) that invades the posterior wall of the stomach. Atrophy of the pancreatic tail with ductal dilatation (arrow, *a*) is well shown on the single-shot T2-weighted image (*a*). Heterogeneous minimal enhancement of the tumor is present on the immediate postgadolinium T1-weighted SGE image (*c*). Improved demonstration of the stomach wall invasion was achieved by gastric distension with orally administered water on the interstitial-phase fat-suppressed T1-weighted SGE image (small arrows, *d*). Multiple varices along the greater curvature of the stomach are present due to thrombosis of the splenic vein. Varices are well shown on gadolinium-enhanced T1-weighted fat-suppressed SGE images as high-signal-intensity tubular structures (arrows, *e, f*).

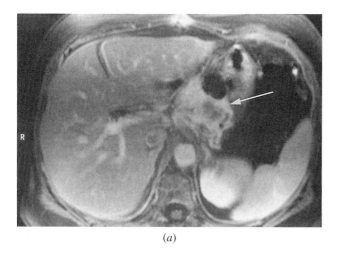

(a)

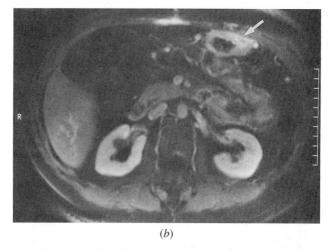

(b)

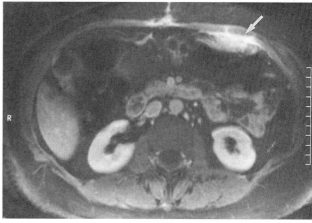

(c)

F IG . 4.30 Staging pancreatic cancer—extension along the transverse mesocolon. Interstitial-phase gadolinium-enhanced fat-suppressed T1-weighted SGE images (*a–c*). A large cancer arises from the body of the pancreas (arrow, *a*) that is adherent to the posterior wall of the stomach. Tumor extends inferiorly along the transverse mesocolon to involve the transverse colon (arrow, *b*), greater omentum, and adjacent peritoneum (arrow, *c*).

that peritoneal abnormalities represent a malignant process.

Lymph nodes are well shown on T2-weighted fat-suppressed images and interstitial-phase gadolinium-enhanced fat-suppressed T1-weighted images. Lymph nodes are moderately high in signal intensity in a background of low-signal-intensity suppressed fat with both of these techniques (figs. 4.28 and 4.32). T2-weighted fat-suppressed imaging is particularly useful for the demonstration of lymph nodes in close approximation to the liver because of the signal intensity difference between moderately high-signal-intensity nodes and moderately low-signal-intensity liver. Both lymph nodes and liver appear moderately enhanced on interstitial-phase gadolinium-enhanced fat-suppressed gradient-echo images, so lymph nodes are not as conspicuous in the region of the porta hepatis with this technique. To detect lymph nodes adjacent to liver it is useful to identify suspicious foci of high signal on the T2-weighted fat-suppressed images and confirm that they have the rounded morphology of lymph nodes on the gadolinium-enhanced fat-suppressed T1-weighted sequences. On nonsuppressed T1-weighted images, lymph nodes

are conspicuous as low-signal-intensity focal masses in a background of high-signal-intensity fat [43], but this technique performs best in the detection of retroperitoneal nodes or mesenteric nodes in the setting of abundant fat in these locations. Coronal plane imaging provides good visualization of the locations.

Liver metastases from pancreatic cancers are generally irregular in shape, are low in signal intensity on conventional or fat-suppressed T1-weighted images and minimally hyperintense on T2-weighted images, and demonstrate irregular rim enhancement on immediate postcontrast gradient-echo images (figs. 4.32–4.34). The low-signal-intensity centers of metastatic lesions reflect the desmoplastic nature of the primary cancer [1]. The low fluid content and hypovascular nature of these metastases permit the distinction between these lesions from cysts and hemangiomas, respectively, even when lesions are 1 cm in diameter. Transient, ill-defined, increased perilesional enhancement in the hepatic parenchyma may be observed on immediate post-gadolinium images. A similar appearance is observed even more commonly for colon cancer metastases. Perilesional enhancement is more typically wedge-shaped

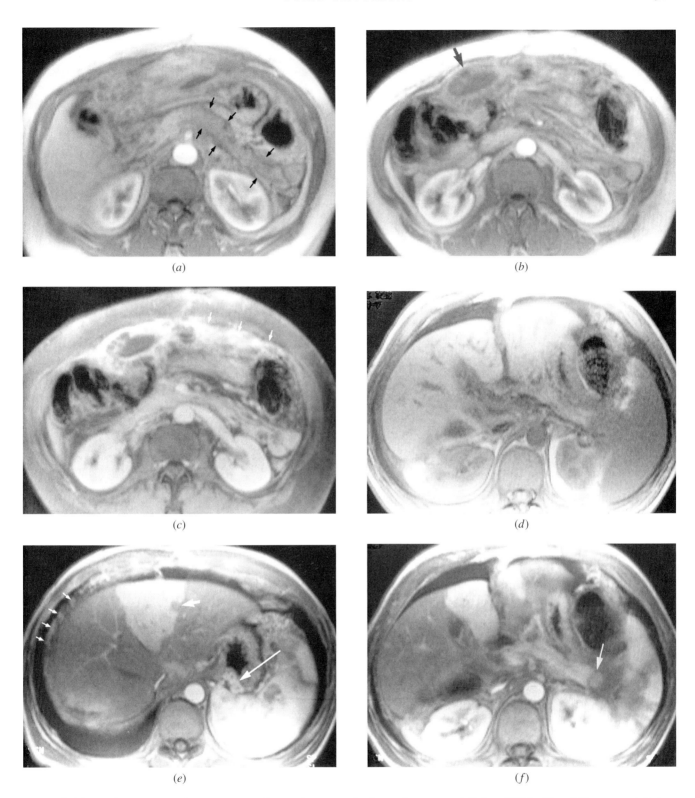

FIG. 4.31 Staging pancreatic cancer—peritoneal metastasis. Immediate postgadolinium SGE (*a*, *b*) and 90-s postgadolinium fat-suppressed SGE (*c*) images. There is normal enhancement of the pancreatic head and neck with an abrupt transition showing hypoenhancement of the body and tail of the pancreas (arrows, *a*). A focal mass is not present, and this is consistent with diffusely infiltrative pancreatic cancer. A large peritoneum-based mass (arrow, *b*) along the anterior abdominal wall is present, which has a multiloculated appearance with peripheral enhancement. There is adjacent peritoneal and omental (arrows, *c*) enhancement. These findings are consistent with diffusely infiltrative pancreatic adenocarcinoma with peritoneal metastasis.

T1-weighted SGE (*d*), immediate postgadolinium T1-weighted SGE (*e*, *f*), and 90-s postgadolinium fat-suppressed SGE (*g*) images at the level of the pancreatic body and tail in a second patient. A 2-cm cancer arises from the pancreatic tail (arrow, *f*), which is

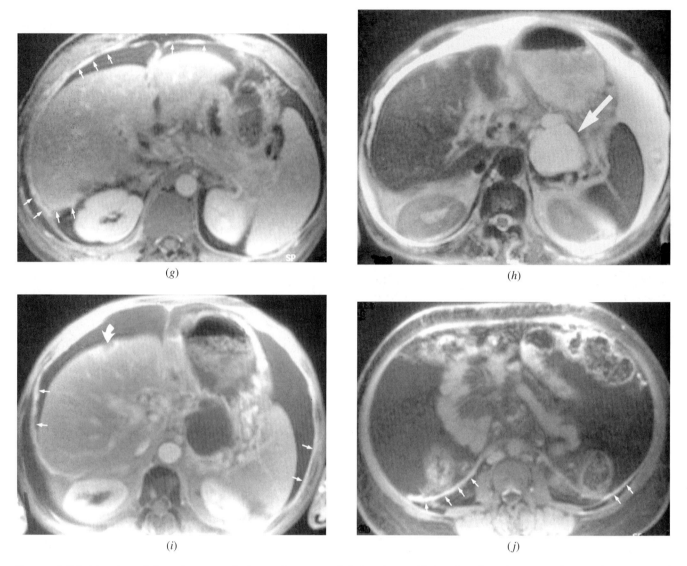

(g)

(h)

(i)

(j)

FIG. 4.31 (*Continued*) best shown on the immediate postgadolinium image (*f*). Wedge-shaped transient hyperenhancement of *segment 4* of the liver on the immediate postgadolinium images is present. Perilesional enhancement is commonly observed with pancreatic cancer liver metastases. A small defect is present in the hyperenhanced liver, which may represent a metastasis (small arrow, *e*). Diminished enhancement centrally in the spleen and a gastric wall varix (long arrow, *e*) reflect splenic vein thrombosis. Ascites and extensive peritoneal metastases are present (very small arrows, *e, g*), which are most conspicuous on interstitial-phase gadolinium-enhanced fat-suppressed SGE images (*g*).

T2-weighted fat suppressed SS-ETSE (*h*) and 90-s postgadolinium fat-suppressed T1-weighted SGE (*i*) images in a third patient who has pancreatic cancer with liver and peritoneal metastases. A 6-cm cystic mass is present in the lesser arc (arrow, *h*). Multiple varices are identified surrounding the cystic lesion (*i*). Ascites is appreciated on both T2 (*h*) and postgadolinium fat-suppressed T1-weighted (*i*) images. Extensive thickening and enhancement of the peritoneum (small arrows, *i*) is only appreciated on the fat-suppressed gadolinium-enhanced images (*i*). A 1.5-cm subcapsular metastasis is identified in *segment 4* (curved arrow, *i*).

Interstitial-phase gadolinium-enhanced fat-suppressed SGE image (*j*) in a fourth patient with pancreatic cancer, ascites, and peritoneal metastases (arrows, *j*).

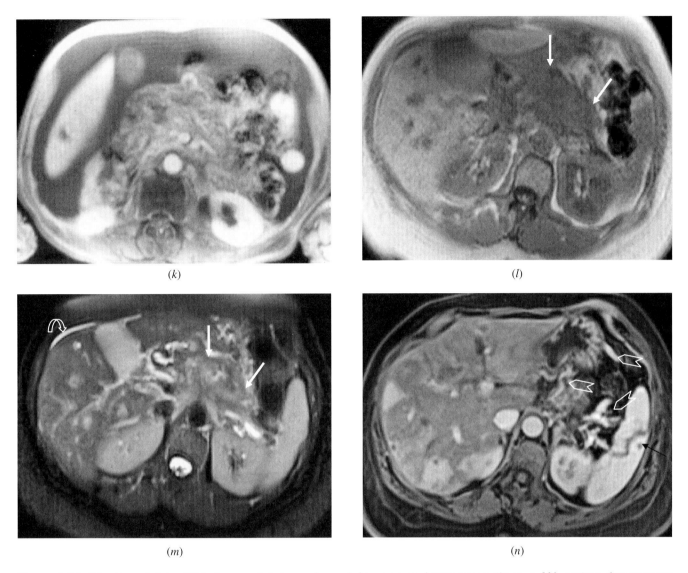

(k)

(l)

(m)

(n)

F I G . 4.31 (*Continued*) Interstitial-phase gadolinium-enhanced fat-suppressed SGE image (*k*) in a fifth patient demonstrates matting of bowel and mesentery due to tumor involvement.

T1-weighted SGE (*l*), T2-weighted single shot echo train spin echo (*m*), T1-weighted postgadolinium hepatic arterial dominant phase (*n, o*) fat-suppressed 3D-GE images demonstrate a large pancreatic adenocarcinoma (white arrows, *l, m*) located in the body in another patient. In the liver, there are multiple metastases showing peripheral enhancement (*n*). Those metastases located peripherally are also associated with wedge type of increased parenchymal enhancement. There is also a metastasis (black arrow, *n*) showing peripheral enhancement in the spleen. The peritoneal surfaces demonstrate plate-like enhancement consistent with peritoneal metastases. Splenic hilar and short gastric—left gastroepiploic varices (hollow arrows; *n*) are also detected due to splenic vein thrombosis. Note that there is free fluid peritoneal thickening (curved arrow, *m*) in the abdomen.

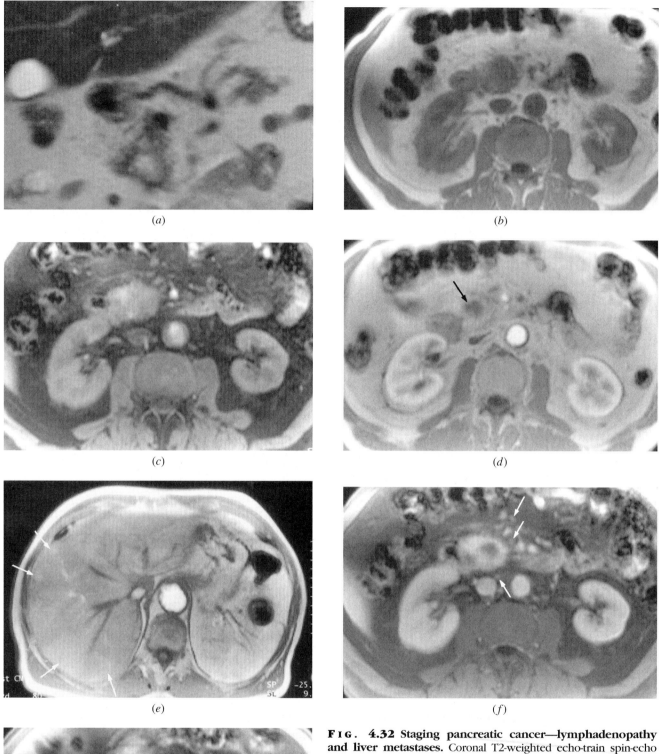

(a)

(b)

(c)

(d)

(e)

(f)

(g)

F I G . 4.32 Staging pancreatic cancer—lymphadenopathy and liver metastases. Coronal T2-weighted echo-train spin-echo (*a*), T1-weighted SGE (*b*), T1-weighted fat-suppressed SGE (*c*), immediate postgadolinium T1 SGE (*d*, *e*), and 90-s postgadolinium T1 weighted fat-suppressed SGE (*f*, *g*) images. There is a 3-cm pancreatic head cancer (arrow, *d*), which is clearly shown on the immediate postgadolinium image (*d*) as a hypoenhancing mass with demarcated borders and adjacent greater-enhancing pancreatic parenchyma. Both tumor and surrounding pancreas are low signal on the fat-suppressed image (*c*) because of changes of chronic pancreatitis in surrounding parenchyma. Liver metastases are present, which measure <1 cm and are predominantly situated in a subcapsular location. These small metastases are best shown on immediate postgadolinium images as uniformly hyperintense or ring enhancing lesions (arrows, *e*). The subcapsular location is quite typical for pancreatic cancer. Associated involved lymph nodes are best seen on interstitial-phase gadolinium-enhanced SGE images as small moderate-signal masses (arrows, *f*, *g*) in a background of suppressed fat. Pancreatic cancer has a propensity to involve nodes without resulting in increased size.

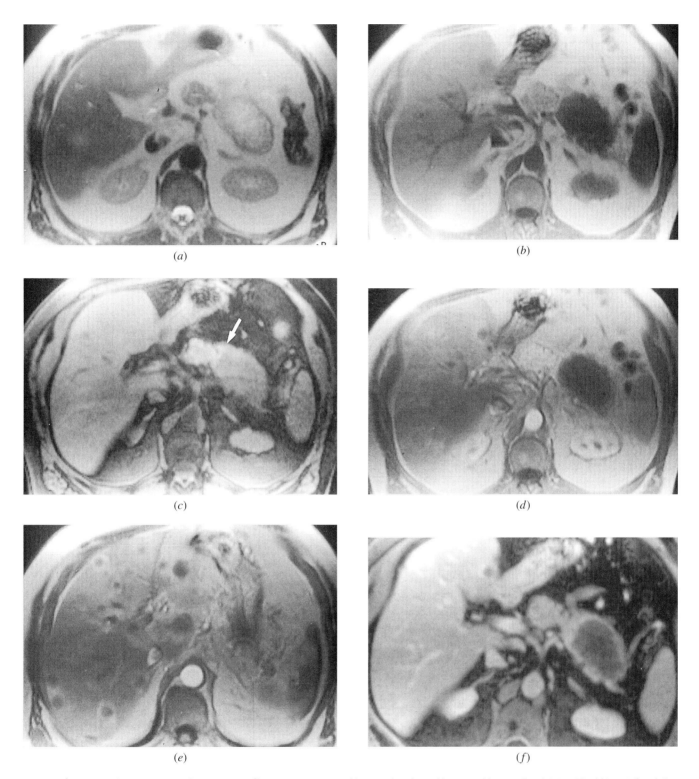

F I G . 4.33 Staging pancreatic cancer—liver metastases. T2-weighted SS-ETSE (*a*), T1-weighted SGE (*b*), T1-weighted fat-suppressed SGE (*c*), immediate postgadolinium T1-weighted SGE (*d, e*), and 90-s postgadolinium fat-suppressed SGE (*f*) images. A 4 × 5-cm tumor arises in the pancreatic tail. Note the shape demarcation of normal pancreas (arrow, *c*) proximal to the large pancreatic cancer. There are multiple liver metastases that are mildly hyperintense on T2 (*a*) and mildly low signal on T1, reflecting a low fluid content. Liver metastases are best seen as ring-enhancing lesions on immediate postgadolinium images (*d, e*) with ring-enhancing metastases involving both lobes. Pancreatic cancer most commonly metastasizes to the liver.

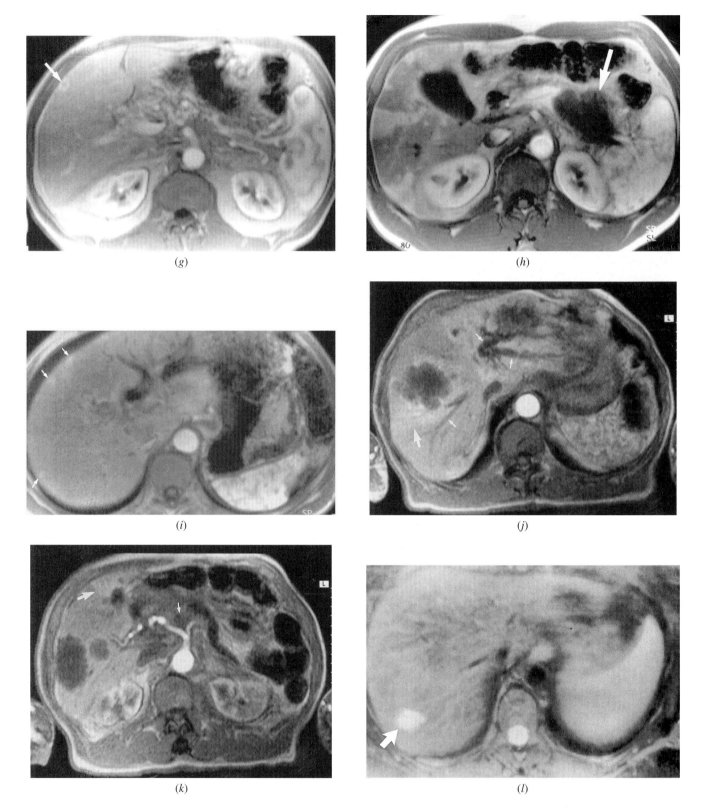

(g)

(h)

(i)

(j)

(k)

(l)

F I G . 4.33 (*Continued*) Immediate postgadolinium SGE image (g) in a second patient demonstrates a 1-cm ring-enhancing metastasis (arrow, g).

Immediate postgadolinium SGE image (h) in a third patient demonstrates a large hypovascular tumor arising from the tail of the tail of the pancreas (arrow, h). Note the beak sign with the proximal pancreatic parenchyma. Multiple hyperenhancing liver metastases are present, the majority <1 cm in size. Wedge-shaped areas of transient increased perilesional enhancement are appreciated surrounding several lesions. Perilesional enhancement is not uncommon in pancreatic ductal adenocarcinoma. The most commonly observed metastases with perilesional enhancement are colon adenocarcinoma.

Immediate postgadolinium T1-weighted SGE image (i) in a fourth patient. Multiple hyperenhancing <1-cm subcapsular liver metastases (arrows, i) are present that were not identifiable on other sequences.

Immediate postgadolinium T1-weighted SGE images (j, k) in a fifth patient. Multiple irregular hepatic metastases with rim enhancement are present. Ill-defined perilesional enhancement (arrow, j, k) is apparent surrounding several metastases. Substantial intrahepatic bile duct dilatation is also identified (small arrows, j) secondary to CBD obstruction by the pancreatic head cancer. Low-signal intensity tissue (small arrows, k) surrounds the celiac axis, a finding consistent with tumor involvement.

Breathing-averaged T2-weighted ETSE (l), immediate postgadolinium SGE (m), and 90-s postgadolinium T1-weighted

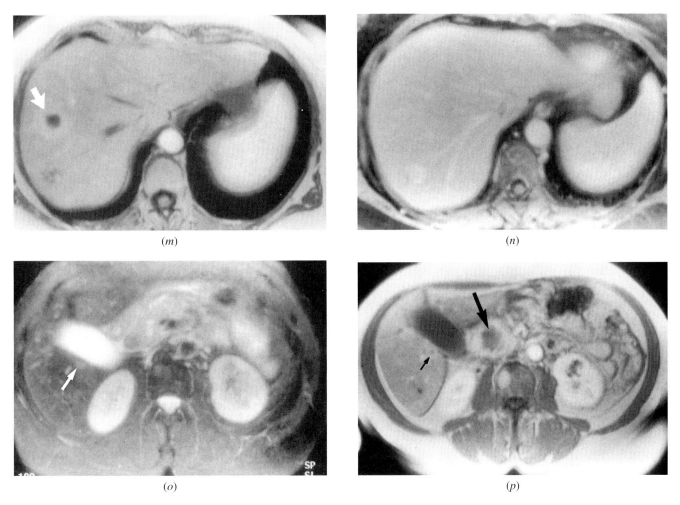

(m)

(n)

(o)

(p)

F I G . 4.33 (*Continued*) fat-suppressed SGE (*n*) images in a sixth patient who has liver metastases and a hemangioma. Hemangiomas and metastases can usually be readily distinguished. The hemangioma (arrow, *l*) is high signal on T2 (*l*) and demonstrates peripheral nodules on the immediate postgadolinium image (*m*) with relatively uniform hyperintense enhancement on delayed images (*n*). In contrast, the 3-cm metastasis is nearly invisible on T2 (*l*) and late postgadolinium images (*n*), with intense ring enhancement (arrow, *m*) on immediate post-gadolinium image (*m*). This constellation of findings is virtually pathognomonic on T2-weighted and postgadolinium images for a liver metastasis coexistent with a hemangioma.

Breathing averaged T2-weighted echo-train spin-echo (*o*) and immediate postgadolinium SGE (*p*) images in a seventh patient. The pancreatic tumor is not well seen on T2, but clearly shown as a hypoenhancing mass (arrow, *p*) on the immediate postgadolinium image (*p*). A <1-cm ring-enhancing lesion (small arrow, *p*) is apparent in a subcapsular location adjacent to the gallbladder in *segment V*. On the T2-weighted image (*o*) the lesion is only mildly hyperintense, consistent with minimal fluid content, characteristic of pancreatic ductal adenocarcinoma metastases.

with pancreatic cancer liver metastases than with colon cancer liver metastases and may have a dramatic appearance. Concomitant liver metastases in the setting of prominent wedge-shaped enhancement abnormalities are commonly small, hypervascular, and subcapsular in location. Small subcapsular hypervascular metastases are observed in over 80% of patients and may be the only pattern of liver mestastases in up to 20% of patients [47]. Optimal utilization of MRI in the investigation of pancreatic carcinoma occurs in the following circumstances: 1) detection of small, non-contour-deforming tumors (due to the high contrast resolution of pre-contrast T1-

weighted fat-suppressed imaging and immediate postgadolinium gradient-echo images), 2) determination of tumor location for imaging-guided biopsy, 3) evaluation of vascular involvement by tumor, 4) determination and characterization of associated liver lesions, and 5) determination of the presence of lymph node and peritoneal metastases. MRI may be particularly valuable in patients who have an enlarged pancreatic head with no definition of a mass on CT images.

Surgery remains the main therapeutic treatment of patients with pancreatic cancer [28, 48]; therefore, earlier detection of potentially curable disease may result in

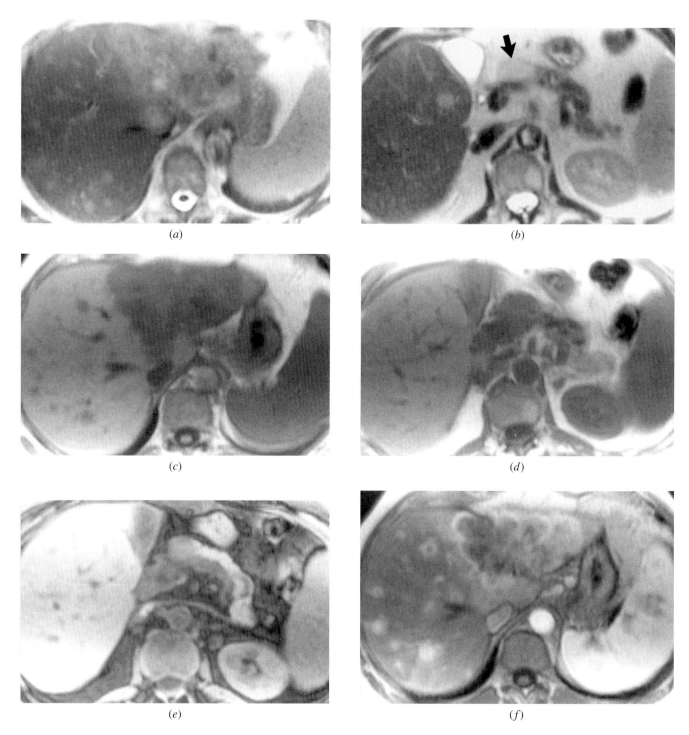

F I G . 4.34 Poorly differentiated carcinoma resembling islet cell tumor. T2-weighted SS-ETSE (*a, b*), T1-weighted SGE (*c, d*), T1-weighted fat-suppressed SGE (*e*), immediate postgadolinium T1-weighted SGE (*f, g*), and 90-s postgadolinium fat-suppressed

improved patient survival. Benassai et al. [48] recently reported on the factors associated with improvement in the 5-year actuarial survival for patients undergoing Whipple procedure (pancreaticoduodenectomy). Five-year survival was greater for node-negative than for node-positive patients (41.7% vs. 7.8%, $P < 0.001$) and

for smaller (<3 cm) than for larger tumors (33.3% vs. 8.8%, $P < 0.006$). The five-year survival for patients with negative surgical margins was 23.3%, whereas no patients with positive surgical margins survived at 13 months ($P < 0.001$). Another recent report by Ariyama et al. [49] demonstrated a 5-year survival of 100% for

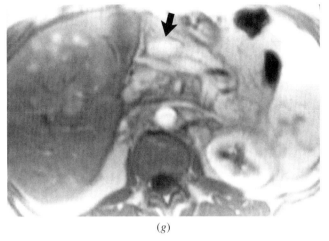

(g)

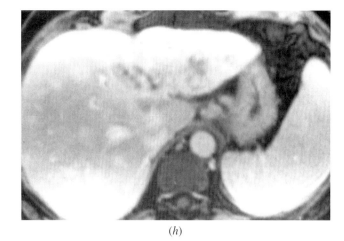

(h)

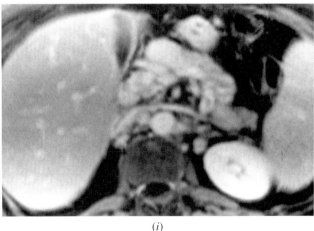

(i)

FIG. 4.34 (*Continued*) SGE (*b*, *i*) images. There is a 3-cm tumor (arrow, *b*) arising in the pancreatic neck, which is moderately hyperintense on T2 (*b*) and moderately hypointense on T1 (*d*, *e*), enhances in a uniform intense fashion immediately after gadolinium administration (arrow, *g*), and retains contrast on interstitial-phase images (*i*). There are multiple liver metastases that are moderately hyperintense on T2 (*a*) and moderately hypointense on T1 (*c*) and show uniform or ring enhancement on immediate postgadolinium images (*f*), mimicking an islet cell tumor.

patients with <1-cm tumors. It may be that MRI, particularly 3.0 T MRI, is best suited to reliably detect these small tumors, and resultant small metastases and subtle vascular and adjacent organ-structure involvement as well.

Poorly Differentiated Carcinoma

Rarely malignant pancreatic cancers may not be classifiable because of too poorly differentiated or anaplastic cytology. These cancers may have an appearance similar to islet cell tumors, with tumors appearing high signal on T2-weighted images and extensive hypervascular liver metastases (see fig. 4.34). The spectrum of appearance for poorly differentiated carcinoma has not been elucidated.

Acinar Cell Carcinoma

Acinar cell carcinoma is a rare primary tumor of the exocrine gland of the pancreas, representing approximately 1% of pancreatic cancers. Tumors generally occur between the fifth and seventh decades. Tatli et al. [50] recently described the appearance of these tumors on CT and MR images. These cancers are gener-

ally exophytic, oval or round, well marginated, and hypovascular. Small tumors are generally solid, whereas larger tumors contain cystic areas representing regions of necrosis.

Chemotherapy/Radiation Therapy-Treated Pancreatic Ductal Adenocarcinoma

After chemotherapy and radiation therapy, morphologic and pathophysiologic changes occur in the tumor, in the pancreas, and in surrounding fatty tissues. In approximately 50% of cases decrease in size of tumor and surrounding fibrogenic response can be demonstrated on MR images that correlate with clinical response. However, in a sizable proportion of cases, the interface is indistinct between tumor margin and surrounding background pancreatic tissue. In these instances, evaluation of tumor dimensions is extremely difficult. In addition, in some cases, posttreatment images may show features consistent with acute on chronic pancreatitis. On imaging, both processes may demonstrate an increase in abnormal pancreatic tissue even though the tumor itself has decreased in size. Assessment of treatment response is challenging (fig. 4.35).

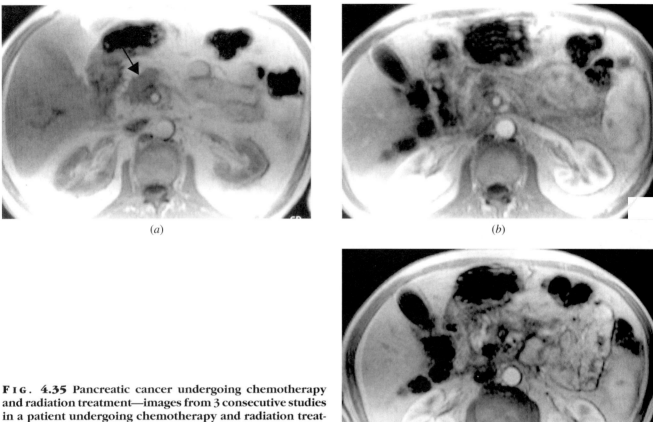

FIG. 4.35 Pancreatic cancer undergoing chemotherapy and radiation treatment—images from 3 consecutive studies in a patient undergoing chemotherapy and radiation treatment. Immediate postgadolinium SGE images from pretherapy (*a*), to 3 months (*b*) and 5 months (*c*) after initiation of treatment. Pancreatic cancer is initially well-defined (arrow, *a*). After the commencement of treatment, both tumor and pancreas become less defined (*b, c*).

Islet Cell Tumors

Islet cell tumors are a subgroup of gastrointestinal neuroendocrine tumors that occur within the endocrine pancreas. These tumors are rare in comparison with tumors arising from the exocrine portion. Islet cell tumors are uncommon, with a reported incidence of less than 1 per 100,000 [51]. Tumors may be nonfunctioning, or, more commonly, they may present with an endocrine abnormality resulting from the secretion of hormones [51]. Histopathologically, only a generic diagnosis of islet cell tumor can be made with routine staining methods. However, islet cell tumors are primarily identified by the peptide they contain, and the tumor itself is named after the hormone it secretes (e.g., an insulin-secreting tumor is termed an insulinoma). Only the results of special immunohistochemical techniques such as fluorescence-labeled antibody specific for a peptide, will permit the designation of a specific islet tumor such as insulinoma, gastrinoma, etc. A certain proportion of islet cell tumors will secrete no identifiable substance and remain uncategorized after special immunohistochemical procedures. The most common pancreatic islet cell tumors are insu-

linomas and gastrinomas [52], followed in frequency by nonfunctional or untyped tumors. In the authors' experience, the majority of clinically or immunohistochemically verified pancreatic neuroendocrine tumors are gastrinomas [53]. Hormonally functional tumors tend to present when they are small because of symptoms related to the hormones secreted by the tumors. Nonfunctional tumors account for at least 15–20% of islet cell tumors and tend to present with symptoms due to large tumor mass or metastatic disease [54]. Malignancy cannot be diagnosed on the basis of the histologic appearance of islet cell tumors. Instead, malignancy is determined by the presence of metastases or local invasion beyond the substance of the pancreas. Insulinomas are most commonly benign tumors, gastrinomas are malignant in approximately 60% of cases, and almost all other types, including nonfunctioning tumors, are malignant in the great majority of cases. The liver is the most common organ for metastatic spread. There is also a modest propensity for splenic metastases.

In the MRI investigation for islet cell tumors, precontrast T1-weighted fat-suppressed images, immediate postgadolinium gradient-echo images, and T2-weighted fat-suppressed images or breath-hold T2-weighted images are useful [1, 55–58]. Because many MR techniques independently demonstrate islet cell tumors well, MR is particularly well suited for the investigation of these tumors. Tumors are low in signal intensity on T1-weighted fat-suppressed images, demonstrate homogeneous, ring, or diffuse heterogeneous enhancement on immediate postgadolinium gradient echo, and are high in signal intensity on T2-weighted fat-suppressed images (figs. 4.36–4.38) [53]. In rare instances, islet cell tumors may be very desmoplastic, appear low in signal intensity on T2-weighted images, and demonstrate negligible contrast enhancement (fig. 4.38). In these cases, the tumors may mimic the appearance of pancreatic ductal adenocarcinoma. Large noninsulinoma islet cell tumors not uncommonly contain regions of necrosis [59].

Features that distinguish the majority of islet-cell tumors from ductal adenocarcinomas include high signal intensity on T2-weighted images, increased homogeneous enhancement on immediate post-gadolinium images, and hypervascular liver metastases [57]. Because islet cell tumors rarely obstruct the pancreatic duct, T1-weighted fat-suppressed images most often show high signal intensity of background pancreas, rendering clear depiction of low-signal-intensity tumors in the majority of cases [56, 57]. Lack of pancreatic ductal obstruction and vascular encasement by tumor are features that differentiate islet cell tumor from pancreatic ductal adenocarcinoma. In contrast to the frequent occurrence of venous thrombosis in pancreatic ductal adenocarcinoma, thrombosis is rare in the setting of islet cell tumors. However, rarely, thromboses may occur and may represent tumor thrombosis (fig. 4.39) [60], unlike the circumstance in pancreatic ductal adenocarcinoma, where the thrombus is usually bland. Peritoneal metastasis and/or regional lymph node enlargement, characteristic features of pancreatic ductal adenocarcinoma, are generally not present in islet cell tumors.

Gastrinomas (G Cell Tumors). The Zollinger–Ellison syndrome is defined by the clinical triad of pancreatic islet cell gastrinoma, gastric hypersecretion, and recalcitrant peptic ulcer disease. Ulcers located in the postbulbar region of the duodenum or in the jejunum, particularly if multiple, suggest the diagnosis of a gastrinoma. Esophagitis is not infrequently observed in these patients.

Gastrinomas occur most frequently in the region of the head of the pancreas including pancreatic head, duodenum, stomach, and lymph nodes in a territory termed the gastrinoma triangle [34]. The anatomic boundaries of the triangle are the porta hepatis as the superior point of the triangle and the second and third parts of the duodenum forming the base. Although gastrinomas are usually solitary, multiple gastrinomas may occur, especially in the setting of multiple endocrine neoplasia syndrome, type 1. In this setting, patients have multiple pancreatic and duodenal islet cell tumors [46, 55, 61].

Gastrinomas are not as frequently hypervascular as insulinomas. Mean size at presentation is 4 cm [59]. CT imaging is able to detect gastrinomas reliably when the tumors measure more than 3 cm in diameter but performs less well in the detection of smaller tumors [62]. Conventional spin-echo MRI also has been limited in the detection of gastrinomas [63, 64]. However, MRI, using current techniques, is very effective at detecting tumors <1 cm in diameter. Gastrinomas are low in signal intensity on T1-weighted fat-suppressed images and high in signal intensity on T2-weighted fat-suppressed images, demonstrating peripheral ringlike enhancement on immediate postgadolinium gradient-echo images (fig. 4.40) [56]. These imaging features are observed in the primary lesion and in hepatic metastases. Central low signal intensity on postgadolinium images reflects central hypovascularity. Occasionally, lesions will be cystic. The enhancing rim of the primary tumor varies substantially in thickness, with the thickness of the rim reflecting the degree of hypervascularity of the tumor. If the enhancing rim is thin, it may appear nearly imperceptible because of similar enhancement of the surrounding pancreatic parenchyma. Gastrinomas may occur outside the pancreas, and fat-suppressed T2-weighted images are particularly effective at detecting these high-signal-intensity tumors in a background of suppressed fat (fig. 4.41). Multiple gastrinomas may be scattered throughout the pancreas and frequently are small. T2-weighted breathing-independent echo-train spin echo may be effective at demonstrating these tumors, because breathing-averaged T2-weighted sequences may result in blurring, which may mask the presence of small tumors (fig. 4.42).

Gastrointestinal imaging findings that may be observed in gastrinomas include enlargement of the rugal folds of gastric mucosa (hypertrophic gastropathy) and intense mucosal enhancement on early post-gadolinium gradient-echo images (fig. 4.43), increased esophageal enhancement, and abnormal enhancement and/or thickness of proximal small bowel. These features are reflective of the inflammatory changes of peptic ulcer disease and gastric hyperplasia due to the effects of gastrin.

In general, islet cell tumor metastases to the liver are well shown on MR images. Gastrinoma metastases frequently are relatively uniform in size and shape [57]. These metastases are generally hypervascular and possess uniform intense rim enhancement on

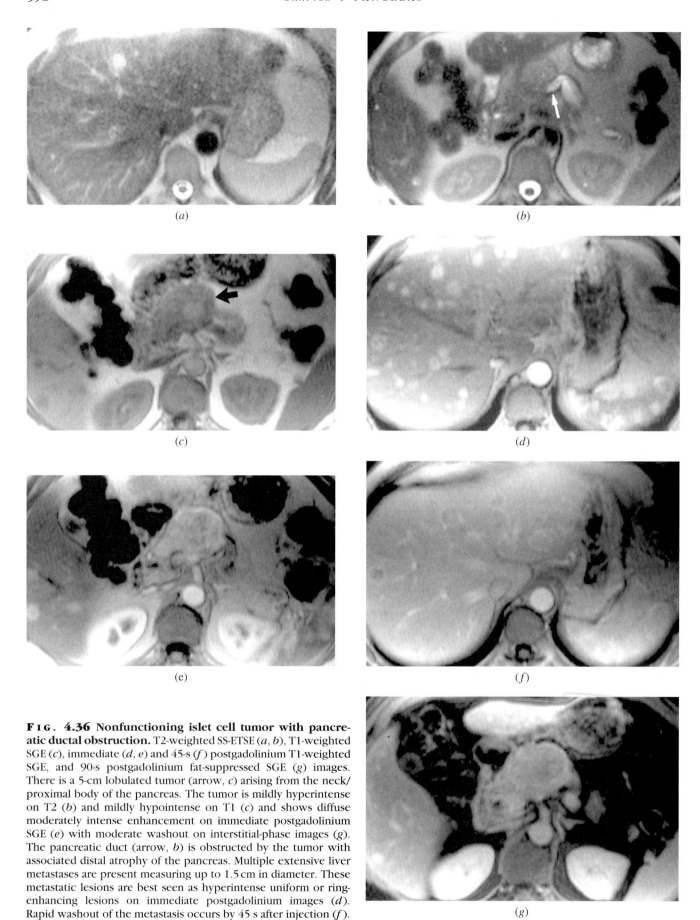

(a)

(b)

(c)

(d)

(e)

(f)

(g)

**F I G . 4.36 Nonfunctioning islet cell tumor with pancre-
atic ductal obstruction.** T2-weighted SS-ETSE (*a, b*), T1-weighted
SGE (*c*), immediate (*d, e*) and 45-s (*f*) postgadolinium T1-weighted
SGE, and 90-s postgadolinium fat-suppressed SGE (*g*) images.
There is a 5-cm lobulated tumor (arrow, *c*) arising from the neck/
proximal body of the pancreas. The tumor is mildly hyperintense
on T2 (*b*) and mildly hypointense on T1 (*c*) and shows diffuse
moderately intense enhancement on immediate postgadolinium
SGE (*e*) with moderate washout on interstitial-phase images (*g*).
The pancreatic duct (arrow, *b*) is obstructed by the tumor with
associated distal atrophy of the pancreas. Multiple extensive liver
metastases are present measuring up to 1.5 cm in diameter. These
metastatic lesions are best seen as hyperintense uniform or ring-
enhancing lesions on immediate postgadolinium images (*d*).
Rapid washout of the metastasis occurs by 45 s after injection (*f*).

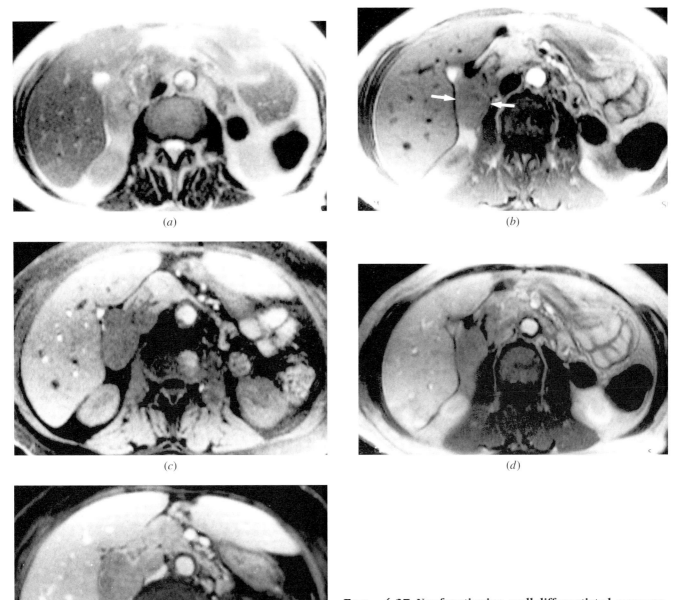

(a)   (b)

(c)   (d)

(e)

FIG. 4.37 Nonfunctioning well-differentiated neuroendocrine carcinoma. T2-weighted SS-ETSE (*a*), T1-weighted SGE (*b*), T1-weighted fat-suppressed SGE (*c*), immediate postgadolinium T1-weighted SGE (*d*), and 90-s postgadolinium fat-suppressed SGE (*e*) images. There is a exophytic mass (arrows, *b*) arising from the head of the pancreas, which is slightly hyperintense relative to the pancreas on T2 (*a*) and moderately hypointense on T1 (*b*, *c*) with mild early (*d*) and late (*e*) enhancement on gadolinium-enhanced images.

immediate postgadolinium gradient-echo images. Unlike pancreatic ductal cancer liver metastases, ill-defined perilesional enhancement is not observed with gastrinoma metastases, despite the substantial hepatic arterial blood supply of these tumors. Typically, lesions are very high in signal intensity on T2-weighted fat-suppressed images and have well-defined margins. This T2-weighted appearance may be confused with hemangiomas, which

are also moderately high signal intensity and well defined. Islet cell tumor liver metastases are differentiated from hemangiomas by their enhancement patterns. Islet cell metastases have uniform ring enhancement on immediate postgadolinium images that fades with time [53], whereas hemangiomas have discontinuous peripheral nodular enhancement on immediate postgadolinium images with centripetal progression of enhancement.

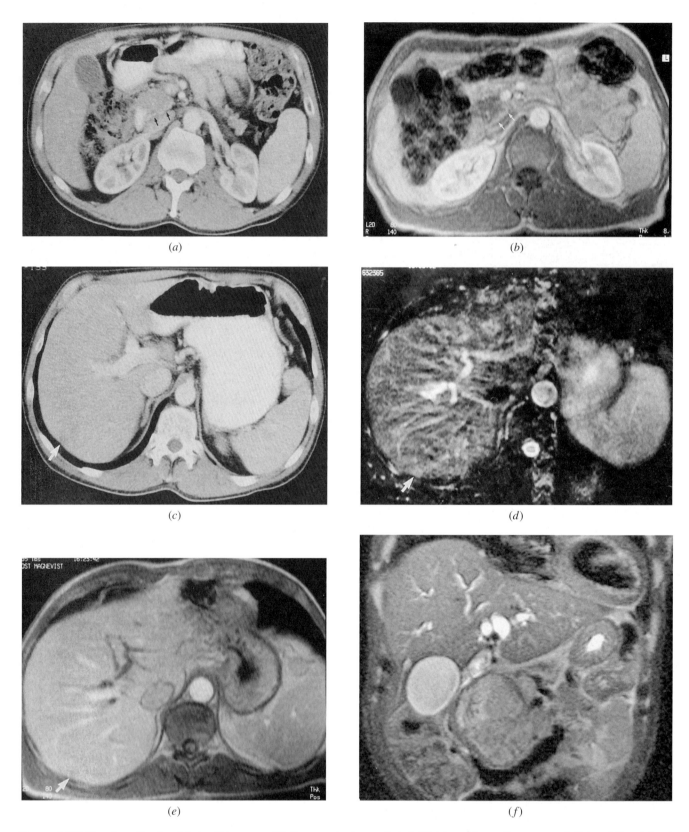

(a) *(b)* *(c)* *(d)* *(e)* *(f)*

F I G . 4.38 Nonfunctioning islet cell tumor with liver metastases. Spiral CT (*a*) and immediate postgadolinium T1-weighted SGE (*b*) images. Low-attenuation/signal intensity tumor is well shown in the head of the pancreas on both spiral CT (*a*) and MR (*b*) images. A thin rim of greater-enhancing normal pancreas is noted posterior to the tumor (small arrows, *a*, *b*). On a higher tomographic section, an ill-defined low-density lesion is noted in the liver on spiral CT image (arrow, *c*) that was considered indeterminate. On the T2-weighted fat-suppressed spin-echo image (*d*), the liver lesion is noted to be low in signal intensity (arrow, *d*), which is not consistent with cyst or hemangioma and is compatible with a hypovascular metastasis. On the 45-s postgadolinium T1-weighted SGE image (*e*), the lesion enhances in a diminished fashion with faint peripheral rim enhancement (arrow, *e*) consistent with a hypovascular metastasis. A cyst would appear nearly signal void, which would be comparable in appearance to the dilated biliary ducts on the postgadolinium image (*e*).The hypovascular nature of this primary tumor is uncommon for islet cell tumors.

Fat-suppressed coronal T2-weighted SS-ETSE (*f*), fat-suppressed T1-weighted gradient-echo (*g*), and immediate (*h*, *i*, *j*) and interstitial-phase (*k*) postgadolinium fat-suppressed T1-weighted gradient-echo images in a second patient with islet cell tumor.

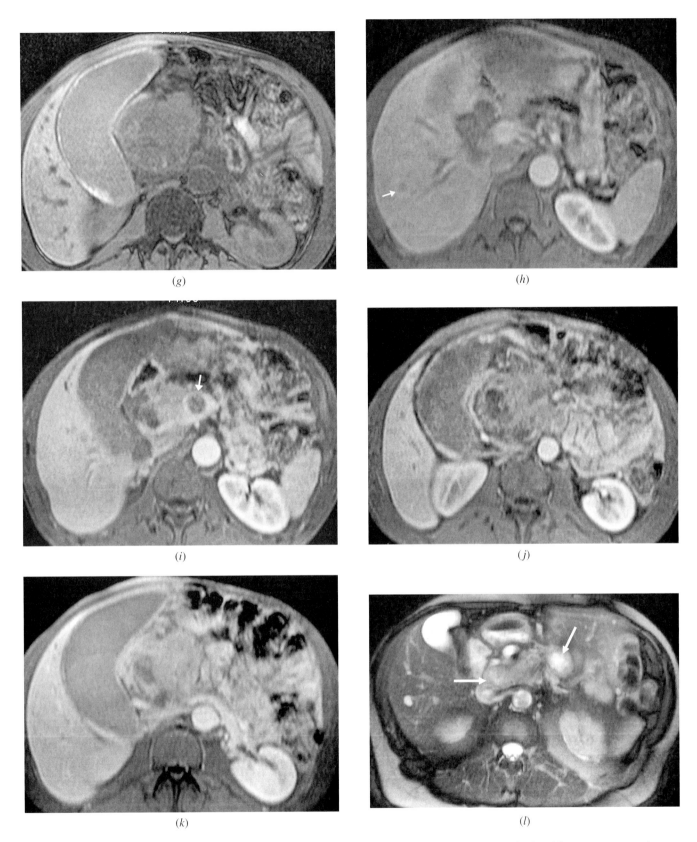

(g)

(h)

(i)

(j)

(k)

(l)

FIG. 4.38 (*Continued*) A 7-cm mass is present in the pancreatic head. The mass shows diminished and heterogeneous enhancement. Bile ducts are dilated secondary to compression by the mass. The gallbladder is markedly dilated. A ring enhancing lesion is seen in the liver on immediate postgadolinium T1-weighted image, consistent with a metastasis (arrow, *h*). The superior mesenteric artery is thrombosed (arrow, *i*).

T2-weighted fat-suppressed single-shot echo-train spin-echo (*l*) and T1-weighted postgadolinium hepatic arterial dominant phase (*m*) and hepatic venous phase (*n*) fat-suppressed 3D-GE images at 3.0 T demonstrate nonfunctioning islet cell tumors (white thick

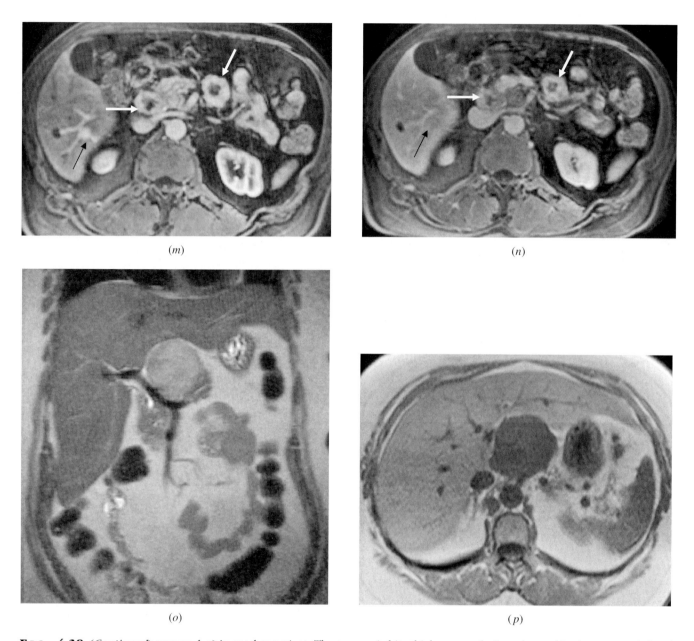

(m)

(n)

(o)

(p)

F I G . 4.38 (*Continued*) arrows, *l–n*) in another patient. The tumors (white thick arrows; *l–n*) are located in the pancreatic head and the pancreatic body. They contain central necrosis. There is also a hypervascular liver metastasis (black arrow, *m, n*) showing intense enhancement on the hepatic arterial dominant phase and fading on the hepatic venous phase. Note the liver cyst located in the right lobe of the liver.

Pancreatic schwannoma. Coronal T2-weighted fat-suppressed single-shot echo-train spin-echo (*o*), transverse T1-weighted SGE (*p*), and transverse T1-weighted postgadolinium hepatic arterial dominant phase (*q*) and hepatic venous phase (*r*) fat-suppressed 3D-GE images demonstrate a pancreatic schwannoma in another patient. The tumor is very well demarcated and shows markedly high signal on T2-weighted image like other neurogenic tumors. The tumor shows progressive heterogeneous enhancement on postgadolinium images. It is located adjacent to the portal vein and between the branches of celiac trunk. The tumor causes widening of the branches of celiac trunk.

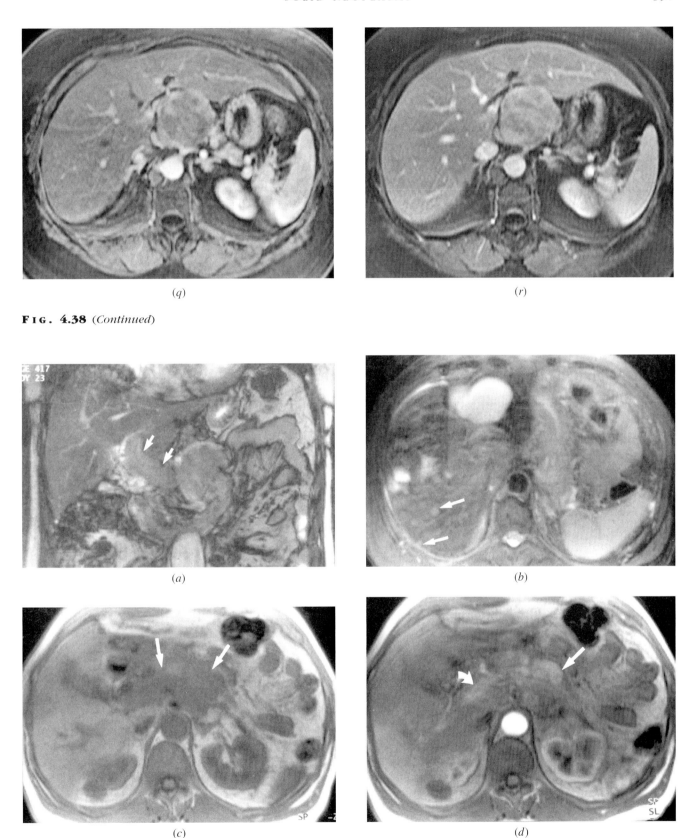

(q)

(r)

FIG. 4.38 (*Continued*)

(a)

(b)

(c)

(d)

FIG. 4.39 Nonfunctioning islet cell tumor with tumor thrombus. Coronal gradient refocused flow-sensitive gradient-echo (*a*), T2-weighted fat-suppressed SS-ETSE (*b*), T1-weighted SGE (*c*), and immediate postgadolinium T1-weighted SGE (*d*) images in a second patient. A 8 × 5-cm mass arises in the pancreatic body (arrows, *c*). Expansible tumor thrombus (arrows, *a*) extending into the intrahepatic portal vein is appreciated on the coronal flow-sensitive gradient-echo image (*a*). Liver cysts and metastases are present, with the <1-cm liver metastases (arrows, *b*) best shown on the T2-weighted image (*b*).The primary tumor exhibits diffuse moderately intense heterogeneous enhancement (arrow, *d*), and enhancement of the tumor thrombus is also appreciated (curved arrow, *d*).

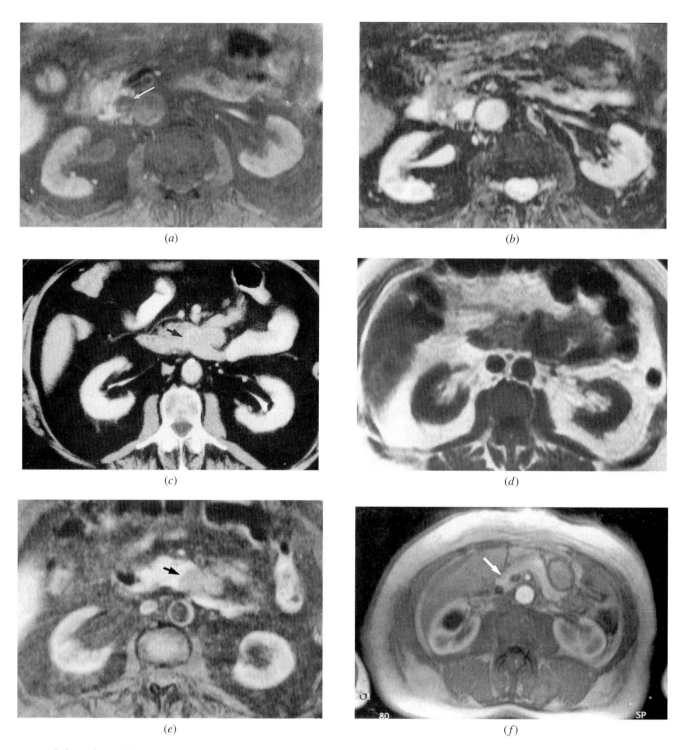

(a)

(b)

(c)

(d)

(e)

(f)

F I G . 4.40 Islet cell tumor—gastrinoma. T1-weighted fat-suppressed spin-echo (*a*) and T2-weighted fat-suppressed spin-echo (*b*) images. Islet cell tumors (arrow, *a*) are usually low in signal intensity in a background of high-signal intensity pancreas on T1-weighted fat-suppressed images (*a*) and high in signal intensity on T2-weighted images (*b*). The uncinate process is a common location for gastrinomas, because it is located in the "gastrinoma triangle."

Dynamic contrast-enhanced CT (*c*), T1-weighted SGE (*d*), and T1-weighted fat-suppressed spin-echo (*e*) images in a second patient. A 2-cm gastrinoma is present arising from the uncinate process of the pancreas (*c–e*).The tumor is most conspicuous on the T1-weighted fat-suppressed spin-echo image with a "beak" sign apparent (arrow, *e*) and was not identified on the CT examination prospectively. An enhancing rim (arrow, *c*) is apparent on the CT image.

Immediate postgadolinium SGE image (*f*) in a third patient demonstrates a 8-mm ring-enhancing tumor (arrow, *f*) in the neck of the pancreas diagnostic for a gastrinoma in the appropriate clinical setting. Gastrinomas most commonly possess uniform ring enhancement in both the primary tumor and liver metastases. This patient had two recent CT examinations that were both negative for gastrinoma.

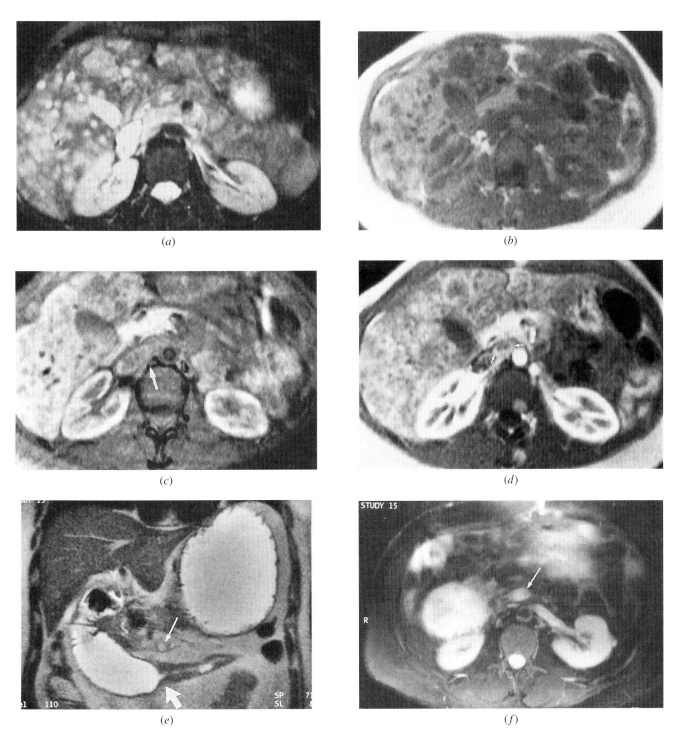

FIG. 4.41 Extrapancreatic gastrinoma. T2-weighted fat-suppressed spin-echo (*a*), T1-weighted SGE (*b*), T1-weighted fat-suppressed spin-echo (*c*), and immediate postgadolinium T1-weighted SGE (*d*) images. On the T2-weighted fat-suppressed image (*a*), multiple high-signal-intensity foci are present throughout the primary tumor, located posterior to the head of the pancreas with an appearance identical to the well-defined high-signal-intensity liver metastases. T1-weighted images (*b, c*) demonstrate the extra-pancreatic gastrinoma multiple <1.5-cm liver metastases that possess similar low signal intensity. The primary tumor (arrow, *c*) is more clearly visible on the T1-weighted fat-suppressed image (*c*) because of the good signal difference between pancreas and tumor. On the immediate postgadolinium image (*d*), multiple ring-enhancing lesions are apparent in both the primary tumor (arrows, *d*) and the liver metastases.

Coronal SS-ETSE (*e*), fat-suppressed breathing-averaged ETSE (*f*), and 90-s postgadolinium fat-suppressed T1-weighted SGE (*g*) images in a second patient demonstrate a gastrinoma (arrows, *e–g*) superior to the fourth portion of the duodenum. The mass is

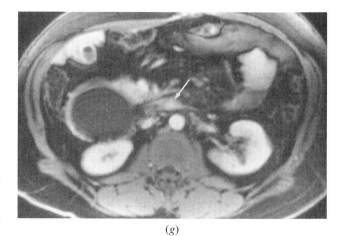

(g)

FIG. 4.41 (*Continued*) uniformly high in signal intensity on T2-weighted (*e, f*) and interstitial-phase gadolinium-enhanced T1-weighted (*g*) images. Stricturing of the fourth part of the duodenum (large arrow, *e*) reflects peptic ulcer disease in Zollinger–Ellison syndrome. Two prior CT imaging examinations were reported as negative.

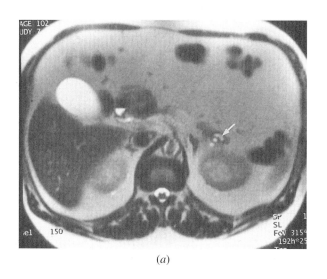

(a)

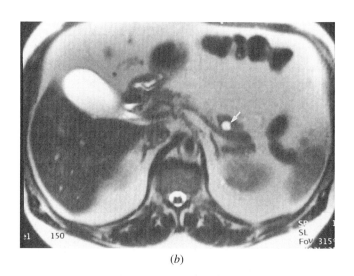

(b)

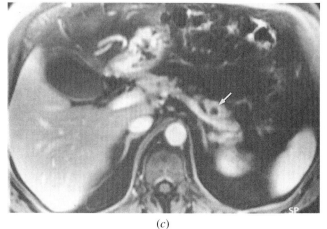

(c)

FIG. 4.42 Multiple gastrinomas. T2-weighted SS-ETSE (*a, b*) and interstitial-phase gadolinium-enhanced fat-suppressed T1-weighted SGE (*c*) images demonstrate multiple high-signal-intensity gastrinomas <1 cm in the tail of the pancreas. The absence of breathing artifact on the SS-ETSE images has resulted in good resolution of the small tumors (arrows, *a, b*). Ring enhancement is apparent on the largest 8-mm tumor (arrow, *c*).

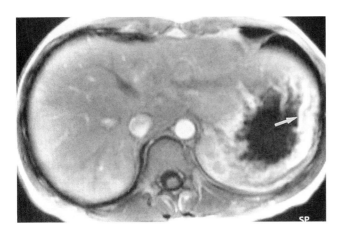

F I G . 4.43 Gastric wall hyperplasia. Immediate postgadolinium T1-weighted SGE image demonstrates intense enhancement of the prominent gastric rugal folds (arrow) in a patient with gastrinoma.

(For a discussion on hemangiomas, see Chapter 2, *Liver.*) These appearances are better shown on MR than CT images because of the higher sensitivity of MRI to contrast enhancement, faster delivery of a compact bolus of intravenous contrast, and greater imaging temporal resolution [53]. The peripheral enhancing rim may be thin or thick, resulting in differences in the degree of vascularity. Occasionally, thick rim enhancement may have a peripherally based spoke-wheel enhancement. Centripetal enhancement of gastrinoma metastases may occur on serial postgadolinium images. Peripheral washout is commonly observed for hypervascular gastrinoma metastases (fig. 4.44).

Insulinomas. Insulinomas are one of the most common islet cell tumors and are frequently functionally active. Tumors frequently come to clinical attention when they are small (<2 cm) because of the severity of the symptomatology [59]. Patients present with signs and symptoms of hypoglycemia. Insulinomas are usually richly vascular. Angiography has been reported as superior to CT imaging in detecting these tumors because of their small size and increased vascularity [65]. MRI may be superior to angiography for the detection of these tumors, reflecting the greater number of different types of data acquisition with MRI and the high sensitivity for contrast enhancement (figs. 4.45 and 4.46).

Insulinomas are low in signal intensity on T1-weighted images and high in signal intensity on T2-weighted images. They are well shown on T1-weighted fat-suppressed images (see fig. 4.45) [56]. Small insulinomas typically enhance homogeneously on immediate postgadolinium gradient-echo images (see fig. 4.45) [57]. Larger tumors, measuring more than 2 cm in diameter, often show ring enhancement. Liver metastases

from insulinomas typically have peripheral ringlike enhancement, although small metastases tend to enhance homogeneously. Enhancement of small metastases frequently occurs transiently in the capillary phase of enhancement and fades on images acquired at 1 min after injection.

Glucagonoma, Somatostatinoma, VIPoma, and ACTHoma. These islet cell tumors are considerably rarer than insulinomas or gastrinomas. They are usually malignant, with liver metastases present at the time of diagnosis (figs. 4.47 and 4.48) [51, 58, 59, 66–69]. The primary pancreatic tumors of glucagonoma and somatostatinoma are large and heterogeneous on MR images [66–69]. They are usually moderately low in signal intensity on T1-weighted fat-suppressed images and moderately high in signal intensity on T2-weighted fat-suppressed images, enhancing heterogeneously on immediate postgadolinium images (see fig. 4.47) [58]. Liver metastases are generally heterogeneous in size and shape, unlike gastrinoma metastases, which are typically uniform (see fig. 4.47) [57]. Metastases possess irregular peripheral rims of intense enhancement on immediate post-gadolinium gradient-echo images (see fig. 4.47). Peripheral spoke-wheel enhancement may be observed in liver metastases on immediate postgadolinium images (fig. 4.49). Hypervascular liver metastases are best shown on immediate postgadolinium gradient-echo images, which are superior to spiral CT images for this determination [58]. Splenic metastases are not uncommon (see fig. 4.47).

ACTHomas may present with a large, heterogeneous enhancing primary tumor and small, hypervascular liver metastases. Their appearance may resemble glucagonomas and somatostatinoma masses.

VIPoma may have a characteristic appearance of a small primary tumor despite large and extensive liver metastases (fig. 4.49). Prior case reports have described ostensibly primary VIPoma of the liver without visualization of a pancreatic primary. The possibility exists that the primary pancreatic tumor may have been extremely small and escaped detection.

Islet Cell Tumors, Untyped or Uncategorized. Islet cell tumors do not receive a specific designation when special immunohistochemical stains or serum assays are negative. Tumors are generally large at presentation because they are clinically silent. The imaging appearance of these tumors resembles glucagonomas and somatostatinomas (see figs. 4.36–4.39). Liver metastases are generally present at the time of diagnosis. Pancreatic schwannomas (fig 4.38) may mimic the appearances of islet cell tumors as well as other pancreatic malignancies.

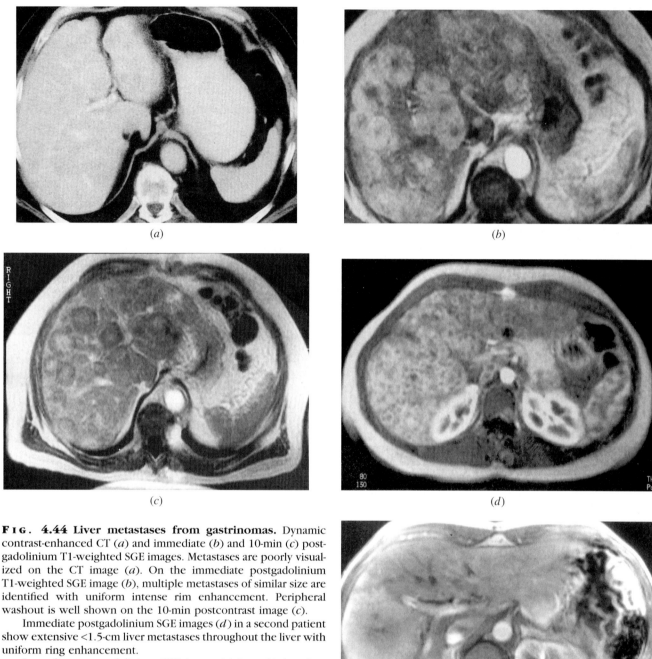

F I G. 4.44 Liver metastases from gastrinomas. Dynamic contrast-enhanced CT (*a*) and immediate (*b*) and 10-min (*c*) postgadolinium T1-weighted SGE images. Metastases are poorly visualized on the CT image (*a*). On the immediate postgadolinium T1-weighted SGE image (*b*), multiple metastases of similar size are identified with uniform intense rim enhancement. Peripheral washout is well shown on the 10-min postcontrast image (*c*).

Immediate postgadolinium SGE images (*d*) in a second patient show extensive <1.5-cm liver metastases throughout the liver with uniform ring enhancement.

Immediate postgadolinium SGE image (*e*) in a third patient show an unusual pattern for gastrinoma liver metastases with varying sized lesions with intense, almost uniform enhancement of a 5-cm metastasis. Often these large hypervascular islet cell metastases that enhance nearly uniformly on immediate postgadolinium images possess a radiating spoke-wheel pattern of bands of lesser-enhancing stroma.

Carcinoid Tumors

Rarely, carcinoid tumors may originate in the pancreas. Pancreatic carcinoids arise from the cells of the gastro-enteropancreatic neuroendocrine system [53]. Carcinoid tumors are generally large at presentation, with coexistent liver metastases (fig. 4.50). Focal and diffuse involvements of the pancreas have been observed. Tumors are generally mildly hypointense on T1 and moderately hyperintense on T2 and show diffuse heterogeneous enhancement on immediate postgadolinium images (fig. 4.51) [53]. Enhancement of the primary tumor may be mild, despite extensive enhancement of

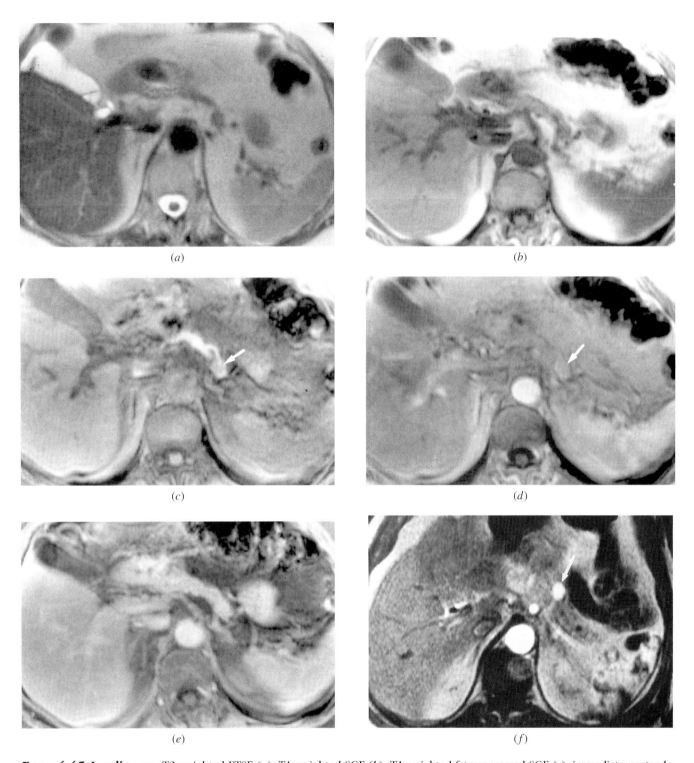

(a)

(b)

(c)

(d)

(e)

(f)

F I G . 4.45 Insulinoma. T2-weighted ETSE (*a*), T1-weighted SGE (*b*), T1-weighted fat-suppressed SGE (*c*), immediate postgado-linium T1-weighted SGE (*d*), and 90-s postgadolinium fat-suppressed SGE (*e*) images. A 1-cm tumor (arrow, *c*) arising in the superior aspect of the midbody of the pancreas is isointense on T2 (*a*) and T1 (*b*)-weighted images and low signal on T1-weighted fat-suppressed image (*c*) and enhances intensely and homogeneously (arrow, *d*) on the immediate postgadolinium image. The lesion fades to isointensity with background pancreas (*e*).

Immediate postgadolinium T1 SGE image (*f*) demonstrates a 1.2-cm uniformly enhancing insulinoma (arrow) arising from the body of the pancreas.

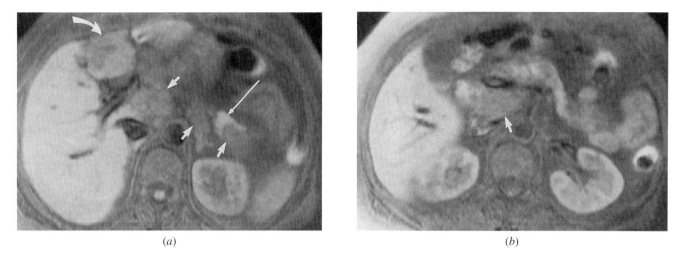

(a)   (b)

F I G . 4.46 Multiple malignant insulinomas. T1-weighted fat-suppressed spin-echo images (*a, b*). Multiple low-signal intensity insulinomas (arrows, *a, b*) ranging in diameter from 1 to 5 cm are present throughout the pancreas. Intervening pancreatic tissue is noted to be normal in signal intensity (long arrow, *a*). Liver metastases are also present (curved arrow, *a*). Multiple insulinomas are uncommon, occurring in <10% of all cases of B cell tumors.

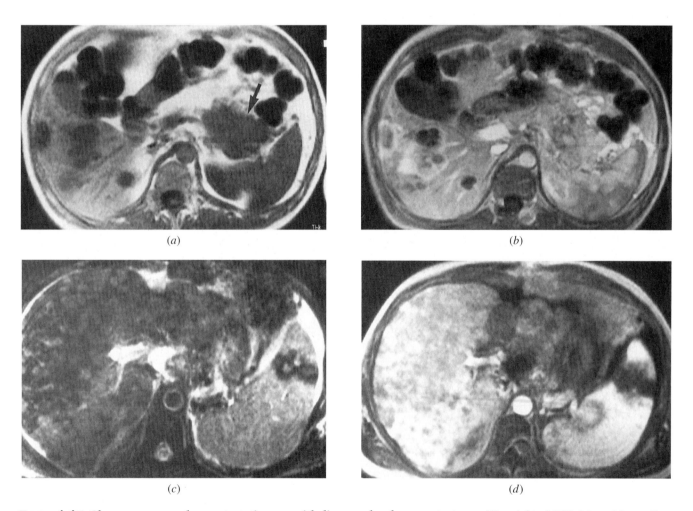

(a)   (b)

(c)   (d)

F I G . 4.47 Glucagonoma and somatostatinoma with liver and spleen metastases. T1-weighted SGE (*a*) and immediate postgadolinium T1-weighted SGE (*b*) images. A 6-cm tumor (arrow, *a*) arises from the tail of the pancreas (*a*). Multiple liver metastases are present, which are low in signal intensity on the precontrast T1-weighted image (*a*). On the immediate postgadolinium T1-weighted SGE image (*b*), the primary tumor enhances heterogeneously. Intense ring enhancement is present in many of the liver metastases, reflecting hypervascularity. Note that the liver metastases are variable in size and shape.

T2-weighted fat-suppressed SS-ETSE (*c*) and immediate postgadolinium T1-weighted SGE (*d*) images. On the T2-weighted image (*c*), multiple small, high-signal-intensity liver metastases and a large, low-signal-intensity splenic metastasis are present. On the immediate postgadolinium image (*d*), the liver metastases enhance intensely and the splenic metastasis is low in signal intensity.

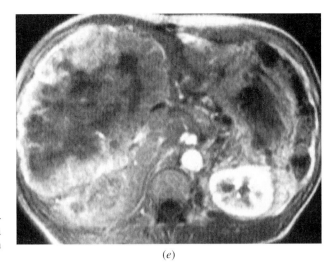

(e)

FIG. 4.47 (*Continued*) Immediate postgadolinium T1-weighted SGE image (*e*) in a second patient with somatostatinoma demonstrates a 14-cm liver metastasis with intense, irregular rim enhancement.

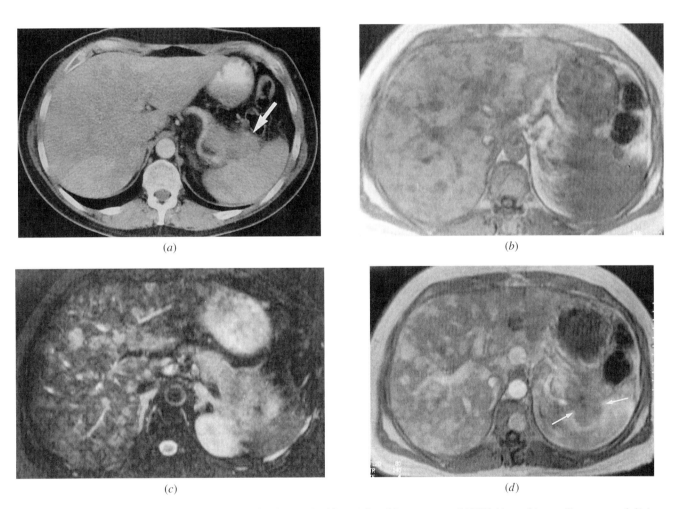

(a)

(b)

(c)

(d)

FIG. 4.48 ACTHoma. Spiral CT (*a*), T1-weighted SGE (*b*), T2-weighted fat-suppressed ETSE (*c*), and immediate postgadolinium T1-weighed SGE (*d*) images. A 4-cm ACTHoma is present in the tail of the pancreas (arrow, *a*). Direct extension of the primary tumor into the spleen is most clearly shown on the immediate postgadolinium T1-weighted SGE image (arrows, *d*). Multiple liver metastases are present, which are poorly seen on the spiral CT image (*a*) but are well shown on the MR images (*b–d*). Liver metastases are most conspicuous on the immediate postgadolinium T1-weighted SGE image (*d*). (Reproduced with permission from Kelekis NL, Semelka RC, Molina PL, Doerr ME: ACTH-secreting islet cell tumor: Appearances on dynamic gadolinium-enhanced MRI. *Magn Reson Imaging* 13: 641–644, 1995.)

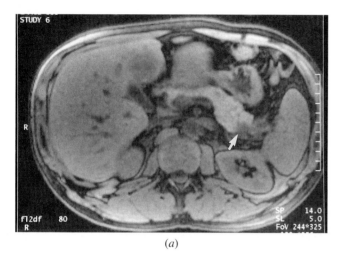

(a)

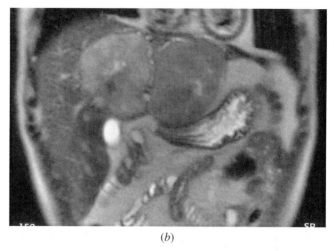

(b)

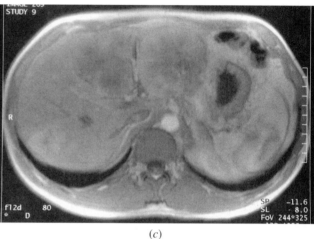

(c)

FIG. 4.49 VIPoma. T1-weighted fat-suppressed SGE (*a*), coronal T2-weighted SS-ETSE (*b*), and immediate postgadolinium T1-weighted SGE (*c*) images in a patient with VIPoma. A 1.5-cm tumor arises from the tail of the pancreas (arrow, *a*) that appears low in signal intensity on the T1-weighted image. Multiple metastases are present that are moderately low signal intensity on the T1-weighted image (*a*) and moderately high signal intensity on the T2-weighted image (*b*) and enhance in a moderately intense peripheral spoke-wheel type radial fashion on the immediate postgadolinium T1-weighted SGE image (*c*).

liver metastases. Liver metastases are variable in size and often exhibit intense enhancement, similar to islet cell tumor liver metastases.

CYSTIC NEOPLASMS

In general, this group of pancreatic tumors arises from the exocrine component of the gland and is much less common than solid exocrine carcinomas. Although secondary cystic change can be seen in most types of pancreatic neoplasms, cystic pancreatic neoplasms are characterized by their consistent, invariably present, cystic configuration.

Serous Cystadenoma

Serous cystadenoma is a benign neoplasm characterized by numerous tiny serous fluid-filled cysts [70]. Serous cystadenomas are usually microcystic and multilocular, and consist of multiple small cysts less than 1 cm in diameter (fig. 4.52). Uncommonly, serous cystadenomas

may be macrocystic (cysts measuring from 1 to 8 cm) including multilocular, oligolocular or unilocular subtypes. This tumor frequently occurs in older patients and has an increased association with von Hippel–Lindau disease [70].

Microcystic serous cystadenoma is well demarcated and occasionally contains a central fibrotic scar. Tumors range in size from 1 to 12 cm, with an average diameter at presentation of 5 cm. The lesion may exhibit either a smooth or a nodular contour. On cut surface, small, closely packed cysts are filled with clear, watery (serous) fluid and separated by fine, fibrous septae, creating a honeycomb appearance. Calcifications may occasionally be present. On MR images, the tumors are well-defined and do not demonstrate invasion of fat or adjacent organs [71]. On T2-weighted images, the small cysts and intervening septations may be well shown as a cluster of small grapelike high-signal-intensity cysts. This appearance is more clearly shown on breath-hold or breathing-independent sequences such as single-shot echo-train spin echo, because the thin septations blur with longer-duration non-breath-hold sequence

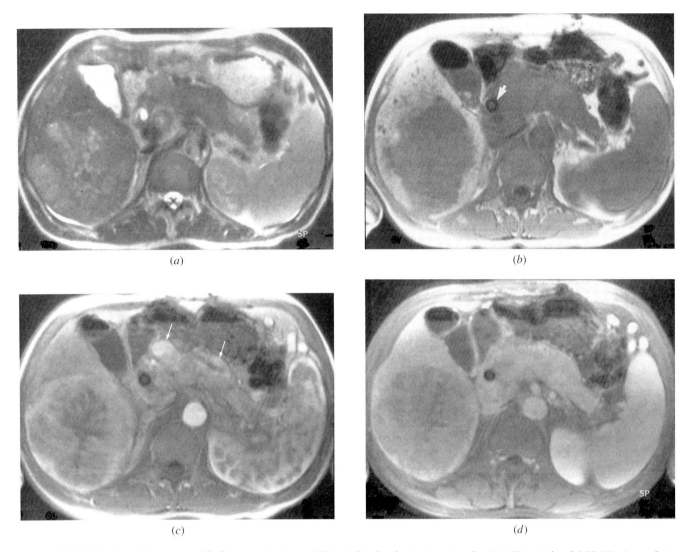

(a)　　　　　(b)

(c)　　　　　(d)

F I G . 4.50 Carcinoid tumor with liver metastases. T2-weighted echo-train spin-echo (*a*), T1-weighted SGE (*b*), immediate postgadolinium T1-weighted SGE (*c*), and 90-s postgadolinium fat-suppressed SGE (*d*) images in a patient with a carcinoid tumor with diffuse involvement of the pancreas and hypervascular liver metastasis. The pancreas is diffusely enlarged with irregular contour and enhances heterogeneously on the immediate postgadolinium image (arrows, *c*). The metastatic liver lesion shows a radial enhancement on gadolinium-enhanced images (*c, d*). Note a biliary stent in the CBD (arrow, *b*).

(fig. 4.52). Relatively thin uniform septations and absence of infiltration of adjacent organs and structures are features that distinguish serous cystadenoma from serous cystadenocarcinoma (see fig. 4.52). Tumor septations usually enhance minimally with gadolinium on early and late postcontrast images, although moderate enhancement on early postcontrast images may occur. Delayed enhancement of the central scar may occasionally be observed [1], and is more typical of large tumors. Delayed enhancement of the central scar on postgadolinium images is apparent in larger tumors, and this enhancement pattern is typical for fibrous tissue in general (see fig. 4.52). The central scar may represent compressed contiguous cyst walls of centrally located cysts.

Macrocystic serous cystadenomas (fig. 4.53) exhibit distinctly different macroscopic features from microcystic lesions and may pose diagnostic difficulties for both radiologist and pathologist. A computed tomography study evaluating these tumors misinterpreted all five cases as mucinous cystic neoplasms or pseudocysts. Microcystic and macrocystic serous tumors represent morphologic variants of the same benign pancreatic neoplasm [71, 72]. They are well demarcated tumors. They have high signal intensity on T2-weighted images and low signal on T1-weighted images. They may be multilocular, oligolocular or unilocular. The cyst wall and septations demonstrate progressive mild to moderate enhancement on postgadolinium T1-weighted images. The central scar is usually absent.

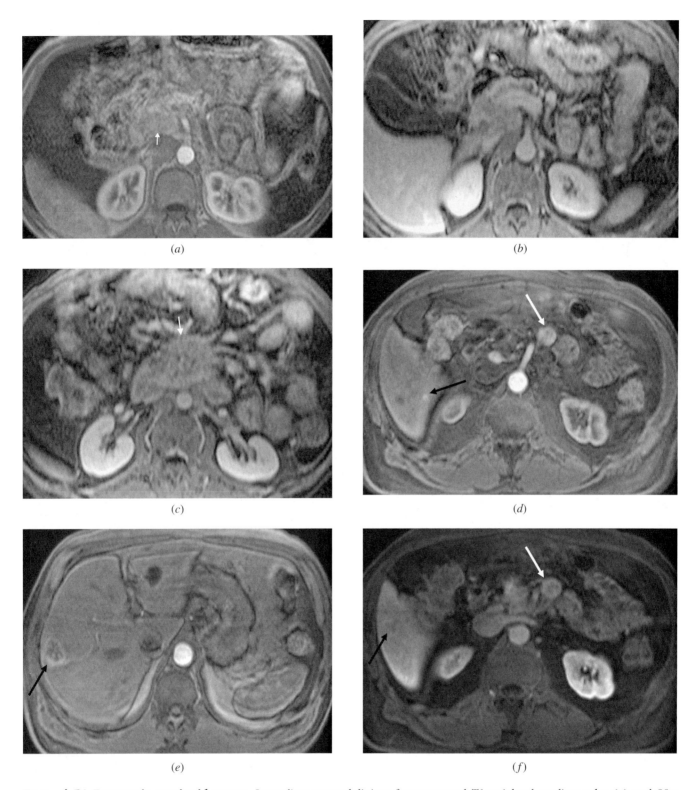

FIG. 4.51 Pancreatic carcinoid tumor. Immediate postgadolinium fat-suppressed T1-weighted gradient-echo (*a*) and 90-s postgadolinium fat-suppressed T1-weighted 3D gradient-echo (*b*, *c*) images from one patient show a large mass arising from the head of the pancreas (arrow, *a*). The mass enhances in a diminished fashion on immediate postgadolinium image (*a*), and "a" pancreatic tumor and a large mesenteric mass (arrow, *c*) are shown on interstitial-phase images. The presence of an associated large mesenteric mass is typical for carcinoid tumors. Lack of pancreatic duct dilation and atrophy of the body of the pancreas in the setting of a large pancreatic head mass are typical of a neuroendocrine tumor and not consistent with pancreatic ductal cancer.

T1-weighted postgadolinium late hepatic arterial phase fat-suppressed 3D-GE (*d*, *e*) and hepatic venous phase fat-suppressed 3D-GE (*f*) images at 3.0 T demonstrate a carcinoid tumor in another patient. The carcinoid tumor (white arrows, *d*, *f*), which shows intense heterogeneous enhancement, is located in the pancreatic body. There are also hypervascular metastases (black arrows, *d–f*) in the liver. Note that there is a liver cyst in the left lobe of the liver.

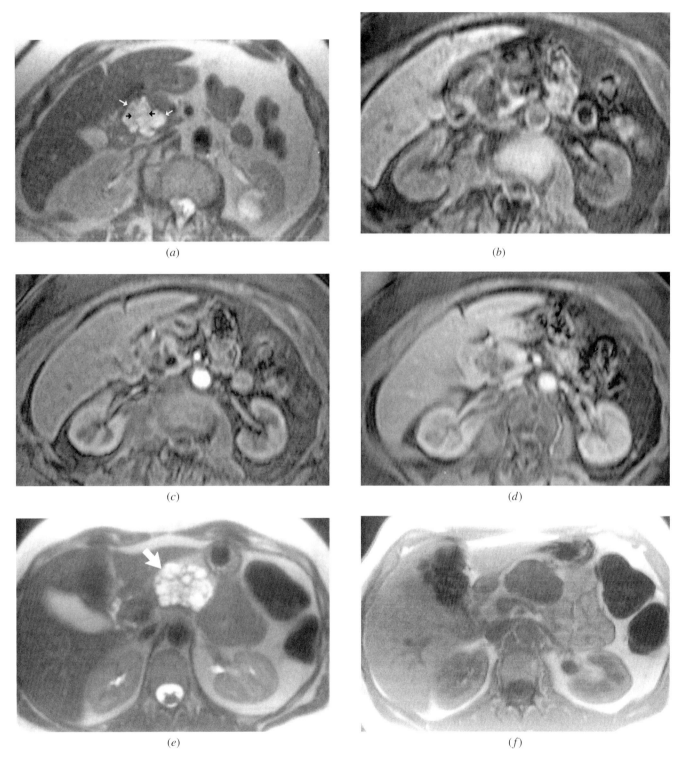

F I G . 4.52 Serous cystadenoma. T2-weighted SS-ETSE (*a*), fat-suppressed T1-weighted gradient-echo (*b*), and immediate (*c*) and interstitial-phase (*d*) postgadolinium fat-suppressed T1-weighted gradient-echo images demonstrate a cystic mass in the pancreatic head. The lesion is well defined and low in signal intensity in a background of high-signal-intensity pancreas. On the T2-weighted image (*a*), definition of fine septations (black arrows, *a*) within the cystic mass (white arrows, *a*) reveals that the cysts are <1 cm in diameter. The serous cystadenoma is high in signal intensity on T2-weighted images (*a*), reflecting their high fluid content.

T2-weighted SS-ETSE (*e*), T1-weighted SGE (*f*), T1-weighted fat-suppressed SGE (*g*), immediate postgadolinium T1-weighted SGE (*h*), and 90-s postgadolinium fat-suppressed SGE (*i*) images in a second patient. There is a 6-cm multicystic mass (arrows, *e*)

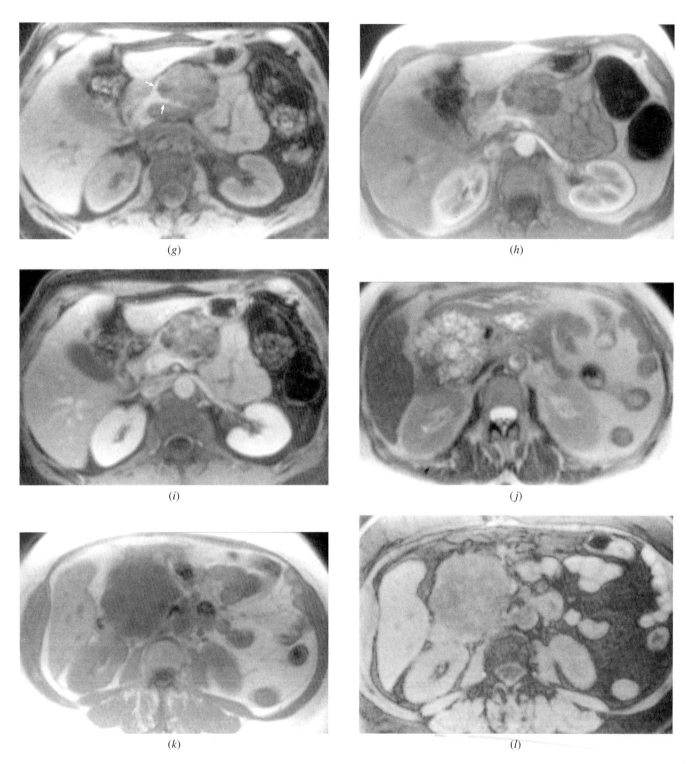

(g)

(h)

(i)

(j)

(k)

(l)

F I G . 4.52 (*Continued*) arising in the pancreatic body with thin septations creating <2-cm cysts. The single-shot T2-weighted sequence (*e*) performs very well at defining the septations in cystic masses. A "beak sign" is demonstrated in the pancreas (arrows, *g*), best shown on the noncontrast T1-weighted fat-suppressed (*g*) and immediate postgadolinium SGE (*h*) images, confirming that the mass originates from this organ. The septations enhance minimally on immediate postgadolinium images (*h*) with progressive enhancement on late images (*i*).

T2-weighted ETSE (*j*), T1-weighted SGE (*k*), T1-weighted fat-suppressed SGE (*l*), immediate postgadolinium T1-weighted SGE (*m*), and 90-s postgadolinium fat-suppressed SGE (*n*) images in a third patient. An 8-cm serous cystadenoma is present in the head

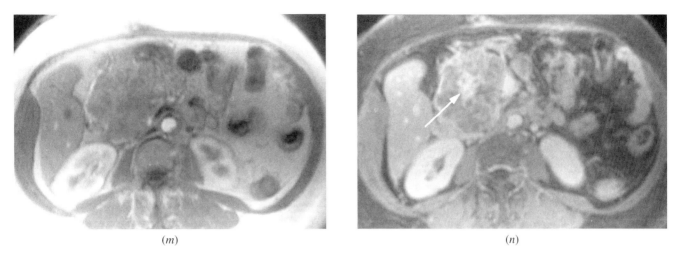

(m)   (n)

F I G . 4.52 (*Continued*) of the pancreas, best shown on the single-shot T2-weighted sequence. There is a central scar, typical for serous cystadenoma, which enhances on late images (arrow, *n*), consistent with fibrosis. Serous cystadenomas occur predominantly in women, as seen in these cases. The importance of the MR study is to differentiate this benign entity from mucinous cystadenomas that are potentially malignant.

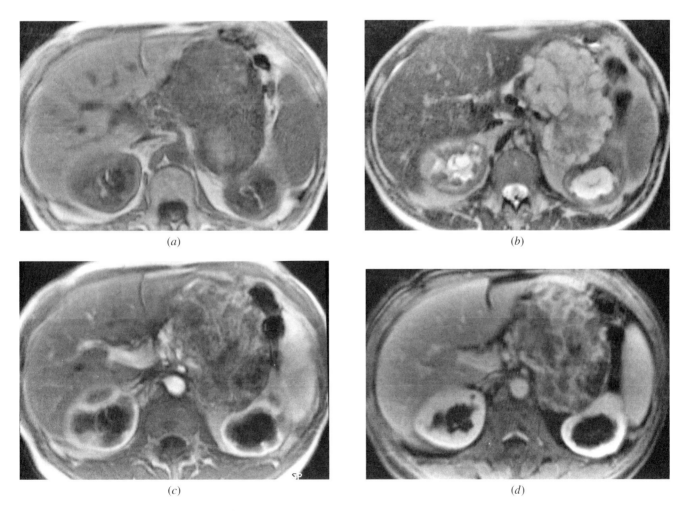

(a)   (b)

(c)   (d)

F I G . 4.53 Macrocystic serous cystadenoma. T1-weighted SGE (*a*), T2-weighted SS-ETSE (*b*), immediate postgadolinium T1-weighted SGE (*c*), and 90-s postgadolinium fat-suppressed SGE (*d*) images. A 10-cm mass arises from the tail of the pancreas. The tumor is mildly hypointense with regions of hyperintensity on precontrast T1-weighted images (*a*). Multiple septations are present throughout the mass, well shown on the breathing-independent T2-weighted image (*b*). Some of the cysts measure >2cm. Moderately intense enhancement of the septations is present on immediate (*c*) and 90-s (*d*) postcontrast images.

Cystic pancreatic masses that contain cysts measuring less than 1 cm in diameter may represent microcystic cystadenoma or side branch type intraductal papillary mucinous tumor (IPMT), which can be difficult to distinguish. The presence of a central scar is a feature distinguishing serous cystadenoma from side branch IPMT, which does not exhibit this finding. Definition of communication with the pancreatic duct on MRCP images establishes the diagnosis of side branch IPMT.

Serous Cystadenocarcinoma

This malignant pancreatic tumor is extremely rare. Distinction from benign serous cystadenoma is difficult on histologic grounds alone and may only be established by the presence of metastatic disease or local invasion. The presence of thick septations and solid components are suggestive signs for serous cystadenocarcinoma.

Mucinous Cystadenoma / Cystadenocarcinoma

Mucinous cystic neoplasms of the pancreas are characterized by the formation of large unilocular or multilocular cysts filled with abundant, thick gelatinous mucin. Histopathologically these tumors are divided into benign (mucinous cystadenoma), borderline, and malignant (mucinous cystadenocarcinoma). However, at many institutions, all cases of mucinous cystic neoplasms are interpreted as mucinous cystadenocarcinomas of low-grade malignant potential to reinforce the need for complete surgical resection and close clinical follow up [70–75]. Mucinous cystic neoplasms occur

more frequently in females (6 to 1), and approximately 50% occur in patients between the ages of 40 and 60 years [76]. These tumors usually are located in the body and tail of the pancreas. They may be large (mean diameter of 10 cm), often multiloculated, and encapsulated [74, 75]. Of these tumors, 10% may have scattered calcifications. There is a great propensity for invasion of local organs and tissues.

On gadolinium-enhanced T1-weighted fat-suppressed images, large, irregular cystic spaces separated by septa are demonstrated [1]. Cyst walls and septations are often thicker in mucinous cystadenocarcinomas than those of mucinous cystadenomas. Mucinous cystadenomas are well circumscribed, and they show no evidence of metastases or invasion of adjacent tissues (fig. 4.54). Mucinous cystadenomas described pathologically as having borderline malignant potential may be very large, but may not show imaging or gross evidence of metastases or local invasion (fig. 4.55). Histopathologically, these tumors show moderate epithelial dysplasia. Mucinous cystadenocarcinoma may be very locally aggressive malignancies with extensive invasion of adjacent tissues and organs (fig. 4.56). Absence of demonstration of tumor invasion into surrounding tissue does not, however, exclude malignancy. The presence of solid component is also suggestive of malignancy. The higher inherent soft-tissue contrast of MRI compared to CT imaging results in superior differentiation between microcystic and macrocystic cystadenomas because of sharp definition of cysts that permits evaluation of cyst size and margins [74]. Breathing-independent T2-weighted images are particularly effective at defining the cysts.

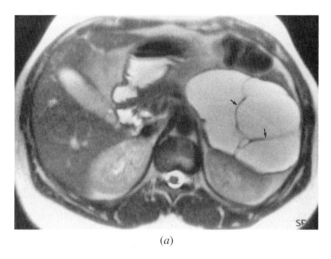
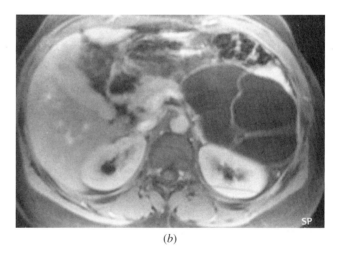

(a)   (b)

F I G. 4.54 Mucinous (macrocystic) cystadenoma. T2-weighted SS-ETSE (*a*) and 90-s postgadolinium fat-suppressed T1-weighed SGE (*b*) images. A well-defined cystic mass arises from the body and tail of the pancreas that is low in signal intensity on the T1-weighted image (not shown) and high in signal intensity on the T2-weighted image (*a*) and demonstrates enhancement of septations on the postgadolinium T1-weighted SGE image (*b*). No evidence of tumor nodules, invasion of adjacent tissue, or liver metastases is appreciated. The uniform thickness of the septations is clearly defined on the breathing-independent SS-ETSE image (arrows, *a*). Mucinous cystadenoma is potentially a low-grade malignant neoplasm.

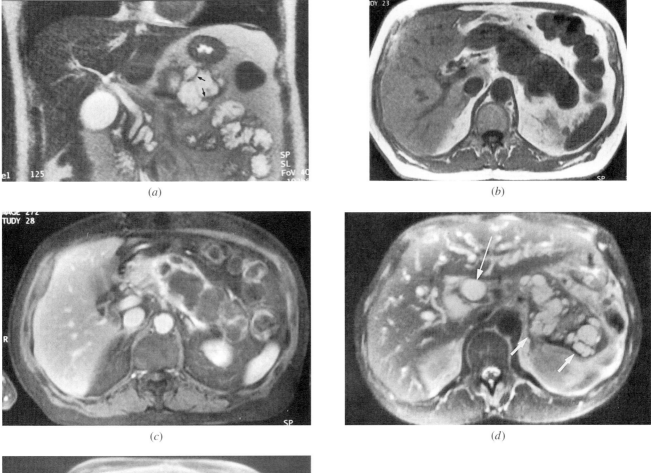

(a)

(b)

(c)

(d)

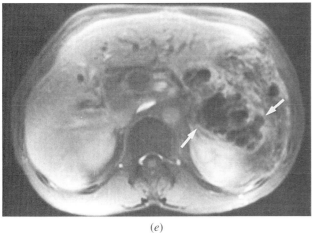

(e)

FIG. 4.55 Mucinous cystadenoma with carcinoma in situ.
Coronal T2-weighted SS-ETSE (*a*), T1-weighted SGE (*b*), and 90-s
postgadolinium fat-suppressed SGE (*c*) images. A multicystic mass
involves the entire body and tail of the pancreas (*a–c*). Septations
are well defined on the breathing-independent T2-weighted image
(arrows, *a*). The moderate irregularity of the septations and the
extent of tumor are features compatible with malignant changes.

T2-weighted SS-ETSE (*d*) and 90-s postgadolinium fat-
suppressed T1-weighted SGE (*e*) images in a second patient demonstrate a mucinous cystadenocarcinoma in the body and tail
(arrows, *d*, *e*). Dilatation of the CBD (long arrow, *d*) and intrahepatic biliary tree are also present.

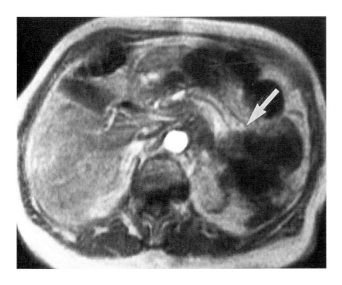

FIG. 4.56 Mucinous cystadenocarcinoma. Immediate postgadolinium T1-weighted SGE image demonstrates a tumor arising
from the tail of the pancreas (arrow) that contains thick septations
and multiple large cysts. The tumor is locally aggressive and
invades into the splenic hilum (not shown).

Mucin produced by these tumors may result in high signal intensity on T1- and T2-weighted images of the primary tumor and liver metastases (figs. 4.57 and 4.58). Liver metastases are generally hypervascular and have intense ring enhancement on immediate gadolinium images. Metastases are commonly cystic and may contain mucin, which results in mixed low and high signal intensity on T1- and T2-weighted images (see fig. 4.58).

Intraductal Papillary Mucinous Neoplasms (Duct-Ectatic Mucin-Producing Tumor)

Intraductal papillary mucinous neoplasms (IPMN) arise in the pancreatic duct epithelium. The lesions can represent a spectrum of abnormalities from simple hyperplasia to dysplasia, papillary adenoma and carcinoma.

This spectrum of abnormalities may coexist. In general hyperplasia, dysplasia and adenoma may undergo malignant transformation and transform into carcinoma; however, these carcinomas have low grade malignancies. Hyperplastic, dysplastic or malignant epithelial lining proliferates and forms papillary projections that protrude into and expand the main pancreatic duct or side branch ducts. Duct obstruction is secondary to tenacious plugs of mucin, elaborated by the epithelium, or ductal compression by cystic masses [77]. Intraductal papillary mucinous neoplasms may be classified into main duct and side branch duct types.

IPMN—Main Duct Type

These tumors are rare. Main pancreatic duct involvement presents as diffuse ductal dilatation, copious mucin production, and papillary growth. These tumors are rare and typically malignant [78]. Clinically these

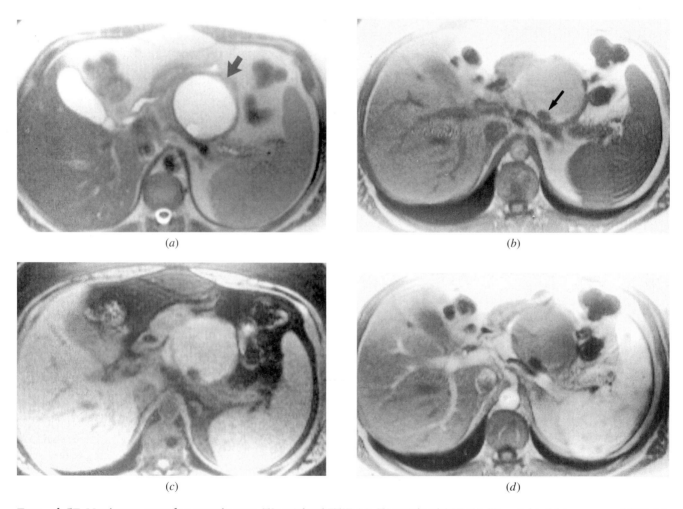

(a)

(b)

(c)

(d)

FIG. 4.57 Mucinous cystadenocarcinoma. T2-weighted ETSE (*a*), T1-weighted SGE (*b*), T1-weighted fat-suppressed SGE (*c*), immediate postgadolinium T1-weighted SGE (*d*), and 90-s postgadolinium fat-suppressed SGE (*e*) images. There is a large cystic

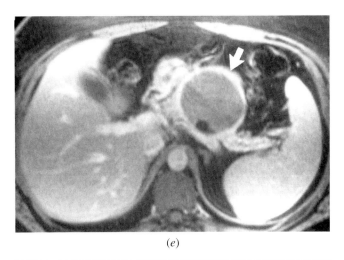

(e)

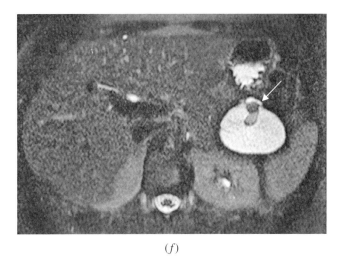

(f)

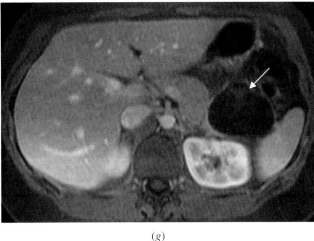

(g)

FIG. 4.57 (*Continued*) mass (arrow, *a*) arising from the pancreatic body, which has a thickened and slightly irregular wall, which demonstrates increased enhancement (arrow, *e*) on interstitial-phase gadolinium-enhanced fat-suppressed images. The cyst is high in signal on T1-weighted images (*b*, *c*), reflecting the presence of high protein content from mucin. The cyst contains a smaller cystic structure (arrow, *b*).

T2-weighted short-tau inversion recovery (STIR) (*f*) and hepatic venous phase fat-suppressed 3D-GE (*g*) images demonstrate mucinous cystadenocarcinoma in another patient. The lesion is a large cystic mass originating from the pancreatic tail. It has a complex structure containing thin septations and internal cystic structures (arrows, *f*, *g*). These internal cystic structures have low signal on T2-weighted image and intermediate signal on postgadolinium image because of their high protein content. While the internal cystic structures do not show appreciable enhancement, the wall of the large cyst shows enhancement.

tumors may result in large volumes of mucin production, which can be appreciated by direct inspection at ERCP investigation.

On MR images, a greatly expanded main pancreatic duct is demonstrated on T2-weighted images or MRCP images (fig. 4.59). Irregular-enhancing tissue along the ductal epithelium is appreciated on post-gadolinium images, confirming that underlying tumor is the cause of the ductal dilatation. Total resection is the treatment for this kind of tumor involving the whole main duct. Local resection may be sufficient for the treatment of tumors involving a segment of the main duct.

IPMN—Side-Branch Type

Intraductal papillary mucinous neoplasms involving predominantly side branch ducts appear as oval-shaped cystic masses in proximity to the main pancreatic duct. Septations are generally present, creating a cluster of grapes appearance. Side-branch type IPMN is usually

a benign process that appears as a localized cystic parenchymal lesion. The majority of side-branch IPMN tumors are located in the head of the pancreas. Unlike the main branch type, side-branch IPMNs are not rare. MRCP images are able to show communication of the cystic tumor with the main pancreatic duct in the majority of cases (figs. 4.60 and 4.61) [73, 79–82]. Another feature distinguishing from microcystic cystadenoma is that central compacted septations are not present in IPMNs.

Side-branch IPMNs which are less than 2.5 cm in size are usually benign and grow very slowly. In our clinical experience, these kind of side-branch IPMNs also pursue a very nonaggressive, indolent course. Annual repeat MRI studies may be the best approach to following these patients, compared to more interventional forms of diagnosis and therapy, especially in elderly patients. Unless these lesions appear to contain soft tissue stromal elements, grow rapidly or more

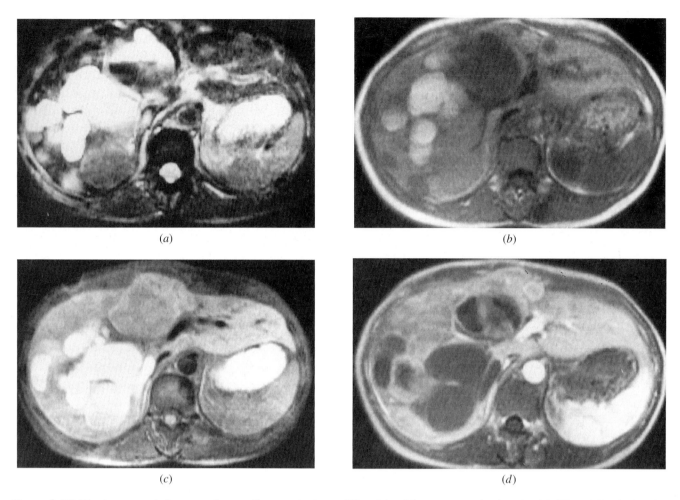

(a)   (b)

(c)   (d)

F I G . 4.58 Mucinous cystadenocarcinoma liver metastases. T2-weighted fat-suppressed spin-echo (*a*), T1-weighted SGE (*b*), T1-weighted fat-suppressed spin-echo (*c*), and immediate postgadolinium T1-weighted SGE (*d*) images. Multiple metastases are present throughout the liver that are mixed low and high signal intensity on T1-weighted (*b*, *c*) and T2-weighted (*a*) images. This appearance is consistent with the presence of mucin in these tumors. On the immediate postgadolinium image (*d*), enhancement of the walls of the cysts is appreciated.

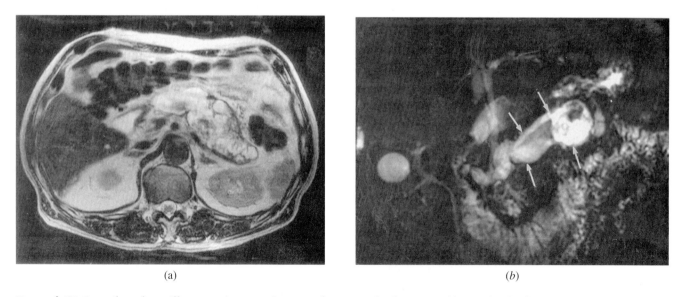

(a)   (b)

F I G . 4.59 Intraductal papillary mucin secreting neoplasm—main duct type. T2-weighted echo-train spin-echo (*a*), thick-slab MRCP (*b*), immediate postgadolinium fat-suppressed SGE (*c*), and interstitial-phase gadolinium-enhanced fat-suppressed

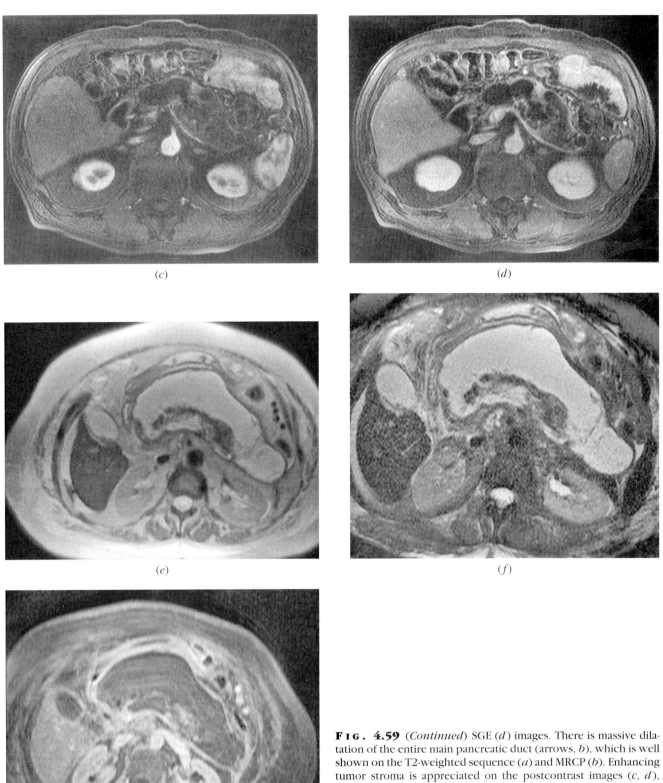

(c)

(d)

(e)

(f)

(g)

FIG. 4.59 (*Continued*) SGE (*d*) images. There is massive dila-tation of the entire main pancreatic duct (arrows, *b*), which is well shown on the T2-weighted sequence (*a*) and MRCP (*b*). Enhancing tumor stroma is appreciated on the postcontrast images (*c, d*), with progressive enhancement on the later interstitial-phase images (*d*). (Courtesy of Masayuki Kanematsu, M.D., Gifu University School of Medicine, Japan.)

T2-weighted SS-ETSE (*e*), fat-suppressed T2-weighted SS-ETSE (*f*), and interstitial phase post-gadolinium fat-suppressed T1-weighted gradient echo (*g*) images in a second patient with main duct type intraductal papillary mucin secreting neoplasm demon-strate similar findings.

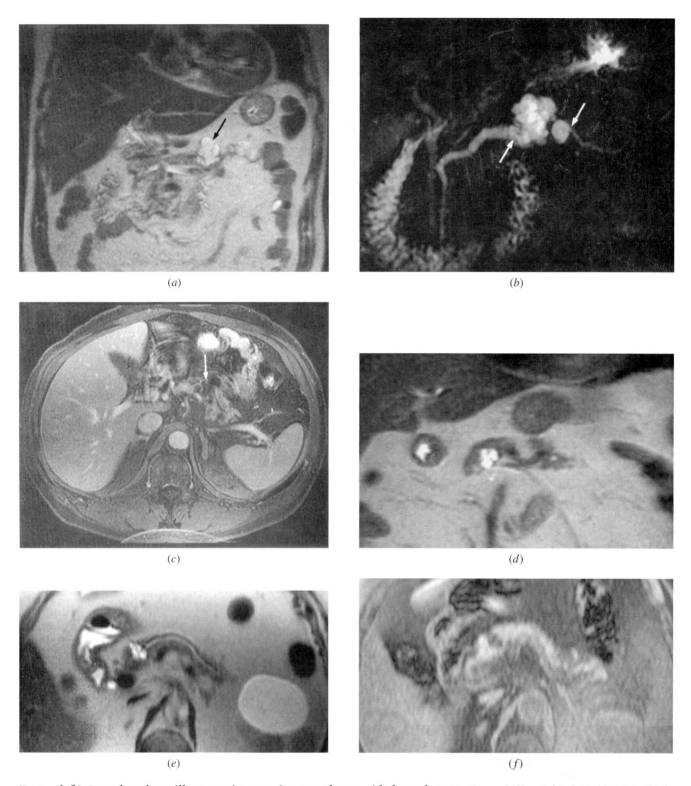

F I G . 4.60 Intraductal papillary mucin-secreting neoplasm—side-branch type. Coronal T2-weighted SS-ETSE (*a*), thick-section MRCP (*b*), and interstitial-phase gadolinium-enhanced fat-suppressed SGE (*c*) images in a patient with branch-type intraductal mucin-producing papillary neoplasm. There are clusters of multiple small cysts (arrow, *a*) in the pancreatic body, which exhibit communication with the main pancreatic duct. Communication with the main duct is well shown on the MRCP image. No apparent tumor stroma (arrow, *c*) is appreciated on postgadolinium images. Branch duct type tumor usually shows cystic paren-chymal lesions and tends to be less aggressive than the main ductal type. (Courtesy of Masayuki Kanematsu, M.D., Gifu University School of Medicine, Japan.) Coronal (*d*) and axial (*e*) T2-weighted SS-ETSE, fat-suppressed T1-weighted gradient-echo (*f*), and

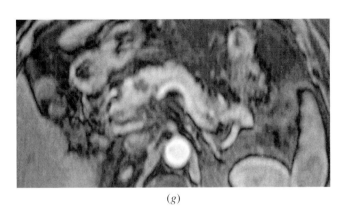

(g)

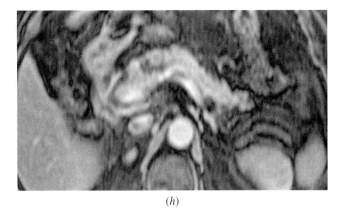

(h)

F I G . 4.60 (*Continued*) immediate (*g*) and interstitial-phase (*h*) postgadolinium fat-suppressed T1-weighted gradient-echo images in a second patient with side-branch IPMT demonstrate similar findings.

than 2.5 cm in size, resection may need to be contemplated.

Solid and Papillary Epithelial Neoplasm (Papillary Cystic Neoplasm)

These tumors are generally considered benign neoplasms, with occasional examples exhibiting low-grade malignant potential. Solid and papillary epithelial neoplasms occur most frequently in women between 20 and 30 years of age [83]. The gross appearance of tumors is an encapsulated mass, which on cut surface reveals areas of hemorrhage, necrosis, and cystic spaces. The capsule and inner portion of tumor may contain calcifications. MRI findings of solid and papillary epithelial neoplasms are virtually diagnostic in the appropriate clinical setting. The MR appearance is a large, well-encapsulated mass, which demonstrates focal signal-void calcification and regions of hemorrhagic degeneration (as evidenced by fluid-debris levels or signal intensities consistent with blood products). A mass with this appearance, discovered in a young female patient, is virtually diagnostic for this entity [84]. A report describing the MRI appearance of solid and papillary epithelial neoplasms found that all tumors were well-demarcated lesions that contained central high signal intensity on T1-weighted images [83]. This central high signal intensity corresponds to hemorrhagic necrosis. The presence of hemorrhage may be related to tumor size because smaller tumors may appear heterogeneous but may not be overtly hemorrhagic (fig. 4.62).

Lymphoma

Non-Hodgkin lymphoma may involve peripancreatic lymph nodes or may directly invade the pancreas

[85]. Intermediate-signal-intensity peripancreatic lymph nodes are distinguished from high-signal-intensity normal pancreas on T1-weighted fat-suppressed images. Invasion of the pancreas is shown by loss of the normal high signal intensity of the pancreas on T1-weighted fat-suppressed images (fig. 4.63).

Burkitt lymphoma has a particular propensity to involve organs and structures within the abdominal cavity, including bowel, gallbladder, peritoneum, and pancreas (see fig. 4.63).

Metastases

Involvement of the pancreas by metastatic tumor may be the result of spread by direct extension or hematogenous metastases. Direct invasion by the extension of cancers arising in neighboring organs is common, particularly carcinoma of the stomach or transverse colon. Hematogenous metastases may occur with carcinomas of the lung, breast, and kidney and malignant melanoma. The MRI appearance of renal cell carcinoma metastases to the pancreas has been described as diffuse micronodular, multifocal, and solitary metastatic deposits [86]. Metastases are low in signal intensity on T1-weighted images and high in signal intensity on T2-weighted images. Small metastases (<1 cm in diameter) enhance uniformly on immediate postgadolinium gradient-echo images, and larger metastases enhance in a ring fashion (fig. 4.64). This appearance is analogous to the appearance of hypervascular metastases to the liver and reflects the pathophysiology of parasitization of host blood supply by metastatic disease. Renal cancer metastases resemble the appearance of islet cell tumors. Clinical history of renal cancer, even if remote, is essential to obtain in order to establish the correct diagnosis. Metastases from other primary tumors generally appear

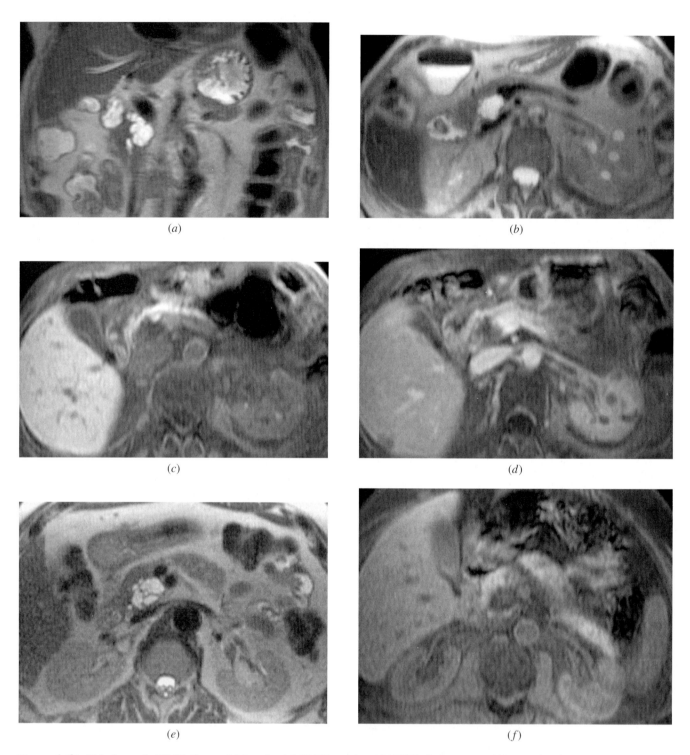

F I G . 4.61 Side-branch IPMN. Coronal (*a*) and axial (*b*) T2-weighted SS-ETSE, fat-suppressed T1-weighted gradient-echo (*c*) and immediate postgadolinium T1-weighted gradient-echo (*d*) images in a patient with side-branch IPMT demonstrate a 3-cm multilocular cystic mass in the pancreatic head. The lesion does not enhance after gadolinium administration (*d*).

T2-weighted SS-ETSE (*e*), fat suppressed T1-weighted gradient-echo (*f*), immediate postgadolinium fat-suppressed T1-weighted

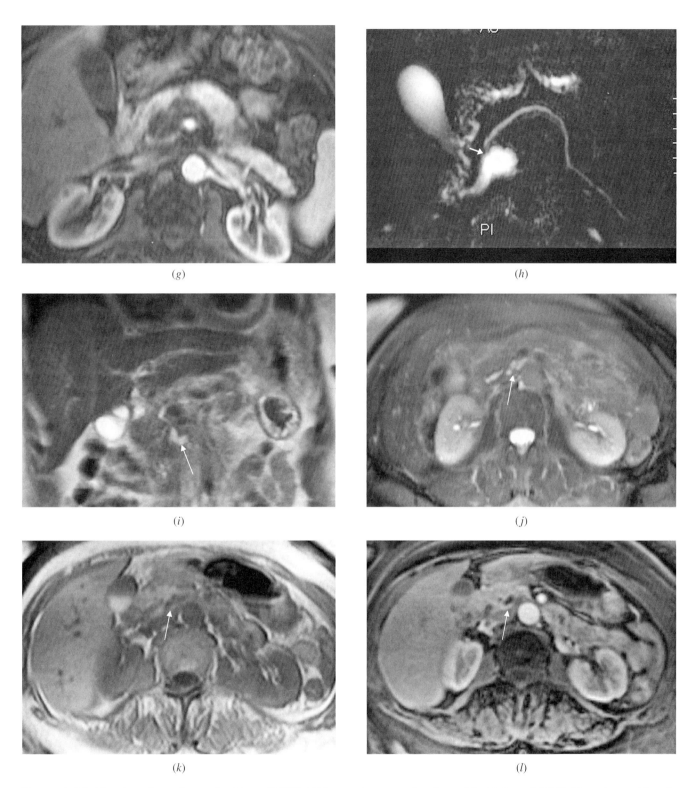

(g)

(h)

(i)

(j)

(k)

(l)

F I G . 4.61 (*Continued*) gradient-echo (*g*), and MRCP (*h*) images in a second patient with side-branch IPMT. There is a multicystic mass in the pancreatic head. Thin-section MRCP image shows that the cystic mass communicates with the main pancreatic duct (arrow, *h*), consistent with a side-branch IPMT. No enhancement of the cystic mass is appreciated on postgadolinium images (*g*).

Coronal T2-weighted single-shot echo-train spin-echo (*i*), transverse fat-suppressed single-shot echo-train spin-echo (*j*), transverse T1-weighted SGE (*k*), and transverse T1-weighted postgadolinium hepatic arterial dominant phase fat-suppressed 3D-GE (*l*) images at 3.0 T demonstrate a small septated cystic structure (arrows, *i–l*) in the pancreatic head in another patient. The diagnosis is consistent with side-branch IPMN.

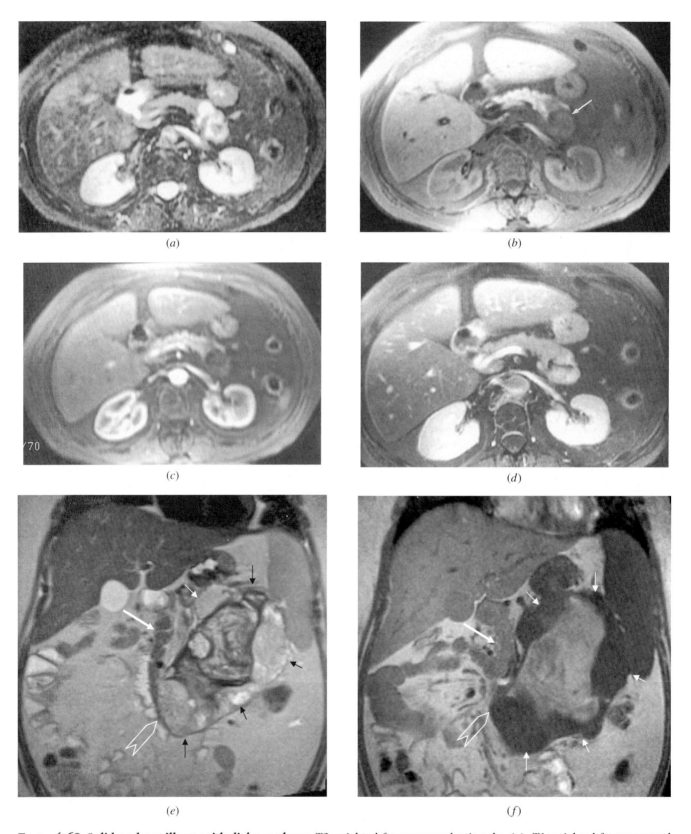

FIG. 4.62 Solid and papillary epithelial neoplasm. T2-weighted fat-suppressed spin-echo (*a*), T1-weighted fat-suppressed SGE (*b*), immediate postgadolinium T1-weighted fat-suppressed SGE (*c*), and 90-s postgadolinium fat-suppressed SGE (*d*) images. A 4-cm tumor mass arises from the tail of the pancreas that is low in signal intensity on the T1-weighted image (arrow, *b*) and heterogeneous on the T2-weighted image (*a*), enhances negligibly on the immediate postgadolinium T1-weighted SGE image (*c*), and shows heterogeneous enhancement on the interstitial-phase image (*d*).This rare low-grade malignant tumor is more frequent in young females and is typically located in the tail of the pancreas. MRI may be useful in these lesions by showing cystic degeneration and hemorrhagic necrosis, which are characteristic of this entity. (Courtesy of Caroline Reinhold, MD, Dept. of Radiology, McGill University.)

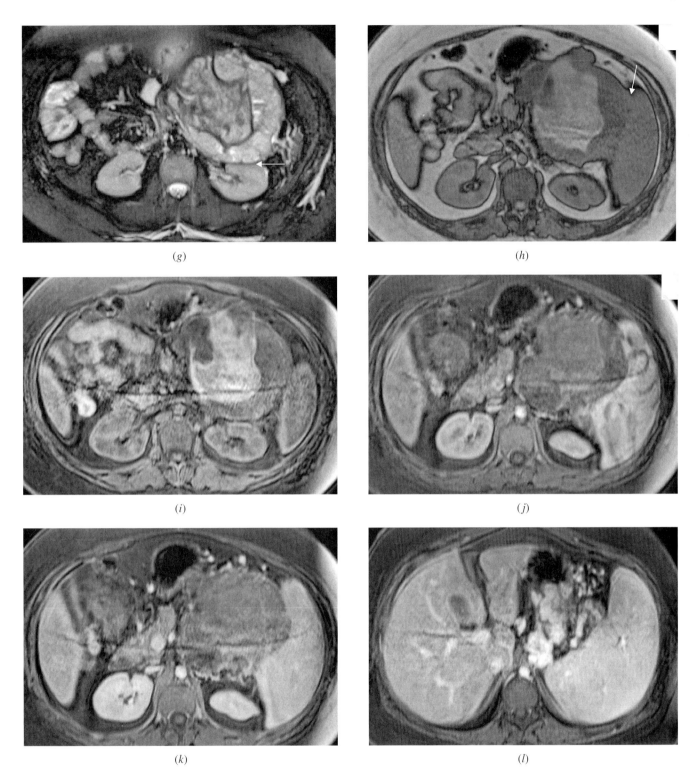

F I G . 4.62 (*Continued*) Coronal T2-weighted single-shot echo-train spin-echo (*e*), coronal T1-weighted SGE (*f*), transverse T2-weighted fat-suppressed single-shot echo-train spin-echo (*g*), transverse T1-weighted out-of-phase SGE (*h*), transverse fat-suppressed T1-weighted SGE (*i*), and transverse postgadolinium hepatic arterial dominant (*j*) and hepatic venous phase (*k, l*) fat-suppressed 3D-GE images in a young pregnant patient with solid and papillary tumor of the pancreas. The tumor (short arrows, *e, f*) is originating from the tail of the pancreas (open arrows, *e, f*) and depresses the whole pancreas (white long arrows, *e, f*) inferomedially. The tumor is well demarcated and compresses the left kidney (white arrow, *g*) and the spleen (white arrow, *h*). The tumor is very heterogeneous. It contains central hemorrhage which demonstrates high signal intensity on out-of-phase (*h*) and fat-suppressed (*i*) T1-weighted SGE images and heterogeneous low signal intensity on T2-weighted images (*e, g*). The tumor also contains cystic and necrotic regions, which show markedly high signal on T2-weighted images (*e, g*). The solid components of the tumor demonstrate intermediate to moderately high signal on T2-weighted images (*e, g*) and low signal on T1-weighted images (*f, h, i*). The tumor shows mild enhancement on postgadolinium images (*j, k*). Note that there are large varices in and around the stomach, and in the splenic hilum due to splenic vein thrombosis. There is an aliasing artifact at the center of transverse T1-weighted images due to the use of parallel imaging. Edema is also detected on the left and posterior body wall (*g*).

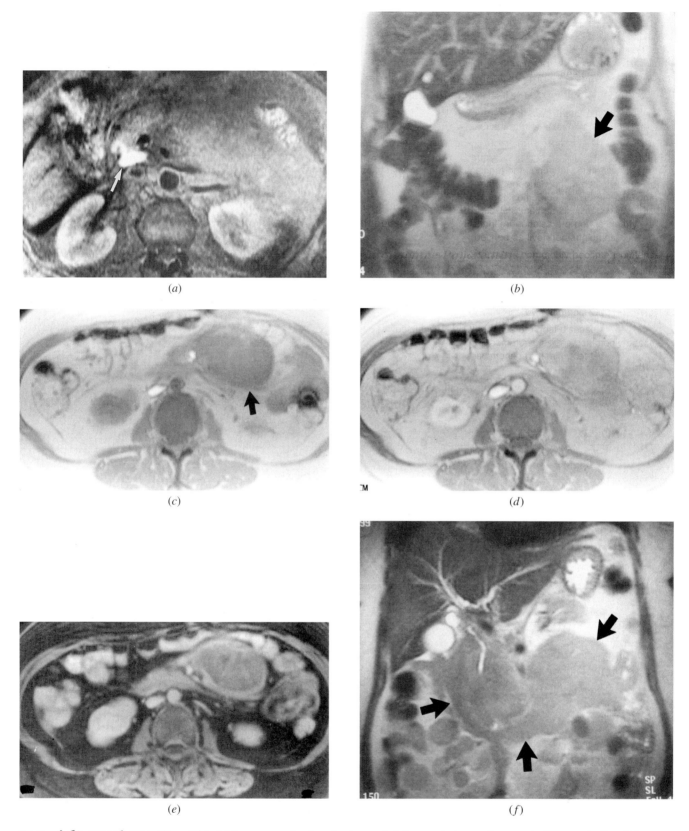

(a)

(b)

(c)

(d)

(e)

(f)

FIG. 4.63 Lymphoma. T1-weighted fat-suppressed spin-echo image (*a*) demonstrates replacement of the majority of the pancreas with intermediate-signal ill-defined lymphomatous tissue. The ventral portion of the pancreatic head is spared (arrow, *a*). (Reproduced with permission from Semelka RC, Shoenut JP, Kroeker MA, Micflikier AB. The Pancreas. In: Semelka RC, Shoenut JP. *MRI of the Abdomen with CT Correlation.* New York: Raven Press, p. 59–76, 1993.)

Coronal T2-weighted SS-ETSE (*b*), T1-weighted SGE (*c*), immediate postgadolinium T1-weighted SGE (*d*), and 90-s postgadolinium fat-suppressed SGE (*e*) images in a second patient, who has Burkitt lymphoma. A 10-cm mass (arrow, *b*, *c*) involves the pancreatic body and tail, which is mildly hypointense in signal intensity on both T1 (*c*)- and T2 (*b*)-weighted images and enhances minimally on early (*d*) and late (*e*) postgadolinium images.

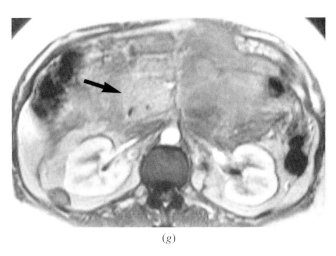
(g)

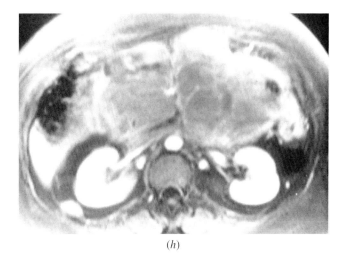
(h)

FIG. 4.63 (*Continued*) Coronal T2-weighted SS-ETSE (*f*), immediate postgadolinium SGE (*g*), and 90-s postgadolinium fat-suppressed SGE (*h*) images in a third patient who has non-Hodgkin lymphoma. A large mass is present in the mesentery, which involves the pancreas as well. Mild enhancement of the mesenteric tumor and tumor involving the pancreatic head (arrow, *g*) is present on early (*g*) and late (*h*) postgadolinium images. As these cases illustrate, lymphoma typically exhibits mild enhancement on early and late postcontrast images.

as focal pancreatic masses that are mildly hypointense on T1-weighted images, moderately hypointense on T1-weighted fat-suppressed images, and mildly hyperintense on T2-weighted images. Metastases to the pancreas often enhance in a ring fashion (figs. 4.65 and 4.66), as observed with liver metastases, and their extent of enhancement generally varies with the angiogenic properties of the primary neoplasms. Ductal obstruction is uncommon, even with larger tumors, which is an important feature distinguishing from pancreatic ductal adenocarcinoma. The lack of ductal obstruction explains why metastases are generally well seen on noncontrast T1-weighted fat-suppressed images. Chronic pancreatitis that arises secondary to ductal obstruction is not present, and therefore background pancreas is moderately high signal intensity, creating sharp contrast with hypointense tumors.

Melanoma metastases may be high in signal intensity on T1-weighted images because of the paramagnetic properties of melanin pigment (fig. 4.67) [1]. Metastatic deposits tend to be focal, well-defined masses (figs. 4.68–4.70).

INFLAMMATORY DISEASE

Pancreatitis

Pancreatitis may occur secondary to chronic alcoholism, gallstones, hypercalcemia, hyperlipoproteinemia, blunt abdominal trauma, penetrating peptic ulcer disease,

viral infections (most frequently Epstein–Barr), and certain drugs [87]. Pancreatitis can also be hereditary and predisposition may be inherited as an autosomal dominant trait [88].

Acute Pancreatitis
Acute pancreatitis is defined as an acute inflammatory condition typically presenting with abdominal pain and associated with elevations in pancreatic enzymes (particularly amylase and lipase). Acute pancreatitis arises in the majority of cases secondary to alcoholism or cholelithiasis [87]. Alcohol-related acute pancreatitis most frequently results in acute recurrent pancreatitis, whereas gallstone-related pancreatitis typically results in a single attack (fig. 4.71). The passage of biliary sludge may also cause acute pancreatitis [89]. At least 95% of patients with acute pancreatitis experience severe midepigastric pain that radiates to the back. Nausea and vomiting occur in 75–85% of patients, and fever occurs in approximately 50%.

Acute pancreatitis results from the exudation of fluid containing activated proteolytic enzymes into the interstitium of the pancreas and leakage of this fluid into surrounding tissue. Trypsin is suspected to be the primary enzyme involved in the coagulative necrosis. Pathologically, acute pancreatitis is characterized by a spectrum of morphologic features, which may be patchy or diffuse. In mild cases, edema predominates, producing so-called edematous or interstitial pancreatitis. There is scattered peripancreatic fat necrosis without parenchymatous or acinar necrosis. In severe cases, extensive

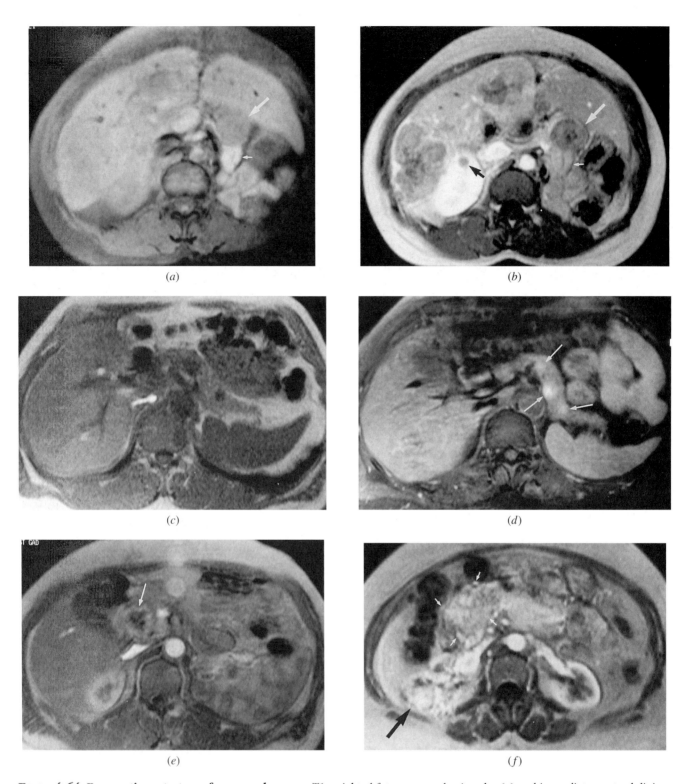

(a)

(b)

(c)

(d)

(e)

(f)

F I G . 4.64 Pancreatic metastases from renal cancer. T1-weighted fat-suppressed spin-echo (*a*) and immediate postgadolinium T1-weighted SGE (*b*) images demonstrate a 3-cm mass in the distal body of the pancreas (arrow, *a*, *b*).The uninvolved tail of the pancreas has a normal high signal intensity (small arrow, *a*, *b*). Multiple liver metastases are present that demonstrate predominant rim enhancement on the immediate postgadolinium image (*b*). Multiple renal cancers are present (black arrow, *b*, only one lesion shown).

T1-weighted SGE (*c*) and interstitial-phase gadolinium-enhanced T1-weighted fat-suppressed spin-echo (*d*) images of the body of the pancreas and immediate postgadolinium T1-weighted SGE image (*e*) in a second patient. Three metastases are present in the body of the pancreas (arrows, *d*) that are low in signal intensity on the precontrast T1-weighted SGE image (*c*) and enhance uniformly and with moderate intensity on the interstitial-phase gadolinium-enhanced image (*d*). A larger 3-cm metastasis is present in the head of the pancreas that demonstrates rim enhancement on the immediate postgadolinium image (arrow, *e*).

Immediate postgadolinium T1-weighted SGE image (*f*) in a third patient demonstrates multiple micronodular metastases to the pancreas <5 mm, which enhance uniformly and intensely on the immediate postgadolinium image (small arrows, *f*). The renal cancer is also shown (arrow, *f*). (Reproduced with permission from Kelekis NL, Semelka RC, Siegelman ES: MRI of pancreatic metastasis from renal cell cancer. *J Comput Assist Tomogr* 20: 249–253, 1996.) Renal cell cancer is among the most common metastatic lesions to the pancreas.

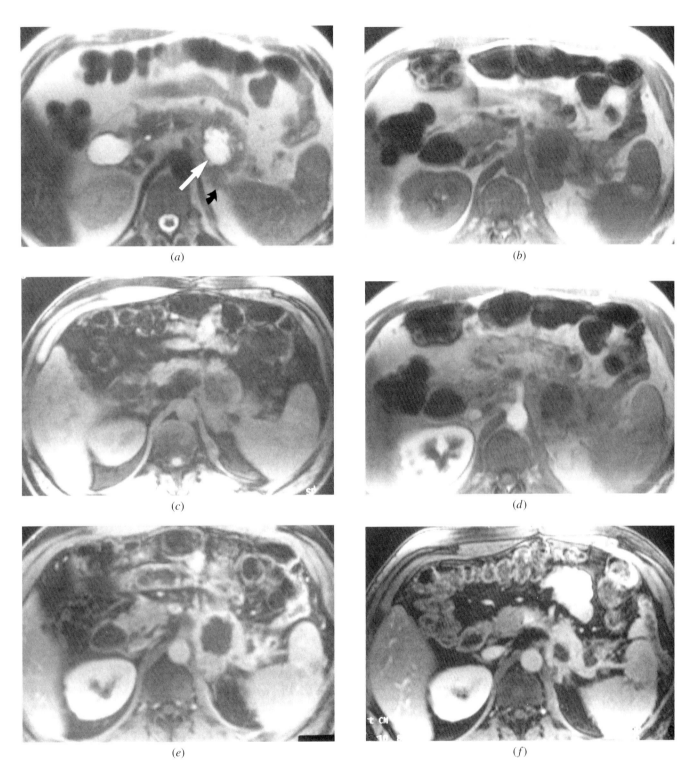

F I G . 4.65 Pancreatic metastasis from transitional cell cancer. T2-weighted ETSE (*a*), T1-weighted SGE (*b*), T1-weighted fat-suppressed SGE (*c*), immediate postgadolinium T1-weighted SGE (*d*), and 90-s postgadolinium fat-suppressed SGE (*e*) images in a patient with recurrent transitional cell cancer, originally from the left kidney. There is a cystic mass (arrow, *a*) that involves the pancreatic tail and the left adrenal gland (curved arrow, *a*). A thick enhancing rim is demonstrated on the interstitial-phase gadolinium-enhanced fat-suppressed image. Interstitial-phase gadolinium-enhanced fat-suppressed SGE image (*f*) obtained after a course of chemotherapy demonstrates substantial decrease in size of the cystic mass.

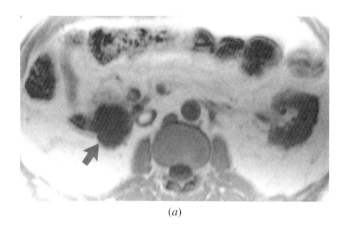

(a)

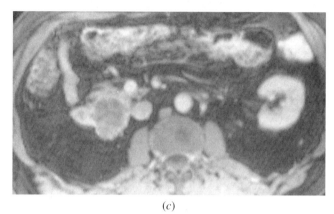

(b)

(c)

F I G .   4.66 Pancreatic metastasis from colon cancer.
T1-weighted SGE (*a*), immediate postgadolinium T1-weighted
SGE (*b*), and 90-s postgadolinium fat-suppressed SGE (*c*) images
in a patient with colon cancer with liver metastases (not
shown). There is a 3.5-cm lobulated mass (arrow, *a*) in the
pancreatic head. The tumor appears hyperintense on T2 (not
shown) and hypointense on T1-weighted image (*a*) and shows
heterogeneous mild enhancement on early (*b*) and late (*c*)
postgadolinium images.

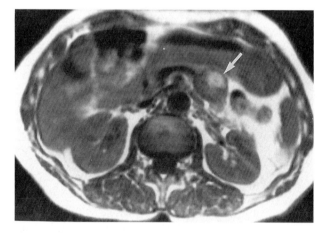

F I G .   4.67 Pancreatic metastasis from melanoma.
T1-SGE image demonstrates a high-signal intensity mass in the
tail of the pancreas (arrow). The high signal intensity of the
mass is due to the paramagnetic effect of melanin. (Reproduced
with permission from Semelka RC, Ascher SM: MRI of the
pancreas—state of the art. *Radiology* 188: 593–602, 1993.)

pancreatic and peripancreatic fat necrosis, parenchymal
necrosis, and hemorrhage occur. In its most devastating
form, severe acute pancreatitis may produce an organ
that resembles oily mud, where degenerative tissue, fat,
and hemorrhage congeal [90].

The signal intensity features of the pancreas in
uncomplicated mild acute pancreatitis resemble those
of normal pancreatic tissue. The pancreas is high in
signal intensity on precontrast T1-weighted fat-suppressed images and enhances in a normal uniform
fashion on immediate postgadolinium images, reflecting
a normal capillary blush (fig. 4.72). The acutely inflamed
pancreas shows either focal or diffuse enlargement,
which may be subtle. Peripancreatic fluid is well shown
on noncontrast or immediate postgadolinium non-fat-
suppressed gradient-echo images and appears as low-
signal-intensity strands of fluid or fluid collections in a
background of high-signal-intensity fat. T2-weighted
single-shot echo-train spin-echo imaging employing fat
suppression is the most sensitive technique for showing
small-volume peripancreatic fluid, which appears as
high signal in a background of intermediate- to low-
signal pancreas and low-signal fat (see fig. 4.72). As a
result, MRI is sensitive for the detection of subtle
changes of acute pancreatitis, particularly minor peripancreatic inflammatory changes even in the setting of
a morphologically normal pancreas. CT imaging examinations appear normal in 15–30% of patients with clinical features of acute pancreatitis [91]. The sensitivity of
MRI exceeds that of CT imaging, suggesting a role
for MRI in the evaluation of patients with suspected

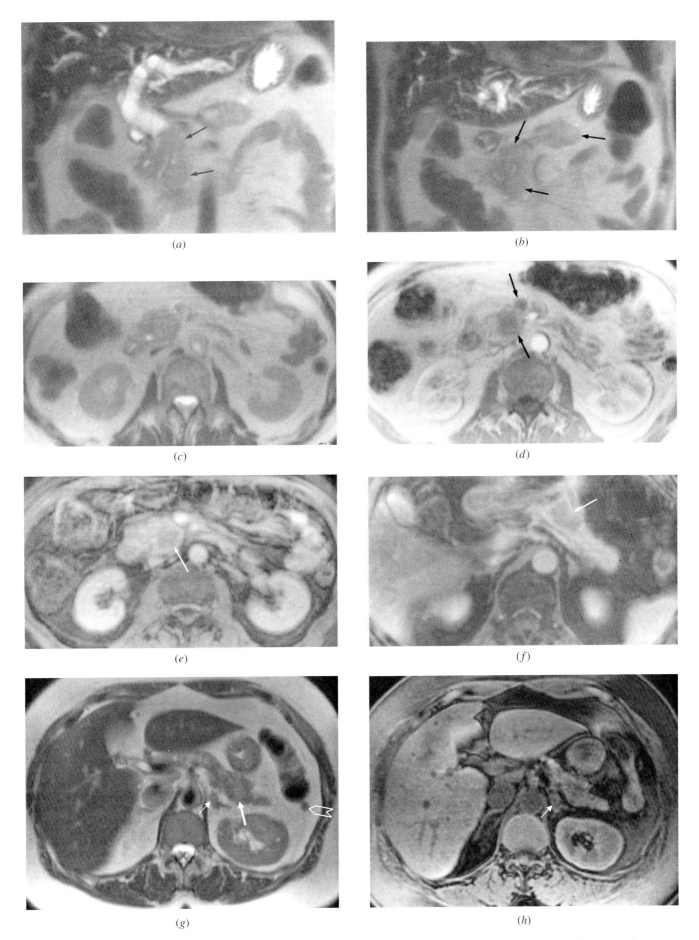

F I G . 4.68 Pancreatic metastasis from lung cancer. Coronal (*a*, *b*) and transverse (*c*) T2-weighted SS-ETSE, immediate post-gadolinium T1-weighed SGE (*d*), and 90-s postgadolinium fat-suppressed SGE (*e*, *f*) images in a patient with small cell lung cancer. Multiple masses (arrows, *a*, *b*) are present throughout the pancreas that are mildly hyperintense on T2 (*a*–*c*) and enhance minimally on early (*d*) and late (*e*, *f*) postgadolinium images.

T2-weighted single-shot echo-train spin-echo (*g*), T1-weighted fat-suppressed SGE (*b*), T1-weighted postgadolinium hepatic

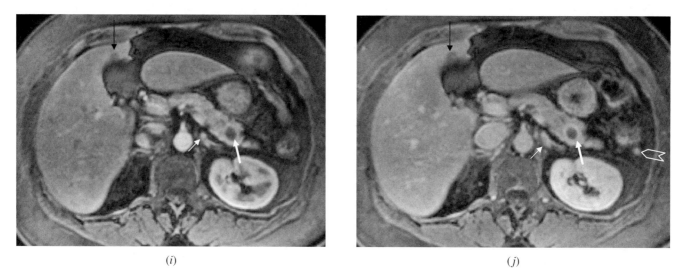

(i) (j)

F I G . 4.68 (*Continued*) arterial dominant phase (*i*), and hepatic venous phase (*j*) fat-suppressed 3D-GE images at 3.0 T demonstrate a metastatic lesion (white long arrows, *g, i, j*) located in the pancreas in another patient with squamous cell lung cancer. The lesion shows peripheral enhancement on postgadolinium images. Note that there are also hypovascular liver metastasis (black arrow, *i, j*), peritoneal metastatic nodule (open arrow, *g, j*) and left adrenal corpus thickening (white short arrow, *g–j*). Lung cancer is among the most common primary tumors that metastasize to the pancreas.

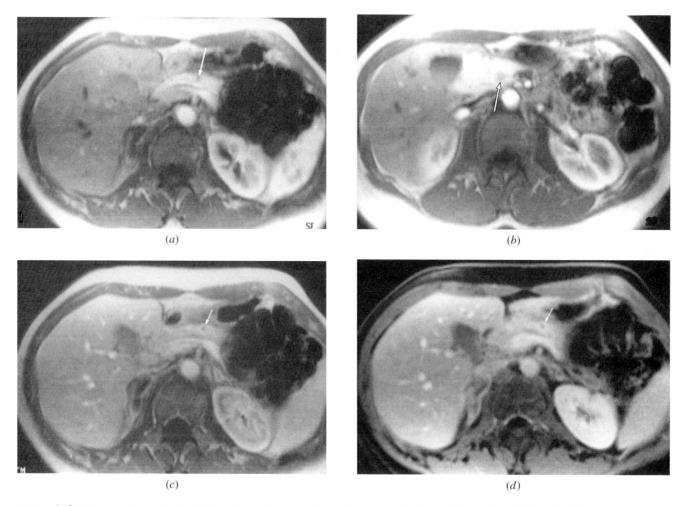

(a) (b)

(c) (d)

F I G . 4.69 Pancreatic metastasis from breast cancer. Immediate postgadolinium T1-weighted SGE (*a, b*), 45-s postgadolinium SGE (*c*), and interstitial-phase gadolinium-enhanced SGE (*d*) images demonstrate multiple <1-cm hypointense metastases (arrow, *a, b*) in the pancreatic head and body. Note ring enhancement of the metastases on the post contrast images (arrows, *c, d*).

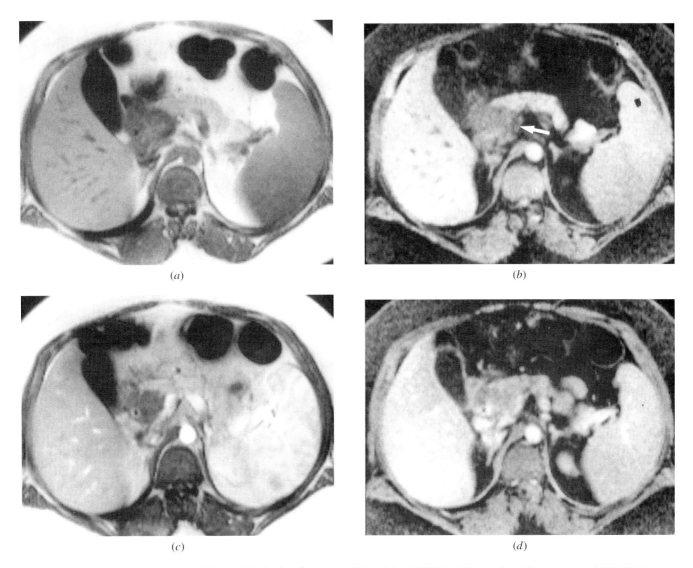

(a)

(b)

(c)

(d)

F I G . 4.70 Pancreatic metastasis from Merkel cell cancer. T1-weighted SGE (*a*), T1-weighted fat-suppressed SGE (*b*), immediate postgadolinium T1-weighted SGE (*c*), and 90-s postgadolinium fat-suppressed SGE (*d*) images in a patient with pancreatic metastasis (arrow, *b*) from a primary neuroendocrine cancer of the skin (Merkel cell carcinoma). There is a well-defined 6-cm mass in the head of the pancreas that is hypointense on T1-weighted images (*a, b*) and enhances minimally on early (*c*) postcontrast images, with progressive enhancement on late images (*d*). Distant metastasis occurs in one-third of patients with Merkel cell cancers.

acute pancreatitis and negative CT imaging examination. As the extent of pancreatitis becomes more severe, the pancreas develops a heterogeneous appearance on pre-contrast T1-weighted fat-suppressed images and enhances in a more heterogeneous, diminished fashion on immediate postgadolinium images (figs. 4.73 and 4.74).

The percentage of pancreatic necrosis has been considered an important prognostic indicator in patients with acute pancreatitis [92, 93]. Dynamic gadolinium-enhanced gradient-echo images may be useful for this determination because MRI is very sensitive for the demonstration of the presence or absence of gadolin-

ium enhancement. Saifuddin et al. [94] described comparable results for dynamic contrast-enhanced CT images and immediate postgadolinium gradient-echo images for determining the presence of pancreatic necrosis. Complications of acute pancreatitis such as hemorrhage, pseudocyst formation, or abscess are clearly shown on MRI (figs. 4.75–4.77). Hemorrhagic fluid collections are high in signal intensity on T1-weighted fat-suppressed images, and depiction of hemorrhage is superior on MR images compared to CT images. Martin et al. [95] demonstrated correlation between the extent of high signal on noncontrast T1-weighted fat-suppressed SGE and severity of acute

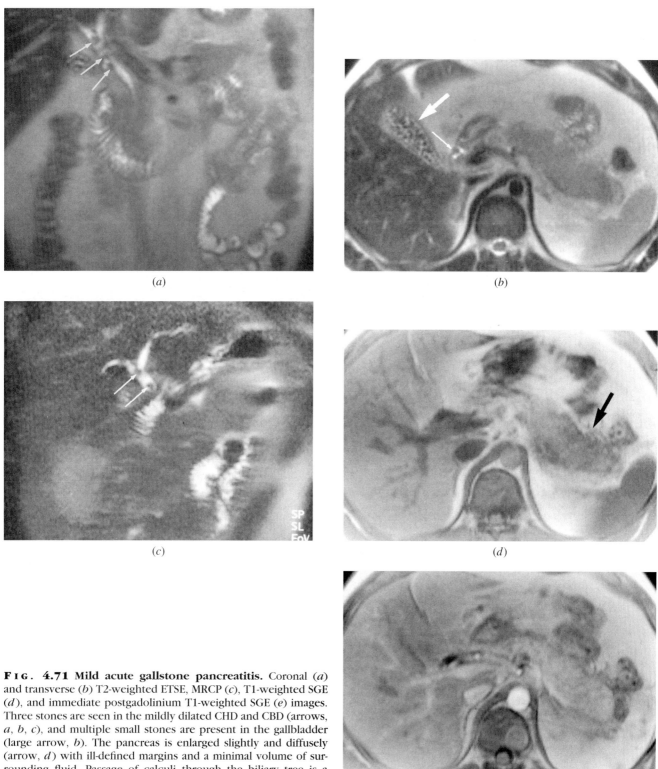

FIG. 4.71 Mild acute gallstone pancreatitis. Coronal (*a*) and transverse (*b*) T2-weighted ETSE, MRCP (*c*), T1-weighted SGE (*d*), and immediate postgadolinium T1-weighted SGE (*e*) images. Three stones are seen in the mildly dilated CHD and CBD (arrows, *a*, *b*, *c*), and multiple small stones are present in the gallbladder (large arrow, *b*). The pancreas is enlarged slightly and diffusely (arrow, *d*) with ill-defined margins and a minimal volume of surrounding fluid. Passage of calculi through the biliary tree is a common cause of single episodes of acute pancreatitis, which, as in this case, is generally of mild severity.

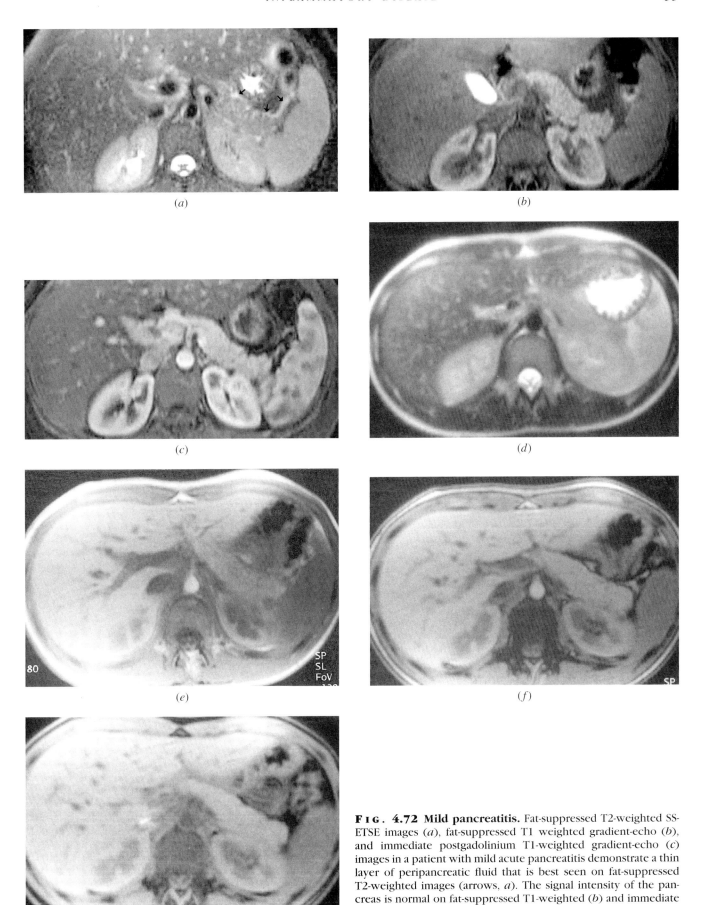

F I G . 4.72 Mild pancreatitis. Fat-suppressed T2-weighted SS-ETSE images (*a*), fat-suppressed T1 weighted gradient-echo (*b*), and immediate postgadolinium T1-weighted gradient-echo (*c*) images in a patient with mild acute pancreatitis demonstrate a thin layer of peripancreatic fluid that is best seen on fat-suppressed T2-weighted images (arrows, *a*). The signal intensity of the pancreas is normal on fat-suppressed T1-weighted (*b*) and immediate postgadolinium T1-weighted (*c*) images.

T2-weighted SS-ETSE (*d*), T1-weighted SGE (*e*), T1-weighted out-of-phase SGE (*f*), T1-weighted fat-suppressed SGE (*g*),

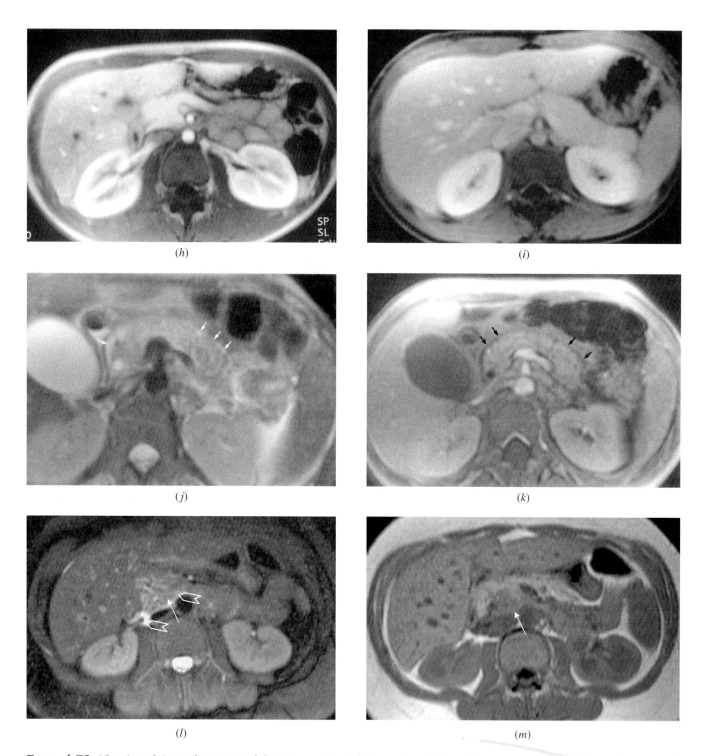

(h)

(i)

(j)

(k)

(l)

(m)

FIG. 4.72 (*Continued*) immediate postgadolinium SGE (*h*), and 90-s postgadolinium fat-suppressed SGE (*i*) images in a second patient.

The pancreas is minimally and diffusely enlarged with subtle loss of lobulated contour. The pancreas is normal in signal on noncontrast T1-weighted fat-suppressed images (*g*) and enhances normally on immediate postgadolinium images (*h*). The appearance is essentially that of normal pancreas, but clinical history and mildly elevated serum amylase were diagnostic for an episode of pancreatitis.

T2-weighted fat-suppressed SS-ETSE (*j*) and early postgadolinium single-shot magnetization-prepared gradient-echo (*k*) images in a third patient demonstrate mild diffuse enhancement of the pancreas and a thin film of peripancreatic fluid surrounding the pancreas (small arrows, *j*, *k*) and throughout the interstices of the marbled pancreatic parenchyma. Fat-suppressed breathing-independent single-shot T2-weighted sequences are very effective at showing small volumes of fluid, as surrounding fat and pancreas are both low signal and only fluid will be high signal (*j*). This case is also noteworthy in that image quality is reasonable despite the fact that the patient was very ill and a noncooperative MR imaging protocol was employed, which uses only breathing-independent single-shot images.

T2-weighted fat-suppressed single-shot echo-train spin-echo (*l*), T1-weighted SGE (*m*), T1-weighted postgadolinium hepatic arterial dominant phase SGE (*n*), and T1-weighted interstitial phase fat-suppressed 3D-GE (*o*) images demonstrate mild focal

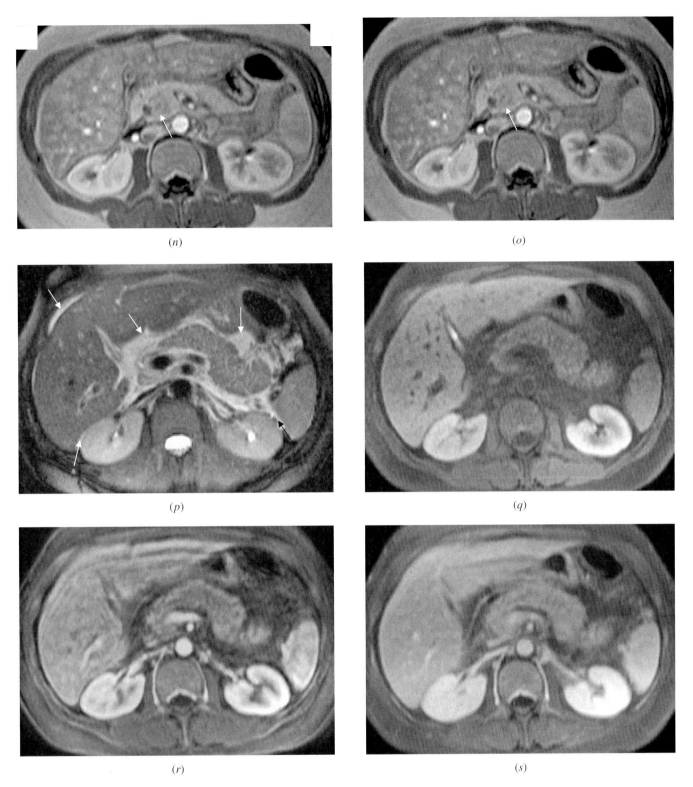

(n)

(o)

(p)

(q)

(r)

(s)

FIG. 4.72 (*Continued*) pancreatitis located in the pancreatic head in another patient. Focal pancreatitis (arrows, *l, m*) shows high signal on T2-weighted image (*l*) and low signal on T1-weighted SGE image (*m*). The pancreatic head is enlarged. There is minimal free fluid (open arrows, *l*) adjacent to the pancreatic head. The lesion (arrows, *n, o*) shows progressive enhancement on postgadolinium images (*n, o*). Additionally, the liver shows heterogeneous transient enhancement on the hepatic arterial dominant phase image due to associated inflammation. The remaining pancreatic parenchyma shows normal signal and enhancement pattern. The lesion can be differentiated from malignancies because it does not cause common bile duct compression although it encircles the common bile duct.

    T2-weighted fat-suppressed single-shot echo-train spin-echo (*p*), T1-weighted fat-suppressed SGE (*q*), T1-weighted hepatic arterial dominant phase (*r*), and hepatic venous phase (*s*) fat-suppressed 3D-GE images in the same patient with focal pancreatitis show the progression of the disease to severe pancreatitis. The pancreas is enlarged, and there is abundant free fluid (arrows, *p*) in the peripancreatic region extending into bilateral anterior pararenal space, perihepatic space, and lesser sac. The signal of pancreas is less than normal on T1-weighted SGE image (*q*). The enhancement of the pancreas is less than normal on postgadolinium images (*r, s*).

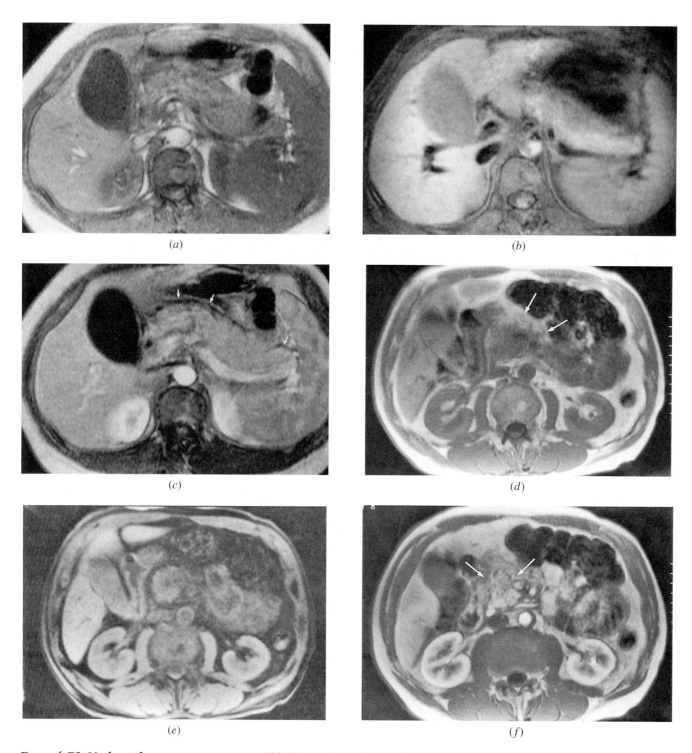

(a)

(b)

(c)

(d)

(e)

(f)

F I G . 4.73 Moderately severe acute pancreatitis. T1-weighted SGE (*a*), T1-weighted fat-suppressed spin-echo (*b*), and immediate postgadolinium T1-weighted SGE (*c*) images. The pancreas is diffusely enlarged (*a–c*). The signal intensity of the pancreas is heterogeneous on the T1-weighted fat-suppressed image (*b*), which suggests a decrease in the proteinaceous fluid content within the acini of the pancreas. Signal-void fluid is shown surrounding the body and tail of the pancreas on the immediate postgadolinium image (arrows, *c*). The intensity of pancreatic enhancement is less than normal for pancreas on the capillary-phase image (*c*).

T1-weighted SGE (*d*), T1-weighted fat-suppressed SGE (*e*), and immediate postgadolinium T1-weighted SGE (*f*) images in a second patient. Peripancreatic fluid is well shown as low-signal intensity stranding in the high-signal intensity fat on the T1-weighted SGE image (arrows, *d*). The anterior portion of the head of the pancreas is lower in signal intensity on the precontrast fat-suppressed image (*e*) and enhances less (arrows, *f*) on immediate postgadolinium images (*f*), reflecting more severe changes of pancreatitis. Relative sparing of either anterior or posterior portions of the head of the pancreas is not uncommon because of separate pancreatic ductal systems. Despite the focal nature of the diminished enhancement of the dorsal head of the pancreas, there is lobular architecture similar to that of the ventral pancreatic head. A pancreatic neoplasm would not exhibit lobular architecture.

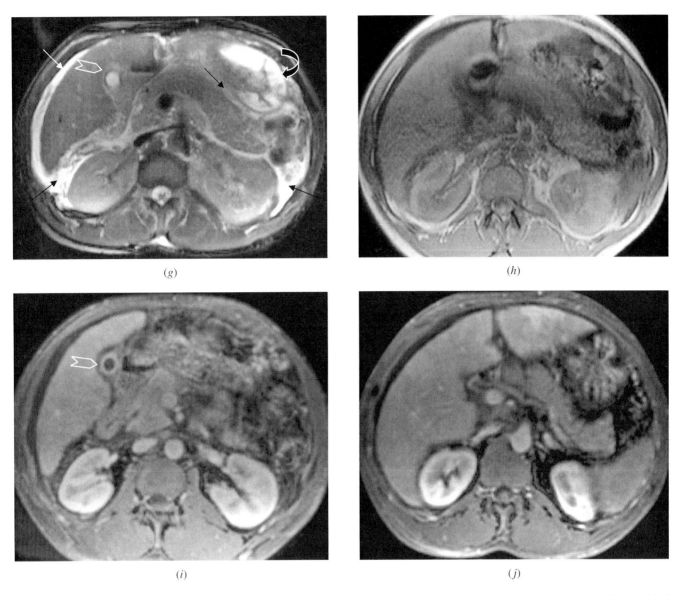

(g)

(h)

(i)

(j)

F I G . 4.73 (*Continued*) **Severe acute pancreatitis.** T2-weighted fat-suppressed single-shot echo-train spin-echo (*g*), T1-weighted fat-suppressed SGE (*h*), and T1-weighted hepatic arterial dominant phase fat-suppressed 3D-GE (*i, j*) images at 3.0 T demonstrate severe pancreatitis in another patient. The pancreas is diffusely enlarged and there is abundant free fluid (arrows, *g*) in the perihepatic space, bilateral anterior pararenal spaces, lesser sac, and left paracolic gutter. The pancreas shows diminished signal on T1-weighted SGE image (*h*). The enhancement of the pancreas is less than normal on postgadolinium images. The gallbladder wall (open arrow, *g*) is also thickened and edematous. The gallbladder wall, particularly the mucosa, (open arrow, *i*) shows intense enhancement on postgadolinium image (*i*). The stomach wall (curved arrow, *g*) is also thickened and edematous. There are regions of heterogeneous enhancement in the liver as well. Associated cholecystitis, gastritis, and inflammation in the liver are not uncommon in the presence of pancreatitis.

pancreatitis, where high signal correlated with hemorrhagic changes. Simple pseudocysts are low in signal intensity or signal void in a background of normal-signal-intensity pancreatic tissue on both noncontrast non-fat-suppressed gradient-echo and T1-weighted fat-suppressed gradient echo images (figs. 4.77–4.80). Extrapancreatic pseudocysts are well shown on breath-

hold gradient-echo images because of high contrast with high-signal-intensity fat. Image acquisition in multiple planes permits determination of pseudocyst location in relation to various organs and structures (see fig. 4.79). Pseudocyst walls enhance minimally on early postgadolinium images and show progressively intense enhancement on 5-min postcontrast images, consistent

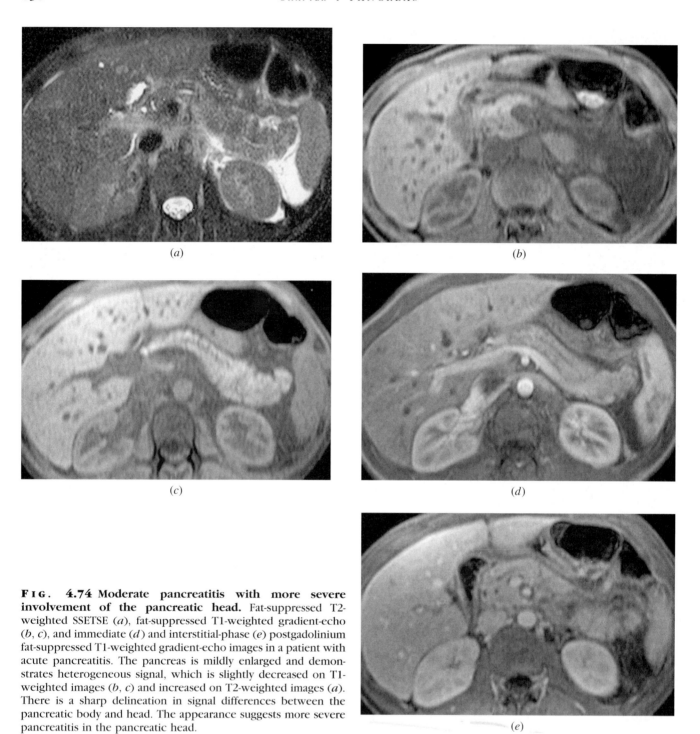

FIG. 4.74 Moderate pancreatitis with more severe involvement of the pancreatic head. Fat-suppressed T2-weighted SSETSE (*a*), fat-suppressed T1-weighted gradient-echo (*b*, *c*), and immediate (*d*) and interstitial-phase (*e*) postgadolinium fat-suppressed T1-weighted gradient-echo images in a patient with acute pancreatitis. The pancreas is mildly enlarged and demonstrates heterogeneous signal, which is slightly decreased on T1-weighted images (*b*, *c*) and increased on T2-weighted images (*a*). There is a sharp delineation in signal differences between the pancreatic body and head. The appearance suggests more severe pancreatitis in the pancreatic head.

with the appearance of fibrous tissue. Simple pseudocysts are relatively homogeneous and high in signal intensity on T2-weighted images. Pseudocysts complicated by necrotic debris, hemorrhage, or infection are heterogeneous in signal intensity on T2-weighted images [94]. Proteinaceous fluid tends to layer in a gradation of concentration with low-signal-intensity

concentrated proteinaceous material in the dependent portion of the cyst. Necrotic material may appear as irregularly shaped regions of low signal intensity in the pseudocyst (see fig. 4.80) [96]. This information may provide both therapeutic and prognostic information because pseudocysts that contain necrotic material may not respond to simple percutaneous drainage

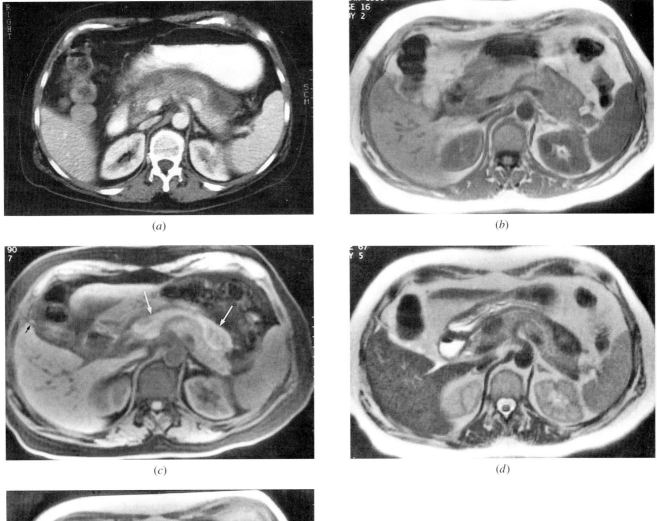

FIG. 4.75 Hemorrhagic pancreatitis. Contrast-enhanced spiral CT (*a*), T1-weighted SGE (*b*), T1-weighted fat-suppressed SGE (*c*), T2-weighted SS-ETSE (*d*), and immediate postgadolinium T1-weighted SGE (*e*) images. The CT image demonstrates an enlarged pancreas with free fluid along its anterior margin, findings consistent with acute pancreatitis. On the T1-weighted SGE image (*b*), the fluid collections are noted to be hyperintense, which is accentuated on the fat-suppressed image (arrows, *c*).

The fluid is low in signal on the T2-weighted image (*d*) and therefore possesses the signal characteristics of intracellular methemoglobin in acute blood. The pancreas enhances relatively uniformly on the immediate postgadolinium image, reflecting the absence of pancreatic necrosis (*e*). A collapsed acutely inflamed gallbladder (arrow, *e*) is present, in which a cholecystostomy catheter was placed (small arrow, *c*, *e*).

and thus require open debridement. Breathing-independent T2-weighted sequences such as single-shot echo-train spin echo may be useful to evaluate these pseudocyst collections, not only because they are the most effective at demonstrating the complexity of fluid but also because many of these patients are very debilitated and unable to cooperate with breath-holding instructions.

Chronic Pancreatitis

Chronic pancreatitis is defined pathologically by continuous or relapsing inflammation of the organ leading to irreversible morphologic injury and typically leading to impairment of function. Chronic pancreatitis is acquired either as a disease process distinct from acute pancreatitis or as a complication of repeated attacks of acute pancreatitis. There is a strong association between

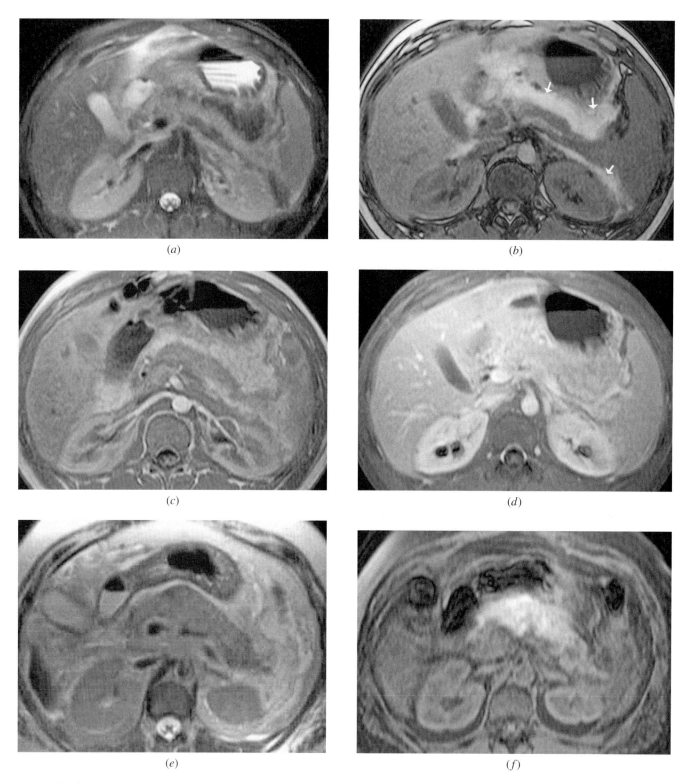

(a)

(b)

(c)

(d)

(e)

(f)

F I G . 4.76 Hemorrhagic pancreatitis. Axial fat-suppressed T2-weighted SS-ETSE (*a*), T1-weighted gradient-echo (*b*), immediate postgadolinium T1-weighted gradient-echo (*c*), and interstitial-phase postgadolinium T1-weighted gradient-echo (*d*) images in a patient with acute pancreatitis. The pancreas demonstrates diffuse hypoenhancement on immediate postgadolinium images, reflecting severe disease. The fluid surrounding the pancreas is hyperintense on T1 (arrows, *b*) and hypointense on T2-weighted images. This appearance is consistent with intracellular methemoglobin seen in subacute hemorrhage. T2-weighted SS-ETSE (*e*), fat-suppressed T1-weighted gradient-echo (*f*), and immediate postgadolinium fat-suppressed T1-weighted gradient-echo (*g*) images

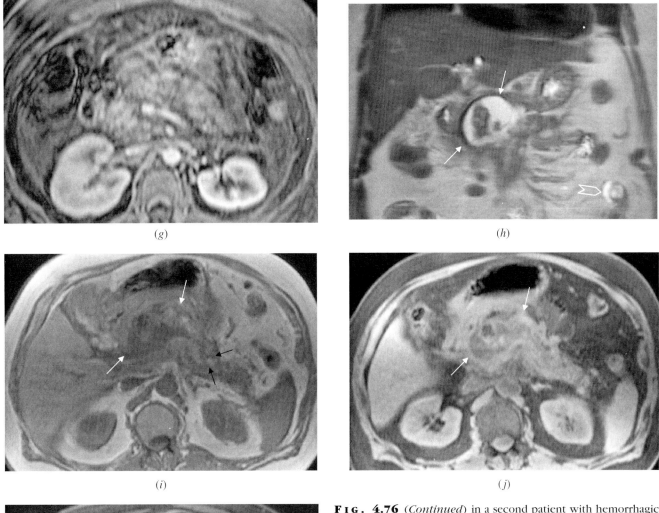

(g)

(h)

(i)

(j)

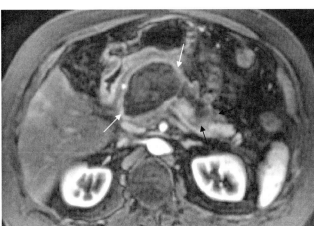

(k)

FIG. 4.76 (*Continued*) in a second patient with hemorrhagic pancreatitis. The pancreas is enlarged (*e*) and shows very high signal intensity on fat-suppressed T1-weighted images (*g*) and low signal on T2-weighted images (*e*), consistent with subacute hemorrhage. The patchy enhancement of the pancreas on immediate postgadolinium images reflects foci of pancreatic necrosis (*g*).

Coronal T2-weighted single-shot echo-train spin-echo (*h*), T1-weighted SGE (*i*), T1-weighted fat-suppressed SGE (*j*), and T1-weighted postgadolinium hepatic arterial dominant phase fat-suppressed 3D-GE (*k*) images at 3.0T demonstrate hemorrhagic necrotizing pancreatitis in another patient. A large pseudocyst (white arrows, *h–k*) containing blood product is located in the pancreatic head and body region. The blood products show low signal on T2-weighted image (*h*) but high signal on T1-weighted precontrast images (*i, j*). There is mild free fluid (open arrow, *h*) in the abdomen. Peripancreatic tissue is low in signal intensity on precontrast images. There are foci of blood products (black arrows, *i*) and necrosis (black arrows, *k*) in the pancreatic parenchyma. Note that there is associated gastric mucosal inflammation and hepatic inflammation, which are characterized by increased enhancement.

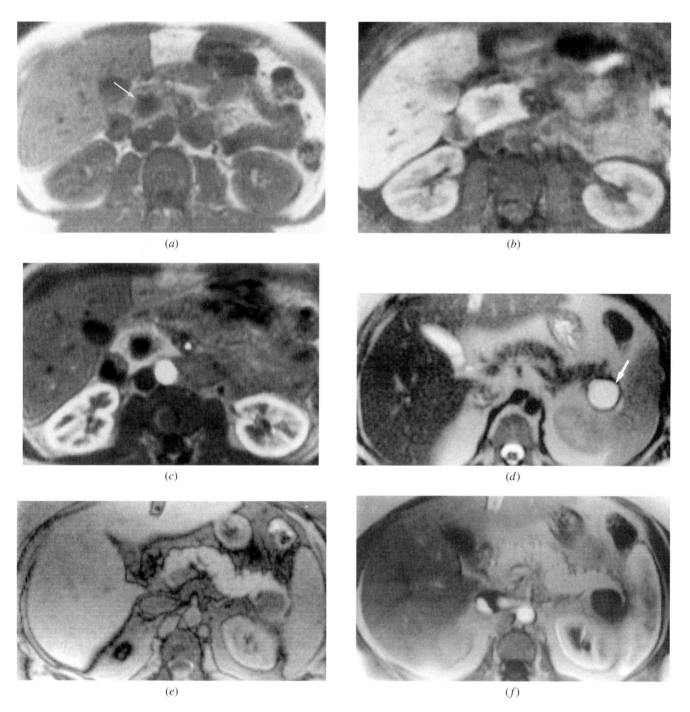

(a)

(b)

(c)

(d)

(e)

(f)

F I G . 4.77 Pseudocyst in acute pancreatitis. T1-weighted SGE (*a*), T1-weighted fat-suppressed spin-echo (*b*), and immediate postgadolinium T1-weighted SGE (*c*) images. A low-signal intensity pseudocyst (arrow, *a*) is present in the head of the pancreas (*a–c*). The pancreas has normal high signal intensity on the T1-weighted fat-suppressed image (*b*), and there is normal uniform enhancement of the pancreas on the immediate postgadolinium image (*c*). These imaging features are consistent with a pseudocyst in the setting of acute pancreatitis because the background pancreas has normal signal intensity features. The lesion did not change in size and shape on delayed images, excluding a poorly vascularized tumor.

T2-weighted SS-ETSE (*d*), T1-weighted fat-suppressed SGE (*e*), immediate postgadolinium T1-weighted SGE (*f*), and 90-s postgadolinium fat-suppressed SGE (*g*) images in a second patient. A 3-cm pseudocyst (arrow, *d*) is in the pancreatic tail. The pancreas

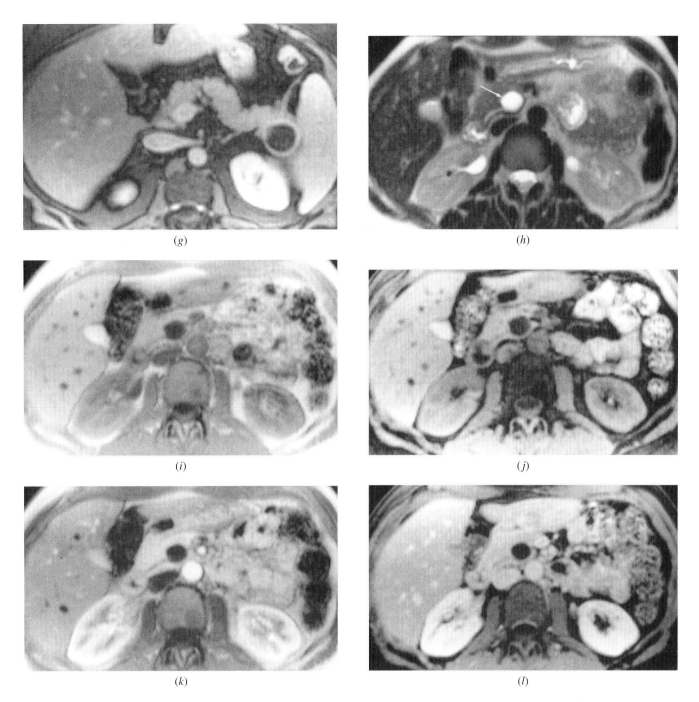

(g)

(h)

(i)

(j)

(k)

(l)

F I G . 4.77 (*Continued*) is normal in signal on noncontrast T1-weighted fat-suppressed images (*e*) and enhances normally on early (*f*) and late (*g*) images, consistent with no substantial parenchymal disease. There is progressive enhancement of the wall of the pseudocyst (*g*), which is typical for fibrous tissue. The pancreas, spleen, and liver are mildly hypointense on T2-weighted images (*d*) secondary to iron deposition from multiple blood transfusions.

T2-weighted SS-ETSE (*h*), T1-weighted SGE (*i*), T1-weighted fat-suppressed SGE (*j*), immediate postgadolinium T1-weighted SGE (*k*), and 90-s postgadolinium fat-suppressed SGE (*l*) images demonstrate a 2-cm pseudocyst (arrow, *h*) in the uncinate process of the pancreas. The normal signal intensity of the pancreas, especially on noncontrast T1-weighted fat-suppressed (*j*) and immediate postgadolinium SGE (*k*) images, shows that background pancreas is not substantially diseased.

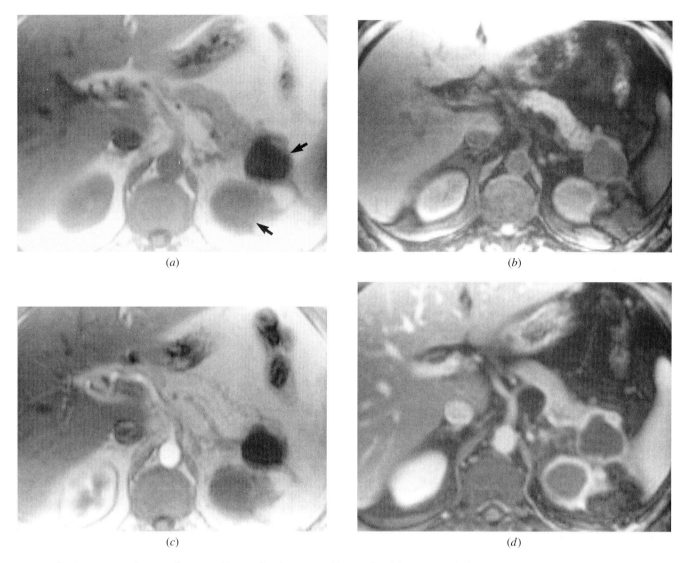

FIG. 4.78 Pancreatic pseudocysts. T1-weighted SGE (*a*), T1-weighted fat-suppressed SGE (*b*), immediate postgadolinium T1-weighted SGE (*c*), and 90-s postgadolinium T1-weighted fat-suppressed SGE (*d*) images. There is a pseudocyst in the tail of the pancreas and a second one adjacent in the upper pole of the left kidney (arrows, *a*). Late enhancement of the pseudocyst walls is appreciated (*d*).

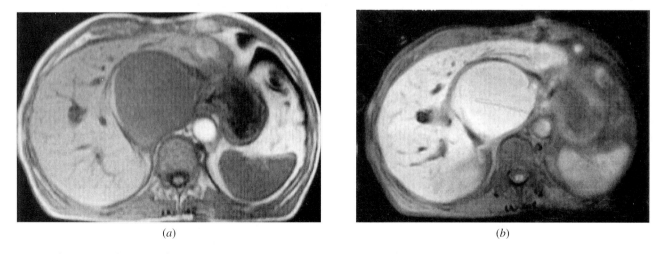

FIG. 4.79 Pseudocysts—large. T1-weighted SGE (*a*), T1-weighted fat-suppressed spin-echo (*b*), T2-weighted fat-suppressed

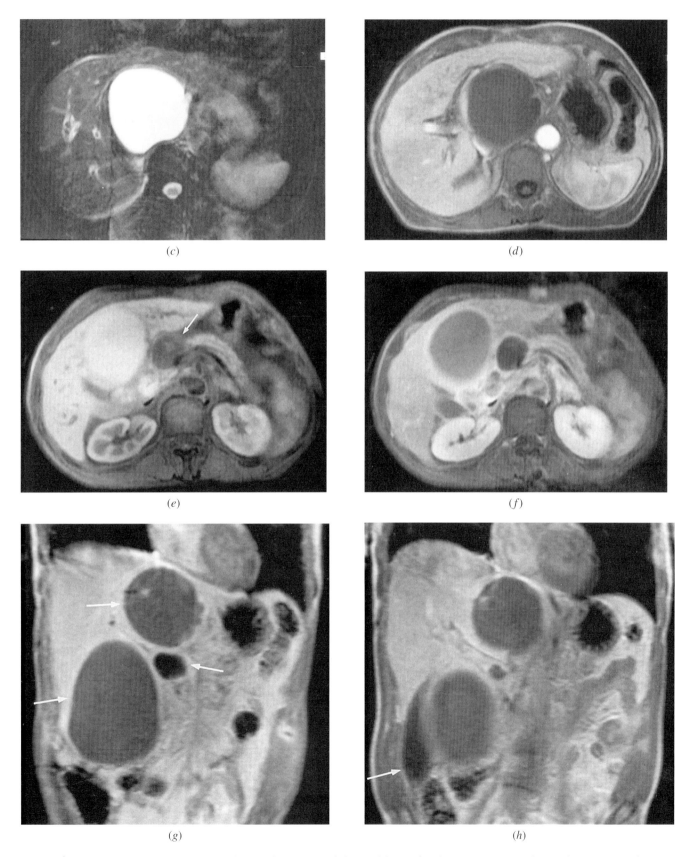

F I G . 4.79 (*Continued*) SSETSE (*c*), and immediate postgadolinium T1-weighted SGE (*d*) images obtained superior to the pancreas, T1-weighted fat-suppressed spin-echo (*e*) and gadolinium-enhanced T1-weighted fat-suppressed spin-echo (*f*) images at the level of the body of the pancreas, coronal gadolinium-enhanced T1-weighted SGE images from midhepatic (*g*) and more anterior (*h*) locations, and sagittal-plane (*i*) T1-weighted SGE images.

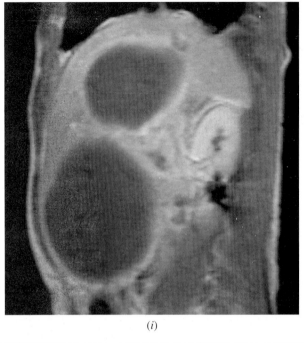

(i)

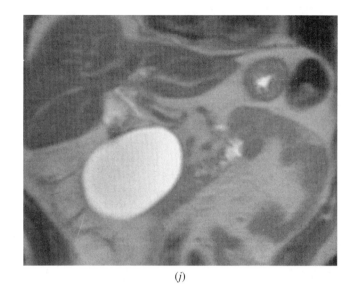

(j)

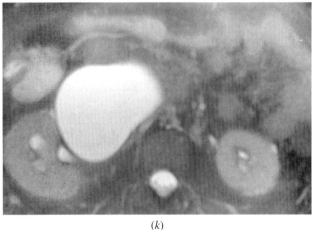

(k)

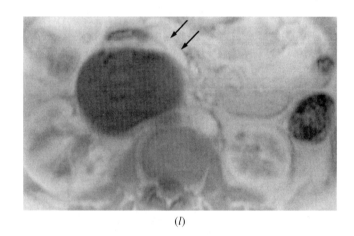

(l)

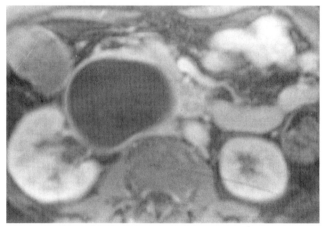

(m)

FIG. 4.79 (*Continued*) An 8-cm pseudocyst is present in the region of the porta hepatis that is mildly high in signal intensity on T1-weighted images (*a, b*) and high in signal intensity on the T2-weighted image (*c*). The mild, high signal intensity on T1-weighted images is more conspicuous with fat suppression (*b*) and consistent with dilute blood or protein. The homogeneous signal intensity on T2-weighted images suggests that the fluid, although proteinaceous, is not complicated by infection or cellular debris. A 3-cm pseudocyst (arrow, *e*) is identified within the body of the pancreas (*e, f*).

Fluid in the pseudocyst is low in signal intensity on the precontrast T1-weighted image (*e*). Capsular enhancement of the pseudocysts is shown on the fat-suppressed gadolinium-enhanced image (*f*). Coronal plane gadolinium-enhanced T1-weighted SGE images (*g, h*) demonstrate the relationship of the pseudocysts to surrounding structures. Three pseudocysts (arrows, *g*) are shown in the coronal plane (*g*). Gallbladder (arrow, *h*) is displaced laterally by the large pseudocyst in the porta hepatis. The sagittal plane image (*i*) demonstrates the anteroposterior orientation of the pseudocysts to other structures.

Coronal SS-ETSE (*j*), transverse fat-suppressed SS-ETSE (*k*), immediate postgadolinium T1-weighted SGE (*l*), and 90-s postgadolinium fat-suppressed SGE (*m*) images in a second patient. A large, 8 × 7 cm, pancreatic pseudocyst is situated between the right kidney and second portion of the duodenum. The pancreatic head is displaced anteriorly (arrows, *l*).

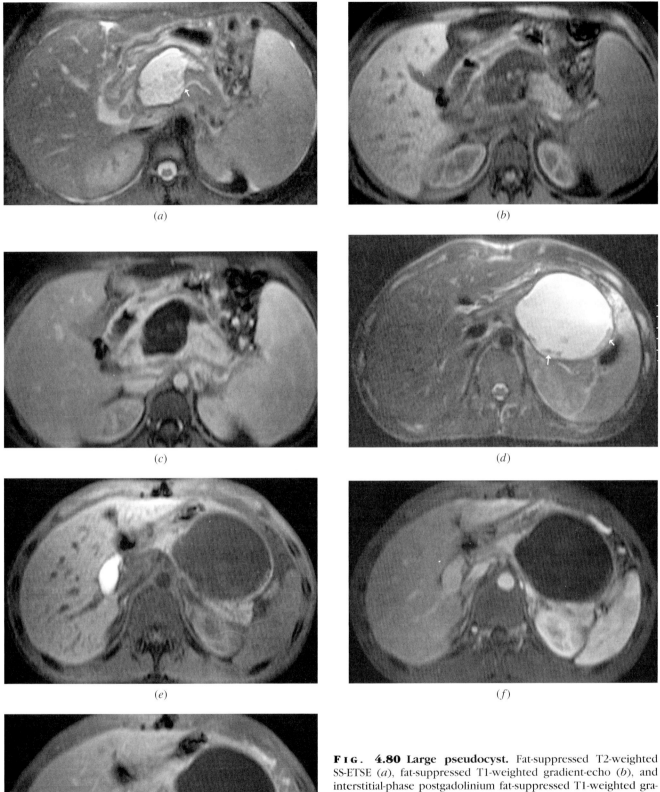

(a)

(b)

(c)

(d)

(e)

(f)

(g)

FIG. 4.80 Large pseudocyst. Fat-suppressed T2-weighted SS-ETSE (*a*), fat-suppressed T1-weighted gradient-echo (*b*), and interstitial-phase postgadolinium fat-suppressed T1-weighted gradient-echo (*c*) images. A large pseudocyst is present in the pancreatic head and neck. The continuity of the cyst with the main pancreatic duct is best seen on the T2-weighted image (arrow, *a*). The heterogeneous signal intensity on the T2-weighted images suggests that the fluid is complicated by infection or cellular debris. Fat-suppressed T2-weighted SS-ETSE (*d*), fat-suppressed T1-weighted gradient-echo (*e*), and immediate (*f*) and interstitial-phase (*g*) postgadolinium fat-suppressed T1-weighted gradient-echo images in a second patient with pancreatic pseudocyst. A large pseudocyst is present in the pancreatic tail. Debris within the pseudocyst is best seen on the T2-weighted image (arrows, *d*).

alcoholism and the development of chronic pancreatitis
[97, 98]. Obstruction of the pancreatic duct from various
causes, including pancreatic ductal cancer, results in
chronic pancreatitis [98]. Acute pancreatitis secondary
to gallstone disease rarely results in chronic
pancreatitis.

Chronic pancreatitis is associated with decreased
endocrine as well as exocrine function [97, 98]. Patients
with chronic pancreatitis have an increased risk of
developing pancreatic cancer [99].

An analysis of patients with chronic pancreatitis
imaged on dynamic contrast-enhanced CT images
showed the following features: 66% had dilatation of
the main pancreatic duct, 54% had parenchymal atrophy,
50% had pancreatic calcifications, 34% had pseudocysts,
32% had focal pancreatic enlargement, 29% had biliary
ductal dilatation, and 16% had densities in peripancreatic fat or fascia. No abnormalities were present in 7%
of patients [100]. Calcification, which is the pathognomonic feature of chronic pancreatitis on CT images, is
a late occurrence following development of fibrosis and
is observed in only half of these patients. CT imaging
is not sensitive at detecting the early changes of fibrosis
in chronic pancreatitis. Focal chronic pancreatitis may
be difficult to distinguish from adenocarcinoma in the
head of the pancreas because both entities may cause
focal enlargement (fig. 4.81), obstruction of the common
bile duct (figs. 4.82 and 4.83) and pancreatic duct,
atrophy of the tail of the pancreas, and obliteration of
the fat plane around the superior mesenteric artery
(SMA) [101–103].

MRI may perform better than CT imaging at detecting changes of chronic pancreatitis in that MRI detects
not only morphologic findings but also the presence of

fibrosis. Fibrosis is shown by diminished signal intensity
on T1-weighted fat-suppressed images and diminished
heterogeneous enhancement on immediate postgadolinium gradient-echo images [104]. Low signal intensity
on T1-weighted fat-suppressed images reflects loss of
the aqueous protein in the acini of the pancreas.
Diminished enhancement on capillary-phase images
reflects disruption of the normal capillary bed and
increased chronic inflammation and fibrous tissue (fig.
4.84). Most cases of chronic pancreatitis show progressive parenchymal enhancement on 5-min postcontrast
images, reflecting the pattern of enhancement of fibrous
tissue. A study that described MRI findings in 13 patients
with chronic calcifying pancreatitis and 9 patients with
acute recurrent pancreatitis demonstrated differences
between these groups on T1-weighted fat-suppressed
images and immediate postgadolinium gradient-echo
images [104]. All patients with pancreatic calcifications
on CT examination had a diminished-signal-intensity
pancreas on T1-weighted fat-suppressed images and an
abnormally low percentage of contrast enhancement on
immediate postgadolinium gradient-echo images (fig.
4.85). Patients with acute recurrent pancreatitis had
signal intensity features of the pancreas comparable to
normal pancreas. Secretin-enhanced MRCP has been
used for the evaluation of patients with pancreatic
pathologies including chronic pancreatitis. Secretin
induces pancreatic duct secretion. Therefore, it has
been reported that it improves the visualization of pancreatic ductal system and associated pathologies.
Secretin-MRCP has been reported to show early ductal
changes (dilatations-strictures) associated with chronic
pancreatitis (fig. 4.85). Secretin-MRCP has also been
reported to evaluate and grade pancreatic exocrine

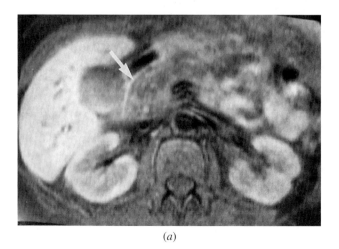

(a)

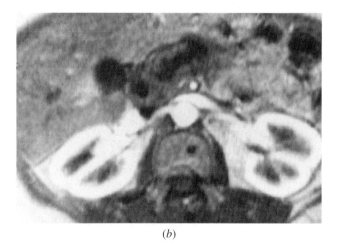

(b)

F I G . 4.81 Chronic pancreatitis with focal enlargement of the head of the pancreas. T1-weighted fat-suppressed spin-echo
(*a*), immediate postgadolinium T1-weighted SGE (*b*), and gadolinium-enhanced T1-weighted fat-suppressed spin-echo (*c*) images.
The head of the pancreas is enlarged (arrow, *a*).The pancreas is diffusely low in signal intensity on the precontrast T1-weighted
fat-suppressed image (*a*). The pancreas shows diffuse diminished enhancement on the immediate postgadolinium image (*b*).

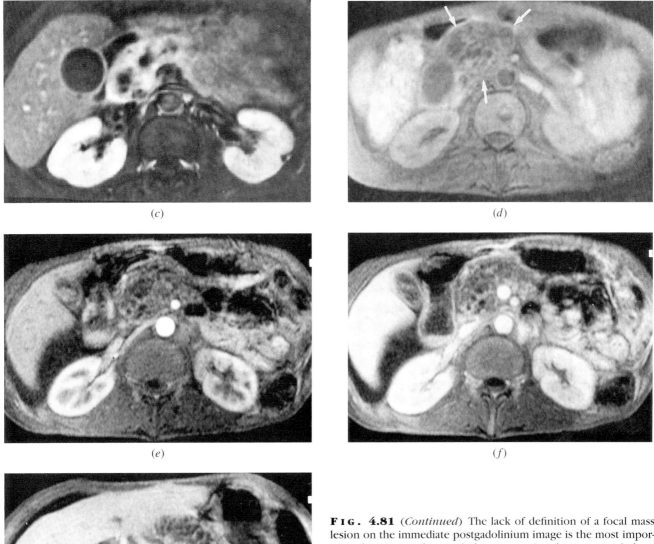

(c)

(d)

(e)

(f)

(g)

FIG. 4.81 (*Continued*) The lack of definition of a focal mass lesion on the immediate postgadolinium image is the most important observation that excludes tumor. On the interstitial-phase gadolinium-enhanced image (*c*), signal-void foci are identified that represent cysts, pseudocysts, dilated pancreatic duct, and calcifications. T1-weighted fat-suppressed spin-echo (*d*) and immediate (*e*) and 90-s (*f*) postgadolinium T1-weighted SGE images in a second patient demonstrate enlargement of the pancreatic head (arrows, *d*). The head enhances in a diminished fashion on immediate (*e*) and 90-s (*f*) postgadolinium images with no definition of a mass lesion and preservation of a marbled texture. Multiple small signal-void foci represent calcifications. The 90-s postgadolinium image (*g*) demonstrates that signal-void foci are also present throughout the body and tail.

function noninvasively (fig. 4.85). Following secretin stimulation, good duodenal filling should be present in the presence of normal exocrine function. Despite its use in routine clinical practice for the last 10 years, the role of secretin-MRCP for the assessment of pancreatic duct pathologies has not been well established yet.

Focal enlargement of the head of the pancreas with chronic pancreatitis may be difficult to distinguish from cancer on CT images [33]. MR images permit distinction between these two entities with greater reliability [33]. Both chronic pancreatitis and carcinoma show similar signal intensity changes of the enlarged region of pancreas on noncontrast T1-weighted fat-suppressed and T2-weighted images: generally mildly hypointense on T1-weighted images and heterogenous and mildly hyperintense on T2-weighted images. On immediate postgadolinium images, focal pancreatitis shows heterogeneous enhancement with the presence of signal-void

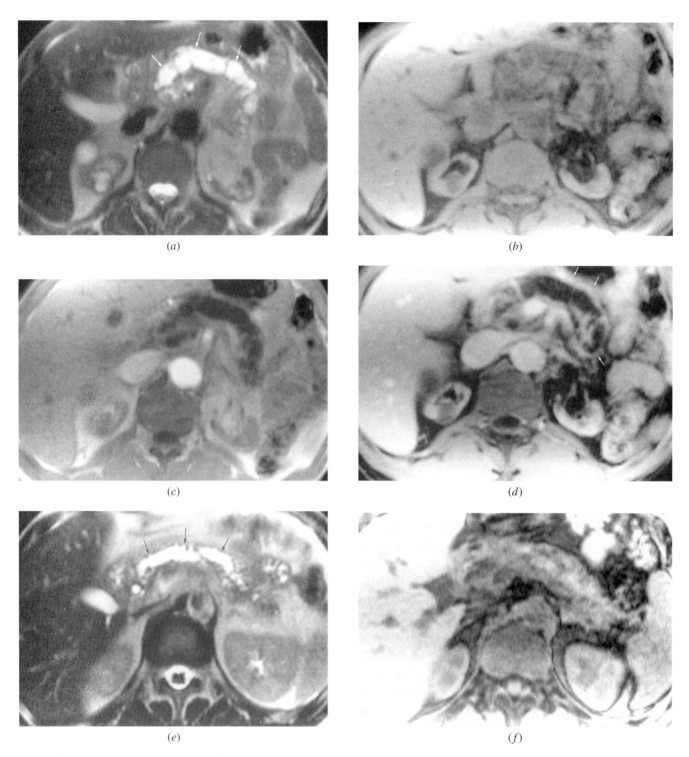

FIG. 4.82 Chronic pancreatitis with moderate to severe pancreatic duct dilatation. T2-weighted SS-ETSE (*a*), T1-weighted fat-suppressed SGE (*b*), immediate postgadolinium T1-weighted SGE (*c*), and 90-s postgadolinium fat-suppressed SGE (*d*) images in a patient with hereditary pancreatitis and recurrent bouts of pancreatitis. The pancreatic ductal is very dilated (arrows, *a*). The pancreatic parenchyma is atrophic and is low signal on noncontrast T1-weighted fat-suppressed SGE (*b*). The thin rim of atrophic pancreas enhances minimally on immediate postgadolinium image (*c*) and shows late enhancement (arrows, *d*) consistent with changes of fibrosis. The pancreas is atrophic for the patient's age (18 years old), and it shows heterogeneous signal intensity on T1-weighted images (*b*) with diminished enhancement on postgadolinium images (*d*). The pancreatic duct is severely dilated.

T2-weighted SS-ETSE (*e*), T1-weighted fat-suppressed SGE (*f*), immediate postgadolinium T1-weighted SGE (*g*), and 90-s postgadolinium fat-suppressed SGE (*h*) images on a second patient demonstrate similar findings. Note moderately severe dilatation of the pancreatic duct (arrows, *e*) and late enhancement of atrophic pancreatic parenchyma (arrows, *h*).

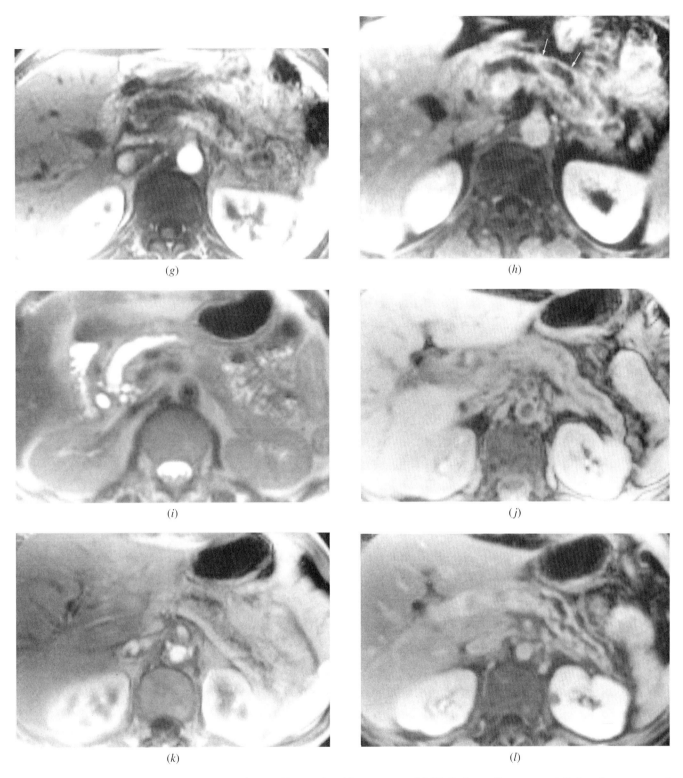

FIG. 4.82 (*Continued*) T2-weighted SS-ETSE (*i*), T1-weighted fat-suppressed SGE (*j*), immediate postgadolinium fat-suppressed SGE (*k*), and 90-s post-gadolinium fat-suppressed SGE (*l*) images in a third patient show the same findings of moderately severe pancreatic ductal dilatation with parenchymal signal intensity changes of chronic pancreatitis.

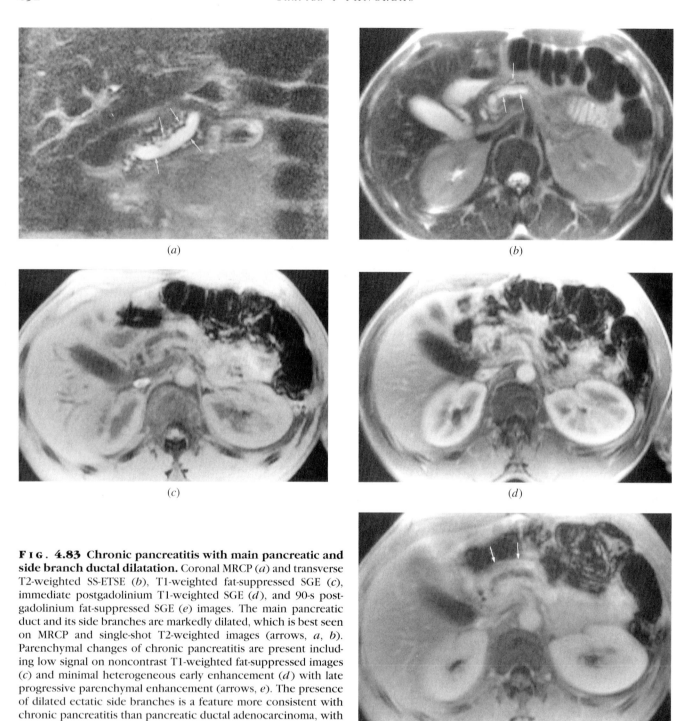

F I G . 4.83 Chronic pancreatitis with main pancreatic and side branch ductal dilatation. Coronal MRCP (*a*) and transverse T2-weighted SS-ETSE (*b*), T1-weighted fat-suppressed SGE (*c*), immediate postgadolinium T1-weighted SGE (*d*), and 90-s postgadolinium fat-suppressed SGE (*e*) images. The main pancreatic duct and its side branches are markedly dilated, which is best seen on MRCP and single-shot T2-weighted images (arrows, *a*, *b*). Parenchymal changes of chronic pancreatitis are present including low signal on noncontrast T1-weighted fat-suppressed images (*c*) and minimal heterogeneous early enhancement (*d*) with late progressive parenchymal enhancement (arrows, *e*). The presence of dilated ectatic side branches is a feature more consistent with chronic pancreatitis than pancreatic ductal adenocarcinoma, with the latter entity more typically causing dilatation of the main pancreatic duct without side branch ectasia.

cysts and calcifications, without evidence of a marginated definable, minimally enhancing mass lesion. Demonstration of a definable, circumscribed mass lesion is most often diagnostic for tumor. In chronic pancreatitis, the focally enlarged portion of the pancreas usually shows preservation of a glandular, feathery, or marbled texture similar to that of the remaining pan-

creas [33]. In contrast, in pancreatic cancer, the focally enlarged portion of the pancreas loses its usual anatomic detail. Tumor disrupts the underlying architecture and generally exhibits irregular, heterogeneous, diminished enhancement. Diffuse low signal intensity of the entire pancreas, similar to and including the area of focal enlargement, on T1-weighted fat-suppressed and

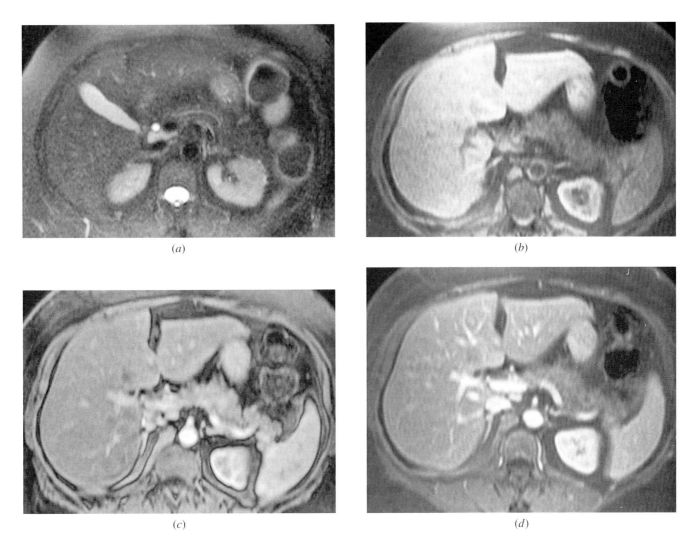

(a)

(b)

(c)

(d)

F I G . 4.84 Early chronic pancreatitis. Fat-suppressed T2-weighted SS-ETSE (*a*), fat-suppressed T1-weighted gradient-echo (*b*), and immediate (*c*) and interstitial-phase (*d*) postgadolinium fat-suppressed T1-weighted gradient-echo images in a patient with early chronic pancreatitis demonstrate mildly diminished signal intensity on fat-suppressed and immediate postgadolinium T1-weighted images. Low signal intensity on T1-weighted fat-suppressed image (*b*) reflects loss of aqueous protein in the acini of the pancreas. Diminished enhancement on capillary-phase image (*c*) reflects disruption of the normal capillary bed due to chronic inflammation and fibrous tissue.

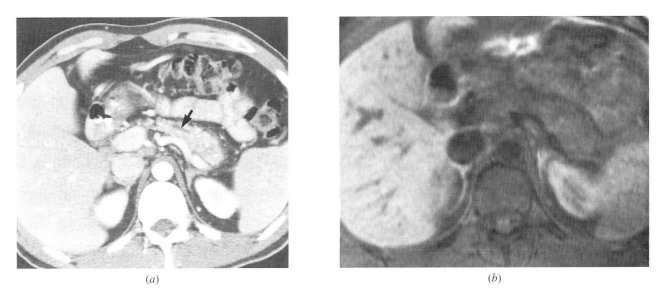

(a)

(b)

F I G . 4.85 Chronic pancreatitis. Contrast-enhanced CT (*a*) T1-weighted fat-suppressed spin-echo (*b*), and immediate postgadolinium

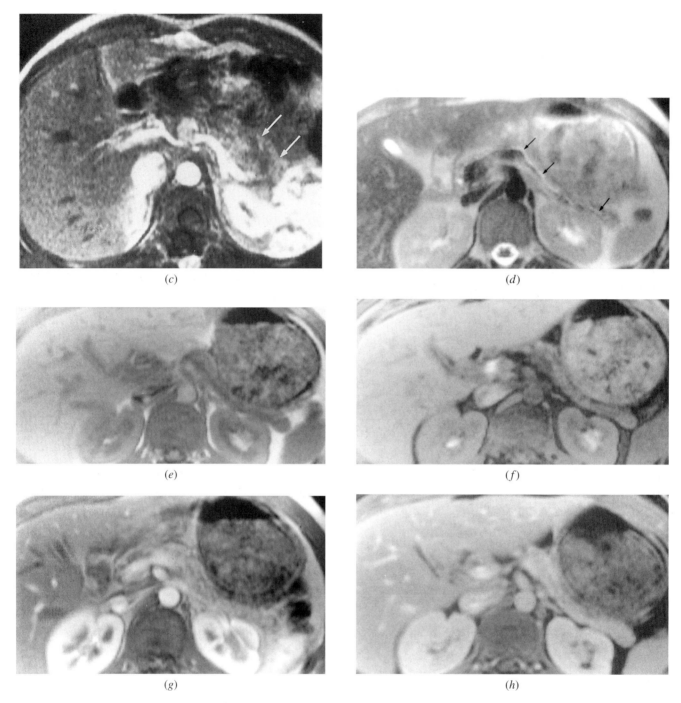

(c)

(d)

(e)

(f)

(g)

(h)

FIG. 4.85 (*Continued*) T1-weighted SGE (*c*) images. The CT image demonstrates pancreatic calcifications, which is diagnostic for chronic pancreatitis. Mild pancreatic ductal dilatation (arrow, *a*) and mild pancreatic enlargement are also present. The pancreas is low in signal intensity on the T1-weighted fat-suppressed image, which is consistent with loss of aqueous protein in the acini. The immediate postgadolinium T1-weighted SGE image demonstrates heterogeneous diminished enhancement of the pancreas (arrows, *c*), reflecting replacement of the normal capillary bed with lesser vascularized fibrotic tissue. (Reproduced with permission from Semelka RC, Kroeker MA, Shoenut JP, Kroeker R, Yaffe CS, Micflikier AB: Pancreatic disease: Prospective comparison of CT, ERCP, and 1.5 T MR imaging with dynamic gadolinium enhancement and fat suppression. *Radiology* 181: 785–791, 1991.)

T2-weighted SS-ETSE (*d*),T1-weighted SGE (*e*), noncontrast T1-weighted fat-suppressed SGE (*f*), immediate postgadolinium T1-weighted SGE (*g*), and 90-s postgadolinium fat-suppressed SGE (*h*) images in a second patient. Moderate dilatation of the pancreatic duct is present (arrows, *d*). There is moderate atrophy of the pancreatic parenchyma, which is low signal on T1-weighted fat-suppressed SGE (*f*) and demonstrates minimal enhancement on immediate postgadolinium images (*g*) with progressive enhancement on 90-s postcontrast images (*h*). These are classic features for chronic pancreatitis.

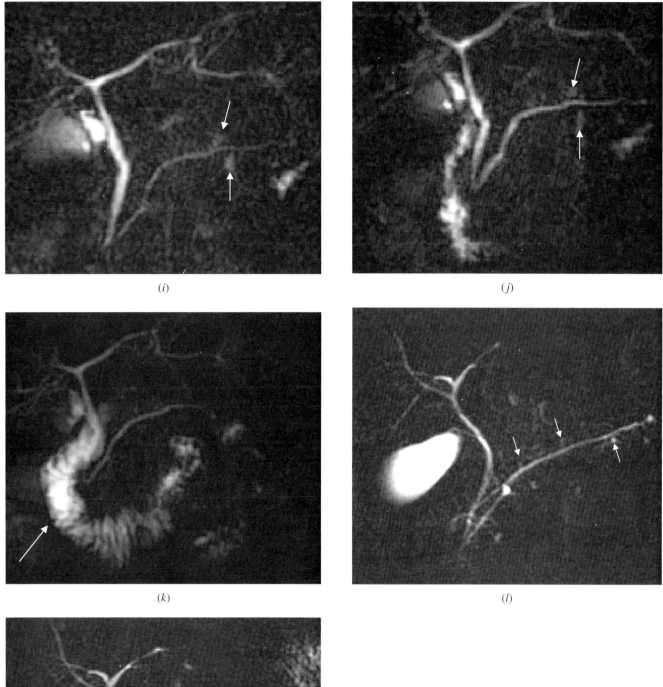

(i)

(j)

(k)

(l)

(m)

F I G . 4.85 (*Continued*) **Chronic pancreatitis—Secretin MRCP.** Presecretin (*i*) and postsecretin MRCP (*j*, *k*) images in a patient with mild chronic pancreatitis. Side branch dilatations (arrows, *i*) are detected on MRCP image (*i*) acquired before secretin administration. After secretin administration, the pancreatic duct and side branch dilatations (arrows, *j*) are seen better. On MRCP image (*k*) acquired at 10 min after the administration of secretin, there is good duodenal filling (arrow, *k*) suggesting normal exocrine function of the pancreas. Presecretin (*l*) and postsecretin MRCP (*m*) images in a patient with mild chronic pancreatitis. Side branch dilatations (arrows, *l*) are detected on MRCP image (*l*) acquired before secretin administration. After secretin administration, more side branch dilatations (arrows, *m*) are detected on MRCP image (*m*) acquired at 10 min. However, duodenal filling is less than normal and consistent with decreased estimated pancreatic exocrine function.

immediate postgadolinium SGE images is typical for chronic pancreatitis (fig. 4.86). In the setting of pancreatic cancer, the enhancement of the tumor is less than adjacent pancreatic parenchyma. Rarely, chronic pancreatitis may involve only the focally enlarged portion of the pancreas, with the reminder of the pancreas having no inflammatory changes. In these cases, the focus of chronic pancreatitis can simulate the appearance of pancreatic ductal adenocarcinoma. The inflammatory process may also be sufficiently destructive that underlying stromal pattern is lost. In these rare cases, diagnosis can only be established by surgical resection and histopathologic examination confirming the absence of malignancy.

Recurrent bouts of acute pancreatitis superimposed on the chronic disease typify the usual clinical course of these patients. Acute on chronic pancreatitis is well shown on MR images (figs. 4.87–4.89). Pancreatic pseu-

docysts observed in patients with chronic pancreatitis often arise as a sequel of episodes of acute inflammation [98]. Small pseudocysts and cysts are well shown on gadolinium-enhanced T1-weighted fat-suppressed images as nearly signal-void oval structures (fig. 4.90). Pseudocysts are generally high in signal intensity on T2-weighted images, but signal intensity varies considerably depending on the presence of blood, protein, infection, and debris (fig. 4.91). Pseudocyst walls generally show minimal early postgadolinium enhancement and progressive enhancement on 5-min postgadolinium images.

Autoimmune Pancreatitis

Most patients presenting with chronic pancreatitis will have alcohol-related disease. In approximately 30% of patients, the nature and course of chronic pancreatitis are unclear, and these cases may be labeled idiopathic.

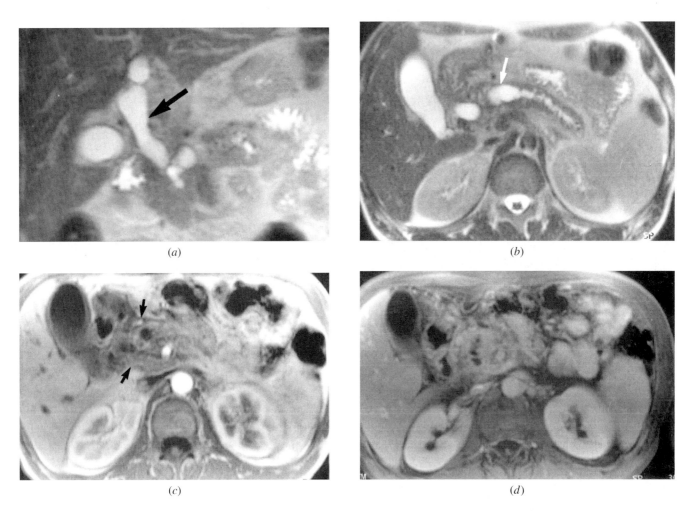

(a)   (b)

(c)   (d)

F I G . 4.86 Chronic pancreatitis simulating pancreatic cancer. Coronal (*a*) and transverse (*b*) T2-weighted SS-ETSE, immediate postgadolinium T1-weighted SGE (*c*), and 90-s postgadolinium fat-suppressed SGE (*d*) images. The CBD (arrow, *a*) and pancreatic (arrow, *b*) ducts are severely dilated, with atrophy of the pancreatic body (*b*) creating the double duct sign. On early (*c*) and late (*d*) postgadolinium images, no demarcated pancreatic mass is observed in the head of the pancreas. Instead, the enlarged pancreas shows a marbled texture (arrows, *c*) comparable in appearance to the remainder of the pancreas.

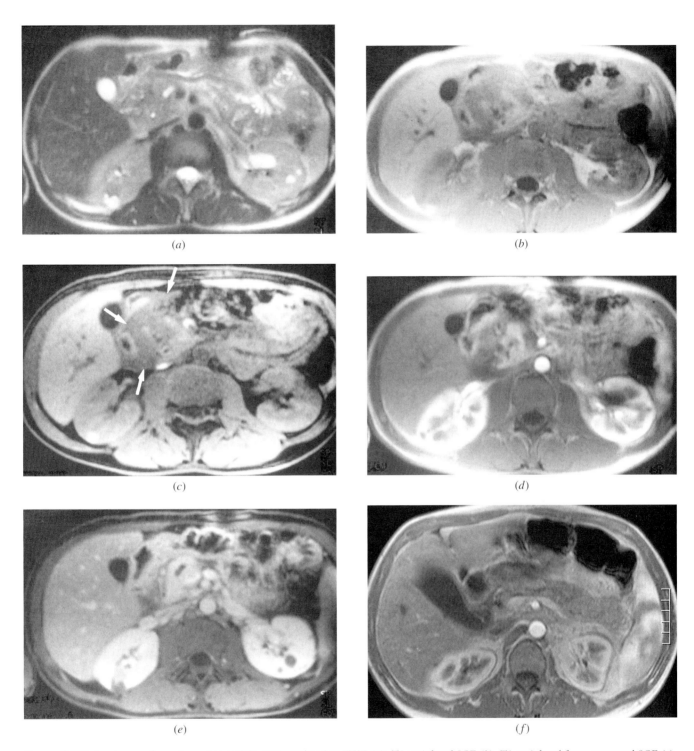

F I G . 4.87 Acute on chronic pancreatitis. T2-weighted SS-ETSE (*a*), T1-weighted SGE (*b*), T1-weighted fat-suppressed SGE (*c*), immediate postgadolinium T1-weighted SGE (*d*), and 90-s postgadolinium fat-suppressed SGE (*e*) images. Complex fluid surrounds the pancreas, predominantly located between the head and the second portion of duodenum (arrows, *c*). The pancreatic head is enlarged and shows decreased signal on noncontrast T1-weighted fat-suppressed SGE (*c*) and heterogeneous and reduced enhancement on immediate postgadolinium images (*d*), which is characteristic of chronic pancreatitis.

Immediate postgadolinium T1-weighted gradient-echo (*f*), interstitial-phase postgadolinium fat-suppressed T1-weighted gradient-echo (*g*), and MRCP (*h*) images in a patient with acute on chronic pancreatitis. The enhancement of the pancreas is

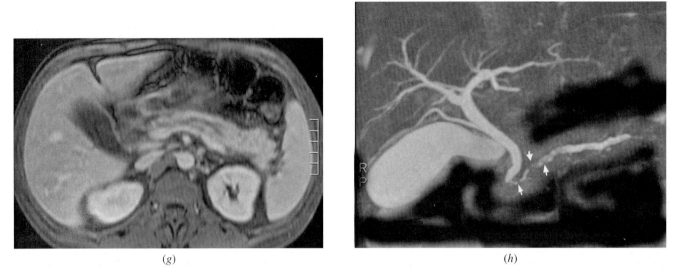

(g)

(h)

FIG. 4.87 (*Continued*) decreased on immediate postgadolinium image (*f*). The main pancreatic duct is mildly dilated and irregular (arrows, *h*).

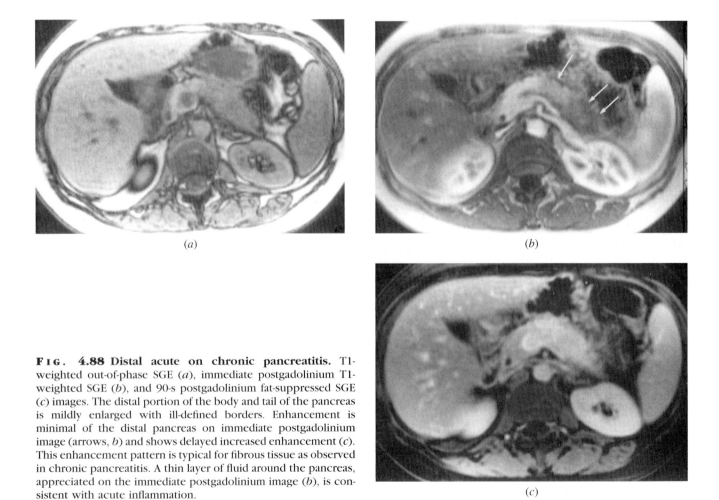

(a)

(b)

(c)

FIG. 4.88 Distal acute on chronic pancreatitis. T1-weighted out-of-phase SGE (*a*), immediate postgadolinium T1-weighted SGE (*b*), and 90-s postgadolinium fat-suppressed SGE (*c*) images. The distal portion of the body and tail of the pancreas is mildly enlarged with ill-defined borders. Enhancement is minimal of the distal pancreas on immediate postgadolinium image (arrows, *b*) and shows delayed increased enhancement (*c*). This enhancement pattern is typical for fibrous tissue as observed in chronic pancreatitis. A thin layer of fluid around the pancreas, appreciated on the immediate postgadolinium image (*b*), is consistent with acute inflammation.

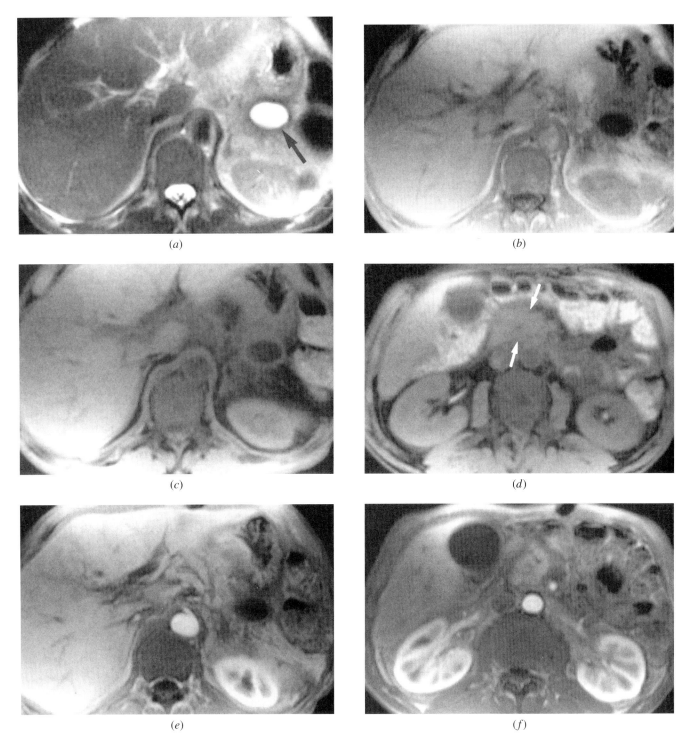

FIG. 4.89 Acute on chronic pancreatitis with pseudocyst formation. T2-weighted SS-ETSE (*a*), T1-weighted SGE (*b*), T1-weighted fat-suppressed SGE (*c*, *d*), immediate postgadolinium T1-weighted SGE (*e*, *f*), and 90-s postgadolinium fat-suppressed

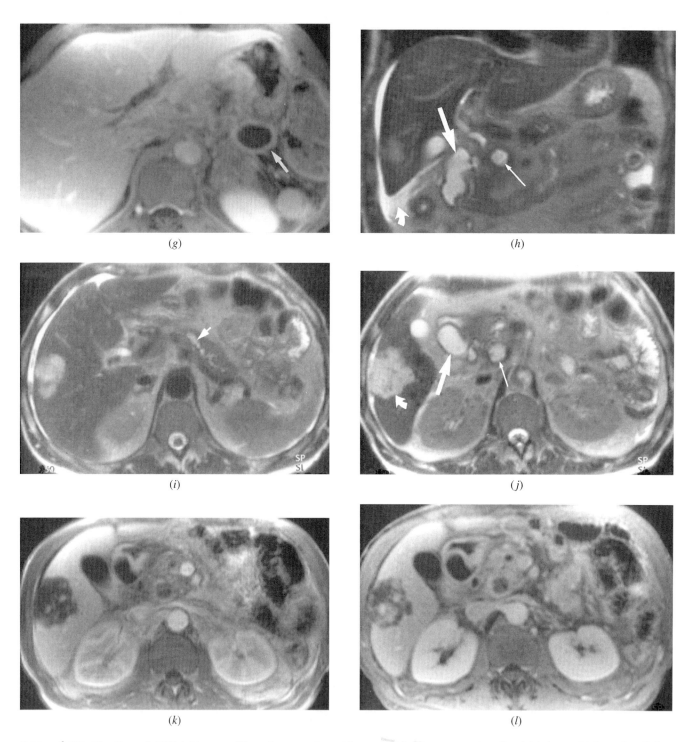

(g)

(h)

(i)

(j)

(k)

(l)

FIG. 4.89 (*Continued*) SGE (*g*) images. There is a pseudocyst (arrow, *a*) in the pancreatic tail, which has a thickened wall that exhibits progressive late enhancement (arrow, *g*). The pancreatic head and neck region (arrows, *d*) are enlarged (*d*, *f*) and exhibit low-signal on noncontrast fat-suppressed images (*d*) and diminished heterogeneous enhancement on immediate postgadolinium SGE images (*f*) consistent with focal acute on diffuse chronic pancreatitis. Note that renal corticomedullary difference is diminished on the noncontrast T1-weighted fat-suppressed image consistent with decreased renal function (*d*).

Coronal (*h*) and transverse (*i*, *j*) T2-weighted SS-ETSE, immediate postgadolinium T1-weighted SGE (*k*), and 90-s postgadolinium fat-suppressed SGE (*l*) images in a second patient. There is mild pancreatic duct dilatation and irregularity (arrow, *i*), which is commonly observed in chronic pancreatitis (*i*). A 2-cm pseudocyst is present in the posterior aspect of the pancreatic head (small arrow, *h*, *j*) and an irregular 4-cm pseudocyst (large arrow, *h*, *j*) adjacent to the second portion of the duodenum. A small volume of ascites is present (curved arrow, *h*). Note an incidental hemangioma in the liver that is high signal on T2 (curved arrow, *j*) demonstrating peripheral nodular enhancement with enlargement and coalescence of the nodules (*k*, *l*).

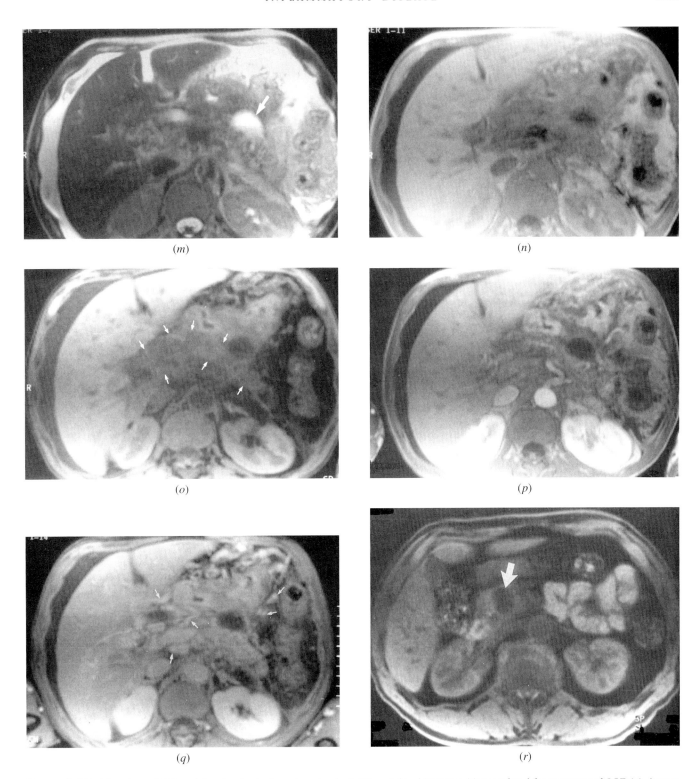

F I G . 4.89 (*Continued*) T2-weighted echo-train spin-echo (*m*), T1-weighted SGE (*n*), T1-weighted fat-suppressed SGE (*o*), immediate postgadolinium T1 SGE (*p*), and 90-s postgadolinium T1-weighted fat-suppressed SGE (*q*) images in a third patient. The pancreas is enlarged and ill-defined with blurring of the adjacent fat. The pancreas is low signal (arrows, *o*) on noncontrast T1-weighted fat-suppressed images (*o*) and on immediate postgadolinium SGE images (*q*) consistent with chronic pancreatitis. The pancreatic parenchyma shows progressive enhancement on late gadolinium-enhanced images (*q*), which is also a feature of chronic pancreatitis. There is a thick-walled pseudocyst anterior to the distal body of the pancreas, which contains a fluid-fluid level (arrow, *m*) on T2 (*m*). Multiple varices (small arrows, *q*) observed on the interstitial-phase gadolinium-enhanced image (*q*) reflect thrombosis of the splenic vein from longstanding severe chronic pancreatitis. T1-weighted fat-suppressed SGE (*r*), immediate postgadolinium

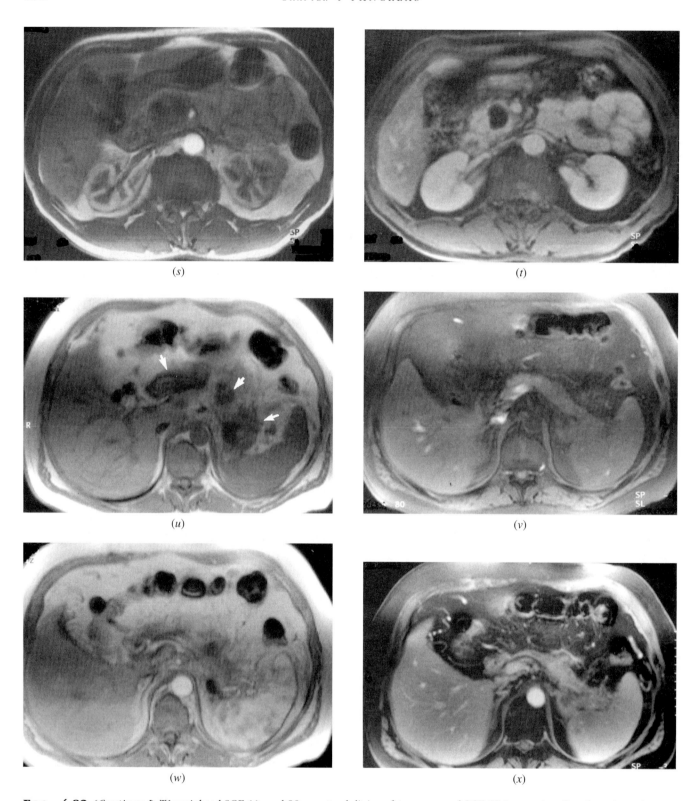

(s)

(t)

(u)

(v)

(w)

(x)

F I G . 4.89 *(Continued)* T1-weighted SGE (*s*), and 90-s postgadolinium fat-suppressed SGE (*t*) images in a fourth patient. A pseudocyst is present in the head of the pancreas (arrow, *r*). Note the decreased signal on the noncontrast T1-weighted fat-suppressed SGE image (*r*), and minimal heterogeneous enhancement on the immediate postgadolinium SGE image (*s*) with progressive enhancement on the parenchyma (*t*), which are imaging features of chronic pancreatitis. Compare this appearance to the pseudocyst in the pancreatic head of patients with acute pancreatitis (fig. 4.77).

T1-weighted SGE (*u*), T1-weighted fat-suppressed SGE (*v*), immediate postgadolinium SGE (*w*), and 90-s postgadolinium fat-suppressed SGE (*x*) images in a fifth patient. Multiple pseudocysts (arrows, *u*) and peripancreatic fluid strands from acute inflammation present superimposed on chronic pancreatitis. The peripancreatic fluid strands are more clearly shown on the non-fat-suppressed images (*u*, *w*) than on the fat-suppressed images (*v*, *x*), because of the excellent contrast between low-signal fluid and high-signal background fat. Background chronic pancreatitis is shown as low signal of a small pancreas on noncontrast T1-weighted fat-suppressed image (*v*) and minimal early enhancement of the pancreas (*w*) with progressive enhancement on late images (*x*).

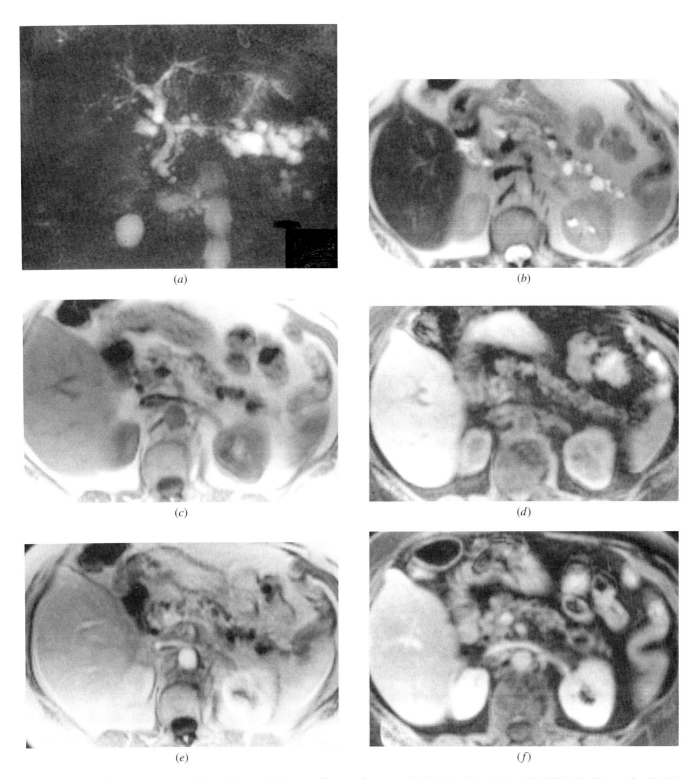

F I G . 4.90 Chronic pancreatitis with multiple small pseudocysts. MRCP (*a*), T2-weighted SS-ETSE (*b*), T1-weighted SGE (*c*), T1-weighted fat-suppressed SGE (*d*), immediate postgadolinium T1-weighted SGE (*e*), and 90-s postgadolinium fat-suppressed SGE (*f*) images. Multiple small pseudocysts are present throughout the atrophic background pancreatic parenchyma and appear hyperintense on T2-weighted images (*a*, *b*) and hypointense on T1-weighted images (*c*, *d*) and show lack of enhancement on early (*e*) and late (*f*) postgadolinium images, consistent with pseudocysts.

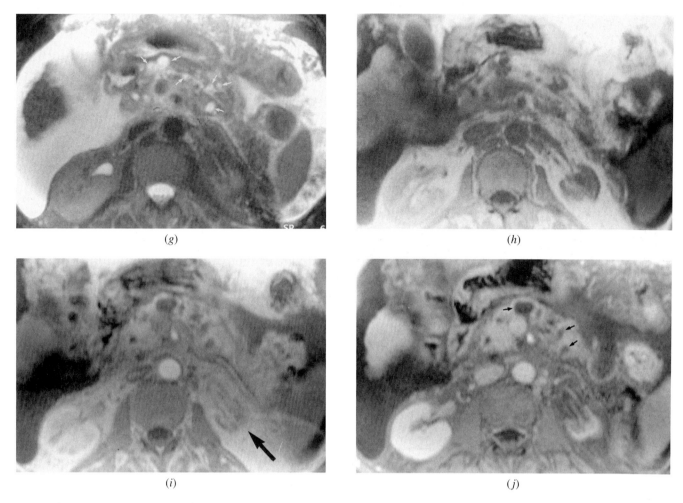

F I G . 4.90 (*Continued*) T2-weighted SS-ETSE (*g*), T1-weighted SGE (*h*), immediate postgadolinium T1-weighted SGE (*i*), and 90-s postgadolinium fat-suppressed SGE (*j*) images in a second patient with alcoholic pancreatitis. There are numerous cysts (arrows, *g*, *j*) scattered throughout the pancreas, and the pancreatic parenchyma enhances poorly on postgadolinium images. There is a large volume of ascites secondary to liver cirrhosis. Note also ischemic nephropathy of the left kidney (arrow, *i*) from main renal artery disease.

A subgroup of these cases has been associated with autoimmune disorders such as Sjögren syndrome, primary biliary cirrhosis, and primary sclerosing cholangitis [105, 106]. Histopathologic examination in cases of chronic nonalcoholic pancreatitis, including associated autoimmune disorders, shows periductal chronic inflammation and fibrosis. This process may result in obstruction or destruction of ducts [107]. Recent studies underscore the importance of diagnosing cases of suspected autoimmune-related chronic pancreatitis because these disorders may have a salutary response to steroid therapy [108]. Recent studies have described the MR appearance of autoimmune chronic pancreatitis as characterized by enlarged pancreas with moderately decreased signal intensity on T1-weighted images, moderately high signal intensity on T2-weighted images, and delayed enhancement of the pancreatic parenchyma after gadolinium administration (fig. 4.92).

Additional findings that may be observed in autoimmune pancreatitis include 1) capsulelike rim surrounding the diseased parenchyma that is hypointense on T2-weighted images and demonstrates delayed enhancement after gadolinium administration [105], 2) absence of parenchymal atrophy, 3) ductal dilatation proximal to the site of stenosis, 4) absence of extra-pancreatic fluid, and 5) clear demarcation of the lesion [106].

Inflammatory Conditions and Infections of the Pancreas

A variety of bacterial, granulomatous, viral, and parasitic diseases may rarely affect the pancreas. Inflammatory diseases may appear as ill-defined focal masses that show irregular infiltration of pancreatic tissue (fig. 4.93). Differentiation between malignant and inflammatory

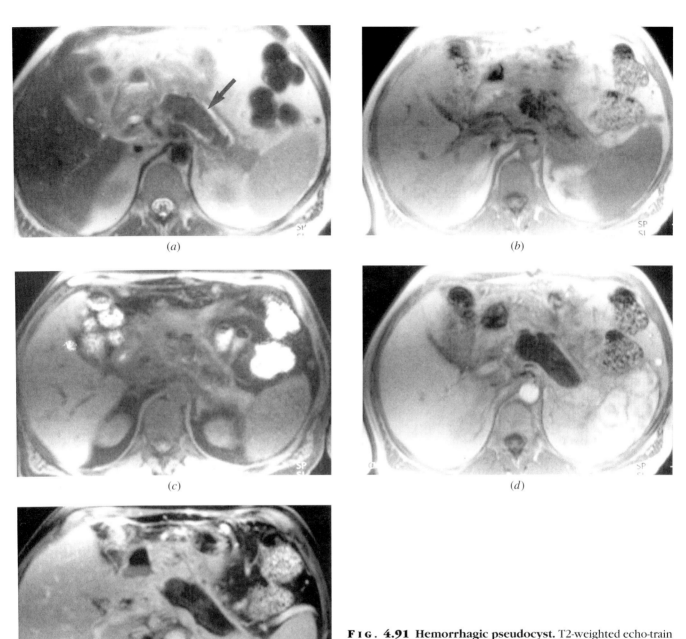

(a)

(b)

(c)

(d)

(e)

FIG. 4.91 Hemorrhagic pseudocyst. T2-weighted echo-train spin-echo (*a*), T1-weighted SGE (*b*), T1-weighted fat-suppressed SGE (*c*), immediate postgadolinium T1-weighted SGE (*d*), and 90-s postgadolinium T1-weighted fat-suppressed SGE (*e*) images. There is a tubule-shaped fluid collection (arrow, *a*) within the pancreas that has heterogeneous signal intensity on T1 (*b*, *c*)- and T2 (*a*)-weighted images compatible with hemorrhage. The pancreas is enlarged and has a blurred contour.

diseases may not, however, be reliably made on imaging studies. Pancreatitis may also arise as a reaction to drugs (fig. 4.94) or toxins.

TRAUMA

Traumatic injury of the pancreas may result in a spectrum of abnormalities from mild contusion to laceration and transection. Stenosis of the pancreatic duct with distal ductal dilatation may be observed as a sequel of trauma (fig. 4.95). A combination of tissue imaging sequences and MR pancreatography can facilitate this diagnosis by the demonstration of ductal dilatation and changes of chronic pancreatitis of the pancreas distal to the stenosis (fig. 4.96). This condition is not rare, and this entity should be entertained when a sharp transition is observed in the midbody of the pancreas, overlying

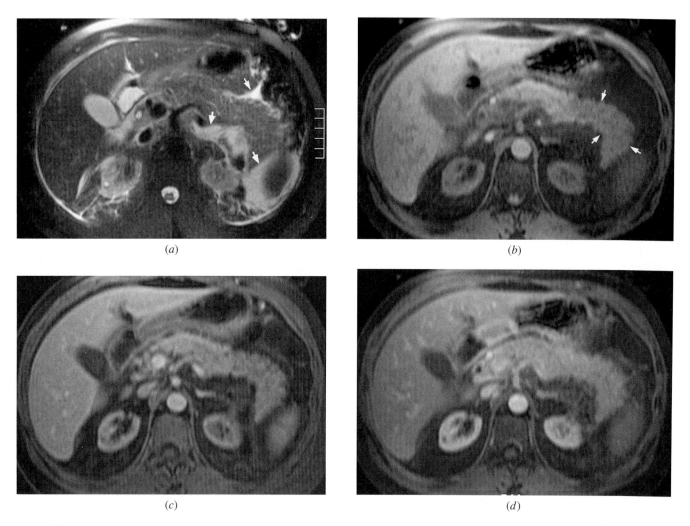

F I G . 4.92 Autoimmune pancreatitis. Fat-suppressed T2-weighted SS-ETSE (*a*), fat-suppressed T1-weighted gradient-echo (*b*), and immediate (*c*) and interstitial-phase (*d*) postgadolinium fat-suppressed T1-weighted images in a patient with autoimmune pancreatitis demonstrate a thin layer of peripancreatic and perisplenic fluid that is best seen on fat-suppressed T2-weighted images (arrows, *a*). The distal body and tail of the pancreas show decreased signal intensity compared to the remainder of the pancreas on fat-suppressed T1-weighted gradient-echo images (arrows, *b*). On immediate postgadolinium image the enhancement of the distal pancreas is less than the proximal portion (*c*). On interstitial-phase image distal pancreas becomes isointense with the rest of the pancreas (*d*).

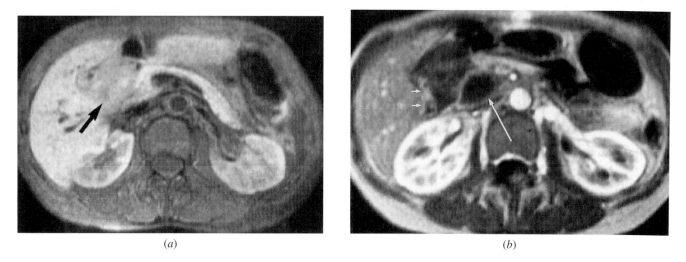

F I G . 4.93 Necrotizing granulomatous pancreatitis. T1-weighted fat-suppressed spin-echo (*a*), immediate postgadolinium T1-weighted SGE (*b*), and gadolinium-enhanced T1-weighted fat-suppressed spin-echo (*c*) images. A heterogeneous low-signal

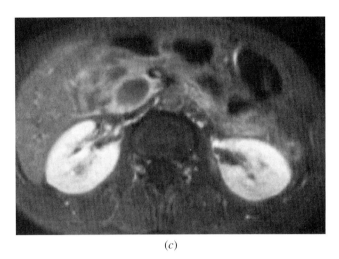

(c)

FIG. 4.93 (*Continued*) intensity mass is present, arising from the lateral aspect of the head of the pancreas (arrow, *a*). The remainder of the pancreas is normal and moderately high in signal intensity on T1-weighted fat-suppressed spin-echo images (*a*). The lesion enhances in a heterogeneous minimal fashion on immediate postgadolinium T1-weighted SGE images (*b*). The duodenum (small arrows, *b*) is displaced laterally by the mass. The mass contains a cystic component (thin arrow, *b*). Heterogeneous enhancement of the mass is also present on the interstitial-phase gadolinium-enhanced T1-weighted fat-suppressed image (*c*).

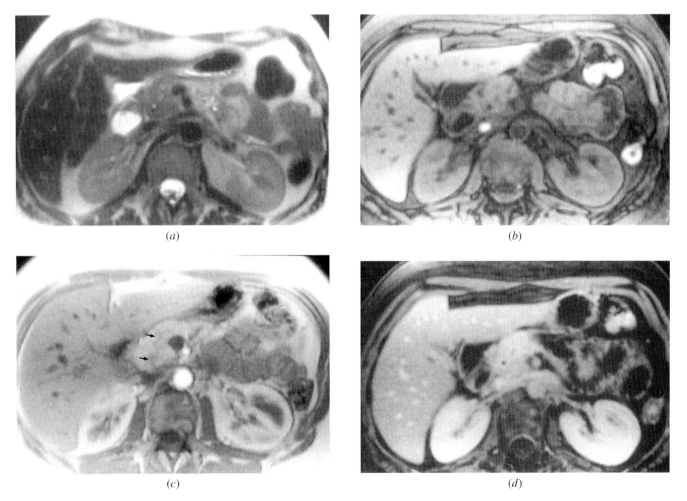

(a)   (b)

(c)   (d)

FIG. 4.94 Chemotherapy-induced pancreatitis. T2-weighted ETSE (*a*), T1-weighted fat-suppressed SGE (*b*), immediate postgadolinium T1-weighted SGE (*c*), and 90-s postgadolinium fat-suppressed SGE (*d*) images. In this patient undergoing chemotherapy for breast cancer, there is a heterogeneous low-signal region in the head of the pancreas on the noncontrast T1-weighted fat-suppressed image (*b*) that also shows heterogeneous decreased enhancement (arrows, *c*) on the immediate postgadolinium SGE image (*c*) consistent with pancreatitis secondary to chemotherapy toxicity.

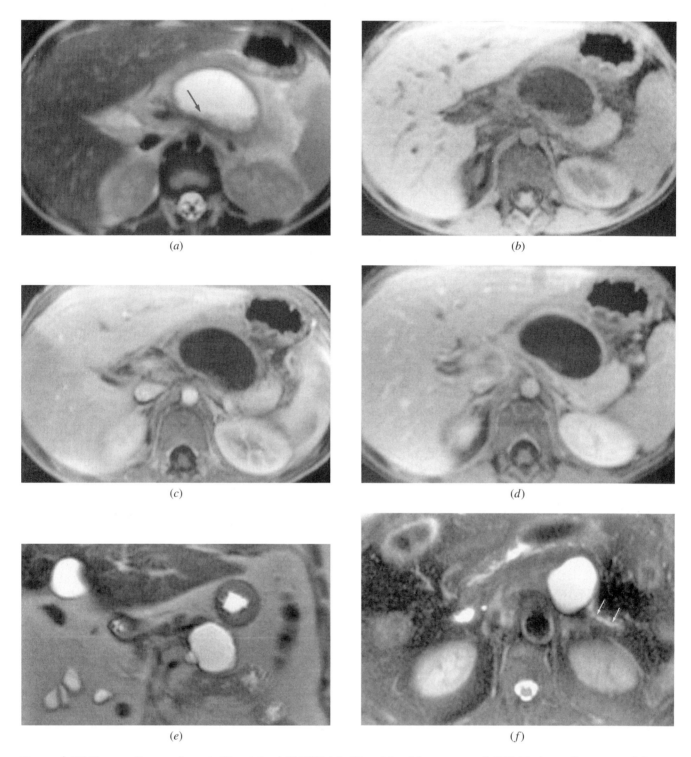

FIG. 4.95 Traumatic pseudocyst. T2-weighted SS-ETSE (*a*), T1-weighted fat-suppressed SGE (*b*), immediate postgadolinium T1-weighted SGE (*c*), and 90-s postgadolinium fat-suppressed SGE (*d*) images in a patient with a history of recent abdominal trauma. There is a pseudocyst in the anterior aspect of the pancreatic body/tail, which contains layering protein/hemoglobin in the dependent portion of the cyst, best appreciated on the T2-weighted image (arrow, *a*). Note transient increased enhancement of the left lobe of the liver on the immediate postgadolinium image (*c*), which reflects compromise of the left portal vein.

Coronal (*e*) and transverse (*f*) T2-weighted SS-ETSE, T1-weighted SGE (*g*), T1-weighted fat-suppressed SGE (*h*), immediate postgadolinium SGE (*i*), and 90-s postgadolinium SGE (*j*) images in a second patient. There is a 4-cm pseudocyst transversing

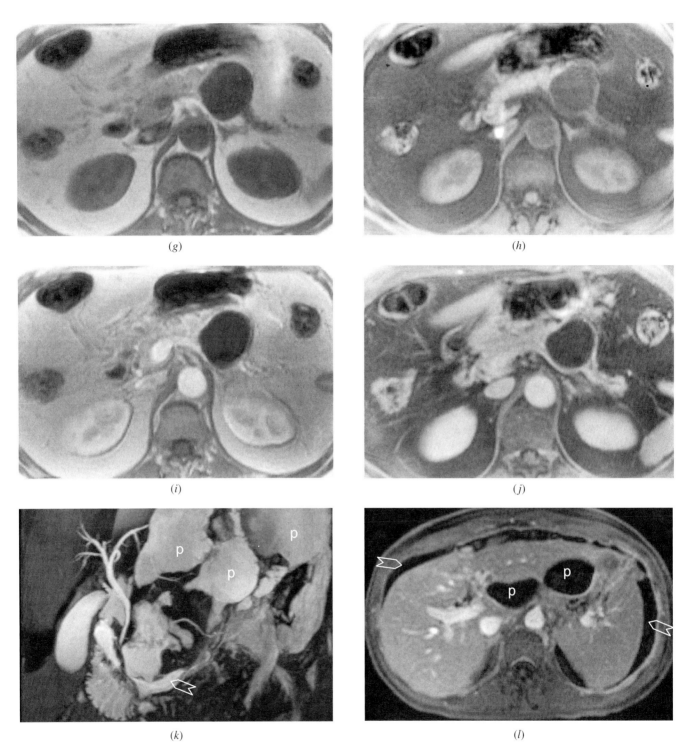

FIG. 4.95 (*Continued*) the pancreas at the junction of the body and tail. The pancreas proximal to the traumatic pseudocyst appears normal. Distal to the pseudocyst, the tail shows ductal dilatation (arrows, *f*) and atrophy consistent with changes of long-term ductal obstruction and resultant chronic pancreatitis, in this patient with a remote history of abdominal trauma. Reconstructed MRCP (*k*), T1-weighted postgadolinium interstitial phase water excitation magnetization prepared rapid gradient echo images (*l-n*) demonstrate traumatic transections located in the pancreatic neck (white arrows, *m, n*) and left lobe of the liver (black arrows, *m, n*).

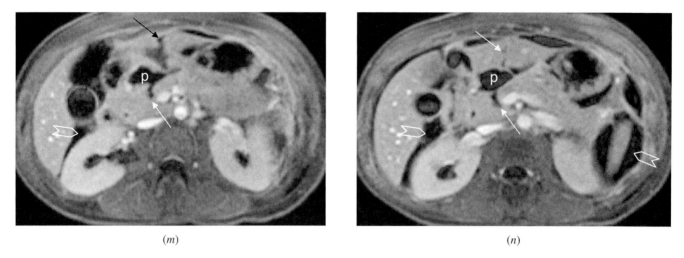

(m)

(n)

FIG. 4.95 (*Continued*) There are multiple pseudocysts (p, *k; l–n*) and free fluid (open arrow; *k–n*) in the abdomen. The peritoneal surfaces also show enhancement due to inflammation.

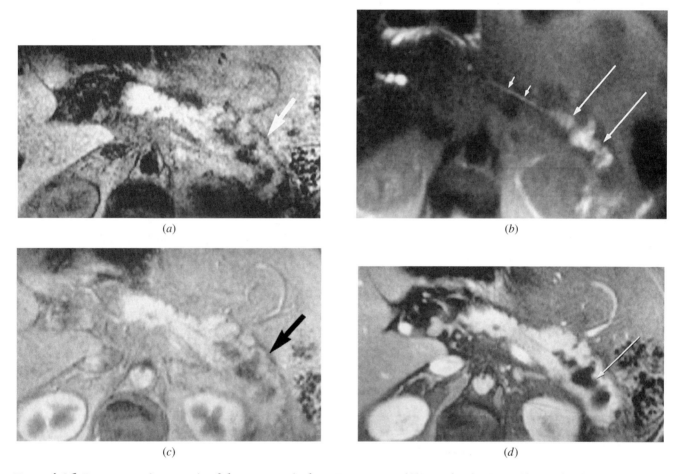

(a)

(b)

(c)

(d)

FIG. 4.96 Posttraumatic stenosis of the pancreatic duct. Fat-suppressed T1-weighted SGE (*a*), T2-weighted SS-ETSE (*b*), and immediate (*c*) and 90-s (*d*) postgadolinium fat-suppressed T1 SGE images in a patient who had undergone abdominal trauma 6 years earlier. A transition is noted in the body of the pancreas between normal-appearing proximal pancreas and abnormal-appearing distal pancreas containing an irregularly dilated pancreatic duct. On the precontrast, fat-suppressed image (*a*), the distal pancreas (arrow, *a*) is noted to be low in signal intensity, consistent with changes of chronic pancreatitis. On the SS-ETSE image (*b*) a transition is well shown between normal-caliber pancreatic duct (small arrows, *b*) and abnormally expanded distal pancreatic duct (long arrows, *b*). The distal pancreas is noted to enhance minimally on the immediate postgadolinium image (arrow, *c*). Enhancement of the pancreas is more uniform on the interstitial phase image (*d*), with clear definition of the irregularly dilated pancreatic duct (long arrow, *d*). (Courtesy of Susan M. Ascher, M.D., Dept. of Radiology, Georgetown University Medical Center.)

the vertebral column, with normal pancreatic head and midbody and distal atrophy and ductal dilatation. History of trauma, typically motor vehicle accident, even if remote, should be sought.

PANCREATIC TRANSPLANTS

Dynamic gadolinium-enhanced MRI has been used to assess rejection of pancreatic transplants (fig. 4.97) [109–

112]. Enhancement in six normal grafts was 98 ± 23% within the first minute compared to 42 ± 20% in six dysfunctional grafts [109]. Inflammation and infection including abscesses can also be well demonstrated with MRI (fig. 4.97). MR angiography also has been used to detect acute vascular compromise, with high sensitivity and specificity (fig. 4.98) [110, 111]. Complications such as venous thrombosis are well shown on gadolinium-enhanced gradient echo, especially 3D-GE imaging, because of the high spatial resolution [112].

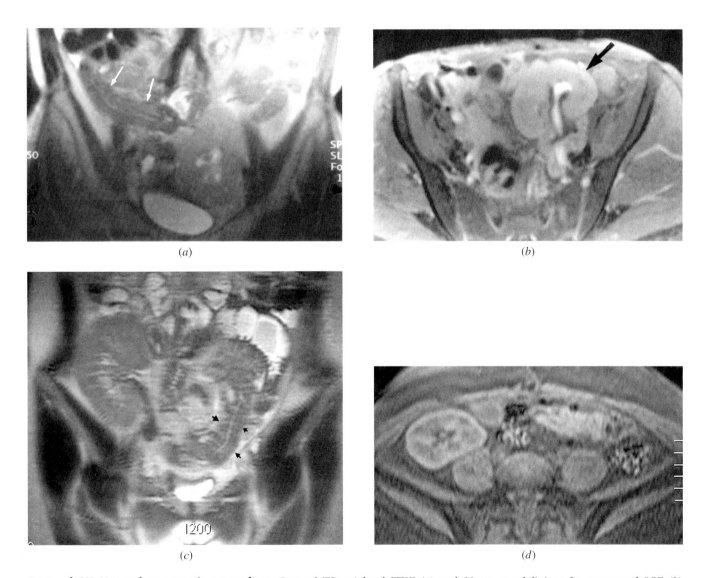

(a)

(b)

(c)

(d)

F I G . 4.97 Normal pancreatic transplant. Coronal T2-weighted ETSE (*a*) and 90-s postgadolinium fat-suppressed SGE (*b*) images in a patient status post-pancreas and renal transplant. The transplanted pancreas is normal in signal intensity and is located in the right lower quadrant (arrows, *a*).The transplanted kidney is in the left lower quadrant (arrow, *b*).
  Transplanted pancreas and kidney. Coronal T2-weighted SS-ETSE (*c*), fat-suppressed T1-weighted gradient-echo (*d*), immediate postgadolinium fat-suppressed T1-weighted gradient-echo (*e*) and interstitial-phase postgadolinium T1-weighted

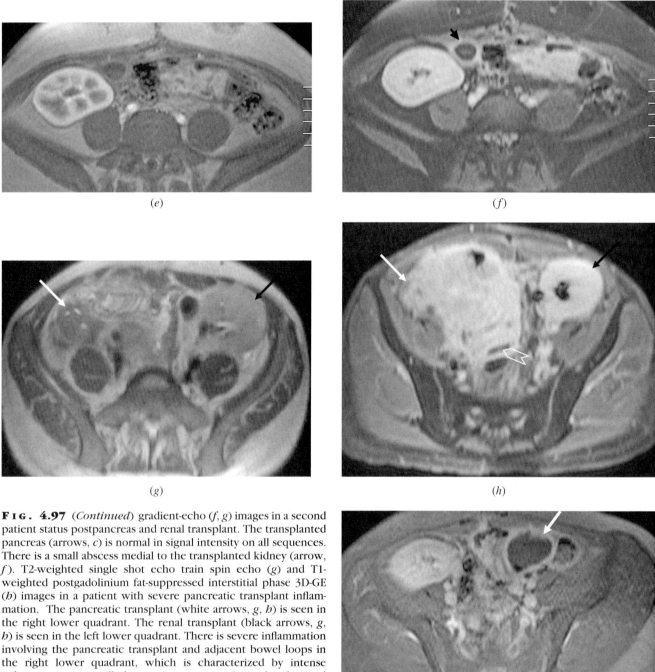

(e)

(f)

(g)

(h)

(i)

FIG. 4.97 (*Continued*) gradient-echo (*f, g*) images in a second patient status postpancreas and renal transplant. The transplanted pancreas (arrows, *c*) is normal in signal intensity on all sequences. There is a small abscess medial to the transplanted kidney (arrow, *f*). T2-weighted single shot echo train spin echo (*g*) and T1-weighted postgadolinium fat-suppressed interstitial phase 3D-GE (*h*) images in a patient with severe pancreatic transplant inflammation. The pancreatic transplant (white arrows, *g, h*) is seen in the right lower quadrant. The renal transplant (black arrows, *g, h*) is seen in the left lower quadrant. There is severe inflammation involving the pancreatic transplant and adjacent bowel loops in the right lower quadrant, which is characterized by intense enhancement. A small abscess (open arrow, *h*) is also detected adjacent to the transplant and bowel loops. The renal transplant (black arrow, *g*) is edematous and enlarged. T1-weighted postgadolinium fat-suppressed interstitial phase 3D-GE (*i*) image in another patient with an abscess adjacent to a pancreatic transplant. A large abscess (arrow, *i*) containing free air is detected in the left lower quadrant adjacent to the pancreatic transplant tissue.

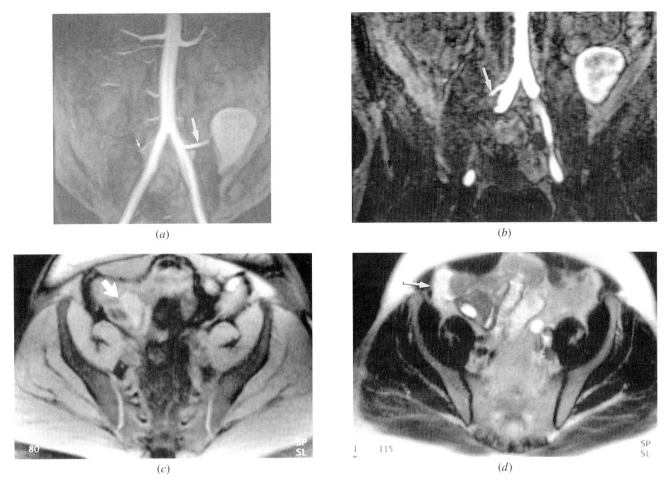

(a)

(b)

(c)

(d)

F I G . 4.98 Pancreatic transplant with arterial thrombosis. Coronal MIP reconstructed MR angiography (MRA) (*a*), gadolinium-enhanced 2-mm 3D gradient-echo source (*b*), T1-weighted fat-suppressed SGE (*c*), and T2-weighted SS-ETSE (*d*) images. The MIP reconstructed MRA image demonstrates a normal artery (arrow, *a*) feeding the renal transplant in the left pelvis and an occluded artery (small arrow, *a*) feeding the pancreas transplant in the right pelvis. To establish the diagnosis of occlusion, examination of the source images is essential; occlusion is confirmed on the source image (arrow, *b*) as abrupt termination of the contrast-enhanced vascular lumen. The transplant is identified in the right side of the pelvis on T1-weighted (arrow, *c*) and T2-weighted (*d*) images. Inflammatory fluid (arrow, *d*) is noted adjacent to the pancreas transplant.

REFERENCES

1. Semelka RC, Ascher SM. MR imaging of the pancreas-state of the art. *Radiology* 188(3): 593–602, 1993.

2. Winston CB, Mitchell DG, Outwater EK et al. Pancreatic signal intensity on T1-weighted fat saturation MR images: clinical correlation. *J Magn Reson Imaging* 5(3): 267–271, 1995.

3. Mitchell DG, Vinitski S, Saponaro S et al. Liver and pancreas: improved spin-echo T1 contrast by shorter echo time and fat suppression at 1.5 T. *Radiology* 178(1): 67–71, 1991.

4. Semelka RC, Kroeker MA, Shoenut JP et al. Pancreatic disease: prospective comparison of CT, ERCP, and 1.5-T MR imaging with dynamic gadolinium enhancement and fat suppression. *Radiology* 181(3): 785–791, 1991.

5. Takehara Y, Ichijo K, Tooyama N et al. Breath-hold MR cholangiopancreatography with a long-echo-train fast spin-echo sequence and a surface coil in chronic pancreatitis. *Radiology* 192(1): 73–78, 1994.

6. Bret PM, Reinhold C, Taourel P et al. Pancreas divisum: evaluation with MR cholangiopancreatography. *Radiology* 199(1): 99–103, 1996.

7. Soto JA, Barish MA, Yucel EK et al. Pancreatic duct: MR cholangiopancreatography with a three-dimensional fast spin-echo technique. *Radiology* 196(2): 459–464, 1995.

8. Zapparoli M, Semelka RC, Altun E et al. 3.0-T MRI evaluation of patients with chronic liver diseases: initial observations. *Magn Reson Imaging* 26(5): 650–660, 2008.

9. Semelka RC, Simm FC, Recht MP et al. MR imaging of the pancreas at high field strength: comparison of six sequences. *J Comput Assist Tomogr* 15(6): 966–971, 1991.

10. Mitchell DG, Winston CB, Outwater EK et al. Delineation of pancreas with MR imaging: multiobserver comparison of five pulse sequences. *J Magn Reson Imaging* 5(2): 193–199, 1995.

11. Fulcher AS, Turner MA. MR pancreatography: a useful tool for evaluating pancreatic disorders. *Radiographics* 19(1): 5–24; discussion 41–24; quiz 148–149, 1999.

12. Catalano C, Pavone P, Laghi A et al. Pancreatic adenocarcinoma: combination of MR imaging, MR angiography and MR cholangio-pancreatography for the diagnosis and assessment of resectability. *Eur Radiol* 8(3): 428–434, 1998.

13. Cruikshank AH, Benbow EW. *Pathology of the Pancreas*. In. 2nd ed. London: Springer; 1995. p. 30.

14. Delhaye M, Engelholm L, Cremer M. Pancreas divisum: congenital anatomic variant or anomaly? Contribution of endoscopic retrograde dorsal pancreatography. *Gastroenterology* 89(5): 951–958, 1985.

15. Delhaye M, Cremer M. Clinical significance of pancreas divisum. *Acta Gastroenterol Belg* 55(3): 306–313, 1992.

16. Rosai J. In: *Ackerman's Surgical Pathology*. 8th ed. St. Louis, MO: Mosby; 1996. p. 1004.

17. Quest L, Lombard M. Pancreas divisum: opinio divisa. *Gut* 47(3): 317–319, 2000.

18. Desai MB, Mitchell DG, Munoz SJ. Asymptomatic annular pancreas: detection by magnetic resonance imaging. *Magn Reson Imaging* 12(4): 683–685, 1994.

19. Applegate KE, Goske MJ, Pierce G et al. Situs revisited: imaging of the heterotaxy syndrome. *Radiographics* 19(4): 837–852; discussion 853–834, 1999.

20. Gayer G, Apter S, Jonas T et al. Polysplenia syndrome detected in adulthood: report of eight cases and review of the literature. *Abdom Imaging* 24(2): 178–184, 1999.

21. Tham RT, Heyerman HG, Falke TH et al. Cystic fibrosis: MR imaging of the pancreas. *Radiology* 179(1): 183–186, 1991.

22. Ferrozzi F, Bova D, Campodonico F et al. Cystic fibrosis: MR assessment of pancreatic damage. *Radiology* 198(3): 875–879, 1996.

23. King LJ, Scurr ED, Murugan N et al. Hepatobiliary and pancreatic manifestations of cystic fibrosis: MR imaging appearances. *Radiographics* 20(3): 767–777, 2000.

24. Siegelman ES, Mitchell DG, Outwater E et al. Idiopathic hemochromatosis: MR imaging findings in cirrhotic and precirrhotic patients. *Radiology* 188(3): 637–641, 1993.

25. Siegelman ES, Mitchell DG, Semelka RC. Abdominal iron deposition: metabolism, MR findings, and clinical importance. *Radiology* 199(1): 13–22, 1996.

26. Hough DM, Stephens DH, Johnson CD et al. Pancreatic lesions in von Hippel-Lindau disease: prevalence, clinical significance, and CT findings. *AJR Am J Roentgenol* 162(5): 1091–1094, 1994.

27. Boring CC, Squires TS, Tong T. Cancer statistics, 1991. *CA Cancer J Clin* 41(1): 19–36, 1991.

28. Warshaw AL, Fernandez-del Castillo C. Pancreatic carcinoma. *N Engl J Med* 326(7): 455–465, 1992.

29. Moossa AR. Pancreatic cancer: approach to diagnosis, selection for surgery and choice of operation. *Cancer* 50(11 Suppl):2689–2698, 1982.

30. Clark LR, Jaffe MH, Choyke PL et al. Pancreatic imaging. *Radiol Clin North Am* 23(3): 489–501, 1985.

31. Rosai J. In: *Ackerman's Surgical Pathology*. 8th ed. St. Louis, MO: Mosby; 1996. p. 976.

32. Baron RL, Stanley RJ, Lee JK et al. Computed tomographic features of biliary obstruction. *AJR Am J Roentgenol* 140(6): 1173–1178, 1983.

33. Kim JK, Altun E, Elias J, Jr. et al. Focal pancreatic mass: distinction of pancreatic cancer from chronic pancreatitis using gadolinium-enhanced 3D-gradient-echo MRI. *J Magn Reson Imaging* 26(2): 313–322, 2007.

34. Wittenberg J, Simeone JF, Ferrucci JT, Jr. et al. Non-focal enlargement in pancreatic carcinoma. *Radiology* 144(1): 131–135, 1982.

35. Megibow AJ, Bosniak MA, Ambos MA et al. Thickening of the celiac axis and/or superior mesenteric artery: a sign of pancreatic carcinoma on computed tomography. *Radiology* 141(2): 449–453, 1981.

36. Gabata T, Matsui O, Kadoya M et al. Small pancreatic adenocarcinomas: efficacy of MR imaging with fat suppression and gadolinium enhancement. *Radiology* 193(3): 683–688, 1994.

37. Semelka RC, Kelekis NL, Molina PL et al. Pancreatic masses with inconclusive findings on spiral CT: is there a role for MRI? *J Magn Reson Imaging* 6(4): 585–588, 1996.

38. Birchard KR, Semelka RC, Hyslop WB et al. Suspected Pancreatic Cancer: Evaluation by Dynamic Gadolinium-Enhanced 3D Gradient-Echo MRI. *AJR Am J Roentgenol* 185(3): 700–703, 2005.

39. Steiner E, Stark DD, Hahn PF et al. Imaging of pancreatic neoplasms: comparison of MR and CT. *AJR Am J Roentgenol* 152(3): 487–491, 1989.

40. Sarles H, Sahel J. Pathology of chronic calcifying pancreatitis. *Am J Gastroenterol* 66(2): 117–139, 1976.

41. Elias J, Jr., Semelka RC, Altun E et al. Pancreatic cancer: correlation of MR findings, clinical features, and tumor grade. *J Magn Reson Imaging* 26(6): 1556–1563, 2007.

42. Vellet AD, Romano W, Bach DB et al. Adenocarcinoma of the pancreatic ducts: comparative evaluation with CT and MR imaging at 1.5 T. *Radiology* 183(1): 87–95, 1992.

43. Pavone P, Laghi A, Passariello R. MR cholangiopancreatography in malignant biliary obstruction. *Semin Ultrasound CT MR* 20(5): 317–323, 1999.

44. Low RN, Semelka RC, Worawattanakul S et al. Extrahepatic abdominal imaging in patients with malignancy: comparison of MR imaging and helical CT in 164 patients. *J Magn Reson Imaging* 12(2): 269–277, 2000.

45. Low RN, Semelka RC, Worawattanakul S et al. Extrahepatic abdominal imaging in patients with malignancy: comparison of MR imaging and helical CT, with subsequent surgical correlation. *Radiology* 210(3): 625–632, 1999.

46. Nishiharu T, Yamashita Y, Abe Y et al. Local extension of pancreatic carcinoma: assessment with thin-section helical CT versus with breath-hold fast MR imaging–ROC analysis. *Radiology* 212(2): 445–452, 1999.

47. Danet IM, Semelka RC, Nagase LL et al. Liver metastases from pancreatic adenocarcinoma: MR imaging characteristics. *J Magn Reson Imaging* 18(2): 181–188, 2003.

48. Benassai G, Mastrorilli M, Quarto G et al. Factors influencing survival after resection for ductal adenocarcinoma of the head of the pancreas. *J Surg Oncol* 73(4): 212–218, 2000.

49. Ariyama J, Suyama M, Satoh K et al. Imaging of small pancreatic ductal adenocarcinoma. *Pancreas* 16(3): 396–401, 1998.

50. Tatli S, Mortele KJ, Levy AD et al. CT and MRI features of pure acinar cell carcinoma of the pancreas in adults. *AJR Am J Roentgenol* 184(2): 511–519, 2005.

51. Mozell E, Stenzel P, Woltering EA et al. Functional endocrine tumors of the pancreas: clinical presentation, diagnosis, and treatment. *Curr Probl Surg* 27(6): 301–386, 1990.

52. Beger HG, Warshaw AL, Carr-Locke D et al. The Pancreas. In. 1st ed. London: Blakwell Science; 1998. p. 1183.

53. Semelka RC, Custodio CM, Cem Balci N et al. Neuroendocrine tumors of the pancreas: spectrum of appearances on MRI. *J Magn Reson Imaging* 11(2): 141–148, 2000.

54. Thompson NW, Eckhauser FE, Vinik AI et al. Cystic neuroendocrine neoplasms of the pancreas and liver. *Ann Surg* 199(2): 158–164, 1984.

55. Mitchell DG, Cruvella M, Eschelman DJ et al. MRI of pancreatic gastrinomas. *J Comput Assist Tomogr* 16(4): 583–585, 1992.

56. Kraus BB, Ros PR. Insulinoma: diagnosis with fat-suppressed MR imaging. *AJR Am J Roentgenol* 162(1): 69–70, 1994.

57. Semelka RC, Cumming MJ, Shoenut JP et al. Islet cell tumors: comparison of dynamic contrast-enhanced CT and MR imaging with dynamic gadolinium enhancement and fat suppression. *Radiology* 186(3): 799–802, 1993.

58. Kelekis NL, Semelka RC, Molina PL et al. ACTH-secreting islet cell tumor: appearances on dynamic gadolinium-enhanced MRI. *Magn Reson Imaging* 13(4): 641–644, 1995.

59. Buetow PC, Parrino TV, Buck JL et al. Islet cell tumors of the pancreas: pathologic-imaging correlation among size, necrosis and cysts, calcification, malignant behavior, and functional status. *AJR Am J Roentgenol* 165(5): 1175–1179, 1995.

60. Smith TM, Semelka RC, Noone TC et al. Islet cell tumor of the pancreas associated with tumor thrombus in the portal vein. *Magn Reson Imaging* 17(7): 1093–1096, 1999.

61. Pipeleers-Marichal M, Donow C, Heitz PU et al. Pathologic aspects of gastrinomas in patients with Zollinger-Ellison syndrome with and without multiple endocrine neoplasia type I. *World J Surg* 17(4): 481–488, 1993.

62. Wank SA, Doppman JL, Miller DL et al. Prospective study of the ability of computed axial tomography to localize gastrinomas in patients with Zollinger-Ellison syndrome. *Gastroenterology* 92(4): 905–912, 1987.

63. Frucht H, Doppman JL, Norton JA et al. Gastrinomas: comparison of MR imaging with CT, angiography, and US. *Radiology* 171(3): 713–717, 1989.

64. Muller MF, Meyenberger C, Bertschinger P et al. Pancreatic tumors: evaluation with endoscopic US, CT, and MR imaging. *Radiology* 190(3): 745–751, 1994.

65. Galiber AK, Reading CC, Charboneau JW et al. Localization of pancreatic insulinoma: comparison of pre- and intraoperative US with CT and angiography. *Radiology* 166(2): 405–408, 1988.

66. Tjon ATRT, Jansen JB, Falke TH et al. MR, CT, and ultrasound findings of metastatic vipoma in pancreas. *J Comput Assist Tomogr* 13(1): 142–144, 1989.

67. Carlson B, Johnson CD, Stephens DH et al. MRI of pancreatic islet cell carcinoma. *J Comput Assist Tomogr* 17(5): 735–740, 1993.

68. Tjon ATRT, Jansen JB, Falke TH et al. Imaging features of somatostatinoma: MR, CT, US, and angiography. *J Comput Assist Tomogr* 18(3): 427–431, 1994.

69. Doppman JL, Nieman LK, Cutler GB, Jr. et al. Adrenocorticotropic hormone–secreting islet cell tumors: are they always malignant? *Radiology* 190(1): 59–64, 1994.

70. Ros PR, Hamrick-Turner JE, Chiechi MV et al. Cystic masses of the pancreas. *Radiographics* 12(4): 673–686, 1992.

71. Lewandrowski K, Warshaw A, Compton C. Macrocystic serous cystadenoma of the pancreas: a morphologic variant differing from microcystic adenoma. *Hum Pathol* 23(8): 871–875, 1992.

72. Khurana B, Mortele KJ, Glickman J et al. Macrocystic serous adenoma of the pancreas: radiologic-pathologic correlation. *AJR Am J Roentgenol* 181(1): 119–123, 2003.

73. Buetow PC, Rao P, Thompson LD. From the Archives of the AFIP. Mucinous cystic neoplasms of the pancreas: radiologic-pathologic correlation. *Radiographics* 18(2): 433–449, 1998.

74. Minami M, Itai Y, Ohtomo K et al. Cystic neoplasms of the pancreas: comparison of MR imaging with CT. *Radiology* 171(1): 53–56, 1989.

75. Friedman AC, Lichtenstein JE, Dachman AH. Cystic neoplasms of the pancreas. Radiological-pathological correlation. *Radiology* 149(1): 45–50, 1983.

76. Compagno J, Oertel JE. Mucinous cystic neoplasms of the pancreas with overt and latent malignancy (cystadenocarcinoma and cystadenoma). A clinicopathologic study of 41 cases. *Am J Clin Pathol* 69(6): 573–580, 1978.

77. Silas AM, Morrin MM, Raptopoulos V et al. Intraductal papillary mucinous tumors of the pancreas. *AJR Am J Roentgenol* 176(1): 179–185, 2001.

78. Traverso LW, Peralta EA, Ryan JA, Jr. et al. Intraductal neoplasms of the pancreas. *Am J Surg* 175(5): 426–432, 1998.

79. Procacci C, Megibow AJ, Carbognin G et al. Intraductal papillary mucinous tumor of the pancreas: a pictorial essay. *Radiographics* 19(6): 1447–1463, 1999.

80. Koito K, Namieno T, Ichimura T et al. Mucin-producing pancreatic tumors: comparison of MR cholangiopancreatography with endoscopic retrograde cholangiopancreatography. *Radiology* 208(1): 231–237, 1998.

81. Onaya H, Itai Y, Niitsu M et al. Ductectatic mucinous cystic neoplasms of the pancreas: evaluation with MR cholangiopancreatography. *AJR Am J Roentgenol* 171(1): 171–177, 1998.

82. Irie H, Honda H, Aibe H et al. MR cholangiopancreatographic differentiation of benign and malignant intraductal mucin-producing tumors of the pancreas. *AJR Am J Roentgenol* 174(5): 1403–1408, 2000.

83. Ohtomo K, Furui S, Onoue M et al. Solid and papillary epithelial neoplasm of the pancreas: MR imaging and pathologic correlation. *Radiology* 184(2): 567–570, 1992.

84. Thompson LD, Becker RC, Przygodzki RM et al. Mucinous cystic neoplasm (mucinous cystadenocarcinoma of low-grade malignant potential) of the pancreas: a clinicopathologic study of 130 cases. *Am J Surg Pathol* 23(1): 1–16, 1999.

85. Zeman RK, Schiebler M, Clark LR et al. The clinical and imaging spectrum of pancreaticoduodenal lymph node enlargement. *AJR Am J Roentgenol* 144(6): 1223–1227, 1985.

86. Kelekis NL, Semelka RC, Siegelman ES. MRI of pancreatic metastases from renal cancer. *J Comput Assist Tomogr* 20(2): 249–253, 1996.

87. Steinberg W, Tenner S. Acute pancreatitis. *N Engl J Med* 330(17):1198–1210, 1994.

88. Kattwinkel J, Lapey A, Di Sant'Agnese PA et al. Hereditary pancreatitis: three new kindreds and a critical review of the literature. *Pediatrics* 51(1): 55–69, 1973.

89. Lee SP, Nicholls JF, Park HZ. Biliary sludge as a cause of acute pancreatitis. *N Engl J Med* 326(9): 589–593, 1992.

90. Shearman DJC, Finlayson N, Camilleri M et al. In: *Diseases of the Gastrointestinal Tract and Liver.* 3rd ed. New York: Churchill Livingstone; 1997. p. 1253.

91. Balthazar EJ. CT diagnosis and staging of acute pancreatitis. *Radiol Clin North Am* 27(1): 19–37, 1989.

92. Balthazar EJ, Robinson DL, Megibow AJ et al. Acute pancreatitis: value of CT in establishing prognosis. *Radiology* 174(2): 331–336, 1990.

93. Johnson CD, Stephens DH, Sarr MG. CT of acute pancreatitis: correlation between lack of contrast enhancement and pancreatic necrosis. *AJR Am J Roentgenol* 156(1): 93–95, 1991.

94. Saifuddin A, Ward J, Ridgway J et al. Comparison of MR and CT scanning in severe acute pancreatitis: initial experiences. *Clin Radiol* 48(2): 111–116, 1993.

95. Martin DR, Karabulut N, Yang M et al. High signal peripancreatic fat on fat-suppressed spoiled gradient echo imaging in acute pancreatitis: preliminary evaluation of the prognostic significance. *J Magn Reson Imaging* 18(1): 49–58, 2003.

96. Morgan DE, Baron TH, Smith JK et al. Pancreatic fluid collections prior to intervention: evaluation with MR imaging compared with CT and US. *Radiology* 203(3): 773–778, 1997.

97. Bank S. Chronic pancreatitis: clinical features and medical management. *Am J Gastroenterol* 81(3): 153–167, 1986.

98. Steer ML, Waxman I, Freedman S. Chronic pancreatitis. *N Engl J Med* 332(22):1482–1490, 1995.

99. Lowenfels AB, Maisonneuve P, Cavallini G et al. Pancreatitis and the risk of pancreatic cancer. International Pancreatitis Study Group. *N Engl J Med* 328(20):1433–1437, 1993.

100. Luetmer PH, Stephens DH, Ward EM. Chronic pancreatitis: reassessment with current CT. *Radiology* 171(2): 353–357, 1989.

101. Aranha GV, Prinz RA, Freeark RJ et al. The spectrum of biliary tract obstruction from chronic pancreatitis. *Arch Surg* 119(5): 595–600, 1984.

102. Lammer J, Herlinger H, Zalaudek G et al. Pseudotumorous pancreatitis. *Gastrointest Radiol* 10(1): 59–67, 1985.

103. Sostre CF, Flournoy JG, Bova JG et al. Pancreatic phlegmon. Clinical features and course. *Dig Dis Sci* 30(10):918–927, 1985.

104. Semelka RC, Shoenut JP, Kroeker MA et al. Chronic pancreatitis: MR imaging features before and after administration of gadopentetate dimeglumine. *J Magn Reson Imaging* 3(1): 79–82, 1993.

105. Irie H, Honda H, Baba S et al. Autoimmune pancreatitis: CT and MR characteristics. *AJR Am J Roentgenol* 170(5): 1323–1327, 1998.

106. Van Hoe L, Gryspeerdt S, Ectors N et al. Nonalcoholic duct-destructive chronic pancreatitis: imaging findings. *AJR Am J Roentgenol* 170(3): 643–647, 1998.

107. Ectors N, Maillet B, Aerts R et al. Non-alcoholic duct destructive chronic pancreatitis. *Gut* 41(2): 263–268, 1997.

108. Ito T, Nakano I, Koyanagi S et al. Autoimmune pancreatitis as a new clinical entity. Three cases of autoimmune pancreatitis with effective steroid therapy. *Dig Dis Sci* 42(7): 1458–1468, 1997.

109. Fernandez MP, Bernardino ME, Neylan JF et al. Diagnosis of pancreatic transplant dysfunction: value of gadopentetate dimeglumine-enhanced MR imaging. *AJR Am J Roentgenol* 156(6): 1171–1176, 1991.

110. Krebs TL, Daly B, Wong JJ et al. Vascular complications of pancreatic transplantation: MR evaluation. *Radiology* 196(3): 793–798, 1995.

111. Krebs TL, Daly B, Wong-You-Cheong JJ et al. Acute pancreatic transplant rejection: evaluation with dynamic contrast-enhanced MR imaging compared with histopathologic analysis. *Radiology* 210(2): 437–442, 1999.

112. Eubank WB, Schmiedl UP, Levy AE et al. Venous thrombosis and occlusion after pancreas transplantation: evaluation with breath-hold gadolinium-enhanced three-dimensional MR imaging. *AJR Am J Roentgenol* 175(2): 381–385, 2000.

CHAPTER 5

SPLEEN

ERSAN ALTUN, JORGE ELIAS, JR., YOUNG HOON KIM,
AND RICHARD C. SEMELKA

To cure the mind's wrong bias, spleen,
some recommend the bowling green,
some, hilly walks;
all exercise
    The Spleen (1737) Matthew Green

Throughout the ages, the human spleen has received attention from poets as the producer of melancholy and ill temper. Long conceived as the seat of negative temper, it was Galen (131–201 A.D.) who believed that the spleen, with its spongy consistency, extracted "melancholy" from the blood or liver before excreting the "humor" via splenogastric veins into stomach. Though couched in the language of antiquity, Galen's theory was a prescient one and prefigured the modern-day, well-established functions of the organ as a specialized filter of blood and in immune surveillance.

NORMAL ANATOMY

The spleen consists of a large encapsulated mass of vascular and lymphoid tissue and is situated posteriorly in the left upper quadrant of the abdomen. It is typically crescent shaped, with a convex lateral border conforming to the abdominal wall and left hemidiaphragm and a concave medial border conforming to the stomach and left kidney. The splenic hilum is directed anteromedially, and the splenic artery and vein enter the spleen at this location. The splenic vein follows a relatively straight course along the posterior surface of the body and tail of the pancreas. The splenic artery is slightly superior to the vein and is often tortuous. The spleen is suspended by diaphragmatic attachments and by the splenorenal, gastrosplenic, and splenocolic ligaments. Veins within these ligamentous structures commonly dilate in the presence of portal hypertension. Isolated dilatation of short gastric veins and left gastro-omental veins along the greater curvature of the stomach may be seen in the presence of splenic vein thrombosis.

The freshly cut surface of an unfixed spleen is a reflection of its underlying microscopic architecture, as one can observe glistening maroon parenchyma, or red pulp, flecked with gray-white nodules, the white pulp. Microscopically, the red pulp consists of numerous, thin-walled vascular sinusoids separated by the splenic cords (Billroth cords). The sinusoids are lined by fenestrated endothelium providing easy passage of cells between sinusoidal lumens and surrounding cords. The splenic cords are spongelike and consist of a labyrinth of macrophages loosely connected by long dendritic process, reticular cells, and reticular fibers. This framework provides a physical and functional filter through which systemic circulatory blood can slowly seep. The white pulp consists of lymphoid follicles containing a central arteriole surrounded by the periarteriolar lymphoid sheath (PALS). The lymphoid cells forming PALS are predominantly T cells, whereas lymphoid follicles consist mainly of B cells. In neonates, the spleen is predominantly composed of red pulp. With age and progressive antigenic stimulation, the volume of white pulp gradually increases to occupy approximately 20% of the splenic parenchyma in the adult.

The white pulp is intimately associated with the arterial tree, whereas the red pulp is associated with the venous system draining the spleen. Splenic microcirculation has long been a subject of controversy because of the complexity of vascular channels and conflicting experimental evidence. Two basic pathways exist for splenic circulation. The closed circulation, which accounts for most of the splenic blood flow and corresponds to the functionally rapid component of the circulation, allows blood to pass from arterioles and capillaries directly into venous sinuses. The open circulation, which corresponds to the functionally slow component, permits blood to percolate through the reticular tissue of the splenic cords before filtering through minute slits in the walls of venous sinuses.

MRI TECHNIQUE

The standard MRI protocol includes precontrast breath-hold T1-weighted spoiled gradient-echo (SGE) sequences including in-phase and out-of-phase SGE sequences, precontrast fat-suppressed three-dimensional gradient echo (3D-GE), T2-weighted sequences including short-tau inversion recovery (STIR), non-fat-suppressed and fat-suppressed single-shot echo-train spin echo (although usually fat-suppressed single-shot echo-train spin echo is sufficient), and immediate and delayed postgadolinium SGE with the delayed images often acquired with fat suppression or immediate and delayed postgadolinium fat-suppressed 3D-GE sequences. The choice between SGE and 3D-GE sequences depends on the type of scanners.

NORMAL

Normal splenic parenchyma is invariably low in signal intensity on T1-weighted images and usually high in signal intensity on T2-weighted images (fig. 5.1).

Signal intensity on T2-weighted images of the spleen may vary and not uncommonly is relatively low. This is usually secondary to prior blood transfusions, which result in iron deposition in the reticuloendothelial system (RES) of the spleen (fig. 5.2). The signal intensity of most forms of benign and malignant disease processes parallels the pattern of low signal intensity on T1-weighted images and high signal intensity on T2-weighted images. As a result, noncontrast MR images are limited in the detection of splenic disease. Differences in blood supply of spleen and diseased tissue permit detection of abnormalities on immediate postgadolinium images.

Immediate postgadolinium breath-hold T1-weighted SGE or 3D-GE sequences demonstrate the different circulations in the normal spleen as regions of transient higher and lower contrast enhancement, usually in an arciform or serpiginous pattern [1–4]. This appears as an alternating pattern of high-signal (closed circulation) and low-signal (open circulation) stroma. Variations of this pattern occur, such as central low and peripheral high signal intensity. This variegated pattern becomes homogeneous and high in signal intensity within 1 min after contrast.

Three variations in splenic enhancement patterns have been described in spleen not infiltrated by disease on immediate postgadolinium image [4]. The most common (79% of patients) is serpiginous enhancement, termed arciform. This pattern has been observed in all normal spleens in nondiseased patients and in some spleens of patients with inflammatory or neoplastic disease (fig. 5.3). The second most common pattern (16% of patients) is homogeneous high-signal-intensity enhancement (fig. 5.4). This has been observed in patients with inflammatory or neoplastic diseases, hepatic focal fatty infiltration, or hepatic enzyme abnormalities. A nonspecific immune response may be responsible for this pattern of enhancement. This appearance may represent the conversion of a mixture of slow and fast channels to only fast channels, reflecting a mechanism to increase transit of immune system cells. The third pattern is uniform low signal intensity (5% of patients) (fig. 5.5). This was found in all patients who had undergone multiple recent blood transfusions. The T2-shortening effects from hemosiderin deposition in the RES supersede the T1-shortening effects of gadolinium [5, 6].

Superparamagnetic iron oxide particles are selectively taken up by the RES and have been used to evaluate the spleen. These particles diminish the signal intensity of the normal spleen on T2-weighted sequences, whereas tumors remain unchanged in signal characteristics [7–9]. Superparamagnetic iron oxide crystals embedded in a starch matrix [magnetic starch microspheres (MSM), Nycomed Imaging, Oslo, Norway] have

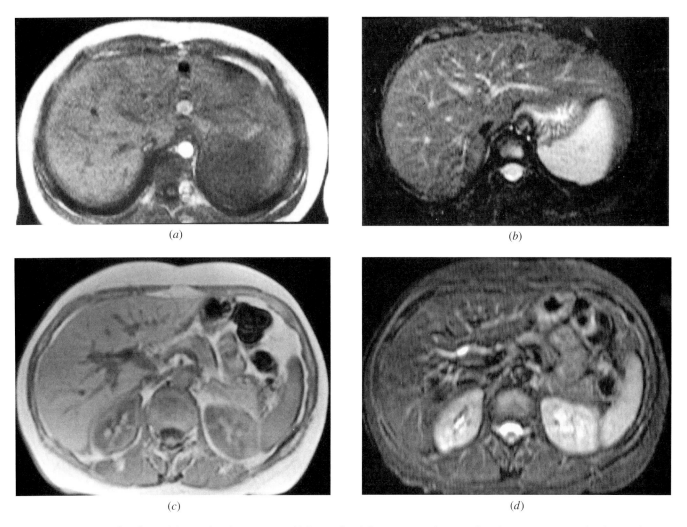

F I G . 5.1 Normal spleen. T1-weighted SGE (*a*) and T2-weighted fat-suppressed spin-echo (*b*) images. Normal spleen is low in signal intensity on T1-weighted image (*a*) and high in signal intensity on T2-weighted image (*b*). Liver is higher in signal intensity on T1-weighted images and lower in signal intensity on T2-weighted images than spleen, which results in a clear distinction between the elongated lateral segment of the liver and the adjacent spleen in this patient. T1-weighted SGE (*c*) and T2-weighted short-tau inversion recovery (STIR) (*d*) images at 3.0 T in a second patient with normal findings demonstrate similar signal characteristics for the spleen and liver compared to 1.5 T.

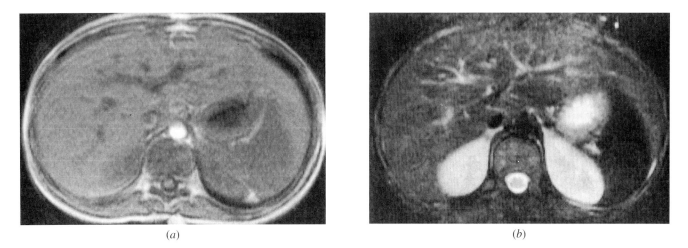

F I G . 5.2 Iron deposition in the spleen. T1-weighted SGE (*a*) and T2-weighted fat-suppressed spin-echo (*b*) images. Signal intensity of the spleen is only slightly lower than normal on the T1-weighted image (*a*), which is consistent with mild iron deposition in the RES. Signal intensity of the spleen is noted to be nearly signal void on the T2-weighted image (*b*), with low signal intensity also noted of liver and bone marrow due to iron deposition in the RES in these organs.

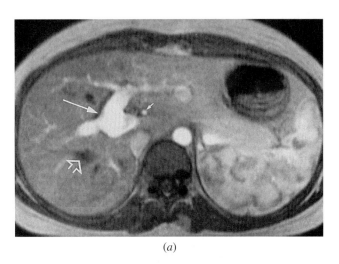

(a)

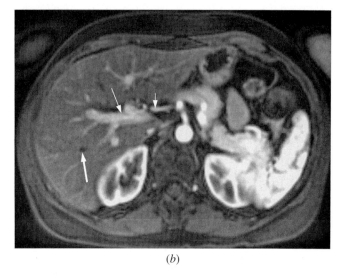

(b)

FIG. 5.3 Arciform enhancement in the normal spleen. Postgadolinium T1-weighted SGE image (a) acquired at 1.5 T on the hepatic arterial dominant phase shows the serpiginous, tubular bands of low signal intensity throughout the splenic parenchyma. Contrast identified in portal vein (long arrow, a) and hepatic arteries (short arrow, a) and lack of contrast in hepatic veins (open arrow, a) define the capillary or hepatic arterial dominant phase of enhancement. Postgadolinium fat-suppressed T1-weighted 3D-GE image (b) acquired at 3.0 T on the hepatic arterial dominant phase, which is again characterized by the presence of contrast in the hepatic artery (short thin arrow, b) and portal vein (long thin arrow, b) and by the absence of contrast in the hepatic veins (thick arrow, b), demonstrates arciform enhancement pattern of the normal spleen.

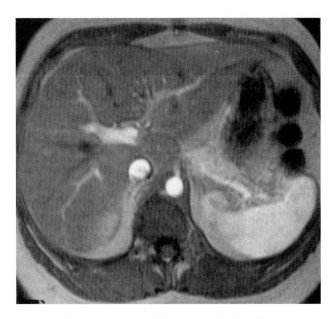

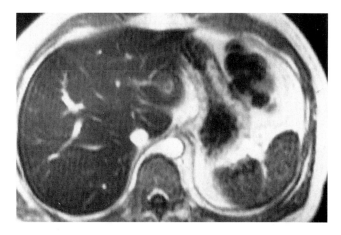

FIG. 5.5 Homogeneous low-signal-intensity splenic enhancement. The spleen is low in signal intensity on immediate postgadolinium images because of the predominant T2-shortening effects of iron in the spleen.

FIG. 5.4 Homogeneous intense splenic enhancement. The spleen is noted to enhance intensely and uniformly in the capillary phase of enhancement. Contrast in hepatic arteries and portal veins and lack of contrast in hepatic veins demonstrate that the image was acquired in the capillary phase of enhancement.

been studied in animal models and have been shown to increase conspicuity of both focal and diffuse splenic lesions [9]. Normal spleen diminishes in signal on T2-weighted or T2*-weighted images, whereas focal or diffuse disease retains signal, which renders disease

conspicuous by being relatively high in signal intensity.

In the neonate and until the infant is approximately 8 months old, the spleen signal intensity is isointense to the liver on T1-weighted images and varies from iso- to hypointense relative to the liver on T2-weighted images (fig. 5.6). As the RES matures, the spleen displays a hypointense signal relative to the liver on T1-weighted images, with a gradual increase in the spleen signal relative to the liver on T2-weighted images, approaching the normal appearance of the adult spleen [10].

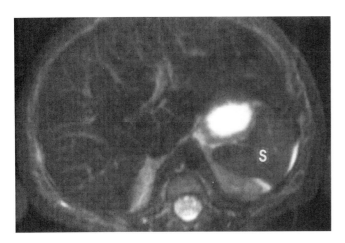

F I G . 5.6 Normal spleen in a 1-month-old patient. T2-weighted fat-suppressed spin-echo image. Normal spleen (S) is low signal intensity, comparable to liver on T2-weighted image.

Normal Variants and Congenital Disease

Accessory Spleens and Wandering Spleen

Accessory spleens, or "spleniculi," are congenital ectopic foci of splenic tissue that fail to fuse with the spleen. This anatomic variant is found in about 10–30% of non-selected autopsy cases. Because of its congenital origin, the accessory spleens are located within the embryological dorsal mesentery of stomach and pancreas. The majority of spleniculi are located in close proximity to the splenic hilum. One in six accessory spleens is located in or adjacent to the tail of the pancreas, which may resemble the appearance of an islet cell tumor (fig. 5.7) [11]. Most intrapancreatic accessory spleens are well marginated and have rounded morphology similar to other pancreatic lesions, especially like pancreatic neuroendocrine tumors [11]. Superparamagnetic iron oxide (SPIO) particles can be used for the differentiation of intrapancreatic accessory spleens from these tumors. Intrapancreatic accessory spleens take up SPIO and show decreased signal on postcontrast T2-weighted images (fig 5.7), but the tumors do not take up the agent [11]. Other accessory spleen locations include the suspensory ligament of spleen, left kidney, left testis, or elsewhere in retroperitoneum (fig. 5.8a–c). Their size varies from microscopic deposits to nodules with a diameter ranging from a few millimeters to 3 cm. After splenectomy they may enlarge considerably in size [12]. The diagnosis of accessory spleen should be considered when a mass has pre- and postcontrast imaging characteristic similar to those of spleen. They are clinically important insofar as they must be differentiated from other mass lesions. Spleniculi may also be confidently characterized in the patient who has undergone repeated blood transfusions because they will be nearly signal void on T2- or T2*-weighted sequences because of iron deposition within the RES of the splenules [13].

Wandering spleen is a condition in which the spleen is free to move if the ligamentous attachments of the spleen are lax or absent [10]. The spleen is not located in the left upper quadrant and may be found in the center of the abdomen or pelvis (fig. 5.8d–g). This condition is usually seen in patients with deficient musculature of the anterior abdominal wall such as prune-belly syndrome [10]. The splenic hilum is usually located anteriorly. Patients with wandering spleen may present with acute abdominal symptoms due to torsion about an elongated pedicle [14]. Splenic ischemia, infarction, and twisted elongated pedicle can be detected with MRI, particularly on postgadolinium images [14]. Edema may be seen as increased signal in the splenic parenchyma on T2-weighted images, and decreased enhancement or the lack of enhancement in the splenic parenchyma may be seen on postgadolinium images.

Asplenia

Asplenia syndrome, right isomerism (situs ambiguous with asplenia, bilateral right-sidedness), or Ivemark syndrome is a congenital syndrome characterized by absence of the spleen associated with thoracoabdominal abnormalities (fig. 5.9). The majority of patients die in infancy, with few surviving longer than 1 year. The mortality in the first year of life approaches 80% because of complex and severe cardiovascular anomalies and a compromised immune system. In cardiac MRI studies in which cardiovascular anomalies raise the possibility of asplenia, a limited abdominal MRI should be performed at the same time to evaluate abdominal situs ambiguous and associated abnormalities, abdominal vessels, and the presence of the spleen, because asplenic patients are at risk of sepsis [15–17]. Associated abnormalities include the liver located in the midline, ipsilateral inferior vena cava and aorta, dextrocardia or levocardia, and variable forms of intestinal malrotation.

Polysplenia

Polysplenia syndrome is a congenital syndrome characterized by multiple small splenic masses and left isomerism (situs ambiguous with polysplenia, bilateral left-sidedness). The splenic masses vary from 2 to 16 in number and are distributed along the greater curvature of the stomach (fig. 5.10). Other associated abnormalities include cardiopulmonary anomalies, malrotation of the intestinal tract, absence of the hepatic segment of the inferior vena cava with azygous or hemiazygous continuation, duplicated inferior vena cava, midline or left-sided liver, right-sided aorta, and a short pancreas. Polysplenia has also been associated with cystic kidney

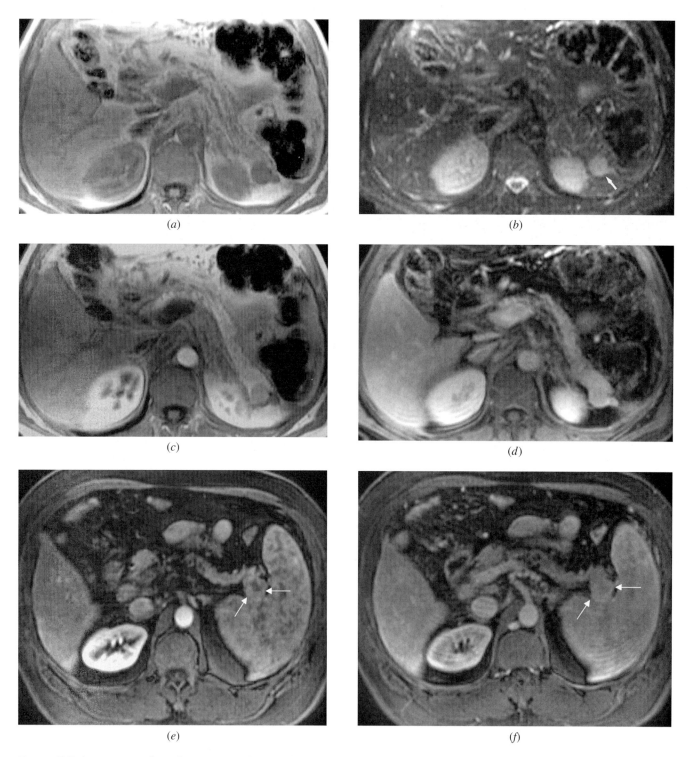

(a)

(b)

(c)

(d)

(e)

(f)

F I G . 5.7 Accessory spleen in pancreas. T1-weighted SGE (*a*), T2-weighted fat-suppressed echo-train single-shot (*b*), immediate postgadolinium T1-weighted SGE (*c*), and delayed T1-weighted fat-suppressed SGE (*d*) images. T1-weighted SGE demonstrates a mass in the pancreatic tail that is homogeneously hypointense compared to background pancreas (*a*). T2-weighted fat-suppressed image shows a round mass in the tail of the pancreas that demonstrates moderate homogeneous hyperintensity (arrow, *b*). Immediate postgadolinium-enhanced T1-weighted SGE demonstrates homogeneous enhancement of the mass (*c*). Ninety-second gadolinium-enhanced T1-weighted fat-saturated SGE demonstrates lower enhancement of the mass compared with surrounding pancreatic tissue (*d*). Immediate (*e*) and 45-s (*f*) postgadolinium T1-weighted fat-suppressed 3D-GE images, precontrast T2-weighted single-shot echo-train spin-echo (*g*), and post-superparamagnetic iron oxide (SPIO) T2-weighted single-shot echo-train spin-echo (*h*) images in a second patient with intrapancreatic accessory spleen. The lesion (arrows) is located in the pancreatic tail and demonstrates enhancement pattern similar to the spleen, which is seen as a serpiginous enhancement pattern on immediate and 45-s 3D-GE images (*e, f*). The lesion (arrows), which shows similar signal intensity to the spleen on precontrast T2-weighted image (*g*),

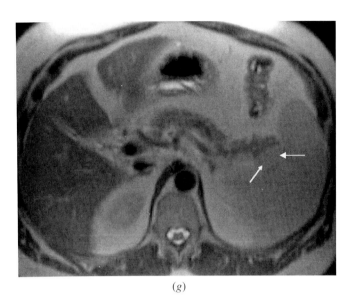
(g)

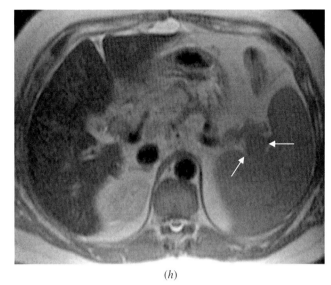
(h)

F I G . 5.7 (*Continued*) demonstrates signal drop on post-SPIO T2-weighted image (*h*) similar to the spleen, due to the presence of RES cells.

diseases. In comparison with asplenia, polysplenia has a lower mortality, and serious cardiac malformations are less common. MRI can demonstrate the situs ambiguous, abdominal vessels, and the number of spleens together with such complications as splenic hemorrhages or infarcts [16, 17].

Gaucher Disease

Gaucher disease is an autosomal recessive lysosomal multisystem hereditary disease caused by deficient glucocerebrosidase activity. Glucocerebroside, a glycolipid, accumulates in the mononuclear phagocytic cells of organs [18]. The abdominal manifestations of Gaucher disease in a population of 46 patients have been described with conventional spin-echo technique [18]. All patients had hepatosplenomegaly. Splenic nodules of variable signal intensity were present in 14 patients (30%). Fifteen patients (33%) had splenic infarcts with or without associated subcapsular fluid collections, and four patients (9%) had both infarcts and nodules. Focal areas of abnormal signal intensity were noted in the livers of nine patients (20%).

Sickle Cell Disease

The manifestations of sickle cell anemia vary and depend on whether the patient is homozygous or heterozygous for the hemoglobinopathy. The spleen shows low signal because of iron deposition from blood transfusions. In patients with homozygous disease, the spleen is nearly and diffusely signal void because of the sequela of iron deposition coupled with microscopic perivascular and parenchymal calcifications [19] (fig.

5.11*a*). Regions of scarring and infarcts are also common (fig. 5.11*b–d*).

MASS LESIONS

The appearance of common splenic lesions on T1-weighted, T2-weighted, and early and late postgadolinium images is presented in Table 5.1.

Benign Masses

Cysts

Cysts are the most common of the benign splenic lesions. Three types of nonneoplastic cysts exist: posttraumatic or pseudocyst, epidermoid cysts, and hydatid cysts [20]. Most splenic cysts are posttraumatic in origin. They are not lined by epithelium and thus are pseudocysts. Epidermoid cysts are true cysts discovered in childhood or early adulthood that may have trabeculations or septations in their walls with occasional peripheral calcification [20, 21] (fig. 5.12). Hydatids, or echinococcal cysts, are rare. They are characterized by extensive wall calcification. The MRI features of cysts include sharp lesion margination, low signal intensity on T1-weighted images, and very high signal intensity on T2-weighted images. Cysts complicated by proteinaceous fluid or hemorrhage may have regions of high signal intensity on T1-weighted images, regions of mixed signal intensity on T2-weighted images, or both. Cysts do not enhance on postgadolinium images. Pseudocysts may be complicated by hemorrhage, particularly early in their evolution, and thus may contain

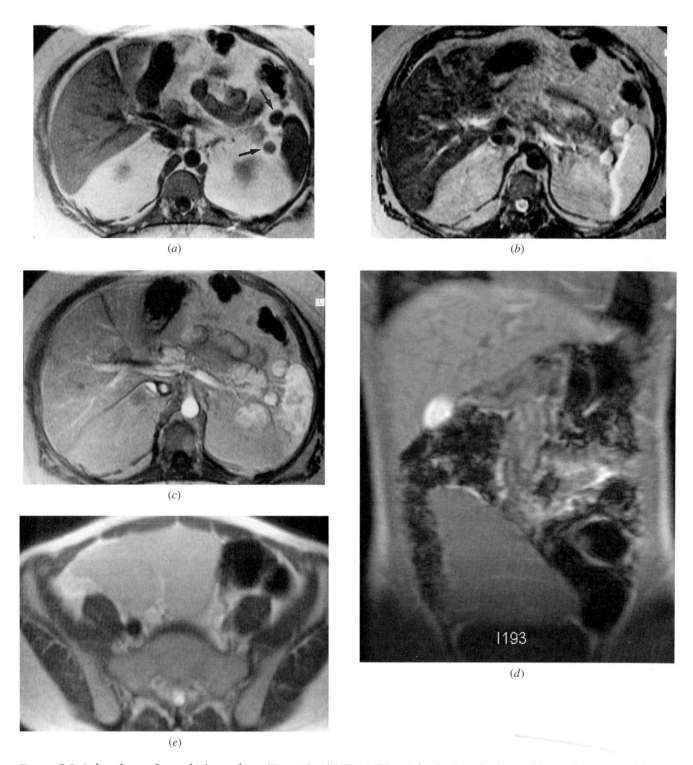

F I G . 5.8 Splenules and wandering spleen. T1-weighted SGE (*a*), T2-weighted spin-echo (*b*), and immediate postgadolinium SGE (*c*) images. Two splenules are identified (arrows, *a*) that parallel the signal intensity of the spleen. They are low in signal intensity on T1-weighted images (*a*) and high in signal intensity on T2-weighted images (*b*) and enhance intensely on immediate postgadolinium image (*c*).The splenules show heterogeneous enhancement on immediate postcontrast images, which suggests that they have architecture similar to that of the spleen. T1-weighted coronal SGE (*d*), T2-weighted single-shot echo-train spin-echo (*e*),

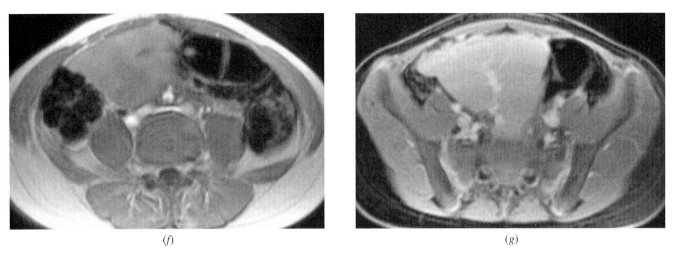

(f) *(g)*

F I G. 5.8 (*Continued*) immediate postgadolinium T1-weighted SGE (*f*), and delayed postgadolinium fat-suppressed T1-weighted SGE (*g*) images demonstrate the wandering spleen located in the pelvis in another patient.

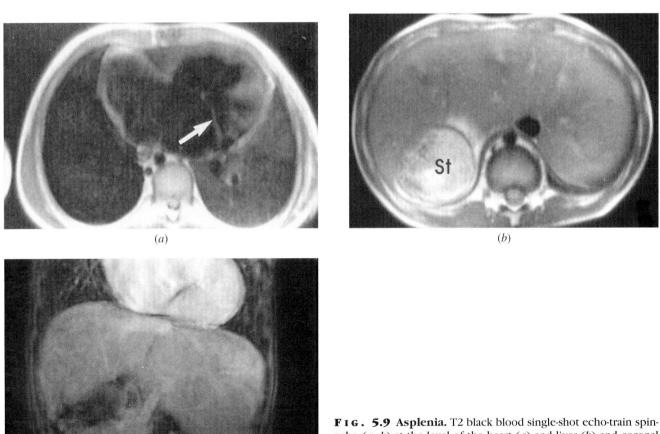

(a) *(b)*

(c)

F I G. 5.9 Asplenia. T2 black blood single-shot echo-train spin-echo (*a, b*) at the level of the heart (*a*) and liver (*b*) and coronal source MRA (*c*) images. Eight-month-old patient with endocardial cushion defect, common AV valve (arrow, *a*), and situs ambiguous, with the stomach (St, *b*) on the right side. No spleen is present.

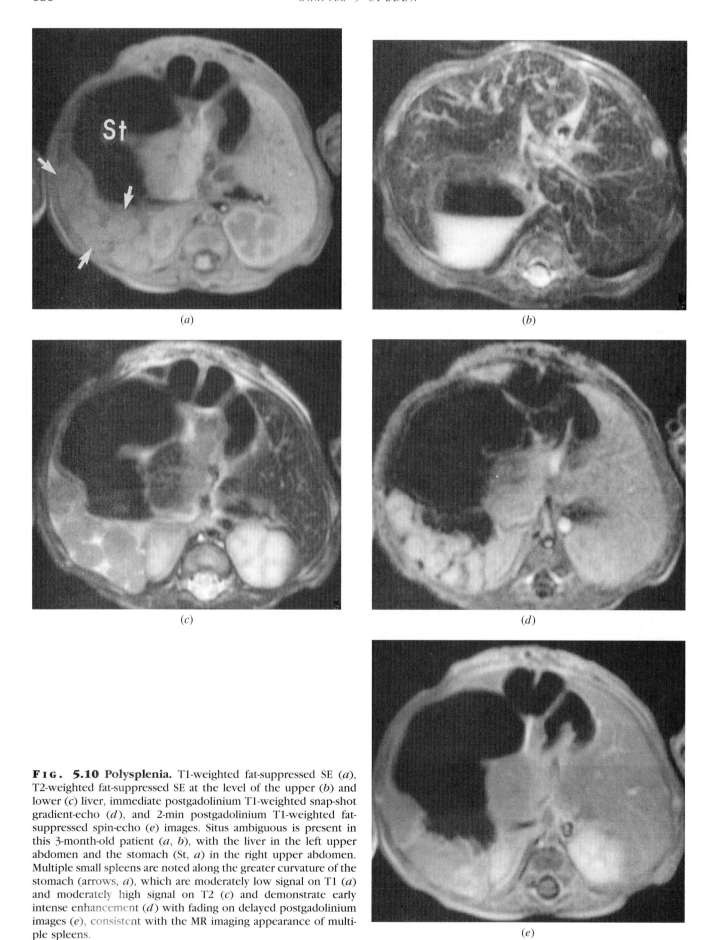

FIG. 5.10 Polysplenia. T1-weighted fat-suppressed SE (*a*), T2-weighted fat-suppressed SE at the level of the upper (*b*) and lower (*c*) liver, immediate postgadolinium T1-weighted snap-shot gradient-echo (*d*), and 2-min postgadolinium T1-weighted fat-suppressed spin-echo (*e*) images. Situs ambiguous is present in this 3-month-old patient (*a, b*), with the liver in the left upper abdomen and the stomach (St, *a*) in the right upper abdomen. Multiple small spleens are noted along the greater curvature of the stomach (arrows, *a*), which are moderately low signal on T1 (*a*) and moderately high signal on T2 (*c*) and demonstrate early intense enhancement (*d*) with fading on delayed postgadolinium images (*e*), consistent with the MR imaging appearance of multiple spleens.

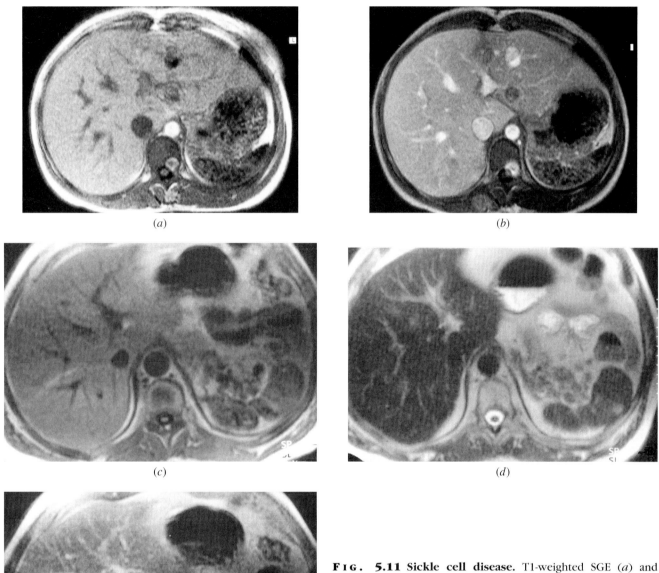

(a)   (b)

(c)   (d)

FIG. 5.11 Sickle cell disease. T1-weighted SGE (*a*) and hepatic venous phase postgadolinium T1-weighted SGE (*b*) images. The spleen is noted to be small and low in signal intensity on all MR images (*a, b*). On the precontrast T1-weighted SGE image (*a*), multiple 1-cm signal-void foci are noted in the small, low-signal-intensity spleen. These foci are better demarcated after contrast administration (*b*) because of enhancement, although minimal, of surrounding splenic parenchyma. T1-weighted SGE (*c*), T2-weighted echo-train spin-echo (*d*), and hepatic venous phase postgadolinium T1-weighted SGE (*e*) images in a second patient. The spleen is small and irregular with extensive low-signal iron deposition, regions of scarring, and infarction.

(e)

foci of high signal intensity on precontrast T1-weighted images (fig. 5.13).

Hemangiomas

Hemangiomas are the most common of the benign splenic neoplasms [22, 23]. Lesions may be single or multiple. Splenic hemangiomas are mildly low to isointense on T1-weighted images and mildly to moderately hyperintense on T2-weighted images, similar to hepatic hemangiomas. Hemangiomas are minimally hypointense to isointense with background spleen on T1-weighted images, because of the relatively low signal intensity of spleen on these images, and minimally hyperintense relative to spleen on T2-weighted images, because of the moderately high signal intensity of spleen on T2-weighted images. Three patterns of contrast

Table 5.1 Pattern Recognition of the Most Common Splenic Lesions

	T1	T2	Early Gd	Late Gd	Other Features
Cyst	↓–Ø	↑↑	None	None	Well-defined
Hamartoma	Ø	Ø–↑	Heterogeneous intense	Homogeneous enhancement, isointense to the spleen	Usually >4 cm and arise from the medial surface of the spleen
Hemangioma	↓–Ø	↑	Peripheral nodules or homogeneous	Centripetal enhancement; retain contrast	Usually <2 cm Lesion more commonly enhances homogeneously on immediate post-Gd images compared to liver hemangiomas, reflecting their small size Peripheral nodules are not as clearly defined as liver hemangiomas
Metastases	↓–Ø	Ø–↑	Focal lesions with minimal enhancement	Isointense or hypointense	Metastases commonly become isointense by 1 min post-Gd
Lymphoma —focal	↓–Ø	↓–↑	Focal lesions with minimal enhancement	Isointense or hypointense	Other sites of nodal disease Lymphomatous lesions commonly become isointense by 1 min post-Gd
Lymphoma —diffuse	↓–Ø	↓–↑	Irregular regions with minimal enhancement	Isointense or hypointense	Other sites of nodal disease Lymphomatous lesions commonly become isointense by 1 min post-Gd

Keys: ↓↓: moderately to markedly decreased; ↓: mildly decreased; Ø: isointense; ↑: mildly increased; ↑↑: moderately to markedly increased.

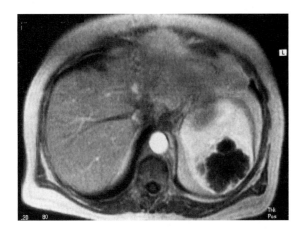

FIG. 5.12 Epidermoid cyst. Immediate postgadolinium T1-weighted SGE image demonstrates a signal-void cystic lesion with peripheral septations.

enhancement are observed: 1) immediate homogeneous enhancement with persistent enhancement on delayed images, 2) peripheral enhancement with progression to uniform enhancement on delayed images (fig. 5.14), and 3) peripheral enhancement with centripetal progression but persistent lack of enhancement of central scar. These patterns are similar to those observed for hepatic hemangiomas. However, unlike hepatic hemangiomas, splenic hemangiomas generally do not demonstrate well-defined nodules on early postgadolinium images. This may, in part, reflect the blood supply from the background organ. Uniform high signal on immediate

postgadolinium SGE images is a common appearance for small (<1.5 cm) hemangiomas, as it is with hepatic hemangiomas. Rarely, hemangiomas with a very large central scar can appear hypointense on T2-weighted images, reflecting the lower fluid content of the central scar (fig. 5.15). These may be termed sclerosing hemangiomas.

Littoral Cell Angioma
Littoral cell angioma (LCA) is a vascular lesion that was first described in 1991 as a benign vascular tumor arising from littoral cells, which line the splenic sinus of the red pulp [24]. LCA is composed of multiple blood-filled vascular channels. Macroscopically, the spleen is enlarged, and these tumors are usually multiple and nodular, with their size ranging from 0.2 to 9 cm. They are well defined and compress the adjacent splenic tissue. Patients with LCA commonly present with signs of hypersplenism (anemia, thrombocytopenia). LCA are thought to be benign tumors, but the malignant potential of LCA has not yet been ascertained. MRI shows the tumor to be multiple with regular well-defined margins and mildly low signal to isointensity on T1-weighted SGE images, low to moderately high signal intensity on T2-weighted images, mild heterogeneous enhancement on arterial dominant phase, and homogenous enhancement on delayed phase [25, 26] (fig. 5.16). Homogenous delayed enhancement and absence of underlying disease such as lymphoma, metastatic diseases, sarcoidosis, or tuberculosis help to establish the correct diagnosis.

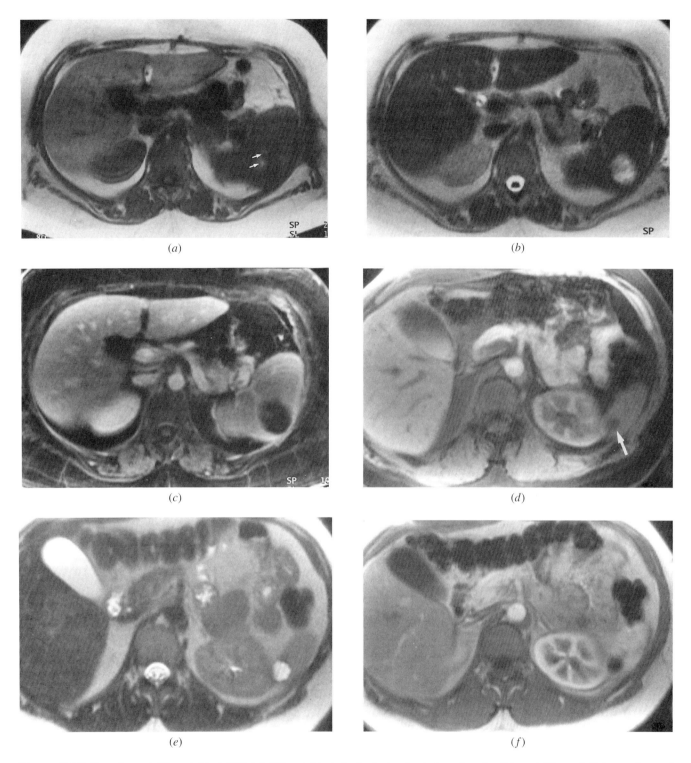

F I G . 5.13 Pseudocyst. T1-weighted SGE (*a*), T2-weighted single-shot echo-train spin-echo (*b*), and 90-s gadolinium-enhanced fat-suppressed SGE (*c*) images. High-signal-intensity foci are identified in the cyst on the precontrast SGE image (arrows, *a*), a finding consistent with hemorrhage. Slight heterogeneity of the cyst on the T2-weighted image (*b*) also reflects the presence of blood degradation products. The cyst is sharply demarcated after gadolinium administration (*c*).The foci of blood remain high in signal intensity on postgadolinium images. T1-weighted fat-suppressed SGE (*d*), T2-weighted single-shot echo-train spin-echo (*e*), immediate postgadolinium T1-weighted SGE (*f*), and 90-s gadolinium-enhanced T1-weighted fat-suppressed SGE (*g*) images in

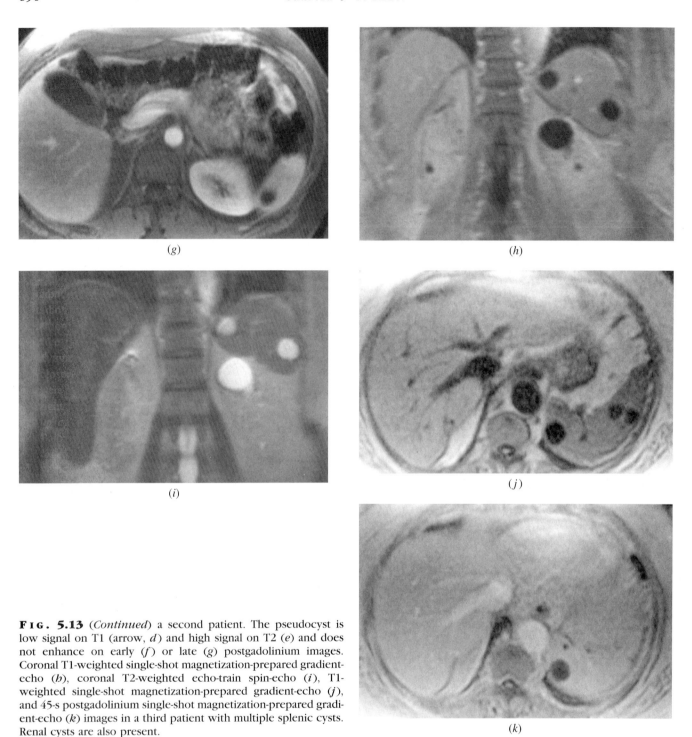

(g)

(h)

(i)

(j)

(k)

FIG. 5.13 (*Continued*) a second patient. The pseudocyst is low signal on T1 (arrow, *d*) and high signal on T2 (*e*) and does not enhance on early (*f*) or late (*g*) postgadolinium images. Coronal T1-weighted single-shot magnetization-prepared gradient-echo (*h*), coronal T2-weighted echo-train spin-echo (*i*), T1-weighted single-shot magnetization-prepared gradient-echo (*j*), and 45-s postgadolinium single-shot magnetization-prepared gradient-echo (*k*) images in a third patient with multiple splenic cysts. Renal cysts are also present.

Hamartomas

Hamartomas are rare and composed of structurally disorganized mature splenic red pulp elements. The lesions tend to be single, spherical, and predominantly solid. They are most likely to occur in the midportion of the spleen, arising from the anterior or posterior aspect of the convex surface. These tumors are mildly low to isointense on T1-weighted images and moderately high in signal intensity on T2-weighted images [23, 27, 28]. They frequently are moderately heterogeneous, in part because of the presence of cystic spaces of varying size. If the composition of fibrous tissue is substantial, hamartomas may have regions of low signal intensity on T2-weighted images [27]. They enhance on immediate

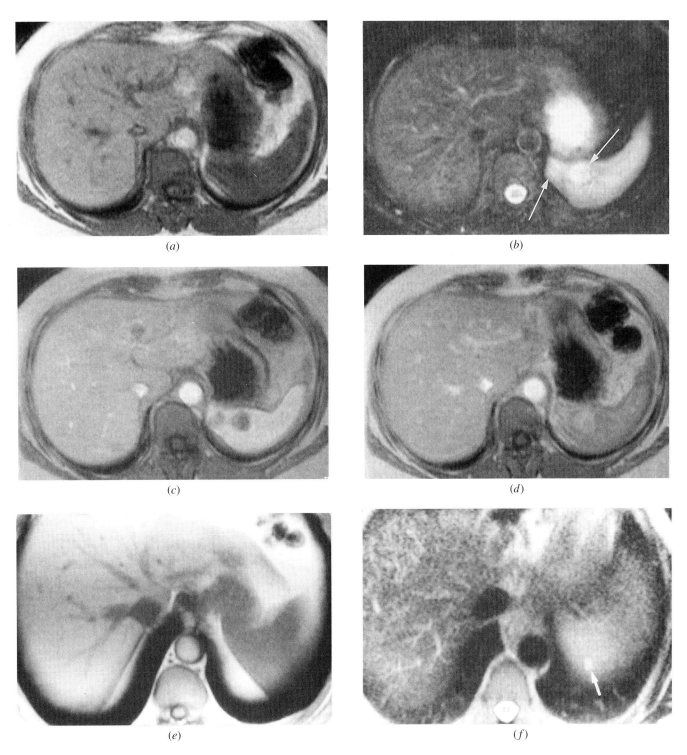

FIG. 5.14 Hemangiomas. T1-weighted SGE (*a*), T2-weighted fat-suppressed spin-echo (*b*), and 45-s (*c*) and 10-min (*d*) postgadolinium SGE images. Two small, <1.5 cm, hemangiomas are present that are minimally hypointense on T1-weighted images (*a*) and moderately hyperintense on T2-weighted images (arrows, *b*). Peripheral nodules are present on early postgadolinium images (*c*), and enhancement progresses to uniform high signal intensity by 10 min (*d*). T1-weighted SGE (*e*), T2 fat-suppressed spin-echo (*f*), immediate postgadolinium T1 SGE (*g*), and 90-s postgadolinium T1-fat-suppressed SGE (*h*) images in a second patient.

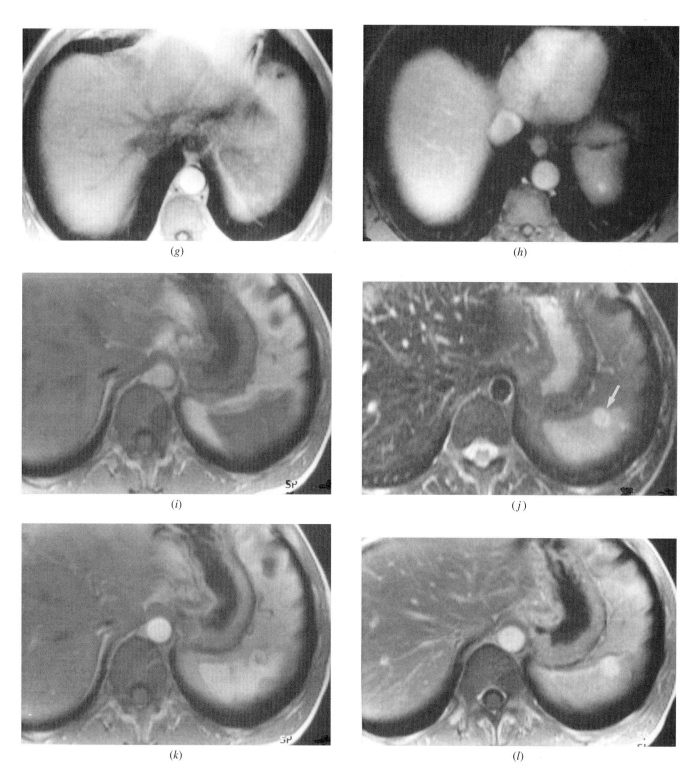

(g)   *(h)*

(i)   *(j)*

(k)   *(l)*

F I G. 5.14 (*Continued*) The small hemangioma in the superior aspect of the spleen is isointense on T1 and moderately hyper-intense on T2 (arrow, *f*) and shows early uniform enhancement (*g*) that persists on the late postgadolinium image (*h*). The hem-angioma is better demonstrated on the later postgadolinium image as background splenic enhancement has diminished and is uniform. Early uniform enhancement is common in <1.5-cm hemangiomas.

T1-weighted SGE (*i*), T2-weighted fat-suppressed spin-echo (*j*), immediate postgadolinium T1-weighted SGE (*k*), and 90-s gadolinium-enhanced T1-weighted SGE (*l*) images in a third patient. The lesion is isointense on T1(*i*) and moderately hyperintense on the T2-weighted image (arrow, *j*). Note centripetal (*k, l*) progressive enhancement of the hemangioma resembling the pattern of a hepatic hemangioma.

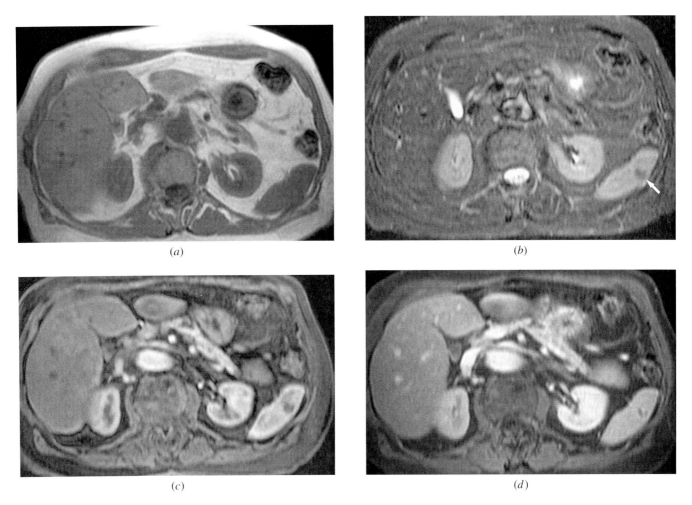

F I G . 5.15 Sclerosing hemangioma. T1-weighted SGE (*a*), T2-weighted fat-suppressed single-shot echo-train spin-echo (*b*), and immediate and 90-s postgadolinium T1-weighted fat-suppressed 3D GRE (*c, d*) images demonstrate a 1-cm hemangioma that is isointense with spleen on the T1-weighted image (*a*) and markedly hypointense on the T2-weighted image (arrow, *b*). Peripheral nodule of enhancement is present on the early postgadolinium image (*c*), with moderate progressive enhancement on the delayed postgadolinium image (*d*). The combination of hypointensity on T2-weighted image with only moderate progression of nodular enhancement on postcontrast T1-weighted image is consistent with a sclerosing hemangioma.

postgadolinium SGE images in an intense diffuse heterogeneous fashion [23, 27, 28] (fig. 5.17). Diffuse enhancement on immediate postgadolinium images is generally observed in tumors that are native to the organ in which they occur. Lesion size and enhancement pattern may mimic a more aggressive lesion. Lesions may also resemble normal splenic parenchyma (fig. 5.17). Enhancement becomes homogeneous on more delayed images, with signal intensity slightly greater than in background spleen. The early diffuse heterogeneous enhancement permits distinction from hemangioma [23].

Lymphangiomas
Lymphangiomas are composed of collections of small and cystically dilated lymphatic channels. Splenic lymphangiomatosis is rare and usually appears as a subcapsular multiloculated mass with increased signal intensity on T2-weighted images and enhancing septa on late-phase gadolinium-enhanced imaging [29].

Malignant Masses

Lymphoma and Other Hematologic Malignancies
Hodgkin and non-Hodgkin lymphomas often involve the spleen [30–32]. Lymphomatous deposits in the spleen frequently parallel the signal intensity of splenic parenchyma on T1- and T2-weighted images. Therefore, conventional unenhanced spin-echo MRI has had only limited success in imaging lymphomatous involvement of the spleen [31]. Immediate postgadolinium SGE images, however, surpass CT images for the evaluation of lymphoma [4]. This is explained by the higher sensitivity of MRI for gadolinium and its ability to acquire

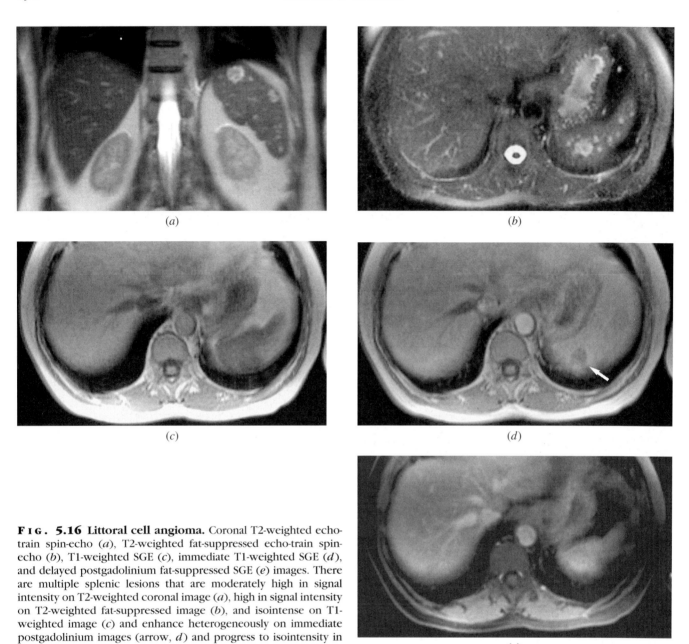

FIG. 5.16 Littoral cell angioma. Coronal T2-weighted echo-train spin-echo (*a*), T2-weighted fat-suppressed echo-train spin-echo (*b*), T1-weighted SGE (*c*), immediate T1-weighted SGE (*d*), and delayed postgadolinium fat-suppressed SGE (*e*) images. There are multiple splenic lesions that are moderately high in signal intensity on T2-weighted coronal image (*a*), high in signal intensity on T2-weighted fat-suppressed image (*b*), and isointense on T1-weighted image (*c*) and enhance heterogeneously on immediate postgadolinium images (arrow, *d*) and progress to isointensity in late images (*e*).

images of the entire spleen in a rapid fashion after a compact bolus of contrast.

Splenic involvement may have various appearances on immediate postgadolinium images. Diffuse involvement may appear as large, irregularly enhancing regions of high and low signal intensity (fig. 5.18), in contrast to the uniform bands that characterize normal arciform enhancement. Multifocal disease is also common, appearing as focal low-signal-intensity mass lesions scattered throughout the spleen [4]. Focal lesions may occur in a background of arciform-enhancing spleen or in a background of uniformly enhancing spleen. Focal involvement appears as spherical lesions, in distinction

to the wavy tubular pattern of arciform enhancement of uninvolved spleen. Focal lymphomatous deposits may be low in signal intensity compared to background spleen on T2-weighted images (fig. 5.19), which is a feature distinguishing lymphomas from metastases, which are rarely low in signal intensity and usually isointense to hyperintense. Although splenomegaly is most often present, lymphoma may involve normal-sized spleens (fig. 5.20). Lymphoma also may appear as a large mass involving spleen and contiguous organs such as stomach, adrenal, or kidney. Bulky lymphadenopathy is frequently, but not invariably, present. It is critical to acquire SGE images within the first 30s after

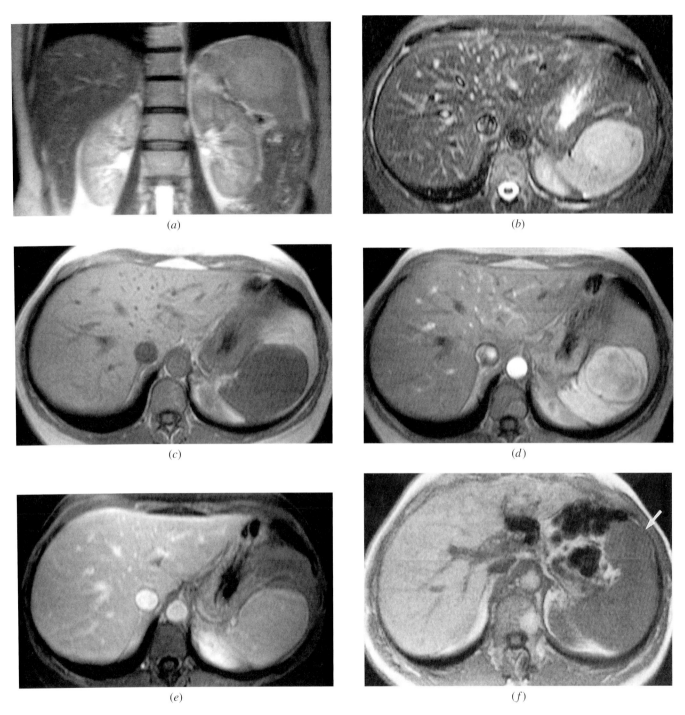

FIG. 5.17 Hamartoma. Coronal T2-weighted single-shot echo-train spin-echo (*a*), T2-weighted fat-suppressed single-shot echo-train spin-echo (*b*), T1-weighted SGE (*c*), immediate postgadolinium T1-weighted SGE (*d*), and late postgadolinium T1-weighted fat-suppressed spin-echo (*e*) images demonstrate a lesion in the spleen that is moderately high in signal intensity on T2-weighted images (*a, b*) and isointense on T1-weighted image (*c*). The lesion enhances heterogeneously on immediate postgadolinium SGE image (*d*). On delayed image (*e*) enhancement becomes more homogeneous and is greater than that of background spleen. T1-weighted SGE (*f*), T2-weighted fat-suppressed spin-echo (*g*), and immediate (*h*), 90-s (*i*), and 10-min (*j*) postgadolinium images

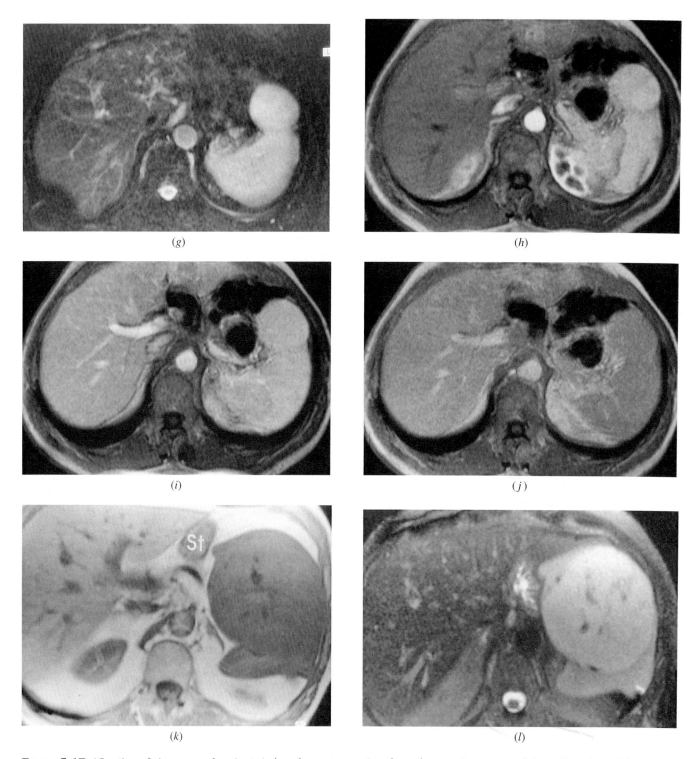

(g)

(h)

(i)

(j)

(k)

(l)

FIG. 5.17 (*Continued*) in a second patient. A 4-cm hamartoma arises from the anterior aspect of the midportion of the spleen (arrow, *f*). The signal intensity of the hamartoma is very similar to that of background spleen on all imaging sequences. A cleavage plane from spleen is noted on the T2-weighted image (*g*). On the immediate postgadolinium image (*h*), the tumor has intense, uniform enhancement, which is different from the arciform enhancement of the normal splenic parenchyma.

T1-weighted SGE (*k*),T2-weighted fat-suppressed echo-train spin-echo (*l*), immediate postgadolinium T1-weighted SGE (*m*), and 90-s gadolinium-enhanced T1-weighted fat-suppressed SGE (*n*) images in a third patient. A large hamartoma in the anterior

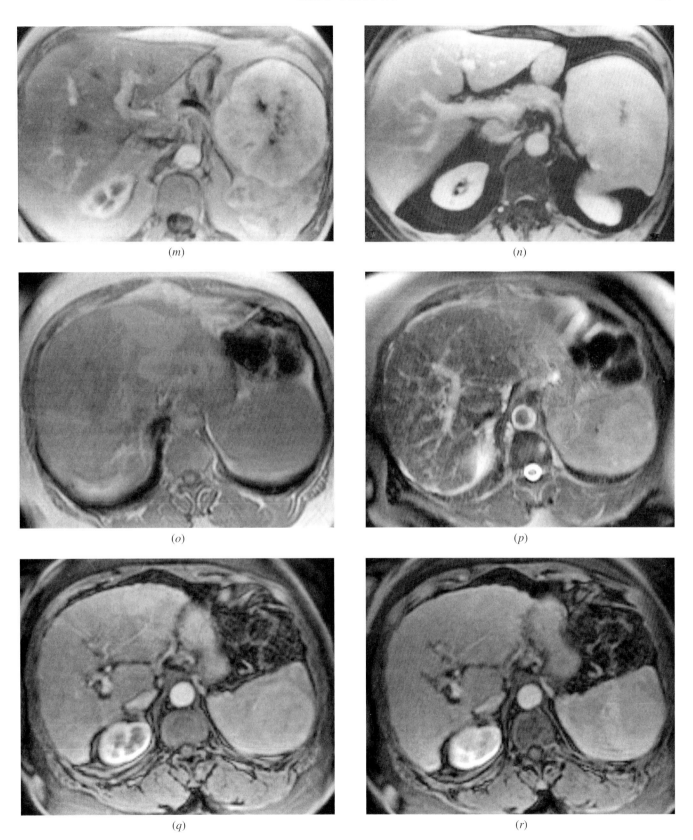

FIG. 5.17 (*Continued*) aspect of the spleen displaces the stomach (St, *k*) medially. The mass is near-isointense to the spleen on all sequences. It shows intense heterogeneous enhancement on the immediate postgadolinium image, similar to the intensity of spleen but with a different pattern. T1-weighted SGE (*o*), T2-weighted fat-suppressed single-shot echo-train spin-echo (*p*), and immediate (*q*) and delayed (*r*) postgadolinium T1-weighted fat-suppressed 3D-GE images at 3.0 T show splenic hamartoma demonstrating similar findings in another patient with cirrhosis and portal hypertension.

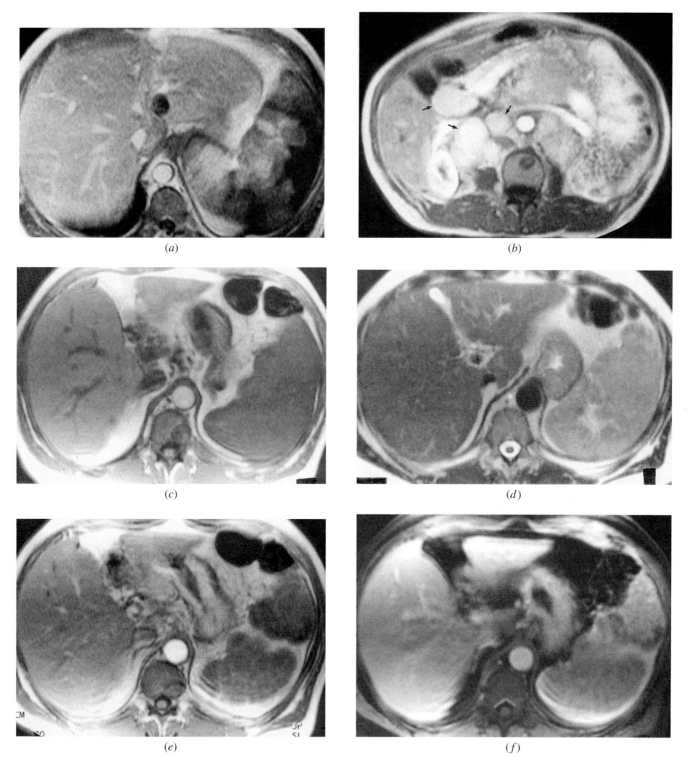

(a)

(b)

(c)

(d)

(e)

(f)

F I G . 5.18 Diffuse infiltration with lymphoma. Immediate postgadolinium T1-weighted SGE image (*a*) demonstrates irregular regions of high and low signal intensity in the spleen in this patient with non-Hodgkin lymphoma. Irregular enhancement is observed in the setting of diffuse infiltration. Immediate postgadolinium SGE image (*b*) in a second patient with non-Hodgkin lymphoma demonstrates irregular enhancement of the spleen consistent with diffuse infiltration. Enhancing lymph nodes (arrows, *b*) are also noted. T1-weighted SGE (*c*), T2-weighted echo-train spin-echo (*d*), immediate postgadolinium T1-weighted SGE (*e*), and 90-s postgadolinium T1-weighted fat-suppressed SGE (*f*) images in a third patient with B cell lymphoma infiltrating the spleen. The spleen is homogeneous in signal intensity on T1 (*c*) and is heterogeneous on the T2-weighted image (*d*). Diffuse heterogeneous enhancement with large irregular foci of decreased enhancement is appreciated on the immediate postgadolinium image (*e*) that persists on the late image (*f*).

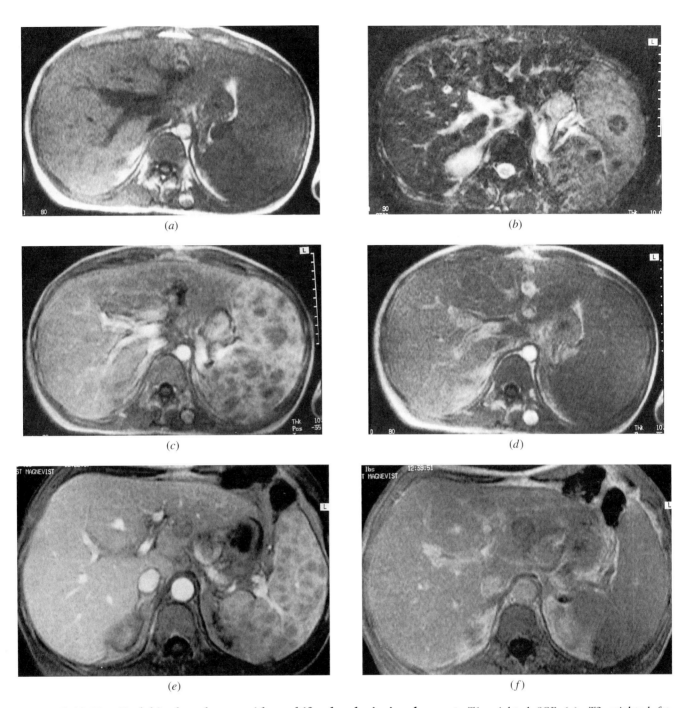

FIG. 5.19 Non-Hodgkin lymphoma with multifocal splenic involvement. T1-weighted SGE (*a*), T2-weighted fat-suppressed spin-echo (*b*), and immediate (*c*) and 2-min (*d*) postgadolinium SGE images. Splenomegaly is present. Lesions are not apparent on the precontrast SGE image. Several low-signal-intensity focal mass lesions are identified on T2-weighted images, an appearance that is not uncommon for lymphoma but rare for other malignant tumors. Multiple focal masses are most clearly demonstrated on immediate postgadolinium images (*c*). Lymphomatous foci become isointense with background spleen by 2 min after contrast (*d*). Immediate (*e*) and 90-s (*f*) postgadolinium SGE images in a second patient. Multiple low-signal-intensity masses are identified on the immediate postgadolinium image (*e*). Lesions become isointense with background spleen by 90 s.

contrast administration because foci of lymphoma equilibrate early, becoming isointense with normal splenic tissue within 2 min and frequently earlier [2, 4]. A rare appearance is that of a solitary mass involving the spleen, which may also show relatively internal diffuse

and mildly heterogeneous enhancement on immediate postgadolinium SGE images (fig. 5.21). This appearance may mimic that of splenic hamartomas. The presence of symptoms and signs of systemic disease may suggest the diagnosis of lymphoma.

Superparamagnetic particles also improve the accuracy of diagnosing splenic lymphoma [9, 10]. These particles are selectively taken up by the RES cells and cause a decrease in signal intensity. By contrast, malignant cells do not take up superparamagnetic particles. Therefore, splenic lymphoma remains hyperintense compared to the normal spleen, improving tumor-spleen contrast [9, 10].

Chronic lymphocytic leukemia frequently involves the spleen and may result in massive splenomegaly. Focal deposits are more infiltrative and less well-defined than lymphoma. Deposits are well shown after gadolinium administration and appear as irregular hypointense masses on early postcontrast images (fig. 5.22). Malignancies related to leukemia, such as angioimmunoblastic lymphadenopathy with dysproteinemia, have a similar appearance, with irregular regions of low signal intensity within the spleen on immediate postgadolinium images (fig. 5.23). Lymphadenopathy is frequently present.

Chemotherapy-treated lymphomatous deposits in the spleen can appear as fibrotic nodules that are low signal intensity on T1-weighted and T2-weighted images and demonstrate negligible enhancement on early and late postgadolinium images (fig. 5.24). These imaging features may be correlated clinically with a favorable response to therapy.

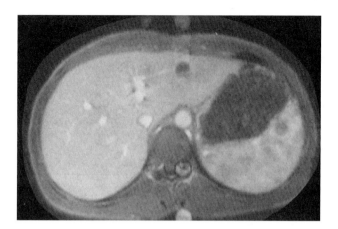

FIG. 5.20 Hodgkin lymphoma. Immediate postgadolinium image demonstrates multiple low-signal-intensity masses within a normal-sized spleen. Rounded lesions are present in a background of arciform-enhancing spleen.

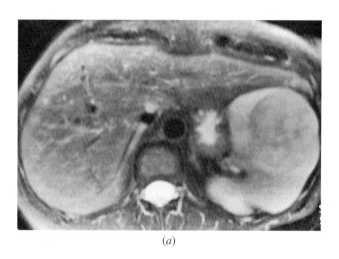

(a)

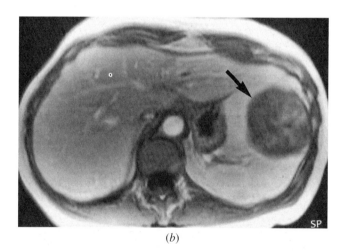

(b)

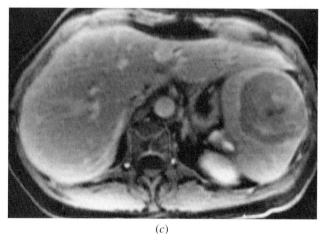

(c)

FIG. 5.21 Splenic lymphoma presenting as a solitary mass. T2-weighted fat-suppressed echo-train spin-echo (a), immediate postgadolinium T1-weighted SGE (b), and 90-s postgadolinium fat-suppressed SGE (c) images. A 6-cm solitary mass arises from the spleen that is mildly heterogeneous and hyperintense on the T2-weighted image (a). The mass enhances moderately in a diffuse heterogeneous fashion on the immediate postgadolinium image (arrow, b), with slightly increased signal intensity by 90 s after contrast (c). The appearance resembles a hamartoma, with diffuse heterogeneous enhancement. Substantially less enhancement is present of this lymphomatous mass than is typically seen with a hamartoma. The patient presented with systemic symptoms, which is a picture in keeping with lymphoma and not hamartoma. The patient did not have retroperitoneal adenopathy, which is another uncommon feature of splenic lymphoma.

Metastases

Although tumors may invade the spleen from contiguous viscera, true tumor metastasis to the spleen is rare, usually occurring only in the setting of disseminated

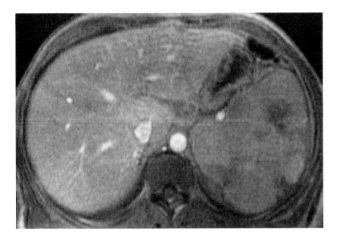

FIG. 5.22 Chronic lymphocytic leukemia. The spleen is noted to be massively enlarged and contains irregularly marginated focal low-signal-intensity masses on the 45-s postgadolinium T1-weighted SGE image.

disease in the terminal stage. Breast cancer, lung cancer, and melanoma are the most common primary tumors [33]. The most generally accepted theory to account for the relative scarcity of splenic metastasis is based on the absence of afferent lymphatic channels within the spleen [34]. Metastases tend to be in the form of nodules or aggregates of tumor, and they are particularly prone to disrupt the normal splenic architecture. Splenic metastases often are occult on conventional spin-echo imaging [32]. One notable exception is melanoma, because its paramagnetic properties may result in a mixed population of high- and low-signal-intensity lesions on both T1- and T2-weighted images. Lesion detection is improved by acquiring immediate postgadolinium SGE images [3] (fig. 5.25). Metastases are lower in signal intensity than normal splenic tissue on these images. Images must be acquired within the first 30 s after gadolinium administration because metastases rapidly equilibrate with splenic parenchyma. Image acquisition with superparamagnetic iron oxide particles renders metastases higher in signal intensity than normal spleen [7, 9]. An attractive feature of iron oxide particles is that the imaging window is longer (60 min) than for gadolinium (<1 min) [7, 9].

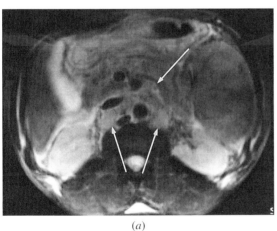

(a)

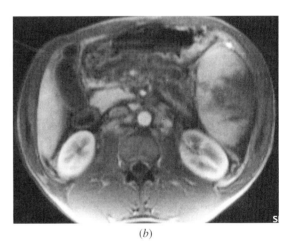

(b)

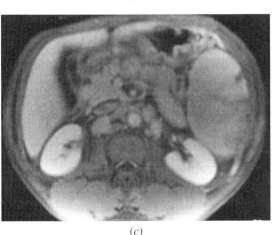

(c)

FIG. 5.23 Angioimmunoblastic lymphadenopathy with dysproteinemia. T2-weighted fat-suppressed spin-echo (a), immediate postgadolinium T1-weighted SGE (b), and 90-s postgadolinium fat-suppressed SGE (c) images. The spleen is noted to be markedly enlarged. Lymphadenopathy is moderately high in signal intensity on T2-weighted images and is rendered conspicuous because of the suppression of fat signal intensity (arrows, a). Mild enhancement of lymph nodes is noted on immediate postgadolinium SGE (b). Lymph nodes enhance more intensely in the interstitial phase and are more clearly defined by the suppression of fat signal intensity (c). Splenic involvement is demonstrated by irregular, poorly marginated, large regions of diminished enhancement on the immediate postgadolinium image (b). Enhancement of the spleen is more uniform by 90 s after contrast (c), and signal intensity is mildly heterogeneous on the T2-weighted image.

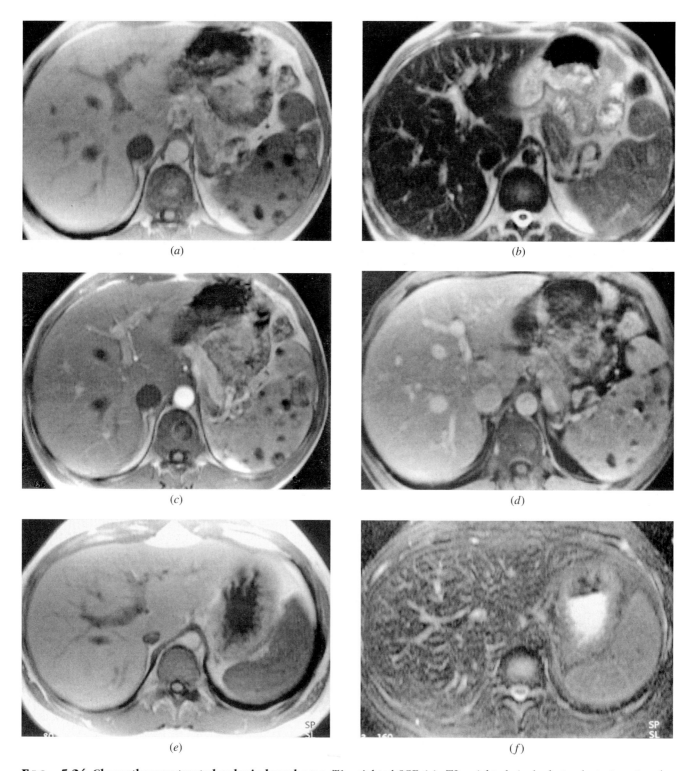

(a)

(b)

(c)

(d)

(e)

(f)

F I G . 5.24 Chemotherapy-treated splenic lymphoma. T1-weighted SGE (*a*), T2-weighted single-shot echo-train spin-echo (*b*), immediate postgadolinium T1-weighted SGE (*c*), and 90-s postgadolinium T1-weighted fat-suppressed SGE (*d*) images. Foci of treated lymphoma are hypointense on T1 (*a*) and hypo- to isointense on T2 (*b*) and demonstrate negligible enhancement on early (*c*) and late (*d*) postgadolinium images. The low signal on T2 reflects a diminished fluid content, and fibrous changes result in the diminished enhancement. T1-weighted SGE (*e*), breath-hold STIR (*f*), immediate postgadolinium SGE (*g*), and 90-s postgadolinium

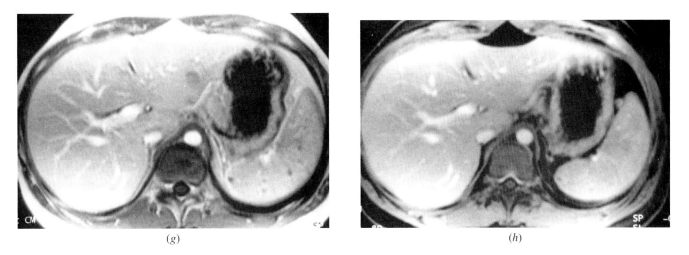

(g)   (h)

FIG. 5.24 (*Continued*) SGE (*b*) images in a second patient with Hodgkin lymphoma receiving chemotherapy. There are multiple small hypointense lesions on T1 (*e*)- and T2 (*f*)-weighted images, which shows peripheral or diffuse enhancement after contrast administration (*g, h*) reflecting the different stages of the fibrotic process. These lesions remained stable in appearance in follow-up MRI exams (not shown).

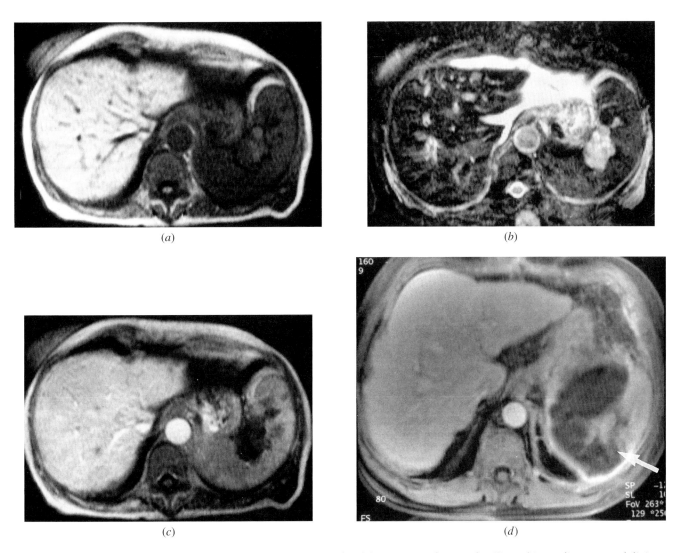

(a)   (b)

(c)   (d)

FIG. 5.25 Splenic metastases. T1-weighted SGE (*a*), T2-weighted fat-suppressed spin-echo (*b*), and immediate postgadolinium T1-weighted SGE (*c*) images in a woman with endometrial cancer. Metastases are noted throughout the spleen that are mixed hypointense and isointense on the T1-weighted image (*a*), mixed isointense and hyperintense on the T2-weighted image (*b*), and low in signal intensity on the immediate postgadolinium image (*c*). Note that metastases are best shown on the immediate post-gadolinium image. The largest metastasis is distinctly demonstrated on the T2-weighted image (*b*). The smaller lesions are poorly shown, despite the presence of iron deposition. Ascites is also present and is low in signal intensity on pre- and postcontrast T1-weighted images and high in signal intensity on the T2-weighted image. Transverse 90-s postgadolinium fat-suppressed SGE image (*d*) in a second patient demonstrates an expansive destructive lesion (arrow, *d*) in the posterior aspect of the spleen associated

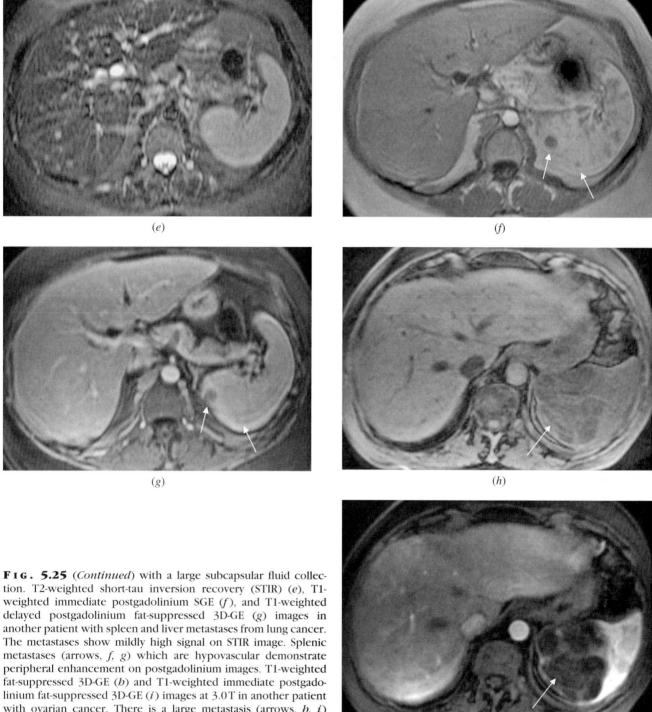

(e)

(f)

(g)

(h)

(i)

FIG. 5.25 (*Continued*) with a large subcapsular fluid collection. T2-weighted short-tau inversion recovery (STIR) (*e*), T1-weighted immediate postgadolinium SGE (*f*), and T1-weighted delayed postgadolinium fat-suppressed 3D-GE (*g*) images in another patient with spleen and liver metastases from lung cancer. The metastases show mildly high signal on STIR image. Splenic metastases (arrows, *f, g*) which are hypovascular demonstrate peripheral enhancement on postgadolinium images. T1-weighted fat-suppressed 3D-GE (*h*) and T1-weighted immediate postgadolinium fat-suppressed 3D-GE (*i*) images at 3.0 T in another patient with ovarian cancer. There is a large metastasis (arrows, *h, i*) located in the spleen demonstrating heterogeneous enhancement on immediate postgadolinium 3D-GE image (*i*).

Direct Tumor Invasion

Direct tumor invasion is most commonly observed with pancreatic cancers including ductal adenocarcinoma, islet cell tumor, and macrocystic cystadenocarcinoma (fig. 5.26). Direct extension from tumors of gastric, colonic, renal, and adrenal origins, in decreasing order of frequency, is also observed. Lymphoma has a par-

ticular propensity to involve the spleen in continuity with other organs.

Angiosarcoma

Angiosarcoma is rare but represents the most common primary nonlymphoid malignant tumor of the spleen. Tumors may be single or multiple and demonstrate an

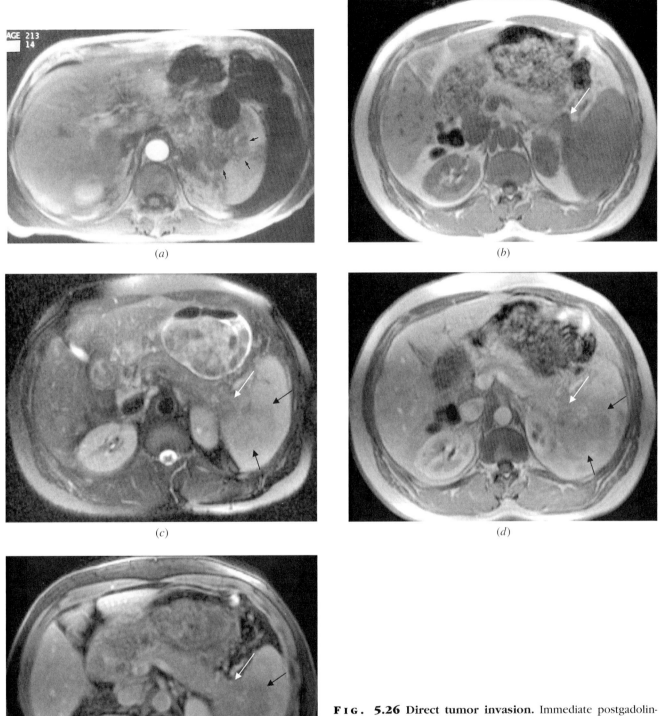

(a)

(b)

(c)

(d)

(e)

FIG. 5.26 Direct tumor invasion. Immediate postgadolinium T1-weighted SGE (*a*) image demonstrates invasion of the splenic hilum by a large infiltrative pancreatic ductal adeno-carcinoma (arrows, *a*). T1-weighted SGE (*b*), T2-weighted fat-suppressed single-shot echo-train spin-echo (*c*), T1-weighted postgadolinium 45-s SGE (*d*) and 90-s fat-suppressed 3D-GE (*e*) images in another patient with pancreatic neuroendocrine tumor. The tumor (white arrows, *b*–*e*) is located in the pancreatic tail and invades the spleen (black arrows, *c*–*e*).

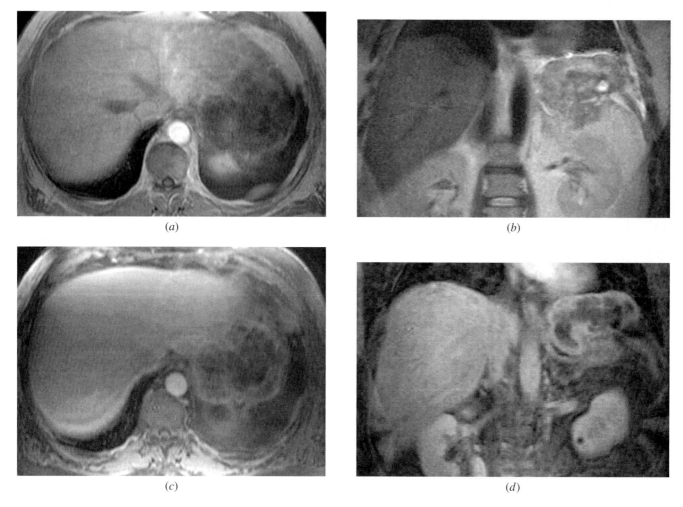

(a)

(b)

(c)

(d)

FIG. 5.27 Angiosarcoma of the spleen. T1-weighted SGE (*a*), coronal T2-weighted single-shot echo-train spin-echo (*b*), immediate postgadolinium T1-weighted fat-suppressed 3D GRE (*c*), and delayed postgadolinium coronal T1-weighted fat-suppressed 3D GRE (*d*) images demonstrate a large splenic mass that is hypointense on T1-weighted image (*a*) and mildly high in signal intensity on T2-weighted image (*b*). The mass enhances heterogeneously on immediate postgadolinium images (*c*), and enhancement progresses on delayed images (*d*).

aggressive growth pattern [35, 36]. Rupture is not uncommon, and hemorrhage is a frequent finding. Angiosarcomas commonly demonstrate a variety of signal intensities on T1-weighted images because of the varying ages of blood products [37]. Tumors are usually highly vascular and enhance intensely with gadolinium [37] (fig. 5.27).

MISCELLANEOUS

Splenomegaly and Vascular Pathologies

Splenomegaly may be observed in a number of disease states including venous congestion (portal hypertension), leukemia, lymphoma, metastases, and various infections. In North America, the most common cause of splenomegaly is secondary to portal hypertension.

On immediate postgadolinium images, demonstration of arciform or uniform high-signal-intensity enhancement is consistent with portal hypertension and excludes the presence of malignant disease (fig. 5.28).

Perisplenic varices and splenorenal shunts are also seen commonly in patients with portal hypertension in combination with splenomegaly (fig. 5.28).

Splenic vein thrombosis can be bland or malignant. Bland splenic vein thrombosis is commonly seen in patients with portal hypertension (for an in-depth discussion, see Chapter 2, *Liver*, and fig. 2.249). Malignant splenic vein thrombosis is usually seen in patients with pancreatic adenocarcinoma (for an in-depth discussion, see Chapter 4, *Pancreas*, and fig. 4.29).

Splenic artery aneurysms are the most common visceral artery aneurysms [38]. The prevalence of splenic artery aneurysm has been reported as 0.04–0.10% at autopsy [38]. Most aneursyms are small (usually less

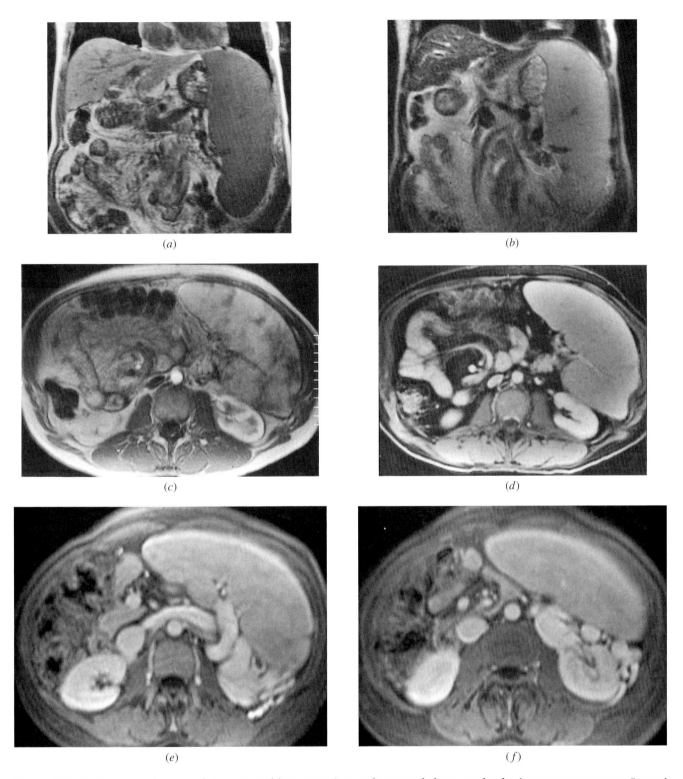

FIG. 5.28 Splenomegaly secondary to portal hypertension, splenorenal shunt, and splenic artery aneurysm. Coronal T1-weighted SGE (*a*), coronal T2-weighted echo-train spin-echo (*b*), immediate postgadolinium T1-weighted SGE (*c*), and 90-s post-gadolinium fat-suppressed SGE (*d*) images. Massive splenomegaly is demonstrated on all MR images. No focal lesions are present on precontrast T1 (*a*) or T2-weighted (*b*) images. The presence of arciform enhancement on the immediate postgadolinium SGE image (*c*) excludes the presence of malignant disease. At 90 s, the spleen becomes homogeneous in signal (*d*). T1-weighted delayed postgadolinium 3D-GE images (*e, f*) demonstrate splenomegaly, splenorenal shunt, and portosystemic collaterals in another patient with portal hypertension. Axial T1-weighted 45-s postgadolinium fat-suppressed 3D-GE images (*g, h*) and coronal reformatted 3D-GE

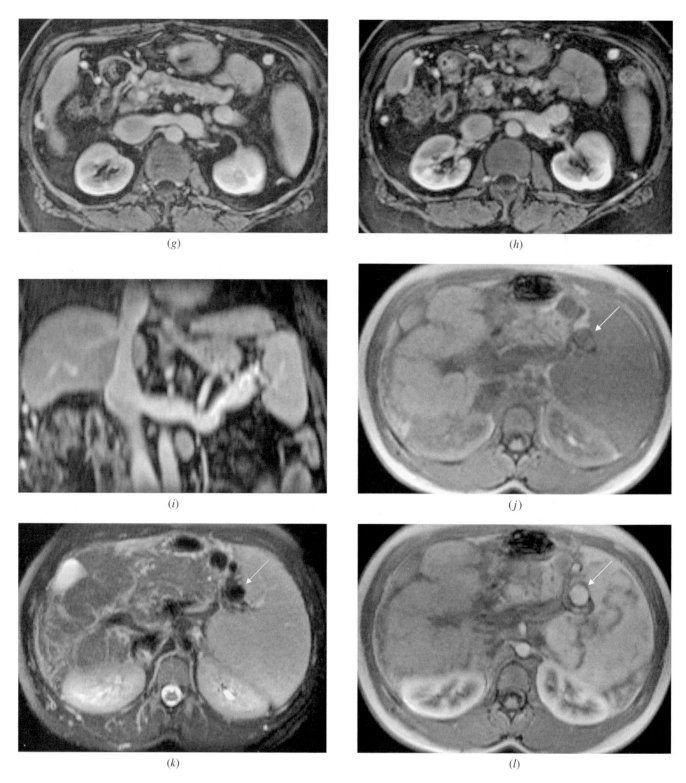

(g)

(h)

(i)

(j)

(k)

(l)

FIG. 5.28 (*Continued*) image (*i*) at 3.0 T demonstrate the splenorenal shunt in another patient with portal hypertension. T1-weighted SGE (*j*), T2-weighted fat-suppressed single-shot echo-train spin-echo (*k*), T1-weighted immediate postgadolinium SGE (*l*),

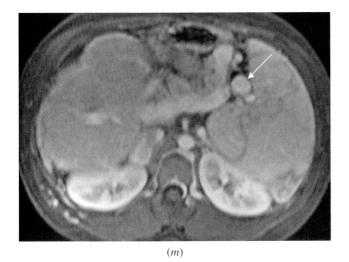

(m)

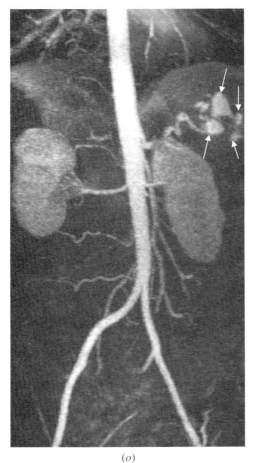

(o)

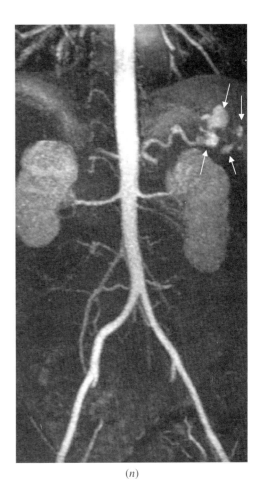

(n)

FIG. 5.28 (*Continued*) and 45-s fat-suppressed 3D-GE (*m*) images in another patient with primary sclerosing cholangitis, splenomegaly, and portal hypertension demonstrate splenic artery aneurysm (arrows). The aneurysm is signal void on T2-weighted image (*k*) and enhances earlier on the arterial phase image (*l*). Reconstructed 3D-MR angiography images (*n, o*) demonstrate distal splenic artery aneurysms in another patient (arrows).

than 2 cm) and saccular. They are located in the middle or distal segment of the splenic artery. They can be multiple in 20% of cases and substantially more common in patients with portal hypertension and cirrhosis (fig. 5.28). Splenic artery pseudoaneurysms may also be seen secondary to digestion of the arterial wall by proteolytic pancreatic enzymes in patients with pancreatitis. Splenic artery aneurysms are usually detected incidentally. Their rupture is rare; however, it may be associated with high mortality rate [38].

Infection

Viral infection may result in splenomegaly. The three most common viruses to involve the spleen are Epstein–Barr, varicella, and cytomegalovirus. Nonviral infectious agents that involve the spleen in patients with normal immune status cause histoplasmosis, tuberculosis, and echinococcosis [39]. These infectious agents are observed in immunocompromised patients with an even greater frequency (fig. 5.29). In the immunocompromised patient, the most common hepatosplenic infection is fungal infection with *Candida albicans* and *Cryptococcus* [40, 41]. Patients with acute myelogenous leukemia are at particular risk for developing fungal infections. Multiorgan involvement is common. The gastrointestinal tract is almost invariably involved, and although esophageal disease is well shown on MR images, involvement of the intestines is frequently not visible. Esophageal candidiasis is common and rarely associated with hepatosplenic candidiasis, whereas small intestine candidiasis is more frequently associated with this infection. Lesions are most commonly observed in the spleen and liver, whereas renal disease is somewhat uncommon. MR images can demonstrate lesions in the acute phase, subacute treated phase, and chronic healed phase [40, 42]. Lesions in each of these phases have distinctive MRI appearances. These varying appearances are more distinct for liver lesions. (For an in-depth discussion, see Chapter 2, *Liver*.) Acute lesions are generally more apparent in the spleen than in the liver, whereas the reverse is true for subacute-treated and chronic-healed lesions. In the acute phase, hepatosplenic candidiasis results in small (<1 cm), well-defined abscesses in the spleen and liver. They are well shown on T2-weighted fat-suppressed images as high signal-intensity rounded foci (fig. 5.30). Lesions also may be visible postgadolinium images, but they usually are not visualized on precontrast SGE images.

MRI has been shown to be superior to contrast-enhanced CT imaging for the detection of fungal micro-abscesses [40]. MRI should be used routinely in the investigation of hepatosplenic candidiasis because patient survival depends on swift pharmacologic intervention with antifungal agents.

Bacterial and fungal abscesses are rare in the spleen. Abscesses appear slightly hypo- to isointense on T1-weighted images and heterogeneous and mildly to moderately hyperintense on T2-weighted images. These lesions show intense mural enhancement on early gadolinium-enhanced images. This pattern persists on later postgadolinium images, accompanied by the pres-

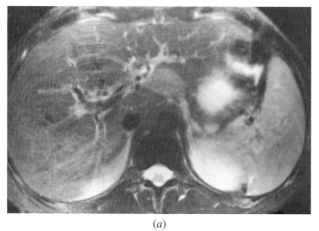

(a)

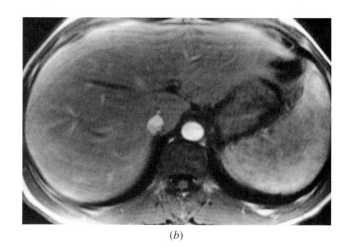

(b)

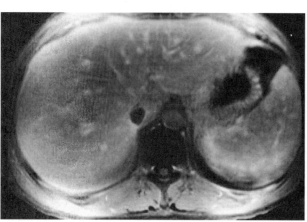

(c)

FIG. 5.29 Hepatosplenorenal histoplasmosis. T2-weighted fat-suppressed echo-train spin-echo (*a*), immediate postgadolinium T1-weighted SGE (*b*), and 90-s postgadolinium fat-suppressed SGE (*c*) images in a patient with human immunodeficiency virus (HIV) infection. Multiple lesions <1 cm are demonstrated in the liver, spleen, and kidneys. Lesions are poorly visualized on T2-weighted images and appear as small minimally hyperintense lesions (*a*). On immediate postgadolinium image, lesions appear low in signal intensity (*b*). By 90 s after gadolinium, lesions enhance more than background tissue.

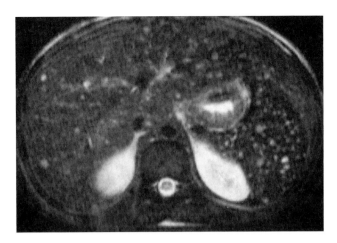

F I G . 5.30 Hepatosplenic candidiasis. T2-weighted fat-suppressed echo-train spin-echo image demonstrates multiple, well-defined, high-signal-intensity candidiasis abscesses <1 cm in the liver and spleen.

ence of periabscess increased enhancement of surrounding tissue on immediate postgadolinium images (fig. 5.31).

Sarcoidosis

Lesions of sarcoidosis are small (<1 cm) and hypovascular. Because of their hypovascularity, the lesions are low in signal intensity on T1- and T2-weighted images and enhance on gadolinium-enhanced images in a minimal and delayed fashion [43] (fig. 5.32). Low signal intensity on T2-weighted images is a feature that distinguishes these lesions from acute infective lesions.

Gamna–Gandy Bodies

Foci of iron deposition occur commonly in patients with cirrhosis and portal hypertension due to microhemorrhages in the splenic parenchyma. On occasion, such foci are observed in patients receiving blood transfusions [44, 45]. Lesions vary in size but are generally smaller than 1 cm. Lesions appear signal void on all pulse sequences [44, 45] (fig. 5.33). Susceptibility artifact is demonstrated on gradient-echo images as blooming artifact, and this artifact is pathognomonic for this entity. An imaging feature that is helpful to distinguish Gamna–Gandy bodies from fibrotic nodules is that Gamna–Gandy bodies appear smaller on shorter TE sequences because of a diminution of susceptibility artifact (e.g., smaller on TE = 2 ms sequence compared to TE = 4 ms sequence at 1.5 T) whereas the size of fibrotic nodules is unchanged on shorter TE sequences.

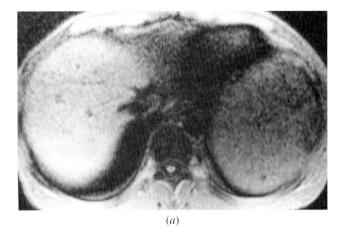

(a)

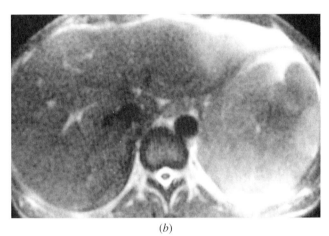

(b)

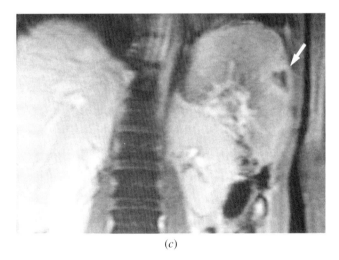

(c)

F I G . 5.31 Cryptococcal abscess. T1-weighted magnetization-prepared gradient-echo (*a*), T2 fat-suppressed single-shot echo-train spin-echo (*b*), and coronal 3-min postgadolinium T1-weighted magnetization-prepared gradient-echo (*c*) images in an immunocompromised patient with HIV and generalized cryptococcal infection. The abscess appears mildly hypointense on T1 (*a*) and mildly hyperintense on T2 (*b*), with subtle signal difference compared to spleen. Lack of enhancement and peripheral ring enhancement (arrow, *c*) present on the postgadolinium image (*c*) are features of bacterial and some fungal abscesses.

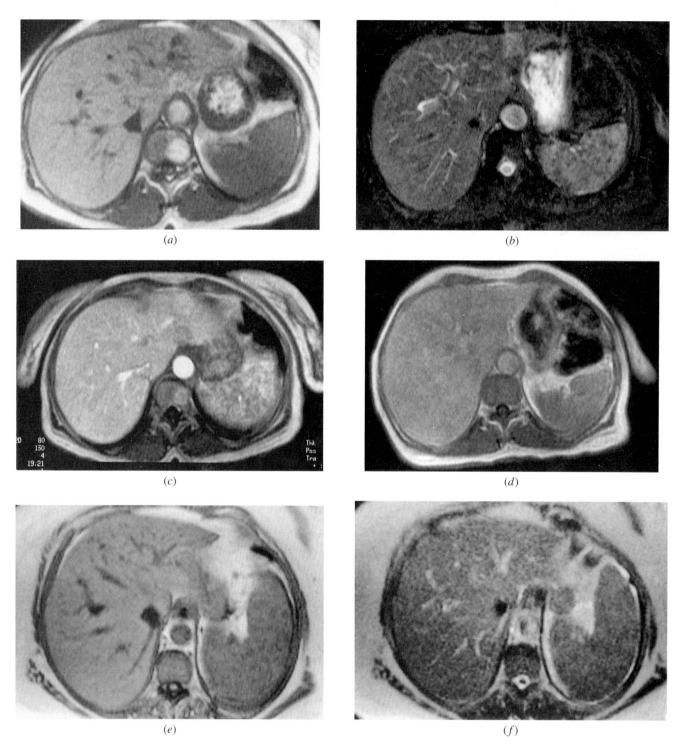

(a)

(b)

(c)

(d)

(e)

(f)

F I G . 5.32 Sarcoidosis. T1-weighted SGE (*a*), T2-weighted fat-suppressed spin-echo (*b*), and immediate (*c*) and 10-min (*d*) postgadolinium T1-weighted SGE images. Multiple sarcoidosis **granulomas**, smaller than 1 cm, are present in the spleen. Lesions are mildly hypointense to isointense on T1-weighted images (*a*), moderately hypointense on T2-weighted images (*b*), and hypointense on immediate postgadolinium images (*c*), gradually enhancing to near isointensity on delayed postgadolinium images (*d*). Hypointensity on T2-weighted images distinguishes these lesions from those of infectious etiologies. (Reproduced with permission from Warshauer DM, Semelka RC, Ascher SM: Nodular sarcoidosis of the liver and spleen: appearance on MR images. *J Magn Reson Imaging* 4: 553–557, 1994.) T1-weighted SGE (*e*), T2-weighted single-shot echo-train spin-echo (*f*), immediate postgadolinium

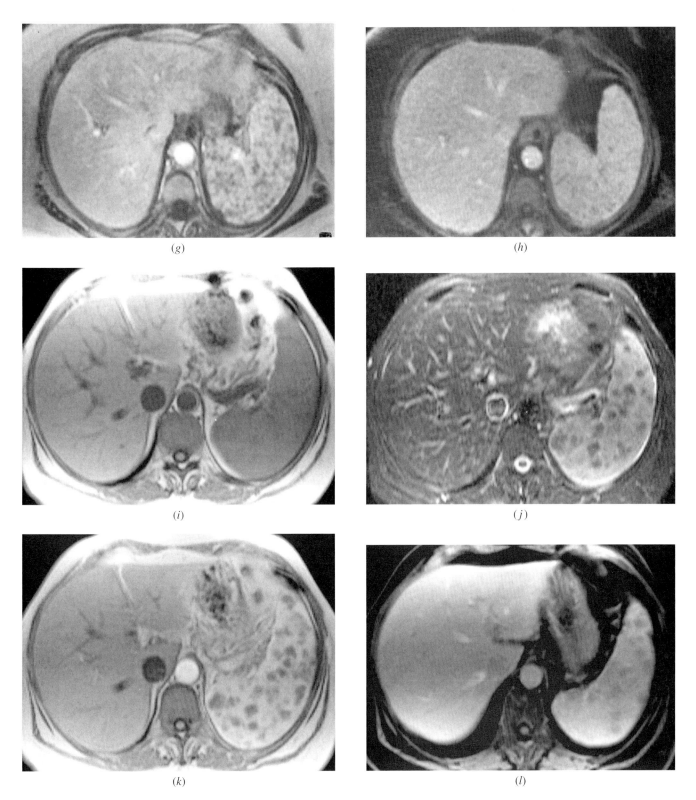

(g)

(h)

(i)

(j)

(k)

(l)

FIG. 5.32 (*Continued*) T1 single-shot magnetization-prepared gradient-echo (*g*), and 90-s postgadolinium T1-weighted fat-suppressed spin-echo (*h*) images in a second patient. The imaging features are comparable to those for the above-described patient. T1-weighted SGE (*i*), T2-weighted fat suppressed single-shot echo-train spin-echo (*j*), immediate postgadolinium T1-weighted SGE (*k*), and 90-s postgadolinium T1-weighted fat-suppressed SGE (*l*) images in a third patient demonstrate similar findings.

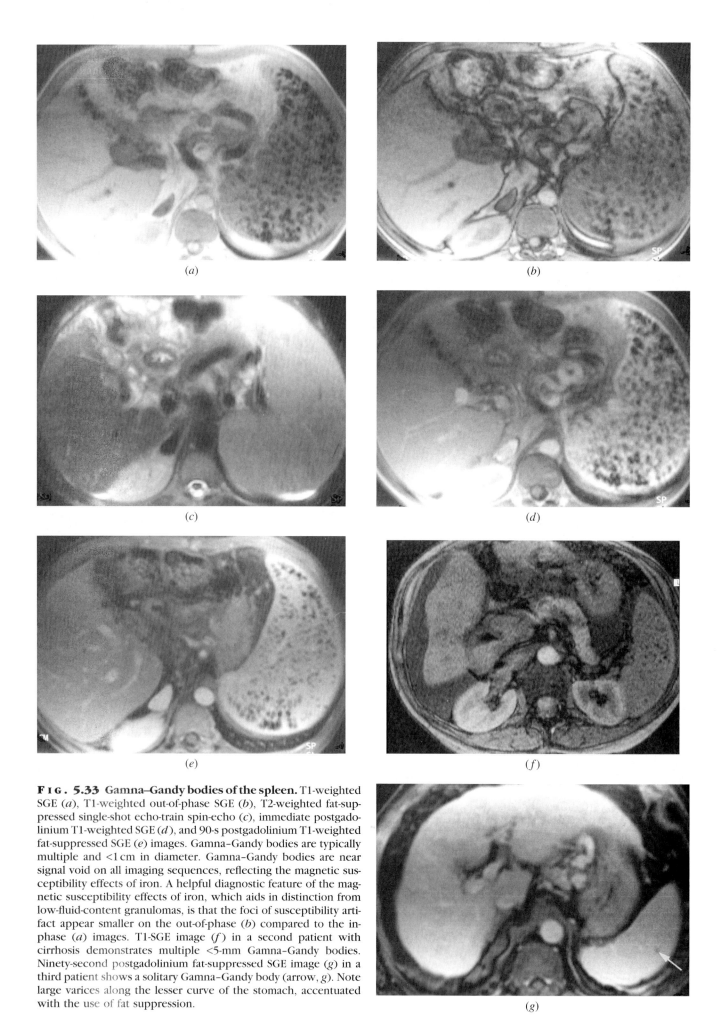

FIG. 5.33 Gamna–Gandy bodies of the spleen. T1-weighted SGE (*a*), T1-weighted out-of-phase SGE (*b*), T2-weighted fat-suppressed single-shot echo-train spin-echo (*c*), immediate postgadolinium T1-weighted SGE (*d*), and 90-s postgadolinium T1-weighted fat-suppressed SGE (*e*) images. Gamna–Gandy bodies are typically multiple and <1 cm in diameter. Gamna–Gandy bodies are near signal void on all imaging sequences, reflecting the magnetic susceptibility effects of iron. A helpful diagnostic feature of the magnetic susceptibility effects of iron, which aids in distinction from low-fluid-content granulomas, is that the foci of susceptibility artifact appear smaller on the out-of-phase (*b*) compared to the in-phase (*a*) images. T1-SGE image (*f*) in a second patient with cirrhosis demonstrates multiple <5-mm Gamna–Gandy bodies. Ninety-second postgadolinium fat-suppressed SGE image (*g*) in a third patient shows a solitary Gamna–Gandy body (arrow, *g*). Note large varices along the lesser curve of the stomach, accentuated with the use of fat suppression.

Trauma

The spleen is the most commonly ruptured abdominal organ in the setting of trauma. Injury to the spleen may take several forms: subcapsular hematoma, contusion, laceration, and devascularization/infarct. Subcapsular or intraparenchymal hematoma secondary to contusion or laceration demonstrates a time course of changes in signal intensity due to the paramagnetic properties of the degradation products of hemoglobin (fig. 5.34). Subacute hemorrhage is particularly conspicuous because of its distinctive high signal intensity on T1- and T2-weighted images (fig. 5.35). Traumatic injury of the spleen, especially devascularization, is well shown on immediate postgadolinium SGE images. Areas of devascularization are nearly signal void compared to the high signal intensity of vascularized tissue.

Subcapsular Fluid Collections

Multiple causes for subcapsular fluid collections exist, the most common being sequelae to trauma. Enhancement of the capsule and surface of the spleen may be observed on postgadolinium images, which confirms the location of these fluid collections (fig. 5.36).

Splenosis

Splenosis is the term used for ectopic tissue resulting from splenic injury. The most common appearance of splenosis on magnetic resonance imaging is solid, well-circumscribed nodules in the abdominal cavity, with signal intensity similar to that of the normal spleen (fig. 5.37).

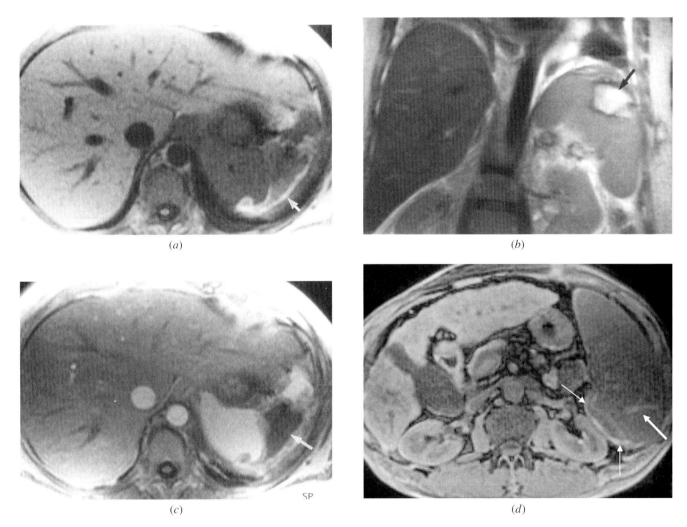

(a) (b) (c) (d)

F I G . 5.34 Splenic laceration with subcapsular hematoma. T1-weighted single-shot magnetization-prepared gradient-echo (*a*), coronal T2-weighted single-shot echo-train spin-echo (*b*), and immediate postgadolinium single-shot magnetization-prepared gradient-echo (*c*) images. Subcapsular blood (arrow, *a*) is appreciated as high-signal fluid on the precontrast T1-weighted image (*a*).The laceration is isointense on T1 (*a*) and high signal on T2 (arrow, *b*) and demonstrates lack of enhancement (arrow, *c*) on the postgadolinium image (*c*). T1-weighted fat-suppressed 3D-GE (*d*), T2-weighted short-tau inversion recovery (STIR) (*e*), and

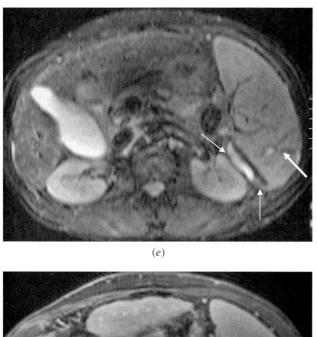

(e)

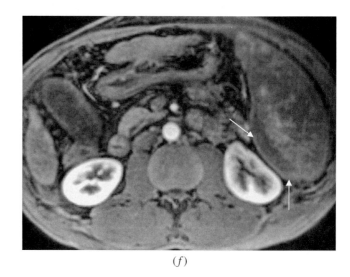

(f)

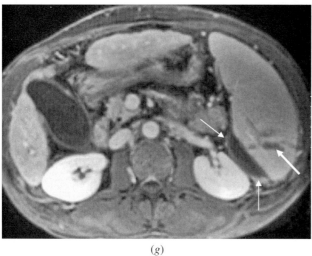

(g)

FIG. 5.34 (*Continued*) T1-weighted fat-suppressed immediate (*f*) and 90-s (*g*) postgadolinium 3D-GE images at 3.0T in another patient with cirrhosis, splenomegaly, splenic laceration, and subcapsular hematoma (thin arrows, *d–g*). The subcapsular hematoma is in a subacute stage, and it has high peripheral signal intensity on T1- and T2-weighted images. The lacerations (thick arrows, *d, e, g*) also show high signal on T1-weighted and mixed signal on T2-weighted images, consistent with subacute blood products.

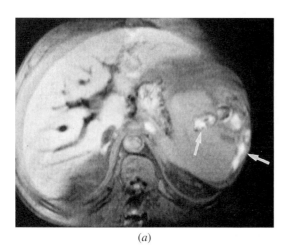

(a)

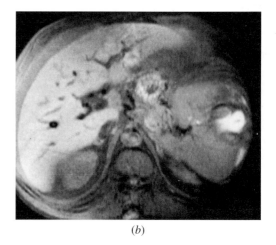

(b)

FIG. 5.35 Splenic laceration. T1-weighted fat-suppressed spin-echo images from adjacent cranial (*a*) and caudal (*b*) transverse sections. Mixed, predominantly high-signal-intensity fluid is present in an intraparenchymal and subcapsular location (arrows, *a*) in the spleen, which represents subacute blood.

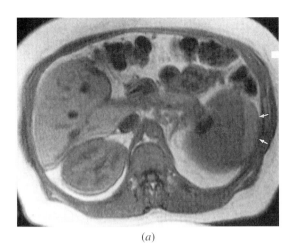

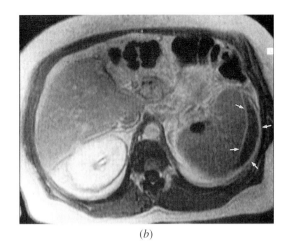

(a)   (b)

FIG. 5.36 Subcapsular fluid collection secondary to pancreatitis. T1-weighted SGE (*a*) and 90-s postgadolinium SGE (*b*) images. A subcapsular fluid collection is present that is slightly high in signal intensity on the T1-weighted image, a finding consistent with the presence of blood or protein (arrows, *a*). Enhancement of the capsule and surface of the spleen on the postgadolinium image (arrows, *b*) confirms the subcapsular location of the fluid collection.

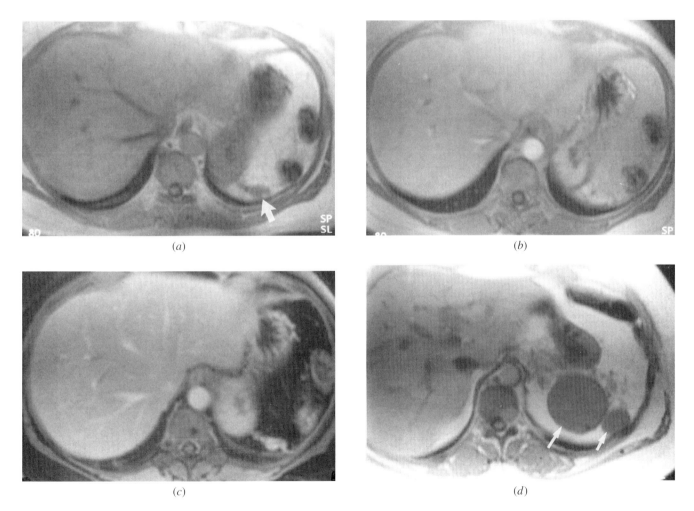

(a)   (b)
(c)   (d)

FIG. 5.37 Splenosis. T1-weighted SGE (*a*), immediate postgadolinium T1-weighted SGE (*b*), and 90-s postgadolinium T1-weighted fat-suppressed SGE (*c*) images. A small, elongated mass is present in the left upper abdominal quadrant in a patient with prior splenectomy. The mass is slightly hypointense to the liver on the T1-weighted image (arrow, *a*), with intense enhancement on the immediate postgadolinium image (*b*) and persistent enhancement on the delayed postgadolinium image (*c*). T1-weighted SGE (*d*), coronal T2-weighted echo-train spin-echo (*e*), breath-hold STIR (*f*), immediate postgadolinium T1-weighted SGE (*g*), and

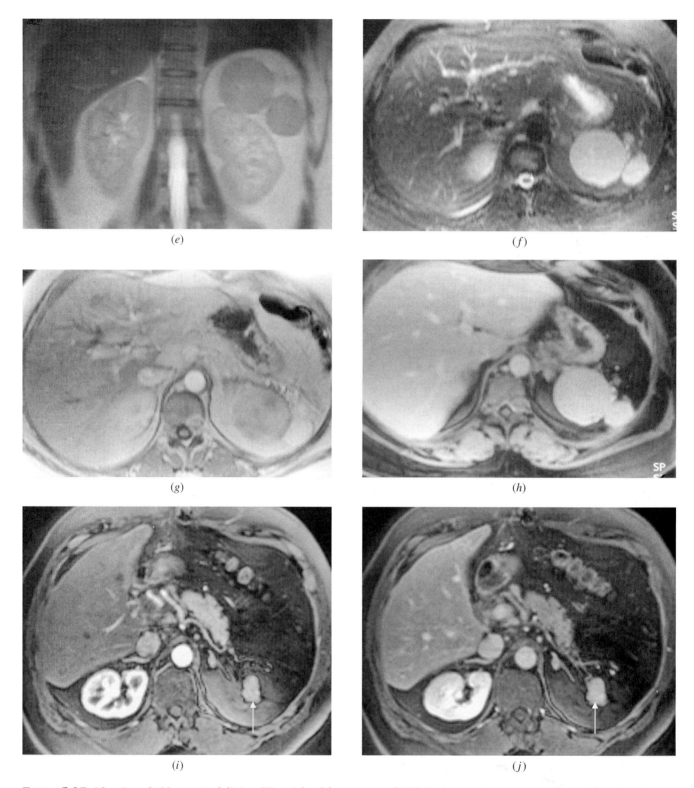

(e) *(f)* *(g)* *(h)* *(i)* *(j)*

FIG. 5.37 (*Continued*) 90-s postgadolinium T1-weighted fat-suppressed SGE (*h*) images in a second patient with prior splenectomy. Two splenules are present in the left upper abdomen (arrows, *d*). The masses have an appearance similar to normal spleen, with mild hypointensity on T1 (*d*), moderate hyperintensity on T2 (*e*), and early heterogeneous enhancement (*g*), which becomes more homogeneous on delayed images (*h*). Note that the enhancement of the larger mass is less than that of the smaller mass, presumably reflecting a smaller feeding arterial supply. T1-weighted fat-suppressed immediate (*i*) and delayed (*j*) postgadolinium 3D-GE images at 3.0T show an enhancing mass (arrows) consistent with splenosis in another patient with prior splenectomy. The mass shows serpiginous enhancement pattern on immediate postgadolinium 3D-GE image (*i*) and homogenous enhancement on postgadolinium delayed 3D-GE image (*j*). T1-weighted fat-suppressed immediate postgadolinium 3D-GE images (*k, l, m*) show

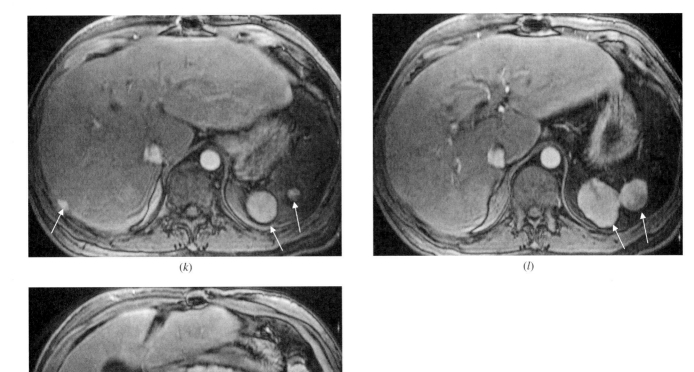

(k)

(l)

(m)

FIG. 5.37 (*Continued*) enhancing masses (arrows), which are located in the liver capsule and the retroperitoneum at both sides, in another patient with prior splenectomy. The bigger lesions demonstrate serpiginous enhancement pattern, and the lesions are consistent with splenosis.

Infarcts

Splenic infarcts are a common occurrence in the setting of obstruction of the splenic artery or one of its branches. The most common cause is cardiac emboli, but local thrombosis, vasculitis, and splenic torsion are also described. Infarcts appear as peripheral wedge-shaped, round, or linear defects that are most clearly defined on 1- to 5-min postgadolinium images as low-signal-intensity wedge-shaped regions (fig. 5.38).

The splenic capsule is commonly observed as a thin peripheral, enhancing linear structure. Massive splenic infarcts may appear as diffuse low signal intensity on T1-weighted images and inhomogeneous high signal on T2-weighted images. Lack of enhancement on early and late postgadolinium images of wedge-shaped regions is the most diagnostic feature (fig. 5.39).

CONCLUSION

MRI is a valuable tool in the evaluation of the spleen and surpasses CT imaging in many clinical settings. One of the major indications for MRI is the investigation of hepatosplenic candidiasis. Other circumstances in which MRI may be of value include the detection of malignant lesions (metastases or lymphoma) and infections, and the characterization of lesions such as hemangiomas or hamartomas. MRI is useful in the further investigation of patients with a CT diagnosis of splenomegaly to determine whether underlying tumor infiltration is present. Superparamagnetic iron oxide particles can be used as a problem-solving approach in selected cases for definitive splenic lesion characterization when not achieved by standard dynamic gadolinium-enhanced MRI.

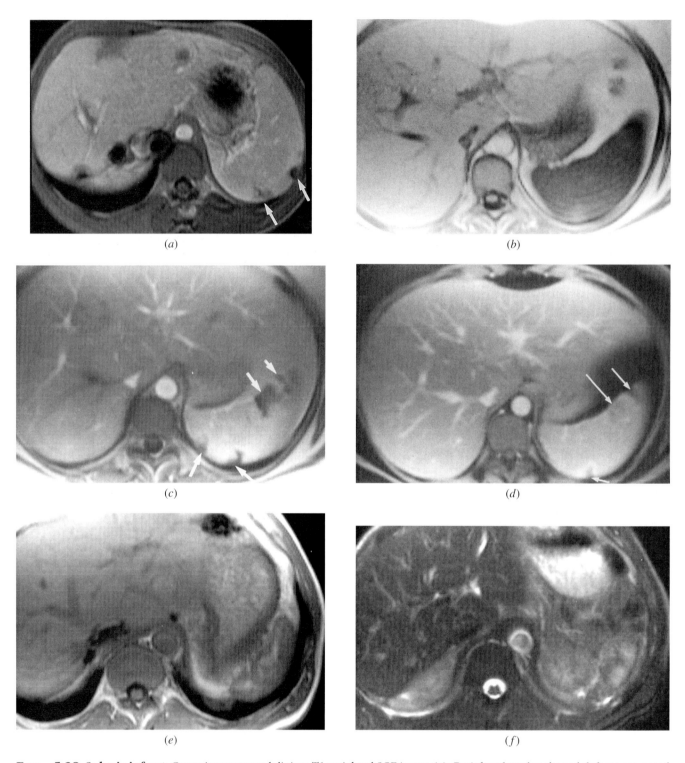

FIG. 5.38 Splenic infarct. One-minute postgadolinium T1-weighted SGE image (*a*). Peripheral wedge-shaped defects are noted in the spleen (arrows, *a*) secondary to infarcts. T1-weighted SGE (*b*), immediate postgadolinium T1-weighted SGE (*c*), and 90-s postgadolinium T1-weighted fat-suppressed SGE (*d*) images in a second patient. An ill-defined posterior subcapsular hyperintensity is present on the T1-weighted image (*b*). Infarct regions are best seen on postgadolinium images (*c*, *d*) and appear as well-defined wedge-shaped defects (arrows, *c*, *d*). Peripheral linear enhancement of the capsule may also be appreciated. Note that some of the regions that have no enhancement on the immediate postgadolinium images show delayed enhancement. These are consistent with areas of ischemia. T1-weighted SGE (*e*), T2-weighted fat-suppressed single-shot echo-train spin-echo (*f*), immediate T1-weighted

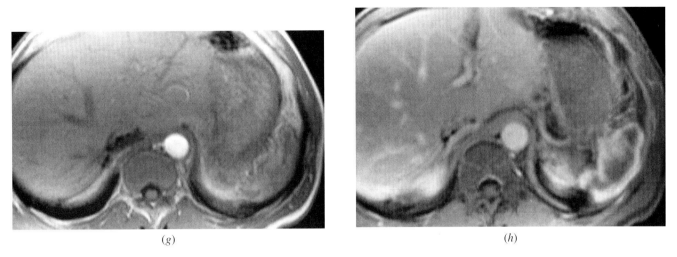

(g)   (h)

F I G . 5.38 (*Continued*) SGE (*g*), and 90-s T1-weighted fat-suppressed SGE (*b*) images in a third patient demonstrate similar findings.

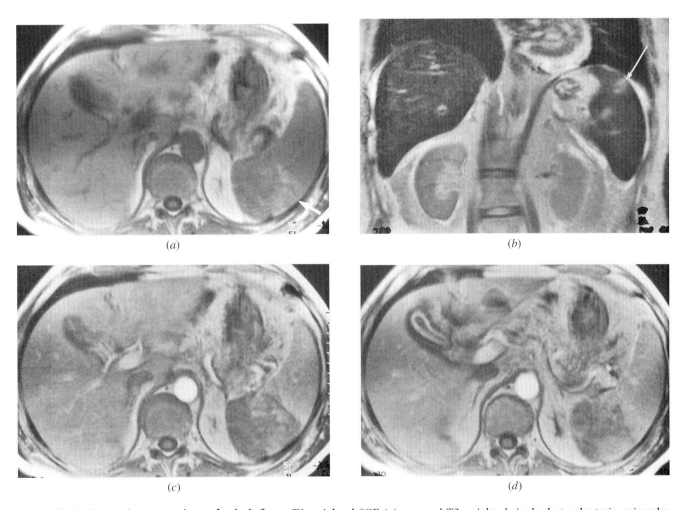

(a)   (b)

(c)   (d)

F I G . 5.39 Extensive posterior splenic infarct. T1-weighted SGE (*a*), coronal T2-weighted single-shot echo-train spin-echo (*b*), immediate (*c*) and 45-s (*d*) postgadolinium T1-weighted SGE, and 90-s postgadolinium T1-weighted fat-suppressed SGE (*e*) images. The splenic infarcts appear heterogeneous and mildly high signal on T1-weighted (arrow, *a*) and heterogeneous and moderately high signal on T2-weighted (arrow, *b*) images. On the immediate (*c*), 45-s (*d*), and 90-s (*e*) postgadolinium images there is

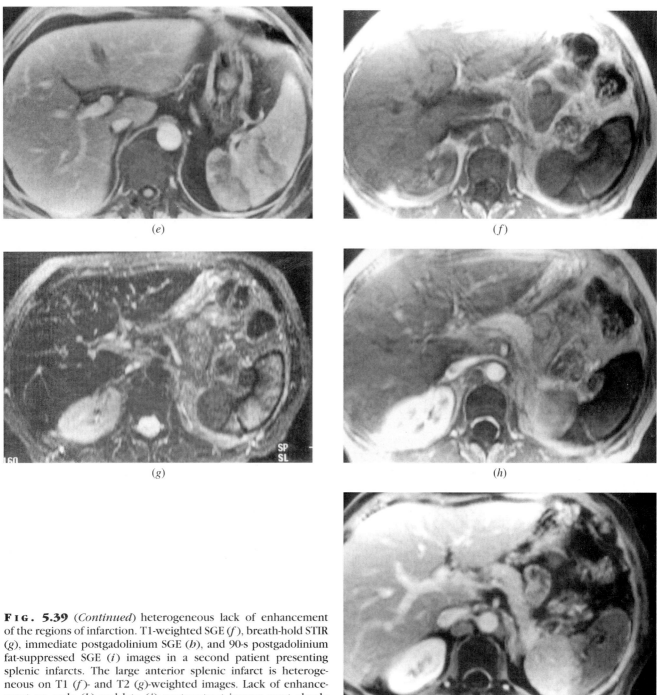

(e)

(f)

(g)

(h)

(i)

F I G . 5.39 (*Continued*) heterogeneous lack of enhancement of the regions of infarction. T1-weighted SGE (*f*), breath-hold STIR (*g*), immediate postgadolinium SGE (*h*), and 90-s postgadolinium fat-suppressed SGE (*i*) images in a second patient presenting splenic infarcts. The large anterior splenic infarct is heterogeneous on T1 (*f*)- and T2 (*g*)-weighted images. Lack of enhancement on early (*h*) and late (*i*) postcontrast images most clearly demonstrates that this region has undergone infarction. Lack of enhancement is more apparent on the later postcontrast image.

REFERENCES

1. Mirowitz SA, Brown JJ, Lee JK et al. Dynamic gadolinium-enhanced MR imaging of the spleen: normal enhancement patterns and evaluation of splenic lesions. *Radiology* 179(3): 681–686, 1991.
2. Mirowitz SA, Lee JK, Gutierrez E et al. Dynamic gadolinium-enhanced rapid acquisition spin-echo MR imaging of the liver. *Radiology* 179(2): 371–376, 1991.
3. Semelka RC, Shoenut JP, Lawrence PH et al. Spleen: dynamic enhancement patterns on gradient-echo MR images enhanced with gadopentetate dimeglumine. *Radiology* 185(2): 479–482, 1992.
4. Hamed MM, Hamm B, Ibrahim ME et al. Dynamic MR imaging of the abdomen with gadopentetate dimeglumine: normal enhancement patterns of the liver, spleen, stomach, and pancreas. *AJR Am J Roentgenol* 158(2): 303–307, 1992.
5. Siegelman ES, Mitchell DG, Rubin R et al. Parenchymal versus reticuloendothelial iron overload in the liver: distinction with MR imaging. *Radiology* 179(2): 361–366, 1991.

6. Siegelman ES, Mitchell DG, Semelka RC. Abdominal iron deposition: metabolism, MR findings, and clinical importance. *Radiology* 199(1): 13–22, 1996.

7. Weissleder R, Hahn PF, Stark DD et al. Superparamagnetic iron oxide: enhanced detection of focal splenic tumors with MR imaging. *Radiology* 169(2): 399–403, 1988.

8. Weissleder R, Elizondo G, Stark DD et al. The diagnosis of splenic lymphoma by MR imaging: value of superparamagnetic iron oxide. *AJR Am J Roentgenol* 152(1): 175–180, 1989.

9. Kreft BP, Tanimoto A, Leffler S et al. Contrast-enhanced MR imaging of diffuse and focal splenic disease with use of magnetic starch microspheres. *J Magn Reson Imaging* 4(3): 373–379, 1994.

10. Paterson A, Frush DP, Donnelly LF et al. A pattern-oriented approach to splenic imaging in infants and children. *Radiographics* 19(6): 1465–1485, 1999.

11. Heredia V, Altun E, Bilaj F et al. Gadolinium- and superparamagnetic-iron-oxide-enhanced MR findings of intrapancreatic accessory spleen in five patients. *Magn Reson Imaging* 26(9): 1273–1278, 2008.

12. Beahrs JR, Stephens DH. Enlarged accessory spleens: CT appearance in postsplenectomy patients. *AJR Am J Roentgenol* 135(3): 483–486, 1980.

13. Storm BL, Abbitt PL, Allen DA et al. Splenosis: superparamagnetic iron oxide-enhanced MR imaging. *AJR Am J Roentgenol* 159(2): 333–335, 1992.

14. Deux JF, Salomon L, Barrier A et al. Acute torsion of wandering spleen: MRI findings. *AJR Am J Roentgenol* 182(6): 1607–1608, 2004.

15. Applegate KE, Goske MJ, Pierce G et al. Situs revisited: imaging of the heterotaxy syndrome. *Radiographics* 19(4): 837–852; discussion 853–834, 1999.

16. Franco V, Aragona F. Association of specific syndromes with renal cystic disease. *Hum Pathol* 20(5): 496, 1989.

17. Fulcher AS, Turner MA. Abdominal manifestations of situs anomalies in adults. *Radiographics* 22(6): 1439–1456, 2002.

18. Hill SC, Damaska BM, Ling A et al. Gaucher disease: abdominal MR imaging findings in 46 patients. *Radiology* 184(2): 561–566, 1992.

19. Adler DD, Glazer GM, Aisen AM. MRI of the spleen: normal appearance and findings in sickle-cell anemia. *AJR Am J Roentgenol* 147(4): 843–845, 1986.

20. Urrutia M, Mergo PJ, Ros LH et al. Cystic masses of the spleen: radiologic-pathologic correlation. *Radiographics* 16(1): 107–129, 1996.

21. Shirkhoda A, Freeman J, Armin AR et al. Imaging features of splenic epidermoid cyst with pathologic correlation. *Abdom Imaging* 20(5): 449–451, 1995.

22. Disler DG, Chew FS. Splenic hemangioma. *AJR Am J Roentgenol* 157(1): 44, 1991.

23. Ramani M, Reinhold C, Semelka RC et al. Splenic hemangiomas and hamartomas: MR imaging characteristics of 28 lesions. *Radiology* 202(1): 166–172, 1997.

24. Levy AD, Abbott RM, Abbondanzo SL. Littoral cell angioma of the spleen: CT features with clinicopathologic comparison. *Radiology* 230(2): 485–490, 2004.

25. Oliver-Goldaracena JM, Blanco A, Miralles M et al. Littoral cell angioma of the spleen: US and MR imaging findings. *Abdom Imaging* 23(6): 636–639, 1998.

26. Bhatt S, Huang J, Dogra V. Littoral cell angioma of the spleen. *AJR Am J Roentgenol* 188(5): 1365–1366, 2007.

27. Ohtomo K, Fukuda H, Mori K et al. CT and MR appearances of splenic hamartoma. *J Comput Assist Tomogr* 16(3): 425–428, 1992.

28. Abbott RM, Levy AD, Aguilera NS et al. From the archives of the AFIP: primary vascular neoplasms of the spleen: radiologic-pathologic correlation. *Radiographics* 24(4): 1137–1163, 2004.

29. Ito K, Mitchell DG, Honjo K et al. MR imaging of acquired abnormalities of the spleen. *AJR Am J Roentgenol* 168(3): 697–702, 1997.

30. Bragg DG, Colby TV, Ward JH. New concepts in the non-Hodgkin lymphomas: radiologic implications. *Radiology* 159(2): 291–304, 1986.

31. Castellino RA. Hodgkin disease: practical concepts for the diagnostic radiologist. *Radiology* 159(2): 305–310, 1986.

32. Hahn PF, Weissleder R, Stark DD et al. MR imaging of focal splenic tumors. *AJR Am J Roentgenol* 150(4): 823–827, 1988.

33. Klein B, Stein M, Kuten A et al. Splenomegaly and solitary spleen metastasis in solid tumors. *Cancer* 60(1): 100–102, 1987.

34. Drinkr CK, Yoffey JM. *Lymphatics, Lymph and Lymphoid Tissue.* Cambridge, MA: Harvard University Press, 1941.

35. Thompson WM, Levy AD, Aguilera NS et al. Angiosarcoma of the spleen: imaging characteristics in 12 patients. *Radiology* 235(1): 106–115, 2005.

36. Vrachliotis TG, Bennett WF, Vaswani KK et al. Primary angiosarcoma of the spleen—CT, MR, and sonographic characteristics: report of two cases. *Abdom Imaging* 25(3): 283–285, 2000.

37. Rabushka LS, Kawashima A, Fishman EK. Imaging of the spleen: CT with supplemental MR examination. *Radiographics* 14(2): 307–332, 1994.

38. Madoff DC, Denys A, Wallace MJ et al. Splenic arterial interventions: anatomy, indications, technical considerations, and potential complications. *Radiographics* 25 Suppl 1: S191–S211, 2005.

39. Fan ZM, Zeng QY, Huo JW et al. Macronodular multi-organs tuberculoma: CT and MR appearances. *J Gastroenterol* 33(2): 285–288, 1998.

40. Semelka RC, Shoenut JP, Greenberg HM et al. Detection of acute and treated lesions of hepatosplenic candidiasis: comparison of dynamic contrast-enhanced CT and MR imaging. *J Magn Reson Imaging* 2(3): 341–345, 1992.

41. Cho JS, Kim EE, Varma DG et al. MR imaging of hepatosplenic candidiasis superimposed on hemochromatosis. *J Comput Assist Tomogr* 14(5): 774–776, 1990.

42. Kelekis NL, Semelka RC, Jeon HJ et al. Dark ring sign: finding in patients with fungal liver lesions and transfusional hemosiderosis undergoing treatment with antifungal antibiotics. *Magn Reson Imaging* 14(6): 615–618, 1996.

43. Warshauer DM, Semelka RC, Ascher SM. Nodular sarcoidosis of the liver and spleen: appearance on MR images. *J Magn Reson Imaging* 4(4): 553–557, 1994.

44. Sagoh T, Itoh K, Togashi K et al. Gamna-Gandy bodies of the spleen: evaluation with MR imaging. *Radiology* 172(3): 685–687, 1989.

45. Minami M, Itai Y, Ohtomo K et al. Siderotic nodules in the spleen: MR imaging of portal hypertension. *Radiology* 172(3): 681–684, 1989.

GASTROINTESTINAL TRACT

DIEGO R. MARTIN, ERSAN ALTUN, JORGE ELIAS, JR.,
MOHAMED ELAZZAZI, MIGUEL RAMALHO, CHANG-HEE LEE,
AND RICHARD C. SEMELKA

ingle-shot echo-train T2-weighted sequences and T1-weighted SGE or 3D GE sequences, combined with intravenous gadolinium enhancement and fat suppression, have resulted in consistent image quality of the gastrointestinal tract. These techniques arrest bowel motion, remove competing high signal of intra-abdominal fat, expand the dynamic range of abdominal tissue signal intensities, decrease susceptibility artifacts, and distinguish between intraluminal bowel contents and bowel wall [1]. The addition of oral or rectal contrast agents may further improve the contrast between lumen and bowel wall to improve the conspicuity of disease. Direct multiplanar imaging has achieved an important role in distinguishing the bowel, which shows a tubular configuration in at least one of two planes, from masses, which do not. Current applications of gastrointestinal MRI include 1) distinguishing type and severity of inflammatory bowel disease (IBD) [1–6]; 2) identifying enteric abscesses and fistulae [7, 8]; 3) preoperative staging of malignant neoplasms, especially rectal carcinoma [5, 9, 10]; and 4) differentiating postoperative and radiation therapy changes from recurrent carcinoma [11–16]. The potential for using MR imaging for screening to detect colonic polyps and early malignancy has also been proposed.

Most recently, reliable 3D-GE T1-weighted sequences (3D VIBE, T1 FAME, 3D THRIVE) have become widely available, permitting volumetric acquisition before and after contrast [17]. Also, newly available True-FISP (FIESTA, BFFE) sequences obtained in the 2D form can be very helpful in delineation of bowel wall pathology, mesentery, and overall bowel anatomy, particularly when combined with a water-based intraluminal distending agent [17]. 3.0 T MR imaging also allows the acquisition of higher-resolution, thinner slices with higher temporal resolution. Therefore, 3.0 T MRI may detect smaller lesions and subtle abnormalities of the GI tract compared to 1.5 T MRI.

THE ESOPHAGUS

Normal Anatomy

The organization of tissues within the esophageal wall follows the general scheme of the entire digestive tract;

namely (from lumen outward) the mucosa with an epithelial lining, submucosa, muscularis externa (propria) with an inner circular and an outer longitudinal muscle layer, and, below the level of the diaphragm, mesothelium-lined serosa instead of adventitia. Except for the portion of the esophagus in the peritoneal cavity, the rest is covered by a layer of loose connective tissue, or adventitia, that blends into surrounding tissue. The lack of a serosal surface explains the rapid spread of esophageal cancer into adjacent mediastinal fat. The esophagus lies posterior to the trachea in the neck. As it enters the thoracic inlet, the esophagus courses toward the left to reside in the posterior mediastinum.

The esophagus then enters the abdomen via the diaphragmatic esophageal hiatus and lies immediately anterior to the aorta. The normal esophageal wall thickness is 3 mm. On cross-sectional images the esophagus tends to be collapsed, although a small amount of air in the lumen is not abnormal.

MRI Technique

Techniques that have been used for MRI of the esophagus include fat saturation, gadolinium enhancement, and cardiac gating (fig. 6.1). The difficulty with T1-weighted ECG-gated fat-suppressed spin-echo imaging is that the sequence is lengthy and the image quality is inconsistent because of the combination of phase artifacts from breathing, patient motion, and cardiac pulsation. The esophagus, therefore, of all bowel segments, suffers the most from image artifacts and uniquely experiences artifacts from cardiac pulsation resulting in severe artifacts on SGE sequences, which form an important component of imaging protocols of other bowel segments. Currently, imaging of the mediastinum and esophagus has been significantly improved with the use of a gadolinium-enhanced 3D GE technique that is acquired during a short breath hold, results in minimized artifacts from motion, and allows excellent depiction of the esophageal wall and mediastinum (fig. 6.2). The 3D GE T1 sequence uses a much shorter TR and TE than utilized with standard fast spin-echo techniques, with the additional benefit of reducing paramagnetic artifacts that arise in the region of gas-soft tissue interfaces, as can be encountered with air within the esophageal lumen or from lung. T1-weighted imaging can be supplemented by T2-weighted imaging using the single-shot echo-train (SSET) technique, acquired during a breath hold. T2-weighted imaging can be used to detect the presence of fluid within cystic masses or collections within the mediastinum around the esophagus. SSET sequences are acquired as a series of individual slices and are very resistant to deterioration from motion. If necessary, this sequence can be combined with respiratory triggering while the patient breathes freely, with

only a minor time penalty and total acquisition times for the chest typically remaining under 45–60 s in duration. Two-dimensional steady-state precession-balanced echo, or true-FISP type, techniques yield images that have both T1- and T2-weighted properties but may be used as a substitute for or in conjunction with SSET images. The images can appear to have good edge sharpness, partly due to these sequences having an out of- phase TE yielding a thin black signal cancellation border at the esophageal border with adjacent mediastinal fat, particularly if combined with cardiac triggering. However, the role for routine evaluation of the esophagus is not established.

Congenital Lesions

Duplication Cysts

Gastrointestinal duplication cysts may occur throughout the alimentary tube. The cysts occur in or adjacent to the wall of a portion of the gastrointestinal tract, and, although they are lined by epithelium, it may not be of the same histologic type as that of the involved segment. Duplication cysts usually are discovered in childhood or infancy secondary to mass effect, hemorrhage, and/or infection resulting from intestinal stasis combined with bowel communication [18]. Patients may also present later in life with peptic ulcers or pancreatitis if the cysts contain gastric or pancreatic epithelium, respectively. In the esophagus, they tend to be small, ovoid, fluid-filled structures in the lower one-third of the esophagus located posteriorly in a periesophageal location or within the esophageal wall. Cysts have variable signal intensity on T1-weighted images, depending on the concentration of mucin or protein within the cyst. Duplication cysts are generally high in signal intensity on T2-weighted images (fig. 6.2) [19]. The cyst wall typically is thin and may enhance after intravenous gadolinium administration, whereas the fluid-filled lumen does not enhance and may appear near signal void on fat-suppressed gadolinium-enhanced delayed-phase images. Relatively intense cyst wall enhancement may reflect the presence of gastric mucosa or inflammatory changes.

Mass Lesions

Benign Masses

Leiomyomas. Leiomyomas are the most common benign tumors of the esophagus. These tumors are composed of smooth muscle and arise from the muscularis externa. They most frequently occur in the distal esophagus and may be single or multiple [20, 21]. Esophageal leiomyomas appear as small, oval masses that may be pedunculated on MRI images. They are often close to isointensity with surrounding bowel wall on T1- and

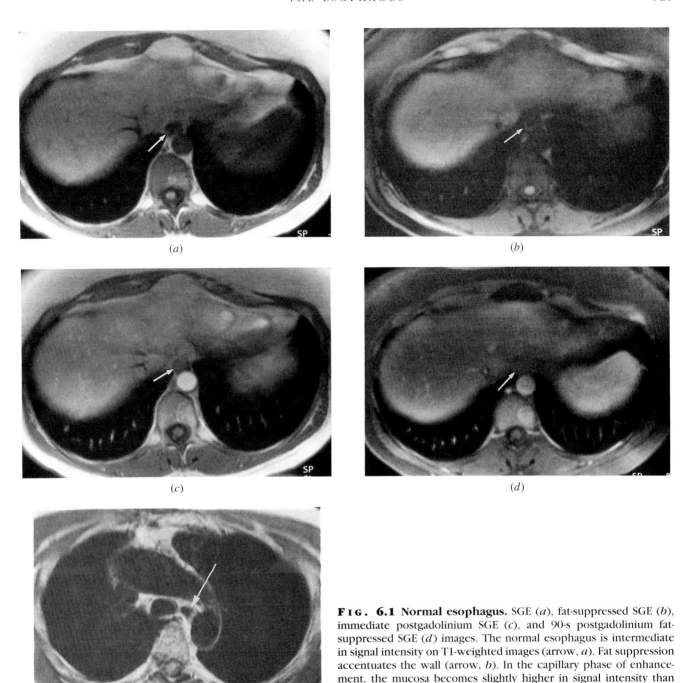

(a)

(b)

(c)

(d)

(e)

FIG. 6.1 Normal esophagus. SGE (*a*), fat-suppressed SGE (*b*), immediate postgadolinium SGE (*c*), and 90-s postgadolinium fat-suppressed SGE (*d*) images. The normal esophagus is intermediate in signal intensity on T1-weighted images (arrow, *a*). Fat suppression accentuates the wall (arrow, *b*). In the capillary phase of enhancement, the mucosa becomes slightly higher in signal intensity than the remainder of the esophageal wall (arrow, *c*). During the interstitial phase, there is equilibration (arrow, *d*). Cardiac-gated T1-weighted spin-echo image (*e*) in a second patient shows a small amount of air in the lumen of a normal esophagus (arrow, *e*).

T2-weighted images; however, with gadolinium, leiomyomas will enhance in a uniform fashion and to a greater degree than adjacent bowel wall in the interstitial phase of enhancement (fig. 6.3). Leiomyomas belong to the gastrointestinal stromal tumor (GIST) classification.

Varices. Varices, or tortuous, dilated submucosal veins, develop in the setting of portal hypertension or splenic vein thrombosis. They occur along the lower esophagus, the stomach, and other locations with portosystemic communications. Varices are best demonstrated on fat-suppressed 3D T1-weighted gadolinium-enhanced delayed-phase imaging (fig. 6.4) but may be demonstrated on SGE postgadolinium images or as signal-void tubular structures on spin-echo images. True-FISP imaging may display varices as tubular

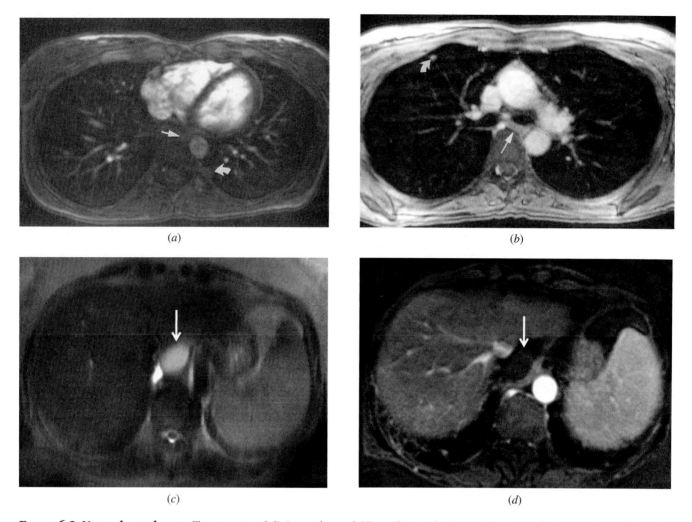

(a)   (b)

(c)   (d)

FIG. 6.2 Normal esophagus. Transverse gadolinium-enhanced 3D gradient-echo (*a* and *b*) images in two patients. On gadolinium-enhanced 3D images, the esophagus is well shown (short arrows, *a, b*) and is free of cardiac motion artifact. Note also a subtle pleura-based density along the posterior left hemithorax (curved arrow, *a*) and pulmonary metastasis (curved arrow, *b*). **Duplication cyst.** T2-weighted single-shot echo-train spin-echo (*c*) and T1-weighted postgadolinium hepatic venous phase fat-suppressed 3D-GE (*d*) images at 3.0 T demonstrate a paraesophageal cyst (arrows, *c, d*), which shows high signal on T2-weighted image (*c*) and no appreciable enhancement on postgadolinium image (*d*).

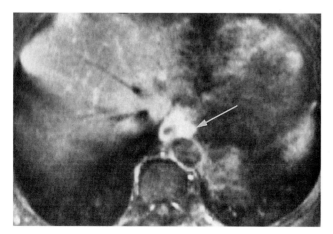

FIG. 6.3 Esophageal leiomyoma. Gadolinium-enhanced T1-weighted fat-suppressed spin-echo image shows a 2-cm leiomyoma (arrow) arising from the lateral aspect of the distal esophagus. Leiomyomas are the most common benign tumors of the esophagus. (Reprinted with permission from Shoenut JP, Semelka RC, Silverman R, Yaffe CS, Mickflikier AB: The gastrointestinal tract. In Semelka RC, Shoenut JP (eds.), *MRI of the Abdomen with CT Correlation.* New York: Raven Press, 1993, pp. 119–143.)

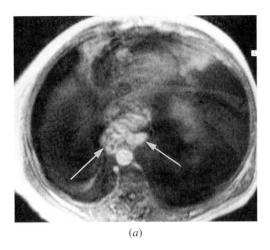
(a)

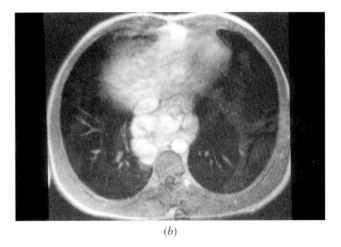
(b)

F I G . 6.4 Esophageal varices. Transverse 45-s postgadolinium SGE image (*a*) in a patient with portal hypertension. Enhancing serpiginous tubular structures (arrows) in the lower esophagus represent varices. Transverse gadolinium-enhanced T1-weighted SGE image (*b*) in a second patient with congenital hepatic fibrosis demonstrates massive esophageal varices.

structures with high internal signal from blood and can be used in situations where gadolinium enhancement may not be possible, such as inadequate venous access or end-stage renal disease.

Malignant Masses

Before 1975, squamous cell carcinoma accounted for 95% of all cases of esophagus cancer. Since that time there has been a marked increase in the incidence of adenocarcinomas among esophagus cancers. At the present time, the overall relative incidence between squamous cell carcinoma and adenocarcinoma is about equal in the United States [22].

The etiology of squamous cell carcinoma is unknown, but there is an association with alcohol consumption and tobacco use [23]. It occurs more commonly in males (3 to 1) and African Americans [24]. Primary adenocarcinoma of the esophagus may arise de novo in Barrett esophagus, or it may arise in the stomach and cross the gastroesophageal junction to involve the distal esophagus and simulate achalasia [25]. It is more common in Caucasian males. Tumors that commonly metastasize to the esophagus include breast and lung carcinoma and melanoma. Gadolinium-enhanced fat-suppressed SGE and 3D-GE techniques delineate primary tumors of the distal esophagus, whereas SGE with cardiac gating or 3D-GE with or without cardiac gating is useful to image midesophageal cancers posterior to the heart (fig. 6.5) [26]. Squamous cell cancers (see fig. 6.5) and adenocarcinomas (fig. 6.6) appear similar on MR images. Predisposing factors such as Barrett esophagus or tumor location, with more proximal tumors mostly represented by squamous cell origin, may aid in making this distinction. The success of MRI in staging esophageal cancer has been inconsistent,

reflecting the variable image quality of breathing-averaged, cardiac-gated sequences [27, 28]. At present, there is no reported series describing the use of gadolinium-enhanced 3D GE in the evaluation of esophageal cancers. This may prove to be the most consistent MR technique to investigate these tumors. The combined use of fat suppression and intravenous gadolinium may facilitate identification of mediastinal involvement. The presence of multiple (more than 5) paraesophageal normal-sized lymph nodes is worrisome for tumor involvement; however, accurate determination awaits the use of contrast agents that can define the presence of tumor in normal-sized lymph nodes. A comprehensive exam for staging patients with esophageal carcinoma should include a metastatic survey of the liver.

Metastases to the esophagus may appear indistinguishable from a primary esophageal tumor, and clinical history helps to establish the diagnosis (fig. 6.7).

Inflammatory and Infectious Disorders

Reflux Esophagitis

Gastroesophageal reflux is defined as the retrograde flow of gastric and sometimes duodenal contents into the esophagus. In general, reflux esophagitis refers to esophageal inflammation resulting from gastroesophageal reflux. Reflux esophagitis may result from several disease entities and/or their treatments: hiatal hernia, achalasia, and scleroderma. Gastroesophageal reflux is common in the setting of hiatal hernia. (For a more complete discussion of hiatal hernia see Chapter 7, *Peritoneal Cavity.*) Achalasia is a primary esophageal disorder that results in failure of relaxation of the lower esophageal sphincter (LES) coupled with nonperistaltic

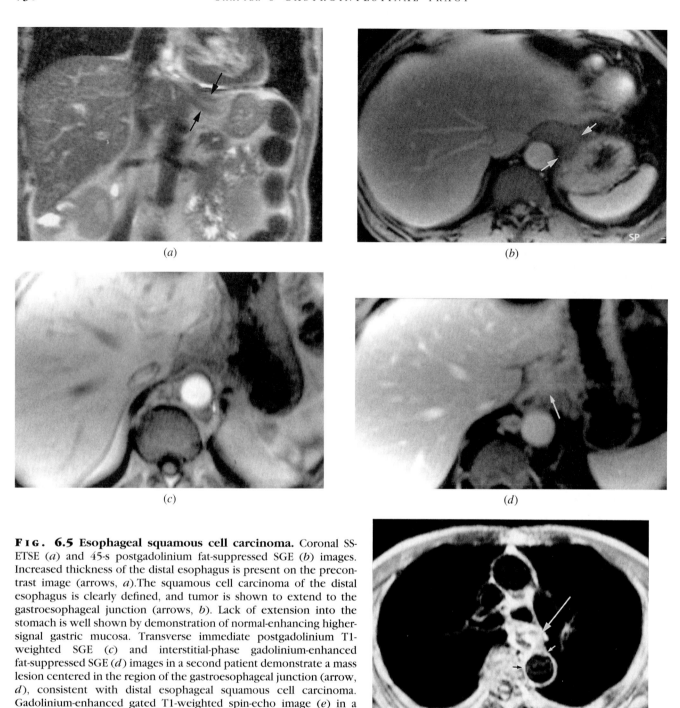

F I G . 6.5 Esophageal squamous cell carcinoma. Coronal SS-ETSE (*a*) and 45-s postgadolinium fat-suppressed SGE (*b*) images. Increased thickness of the distal esophagus is present on the precontrast image (arrows, *a*).The squamous cell carcinoma of the distal esophagus is clearly defined, and tumor is shown to extend to the gastroesophageal junction (arrows, *b*). Lack of extension into the stomach is well shown by demonstration of normal-enhancing higher-signal gastric mucosa. Transverse immediate postgadolinium T1-weighted SGE (*c*) and interstitial-phase gadolinium-enhanced fat-suppressed SGE (*d*) images in a second patient demonstrate a mass lesion centered in the region of the gastroesophageal junction (arrow, *d*), consistent with distal esophageal squamous cell carcinoma. Gadolinium-enhanced gated T1-weighted spin-echo image (*e*) in a third patient with squamous cell carcinoma of the midesophagus. A 2-cm cancer (arrow, *e*) is present that shows heterogeneous extension into the aortic wall (small arrows, *e*).

esophageal contractions. Balloon dilation of the LES is the mainstay of treatment and may lead to reflux esophagitis. Scleroderma involvement of the esophagus results in a patulous gastroesophageal junction with substantial reflux of gastric contents. In all of these conditions, MRI demonstrates a thickened esophageal wall, and, after the administration of gadolinium, the inflamed and

possibly fibrosed wall shows marked enhancement on delayed images (fig. 6.8).

Radiation Esophagitis

Patients undergoing radiation therapy to the thorax are at risk of developing radiation damage to the esophagus. In the early period, 4–6 weeks after treatment,

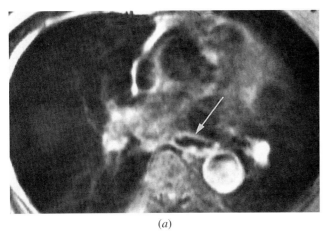

(a)

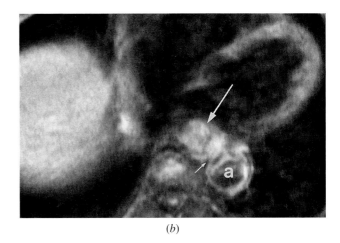

(b)

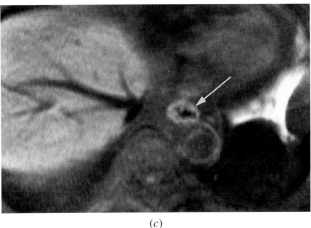

(c)

F I G . 6.6 Esophageal adenocarcinoma. Gadolinium-enhanced T1-weighted fat-suppressed (*a, b*) and T1-weighted fat-suppressed (*c*) spin-echo images in a patient with esophageal adenocarcinoma. Above the tumor at the level of the midthorax, the esophagus has a normal-appearing thin wall (arrow, *a*). More inferiorly at the level of the mitral valve, a 2.5-cm tumor (long arrow, *b*) is identified in the esophagus. Note that the interface of the tumor with the descending aorta (a, *b*) is less than 90° (short arrow, *b*). Below the tumor the esophagus once again has a normal thin wall (arrow, *c*). (Reprinted with permission from Shoenut JP, Semelka RC, Silverman R, Yaffe CS, Mickflikier AB: The gastrointestinal tract. In Semelka RC, Shoenut JP (eds.), *MRI of the Abdomen with CT Correlation.* New York: Raven Press, 1993.)

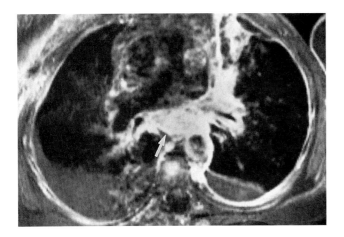

F I G . 6.7 Esophageal metastases. Gadolinium-enhanced T1-weighted fat-suppressed image in a woman with metastatic breast carcinoma. Enhancing tumor (arrow) encases the esophagus, extends along the left hilum and left mediastinum, and invades the chest wall. (Reprinted with permission from Shoenut JP, Semelka RC, Silverman R, Yaffe CS, Mickflikier AB: The gastrointestinal tract. In Semelka RC, Shoenut JP (eds.), *MRI of the Abdomen with CT Correlation.* New York: Raven Press, 1993, pp. 119–143.)

mucosal edema may be seen. Approximately 6–8 months after treatment, strictures may begin to develop.

Corrosive Esophagitis

Ingestion of caustic material such as strong alkaline or acidic agents or very hot liquids may cause esophagitis. Damage to tissue is most severe after ingestion of strongly alkaline agents. These substances cause a liquefactive necrosis that penetrates the entire esophageal wall rapidly. Acute changes include edema and ulceration. Stricture formation occurs later, and there is a strong association between corrosive stricture and the development of carcinoma.

Infectious Disease

Esophageal infection by *Candida albicans,* cytomegalovirus (CMV), and herpes simplex virus (HSV) is commonly observed in association with immunocompromised conditions. *Candida albicans* may be found in the esophagus of normal patients but is frequently pathological in patients who have bone marrow transplantation, chemotherapy, acquired immunodeficiency

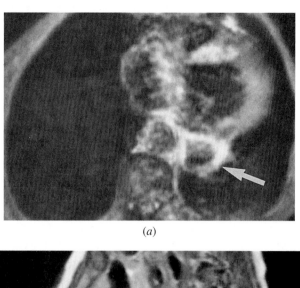

(a)

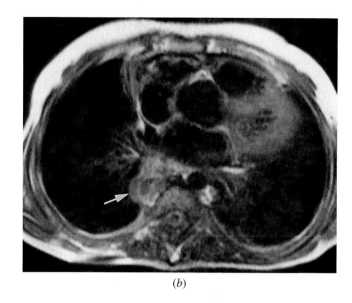

(b)

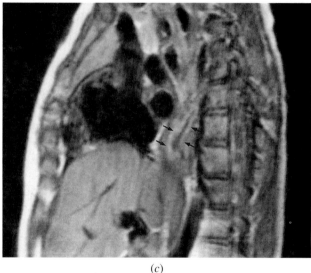

(c)

FIG. 6.8 Reflux esophagitis. Gadolinium-enhanced T1-weighted fat-suppressed spin-echo (a), gadolinium-enhanced gated transverse (b), and sagittal (c) T1-weighted spin-echo images in two patients [(a) and (b, c)] with reflux esophagitis. In a patient with achalasia (a), balloon dilation for achalasia predisposes to reflux esophagitis. The esophagus appears dilated, and the wall is thickened with increased mural enhancement. The esophagus in a second patient with reflux esophagitis due to hiatal hernia shows increased thickness of the esophageal wall (arrow, b) and increased signal intensity of the mucosa. The superior extent of inflamed mucosa (small arrows) is well shown on the sagittal image (c).

syndrome (AIDS), administration of exogenous steroids, or blood dyscrasias. Infection is diffuse, with white-colored plaques coating the mucosa. The mucosa becomes friable, and ulceration results. MRI demonstrates a high-signal-intensity thickened esophageal wall on T2-weighted images. Hyperemia and capillary leakage account for the marked enhancement after intravenous gadolinium injection (fig. 6.9).

Achalasia

The underlying defect in achalasia results from altered nervous control of esophageal coordinated contraction and relaxation with development of an inability to relax the circular muscle at the gastroesophageal junction that interferes with the passage of esophageal contents into the stomach. There is associated impaired primary peri-

staltic contraction of the esophagus, and the esophagus typically becomes markedly dilated, with development of beaklike narrowing at the closed gastroesophageal junction (fig. 6.10). Treatment involves balloon dilation, but this often results in only transient improvement, or distal esophagomyotomy. MR imaging provides an alternative to standard fluoroscopic techniques and provides the advantage of allowing visualization of the soft tissues in and adjacent to the wall of the distal esophagus and cardia of the stomach. Primary achalasia may develop from causes including infection, such as Chagas disease, but may also occur secondary to neoplasm. When considering the diagnosis of achalasia, cross-sectional imaging should be performed in every case to exclude the possibility of a secondary etiology.

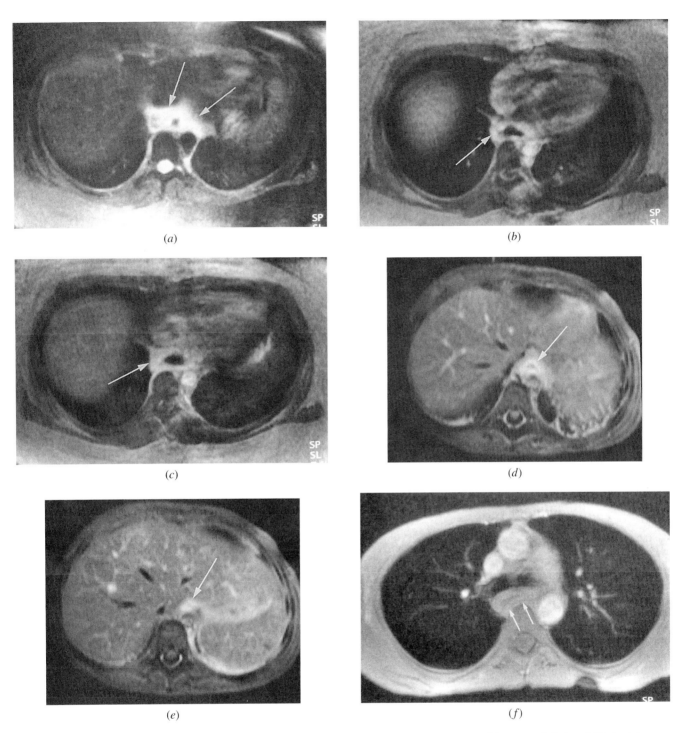

(a) *(b)*

(c) *(d)*

(e) *(f)*

FIG. 6.9 Esophagitis. T2-weighted fat-suppressed echo-train spin-echo (*a*) and contiguous 45-s postgadolinium SGE (*b, c*) images in a patient with AIDS and esophageal candidiasis. The high signal intensity on the T2-weighted images reflects both the fungal plaques that coat the esophagus and the underlying inflamed wall (arrows, *a*). After contrast, the thickened esophageal wall enhances (arrows, *b, c*). Gadolinium-enhanced T1-weighted fat-suppressed spin-echo images (*d, e*) in a second immunocompromised patient with acute myelogenous leukemia on chemotherapy. Capillary leakage associated with inflammation leads to marked mucosal enhancement (arrows, *d, e*) in this patient with *Candida albicans* esophageal invasion. Transverse gadolinium-enhanced SGE (*f*) image in a third patient who has AIDS and dysphagia shows diffuse esophageal wall thickening (arrows, *f*) consistent with inflammatory changes.

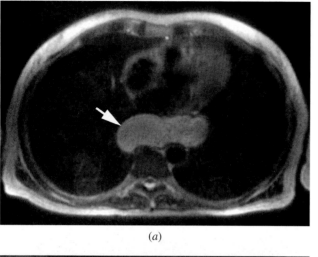

(a)

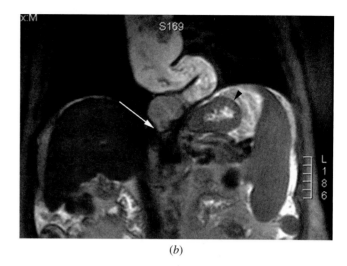

(b)

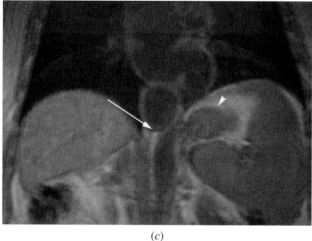

(c)

FIG. 6.10 Achalasia. Axial (*a*) and coronal (*b*) T2-weighted single-shot spin-echo and coronal T1-weighted gradient-echo (*c*) images show marked dilatation of the fluid-filled esophagus (arrow, *a*) with abrupt tapered narrowing at the gastroesophageal junction (arrows, *b, c*). The fundal portion of the stomach is normal (arrowheads, *b, c*), with no evidence of mass demonstrated.

THE STOMACH

Normal Anatomy

The stomach serves as a reservoir for ingested food and continues the process of mechanical and chemical breakdown. Although the stomach is typically J-shaped and resides in the posterior aspect of the left upper quadrant, its position varies with degree of distension and body habitus. Gross inspection shows four anatomic regions: cardia, fundus, body, and antrum. The antrum ends at the pylorus, from the Greek *pyl ros*, or gatekeeper, a narrow channel that connects the stomach to the duodenum. The stomach's curved morphology also gives rise to a greater (caudal) and a lesser (cephalic) curvature in addition to anterior and posterior walls. Four distinct layers comprise the stomach wall: mucosa, submucosa, muscularis, and serosa. Subdivisions exist within each layer. The mucosa is composed of distinct populations of endocrine and exocrine cells. The muscularis externa has three differ-

ent muscle groups: inner oblique, middle circular, and outer longitudinal.

MRI Technique

Imaging the stomach achieves best results with distension and hypotonia. MRI examinations of the stomach may benefit from administration of water in an approximate volume of 1 liter and intravenous glucagon, with 0.5 mg administered intravenously immediately before the start of the examination and 0.5 mg before the administration of gadolinium [29].

A recommended imaging protocol includes: 1) T1-weighted fat-suppressed SGE or 3D-GE imaging before and after intravenous gadolinium, 2) unenhanced T1-weighted SGE imaging, and 3) T2-weighted non-fat-suppressed and fat-suppressed single-shot echo-train spin-echo [e.g., half-Fourier single-shot turbo spin-echo (HASTE)] imaging (fig. 6.11). Gastric mucosa enhances more intensely than other bowel mucosa after intravenous gadolinium [30]. This observation may be helpful

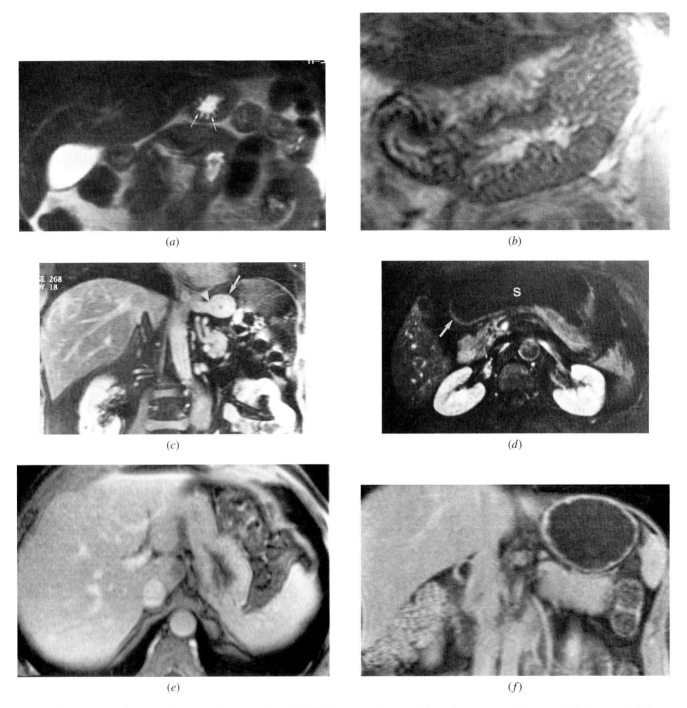

FIG. 6.11 Normal stomach. Coronal T2-weighted SS-ETSE (*a*, *b*) and coronal (*c*) and transverse (*d*) interstitial-phase gadolinium-enhanced fat-suppressed SGE images in four patients with a normal stomach. T2-weighted SS-ETSE is well-suited for imaging the rugal folds (arrows, *a*, *b*). After intravenous contrast the stomach wall shows marked enhancement (arrows, *c*, *d*). The normal gastroesophageal junction (arrowhead, *c*) is frequently well-defined by imaging in transverse and coronal planes. Optimal stomach (s, *d*) distension was obtained after ingestion of a negative oral contrast agent. Transverse gadolinium-enhanced fat-suppressed SGE (*e*) and coronal gadolinium-enhanced fat-suppressed SGE (*f*) images in a another patient before and after water ingestion. Optimal gastric distension can also be achieved with water.

for the detection of a gastric mucosa-lined duplication cyst or Meckel diverticulum.

Congenital Lesions

Congenital lesions, except for hypertrophic pyloric stenosis, are rare in the stomach.

Gastric Duplication Cysts

Gastric duplication cysts account for less than 4% of duplications of the gastrointestinal tract. They occur along the greater curvature and are more common in females. Occasionally, gastric duplication cysts calcify, and in 15% the cysts communicate with the gastric lumen. Although gastric duplication cysts are uncommon, they are important to recognize because 35% of these patients will have other congenital anomalies [31].

Congenital Heterotopias

Congenital heterotopias result from cellular entrapment during the morphogenic movements throughout embryogenesis. Pancreatic rests occur throughout the alimentary tract but are most common along the greater curvature or posterior antral wall of the stomach. Heterotopic pancreas usually appears as a solitary, submucosal globoid mass with a central nipplelike structure representing ductal openings into the gastric lumen [32].

Congenital Diverticula

Congenital diverticula may also be demonstrated in the stomach (fig. 6.12) [29]. Gastric diverticula are rare, and more than 75% of them occur in a juxtacardiac position high on the posterior wall of the stomach, approximately 2 cm below the gastroesophageal junction and 3 cm from the lesser curvature of the stomach [33]. Congenital diverticula are characterized as solitary, well-defined, oval or pear-shaped pouches that communicate with the gastric lumen via a narrow or broad-based opening [34]. The clinical presentation depends on location, size, type of mucosa of the diverticulum, and presence or absence of communication with the stomach.

Mass Lesions

Benign Masses

Polyps. Gastric polyps may be hyperplastic, adenomatous, or hamartomatous. They may be isolated findings or associated with a polyposis syndrome. Eighty to ninety percent of gastric polyps are hyperplastic and benign, whereas approximately 10% are adenomatous. Hyperplastic polyps are nonneoplastic lesions that result from an exaggerated regenerative response to injury, namely ulcers, gastroenterostomy stomas, or a background of chronic gastritis. In contrast to hyperplastic polyps, adenomatous polyps are true neoplasms, morphologically similar to those seen in the colon. Microscopic features show close-packed glandular structures lined by neoplastic cells with cytologic atypia. Approximately one-third of adenomatous polyps contain a focus of adenocarcinoma [35]. Malignant potential is related to size, with up to 46% of adenomas larger than 2 cm containing carcinoma [36]. Both hyperplastic and adenomatous polyps are found in patients with chronic atrophic gastritis and Gardner and familial polyposis syndromes, conditions associated with an increased incidence of malignancy. (For a more complete discussion on polyposis syndromes, see the section on the large intestine in this chapter.) Although most polyps are asymptomatic, anemia related to chronic blood loss, iron deficiency, or malabsorption of vitamin B12 may be present. Hamartomatous gastric polyps are lesions produced by excessive, disorganized overgrowth of mature normal cells and tissues indigenous to the stomach. Hamartomatous polyps may be an isolated finding or can occur in patients with Peutz–Jeghers syndrome. Although both isolated hamartomatous polyps and those associated with Peutz–Jeghers syndrome are benign lesions, patients with Peutz–Jeghers syndrome have an increased risk of developing carcinomas of the gastrointestinal tract, pancreas, breast, lung, ovary, and uterus.

Benign polyps are generally isointense with the gastric wall on unenhanced MR images. Adequate distension of the stomach is mandatory to distinguish a polyp from a prominent rugal fold. Benign polyp enhancement is usually isointense to slightly hyperintense compared to normal gastric mucosa on early postgadolinium images and mildly hyperintense on 2-min postgadolinium images, reflecting retention of contrast in the interstitial space (fig. 6.13). In polyps complicated by invasive adenocarcinoma, more heterogeneous gadolinium enhancement and disruption of the underlying gastric wall may be observed.

Leiomyomas. Leiomyomas are the most common benign nonepithelial tumors of the stomach. They arise from the smooth muscle of the gastric wall. They may grow inward toward the lumen and mimic a polyp or extend to the serosa and present as an exophytic mass. When large, the overlying gastric mucosa may ulcerate, leading to gastrointestinal bleeding.

Neurogenic Tumors and Lipomas. Other mesenchymal gastric wall elements may give rise to benign neoplasms: neurogenic tumors (fig. 6.13), lipomas (fig. 6.13), fibromas, and hemangiomas. Except for lipomas, these mesenchymal tumors are indistinguishable from each other on MRI. Similar to fatty lesions elsewhere in

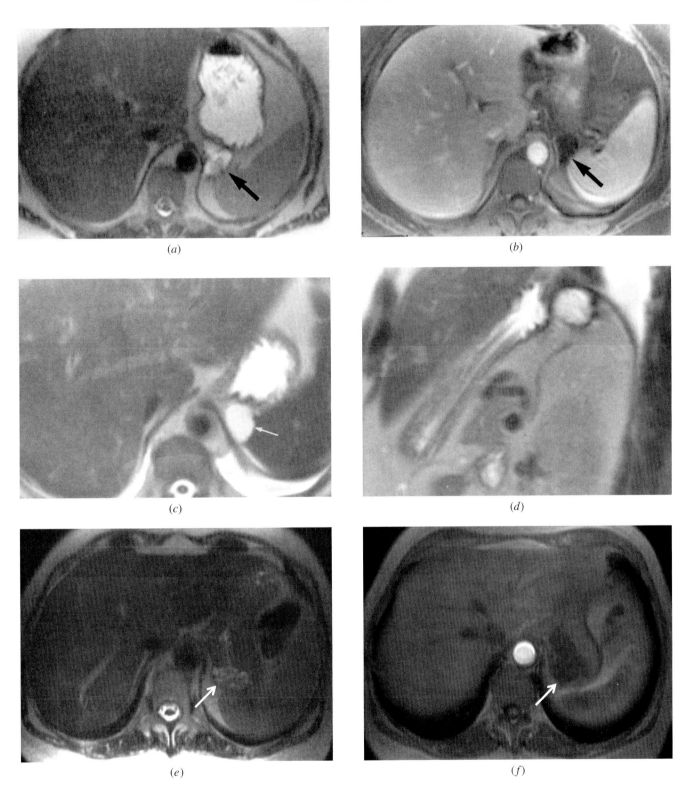

F I G . 6.12 Gastric diverticulum. Transverse T2-weighted SS-ETSE (*a*) and 90-s postgadolinium fat-suppressed SGE (*b*) images. A small cystic thin-walled mass (arrow, *a*) is shown, which is high signal intensity and intimately related to the posterior aspect of the cardiac portion of the stomach. On the 90-s postgadolinium image (*b*), the diverticulum appears signal void with a thin enhancing wall (arrow, *b*). (Reprinted with permission from Marcos HB, Semelka RC: Stomach diseases: MR evaluation using combined T2-weighted single-shot echo train spin-echo and gadolinium-enhanced spoiled gradient-echo sequences. *J Magn Reson Imaging* 10: 950–960, 1999.) Transverse (*c*) and coronal (*d*) T2-weighted SS-ETSE in a second patient. A small posterior gastric diverticulum (arrow, *c*) is seen in the fundus of the stomach. T2-weighted single-shot echo-train spin-echo (*e*), T1-weighted postgadolinium early arterial-phase SGE (*f*) and T1-weighted postgadolinium fat-suppressed interstitial- phase 3D-GE (*g*) images demonstrate a broad-based gastric diverticulum (arrows, *e*–*g*) in the posterior aspect of the cardia portion of the stomach in another patient. The diverticulum shows high signal on T2-weighted image (*f*), and thin enhancing wall is appreciated on the interstitial phase (*g*).

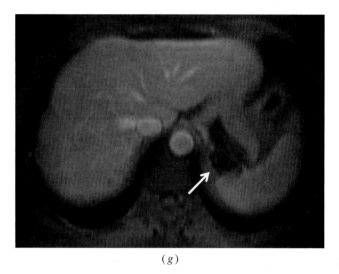

(g)   FIG. 6.12 (Continued)

the body, lipomas will be high in signal intensity on T1-weighted images and decreased in signal intensity on fat-suppressed images.

Varices. Portal hypertension and splenic vein thrombosis lead to gastric varices. Varices restricted to the short gastric veins along the greater curvature of the stomach should raise the suspicion of splenic vein thrombosis (fig. 6.14).

Bezoar. The word bezoar derives from the Arabic *bazahr* or *badzeahr*, meaning antidote. Bezoars were valued for their medicinal qualities and were thought to be imbued with magical powers and to be effective antidotes for poisoning [37].

The term bezoar is used to refer to an intragastric mass composed of accumulated ingested material. It may be composed of hair (trichobezoar), fruit or vegetable products (phytobezoar), or concretions such as resins, asphalt, or other material. Factors that predispose to bezoar development include psychiatric illness, lack of teeth, previous vagotomy or gastric surgery, and diseases such as diabetes and muscular dystrophies. Altered gastric motility or anatomy that causes retention of material in the stomach underlies most of the risk factors (fig. 6.15).

Malignant Masses

Carcinoma is the most important and the most common tumor of the stomach. Most gastric carcinomas are adenocarcinomas [38].

Adenocarcinoma. The incidence of gastric adenocarcinoma is on the decline. At present, 22,800 Americans are diagnosed with gastric cancer each year [39]. Males are affected twice as often as females. Predisposing

conditions include atrophic gastritis, pernicious anemia, adenomatous polyps, dietary nitrates, and Japanese heritage [40, 41]. The tumors show a predilection for the lesser curvature of the antropyloric region. Grossly, adenocarcinomas of the stomach can be divided generally into three forms: 1) exophytic or polypoid, projecting into the lumen; 2) ulcerated, with a shallow or deeply erosive crater; and 3) diffusely infiltrative. The last-named form of adenocarcinoma creates a rigid, thickened "leather" stomach wall termed linitis plastica carcinoma. Gastric cancer may spread hematogenously to the liver and lung, contiguously to adjacent organs, lymphatically to regional and remote lymph nodes, and/ or intraperitoneally to the abdominal lining, mesentery, and serosa. The overall prognosis is poor. A TNM system is used for staging (Table 6.1).

Early in the disease, symptoms are vague and include dyspepsia, anorexia, and weight loss. Later, vomiting and hematemesis may occur in association with a palpable epigastric mass and anemia.

The goals of MRI in patients with gastric cancer are to demonstrate the primary tumor, assess the depth of invasion, and detect extragastric disease. Adequate distension is necessary for surveying the gastric wall. On T1-weighted sequences, gastric adenocarcinoma is isointense to normal stomach and may be apparent as focal wall thickening. On T2-weighted images, tumors usually are slightly higher in signal intensity than adjacent normal stomach [42].

An important observation on gadolinium-enhancement MRI images is that collapsed normal gastric wall enhances identically to the remainder of the wall on early and late postgadolinium images (fig. 6.16), whereas tumors show more heterogeneous enhancement that may be decreased or increased relative to the gastric wall on early, late, or both sets of images [29].

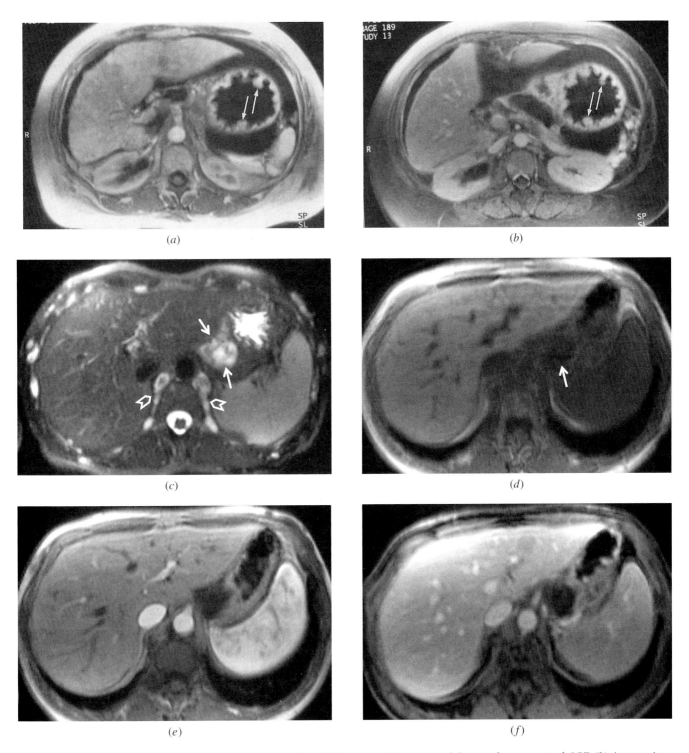

(a)   (b)

(c)   (d)

(e)   (f)

FIG. 6.13 Gastric polyps. Immediate postgadolinium SGE (*a*) and 90-s postgadolinium fat-suppressed SGE (*b*) images in a patient with Gardner syndrome demonstrate multiple enhancing gastric polyps (arrows, *a, b*). The polyps possess intense enhancement. **Gastric neurofibromas.** T2-weighted single-shot echo-train spin-echo (*c*), T1-weighted SGE (*d*), T1-weighted postgadolinium hepatic arterial dominant-phase SGE (*e*), and T1-weighted postgadolinium fat-suppressed hepatic venous-phase SGE (*f*) images demonstrate neurofibromas (arrows, *c, d*) located in the cardia portion of the stomach. The lesions show heterogeneous high signal on T2-weighted image (*c*) and low signal on T1-weighted image (*d*). The lesions show negligible enhancement on postgadolinium images (*e, f*). Note that paravertebral neurofibromas (open arrows, *c*) are present. **Gastric schwannoma.** Coronal T2-weighted

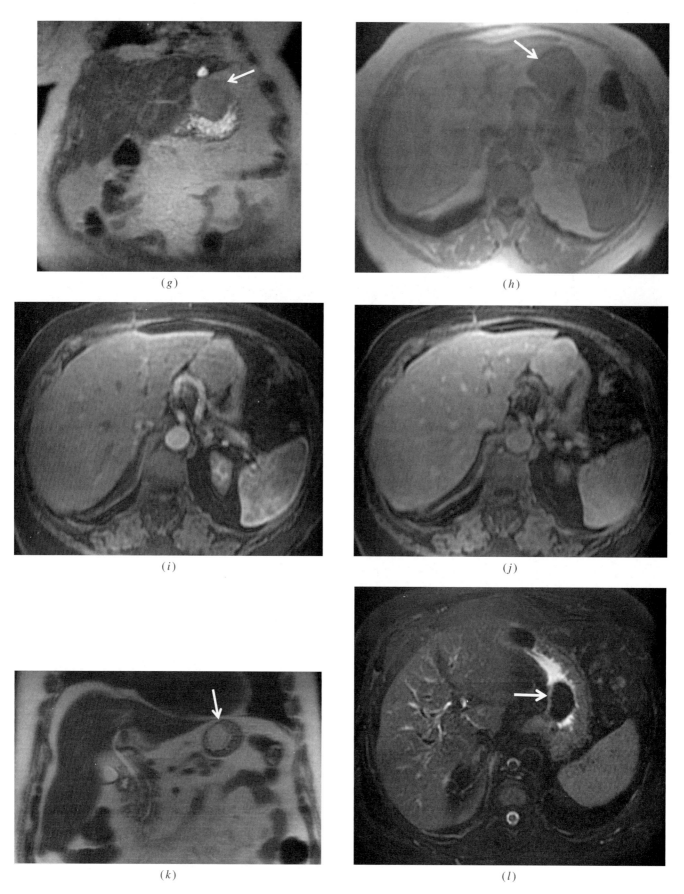

(g)

(h)

(i)

(j)

(k)

(l)

FIG. 6.13 (*Continued*) single-shot echo-train spin-echo (*g*), transverse T1-weighted SGE (*h*), transverse T1-weighted postgado-linium fat-suppressed hepatic arterial dominant-phase (*i*), and hepatic venous-phase (*j*) 3D-GE images demonstrate a gastric schwannoma (arrows, *g*, *h*) located in the lesser curvature. Exophytic lesion shows intermediate signal on precontrast sequences and homogeneous enhancement on postgadolinium images. Note that there is a cyst in the left liver lobe. **Gastric lipoma.** Coronal

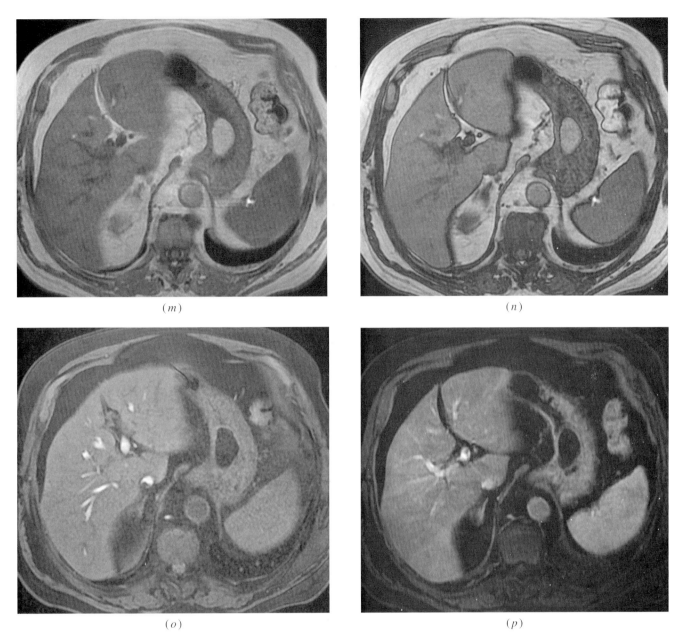

(m) (n)

(o) (p)

FIG. 6.13 (*Continued*) T2-weighted single-shot echo-train spin-echo (*k*), transverse T2-weighted fat-suppressed single-shot echo-train spin-echo (*l*), transverse T1-weighted in-phase (*m*) and out-of-phase (*n*) SGE, transverse T1-weighted fat-suppressed 3D-GE (*o*), and transverse T1-weighted postgadolinium hepatic venous-phase 3D-GE (*p*) images demonstrate a lipoma in the stomach lumen. The lesion shows high signal on precontrast non-fat-suppressed images (*k*, *m*, *n*). The lesion shows low signal on fat-suppressed images (*l*, *o*). Note that phase-cancellation artifact is present around the lipoma on out-of-phase image (*n*). The capsule of lipoma shows enhancement, and no enhancement is detected in the lipoma (*p*).

Tumors that originate in the cardia (fig. 6.17), body (fig. 6.18), antrum (fig. 6.19), and pylorus (fig. 6.20) are all well shown. Diffusely infiltrative carcinoma (linitis plastica carcinoma) tends to be lower in signal intensity than normal adjacent stomach on T2-weighted images because of its desmoplastic nature. Linitis plastic carcinoma enhances only modestly after intravenous contrast (fig. 6.21). In contradistinction, the other morphologic types of gastric carcinoma enhance more intensely with intravenous gadolinium. Gadolinium-enhanced fat-suppressed SGE or 3D-GE imaging aids in identification of transmural spread including peritoneal disease (fig. 6.22) and tumor involvement of lymph nodes. In vitro work with resected gastric cancer specimens at high field strength has demonstrated mucosal, submucosal, and muscle invasion [42].

Metastases enhance conspicuously against a background of low-signal-intensity fat. Detection of hepatic

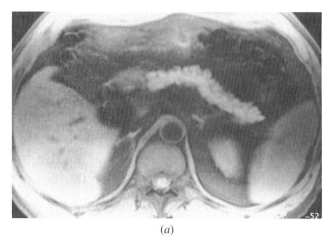

(a)

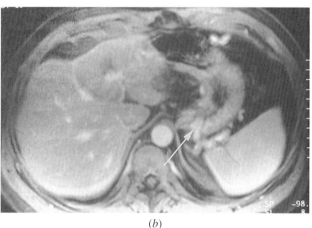

(b)

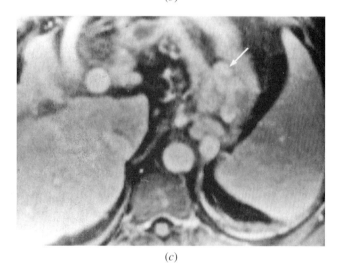

(c)

FIG. 6.14 Gastric varices. Fat-suppressed SGE (*a*) and 90-s postgadolinium fat-suppressed SGE (*b*) images. No splenic vein is identified posterior to the pancreas (*a*). After intravenous gadolinium administration (*b*), gastric varices enhance. These veins are part of the portosystemic circulation that are recruited to provide alternative venous channels in the presence of splenic vein thrombosis. A prominent varix is identified in the gastric wall (arrow, *b*). Transverse interstitial-phase gadolinium-enhanced fat-suppressed SGE image (*c*) in a second patient with hepatic cirrhosis. Large-caliber varices (arrow, *c*) are seen within the posterior wall stomach, immediately distal to the GE junction.

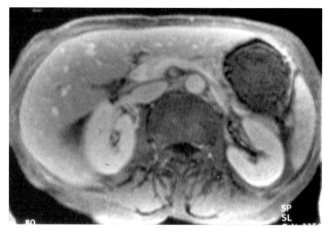

FIG. 6.15 Gastric bezoar. Transverse interstitial-phase gadolinium-enhanced fat-suppressed SGE image. The stomach is distended and filled with debris, which demonstrates a rounded configuration that represents a bezoar.

Table 6.1 TNM Staging for Cancer of the Stomach

T—Primary tumor

Tx Primary tumor cannot be assessed

T0 No evidence of primary tumor

Tis Pre-invasive carcinoma (carcinoma in situ)

T1 Tumor limited to the mucosa, or mucosa and submucosa regardless of extent and location

T2 Tumor with deep infiltration occupying not more than one-half of one region

T3 Tumor with deep infiltration occupying more than one-half but not more than one region

T4 Tumor with deep infiltration occupying more than one-half but not more than one region or extending to neighboring structures

N—Regional lymph nodes

Nx Regional lymph nodes cannot be assessed

N0 No evidence of regional lymph node metastasis

N1 Metastasis in lymph node(s) within 3 cm of the primary tumor along the greater or lesser curvatures

N2 Evidence of lymph node metastasis more than 3 cm from the primary tumor including those along the left gastric, splenic, celiac, and common hepatic arteries

N3 Evidence of involvement of the para-aortic and hepatoduodenal lymph nodes and/or other intra-abdominal lymph nodes

M—Metastases

Mx Distant metastases cannot be assessed

M0 No distant metastases

M1 Distant metastases

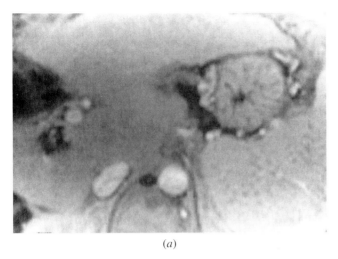

(a)

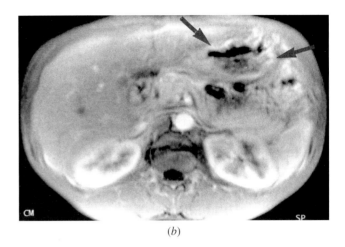

(b)

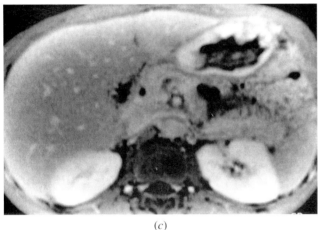

(c)

FIG. 6.16 Comparison between normal collapsed gastric wall and tumor. Transverse interstitial-phase gadolinium-enhanced fat-suppressed SGE image (*a*) in a normal patient. Note that the stomach is collapsed and the gastric wall enhancement is homogeneous. Note the symmetric radial fold pattern of the gastric rugae in the collapsed stomach. Transverse immediate postgadolinium (*b*) and interstitial-phase gadolinium-enhanced fat-suppressed SGE (*c*) images in a second patient with gastric cancer show diffuse gastric wall thickening and heterogeneous enhancement of the gastric wall. (Reprinted with permission from Marcos HB, Semelka RC: Stomach diseases: MR evaluation using combined T2-weighted single-shot echo train spin-echo and gadolinium-enhanced spoiled gradient-echo sequences. *J Magn Reson Imaging* 10: 950–960, 1999.)

involvement is facilitated by T2-weighted fat-suppressed sequences and dynamic gadolinium-enhanced SGE or 3D-GE techniques. This combined approach is superior to conventional CT imaging [43].

Marcos and Semelka reported on the detection and staging of gastric carcinoma [29]. In five of eight patients, focal, asymmetric gastric wall thickening or mass, consistent with gastric adenocarcinoma, was well demonstrated on MR evaluation. Failure of detection was related to small tumor size (<1–2 cm), lack of gastric distension, tumor enhancement similar to stomach wall, and tumoral isointensity on T2-weighted images. Staging accuracy was good, reflecting the adequate display of tumor and tumor extent on gadolinium-enhanced fat-suppressed SGE or 3D-GE images.

Gastrointestinal Stromal Tumors (GISTs).
Gastrointestinal mesenchymal neoplasms can be divided into two broad categories, those that represent clear-cut diagnostic entities (such as leiomyomas and lipomas) and those that are difficult to classify into any specific cell lineage, that is, ultrastructural or immunohistochem-

ical studies are not able to determine the histogenesis of the neoplastic cell population. The latter group of tumors falls into the category of gastrointestinal stromal tumors (GISTs). Although rare, GISTs most commonly occur in the stomach. All symptomatic GISTs are potentially malignant. These tumors are divided pathologically into lesions of 1) uncertain malignant potential, 2) low-grade malignant GIST, and 3) high-grade GIST. Grossly, these tumors differ from adenocarcinoma and lymphoma in that they often have a large exophytic component. Liquefactive necrosis and intratumoral hemorrhage are common. Spread is via direct extension and hematogenous metastases. High-grade GISTs are heterogeneous and high in signal on T2-weighted and gadolinium-enhanced fat-suppressed SGE or 3D-GE images because of their increased vascularity (figs. 6.23–6.26). During the capillary phase of imaging, they show marked enhancement that persists throughout the interstitial phase. Hasegawa et al. [44] reported that high-grade tumors have ill-defined tissue planes with adjacent tissues and organs, reflecting invasion, whereas low-grade tumors have well-defined planes, reflecting less

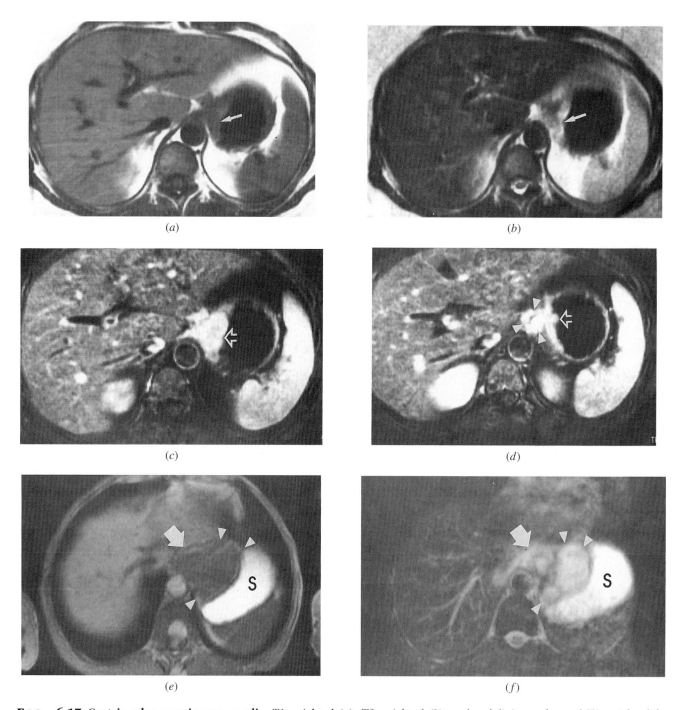

FIG. 6.17 Gastric adenocarcinoma, cardia. T1-weighted (*a*), T2-weighted (*b*), and gadolinium-enhanced T1-weighted fat-suppressed spin-echo (*c, d*) images in a patient with gastric cancer. The stomach has been distended with negative oral contrast agent. The gastric adenocarcinoma causes wall thickening medially, which is intermediate in signal intensity on the T1-weighted image (arrow, *a*) and heterogeneous and slightly hyperintense on the T2-weighted image (arrow, *b*). After intravenous gadolinium administration, the tumor (open arrows, *c, d*) enhances more than the normal stomach. The distal esophagus is also abnormally thickened with increased enhancement (arrowheads, *d*), which is consistent with spread across the gastroesophageal junction. SGE (*e*), T2-weighted fat-suppressed echo-train spin-echo (*f*), and immediate postgadolinium SGE (*g*) images in a second patient. The stomach (S, *e–g*) has been distended with a positive oral contrast agent. A large tumor in the cardia of the stomach (arrowheads, *e–g*) causes mass effect on the lumen. The cancer is low in signal intensity on the T1-weighted image (*e*) and heterogeneous and high in signal intensity on the T2-weighted image (*f*) and enhances heterogeneously after intravenous contrast (*g*). Note that

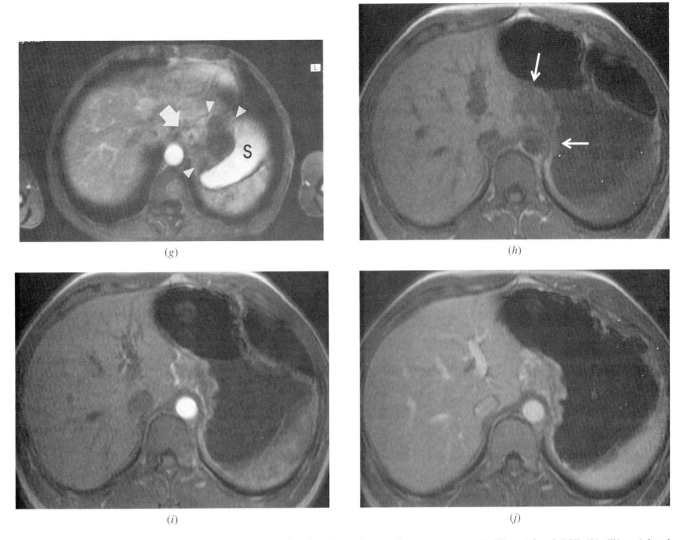

FIG. 6.17 (*Continued*) the tumor also involves the distal esophagus (large arrow, *e–g*). T1-weighted SGE (*h*), T1-weighted hepatic arterial phase (*i*), and hepatic venous phase (*j*) SGE images demonstrate ulcerated gastric adenocarcinoma (arrow, *h*) located in the cardia of the stomach in another patient. The tumor shows progressive enhancement on postgadolinium images.

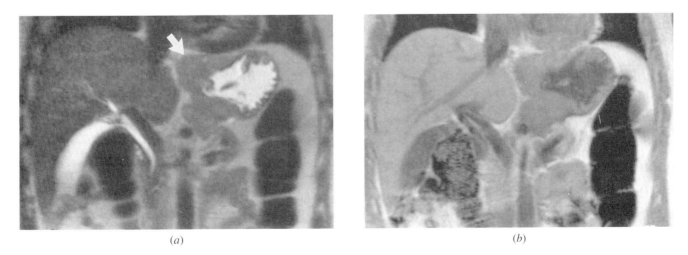

FIG. 6.18 Gastric adenocarcinoma, body. Coronal T2-weighted SS-ETSE (*a*), coronal precontrast SGE (*b*), transverse immediate postgadolinium SGE (*c*), and transverse 2-min postgadolinium fat-suppressed SGE (*d*) images. A circumferential low-signal-intensity mass is demonstrated in the body of the stomach. The high-signal-intensity fluid contents of the stomach permit good delineation of the low-signal-intensity mass on the T2-weighted SS-ETSE image (arrow, *a*). The mass is isointense to the stomach wall on the precontrast T1-weighted image (*b*). On the immediate postgadolinium image, the tumor (arrows, *c*) shows mild

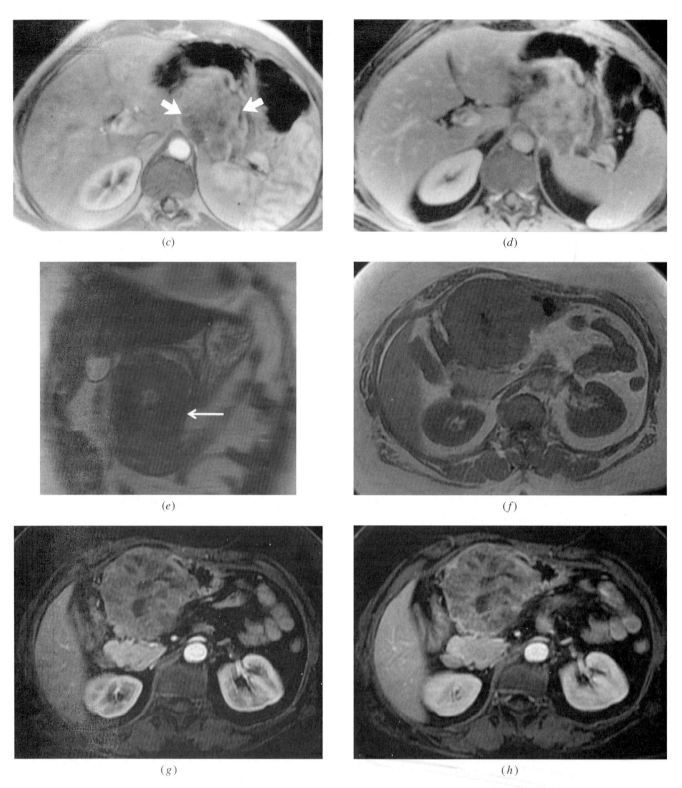

(c)

(d)

(e)

(f)

(g)

(h)

FIG. 6.18 (*Continued*) heterogeneous enhancement. On 2-min postgadolinium image (*d*), the tumor continues to enhance but to a lesser extent and heterogeneously compared to the remainder of the gastric wall. Note the intense enhancement of the normal renal cortex, which is greater than the enhancement of gastric wall or tumor. (Reprinted with permission from Marcos HB, Semelka RC: Stomach diseases: MR evaluation using combined T2-weighted single-shot echo train spin-echo and gadolinium-enhanced spoiled gradient-echo sequences. *J Magn Reson Imaging* 10: 950–960, 1999.) Coronal T2-weighted single shot echo train spin echo (*e*), transverse T1-weighted SGE (*f*), transverse postgadolinium fat-suppressed hepatic arterial dominant phase (*g*) and hepatic venous phase (*h*) 3D-GE images demonstrate a large adenocarcinoma (arrow, *e*) located in the body of the stomach in another patient. The exophytic tumor shows continuity with the stomach wall, and it displaces the transverse colon along its interface with transverse colon. The tumor is also adjacent to the pancreatic head, which is located posteriorly. The tumor demonstrates low signal on precontrast images (*e, f*). Progressive heterogeneous enhancement of the tumor is detected on postgadolinium images (*g, h*). Central necrosis is also present. Note that the tumor mimics gastrointestinal stromal tumor.

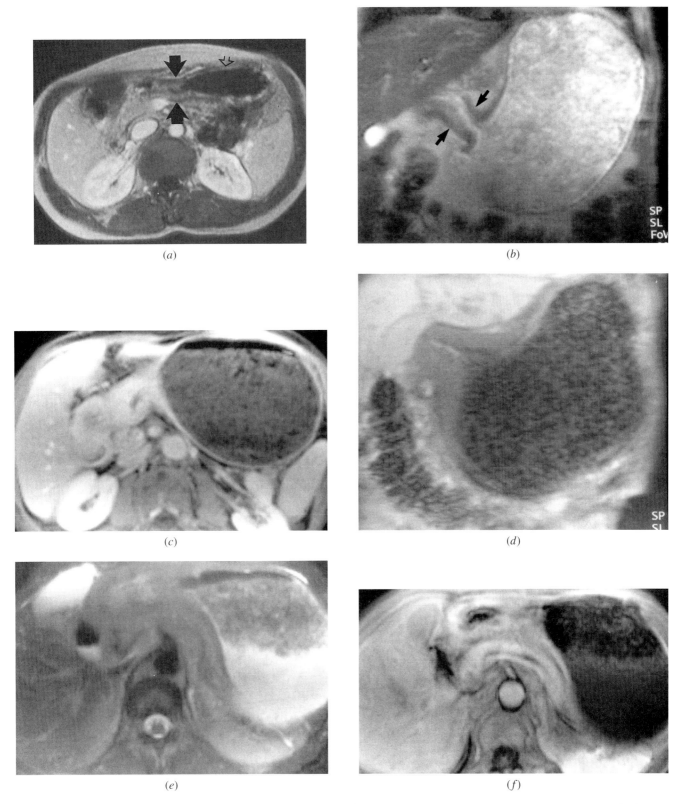

FIG. 6.19 Gastric adenocarcinoma, antrum. Transverse 45-s postgadolinium SGE image (*a*) demonstrates thickening and increased enhancement of the antrum secondary to gastric carcinoma (solid arrows, *a*). The remaining normal stomach has a thin wall (open arrow, *a*). Coronal SS-ETSE (*b*) and transverse interstitial-phase gadolinium-enhanced SGE (*c*) images in a second patient with antral tumor demonstrate a large, distended, debris-filled stomach secondary to gastric outlet obstruction. Note the substantial thickening and increased enhancement with gadolinium (*c*) of the antrum (arrows, *b*). Coronal (*d*) and transverse (*e*) T2-weighted SS-ETSE and transverse interstitial-phase gadolinium-enhanced fat-suppressed SGE (*f*) images in a third patient also show circumferential thickening and increased enhancement of the gastric antrum, with marked distension of the stomach.

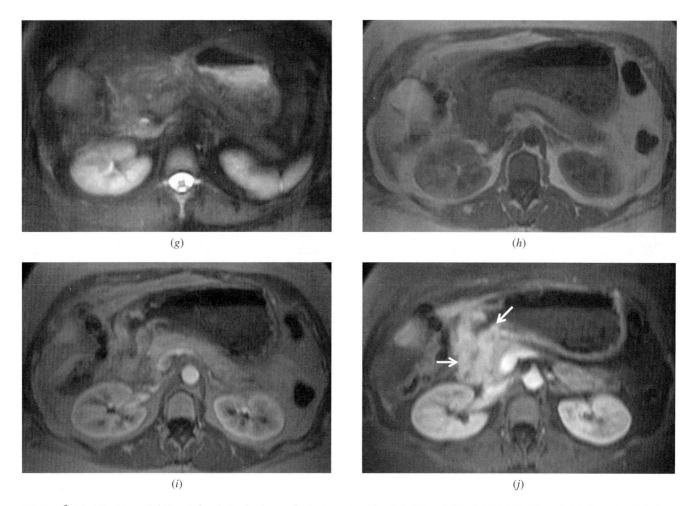

FIG. 6.19 (*Continued*) T2-weighted single-shot echo-train spin-echo (*g*), T1-weighted SGE (*h*), T1-weighted postgadolinium hepatic arterial dominant-phase SGE (*i*), and T1-weighted postgadolinium hepatic venous phase fat-suppressed 3D-GE (*j*) images demonstrate gastric adenocarcinoma (arrows, *j*) in the antrum in another patient. The wall of the antrum is thickened and shows intense enhancement due to tumoral involvement. The tumor extends into the duodenal wall. Note that the stomach is moderately dilated because of outlet obstruction.

aggressive tumor behavior. The necrotic portions of the tumor remain signal void on postcontrast images. Dynamic gadolinium-enhanced T1-weighted imaging also detects hepatic metastases. The hypervascular lesions show early ring or uniform enhancement, which rapidly becomes isointense with normal hepatic parenchyma. Low-grade tumors enhance to a lesser extent than higher-grade tumors (fig. 6.27). GIST of the stomach may be submucosal, intramural, or subserosal; subserosal lesions may be predominantly exophytic, and their origin from the gastric wall may not be apparent on radiologic evaluation [45]. In the Hasegawa series, the gastric origin of the tumor was uncertain in three of nine cases because of the large exophytic component, relatively small gastric pedicle, and absence of mucosal invasion. It is therefore prudent to consider the possibility of GIST for any large tumor with central necrosis

and hemorrhage that may appear radiologically to only abut the stomach.

Kaposi Sarcoma. Kaposi sarcoma most commonly occurs in immunocompromised patients, usually AIDS patients or recipients of organ transplantation. Grossly, the lesions of gastrointestinal tract Kaposi sarcoma consist of solitary, but frequently multiple, submucosal nodules. Microscopically, tumor is characterized by proliferation of spindle cells admixed with numerous vascular channels and red blood cell extravasation. Although approximately 50% of patients with AIDS-related Kaposi sarcoma will have gastrointestinal lesions at autopsy, most patients are asymptomatic. In rare instances, gastrointestinal Kaposi sarcoma may cause obstruction, intussusception, or hemorrhage. The stomach is the most common site of gut involvement,

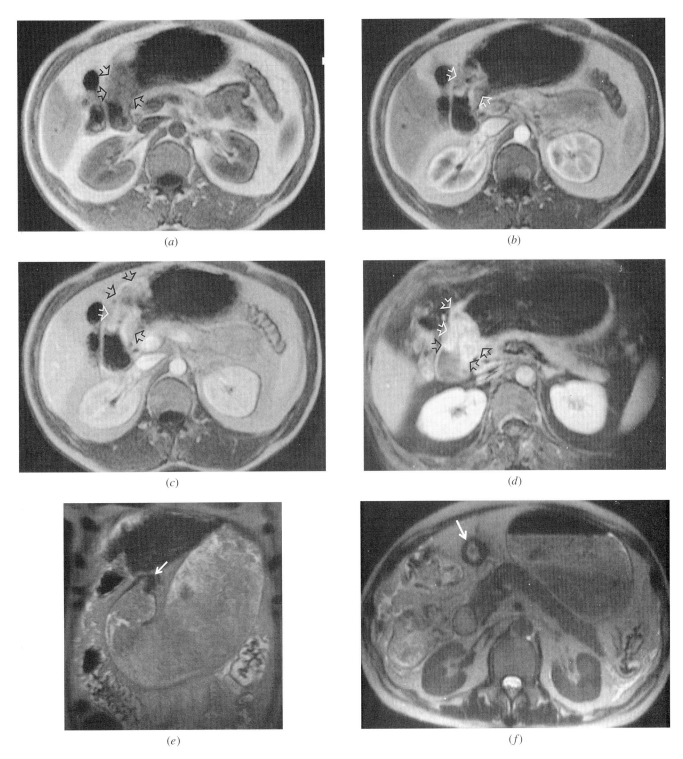

F I G . 6.20 Gastric adenocarcinoma, pylorus. SGE (*a*), 1-s (*b*) and 45-s (*c*) postgadolinium SGE, and interstitial-phase gadolinium-enhanced T1-weighted fat-suppressed spin-echo (*d*) images. A circumferential pyloric channel adenocarcinoma with duodenal extension (arrows, *a–d*) is present. The tumor enhances heterogeneously (*b*) and increases in signal intensity on the 3-min interstitial-phase image (*d*). This reflects accumulation of contrast in the interstitial space of the tumor. Coronal (*e*) and transverse (*f*) T2-weighted single-shot echo-train spin-echo images demonstrate gastric adenocarcinoma of the pylorus in another patient. The wall of the pylorus is thickened (arrows; *e, f*) because of tumoral involvement. Note that the stomach is dilated because of outlet obstruction and there is small amount of free fluid in the abdomen.

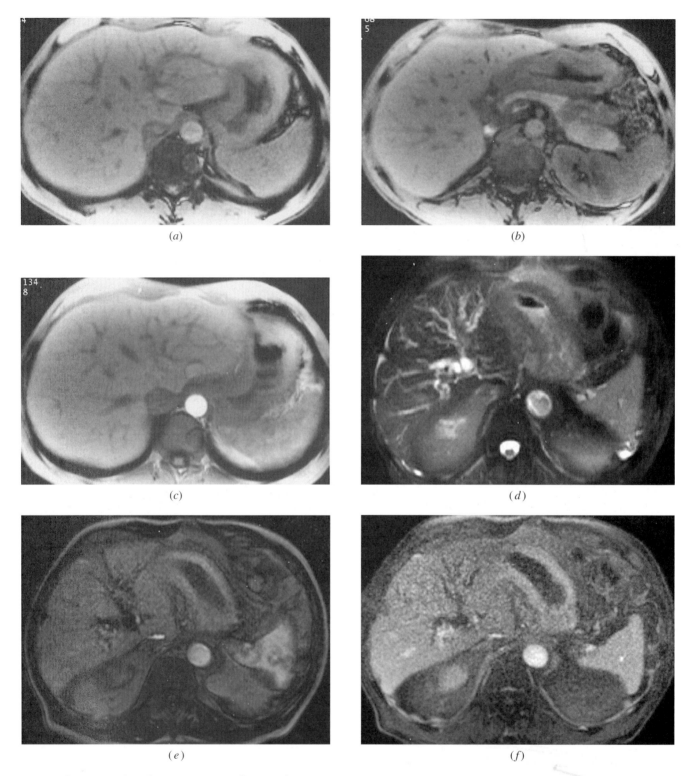

(a)

(b)

(c)

(d)

(e)

(f)

FIG. 6.21 Gastric adenocarcinoma, linitis plastica. Fat-suppressed SGE (*a*, *b*) and immediate postgadolinium SGE (*c*) images. Diffuse relatively homogeneous gastric wall thickening is present (*a*, *b*). Minimal enhancement is appreciated on the immediate postgadolinium SGE image (*c*). Transverse T2-weighted single-shot echo-train spin-echo (*d*) and T1-weighted postgadolinium magnetization-prepared gradient-echo (MPRAGE) transverse (*e*, *f*) and coronal (*g*) images demonstrate linitis plastica in

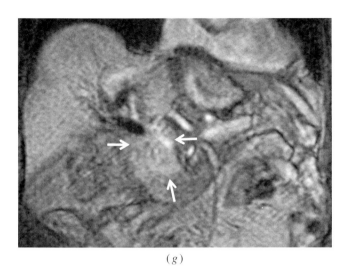

(g)

FIG. 6.21 (*Continued*) another patient. The gastric wall is diffusely thickened and shows diffuse enhancement. Note that the bile ducts are dilated because of the tumor (arrows, g) invasion.

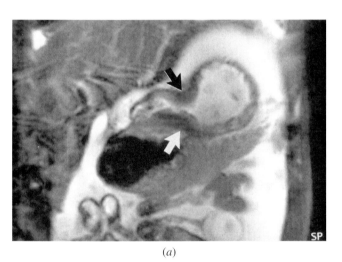

(a)

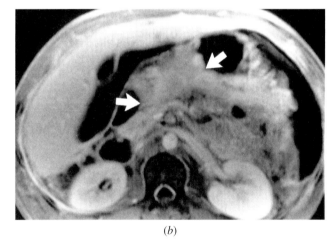

(b)

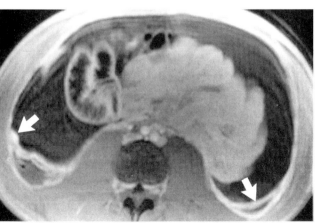

(c)

FIG. 6.22 Gastric adenocarcinoma with extensive carcinomatosis. Coronal T2-weighted SS-ETSE (*a*) image and transverse 2-min postgadolinium fat-suppressed SGE images at more superior (*b*) and inferior (*c*) tomographic levels. Diffuse thickening of a low-signal-intensity gastric wall is appreciated (arrows, *a*). Ascites is shown as high-signal-intensity intraperitoneal fluid on the T2-weighted image (*a*). The gastric tumor (arrows, *b*) is mildly enhanced on the 2-min postgadolinium image (*b*) compared to gastric wall. At a lower tomographic level (*c*), intense peritoneal enhancement (arrows, *c*) with nodules is shown, representing peritoneal metastases. (Reprinted with permission from Marcos HB, Semelka RC: Stomach diseases: MR evaluation using combined T2-weighted single-shot echo train spin-echo and gadolinium-enhanced spoiled gradient-echo sequences. *J Magn Reson Imaging* 10: 950–960, 1999.)

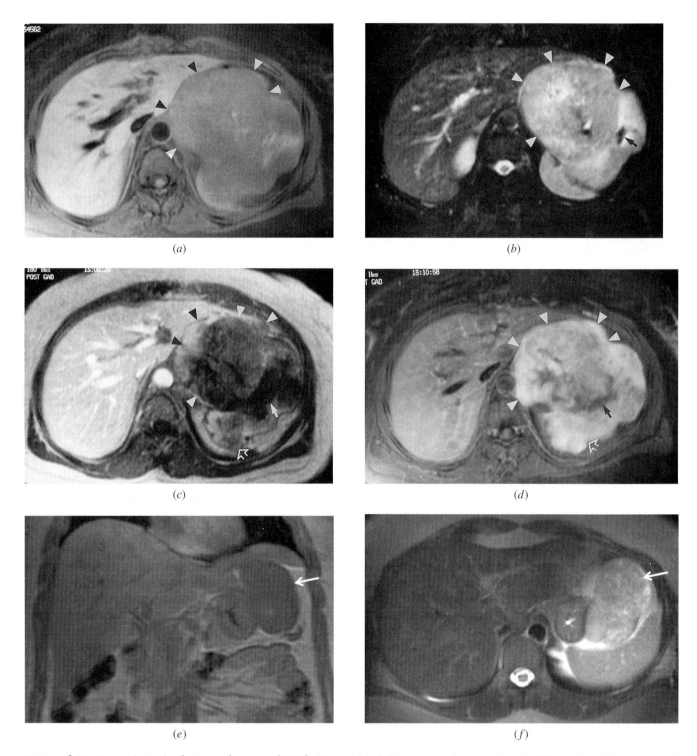

F I G . 6.23 Gastrointestinal stromal tumor (GIST). T1-weighted fat-suppressed spin-echo (*a*), T2-weighted fat-suppressed spin-echo (*b*), 45-s postgadolinium SGE (*c*), and gadolinium-enhanced fat-suppressed spin-echo (*d*) images. A large exophytic GIST arises from the lesser curvature (arrowheads, *a–d*) and is contiguous with the spleen. The tumor is heterogeneous and high in signal intensity on the T2-weighted image (*b*) and enhances intensely (*c, d*). Enhancing tumor extends adjacent to the spleen (open arrow, *c, d*). Signal-void areas within the tumor are consistent with necrosis. Air within the gastric lumen is also signal void (solid arrow, *b–d*). Coronal T1-weighted SGE (*e*), transverse T2-weighted single-shot echo-train spin-echo (*f*), and transverse T1-weighted postgadolinium hepatic venous phase fat-suppressed 3D-GE (*g*) images at 3.0 T demonstrate an exophytic GIST (arrows, *e–g*) arising from the greater curvature of the stomach in another patient. The tumor shows low signal on T1-weighted image (*e*), mildly high signal on T2-weighted image (*f*), and mild enhancement on postgadolinium image (*g*). CT (*h*), T2-weighted fat-suppressed

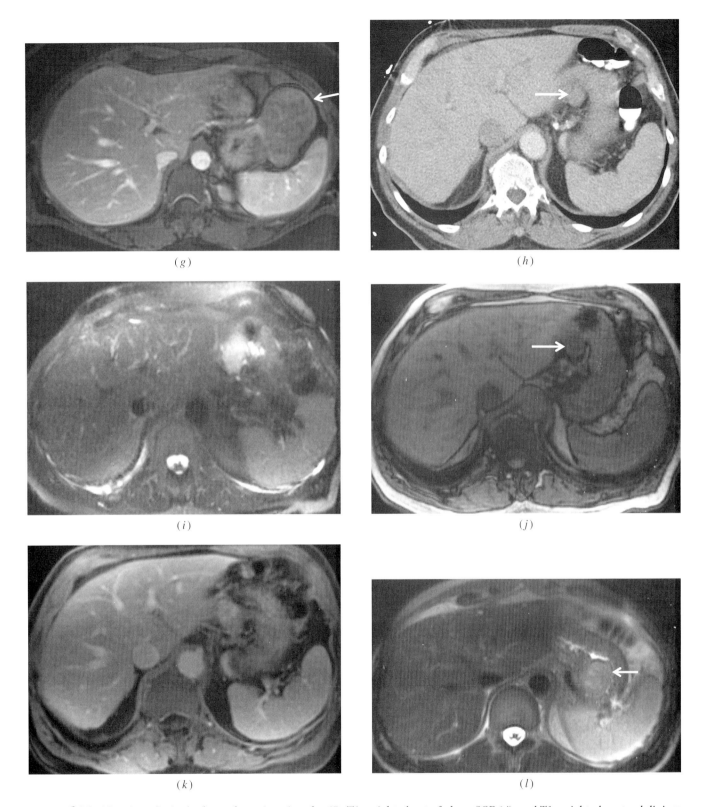

(g)

(h)

(i)

(j)

(k)

(l)

F I G . 6.23 (*Continued*) single-shot echo-train spin-echo (*i*), T1-weighted out-of-phase SGE (*j*), and T1-weighted postgadolinium hepatic venous phase fat-suppressed 3D-GE (*k*) images demonstrate subserosal GIST (arrows, *b, j*) arising from the lesser curvature in another patient. The tumor shows high signal on T2-weighted image (*i*), low signal on T1-weighted image (*j*), and prominent enhancement on postgadolinium image (*k*). T2-weighted single-shot echo-train spin-echo (*l*), T1-weighted SGE (*m*), T1-weighted

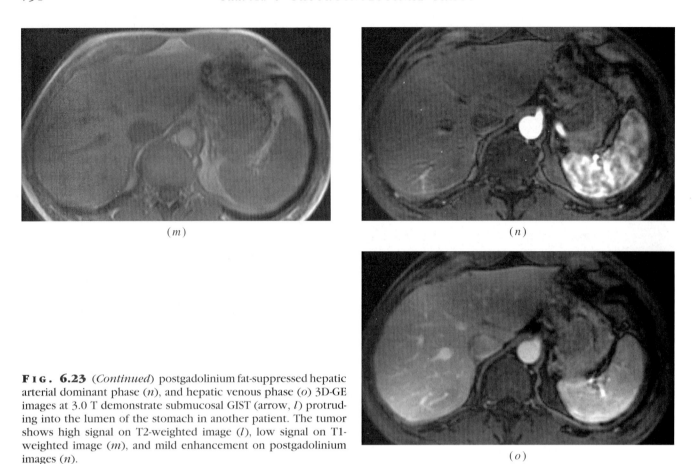

FIG. 6.23 (*Continued*) postgadolinium fat-suppressed hepatic arterial dominant phase (*n*), and hepatic venous phase (*o*) 3D-GE images at 3.0 T demonstrate submucosal GIST (arrow, *l*) protruding into the lumen of the stomach in another patient. The tumor shows high signal on T2-weighted image (*l*), low signal on T1-weighted image (*m*), and mild enhancement on postgadolinium images (*n*).

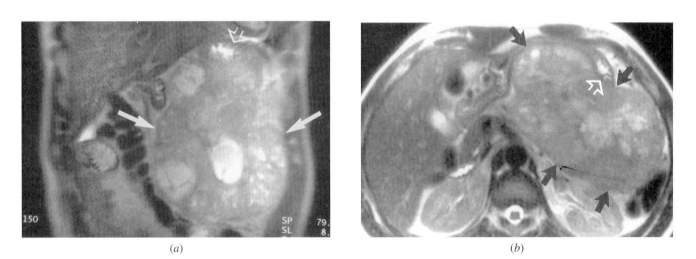

FIG. 6.24 Gastrointestinal stromal tumor (GIST). Coronal (*a*) and transverse (*b*) T2-weighted SS-ETSE, immediate postgadolinium SGE (*c*), and 90-s postgadolinium fat-suppressed SGE (*d*) images. A large multilobulated tumor (arrows, *a*, *b*) measuring 18 × 16 × 13 cm is shown arising from the gastric wall (open arrow, *a*, *b*). Multiple internal foci of high signal intensity are seen, representing areas of hemorrhage and necrosis. On the immediate postgadolinium image (*c*), the tumor enhances heterogeneously

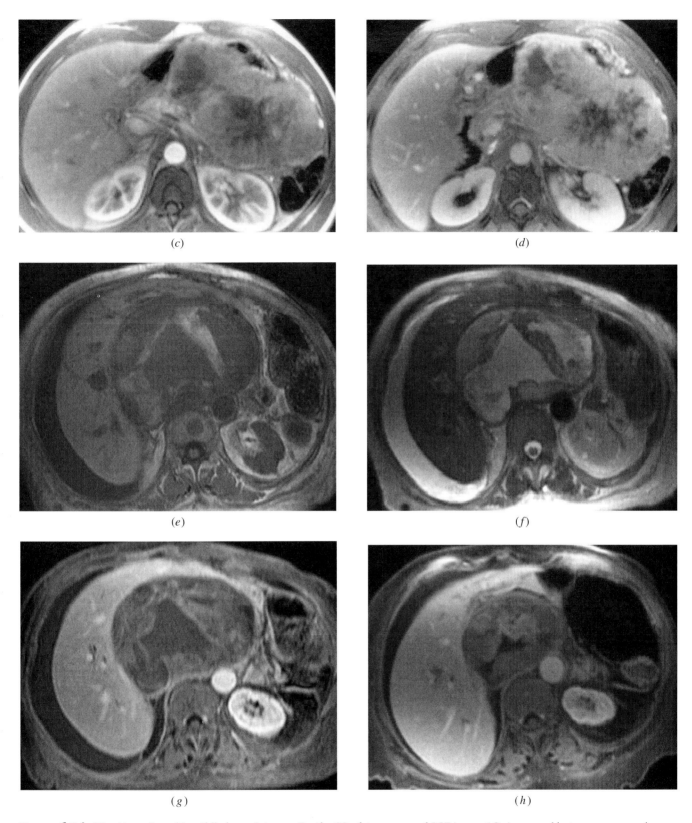

(c)

(d)

(e)

(f)

(g)

(h)

F I G. 6.24 (*Continued*) and is mildly hyperintense. On the 90-s fat-suppressed SGE image (*d*), increased heterogeneous enhancement of the mass is shown, which contains nonenhancing areas of necrosis and hemorrhage. (Reprinted with permission from Marcos HB, Semelka RC: Stomach diseases: MR evaluation using combined T2-weighted single-shot echo train spin-echo and gadolinium-enhanced spoiled gradient-echo sequences. *J Magn Reson Imaging* 10: 950–960, 1999.) T1-weighted SGE (*e*), T2-weighted single-shot echo-train spin-echo (*f*) and T1-weighted postgadolinium fat-suppressed interstitial-phase 3D-GE (*g*) images demonstrate a GIST arising from the stomach in another patient. The tumor is very heterogeneous and contains hemorrhagic and necrotic foci. Hemorrhagic foci show high signal on T1-weighted image (*e*) and heterogeneously low signal on T2-weighted image (*f*). Necrotic foci show low signal on T1-weighted image (*e*) and high signal on T2-weighted image (*f*). The tumor shows heterogeneous enhancement on postgadolinium image (*g*). Note that there is peritoneal enhancement and ascites, which are consistent with metastatic peritoneal disease. The tumor displaces the IVC and aorta laterally and the liver anteriorly. After chemotherapy, the tumor shows decrease in size (*h*).

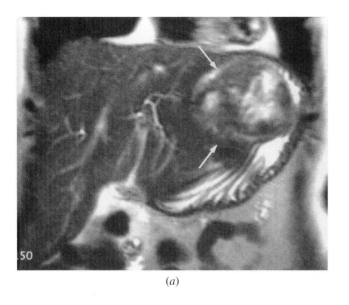

(a)

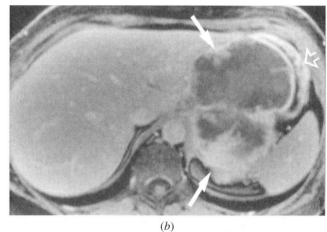

(b)

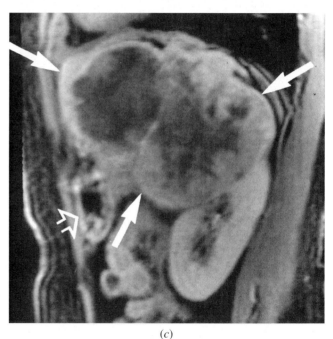

(c)

F I G . 6.25 High-grade GIST. Coronal T2-weighted SS-ETSE (a) and transverse (b) and sagittal (c) 2- to 3-min gadolinium-enhanced fat-suppressed SGE images. A large, heterogeneous tumor (arrows, a–c) arises from the gastric fundus and body. The lesion has ill-defined margins that correspond to high-grade cellular features seen at histopathologic examination. The stomach (open arrow, b, c) is compressed and deviated by the mass.

but lesions may occur throughout the gastrointestinal tract. Kaposi sarcoma should be considered in an AIDS patient who has gastrointestinal lesions in concert with bulky retroperitoneal lymphadenopathy, hepatic and splenic lesions, and infiltration of the psoas or abdominal wall [46].

Lymphoma. Primary gastric lymphoma is rare. Hodgkin lymphomas and non-Hodgkin lymphomas (NHL) are more commonly observed in the context of disseminated disease. Approximately 50% of gastrointestinal NHL arise in the stomach, 40% in the small intestine, and 10% in the colon [47]. Infiltration of the gastric wall by tumor cells results in diffuse mural thick-

ening [48, 49]. Non-Hodgkin lymphoma often preserves gastric distensibility, whereas Hodgkin lymphoma mimics the diffusely infiltrating form of primary gastric adenocarcinoma (linitis plastica): a desmoplastic reaction predominates, leading to a noncompliant aperistaltic viscus. Diffuse gastric wall thickening is best seen on single-shot echo-train spin-echo and gadolinium-enhanced fat-suppressed SGE or 3D-GE images (fig. 6.28). Involved regional lymph nodes also can be identified with these techniques.

Carcinoid. These tumors were first described by Obendorfer in 1907 as *karzinoide* (resembling carcinoma) because, despite their malignant potential, they

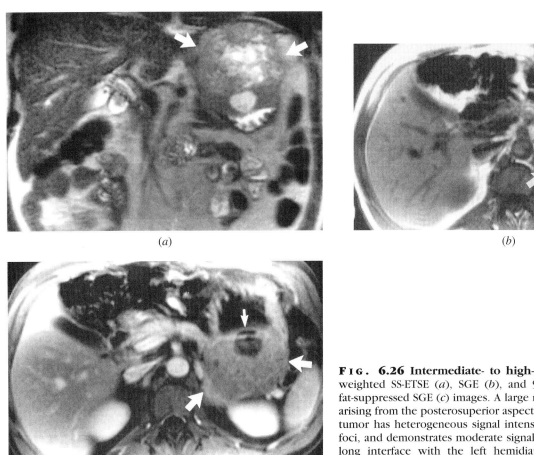

(a)

(b)

(c)

FIG. 6.26 Intermediate- to high-grade GIST. Coronal T2-weighted SS-ETSE (*a*), SGE (*b*), and 90-s gadolinium-enhanced fat-suppressed SGE (*c*) images. A large mass is seen (arrows, *a–c*) arising from the posterosuperior aspect of the gastric fundus. The tumor has heterogeneous signal intensity, contains hemorrhagic foci, and demonstrates moderate signal intensity. The mass has a long interface with the left hemidiaphragm and surrounding organs, but there is no evidence of deep invasion. A dominant necrotic focus is evident that represents an ulcer crater (small arrow, *c*).

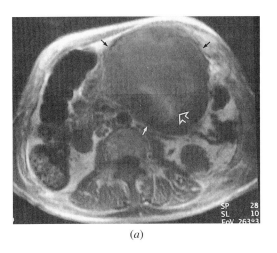

(a)

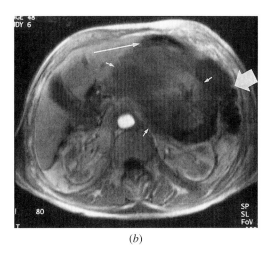

(b)

FIG. 6.27 Gastrointestinal stromal tumor (GIST), low grade. Transverse SGE (*a*), immediate postgadolinium SGE (*b*), and 90-s postgadolinium fat-suppressed SGE (*c*, *d*) images in a low-grade GIST (short arrows, *a–d*). On the precontrast image, high signal within the tumor represents hemorrhage (open arrow, *a*). Low-grade GISTs enhance minimally after intravenous contrast. The tumor causes mass effect on the remaining stomach (long arrows, *b*, *c*) and the adjacent colon (large arrows, *b*, *c*).

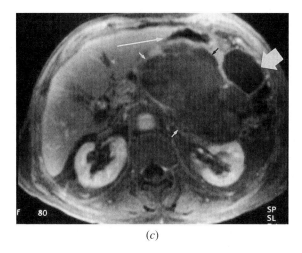

(c)

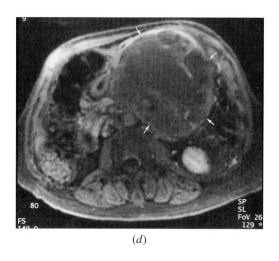

(d)

F I G . 6.27 (*Continued*)

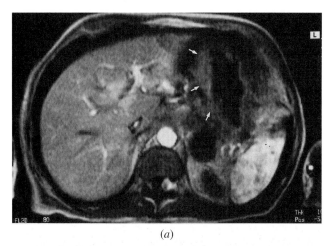

(a)

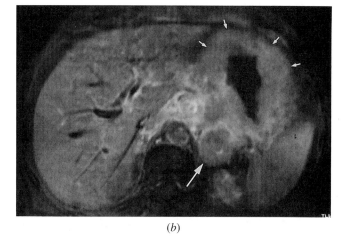

(b)

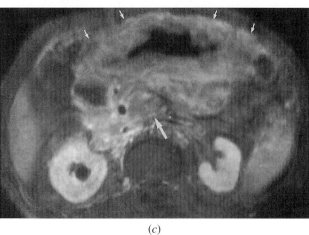

(c)

F I G . 6.28 Non-Hodgkin lymphoma of the stomach.
Immediate postgadolinium SGE (*a*) and gadolinium-enhanced T1-weighted fat-suppressed spin-echo (*b*, *c*) images. There is diffuse circumferential lymphomatous infiltration of the stomach wall (short arrows, *a–c*). Lymphoma extends to the left adrenal gland (long arrow, *b*). At a lower tomographic section, prominent retroperitoneal lymphadenopathy is present (arrow, *c*), which is commonly observed in the setting of gastric lymphoma.

exhibited slow growth patterns and were slow to metastasize. Carcinoids are best characterized as well-differentiated neuroendocrine neoplasms that occur most commonly in the appendix and small intestine (see discussion under small intestine). Gastric carcinoids are divided into two basic clinicopathologic categories, depending on whether they arise in the presence or absence of chronic atrophic gastritis [50].

Gastrin is secreted in a normal physiologic state by G cells in the gastric antrum. Secretion rates are normally controlled by gastric acid levels (mainly hydrochloric acid secretion by parietal cells in the fundus). When hydrochloric acid levels decrease, as occurs in the setting of chronic atrophic gastritis, increased secretion by G cells causes hypergastrinemia. Gastrin acts as a trophic factor to neuroendocrine-like cells in the fundic mucosa, resulting in hyperplasia progressing to carcinoid tumors. These tumors arise in situations of hypergastrinemia in conditions such as chronic autoimmune atrophic gastritis (pernicious anemia), chronic atrophic gastritis associated with *Helicobacter pylori* infection, and prolonged iatrogenic acid suppression with proton pump inhibitors (such as omeprazole) [51]. Hypergastrinemia may also occur in patients with Zollinger–Ellison syndrome and multiple endocrine neoplasia (MEN) type I. Gastric carcinoid tumors associated with chronic atrophic gastritis tend to occur in the fundus and are multiple, limited to the mucosa and submucosa. Lesions are rarely malignant and regress when gastrin levels are decreased, usually after antrectomy (gastrin-producing cells reside predominantly in the antrum). This situation is in sharp contrast to gastric carcinoid tumors that arise sporadically in a normogastrinemic state. Sporadic gastric carcinoid tumors arise anywhere in the stomach and may be small (<2-cm diameter) submucosal nodules or large tumors that invade deeply and promote prominent fibrosis in surrounding tissues. Sporadic gastric carcinoids should be regarded as malignant neoplasms and should be completely surgically resected.

On MR images, carcinoid tumors are near-isointense on T1 and mildly hyperintense and heterogeneous on T2 and often show increased enhancement on early and later postgadolinium images (fig. 6.29).

Metastases. Metastatic involvement of the stomach is uncommon. Gastric metastatic lesions are generally

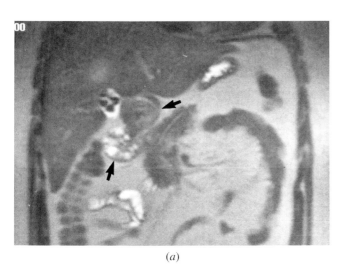

(*a*)

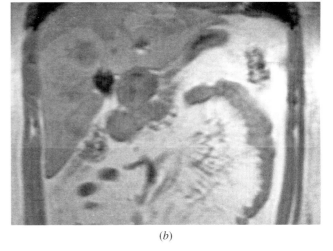

(*b*)

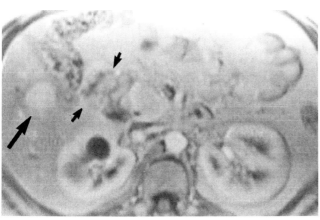

(*c*)

FIG. 6.29 Gastric carcinoid. Coronal T2-weighted SS-ETSE (*a*), coronal SGE (*b*), and transverse immediate postgadolinium SGE (*c*) images. This primary carcinoid tumor of the stomach appears as a mass in the wall of the antrum that invades the duodenum and pancreas. The tumor is mixed solid with cystic spaces (arrows, *a*) on T2 and isointense on T1 (*b*) and enhances heterogeneously after contrast administration (arrows, *c*). There are also hepatic metastases that are moderately hyperintense on T2-weighted image and hypointense on precontrast SGE image (*b*) and show homogeneous early enhancement (large arrow, *c*). A simple cyst is also seen in the right kidney.

submucosal. Tumors of neighboring organs, such as esophagus, pancreas, and transverse colon, may involve the stomach by direct extension. Specifically, colon carcinoma arising in the transverse colon invades the stomach via the gastrocolic ligament, whereas pancreatic carcinoma invades the posterior wall of the gastric body and antrum via the transverse mesocolon.

Carcinomas of lung and breast and melanoma are the most common primary malignancies that result in hematogenous gastric metastases (fig. 6.30). Breast cancer metastases are noteworthy in that submucosal involvement with diffuse thickening of gastric wall may be indistinguishable from diffusely infiltrative gastric adenocarcinoma (linitis plastica) (fig. 6.30).

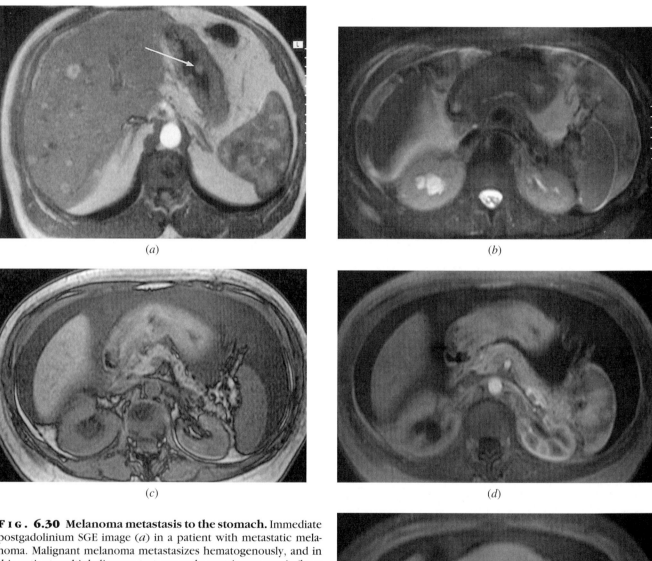

(a)

(b)

(c)

(d)

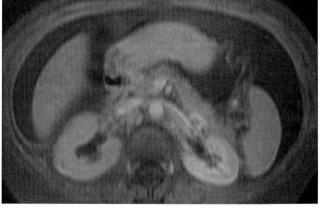

(e)

F I G. 6.30 Melanoma metastasis to the stomach. Immediate postgadolinium SGE image (*a*) in a patient with metastatic melanoma. Malignant melanoma metastasizes hematogenously, and in this patient multiple liver metastases and a gastric metastasis (long arrow, *a*) are identified. The metastases are high in signal on this T1-weighted image because of the paramagnetic properties of melanin. **Breast cancer metastases to the stomach and peritoneum.** T2-weighted single-shot echo-train spin-echo (*b*), T1-weighted out-of-phase SGE (*c*), T1-weighted postgadolinium hepatic arterial dominant-phase SGE (*d*), and T1-weighted postgadolinium interstitial-phase fat-suppressed 3D-GE (*e*) images demonstrate hematogenous metastases in the stomach and peritoneum from breast cancer in another patient. The gastric wall is diffusely thickened and shows diffuse prominent enhancement due to metastatic involvement. Note that there is peritoneal enhancement and ascites, which are consistent with metastatic peritoneal disease. Parapelvic cysts are present in the right kidney.

Inflammatory and Infectious Disorders

Gastric Ulceration and Gastritis

Ulcers are defined pathologically as localized, destructive lesions involving full-thickness mucosa. Ulcer craters may extend into submucosa or deeper aspects of the gut wall. The two most important factors involved in the etiology of chronic peptic ulcer disease are the amount of gastric acid and the mucosal resistance. An almost invariable feature of gastric ulcer disease is evidence of diffuse inflammation of surrounding mucosa, indicative of chronic antral gastritis that is mainly caused by *H. pylori* infection. In some cases, gastritis may result from repeated exposure to toxic substances including alcohol, drugs, and bile salts. Approximately 10% of patients have ulcers in both the antrum and the duodenum [52].

Benign gastric ulcers most commonly occur along the lesser curvature in the region of the border zone between the corpus and antral mucosa.

Marcos and Semelka reported on the MR appearance of gastric ulcers [29]. Gastric inflammatory disease in general results in increased mural enhancement on both early and late gadolinium images (fig. 6.31). Ulcer craters may be demonstrated on both single-shot echo-train spin-echo and gadolinium-enhanced fat-suppressed SGE or 3D-GE images (fig. 6.31).

Gastritis is defined as inflammation of the gastric mucosa. Inflammation may be acute, consisting predominantly of neutrophils, or chronic, with a preponderance of lymphocytes or plasma cells.

Acute gastritis is usually transient in nature and may be associated with a variety of factors including heavy use of drugs, especially NSAIDs, excessive alcohol consumption, smoking, and severe stress (e.g., trauma, burns, surgery). Severe acute gastritis is often characterized pathologically by the presence of erosions and hemorrhage. The term "erosion" denotes the loss of superficial epithelium, in contrast to ulcers, which involve the full-thickness mucosa. Gastritis causes mural edema, which is seen as high signal intensity in the submucosa (fig. 6.31). Gastritis also results in increased mural enhancement on both early and late gadolinium images (fig. 6.31).

Chronic gastritis is characterized by the presence of chronic inflammation leading to mucosal atrophy and abnormal changes in the epithelium (fig. 6.32). Erosions generally do not occur in this setting. The major etiologies of chronic gastritis include immunologic (pernicious anemia), chronic infection, especially with *Helicobacter pylori*, and toxic, as in alcohol consumption and cigarette smoking.

Both acute and chronic gastritis may occur in patients receiving high-dose radiation therapy. A chronic ulcer may develop months to several years after radiation exposure. Gastric inflammation, fibrosis, and stricture formation may lead to outlet obstruction (fig. 6.33) [53].

Gastric Wall Edema

Mural edema without substantial inflammatory changes is shown by the combination of mural high signal on single-shot T2-weighted images in combination with the lack of substantial enhancement on postgadolinium fat-suppressed T1-weighted gradient-echo images. A useful internal standard is to compare the extent of enhancement of the gastric wall with nearby renal cortex. The wall should not enhance more than renal cortex to establish the diagnosis of gastric wall edema. A variety of disease processes may result in gastric wall edema, including food allergies (fig. 6.33).

Hypertrophic Rugal Folds

Localized or diffuse thickening and gross enlargement of rugal folds ("cerebriform") may result from discrete hyperplasia of one of the epithelial mucosal components, inflammatory diseases, or tumors, most notably lymphoma or carcinoma. Causes of diffuse mucosal hypertrophy include hyperplasia of the parietal cells in Zollinger–Ellison syndrome (fig. 6.34) or of surface foveolar mucous cells in Menetrier disease. Types of specific inflammatory conditions that may cause rugal enlargement, often localized to the antrum, include infections such as tuberculosis and syphilis, chronic granulomatous diseases, and sarcoidosis [54].

The use of the single-shot echo-train spin-echo technique coupled with adequate distension permits detection of rugal thickening. The hyperemia and capillary leakage that accompany inflammation are highlighted on T1-weighted fat-suppressed SGE or 3D-GE images. The inflamed tissue demonstrates early marked enhancement, which persists as the contrast pools in the interstitium. The inflammatory nature of some of these gastric diseases is best shown on gadolinium-enhanced images.

The Postoperative Stomach

A spectrum of surgical procedures involves the stomach. These procedures may be categorized as drainage with or without partial gastric resection, antireflux operations, gastroplasty, resection, band surgery (fig. 6.35), and feeding gastrostomy (fig. 6.35). Familiarity with the exact surgical procedure performed aids radiologic investigation. The single-shot T2-weighted technique allows visualization of the anatomic changes following surgery, such as bowel anastomoses (fig. 6.35). Evaluation of inflammatory changes is accomplished with gadolinium-enhanced images.

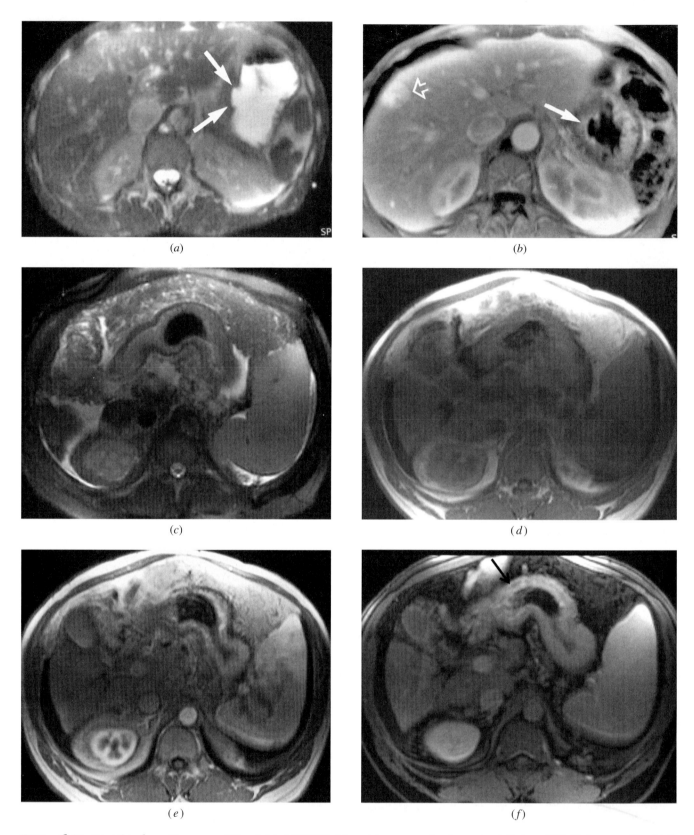

(a)

(b)

(c)

(d)

(e)

(f)

FIG. 6.31 Gastric ulcer. Transverse T2-weighted SS-ETSE (*a*) and transverse 1-min postgadolinium SGE (*b*) images. The high signal intensity of gastric contents (orally administered water) delineates the ulcer crater (arrows, *a*) on the mucosal surface of the lesser curvature. On the 1-min postgadolinium SGE image (*b*), the ulcer shows mildly increased enhancement (arrow). A 2-cm hemangioma is incidentally noted as an intensely enhancing mass lesion in the liver on the 1-min postgadolinium image (open arrow, *b*). (Reprinted with permission from Marcos HB, Semelka RC: Stomach diseases: MR evaluation using combined T2-weighted single-shot echo train spin-echo and gadolinium-enhanced spoiled gradient-echo sequences. *J Magn Reson Imaging* 10: 950–960, 1999.) **Gastritis.** T2-weighted single-shot echo-train spin-echo (*c*), T1-weighted SGE (*d*), T1-weighted postgadolinium hepatic arterial dominant-phase SGE (*e*), and T1-weighted postgadolinium hepatic venous phase fat-suppressed 3D-GE (*f*) images demonstrate diffuse gastritis in another patient. The gastric wall is diffusely thickened, but the rugal folds are regularly seen. The gastric wall shows diffuse prominent enhancement on postgadolinium images (*e, f*). Bilaminar enhancement of the gastric wall (arrow, *f*), which is due to the presence of edema, is seen on the hepatic venous phase (*f*). Note that portal hypertension findings including splenomegaly, ascites, and varices are present.

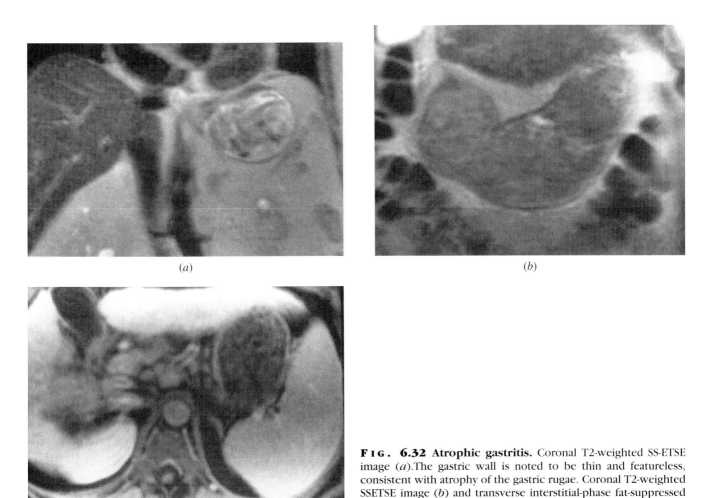

(a)

(b)

(c)

FIG. 6.32 Atrophic gastritis. Coronal T2-weighted SS-ETSE image (*a*).The gastric wall is noted to be thin and featureless, consistent with atrophy of the gastric rugae. Coronal T2-weighted SSETSE image (*b*) and transverse interstitial-phase fat-suppressed postgadolinium SGE image (*c*) in a second patient show similar features of gastric wall atrophy.

(a)

(b)

FIG. 6.33 Radiation gastritis. Transverse T2-weighted SSETSE (*a*), SGE (*b*), and 90-s postgadolinium fat-suppressed SGE (*c*) images in a patient after radiation therapy for pancreatic cancer. There is marked wall thickening of the stomach with submucosal edema. Note the high signal of the thickened submucosa on the T2-weighted image (arrows, *a*), reflecting edema. After contrast administration, mucosal enhancement is noted. **Gastric wall edema secondary to food allergy.** Coronal T2-weighted single-shot

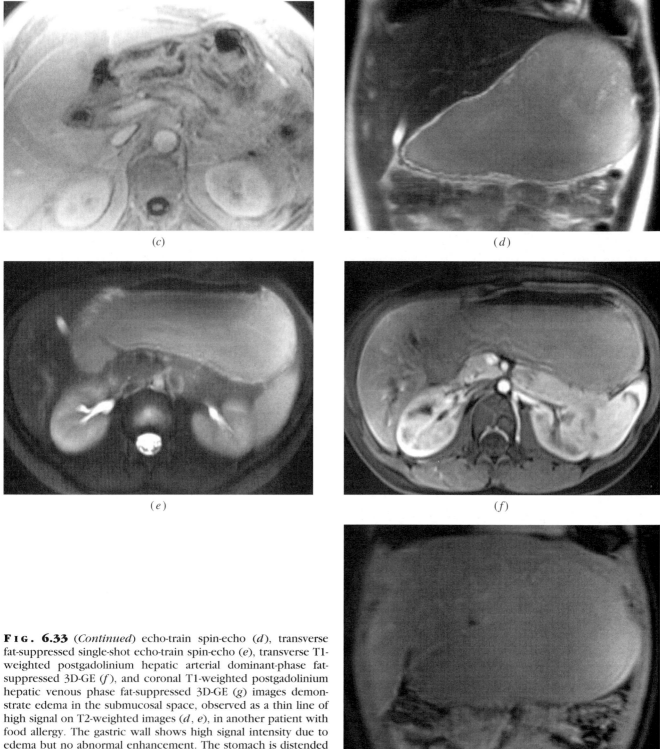

FIG. 6.33 (*Continued*) echo-train spin-echo (*d*), transverse fat-suppressed single-shot echo-train spin-echo (*e*), transverse T1-weighted postgadolinium hepatic arterial dominant-phase fat-suppressed 3D-GE (*f*), and coronal T1-weighted postgadolinium hepatic venous phase fat-suppressed 3D-GE (*g*) images demonstrate edema in the submucosal space, observed as a thin line of high signal on T2-weighted images (*d*, *e*), in another patient with food allergy. The gastric wall shows high signal intensity due to edema but no abnormal enhancement. The stomach is distended due to oral administration of one L of water to achieve adequate visualization of the gastric wall.

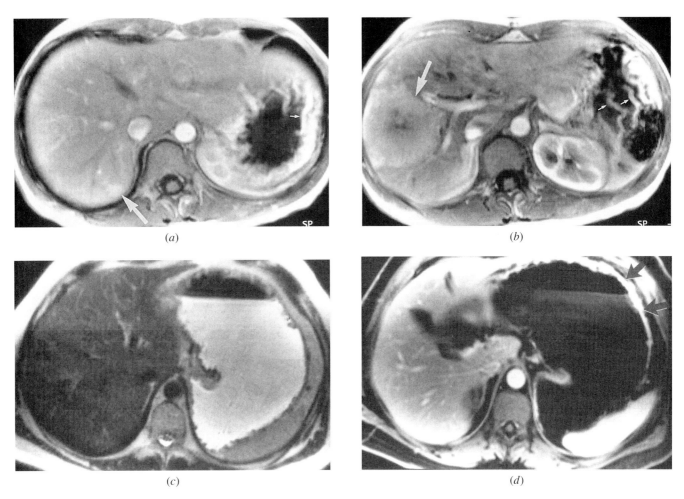

F I G . 6.34 Zollinger–Ellison syndrome. Immediate postgadolinium SGE images (*a, b*). Intense enhancement and increased thickness of gastric rugae are appreciated (small arrows, *a, b*). Hypervascular liver metastases are also present (large arrow, *a, b*). Transverse T2-weighted SS-ETSE (*c*) and transverse 90-s fat-suppressed postgadolinium SGE (*d*) images in a second patient. There is a marked distension of the stomach and duodenum, and the anterior gastric wall is thickened. On the 90-s postgadolinium fat-suppressed SGE image (*d*), the gastric wall shows intense enhancement (arrows, *d*). (Reprinted with permission from Marcos HB, Semelka RC: Stomach diseases: MR evaluation using combined T2-weighted single-shot echo train spin-echo and gadolinium-enhanced spoiled gradient-echo sequences. *J Magn Reson Imaging* 10: 950–960, 1999.)

THE SMALL INTESTINE

Normal Anatomy

The small bowel measures approximately 20–22 feet from the ligament of Treitz to the ileocecal valve. On gross inspection, the lining of the small intestine shows a series of permanent circular folds, plicae circulares. Each fold is covered by mucosa and contains a core of submucosa. The mucosal surface covered by villi, and the plicae circulares, increase the surface area and act as partial barriers that attenuate the forward flow of intraluminal contents, thus increasing the time of contact with absorptive surfaces. The duodenum is in continuation with the pylorus. It extends in a C shape to curve around the pancreatic head to end at the duodenal-jejunal flexure in the left upper quadrant. The duodenum is divided into four parts: bulb, descending, horizontal, and ascending segments. The bulb is the only intraperitoneal portion of the duodenum and is the most mobile. The second portion is in close proximity to the head of the pancreas, and both the pancreatic and common bile ducts converge to enter the postero-medial aspect forming the ampulla. The mesenteric small intestine begins at the jejunum. The jejunum occupies the superior and left abdomen, and the ileum occupies the inferior and right abdomen. Their mesenteric attachment gives rise to two distinct borders, the concave or mesenteric border and the convex or antimesenteric border. The ileum has a narrower lumen and, migrating from jejunum to distal ileum, has progressively fewer mucosal folds and a greater number of

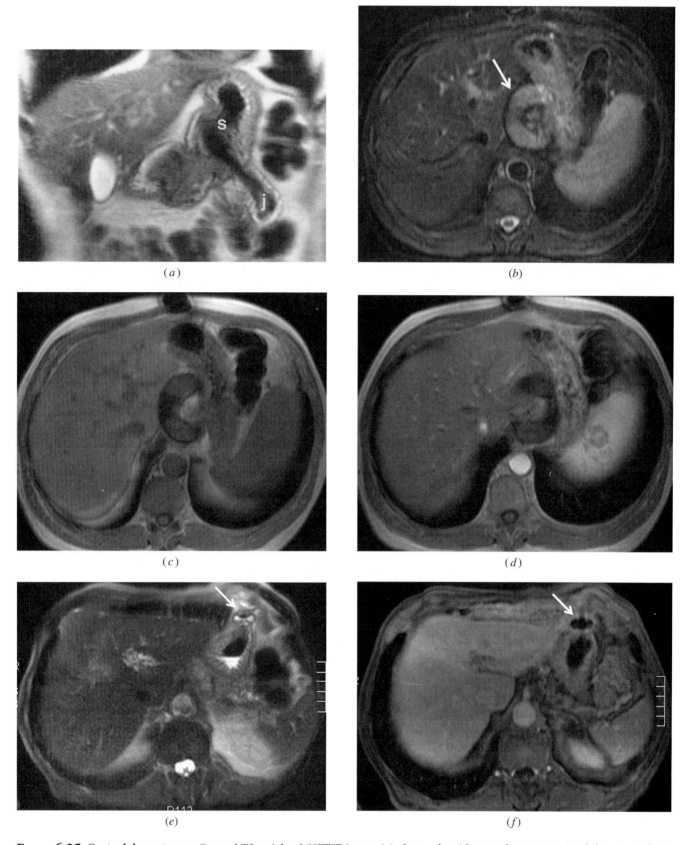

(a)

(b)

(c)

(d)

(e)

(f)

FIG. 6.35 Gastrojejunostomy. Coronal T2-weighted SSETSE image (*a*) shows the side-to-end anastomosis of the stomach (s) to the jejunum (j) in this patient status post gastrointestinal bypass surgery. **Gastric band.** T2-weighted short-tau inversion recovery (*b*), T1-weighted SGE (*c*), and T1-weighted postgadolinium hepatic arterial dominant phase SGE (*d*) images show gastric band (arrow, *b*) secondary to the operation. **Percutaneous gastrostomy tube.** T2-weighted single-shot echo-train spin-echo (*e*) and T1-weighted hepatic venous phase fat-suppressed 3D-GE (*f*) images demonstrate that the percutaneous gastrostomy tube is not located in the gastric lumen.

mesenteric arcades. Normal bowel wall thickness should not exceed 3–4 mm.

MRI Technique

Previously, MRI had a limited role in assessing the small bowel because of poor intrinsic contrast resolution and motion artifacts caused by peristalsis. The combination of single-shot echo-train spin-echo images that are less sensitive to motion deterioration and pre- and postgadolinium fat-suppressed breath-hold SGE or 3D-GE images is an effective approach for imaging the bowel (fig. 6.36). As a routine, patients should fast for at least 5 hours before the exam to decrease bowel motion and peristalsis with the resulting blurring artifact. Ingested water coupled with the single-shot echo-train spin-echo technique provides high-quality images of the small bowel (see fig. 6.36). Images of the upper and midabdomen should be obtained in the axial and coronal planes to distinguish bowel, which will show tubular-shaped configuration in at least one plane, from masses, which will not. Unenhanced SGE images with and without fat suppression followed by gadolinium-enhanced T1-weighted fat-suppressed SGE or 3D-GE images are necessary for a comprehensive exam. Normal bowel has a feathery appearance on unenhanced images because of the plicae circulares and after intravenous gadolinium enhances in a moderate and uniform fashion [55] (see fig. 6.36). Small bowel enhances less than the gastric wall (see fig. 6.36) and pancreas. Use of 3D-GE fat-suppressed gadolinium-enhanced images provide an optimal technique for T1-weighted imaging. The shorter TR and TE result in decreased image deterioration from paramagnetic effects from intraluminal gas, and the short TR allows faster imaging, resulting in more coverage with higher resolution during a shorter breath hold period than can be achieved with SGE technique. Combined with parallel processing, such as sensitivity-enhanced (SENSE) methods, rapid breath-hold examination of the abdomen and pelvis has become more feasible. In addition, development of coil and software-hardware schemes, including multistep table technology, has facilitated optimization of the signal-to-noise ratio of the images through utilization of surface coils that can cover larger fields of view and allow evaluation of the abdomen and pelvis without having to pause the examination to readjust coils or reacquire preparation scans. The lesser enhancement of small bowel compared to pancreas generally allows clear distinction between these two organs on immediate postgadolinium images. The administration of intravenous gadolinium in combination with fat-suppressed 3D-GE T1-weighted sequences permits evaluation of the bowel wall and assessment of mesenteric and retroperitoneal lymphadenopathy, peritoneal disease, and accompanying fistula, if present. The use of true-FISP sequence is also helpful for the evaluation of small bowel and mesentery.

MR Small Bowel Follow-Through and Enteroclysis
Recent studies have described small bowel follow-through and small bowel enema performed as MR

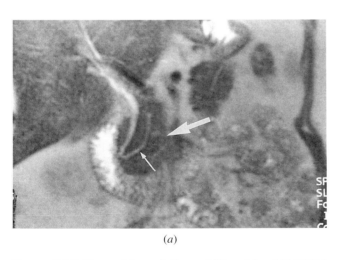

(a)

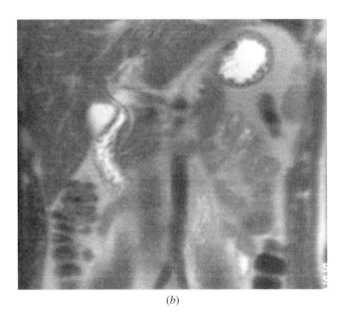

(b)

F I G . 6.36 Normal bowel. Coronal T2-weighted SS-ETSE images (*a–e*) in five patients. The valvulae conniventes of the C loop of the duodenum (*a–c*) and of multiple loops of jejunum and ileum are well shown as low-signal-intensity bands on the T2-weighted images (arrows, *e*) and stand out in relief against the high-signal-intensity intraluminal contents and moderately high-signal-intensity fat. Normal head of pancreas (large arrow, *a*), and pancreatic duct (thin arrow, *a*) are demonstrated. Fat-suppressed SGE (*f*) and

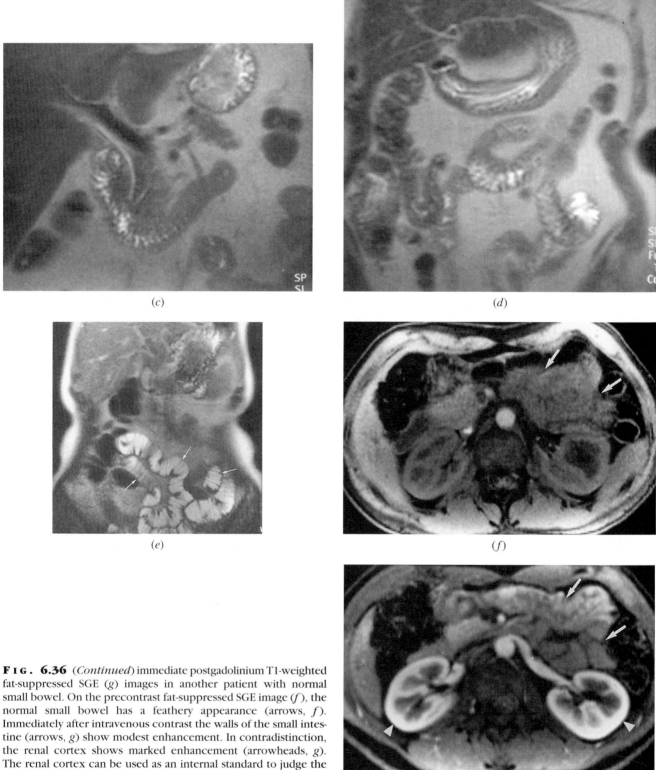

(c)

(d)

(e)

(f)

F I G. 6.36 (*Continued*) immediate postgadolinium T1-weighted fat-suppressed SGE (*g*) images in another patient with normal small bowel. On the precontrast fat-suppressed SGE image (*f*), the normal small bowel has a feathery appearance (arrows, *f*). Immediately after intravenous contrast the walls of the small intestine (arrows, *g*) show modest enhancement. In contradistinction, the renal cortex shows marked enhancement (arrowheads, *g*). The renal cortex can be used as an internal standard to judge the severity of inflammatory bowel disease because severe disease enhances comparably to renal cortex.

(g)

studies. The technique involves administering a large volume of fluid by mouth or enteric tube and acquiring thick-section (5–8 cm) single-shot echo-train spin-echo images with strong T2 weighting, to obtain images that resemble fluoroscopic small bowel images (fig. 6.37). Although both bright and dark lumen contrast agents have been proposed, water-based methods may be relatively easy to implement and may provide excellent signal characteristics, resulting in bright lumen on T2-weighted and dark lumen on T1-weighted images. In addition, to slow absorption of the water, which normally would occur rapidly in the jejunum, osmotic and viscosity agents may be added.

The use of a naso-jejunal tube for administration of intraluminal contrast may provide superior small bowel distension; oral administration may provide sufficient advantage for visualization of disease, particularly for demonstration of inflammatory bowel disease and related complications. Furthermore, enteroclysis requires fluoroscopic assistance and is an invasive procedure for which patient compliance may be less favorable compared to an MR small bowel follow-through technique. The addition of 2.5% mannitol, a nondigested carbohydrate, provides an osmotic load that slows water absorption. The

further addition of a viscosity agent has been shown to further improve small bowel distension. This approach may be preferable to methylcellulose and water, as used for conventional fluoroscopic small bowel examinations, as the degree of reflux emesis is felt to be a drawback particular to methylcellulose. Between 1000 and 1200 ml of the water-based contrast can be given to the patient for oral ingestion 20 to 30 minutes before the examination and 20 mg of metoclopromide or 100 mg of erythromycin given intravenously to promote gastric emptying. Metoclopromide is well tolerated, whereas erythromycin can generate nausea, although generally well-tolerated at the low dose used here.

Initial images can be obtained with both single-shot T2 and true-FISP, both acquired with breath hold or respiratory gated and both providing high contrast and resistant to deterioration from bowel motion. These images can give information regarding the degree and location of optimal small bowel distension. Fat-suppressed single-shot T2 technique may yield key images for visualization of edema and abnormal fluid collections outside of the bowel. In addition, a coronal MRCP heavily T2-weighted single-shot slab technique can be used to produce a single slice within 2 to 5 s,

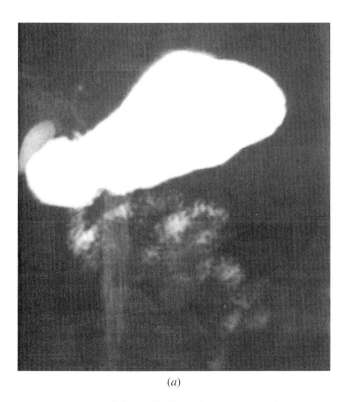

(a)

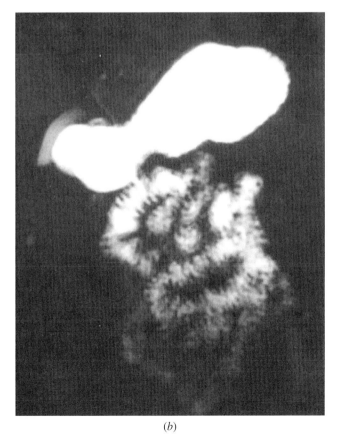

(b)

F I G . 6.37 Small bowel follow-through. SS-ETSE images with strong T2-weighting. Thick-slab (6 cm) images obtained 5 (a) and 20 (b) min after ingestion of a large volume of water resemble fluoroscopic small bowel images.

resulting in an image that is similar to a small bowel fluoroscopic view. However, without concerns for radiation dose, these slab images can be obtained serially over time to monitor progression of the oral contrast and these images then can scrolled together into a single series of images that, when viewed one after the other, may generate information regarding bowel motion and reveal subtle areas of abnormalities such as fixed narrowing from adhesion or hernia. Once the distal ileum is distended, gadolinium-enhanced 3D-GE T1-weighted images are acquired in both the coronal and axial planes. A 20-s delay image set through the liver and upper abdomen can be obtained and then followed by 70- and 90-s acquisitions in the coronal and axial planes through the abdomen and pelvis. This provides comprehensive examination of the abdominal solid organs. Just before gadolinium administration, 1 mg of glucagon or 20 mg of Buscopan may be injected intravenously to produce bowel paralysis and improve image quality. This will also slow progression of the oral contrast. Advantages and specific applications for disease visualization are discussed in the corresponding sections that follow.

Congenital Lesions

Rotational Abnormalities

Intestinal malrotations or nonrotations result from disordered or interrupted embryonic intestinal counterclockwise rotations around the axis of the superior mesenteric artery. In rotational abnormalities, the normal rotations and fixations are either incomplete or occur out of sequence [56]. The most common form, nonrotation, is readily apparent on tomographic images, demonstrated by the lack of normal passage of the third and fourth parts of the duodenum from right to left of midline. The other types of malrotation occur less frequently and include incomplete rotation, reversed rotation, and anomalous fixation or fusion of the mesenteries. Marcos et al. [57] have shown that rotational abnormalities can be well visualized on snap-shot echo-train spin-echo images (fig. 6.38).

Diverticulum

A diverticulum is defined as a mucosal outpouching emanating from the alimentary tract that communicates with the gut lumen. Congenital diverticula usually contain all three layers with a complete muscularis externa in the outpouching; in contrast, acquired diverticula lack a muscularis externa. Diverticula of the jejunum and ileum involve the mesenteric side of the bowel. In the small intestine muscular wall, points at which mesenteric vessels and nerves enter provide potential sites of weakness where mucosa may herniated into the mesentery.

Small bowel diverticula occur most commonly in the duodenum. Multiple small bowel diverticula may be associated with intestinal bacterial overgrowth and resultant metabolic complications. Diverticula may be demonstrated on MR images as air or air fluid-containing structures that arise from the bowel (fig. 6.39). Change in size of the diverticulum may be observed between sequences in an MRI examination, reflecting contraction and expansion. Single-shot echo-train spin echo is effective at demonstrating this entity. The absence of appreciable susceptibility artifact from air in the diverticula with this technique allows clear delineation of diverticula and their origin from bowel [57].

Meckel Diverticulum

Meckel diverticulum is a remnant of the omphalomesenteric duct (vitelline duct). Normally, this duct is obliterated by the fifth week of gestation. Meckel diverticulum is common, with a prevalence of about 2% in the general population. It occurs within 25 cm of the ileocecal valve along the antimesenteric border. Most patients with Meckel diverticulum are asymptomatic. If the diverticulum contains acid-secreting epithelium of gastric mucosa, ulceration and bleeding may result. Intussusception and inflammation may also occur, irrespective of the type of mucosa present. The mainstay of diagnosis has been ^{99m}Tc-pertechnetate scintigraphy and enteroclysis. MRI, like scintigraphy, exploits the presence of gastric mucosa in making the diagnosis. Because gastric mucosa enhances more than any other segment of bowel, a gastric-lined Meckel diverticulum will demonstrate marked enhancement on immediate (capillary phase) and interstitial-phase postgadolinium images (fig. 6.40) [58, 59].

Atresia and Stenosis

Intestinal atresia results in complete absence of a portion of bowel or closure by an occluding mucosal diaphragm, whereas congenital stenosis implies a narrowing of an intestinal segment by fibrosis or stricture. Both may cause intestinal obstruction. Duodenal atresia represents the most common gastrointestinal atresia; jejunal and ileal atresia are rare and occur with equal frequency.

Approximately 25% of cases will have associated congenital anomalies including malrotation of the gut and Meckel diverticulum. Although the precise etiology of congenital atresia and stenosis is not known, lesions appear to arise from developmental failure, intrauterine vascular accidents, or intussusceptions occurring after the intestine has developed. Barium studies are the most common means of diagnosis, although T2-weighted single-shot echo-train spin-echo images can highlight the atretic/stenotic segment and proximal dilatation (fig. 6.41).

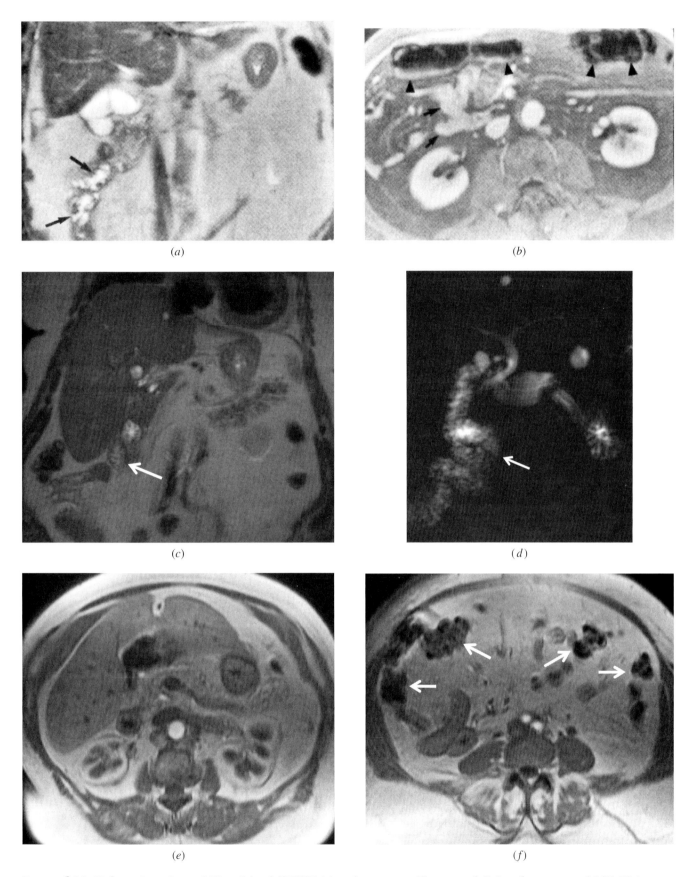

(a)

(b)

(c)

(d)

(e)

(f)

F I G . 6.38 Malrotation. Coronal T2-weighted SS-ETSE (*a*) and transverse 90-s postgadolinium fat-suppressed SGE (*b*) images. Coronal T2 image (*a*) demonstrates that small bowel is predominantly located in the right side of the abdomen (arrows). The 90-s postgadolinium fat-suppressed SGE image (*b*) demonstrates that the third and fourth portions of the duodenum are located to the right of midline (arrows, *b*). Note that the large bowel is in a normal location (arrowheads). (Reprinted with permission from Marcos HB, Semelka RC, Noone TC, Woosley JT, Lee JKT: MRI of normal and abnormal duodenum using half-Fourier single-shot RARE and gadolinium-enhanced spoiled gradient-echo sequences. *Magn Reson Imaging* 17: 869–880, 1999.) Coronal T2-weighted single-shot echo-train spin-echo (*c*), coronal fast spin-echo thick-section MRCP (*d*), and transverse T1-weighted postgadolinium arterial-phase SGE (*e, f*) images demonstrate malrotation of the small bowel in another patient. The duodenum does not form its normal C loop, and the 4th part of duodenum and jejunal loops are located at the right side of the abdomen (arrows, *c*, *d*). These findings are consistent with malrotation. Note that the colon is located in its normal position (arrows, *f*).

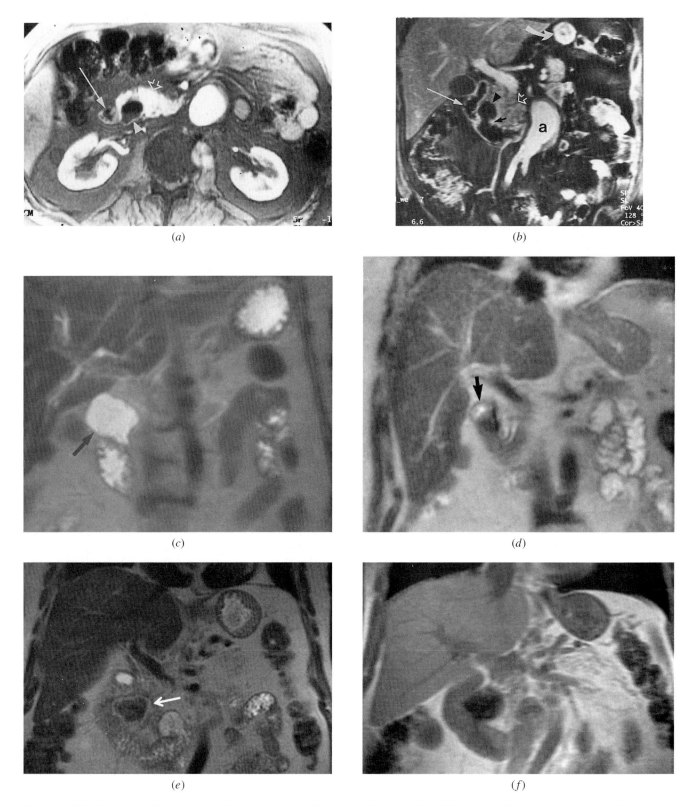

FIG. 6.39 Duodenal diverticulum. Transverse immediate (*a*) and coronal 90-s (*b*) postgadolinium fat-suppressed SGE images. An air- and fluid-containing diverticulum (arrowheads, *a*, *b*) is interposed between the duodenum (long arrows, *a*, *b*) and the head of the pancreas (open arrows, *a*, *b*). On the coronal image, a neck (short arrow, *b*) connecting the diverticulum to the duodenum is well shown, which confirms that the lesion represents a diverticulum and not a cystic mass in the head of the pancreas. Duodenal diverticula are common and usually incidental findings. The normal gastric wall (curved arrow, *b*) enhances more intensely than normal small bowel. An abdominal aortic aneurysm (a, *b*) is also present. Coronal T2-weighted SS-ETSE images (*c*, *d*) in two other patients demonstrate fluid-containing duodenal diverticula (arrow, *c*, *d*). Coronal T2-weighted single shot-echo-train spin-echo (*e*), coronal T1-weighted SGE (*f*), transverse T1-weighted SGE (*g*), and transverse T1-weighted postgadolinium hepatic venous phase

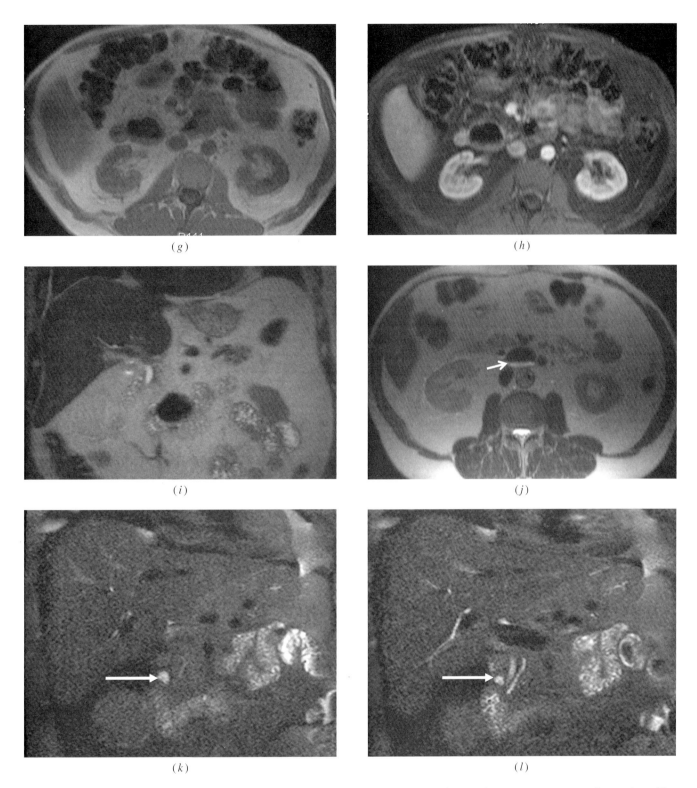

(g)

(h)

(i)

(j)

(k)

(l)

F I G . 6.39 (*Continued*) fat-suppressed SGE (*h*) images demonstrate a duodenal diverticulum (arrow, *e*) in another patient. The duodenal diverticulum is located at the medial side of the second portion of the duodenum. It contains air and therefore shows low signal on both on T2-weighted and T1-weighted images. The duodenal wall shows regular enhancement on postgadolinium image (*h*). Note that an air-fluid level is seen in the diverticulum on postgadolinium image (*h*). Coronal (*i*) and transverse (*j*) T2-weighted single-shot echo-train spin-echo images demonstrate a duodenal diverticulum in another patient. The diverticulum is located in the 3rd to 4th portion of the duodenum. Note that an air-fluid level (arrow, *j*) is seen on transverse image (*j*). Coronal T2-weighted thin-section single-shot echo-train spin-echo MRCP (*k*, *l*) and reconstructed 3D MIP MRCP (*m*) images demonstrate a small duodenal diverticulum (arrows, *k–m*) located at the medial aspect of the 2nd portion of the duodenum adjacent to the major papilla in another patient. The diverticulum does not have any connection with the common bile duct and shows high signal because of its fluid content.

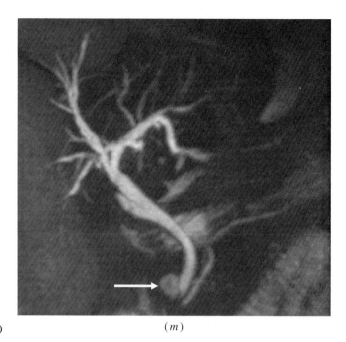

F I G . 6.39 (*Continued*)   (*m*)

F I G . 6.40 Meckel diverticulum. Gadolinium-enhanced T1-weighted fat-suppressed spin-echo image in a patient with lower gastrointestinal bleeding. A teardrop-shaped Meckel diverticulum (arrow) extends from a loop of mildly dilated ileum. The inner wall of the diverticulum enhances to a greater extent than adjacent small bowel and colon. This allows detection of the diverticulum, and the degree of enhancement is consistent with the presence of gastric mucosa.

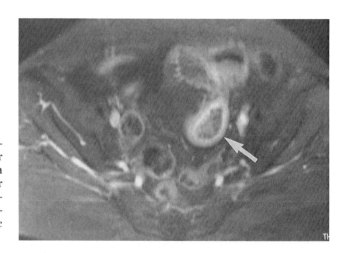

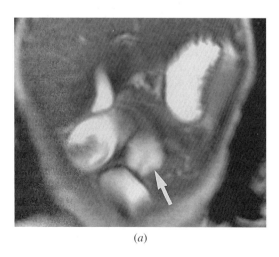

(*a*)

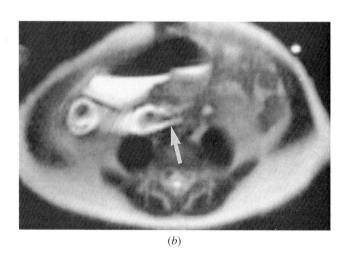

(*b*)

F I G . 6.41 Congenital stenosis, duodenum. Coronal (*a*) and transverse (*b*) T2-weighted SS-ETSE images. The coronal image demonstrates dilatation of the third part of the duodenum (arrow, *a*). The duodenum is noted to narrow (arrow, *b*) at the crossing of the superior mesenteric artery on the transverse image (*b*).

Choledochocele

Choledochocele is a congenital anomaly characterized by cystic dilatation of the distal common bile duct in the region of the papilla. Clinically, it may be associated with abdominal pain, bleeding, jaundice, and pancreatitis. The diverticulum can contain calculi. On imaging examinations, these may appear as polypoid masses indistinguishable from papillary edema or carcinoma. When large enough, they can protrude into the duodenum and even occlude it. MR cholangiopancreatography (MRCP) (see Chapter 3, *Gallbladder and Biliary System*) and single-shot echo-train spin-echo images facilitate establishing the correct diagnosis (fig. 6.42).

Mass Lesions

Benign and malignant small intestinal tumors are uncommon. Adenomas, leiomyomas, and lipomas constitute the three most common primary benign small intestinal tumors [60]. In general, benign tumors occur less commonly in the duodenum and increase in frequency toward the ileum.

Benign Masses

Polyps. The term "polyp" is a clinical term for any tumorous mass that projects above the surrounding normal mucosa. Hamartomatous, hyperplastic, and inflammatory polyps are benign, nonneoplastic lesions; adenomatous polyps (fig. 6.43) are true neoplastic tumors containing dysplastic epithelium and are precursors of carcinoma.

Polyps are infrequently symptomatic and are usually incidental findings at autopsy. Clinically evident polyps present with pain, obstruction, or bleeding. Polyps are the most common lead points for intussusceptions in adults. Except in hereditary polyposis syndrome, adenomatous polyps of the small intestine are rare, with <0.05% of all intestinal adenomas arising in the small intestine [61]. Overall, the frequency of cancer in adenomas ranges from 45% to 63% [62]. Multiple adenomas predominate in the setting of Gardner and familial polyposis syndromes. Small bowel hamartomas occur commonly in Peutz–Jeghers syndrome and rarely in juvenile polyposis syndromes.

Similar to polyps elsewhere in the gastrointestinal tract, small bowel polyps appear as enhancing masses on gadolinium-enhanced fat-suppressed SGE or 3D-GE images (fig. 6.44). On single-shot echo-train spin-echo images, polyps appear as rounded low-signal-intensity masses. Polyps are termed pedunculated when they are anchored by a slender stalk and sessile when they are attached by a broad base. Although it may not be possible to exclude a focus of carcinoma within the polyp, extraserosal extension of a polyp is compatible with malignant degeneration.

Neurofibromas. Primary neurogenic tumors of the gastrointestinal tract are rare. Pathologically, neurofibromas consist of neoplastic cells arising from the nerve sheath.

Gastrointestinal involvement in neurofibromatosis type 1, or Von Recklinghausen disease, is well recognized, and solitary or multiple gastrointestinal tumors have been reported in 11–25% of patients with this disease [63, 64].

Neurofibromatosis type 1 predisposes individuals to an increased risk of a variety of gastrointestinal lesions, including neurofibromas, schwanomas, smooth muscle tumors, and neuroendocrine tumors of the duodenum and ampullary region [63].

The detection of these tumors by MRI depends essentially on their size [65]. They appear as intraluminal masses that enhance to the same extent as bowel wall (fig. 6.45).

Leiomyomas. Leiomyomas are common tumors of the small bowel, but the majority are subcentimetric and not visible on imaging studies. The frequency of small bowel leiomyoma is comparable to that of adenoma. Leiomyomas are smooth muscle proliferations that usually originate in the submucosa or muscularis externa. Depending on their location, they may protrude into the lumen or produce a mass effect on adjacent bowel. In general, leiomyomas are usually solitary lesions. As leiomyomas enlarge, they may undergo central necrosis and bleeding. Features of small bowel leiomyoma include the following: They are mural-based and do not encroach substantially on the lumen, they are well-defined and oval, enhancement is relatively uniform, and they exhibit delayed relatively increased enhancement at 2–5 min after contrast (fig. 6.46).

Lipomas. Lipomas are mature adipose tissue proliferations that arise in the submucosa and occur predominantly in the duodenum and ileum. Similar to leiomyomas, they may ulcerate and bleed. Lipomas are high in signal intensity on T1-weighted images and have signal intensity comparable to intra-abdominal fat on T2-weighted images. On T1-weighted fat-suppressed images these lesions show a characteristic loss of signal intensity.

Varices. Duodenal varices may be seen in isolation or in conjunction with portal vein obstruction. SGE or fat-suppressed SGE gadolinium-enhanced images obtained during the venous phase or further delayed phase demonstrate varices as thin tubular structures within the bowel wall (fig. 6.47). 3D-GE T1-weighted gadolinium-enhanced fat suppressed technique provides optimal visualization; however, varices can also be visualized with a steady-state precession true-FISP sequence.

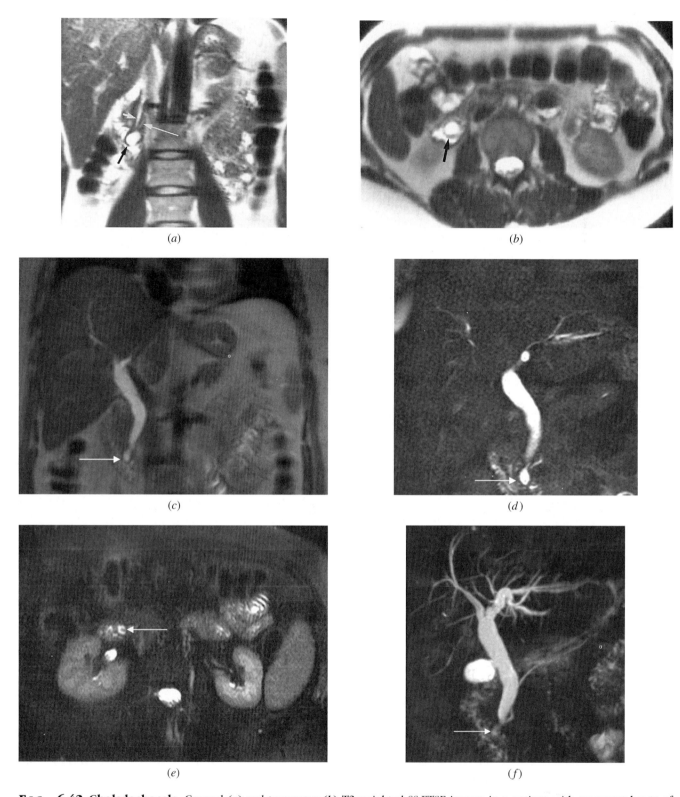

F I G . 6.42 Choledochocele. Coronal (*a*) and transverse (*b*) T2-weighted SS-ETSE images in a patient with recurrent bouts of pancreatitis. A high-signal-intensity choledochocele (black arrow, *a*, *b*) protrudes into the duodenum. The HASTE image clearly defines the cystic nature of the lesion, which excludes an ampullary tumor, and demonstrates the relationship to the common bile duct (small arrow, *a*) and the pancreatic duct (long arrow, *a*). Coronal T2-weighted single-shot echo-train spin-echo (*c*), coronal (*d*) and transverse (*e*) thin-section T2-weighted single-shot echo-train spin-echo MRCP, and reconstructed 3D MIP MRCP (*f*) images demonstrate the protrusion of choledochocele (arrows, *c*-*f*) into the duodenum in another patient.

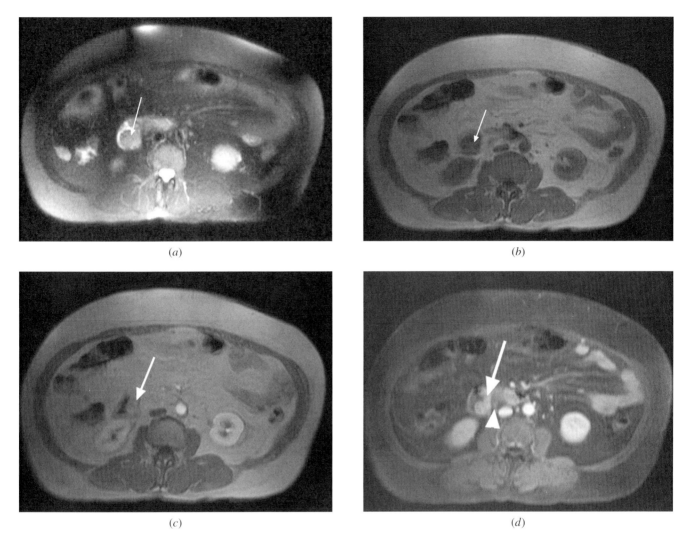

F I G . 6.43 Duodenal adenoma. Axial T2 (*a*),T1 gradient-echo (*b*), and early (*c*) and late (*d*) gadolinium-enhanced T1 images show a discrete mass and thickening of the medial wall of the second part of the duodenum. The pancreas can be clearly seen separate from this mass (arrowhead, *d*).

Malignant Masses

Adenocarcinomas. Small bowel tumors account for only 1% of all gastrointestinal malignancies, and one-half are adenocarcinomas [27]. The most common site for small bowel adenocarcinoma is the duodenum. This tumor frequently occurs in close proximity to the ampulla and as a result may cause obstructive jaundice [66]. Other symptoms, regardless of location, include intestinal obstruction, chronic blood loss, or both. Patients usually are asymptomatic early in the course of their disease; as a result, presentation is often late with advanced disease [27]. The combined use of T2-weighted single-shot echo-train spin-echo and gadolinium-enhanced fat-suppressed SGE or 3D-GE imaging has resulted in reproducibly high image quality for the evaluation of small bowel neoplasms [67]. Duodenal neoplasms are particularly well shown because of the

relatively fixed position of the duodenum in the anterior pararenal space. The most consistent MR imaging feature that permits their detection is that tumors enhance heterogeneously on interstitial-phase gadolinium-enhanced images (fig. 6.48). T2-weighted single-shot echo-train spin-echo images provide information about the tumor itself and can be performed as an MRCP study to evaluate the biliary tree. Immediate postgadolinium SGE or 3D-GE images may be used to survey the liver for metastatic disease, whereas 2-min postgadolinium fat-suppressed SGE or 3D-GE images may be obtained to determine the presence of lymphadenopathy and intraperitoneal spread.

Gastrointestinal Stromal Tumor (GIST).
Although the stomach is the principal site for approximately two-thirds of all gut stromal tumors (see

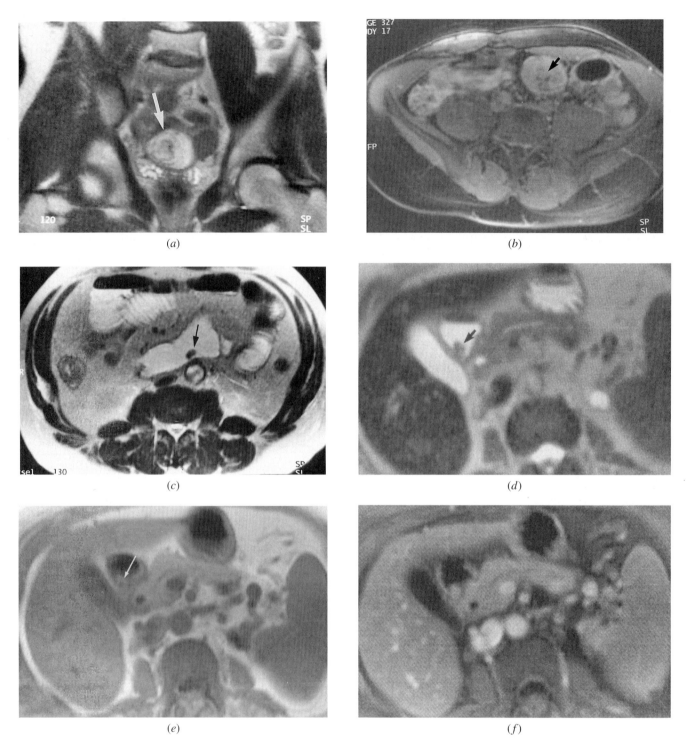

F I G . 6.44 Small bowel polyps. T2-weighted SS-ETSE (*a*) and gadolinium-enhanced fat-suppressed SGE (*b*) images of a hamartoma in Peutz–Jeghers syndrome. A bowel-within-bowel appearance (arrow, *a*) is identified on the T2-weighted image (*a*) in the proximal jejunum because of intussusception. The intussusception is caused by a hamartomatous polyp that has acted as a lead point. The hamartoma is shown as a 1-cm uniformly enhancing mass (arrow) on the gadolinium-enhanced fat-suppressed SGE image (*b*). T2-weighted image (*c*) in a second patient demonstrates a 1-cm polyp (arrow) within a slightly dilated loop of duodenum. T2-weighted SS-ETSE (*d*), SGE (*e*), and 90-s postgadolinium fat-suppressed SGE (*f*) images in a third patient. T2 image shows a low-signal-intensity mass (arrow, *d*) measuring 1.5 cm located in the descending portion of the duodenum. Note that the high signal intensity of intraluminal fluid within the duodenum clearly delineates the polyp, which appears moderately low in signal intensity. Comparing precontrast (*e*) and postgadolinium (*f*) images, enhancement of the polyp is demonstrated, showing it to remain comparable in signal to the duodenal wall, reflecting the tissue nature of the polyp. (Reprinted with permission from Marcos HB, Semelka RC, Noone TC, Woosley JT, Lee JKT: MRI of normal and abnormal duodenum using half-Fourier single-shot RARE and gadolinium-enhanced spoiled gradient-echo sequences. *Magn Reson Imaging* 17: 869–880, 1999.)

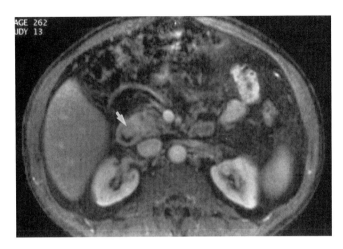

F I G . 6.45 Neurofibroma of duodenum. Transverse 90-s postgadolinium fat-suppressed SGE image in a patient with type 1 neurofibromatosis. A 1-cm intraluminal mass (arrow) arises in the second part of the duodenum. This mass enhances to the same extent as the duodenal wall, reflecting the tissue composition of the neurofibroma. The patient expired, and at autopsy multiple cutaneous and gastrointestinal neurofibromas were found. (Reprinted with permission from Semelka RC, Marcos HB: Polyposis syndromes of the gastrointestinal tract. *J Magn Reson Imaging* 11: 51–55, 2000.)

description above), the small intestine accounts for about 25% of these tumors. As in the stomach, these may be large and ulcerating. Gadolinium-enhanced SGE/3D-GE or fat-suppressed SGE/3D-GE images demonstrate heterogeneous and substantial enhancement of the primary tumor (fig. 6.49). Local or intraperitoneal recurrence may occur after surgical resection (fig. 6.50) and is relatively common, and fat-suppressed gadolinium-enhanced SGE or 3D-GE images are optimal in order to develop maximized contrast between the enhancing tumor and the surrounding retroperitoneal or mesenteric fat. MRI using immediate postgadolinium SGE or 3D-GE is particularly effective at detecting liver metastases because these tend to be hypervascular and often are small.

Lymphoma. Throughout the small intestine and colon are nodules of lymphoid tissue within the mucosa and submucosa. Primary gastrointestinal non-Hodgkin lymphomas are most commonly of the B cell type and appear to arise from B cells of mucosa-associated lymphoid tissue (MALT) (fig. 6.51). In the small intestine, the terminal ileum is the most common site affected (fig. 6.52), which may reflect the relatively greater amount of lymphoid tissue present in this segment compared to the duodenum and jejunum [68]. Gastrointestinal lymphomas comprise 1–2% of all gastrointestinal malignancies and can assume different gross appearances: 1) diffusely infiltrating lesions that often produce full-thickness mural thickening with effacement of overlying mucosal folds, 2) polypoid lesions that protrude into the lumen, and 3) large, exophytic, fungating masses that are prone to ulceration and fistula formation. The small intestine is involved in up to 50% of patients with widespread primary nodal non-Hodgkin lymphoma. The MRI features of small intestine lymphoma include moderately enhancing thickened loops of bowel and large tumor masses that invade the bowel but usually do not result in obstruction (fig. 6.53). In the setting of diffusely infiltrating lesions, the bowel may appear dilated, possibly because of interference with the normal innervation and regulation of smooth muscle bowel wall contraction. The presence of bowel wall mass and dilation without proximal bowel obstruction is suggestive of lymphoma. The presence of splenic lesions or diffuse splenomegaly and mesenteric and retroperitoneal lymphadenopathy supports the diagnosis.

Carcinoid. Carcinoids are the most common primary neoplasm of the small bowel. Tumors are well-differentiated neuroendocrine neoplasms that occur primarily in the distal ileum, in which location they are almost always malignant. Men and women are affected with equal frequency. Most patients present with tumor-related symptoms of bleeding and bowel obstruction or intussusception. Particular to ileal carcinoids are regional mesenteric metastases and vascular sclerosis. The primary tumor may be quite small, with the accompanying lymphadenopathy and desmoplastic reaction in the root of the mesentery presenting as the only visible manifestation of disease. However, when large enough, the primary tumor causes asymmetric bowel wall thickening and enhances heterogeneously, usually moderate in intensity after intravenous gadolinium (figs. 6.54 and 6.55). The characteristic desmoplastic changes in the mesentery and retroperitoneum that occur in response to the secretion of serotonin and tryptophan are low in signal on both T1- and T2-weighted images and show negligible enhancement after contrast. Liver metastases are responsible for the "carcinoid syndrome," which is characterized by vasomotor instability, intestinal hypermotility, and bronchoconstriction [69]. Liver metastases are often hypervascular and high in signal intensity on T2-weighted images, possessing intense ring or uniform enhancement on immediate postgadolinium SGE or 3D-GE images. In the recent series by Bader et al. [70], 98% of liver metastases were hypervascular. Occasionally, carcinoid liver metastases are hypovascular and appear nearly isointense with liver on T2-weighted images and demonstrate faint ring enhancement on immediate postgadolinium SGE or 3D-GE images.

Metastases. Tumors arising in the mesentery, pancreas, stomach, or colon may involve the small intestine

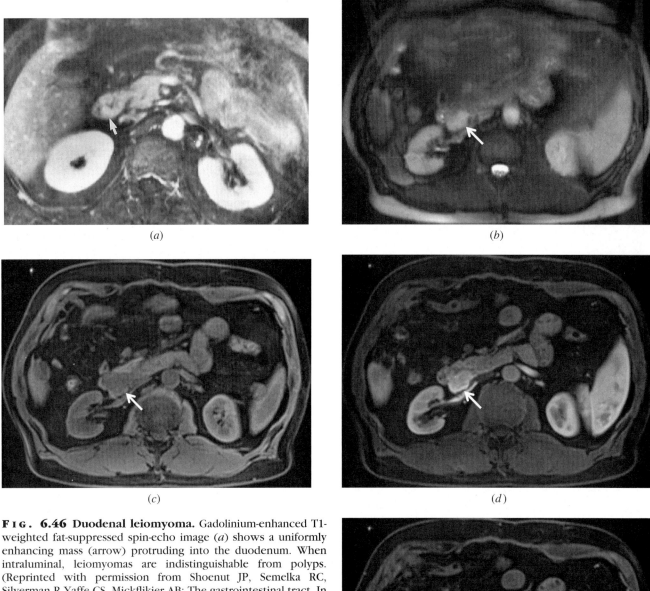

(a)

(b)

(c)

(d)

(e)

F I G . 6.46 Duodenal leiomyoma. Gadolinium-enhanced T1-weighted fat-suppressed spin-echo image (*a*) shows a uniformly enhancing mass (arrow) protruding into the duodenum. When intraluminal, leiomyomas are indistinguishable from polyps. (Reprinted with permission from Shoenut JP, Semelka RC, Silverman R, Yaffe CS, Mickflikier AB: The gastrointestinal tract. In Semelka RC, Shoenut JP (eds.), *MRI of the Abdomen with CT Correlation.* New York: Raven Press, 1993, p. 119–143.) T2 single-shot echo-train spin-echo (*b*), T1-weighted fat-suppressed 3D-GE (*c*), and T1-weighted postgadolinium hepatic arterial dominant-phase (*d*) and interstitial-phase (*e*) fat-suppressed 3D-GE images at 3.0 T demonstrate a duodenal leiomyoma in another patient. A 2-cm well-defined mass (arrows, *b–d*) is evident in the posterior wall of the third part of the duodenum. The mass is homogeneous and mildly high signal on T2 (*b*) and mildly low signal on T1 (*c*) and exhibits mild homogeneous early enhancement (*c*), with progressive enhancement on the interstitial phase (*d*). The uniform moderately intense enhancement of the leiomyoma on the interstitial phase is a typical feature for this entity. Note that the tumor does not prominently extend into the lumen.

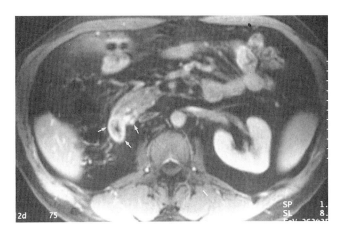

FIG. 6.47 Periduodenal and duodenal varices. Transverse 90-s postgadolinium fat-suppressed SGE image in a patient with splenic vein thrombosis. Periduodenal and duodenal varices are clearly shown as thin enhancing tubular structures adjacent to and within the wall of the duodenum. Venous blood is rerouted to periduodenal and duodenal varices as one of the collateral pathways in the setting of splenic vein thrombosis.

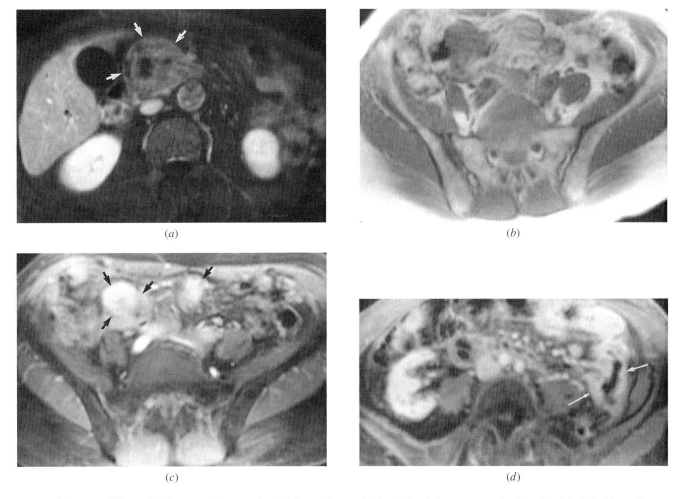

(a) (b) (c) (d)

FIG. 6.48 Small bowel adenocarcinoma. Gadolinium-enhanced T1-weighted fat-suppressed spin-echo (*a*), SGE (*b*), and postgadolinium T1-weighted fat-suppressed spin-echo (*c*) images in two patients with small bowel adenocarcinoma. In the first patient (*a*), the size and extent of a large duodenal tumor (arrows) is well shown on the gadolinium-enhanced fat-suppressed image. In the second patient (*b*, *c*), the neoplasm is difficult to identify on the precontrast SGE image (*b*) because it is isointense with background bowel. On the gadolinium-enhanced fat-suppressed SGE image (*c*), the distal jejunal tumors are conspicuous (*c*) because they are higher in signal intensity and heterogeneous compared to background bowel. Transverse 90-s postgadolinium fat-suppressed SGE image (*d*) in another patient with adenocarcinoma of the jejunum. Irregular thickening and enhancement of a segment of proximal jejunum is apparent (arrows, *d*). Coronal (*e*) and transverse (*f*) T2-weighted single-shot echo-train spin-echo and transverse

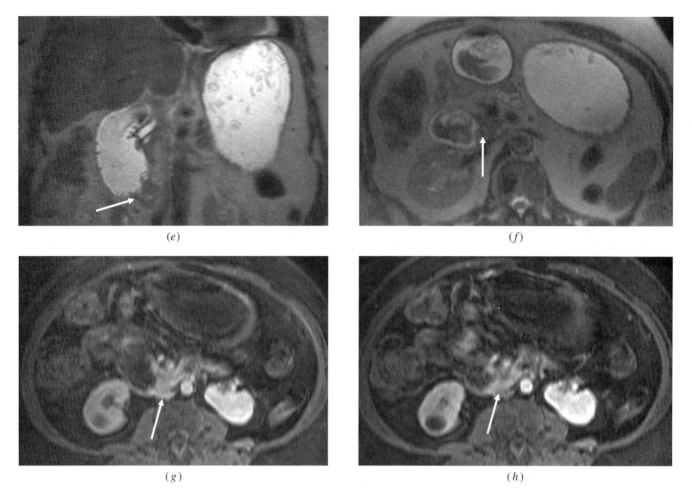

(e)

(f)

(g)

(h)

FIG. 6.48 (*Continued*) T1-weighted postgadolinium interstitial-phase fat-suppressed 3D-GE (*g, h*) images demonstrate a duode-nal adenocarcinoma (arrows, *e–h*) in another patient. The wall of the third portion of the duodenum is diffusely thickened because of adenocarcinoma. The tumor shows intense enhancement and causes obstruction. The stomach and proximal portions of the duodenum is dilated because of the obstruction.

through contiguous extension (fig. 6.56). Metastases to small intestine from melanoma and carcinomas of the lung, testes, adrenal, ovary, stomach, large intestine, uterus, cervix, liver, and kidney have been reported. Of these malignancies, ovarian tumors are the most common cause of disseminated serosal implants in females and colon adenocarcinoma in males (fig. 6.57).

On gadolinium-enhanced fat-suppressed SGE or 3D-GE images, metastases are moderately high in signal intensity in contrast to the low signal intensity of intra-abdominal fat. Malignant peritoneal tissue enhances moderately to substantially on interstitial-phase gadolin-ium-enhanced images and appears as nodular or irregu-larly thickened peritoneal or serosal tissue (fig. 6.58). Gadolinium-enhanced fat-suppressed imaging has been shown to be more sensitive than CT imaging in detect-ing small tumor nodules [71, 72]. Metastatic spread of carcinomas from distal sites such as breast and lung

occur, and lesions often lodge on the antimesenteric border of the small bowel. These lesions may be visual-ized as intramural masses (fig. 6.59). Metastatic tumor may create large submucosal masses and serve as lead points for intussusception, or mechanical obstruction. The use of water-based oral contrast and a MR small bowel follow-through technique may be valuable in exacerbating and demonstrating metastatic disease and obstruction of different degrees (see fig. 6.57).

Inflammatory, Infectious, and Diffuse Disorders

Inflammatory Bowel Disease
Crohn disease and ulcerative colitis are the most common forms of inflammatory bowel disease (IBD). MRI findings correlate well with clinical evaluation, endoscopy, and histologic findings. It is a robust tech-

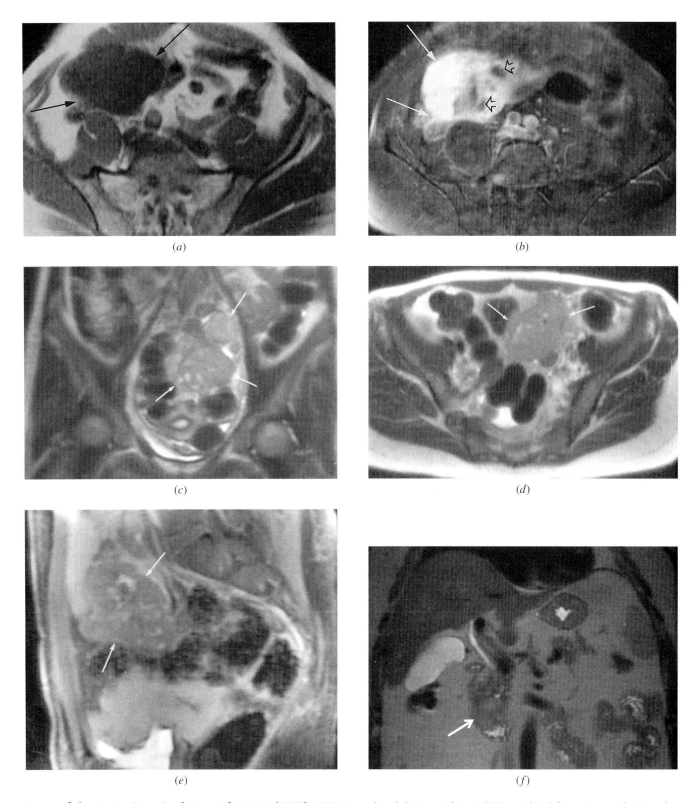

F I G . 6.49 Gastrointestinal stromal tumor (GIST). SGE (*a*) and gadolinium-enhanced T1-weighted fat-suppressed spin-echo (*b*) images. A large exophytic mass (arrows, *a*) arises from the ileum. Lack of proximal bowel obstruction is consistent with its eccentric origin. The tumor's large size coupled with intense enhancement (arrows, *b*) and regions of necrosis (open arrows, *b*) are typical features of GIST. Coronal (*c*) and transverse (*d*) T2-weighted SS-ETSE and sagittal interstitial-phase gadolinium-enhanced fat-suppressed SGE (*e*) images in a second patient with small bowel GIST also show large heterogeneous lobulated masses (arrows, *c–e*) in the pelvis. Coronal T2-weighted single-shot echo-train spin-echo (*f*), transverse T2-weighted fat-suppressed single-shot

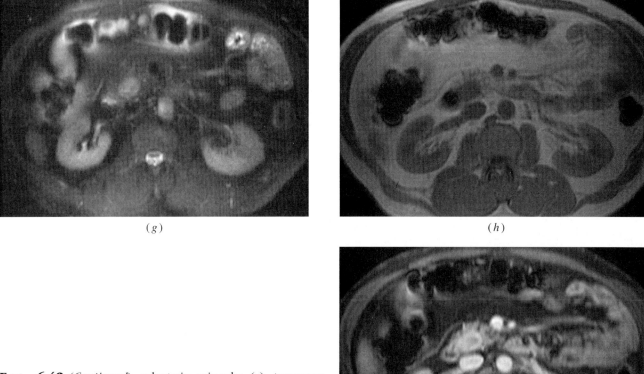

(g)

(h)

(i)

F I G . 6.49 (*Continued*) echo-train spin-echo (*g*), transverse T1-weighted SGE (*h*), and transverse T1-weighted postgadolinium fat-suppressed SGE (*i*) images demonstrate a GIST (arrow, *f*) arising from the second portion of the duodenum in another patient. The tumor shows mildly high signal on T2-weighted images (*f, g*), low signal on T1-weighted SGE (*h*), and intense enhancement on postgadolinium image (*i*). The tumor does not cause luminal obstruction and shows homogeneous internal structure due to its small size.

nique capable of diagnosing type, evaluating severity, and monitoring response to treatment in patients with IBD [1–4]. Conventional fluoroscopic and CT methods of examination of the small bowel may be able to detect disease but have been found to be nonspecific in regard to determining activity of disease. Capsule endoscopy utilizes a miniaturized camera that is ingested and that records the images taken as it passes through the small bowel. This represents another technique sensitive for early mucosal changes. The combination of capsule endoscopy and MR small bowel examination may provide a comprehensive and noninvasive safe approach for detection and characterization of the spectrum of changes associated with IBD, from early to progressed disease.

Crohn Disease. In North America, Crohn disease is the most common inflammatory condition to affect the small bowel. The incidence is greatest in the second and third decades of life, and Crohn disease is most prevalent in urban-dwelling women. There is evidence

for familial associations in Crohn disease, and there is a higher incidence in Ashkenazi Jews. Although the precise etiology of this disease is not fully understood, there is clearly a combination of genetic, immunologic, and infectious factors [73]. Crohn disease usually presents in young adults but can occur in any age group including children and the elderly. Symptoms include watery diarrhea, crampy abdominal pain, weight loss, and fever. Patients with longstanding Crohn disease have a well-documented increased incidence of cancer (approximately 3% of patients) of the gastrointestinal tract, usually involving the colon or ileum.

Although any part of the gastrointestinal tract, from the mouth to the anus, may become involved with Crohn disease, it most commonly involves the terminal ileum, frequently in association with disease in the right colon. Involvement of the terminal ileum occurs in approximately 70% of patients, with combined terminal ileal and cecal disease present in 40% of the total and isolated terminal ileal involvement in the remaining 30%. Five percent of patients will manifest Crohn disease

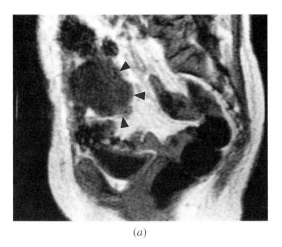

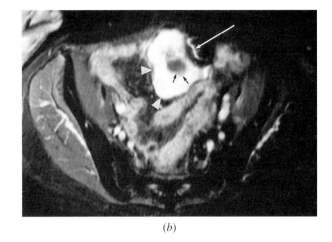

(a)

(b)

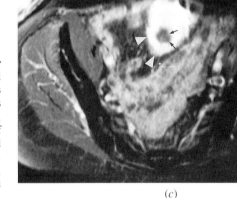

(c)

F I G . 6.50 Recurrent gastrointestinal stromal tumor (GIST). Sagittal SGE (*a*) and gadolinium-enhanced T1-weighted fat-suppressed spin-echo (*b*, *c*) images in a patient with previous surgical resection for GIST. Recurrent GIST exhibits features similar to those of the primary tumor: large size, exophytic growth, hypervascularity, and central necrosis. The eccentric location of the tumor (arrowheads, *a–c*) is seen on all imaging planes. Marked enhancement after intravenous contrast reflects hypervascularity. Necrosis often accompanies these large tumors (short arrows, *b*, *c*). Note the susceptibility artifact (long arrow, *b*) associated with surgical clips from prior resection.

in the duodenum or jejunum. Twenty to thirty percent will have isolated colon involvement [74]. Crohn disease is characterized pathologically by sharply defined areas showing transmural involvement by chronic inflammation, fibrosis, and noncaseating granulomas. Sometimes several well-demarcated lesions are separated by normal bowel, producing what are termed "skip lesions." This particular pattern is not found in ulcerative colitis, which produces instead a confluent or continuous region of inflammation that begins in the rectum and progresses contiguously to involve more proximal large bowel to different degrees. Other features typical of Crohn disease include prominent lymph follicles, lymphangiectasia, and submucosal edema. Grossly, at the beginning stages of Crohn disease, the mucosa may show only small, hyperemic ("aphtoid") ulcerations. In time, the ulcers extend transmurally, often beyond the intestinal serosa to become sinus tracts or fistulae. With the evolution of the disease, the bowel wall becomes thickened and inflexible, secondary to fibrosis. In addition, strictures, abscesses, and lymphoid hyperplasia may complicate the disease. The mesenteric changes include inflammatory stranding, a reflection of dilated vasa rectae and

sinus tracts, reactive lymphadenopathy, and mesenteric fat that becomes stranded and retracted because of development of fibrotic bands, resulting in the descriptive term "creeping" fat. Current therapeutic strategy is based on medical therapy, using a combination of steroid and antibiotics for suppressing acute exacerbations and long-term therapy utilizing immunosuppressants such as 6-mercaptopurine. Surgery is reserved for complicated cases, but anastomotic recurrence is common. Surgery is felt to represent a therapeutic intervention of last resort. Typically, disease will first appear in the second or third decade and subside by the midadult years, allowing eventual weaning from immunosuppressant therapy.

Changes of Crohn disease are well shown on MRI. Severe disease is characterized by wall thickness greater than 1 cm, length of involvement greater than 15 cm, and mural enhancement greater than 100% (fig. 6.60). Mild disease results in subtle findings that may only be appreciated on gadolinium-enhanced fat-suppressed images (fig. 6.61). Multiplanar imaging provides comprehensive information on disease extent and complications. T2-weighted single-shot echo-train spin-echo and

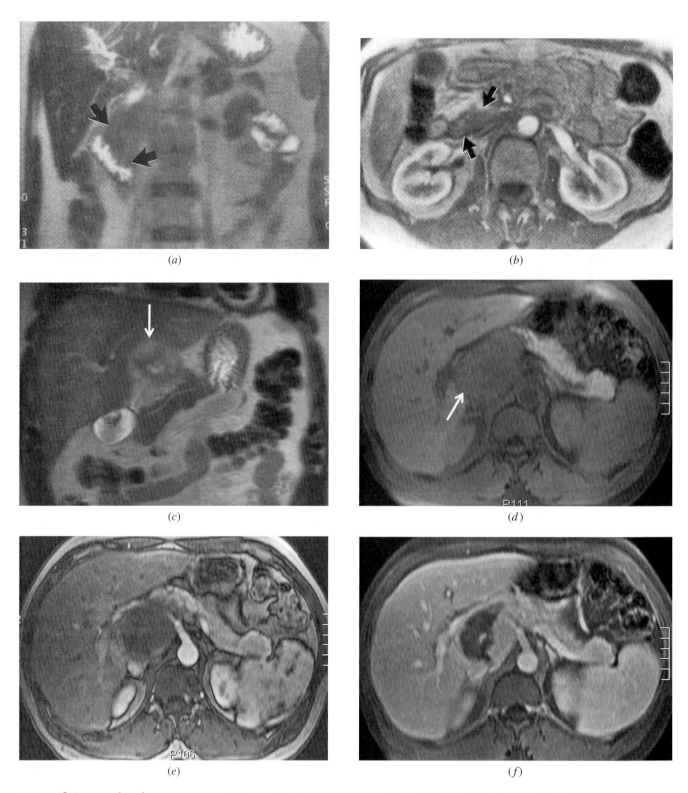

(a)

(b)

(c)

(d)

(e)

(f)

FIG. 6.51 Duodenal MALToma. Coronal T2-weighted SS-ETSE (*a*) and immediate postgadolinium fat-suppressed SGE (*b*) images. T2-weighted image demonstrates irregular thickening of the superior aspect of the duodenal wall caused by a paraduodenal mass (arrows, *a*). Postgadolinium image (*b*) shows a mass that is interposed between the third portion of the duodenum and the head of the pancreas. This mass shows mild heterogeneous enhancement compared to duodenal wall and pancreas, which permits a good distinction between mass and pancreas. Low-grade lymphoma (MALToma type) was proven by endoscopic biopsy. (Reprinted with permission from Marcos HB, Semelka RC, Noone TC, Woosley JT, Lee JKT: MRI of normal and abnormal duodenum using half-Fourier single-shot RARE and gadolinium-enhanced spoiled gradient-echo sequences. *Magn Reson Imaging* 17: 869–880, 1999.) Coronal T2-weighted single-shot echo-train spin-echo (*c*), T1-weighted fat-suppressed SGE (*d*), and T1-weighted postgadolinium hepatic arterial dominant-phase (*e*) and fat-suppressed interstitial-phase (*f*) 3D-GE images demonstrate a large mass originating from the duodenum in another patient. The tumor shows mildly high signal on T2-weighted image (*c*), low signal on T1-weighted image (*d*), and progressive enhancement on postgadolinium images (*e*, *f*). Central necrotic region is detected in the tumor. No biliary or proximal gastrointestinal dilatation is detected. The tumor is located adjacent to the pancreatic head and displaces the IVC posterolaterally and the portal vein anteriorly. The diagnosis is MALToma histopathologically.

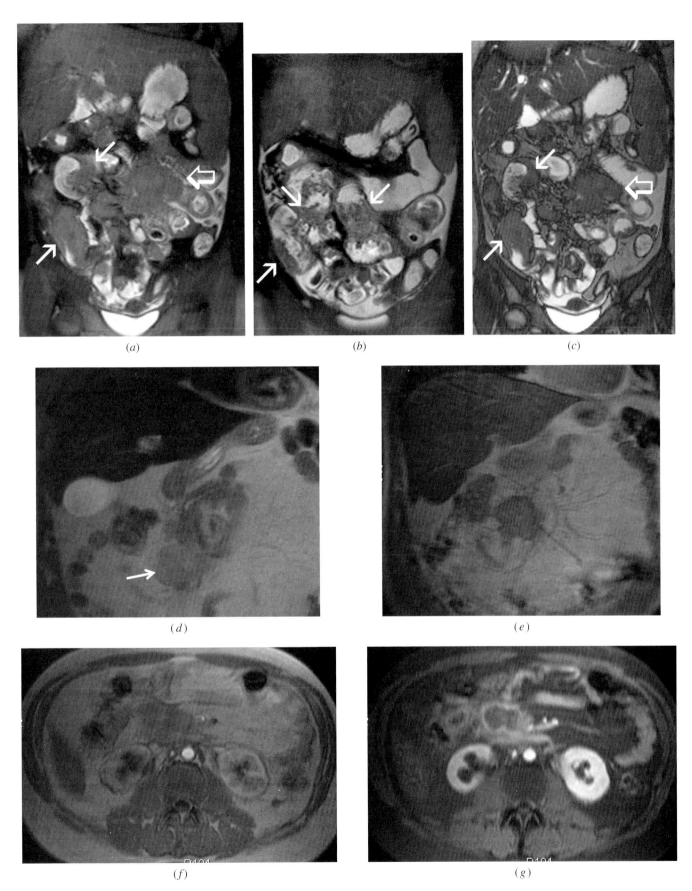

F I G . 6.52 Small bowel lymphoma. A 58-year-old female patient with non-Hodgkin lymphoma of the abdomen. Coronal single-shot echo-train T2 (*a* and *b*) and coronal true-FISP (*c*) images show large mesenteric lymph nodes (open arrows). Lymphoma infiltration of the bowel wall is seen as diffuse wall thickening (arrows, a–c). Coronal T2-weighted single-shot echo-train spin-echo (*d*), coronal T1-weighted SGE (*e*), transverse T1-weighted postgadolinium arterial-phase SGE (*f*), and transverse T1-weighted post-gadolinium interstitial-phase fat-suppressed 3D-GE (*g*) images demonstrate duodenal lymphoma (arrow, *d*) in another patient. The exophytic tumor is located in the third portion of the duodenum. The tumor shows high signal on T2-weighted image and low signal on T1-weighted image. The enhancement is progressive and predominantly peripheral. Note that there is no proximal luminal obstruction. The liver shows low signal on precontrast images because of iron deposition.

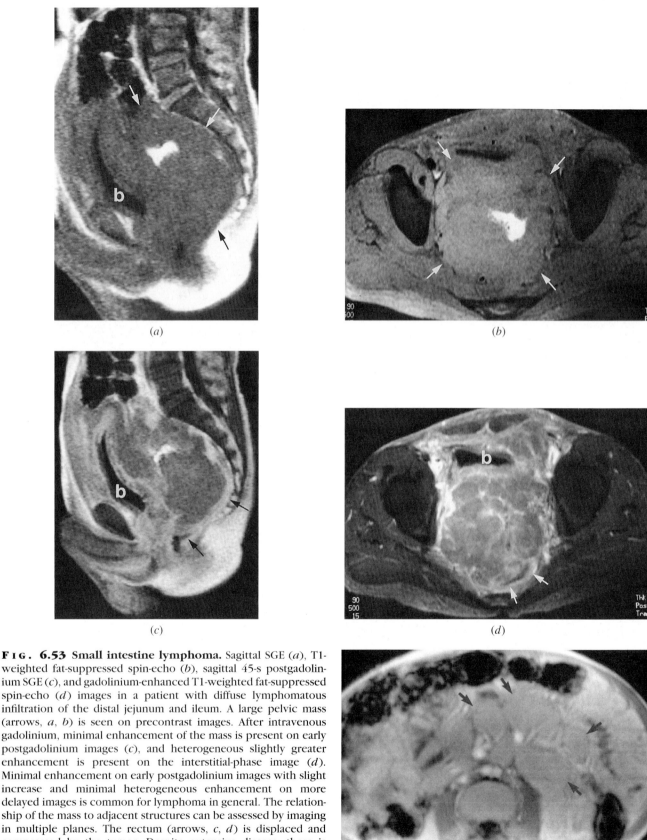

(a)

(b)

(c)

(d)

(e)

FIG. 6.53 Small intestine lymphoma. Sagittal SGE (*a*), T1-weighted fat-suppressed spin-echo (*b*), sagittal 45-s postgadolinium SGE (*c*), and gadolinium-enhanced T1-weighted fat-suppressed spin-echo (*d*) images in a patient with diffuse lymphomatous infiltration of the distal jejunum and ileum. A large pelvic mass (arrows, *a*, *b*) is seen on precontrast images. After intravenous gadolinium, minimal enhancement of the mass is present on early postgadolinium images (*c*), and heterogeneous slightly greater enhancement is present on the interstitial-phase image (*d*). Minimal enhancement on early postgadolinium images with slight increase and minimal heterogeneous enhancement on more delayed images is common for lymphoma in general. The relationship of the mass to adjacent structures can be assessed by imaging in multiple planes. The rectum (arrows, *c*, *d*) is displaced and compressed by the tumor. Despite extensive disease, there is no proximal small bowel obstruction, a characteristic finding with small intestine lymphoma. High signal intensity within the pelvic mass is consistent with hemorrhage. Bladder = b (*a*, *c*, *d*).

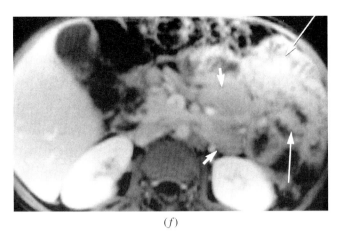

(f)

F I G . 6.53 (*Continued*) Transverse gadolinium-enhanced SGE (*e*) and interstitial-phase gadolinium-enhanced fat-suppressed SGE (*f*) images in a second patient with non-Hodgkin lymphoma. Bulky mesenteric lymphadenopathy (small arrows, *e,f*) is observed as well as thickening of small bowel loops (long arrows, *f*).

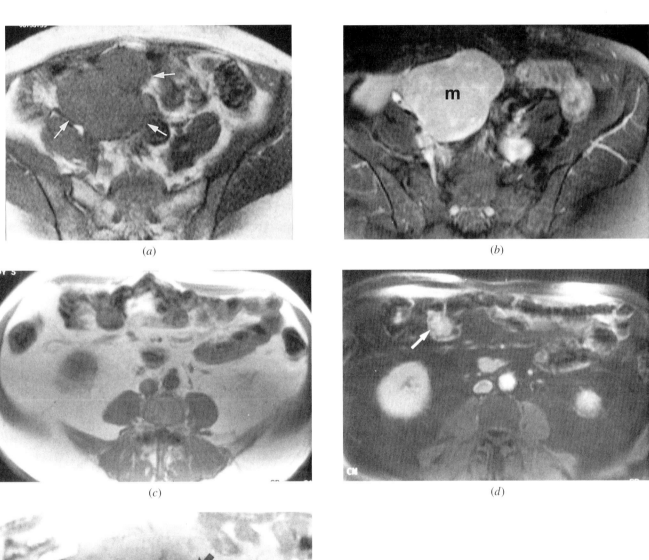

(a)

(b)

(c)

(d)

(e)

F I G . 6.54 Ileal carcinoid. SGE (*a*) and gadolinium-enhanced T1-weighted fat-suppressed spin-echo (*b*) images. The carcinoid tumor (arrows, *a*) causes asymmetric bowel wall thickening, is isointense with bowel on the T1-weighted image (*a*), and enhances heterogeneously and moderately intensely on gadolinium-enhanced interstitial-phase images (*b*). Transverse SGE (*c*) and interstitial-phase gadolinium-enhanced fat-suppressed SGE (*d*) images in a second patient with ileal carcinoid demonstrate a nodular mass originating from the bowel loop that is isointense on the transverse precontrast T1-weighted image and enhances moderately and heterogeneously on the delayed image (arrow, *d*). Transverse T2-weighted SS-ETSE (*e*) in a third patient shows irregular circumferential thickening small bowel consistent with carcinoid tumor.

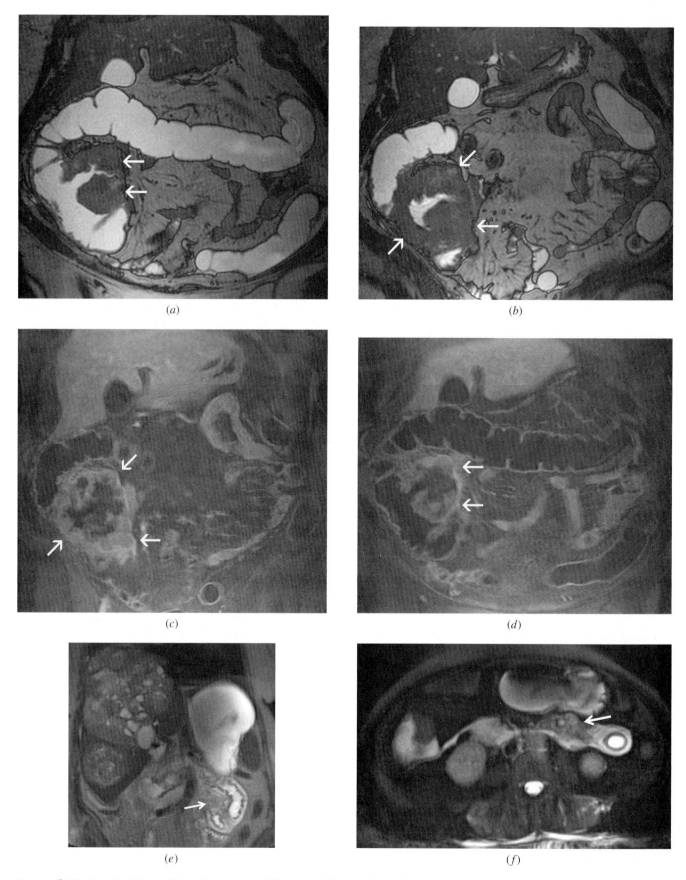

(a)

(b)

(c)

(d)

(e)

(f)

F I G . 6.55 Carcinoid involving the terminal ileum. A 56-year-old man has a large carcinoid tumor demonstrated on coronal true-FISP images (arrows, *a, b*). Central tumor necrosis is best shown on the coronal interstitial-phase gadolinium-enhanced T1-weighted fat-suppressed 3D-GE sequence (arrows, *c, d*). **Jejunal neuroendocrine tumor.** Coronal T2-weighted single-shot echo-train spin-echo (*e*), transverse T2-weighted fat-suppressed single-shot echo-train spin-echo (*f*), transverse T1-weighted fat-suppressed

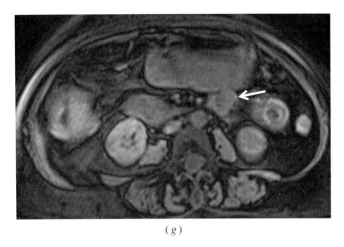

(*g*)

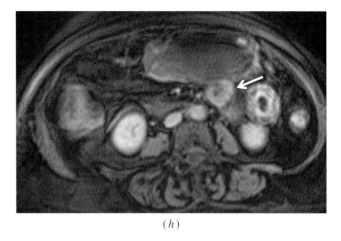

(*h*)

F I G . 6.55 (*Continued*) 3D-GE (*g*), and T1-weighted postgadolinium interstitial phase fat-suppressed 3D-GE (*h*) images demonstrate a small neuroendocrine tumor (arrows, *e–h*) located in the mesentery adjacent to the jejunum. The tumor shows heterogeneous signal on T2-weighted images (*e, f*) and enhances moderately on the interstitial phase (*h*). Multiple liver metastases and ascites are detected. Note that the wall of the jejunal segment adjacent to the tumor shows edema and moderate enhancement.

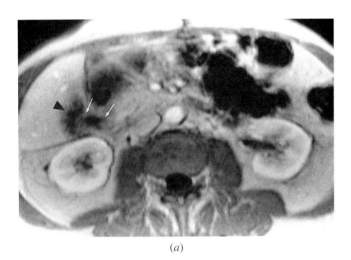

(*a*)

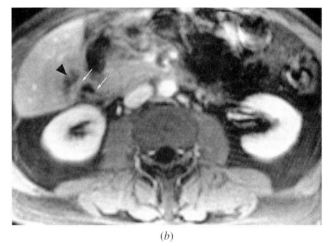

(*b*)

F I G . 6.56 Colon cancer liver metastasis with invasion of the duodenum. Immediate postgadolinium SGE (*a*) and 90-s postgadolinium fat-suppressed SGE (*b*) images in a patient with colon cancer metastasis to liver and duodenum. A peripheral hepatic metastasis (arrowhead, *a, b*) transgresses the liver capsule to directly invade the adjacent duodenum (arrows, *a, b*).

gadolinium-enhanced T1-weighted fat-suppressed SGE or 3D-GE images demonstrate characteristic findings: transmural involvement, skip lesions, and mesenteric inflammatory changes (figs. 6.62–6.64).

Marcos and Semelka evaluated the capability of single-shot echo-train spin-echo and gadolinium-enhanced T1 SGE images for evaluating bowel changes and complications of Crohn disease [75]. The results of this study showed that single-shot echo-train spin-echo image is a very effective technique to demonstrate dilated obstructed bowel, whereas gadolinium-enhanced fat-suppressed SGE is useful in demonstrating inflammatory changes in bowel. Both techniques were effective in showing wall thickening and abscess formation.

Good correlation has been reported between MRI findings and disease activity [2, 4, 5], where demonstration of edema on T2 fat-suppressed images is associated with disease activity (fig. 6.65). These results are in contrast to barium or CT studies, which have limited correlation with symptomatology or response to therapy. It is challenging to discriminate between edema and fibrosis on CT imaging, and it may be largely for this reason that CT findings have not correlated well with disease activity.

Moreover, the potential harm of radiation exposure from serial barium examinations in pregnant women and patients of reproductive age is not inconsequential [74]. MRI may be the modality of choice for evaluation

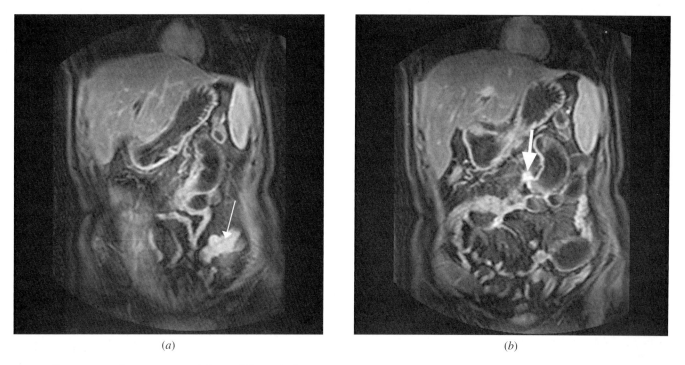

(a)   *(b)*

F I G . 6.57 Serosal metastases with small bowel obstruction. Multiple serosal metastases from large bowel adenocarcinoma resulted in mesenteric metastases and multiple partial small bowel obstructions. Metastases can be identified on gadolinium-enhanced T1 coronal 3D gradient-echo images as abnormal enhancement adjacent to distal (arrow, *a*) and proximal (arrow, *b*) small bowel associated with focal narrowing and proximal dilation of the involved bowel segment. The patient was given oral water-based contrast mixed with mannitol and locust bean gum to achieve better small bowel distension and to increase the conspicuity of partially obstructing lesions.

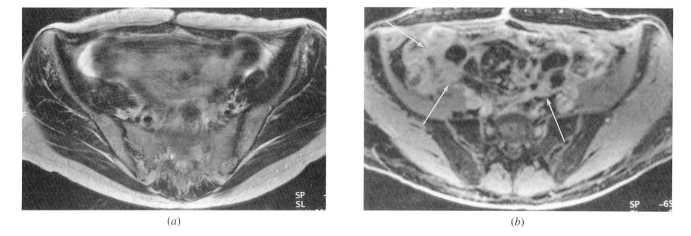

(a)   *(b)*

F I G . 6.58 Ovarian carcinoma metastases to the peritoneal and serosal surfaces. Transverse 512-resolution T2-weighted echo-train spin-echo (*a*) and 90-s postgadolinium fat-suppressed SGE (*b*) images highlight the improvement in disease detection afforded by breath-hold gadolinium-enhanced fat-suppressed SGE. On the high-resolution T2-weighted image, bowel motion degrades image quality; no metastatic disease can be identified. On the gadolinium-enhanced fat-suppressed SGE image, the acquisition during suspended respiration avoids breathing artifact and minimizes bowel motion. Enhancement of irregularly thickened tissue along the peritoneum and serosal surface of bowel (arrows, *b*) is consistent with widespread metastatic disease.

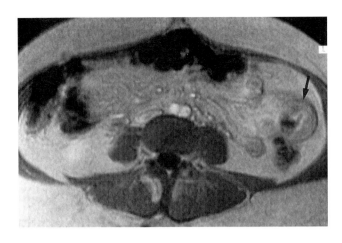

FIG. 6.59 Hematogenous metastases. Transverse 45-s post-gadolinium SGE image demonstrates an eccentric mural tumor in the midjejunum (arrow). This tumor was a hematogenous metastasis from uterine leiomyosarcoma.

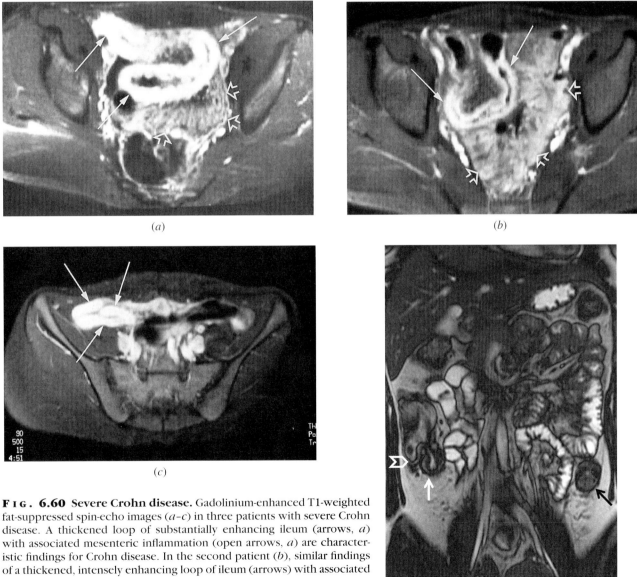

(a)

(b)

(c)

(d)

FIG. 6.60 Severe Crohn disease. Gadolinium-enhanced T1-weighted fat-suppressed spin-echo images (a–c) in three patients with severe Crohn disease. A thickened loop of substantially enhancing ileum (arrows, a) with associated mesenteric inflammation (open arrows, a) are characteristic findings for Crohn disease. In the second patient (b), similar findings of a thickened, intensely enhancing loop of ileum (arrows) with associated mesenteric inflammation (open arrows) are identified. In the third patient (c), multiple thickened loops of intensely enhancing ileum are present (arrows). Coronal T2-weighted true-FISP (d, e) and coronal T1-weighted

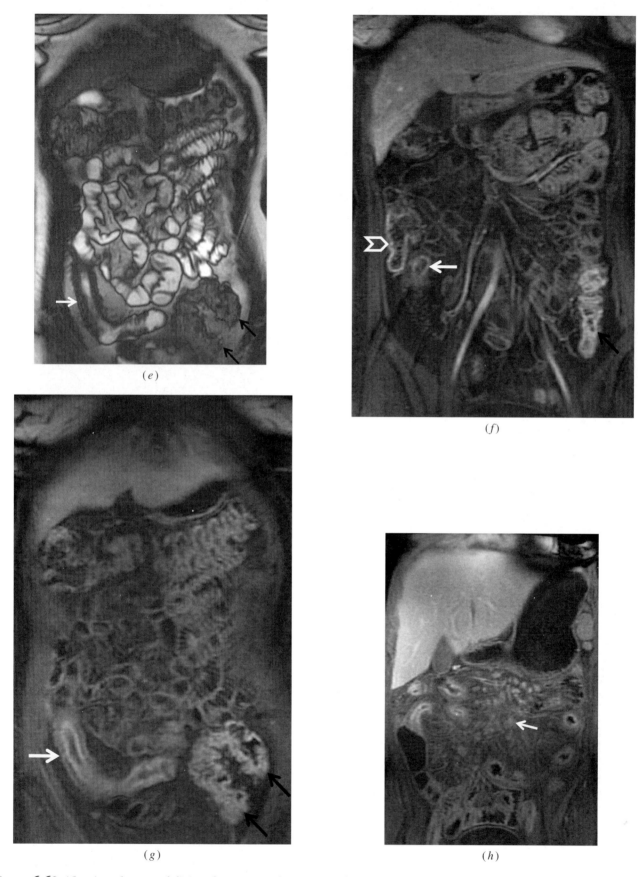

(e)

(f)

(g)

(h)

FIG. 6.60 *(Continued)* postgadolinium fat-suppressed interstitial-phase 3D-GE (*f, g*) images demonstrate severe Crohn disease in another patient. The walls of terminal ileum (white arrows, *d–g*), cecum (open arrows, *d, f*), descending colon (black arrows, *d, f*), and sigmoid colon (black arrows, *e, g*) show thickening and edema (white arrows, *d, e*). Edema is seen as high signal in the wall. Associated mild mesenteric inflammation and fibrofatty proliferation are detected. The wall of terminal ileum shows trilaminar enhancement (white arrow, *g*) pattern due to the presence of submucosal edema, which is seen as low signal intensity. The walls of the cecum and colon show diffuse enhancement (open and black arrows, *f, g*). Coronal T1-weighted postgadolinium interstitial phase fat-suppressed 3D-GE image (*h*) in another patient with severe Crohn disease demonstrates multiple enlarged and enhancing mesenteric lymph nodes (arrow, *h*). Note that the walls ileal and colonic segments show diffuse and mucosal increased enhancement, respectively.

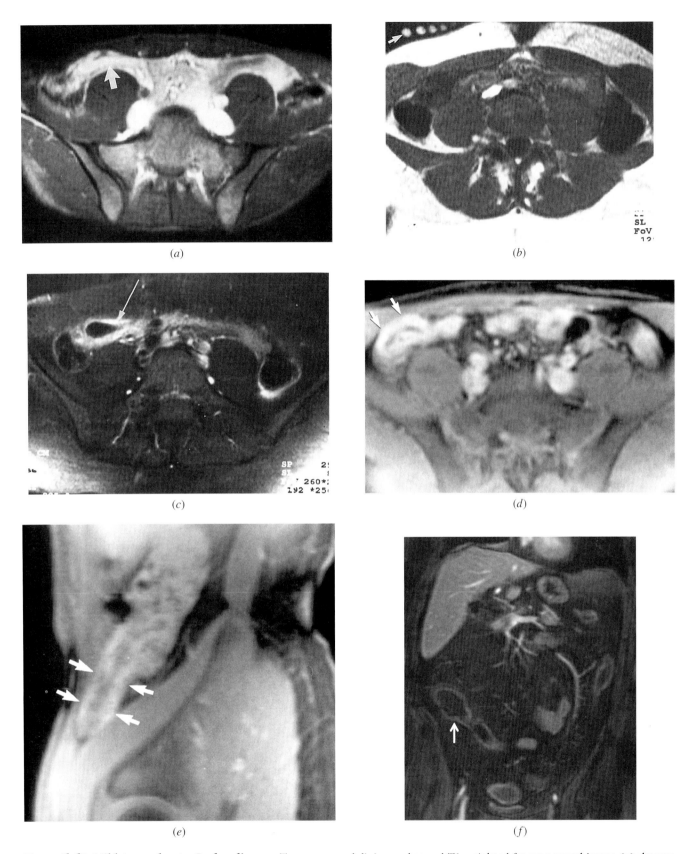

FIG. 6.61 Mild to moderate Crohn disease. Transverse gadolinium-enhanced T1-weighted fat-suppressed image (*a*) demonstrates moderate inflammatory disease of the terminal ileum (arrow, *a*), that has a wall thickness of 5 mm,<10 cm of diseased bowel, and moderate wall enhancement. SGE (*b*) and gadolinium-enhanced T1-weighted fat-suppressed spin-echo (*c*) images in a second patient with mild Crohn disease. The unenhanced image (*b*) appears unremarkable. On the gadolinium-enhanced image, transmural enhancement is apparent with wall thickness of 5 mm, length of involved segment of <10 cm, and moderate mural enhancement. This constellation of imaging findings is consistent with mild disease. Assessment of severity of disease must be determined on the nondependent bowel wall (arrow, *c*) after intravenous contrast administration. Lipid beads (small arrow, *b*) demarcate the area of patient tenderness. Transverse (*d*) and sagittal (*e*) interstitial-phase gadolinium-enhanced fat-suppressed SGE images in a third patient show segmental wall thickening and abnormal enhancement of the distal ileum (arrows, *d, e*). Coronal (*f*) and transverse (*g*) T1-weighted postgadolinium interstitial phase fat-suppressed 3D-GE images at 3.0 T demonstrate mild Crohn disease in another patient.

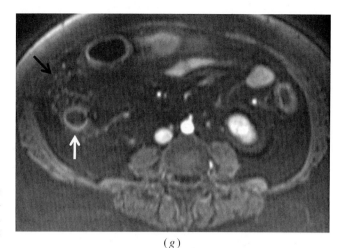

(*g*)

FIG. 6.61 (*Continued*) The wall of terminal ileum (white arrows, *f*, *g*) is thickened and shows diffuse increased enhancement. Adjacent mesenteric inflammation (black arrow, *g*) and inflamed lymph nodes (black arrow, *g*) are detected. Note that fatty proliferation is seen around the terminal ileum.

of Crohn disease in patients with contraindication to barium examinations or CT imaging (fig. 6.66).

The MRI criteria of mild, moderate, and severe disease have been described and are a function of wall thickness, length of diseased segment, and percentage of mural contrast enhancement (Table 6.2). The extent of mural enhancement may also be determined by comparison of bowel enhancement on gadolinium-enhanced fat-suppressed SGE or 3D-GE with that of the renal parenchyma [75]. Bowel should not enhance to the same degree as renal cortex on either early capillary-phase images or >1-min interstitial-phase images. Enhancement equivalent to or greater than renal cortex is abnormal and most often reflects the presence of inflammatory change.

MRI assessment is made on gadolinium-enhanced T1-weighted fat-suppressed images using the nondependent bowel surface. It is critical that the time point for determining percentage of enhancement is standardized. This establishes reproducible measures of disease activity between studies in the same patient. We have used a time point of 2.5 min after injection. Immediate postgadolinium images reflect significant perivascular inflammation and increased capillary blood flow. Commonly, the inner half of the bowel wall enhances most intensely in this phase of enhancement in severely inflamed bowel. Later interstitial-phase images demonstrate more uniform enhancement in diseased bowel, reflecting capillary leakage and decreased venous removal in transmurally inflamed bowel. A pilot study found good correlation between clinical indices to measure Crohn activity [Crohn Disease Activity Index (CDAI) and the modified Index of the International Organization for the Study of Inflammatory Bowel Disease (IOIBD)] and an MRI determinant, the MRI product [wall thickness × length of diseased segment × percentage mural enhancement (MRP)] (fig. 6.67) [4].

This work suggests that MRI may be the best modality for evaluating the severity of Crohn disease. It may provide complementary or confirmatory information to clinical assessment. MRI also may have a role in the evaluation of acute exacerbations of Crohn disease. Specifically, in patients with longstanding disease, marked enhancement of the mucosa with substantially thickened wall and minimal enhancement of the outer layer is suggestive of acute on chronic involvement and may have a role in the evaluation of acute exacerbations of Crohn disease (see fig. 6.67). In patients with nonactive chronic disease, there may remain persistent thickening and abnormal enhancement seen on delayed postgadolinium images. Acute disease results in edema that may be best visualized on fat-suppressed single-shot T2-weighted images. It has been suggested that more detailed evaluation of the bowel wall in patients with longstanding disease may reveal marked enhancement of the mucosa with a thickened and minimally enhancing outer layer, suggestive of acute on chronic involvement (fig. 6.68).

Crohn disease may also result in large patulous segments of small bowel that may contain debris due to the presence of chronic distal small bowel obstruction. Patients may be symptomatic from the effects of bacterial overgrowth. On MR images, greatly dilated segments of bowel are shown that contain substantial debris. Single-shot echo-train spin echo is very effective in delineating the extent of dilatation and gadolinium-enhanced fat-suppressed SGE or 3D-GE technique for showing the inflammation (fig. 6.69), and MR small bowel follow-through technique may also help in this evaluation.

Ulcerative Colitis. Ulcerative colitis is a recurrent acute and chronic ulcero-inflammatory disorder of unknown etiology that affects the large bowel and is discussed in the section on the large intestine. Small

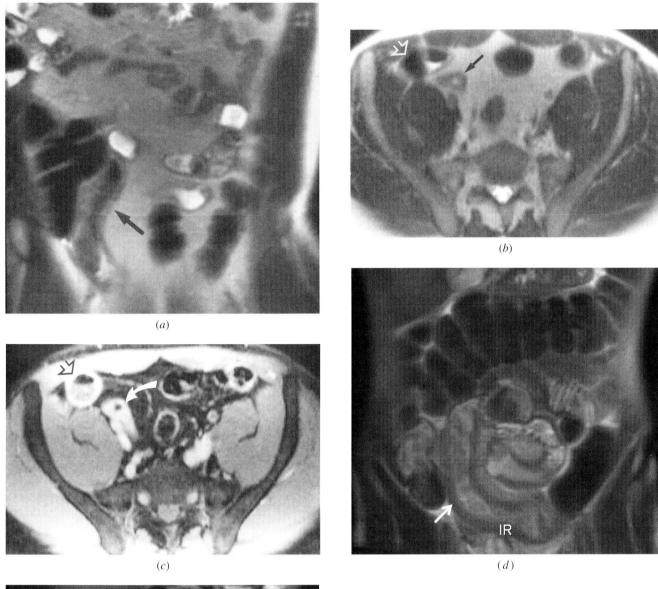

(a)

(b)

(c)

(d)

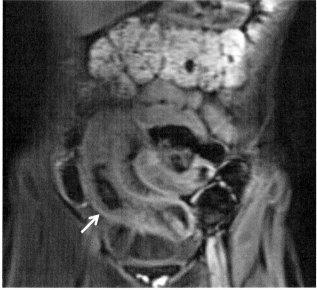

(e)

F I G . 6.62 Moderate Crohn disease. Coronal (*a*) and transverse (*b*) T2-weighted SS-ETSE and 2-min fat-suppressed SGE (*c*) images. The distal terminal ileum (arrow, *a*, *b*) shows increased wall thickness, whereas the ascending colon (open arrow, *b*) demonstrates normal wall thickness. On the 2-min fat-suppressed SGE image (*c*), moderate enhancement of the thickened distal terminal ileum (curved arrow) and ascending colon (open arrow) are present, reflecting moderate severity of the disease. Note that the ascending colon has a normal wall thickness associated with moderately increased enhancement due to Crohn involvement. (Reprinted with permission from Marcos HB, Semelka RC: Evaluation of Crohn's disease using half-Fourier RARE and gadolinium-enhanced SGE sequences: initial results. *Magn Reson Imaging* 18: 263–268, 2000.) Coronal T2-weighted single-shot echo-train spin-echo (*d*) and coronal T1-weighted postgadolinium fat-suppressed interstitial-phase 3D-GE (*e*) images at 3.0 T demonstrate moderate Crohn disease in another patient. The walls of involved ileal segments (arrows, *d*, *e*) are thickened and show increased enhancement. Note that inflammatory stranding is evident in the mesentery.

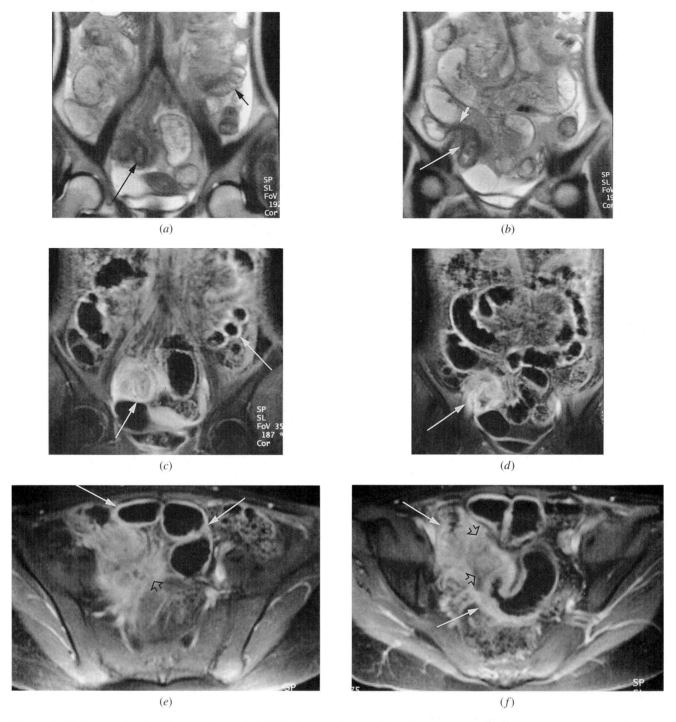

FIG. 6.63 Severe Crohn disease. Coronal SS-ETSE (*a, b*) and coronal (*c, d*) and transverse (*e, f*) 2- to 3-min postgadolinium fat-suppressed SGE images in a patient with severe disease. Coronal T2-weighted images from midabdominal plane (*a*) and 2 cm more anterior (*b*) demonstrate thickened loops of distal small bowel (long arrows, *a, b*). The terminal ileum is well shown at its entry into the cecum (small arrow, *b*). Coronal gadolinium-enhanced fat-suppressed SGE images acquired from similar tomographic sections, respectively, demonstrate substantial enhancement of the thickened loops of bowel and surrounding tissues. An enhancing fistulous tract (arrow, *d*) is apparent close to the ileocecal valve. Transverse gadolinium-enhanced images demonstrate intense enhancement of multiple loops of bowel, including loops with wall thickness of 4 mm (arrows, *e*). On the more inferior tomographic section narrowing of distal ileum is apparent (long arrows, *f*), which accounts for the mild dilation of more proximal loops (arrows, *e*). Inflammatory mesenteric changes are evident (open arrows, *e, f*). Normal-appearing proximal jejunum (small arrow, *a*) is appreciated on the T2-weighted image.

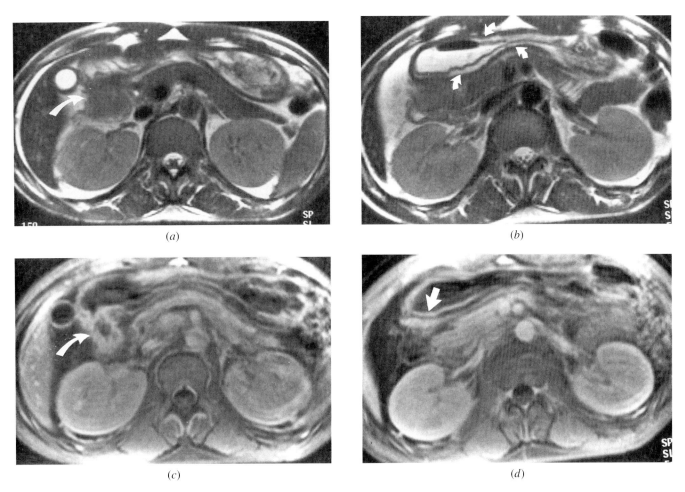

F I G . 6.64 Duodenal Crohn disease and gastric outlet obstruction. Transverse T2-weighted SS-ETSE (*a*, *b*) and 2-min post-gadolinium fat-suppressed (*c*, *d*) images. The stomach and proximal duodenum are dilated a with transition point in the second portion of the duodenum. The duodenum at the level of obstruction shows increased wall thickness on the T2-weighted image (curved arrow, *a*). High signal intensity of the submucosa of the antrum and first portion of the duodenum is identified (curved arrows, *b*). The thickened portion of the duodenum demonstrates moderately increased mural enhancement (curved arrow, *c*), with mucosa and serosa layers of the antrum and proximal duodenum demonstrating enhancement reflecting moderate chronic inflammatory changes (arrow, *d*). Low signal intensity of the submucosa on the postgadolinium T1-weighted images (*c*, *d*) represents submucosal edema and corresponds to high signal intensity on the T2-weighted image. (Reprinted with permission from Marcos HB, Semelka RC: Evaluation of Crohn's disease using half-Fourier RARE and gadolinium-enhanced SGE sequences: initial results. *Magn Reson Imaging* 18: 263–268, 2000.)

bowel involvement ("backwash ileitis") is the sequel of pancolonic disease. Free reflux of colon contents into the ileum via a patulous, incompetent ileocecal valve is believed to be responsible [74]. The lumen of the ileum is moderately dilated, and on MRI the diseased ileal wall is abnormal, showing mild dilatation and moderately increased enhancement with gadolinium, reflective of diffuse inflammation, erosion, and ulcerations (fig. 6.70).

Gluten-Sensitive Enteropathy (Celiac Disease, Celiac Sprue)

Gluten-sensitive enteropathy (GSE) is an immunologically mediated gastrointestinal disease that produces a malabsorption syndrome. GSE likely results from a specific immunologic hyperactivity to a constituent of dietary gluten. The diagnosis is made through jejunal biopsy and is based on the presence of mucosal atrophy with blunting or complete loss of the villi and inflammation within the mucosa of the small intestine. T2-weighted single-shot echo-train spin-echo technique may demonstrate an abnormal mucosal fold pattern of the small bowel, associated with an increase of intraluminal fluid (figs. 6.71 and 6.72) [57]. One recent study showed that MRI is able to demonstrate intra- and extraintestinal features that may lead to the diagnosis of celiac disease in adults [76]. The authors have studied 31 patients with celiac disease and have found that MRI

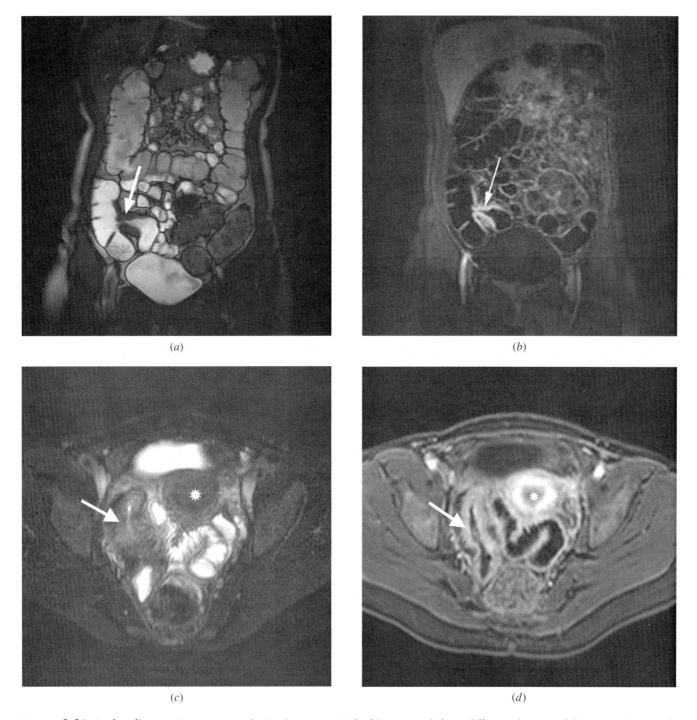

(a) *(b)*

(c) *(d)*

F I G . 6.65 Crohn disease. Images were obtained over a period of 2 years and show different degrees of disease activity, with examples of images obtained during quiescent nonactive disease (*a, b*), 2 years later on acute presentation with active disease (*c, d*), 1 month later while on immunosuppressant and oral antibiotic therapy (*e, f*), and 3 months after therapy with resolution of acute imaging findings and complications (*g–j*).The terminal ileum (TI) is concentrically thickened (*a*) and demonstrates dark signal intensity on coronal T2-weighted imaging (WI) (arrow, *a*), indicating no evidence of edema and consistent with quiescent Crohn disease, whereas coronal gadolinium-enhanced delayed-phase T1-weighted imaging (arrow, *b*) demonstrates that the abnormally thickened tissue enhances. This combination of features is consistent with fibrosis and chronic disease. Two years later, active Crohn disease has developed and is demonstrated by a long segment of distal ileum (*c, d*) that has abnormal wall thickening with high signal on T2-weighted imaging (arrow, *c*) associated with abnormal enhancement (arrow, *d*) in keeping with active inflammation. The uterus is noted within the image as a normal structure (asterisks, *c, d*). One month after immunosuppressive,

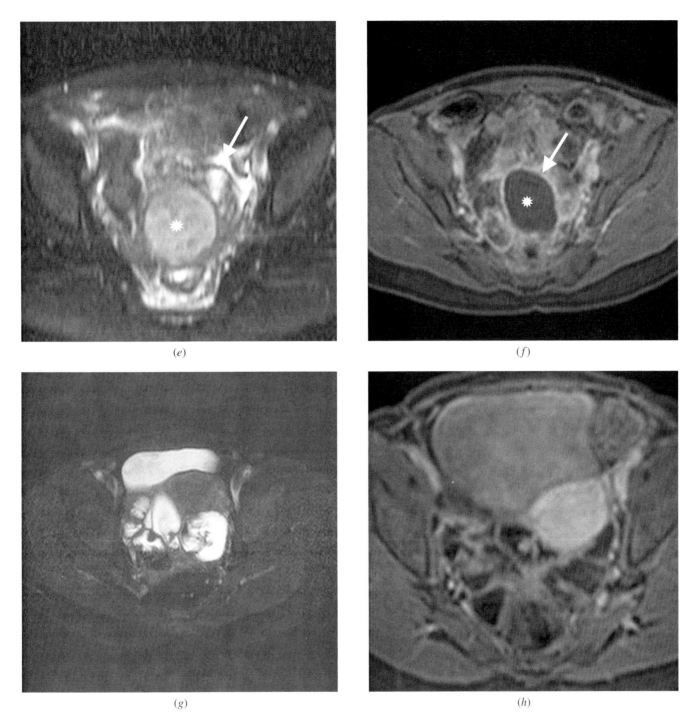

(e)

(f)

(g)

(h)

FIG. 6.65 (*Continued*) anti-inflammatory, and oral antibiotic therapy the patient presented with mild pelvic discomfort and pressure symptoms with imaging demonstrating development of a central pelvic abscess situated in the cul de sac on T2-weighted imaging (star, *e*) and delayed gadolinium-enhanced T1-weighted imaging (asterisk, *f*), with a thickened enhancing abscess wall (arrow, *f*). There remains marked diffuse mesenteric edema and fluid (arrow, *e*). Two months after acute presentation, the abscess has been percutaneously drained with complete resolution of the abscess, inflammation, and pelvic edema on T2-weighted imaging (*g*) and gadolinium enhanced T1-weighted imaging (*h*). The TI has returned to nearly the same appearance as 2 years previously

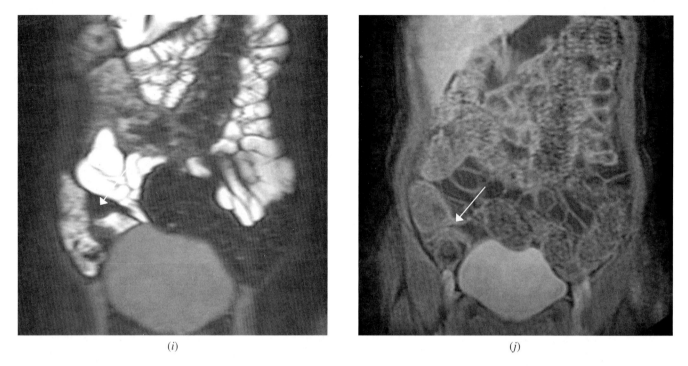

(i)   (j)

F I G . 6.65 (*Continued*) on coronal T2 (*i*)- and gadolinium-enhanced T1 (*j*)-weighted images, consistent with persistent fibrosis and return to quiescent disease.

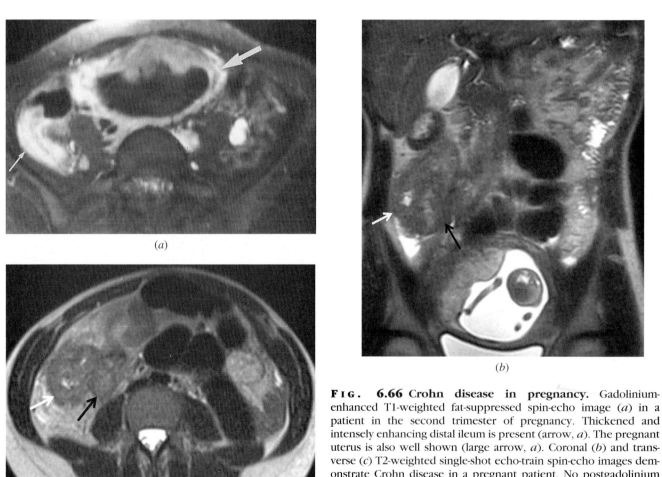

(a)

(b)

(c)

F I G . 6.66 Crohn disease in pregnancy. Gadolinium-enhanced T1-weighted fat-suppressed spin-echo image (*a*) in a patient in the second trimester of pregnancy. Thickened and intensely enhancing distal ileum is present (arrow, *a*). The pregnant uterus is also well shown (large arrow, *a*). Coronal (*b*) and transverse (*c*) T2-weighted single-shot echo-train spin-echo images demonstrate Crohn disease in a pregnant patient. No postgadolinium imaging was performed because of the pregnancy. Diffuse wall thickening is present in the cecum (white arrows, *b, c*) and terminal ileum (black arrows, *b, c*). Inflammatory stranding is detected in the fat tissue around the terminal ileum and cecum. Note that minimal free fluid is also present around the terminal ileum and cecum.

Table 6.2 Crohn Disease Severity Criteria

Severity	Contrast Enhancement (%)	Wall Thickness (mm)	Length of Diseased Segment (cm)
Mild*	<50	<5	<5
Moderate	50–100	5–20	Variable
Severe	>100	>10	>5**

*Bowel-wall thickening must be at least 4 mm, and one of the other 2 criteria must be satisfied.
**Typically >10 cm of affected bowel.
Reprinted with permission from Ascher SM, Semelka RC: MRI of the gastrointestinal tract. In Higgins CB, Hricak H, Helms CA (eds.). *Magnetic Resonance Imaging of the Body*. New York: Raven Press, p. 677–700, 1997.

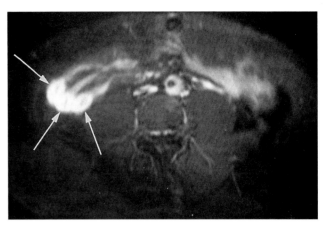

FIG. 6.67 Crohn disease activity assessment. Gadolinium-enhanced T1-weighted fat-suppressed spin-echo image in a patient with active Crohn disease. There is good correlation between clinical indices [CDAI, 185 (active disease 1150); modified IOIBD index, 8 (scale 1–10)] and MRI findings (arrows) of thickened wall, length of diseased segment, and percentage of mural enhancement (MRP, 4,664). (Reprinted with permission from Kettritz U, Isaacs K, Warshauer DM, Semelka RC: Crohn's disease: pilot study comparing MRI of the abdomen with clinical evaluation. *J Clin Gastroenterol* 21: 249-253, 1995.)

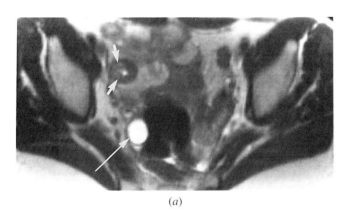

(a)

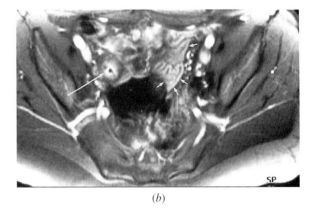

(b)

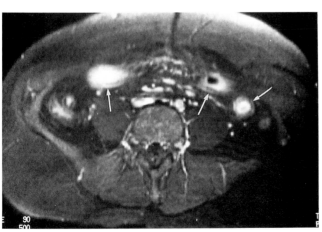

(c)

FIG. 6.68 Acute on chronic Crohn disease. T2-weighted SS-ETSE (*a*) and gadolinium-enhanced T1-weighted fat-suppressed spin-echo (*b*) images in a patient with longstanding disease. Increased thickness of distal ileum is present, which demonstrates increased signal intensity in the inner aspect of the wall (arrow, *a*). Acute exacerbation is characterized by intense mucosal enhancement (long arrow, *b*), with minimal enhancement of the outer wall in substantially thickened bowel. Accompanying hyperemia of the mesentery reflects the active inflammatory process (short arrows, *b*). Incidental note is made of a right adnexal cyst (long arrow, *a*) and free fluid in the pelvis. Gadolinium-enhanced T1-weighted fat-suppressed spin-echo image (*c*) in a second patient with a long history of Crohn disease. Thickened loops of small bowel with intense enhancement of the inner wall are apparent (arrows, *c*). The appearance is that of acute mucosal exacerbation

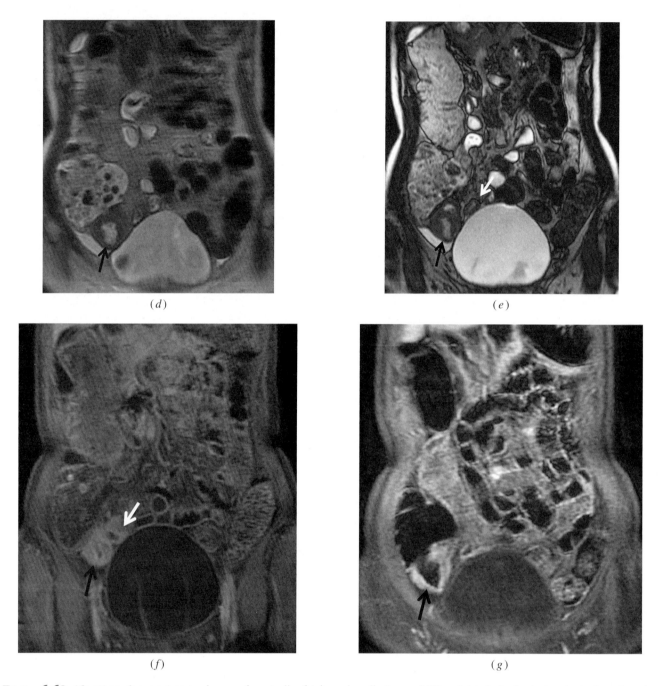

(d)

(e)

(f)

(g)

FIG. 6.68 (*Continued*) superimposed on a chronically thickened wall. Coronal T2-weighted single-shot echo-train spin-echo (*d*), coronal T2-weighted true-FISP (*e*), and coronal T1-weighted fat-suppressed postgadolinium interstitial-phase 3D-GE (*f, g*) images demonstrate acute on chronic Crohn disease in another patient. The cecum (black arrows, *d–g*) is retracted because of fibrosis, and its thickened wall shows progressive enhancement due to fibrosis and inflammation. The wall of the terminal ileum is also thickened and shows increased enhancement (white arrows, *e, f*). Free fluid is also detected in the right lower quadrant. The presence of retracted fibrotic cecum, and thickened and enhancing terminal ileum in combination with free fluid suggests the diagnosis of acute on chronic Crohn disease.

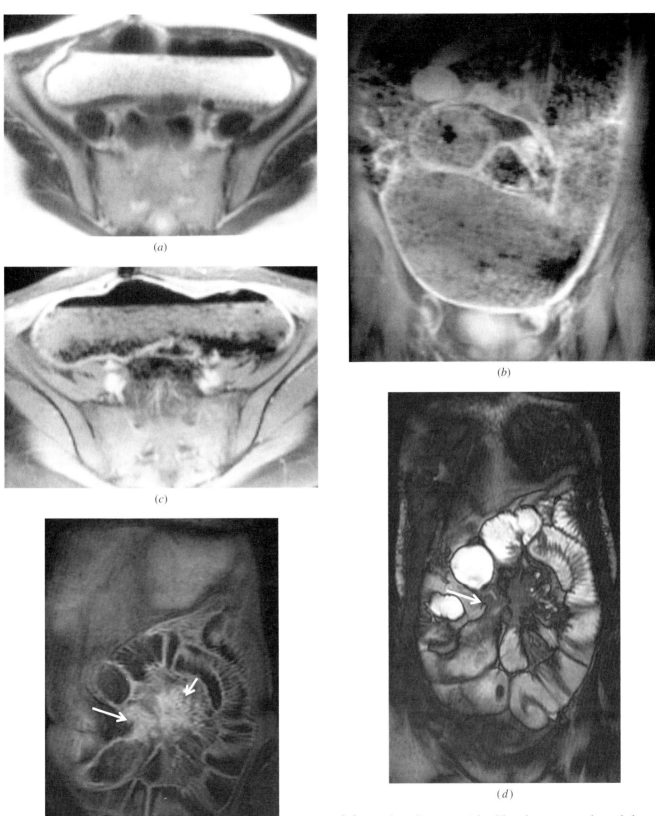

FIG. 6.69 Crohn disease with dilated stagnant bowel loop. Transverse T2-weighted SS-ETSE (*a*) and coronal (*b*) and transverse (*c*) gadolinium-enhanced interstitial-phase fat-suppressed SGE images. An enlarged loop of distal small bowel is present that contains substantial debris. Enlarged stagnant loops of small bowel are a complication of long-standing distal small bowel obstruction as observed in Crohn disease. Coronal T2-weighted true-FISP (*d*) and coronal T1-weighted postgadolinium fat-suppressed 3D-GE (*e*) images demonstrate stenotic small bowel segment (white arrows, *d, e*) and prestenotic dilated bowel segments in another patient with Crohn disease. The wall of stenotic bowel segment is thickened and shows increased enhancement on postgadolinium image (*e*). Note that there is associated enhancing mesenteric inflammation (short arrow, *e*).

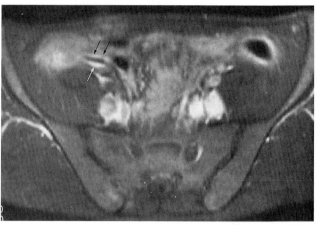

F I G . 6.70 Backwash ileitis. Gadolinium-enhanced T1-weighted fat-suppressed spin-echo image in a patient with ulcerative colitis. Pancolonic involvement with ulcerative colitis results in a patulous ileocecal valve. Reflux of colon contents into the ileum causes inflammatory changes (arrows). (Reprinted with permission from Shoenut JP, Semelka RC, Silverman R, Yaffe CS, Mickflikier AB: The gastrointestinal tract. In Semelka RC, Shoenut JP (eds.), *MRI of the Abdomen with CT Correlation.* New York: Raven Press, 1993, pp. 119–143.)

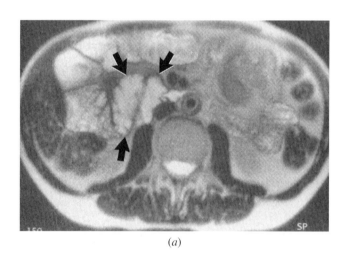

(a)

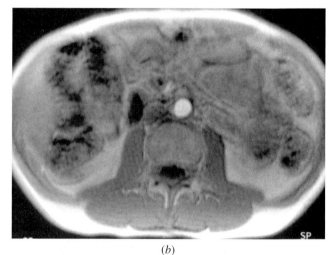

(b)

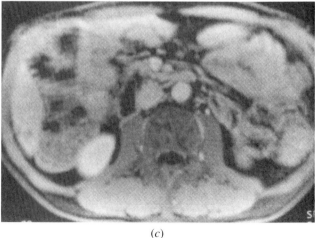

(c)

F I G . 6.71 Gluten-sensitive enteropathy. T2-weighted SSETSE (*a*), immediate postgadolinium SGE (*b*), and 90-s postgadolinium fat-suppressed SGE (*c*) images. T2-weighted image demonstrates an abnormally prominent mucosal pattern in the duodenum associated with an increase in intraluminal fluid (arrows, *a*). The duodenal mucosa enhances normally, which reflects a lack of vascular changes related to the disease process. Upper gastrointestinal endoscopy with biopsy was performed, and histopathologic examination established the diagnosis of gluten-sensitive enteropathy. (Reprinted with permission from Marcos HB, Semelka RC, Noone TC, Woosley JT, Lee JKT: MRI of normal and abnormal duodenum using half-Fourier single-shot RARE and gadolinium-enhanced spoiled gradient-echo sequences. *Magn Reson Imaging* 17: 869–880, 1999.)

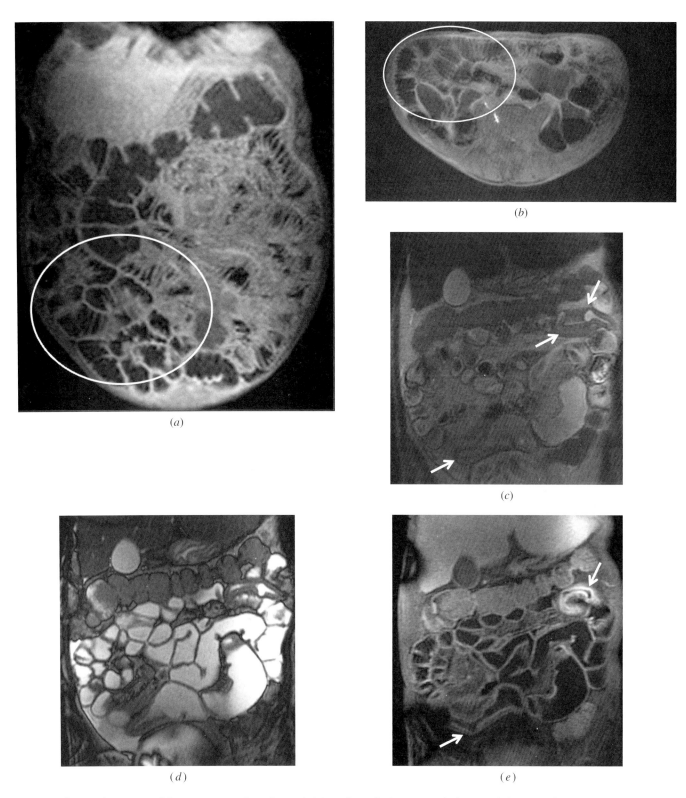

FIG. 6.72 Gluten-sensitive enteropathy. Coronal (*a*) and axial (*b*) interstial-phase gadolinium-enhanced T1-weighted fat-suppressed 3D-GE images in a 61-year-old man demonstrate abnormal ileal fold pattern (small bowel loops shown within circle, *a* and *b*) with increased number and irregularity of folds mimicking the appearance normally associated with the jejunum. Coronal T2-weighted single-shot echo-train spin-echo (*c*), coronal T2-weighted true-FISP (*d*), and coronal T1-weighted postgadolinium inter-stitial phase fat-suppressed 3D-GE (*e,f*) images demonstrate refractory gluten-sensitive enteropathy (RGSE) in another patient. Valvula conniventes of the jejunum are lost due to RGSE. Segmental wall thickening (arrows, *c*) and associated increased enhancement (arrows, *e*) are detected in the jejunum and ileum, suggesting jejunoileitis. Submucosal edema is detected in these segments.

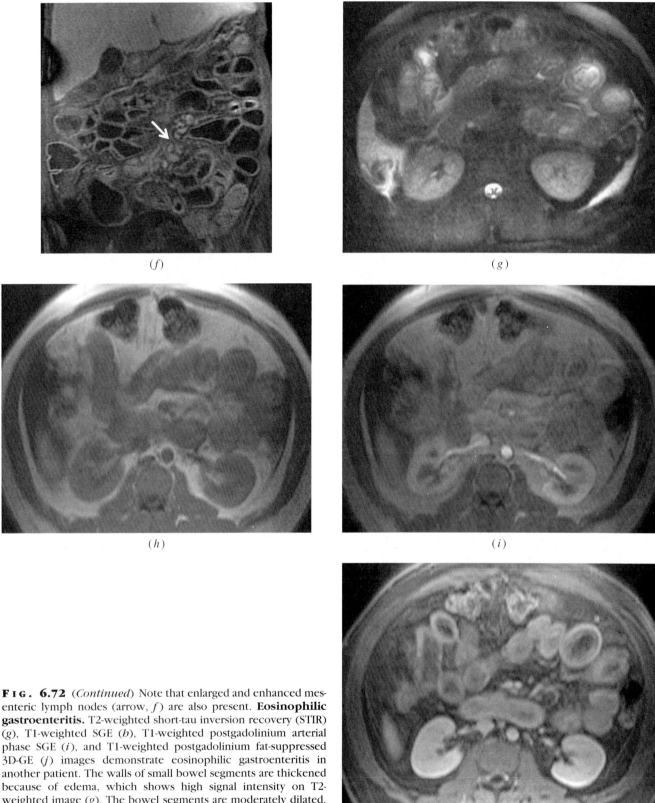

FIG. 6.72 (*Continued*) Note that enlarged and enhanced mesenteric lymph nodes (arrow, *f*) are also present. **Eosinophilic gastroenteritis.** T2-weighted short-tau inversion recovery (STIR) (*g*), T1-weighted SGE (*h*), T1-weighted postgadolinium arterial phase SGE (*i*), and T1-weighted postgadolinium fat-suppressed 3D-GE (*j*) images demonstrate eosinophilic gastroenteritis in another patient. The walls of small bowel segments are thickened because of edema, which shows high signal intensity on T2-weighted image (*g*). The bowel segments are moderately dilated, and their walls show progressive increased enhancement. Note that free fluid is also present in the abdomen.

showed bowel dilatation in 61.3% (*n* = 19), increased number of ileal folds in 48.4% (*n* = 15), reversed fold pattern abnormality in 38.7% (*n* = 12), increased wall thickness in 16.1% (*n* = 5), duodenal stenosis in 6.5% (*n* = 2), intussusception in 12.9% (*n* = 4), mesenteric lymphadenopathy in 41.9% (*n* = 13), mesenteric vascular changes in 22.6% (*n* = 7), ascites in 6.5% (n=2), and no abnormalities in 12.9% (*n* = 4) [76]. The overall specificity and accuracy were 100%, and sensitivity was 79% and 75% for increased number of ileal folders and reversed fold pattern abnormality, respectively [76]. MRI can detect the complications of GSE including jejunoileitis and lymphoma.

Eosinophilic Gastroenteritis

Eosinophilic gastroenteritis is a rare disease affecting both children and adults. It is characterized by the presence of GI symptoms, eosinophilic infiltration in the GI tract, the absence of an identified cause of eosinophilia, and the exclusion of eosinophilic involvement in organs other than the GI tract. Atopy or food allergy history may be present. MR imaging features are nonspecific and include gastric or bowel dilatation, thickened or flattened valvula conniventes, gastric and bowel wall thickening, strictures, ulcerations, enlarged lymph nodes, and ascites. Edema in the bowel wall submucosa can be seen as high-signal-intensity changes on T2-weighted images. Thickened bowel wall shows increased enhancement on postgadolinium images.

Scleroderma

Scleroderma, or progressive systemic sclerosis, is a connective tissue disease that often involves the gastrointestinal tract. There is a patchy destruction of the muscularis propria in the small intestine, mainly involving the duodenum and jejunum. There is also degeneration of both circular and longitudinal muscle layers and replacement by collagen tissue [77]. Dilatation is the most common finding in imaging studies (fig. 6.73), and

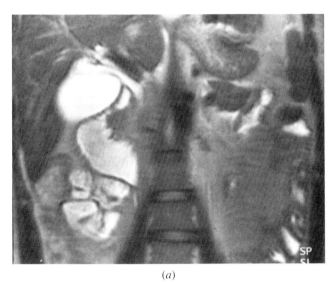

(*a*)

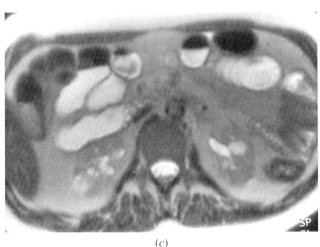

(*c*)

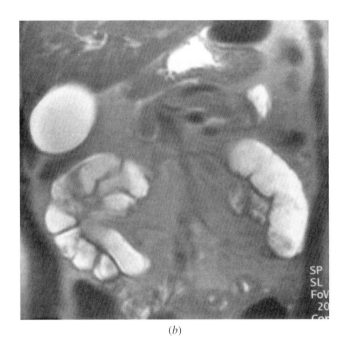

(*b*)

F I G . 6.73 Scleroderma. Coronal (*a*, *b*) and transverse (*c*) T2-weighted SS-ETSE images show dilatation of the duodenum and multiple small bowel loops without evidence of obstruction.

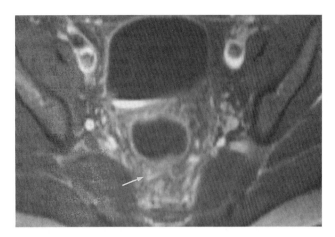

F I G. 6.74 Pouchitis. Gadolinium-enhanced T1-weighted fat-suppressed spin-echo image demonstrates slight thickening of the pouch with stranding in the surrounding fat (arrow).

sacculation with formation of pseudodiverticula also may develop.

Pouchitis

A continent ileostomy ("pouch") is often fashioned for patients after total colectomy. The creation of an ileal pouch changes the usual function of this part of the small intestine from absorption to fecal storage. With fecal storage, stasis and bacterial overgrowth may occur. The most common long-term complication of an ileal reservoir is inflammation known as "pouchitis." This condition is more common in patients with Crohn disease [78], MRI features of which include an enhancing and thickened pouch wall and inflammatory stranding of the "peripouch" fat (fig. 6.74).

Fistula

A fistula is defined as an abnormal passage or communication, generally between two internal organs or leading from an organ to the surface of the body. In the setting of small bowel pathology, fistulas result from compromise in the integrity of the visceral wall and may be sequelae of infection, inflammation, neoplasia, radiation therapy, and ischemia (embolic, thrombotic, or vasoconstrictive). MRI's good contrast and spatial resolution, in conjunction with direct image acquisition in any plane, makes it a very effective modality in the workup of fistulas. The appearance of a fistula will depend on its contents, the degree of inflammation, and the type of sequence employed. Fluid-filled tracts are high in signal intensity on T2-weighted sequences, whereas gas-filled tracts are signal void. Fat suppression combined with intravenous gadolinium highlights the enhancing fistulous tracts amid the surrounding low-signal intensity intra-abdominal fat. Focal discontinuity

of the involved organ at the site of tract penetration is diagnostic (fig. 6.75) [7, 8].

Infectious Enteritis

Active inflammation may be caused by a variety of bacterial, protozoal, fungal, or viral pathogens. *Yersinia enterocolitica* infection may cause acute gastroenteritis, terminal ileitis, mesenteric lymphadenitis, and colitis [79]. *Yersinia* ileitis and *Yersinia* enterocolitis may mimic appendicitis and Crohn disease, respectively. *Campylobacter jejuni* may produce diarrhea, severe gastroenteritis, or colitis [80]. *Giardia lamblia* and *Strongyloides stercoralis* are protozoa that typically involve proximal small bowel. The increasing population of immunocompromised patients has led to an increase in occurrence of infectious granulomatous disease of the bowel. Tuberculosis mycobacteria infection involves the terminal ileum. Patients may be symptomatic from the acute inflammatory response, late fibrotic stenosis, or both. *Mycobacterium avium-intracellulare* favors the colon and is frequently accompanied by bulky retroperitoneal lymphadenopathy. Cytomegalovirus and *Cryptosporidium parvum* are infections common in AIDS patients. In all of these inflammatory conditions, the MRI findings may be nonspecific, demonstrating bowel wall thickening, increased secretions, and mesenteric edema. Gadolinium-enhanced fat-suppressed SGE or 3D-GE imaging demonstrates bowel wall thickening and increased enhancement (fig. 6.76) and detects the presence of abscesses by the identification of encapsulated fluid collections that possess an enhancing rim. Clinical history, coupled with the segment of bowel affected, may suggest the correct diagnosis. For example, in an AIDS patient, small bowel wall thickening and submucosal hemorrhage may be seen in cytomegalovirus infection, whereas focal thickening of the bowel wall and mildly dilated, fluid-filled segments may suggest *Cryptosporidium* infection [46].

Pancreatitis

Small bowel changes also may occur adjacent to an active inflammatory process. Specifically, in patients with pancreatitis, small bowel wall thickening and focal ileus are seen on gadolinium-enhanced SGE or 3D-GE images (fig. 6.77). An MRI colon cutoff sign also may be demonstrated.

Drug Toxicity

Inflammatory changes of small bowel may result from a number of etiologies. Chemotherapy toxicity is one example. Diffuse and circumferential wall thickening with increased enhancement are observed (fig. 6.78).

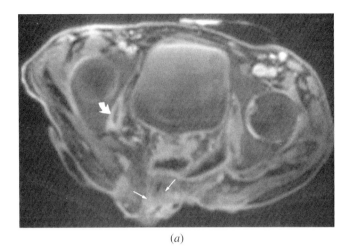

(a)

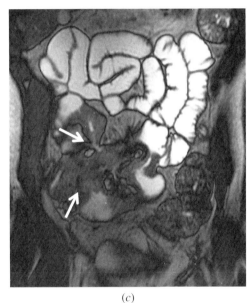

(c)

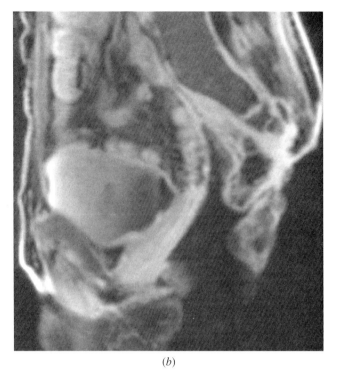

(b)

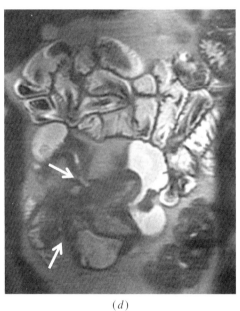

(d)

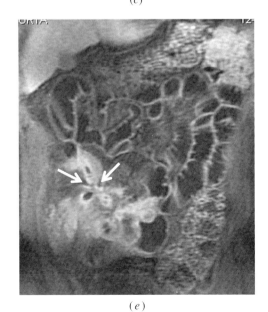

(e)

FIG. 6.75 Pelvic fistulas in a patient with Crohn disease. Transverse (a) and sagittal (b) interstitial-phase gadolinium-enhanced fat-suppressed SGE images. There is a large decubitus ulcer associated with destruction of the coccyx and lower part of the sacrum. Extensive pelvic cutaneous fistulas appear as enhancing track walls (arrows, a). An abscess of the obturator internus muscle is present (curved arrow, a). **Entero-enteric fistulas in patients with Crohn disease.** Coronal T2-weighted true-FISP (c), single-shot echo-train spin-echo (d), and coronal T1-weighted postgadolinium interstitial-phase fat-suppressed 3D-GE (e) images demonstrate several entero-enteric fistulas in another patient with Crohn disease. Several small bowel segments with thickened and abnormally enhancing walls form fistulas (arrows, c–e) with each other. Note the associated

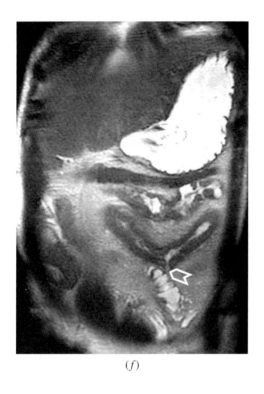

(f)

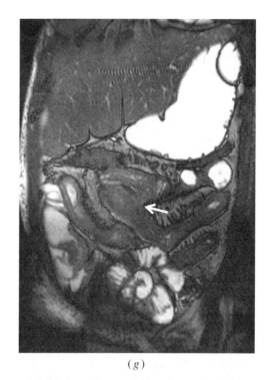

(g)

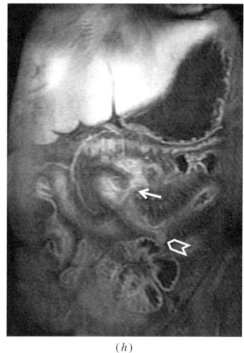

(h)

FIG. 6.75 (*Continued*) mesenteric inflammation adjacent to the fistulas. Coronal T2-weighted single-shot echo-train spin-echo (*f*), coronal T2-weighted true-FISP (*g*), and coronal T1-weighted postgadolinium fat-suppressed interstitial phase 3D-GE (*h*) images demonstrate an entero-enteric fistula (white arrow, *g, h*) and an ulcer (open arrow, *f, h*) in another patient with Crohn disease. The walls of small bowel segments are thickened and show increased enhancement. A fistula (white arrows, *g, h*) is present between two jejunal segments. Note that there is stranding in the mesenteric fat adjacent to the involved segments, which is best seen on true-FISP (*g*) and postgadolinium (*h*) images. An ulcer (open arrow, *f, h*) that is detected in the inferior border of a jejunal segment shows high signal on T2-weighted image (*f*) and increased enhancement on postgadolinium image (*h*) within the wall. **Entero-vesical fistula in**

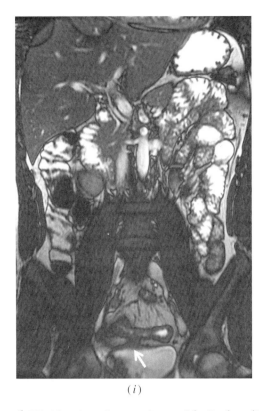

(*i*)

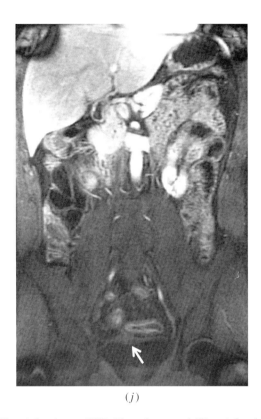

(*j*)

FIG. 6.75 (*Continued*) **a patient with Crohn disease.** Coronal T2-weighted true-FISP (*i*) and coronal T1-weighted post-gadolinium interstitial-phase fat-suppressed 3D-GE (*j*) images demonstrate a fistula (arrow, *i, j*) between an ileal segment and the dome of the bladder. Note that the wall of the ileal segment is thickened and shows increased enhancement.

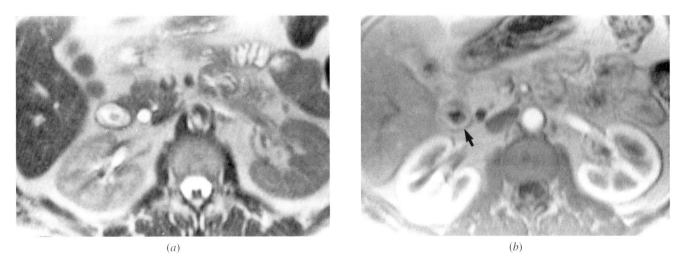

(*a*) (*b*)

FIG. 6.76 **Duodenitis.** Transverse T2-weighted SS-ETSE (*a*), immediate postgadolinium SGE (*b*), and interstitial-phase gadolinium-enhanced fat-suppressed SGE (*c*) images. Diffuse wall thickening and enhancement (arrow, *b*) involving the second part of

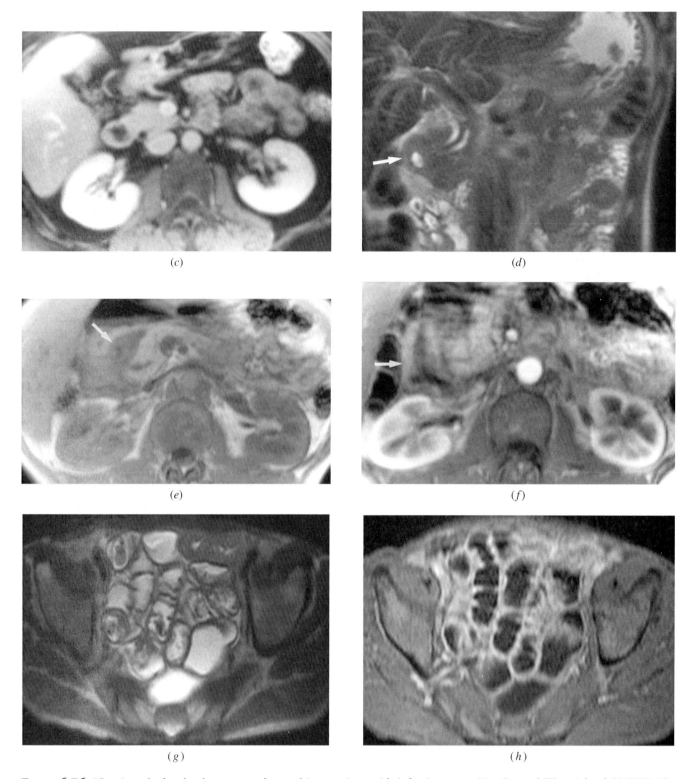

FIG. 6.76 (*Continued*) the duodenum are observed in a patient with infectious enteritis. Coronal T2-weighted SS-ETSE (*d*), transverse SGE (*e*), and immediate postgadolinium T1-weighted SGE (*f*) images in a second patient with eosinophilic enteritis. There is thickening of the first and second portions of the duodenum (arrows, *d*–*f*) with duodenal dilatation. **Infectious enteritis.** T2-weighted single-shot echo-train spin-echo (*g*) and T1-weighted postgadolinium interstitial-phase fat-suppressed 3D-GE (*h*) images demonstrate dilated small bowel loops with intensely enhancing thickened walls in another patient with AIDS.

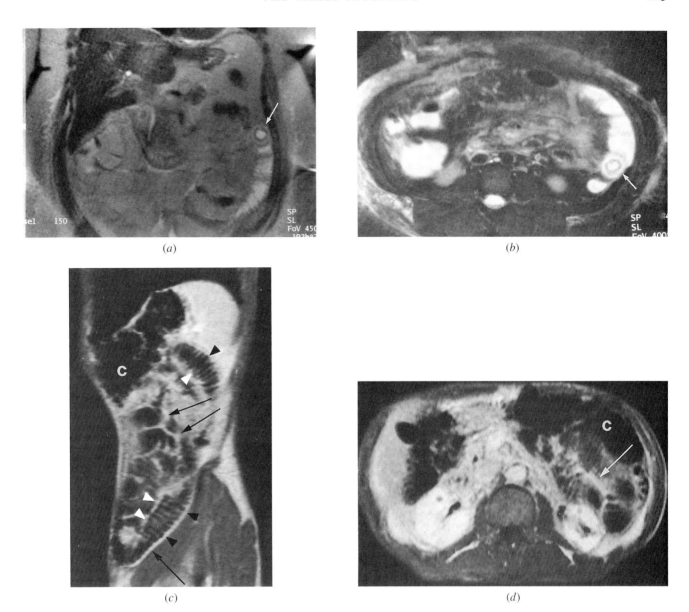

(a)

(b)

(c)

(d)

F I G . 6.77 Small intestine inflammation secondary to pancreatitis. Coronal T2-weighted SS-ETSE (*a*) and T2-weighted fat-suppressed echo-train spin-echo (*b*) images demonstrate circumferential high signal intensity of the wall of the jejunum (arrow, *a*, *b*) secondary to edema caused by inflammatory changes induced by pancreatitis. The outer wall is high in signal intensity, whereas the inner wall is low in signal intensity, reflecting the extrinsic nature of the bowel inflammation. Sagittal (*c*) and transverse (*d*) interstitial-phase gadolinium-enhanced SGE images in a second patient demonstrate dilatation (arrowheads, *c*) of small bowel with increased wall enhancement (arrows, *c*, *d*).The transverse colon (*c*, *c*, *d*) shows a transition from normal caliber to narrowed, which is the transverse colon cutoff sign of pancreatitis.

Radiation Enteritis

In the gastrointestinal tract, the small intestine is the region most sensitive to radiation injury. Radiation therapy for malignant disease may cause an enteritis with tumor doses greater than 45 Gy. The majority of cases are secondary to treatment for female genital tract malignancy. The distal jejunum and ileum are the most common sites affected. Acute injury to the small intestine occurs within hours to days after radiation therapy. Although some damage to the intestinal wall is a regular occurrence, lesions are variable in severity. Microscopic inspection may show sloughed villi with mucosal hemorrhage, edema, focal necrosis, and inflammation. Early postradiotherapy complications include ulceration, necrosis, bleeding, perforation, and abscess formation. The development of chronic radiation enteritis is variable, developing months to years after the radiation event. Chronic radiation enteritis is a progressive disease resulting from underlying vascular damage. Vascular injury includes fibrosis and hyalinization of blood vessel walls leading to obliterative endarteritis within the intestinal wall and mesentery. Progression of the vascular pathology causes ischemia. Normal tissue is replaced by parenchymal atrophy and progressive fibrosis. Complications of chronic radiation enteritis include strictures, fistulas, bowel fixation, and angulation. Varying degrees of small bowel obstruction may result. Gadolinium-enhanced fat-suppressed SGE or 3D-GE imaging is the most effective technique for detecting the diffuse early ischemic and inflammatory changes of radiation enteritis as well as the more focal late fibrotic sequelae. Changes caused by radiation effect are reflected in diffuse symmetric bowel wall thickening and enhancement of multiple loops of small bowel in the same region of the abdomen. Radiation effect can be readily distinguished from recurrent tumor, which demonstrates irregular, nodular bowel wall thickening (fig. 6.79).

Ischemia and Hemorrhage

Ischemia and hemorrhage may occur in tandem or as isolated events. Ischemia, regardless of etiology, leads to wall edema secondary to capillary leakage (fig. 6.80). If prolonged, infarction can result. The MRI findings parallel the severity of blood flow compromise. Early changes include mural thickening and increased enhancement on late postcontrast images (fig. 6.81). Increased enhancement on immediate postgadolinium images reflects leaky capillaries. Necrotic bowel manifests MRI findings consistent with hemorrhage, and in severe cases portal venous gas may be observed (see fig. 6.81). Vascular compromise or thrombosis may be well shown on early (>1 min) postgadolinium images (fig. 6.82) and MRA images (see fig. 6.81). Bowel wall hemorrhage from trauma or ischemia may be diagnosed by high signal intensity within the submucosa on both T1- and T2-weighted sequences due to the presence of extracellular methemoglobin [81]. Noncontrast T1-weighted fat-suppressed images are the most sensitive for the detection of subacute blood (fig. 6.83). One study evaluated the MR appearance of small bowel wall hemorrhage and showed that MR findings was able to distinguish mural-based hematoma from contained perimural small bowel hematoma (fig. 6.83) [81]. The most effective MR feature to make this distinction was demonstration of the lack of involvement of the wall with single-shot T2-weighted images (fig. 6.83) [81].

Hypoproteinemia

Hypoproteinemia may arise from a number of causes, the most common of which are cirrhosis and malnourishment. In the setting of cirrhosis, hypoproteinemia has been postulated as the primary cause of intestinal wall edema of the large and small bowel. It is generally thought that edema is diffuse and results from changes in oncotic pressure [82]. Generalized bowel wall thickening is present, which is best appreciated in the jejunum. Unlike inflammatory conditions, enhancement on gadolinium-enhanced images is negligible (fig. 6.84).

Intussusception

Intussusception is a form of intestinal obstruction characterized by the telescoping of one intestinal segment into another. Predisposing factors include masses and motility disorders [83]. Transient asymptomatic intussusceptions are not uncommon imaging findings, but multiple nonobstructing intussusceptions suggest an underlying bowel disorder such as sprue. The invaginating bowel segment is referred to as the intussusceptum, and the bowel segment into which the prolapse has occurred is referred to as the intussuscipiens. Intussusception is clearly demonstrated on T2-weighted single-shot echo-train spin-echo images because of the sharp anatomic detail of this sequence. In the setting of intussusception, fluid in dilated bowel provides excellent intrinsic contrast for the bowel-within-bowel appearance (fig. 6.85). The use of T2-weighted single-shot echo train spin echo sequences is very helpful in pregnant patients (fig. 6.85) since postgadolinium imaging should be avoided in pregnant patients unless maternal and fetal survival depend on it.

Hernia

Small bowel mechanical obstruction is most commonly related to adhesions (fig. 6.85) or hernias. Small bowel hernias may be classified as internal, as may form from a loop of small bowel passing through an abnormal defect or tear within the mesentery, or as external, as may form from a small bowel loop passing into an inguinal defect (fig. 6.86). Distension of the small bowel with an oral contrast agent may provide additional sensitivity by making even a partially obstructed small bowel segment more conspicuous. A water-based agent can serve well for this purpose by producing high signal (bright lumen) on T2-weighted and low signal (dark lumen) on T1-weighted images (see fig. 6.86) [84–86].

Graft-Versus-Host Disease

Graft-versus-host disease (GVHD) is an immunologic disorder that occurs in any situation in which immunologically competent donor cells are transplanted into an immunologically incompetent recipient. GVHD most commonly follows bone marrow or organ transplantation. The acute form involves the gastric antrum, small bowel, and colon and occurs within days (7–100) in recipients. Histologically, acute GVHD shows loss of normal intestinal mucosal architecture with ulceration, mucosal denudation, and submucosal edema. On MR

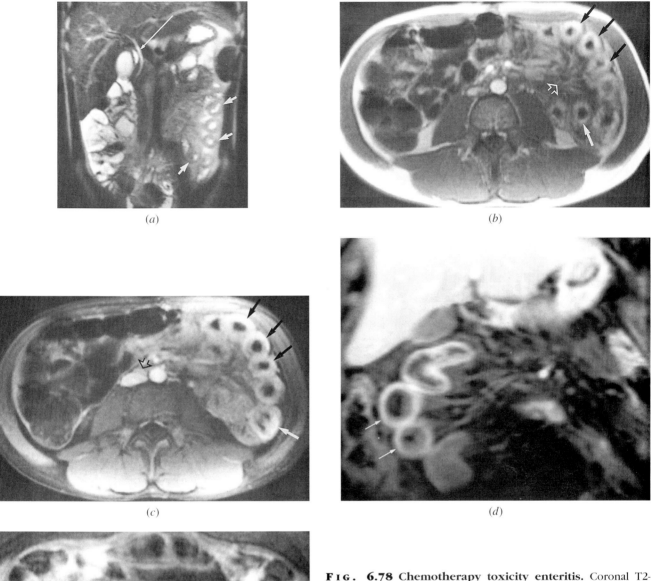

F I G . 6.78 Chemotherapy toxicity enteritis. Coronal T2-weighted SS-ETSE (*a*), immediate postgadolinium SGE (*b*), and 90-s postgadolinium fat-suppressed SGE (*c*) images in a patient with chemotherapy toxicity enteritis. Many etiologic agents may cause inflammation of the small bowel. The findings are nonspecific and include diffuse circumferential wall thickening (short arrows, *a*), marked bowel wall enhancement (arrows, *b*, *c*), mesenteric infiltration and hyperemia (open arrow, *b*), and lymphadenopathy (open arrow, *c*). Note the normal common bile duct on the T2-weighted image (long arrow, *a*). Coronal (*d*) and transverse (*e*) interstitial-phase gadolinium-enhanced fat-suppressed SGE images in a second patient, who underwent chemotherapy for ovarian cancer. There is abnormal enhancement of multiple loops of small bowel (arrows, *d*, *e*) consistent with chemotherapy toxicity enteritis.

images there is diffuse bowel wall thickening with increased enhancement of the inner wall layers (fig. 6.87). The chronic form of GVHD may follow the acute form or occur insidiously and is usually associated with

esophageal involvement. Microscopic examination of the esophagus shows a sloughed and hyperemic mucosa. This desquamative esophagitis may lead to webs and strictures.

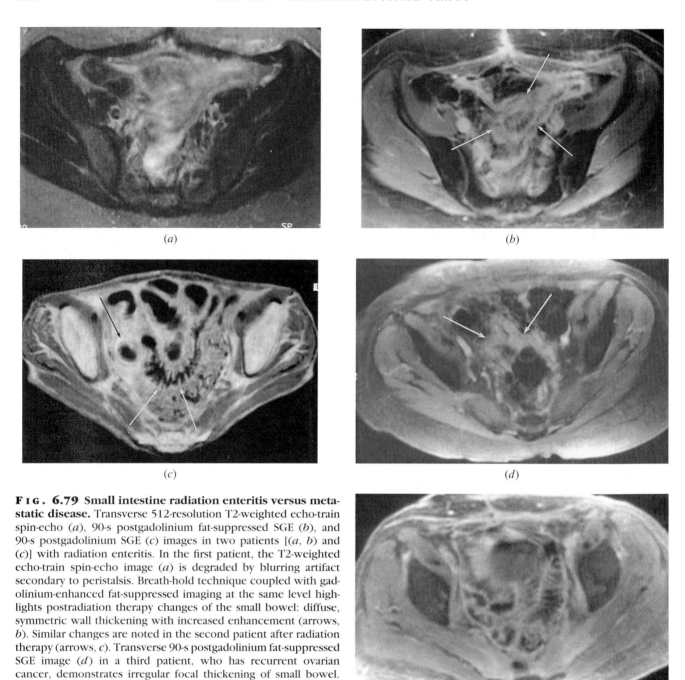

F I G . 6.79 Small intestine radiation enteritis versus metastatic disease. Transverse 512-resolution T2-weighted echo-train spin-echo (*a*), 90-s postgadolinium fat-suppressed SGE (*b*), and 90-s postgadolinium SGE (*c*) images in two patients [(*a*, *b*) and (*c*)] with radiation enteritis. In the first patient, the T2-weighted echo-train spin-echo image (*a*) is degraded by blurring artifact secondary to peristalsis. Breath-hold technique coupled with gadolinium-enhanced fat-suppressed imaging at the same level highlights postradiation therapy changes of the small bowel: diffuse, symmetric wall thickening with increased enhancement (arrows, *b*). Similar changes are noted in the second patient after radiation therapy (arrows, *c*). Transverse 90-s postgadolinium fat-suppressed SGE image (*d*) in a third patient, who has recurrent ovarian cancer, demonstrates irregular focal thickening of small bowel. Note the difference between the symmetric and uniform bowel thickening associated with radiation changes (*b*, *c*) and the more focal and asymmetric changes produced by metastatic disease to the small bowel (arrows, *d*). Transverse gadolinium-enhanced interstitial-phase fat-suppressed SGE (*e*) image in a fourth patient, after radiation therapy for colon cancer, shows circumferential small bowel thickening.

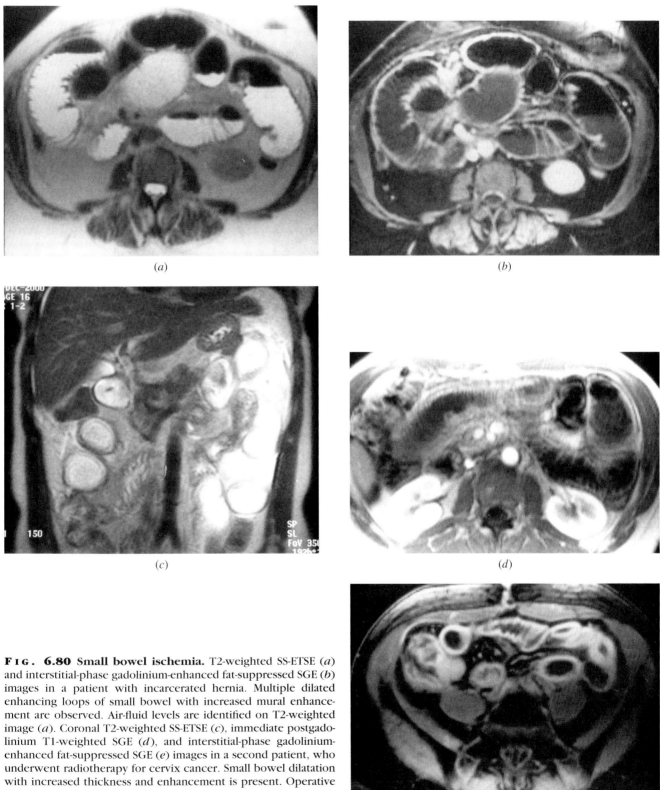

(a)

(b)

(c)

(d)

F I G . 6.80 Small bowel ischemia. T2-weighted SS-ETSE (a) and interstitial-phase gadolinium-enhanced fat-suppressed SGE (b) images in a patient with incarcerated hernia. Multiple dilated enhancing loops of small bowel with increased mural enhancement are observed. Air-fluid levels are identified on T2-weighted image (a). Coronal T2-weighted SS-ETSE (c), immediate postgadolinium T1-weighted SGE (d), and interstitial-phase gadolinium-enhanced fat-suppressed SGE (e) images in a second patient, who underwent radiotherapy for cervix cancer. Small bowel dilatation with increased thickness and enhancement is present. Operative findings were consistent with multiple adhesions and bowel ischemia. Coronal T2-weighted SS-ETSE (f) image in a third patient shows diffuse, markedly dilated small bowel loops.

(e)

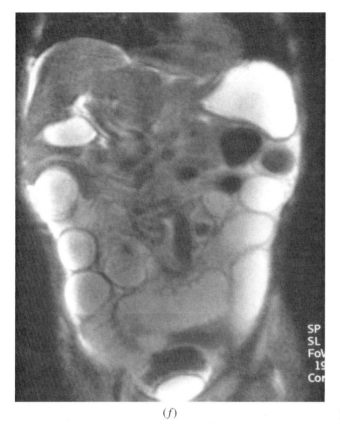

(f)   **FIG. 6.80** (*Continued*)

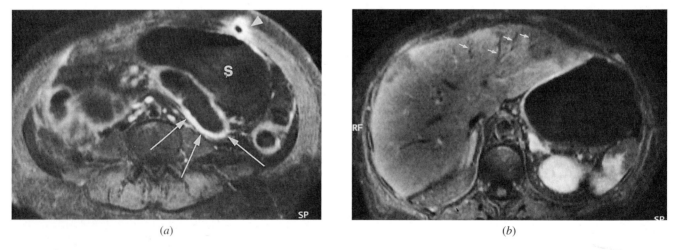

(a)   (b)

FIG. 6.81 Small bowel ischemia. Gadolinium-enhanced T1-weighted fat-suppressed spin-echo images (*a, b*). The patient had undergone previous small bowel resection. Increased enhancement of a loop of proximal small bowel (arrows, *a*) is present. The stomach (s, *a*) also contains regions of increased mural enhancement. Increased enhancement results from leaky capillaries in ischemic bowel disease. Portal venous gas (small arrows, *b*) is an ominous finding suggesting bowel necrosis. Susceptibility artifact (arrowhead, *a*) is noted within the anterior abdominal wall. Coronal T2-weighted single-shot echo-train spin-echo (*c*) and

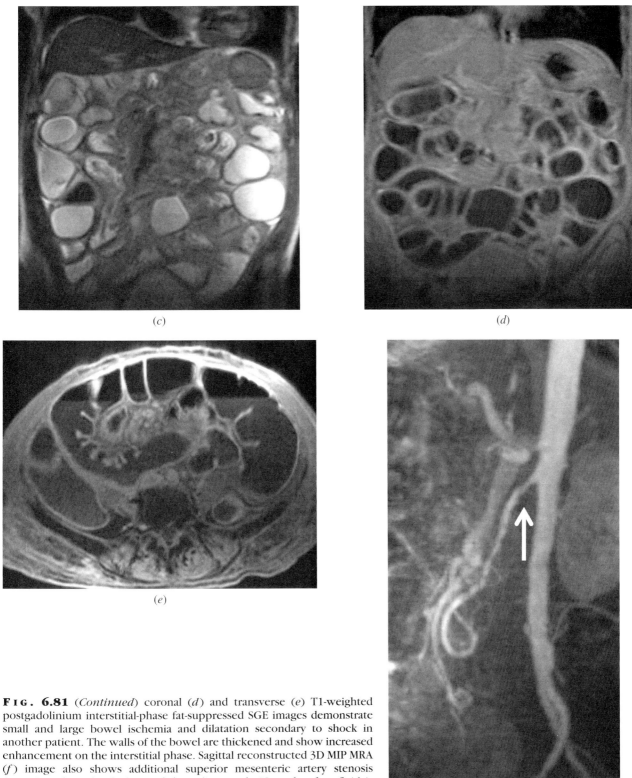

(c)

(d)

(e)

FIG. 6.81 (*Continued*) coronal (*d*) and transverse (*e*) T1-weighted postgadolinium interstitial-phase fat-suppressed SGE images demonstrate small and large bowel ischemia and dilatation secondary to shock in another patient. The walls of the bowel are thickened and show increased enhancement on the interstitial phase. Sagittal reconstructed 3D MIP MRA (*f*) image also shows additional superior mesenteric artery stenosis (arrow) and similar findings of the celiac trunk. Note that free fluid is present in the abdomen.

(f)

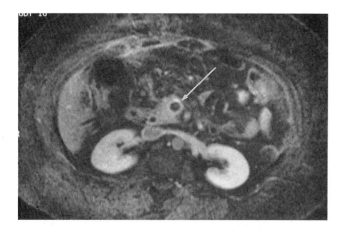

F I G . 6.82 Superior mesenteric vein (SMV) thrombosis. Transverse 90-s postgadolinium fat-suppressed SGE image demonstrates signal-void thrombus in the SMV with increased enhancement of the SMV wall (arrow), which was caused by infection associated with thrombosis.

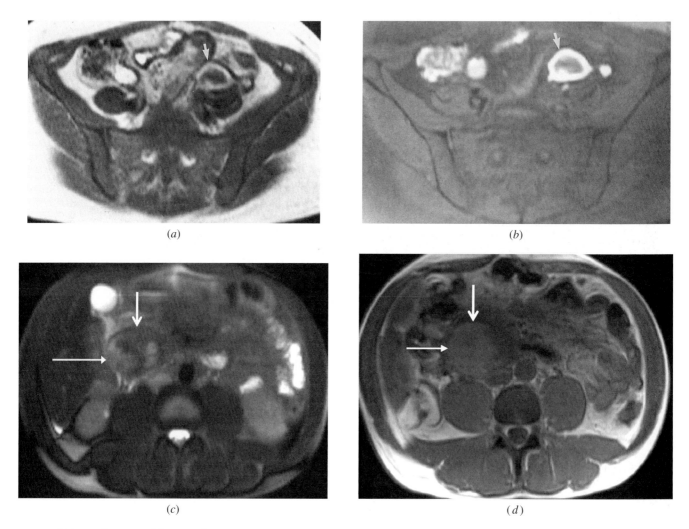

(a)

(b)

(c)

(d)

F I G . 6.83 Submucosal hemorrhage. SGE (*a*) and T1-weighted fat-suppressed spin-echo (*b*) images in a woman status post hysterectomy who had undergone vigorous intraoperative bowel retraction. Increased signal intensity in the bowel wall on the SGE image (arrow, *a*) becomes more conspicuous after fat suppression (arrow, *b*). **Duodenal hematoma.** Transverse T2-weighted single-shot echo-train spin-echo (*c*), transverse T1-weighted SGE (*d*), and coronal T1-weighted postgadolinium interstitial-phase fat-suppressed 3D-GE (*e*) images demonstrate an intramural duodenal hematoma (arrows, *c–e*) in another patient. An eccentrically

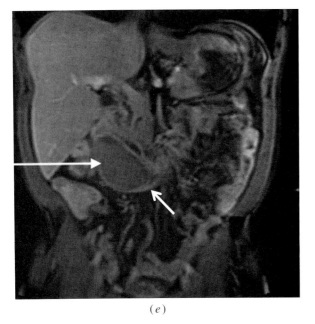

(e)

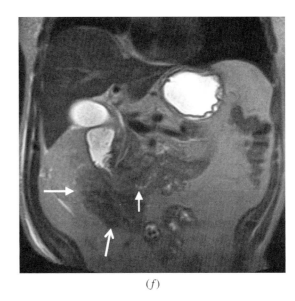

(f)

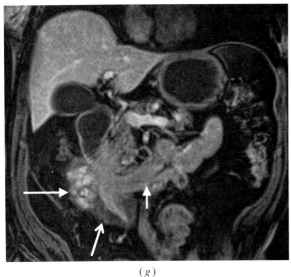

(g)

FIG. 6.83 (*Continued*) located duodenal mass shows heterogeneously high signal on T2-weighted image (*c*) and intermediate signal on T1-weighted image (*d*). No enhancement is detected in the lesion on postgadolinium image (*e*). Note that minimal perihepatic free fluid is detected. Coronal T2-weighted single-shot echo-train spin-echo (*f*) and coronal T1-weighted fat-suppressed interstitial-phase 3D-GE (*g*) images demonstrate periduodenal hematoma in another patient. Periduodenal hematoma (long arrows, *f*, *g*) is present in the mesentery along the 2nd and 3rd portions of the duodenum. The hematoma shows intermediate signal on T2-weighted image (*f*) and high signal on T1-weighted precontrast image (not shown). The hematoma does not show any enhancement on postgadolinium image (*g*). Note that the duodenal wall (short arrow, *f*, *g*) is intact.

THE LARGE INTESTINE

Normal Anatomy

The large bowel measures approximately 4.5 ft in length and is divided into the appendix, cecum, ascending colon, transverse colon, descending colon, sigmoid colon, rectum, and anal canal. Its main functions include absorption of water and electrolytes, storage of fecal matter, and mucus secretion.

The cecum lies below the level of the ileocecal valve. Although the cecum is in the right iliac fossa, it possesses a mesentery and sometimes is freely mobile. This mobility predisposes the cecum to volvulus formation. The ascending and descending colon are retroperi-

toneal and located in the anterior pararenal space. The transverse colon is located anteriorly in the peritoneal cavity suspended by the transverse mesocolon, which originates from the peritoneal covering of the anterior surface of the pancreas. The gastrocolic ligament connects the superior surface of the transverse colon to the greater curvature of the stomach. The sigmoid colon is intraperitoneal and suspended by a mesentery, whereas the rectum is retroperitoneal and relatively fixed. The frontal and lateral surfaces of the rectum are covered with peritoneum, which is then reflected anteriorly, forming the rectovaginal recess in females and the rectovesical recess in males. Below the coccyx, the rectum traverses the levator ani muscles to become the anal canal.

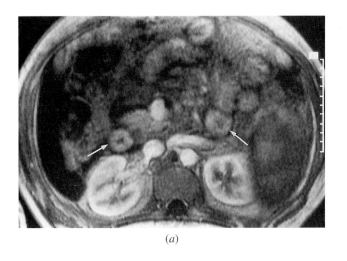

(a)

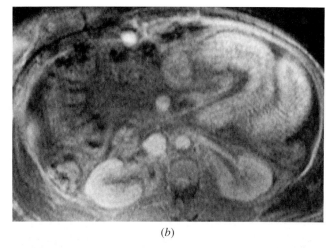

(b)

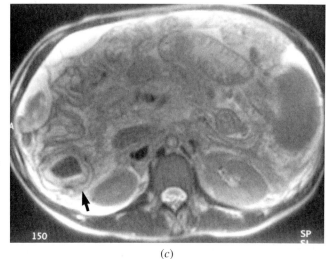

(c)

F I G . 6.84 Small bowel edema in cirrhosis. Immediate post-gadolinium SGE (*a*), 90-s postgadolinium SGE (*b*), and T2-weighted single-shot echo-train spin-echo (*c*) images in three different patients with cirrhosis. Ascites and diffuse thickening of multiple loops of small bowel (arrows, *a*) are present. Third-spacing of fluid secondary to hypoproteinemia accounts for the bowel wall thickening. High-signal submucosal edema is well shown on the single-shot T2-weighted image (arrow, *c*)

Colonic microstructure consists of four layers: mucosa, submucosa, muscularis externa, and serosa. The bowel wall is usually less than 4 mm thick. The muscularis consists of an inner circular and an outer longitudinal layer. Thickened muscular bundles of the outer muscle layer form the taeniae coli. Because the taeniae are shorter in length than the colonic wall itself, taeniae coli gather the wall into sacculations or haustra. Colonic luminal diameter is greatest in the cecum and gradually decreases distally to the level of the rectal ampulla, where the caliber again increases.

MRI Technique

The technique and considerations for studying the large bowel parallel those for the small bowel. Fasting at least 4–6 h before imaging is recommended to reduce peristalsis. Blurring artifact from bowel motion decreases image quality of long-acquisition-time T2-weighted conventional and fast spin-echo techniques. T2-weighted single-shot echo-train spin-echo and True-FISP techniques overcome this limitation and should be performed in the axial and coronal planes for imaging colonic disease, with the sagittal plane reserved for imaging the rectum. Gadolinium-enhanced fat-suppressed SGE or 3D-GE imaging is an important sequence for imaging the colon, as with all other segments of intra-abdominal bowel. Normal colon is thin walled, has haustrations, and enhances minimally with gadolinium (fig. 6.88).

The rectum deserves special mention. Unlike the remaining large intestine, the relatively fixed position of the rectum benefits from high-resolution (512 matrix) T2-weighted echo-train spin-echo imaging. This technique is particularly useful for the evaluation of rectal carcinoma, assessing the extent of bowel wall involvement by tumor, determining the relationship of tumors to adjacent structures, and distinguishing tumor recurrence from fibrosis. Endorectal MRI also may be used to study the rectum. The endoluminal surface coil optimizes

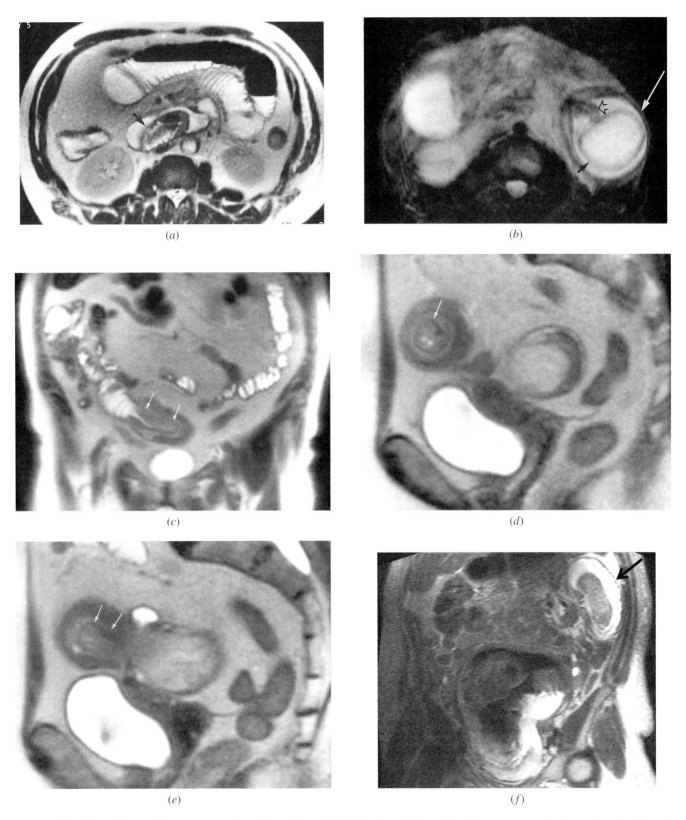

F I G. 6.85 Small bowel intussusception. T2-weighted SS-ETSE (*a*) and T2-weighted fat-suppressed echo-train spin-echo (*b*) images in two patients. In the first patient, the T2-weighted image (*a*) provides clear definition of the bowel-within-bowel appearance (arrow) of intussusception. In the second patient (*b*), respiratory and bowel motion degrades the majority of the peritoneal cavity. However, the dilated, relatively fixed, hypotonic loop of the intussuscipiens (long arrow, *b*) is relatively well shown. The intussusceptum (short arrow, *b*) is clearly shown, and its mesentery (open arrow, *b*) is also appreciated. In this second patient adequate visualization of the intussusception occurred in this non-breath-hold study because of the hypotonicity of the involved bowel segments. Coronal (*c*) and sagittal (*d*, *e*) T2-weighted SSETSE images in a third patient. The bowel-within-bowel appearance (arrows, *a*–*c*) is clearly demonstrated. (Courtesy of N. Cem Balci, Florence Nightingale Hospital, Istanbul, Turkey). **Intussusceptions**

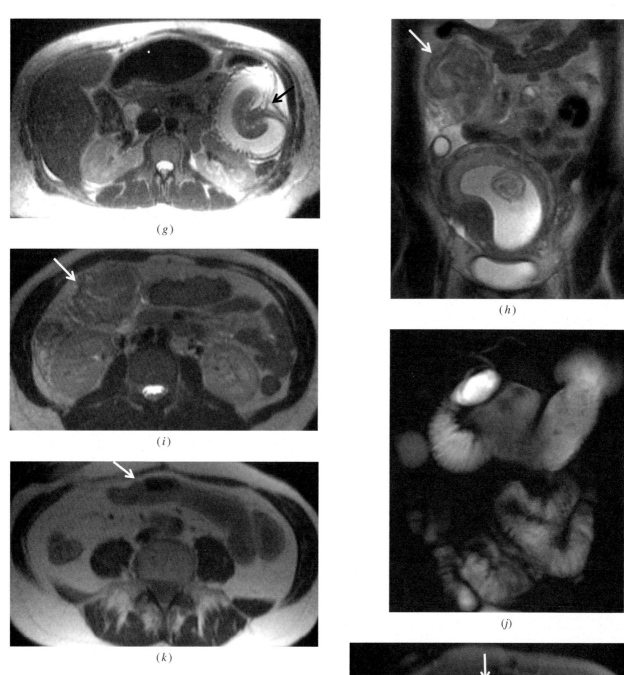

FIG. 6.85 (*Continued*) **in pregnant patients.** Coronal (*f*) and transverse (*g*) T2-weighted single-shot echo-train spin-echo and coronal (*h*) and transverse (*i*) single-shot echo-train spin-echo images demonstrate intussusceptions in two pregnant patients. Bowel-within-bowel appearance (black arrow, *f*, *g*) is detected in the left upper quadrant in a patient with jejuno-jejunal intussusception. Note the pregnancy and free fluid in this patient. Bowel-within-bowel appearance is detected in the right upper quadrant in another patient with colo-colic intussusception. Inflammatory stranding is present around the intussusception. Note the pregnancy and free fluid in this patient. **Small bowel obstruction secondary to adhesion.** T2-weighted thick-section fast spin-echo MRCP (*j*), T1-weighted SGE (*k*), and T1-weighted post-gadolinium fat-suppressed interstitial-phase 3D-GE (*l*) images demonstrate small bowel obstruction secondary to adhesions. Small bowel dilatation in combination with small bowel wall thickening and increased mural enhancement are detected. The transition point (arrows, *k*, *l*) between dilated small bowel segments and normal caliber small bowel segment is shown.

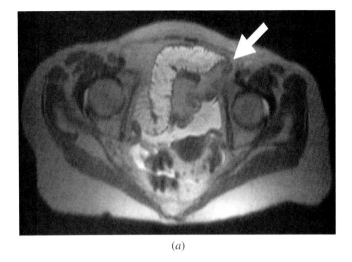

(a)

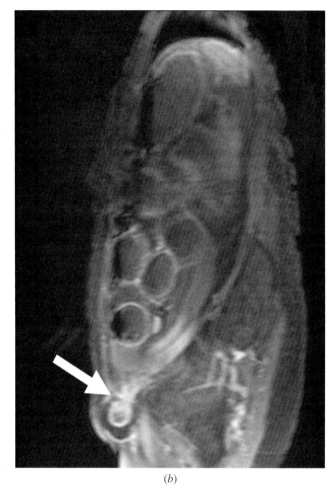

(b)

FIG. 6.86 Small bowel inguinal hernia. Axial single-shot T2 (*a*) and sagittal gadolinium-enhanced delayed-phase gradient-echo fat-suppressed T1 (*b*) images show an inguinal hernia (arrows) with mild dilatation of the small bowel proximal to the involved segment.

spatial resolution and demonstrates the rectal wall layers, anal sphincter complex, and disease processes [9, 10, 87, 88]. The use of intraluminal contrast to distend the colon may improve detection of mucosal abnormalities [89]. The layers of the rectal wall can be visualized on gadolinium-enhanced T1-weighted fat-suppressed images, high-resolution T2-weighted images, and endorectal coil T2-weighted images (see fig. 6.88). The transition between the rectum and the anal canal can be determined by the observation that the rectum contains intraluminal air and the anal canal is collapsed (fig. 6.89). Phased array torso coil imaging is generally used for imaging the rectum due to ease of use and patient acceptive. High-resolution (512 matrix) T2-weighted image combined with gadolinium-enhanced thin section 3D gradient echo is generally recommended.

MR colonography is a relatively recent technique that involves distending the colon with fluid and obtaining coronal thick-slab (5–8 cm) T2-weighted single-shot echo-train spin echo to generate images that resemble fluoroscopic barium enemas [90–92]. Water serves well as an intraluminal contrast agent.

Congenital Anomalies

Malrotation
Nonrotation, the most common rotational abnormality, is discussed above. In this condition the large bowel will occupy the left side of the abdomen (fig. 6.89).

Duplication
Colonic duplications represent a congenital longitudinal division of the developing gut. Grossly, two intestinal lumens are identified. The abnormalities may be limited to a single segment of large bowel, or they can involve the entire colon (fig. 6.90). Symptoms will depend on whether or not there is communication of the duplication with the remainder of the colon. Patients with right colon duplication are at risk for intussusception.

Anorectal Anomalies
Most cases of anorectal anomalies occur in association with other congenital malformations. MRI has been successful in evaluating these patients because it directly demonstrates the rectal pouch and sphincter muscles in

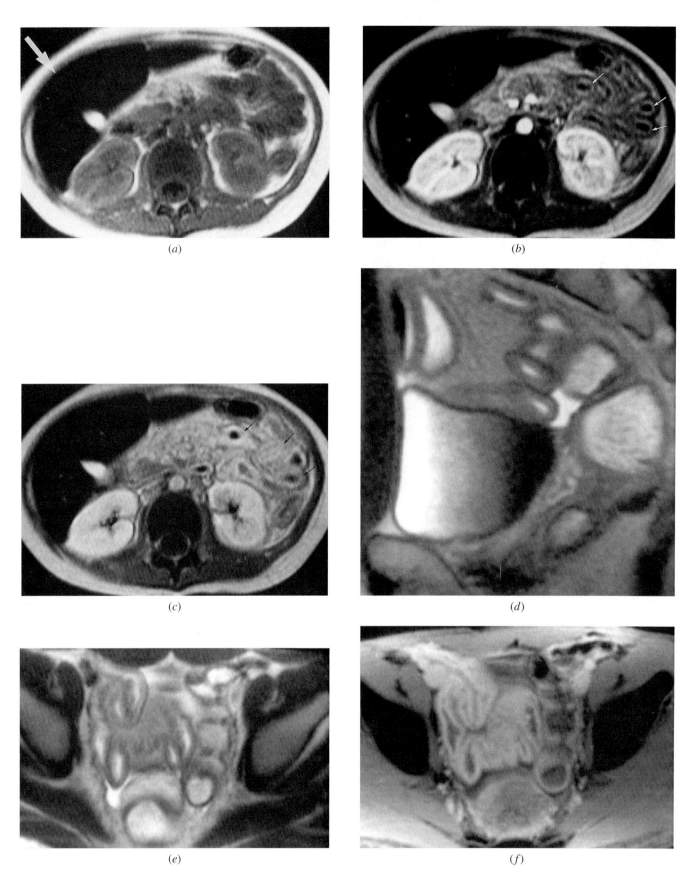

(a)

(b)

(c)

(d)

(e)

(f)

F I G . 6.87 Graft-versus-host disease. SGE (*a*) and immediate (*b*) and 90-s (*c*) postgadolinium SGE images in a patient after bone marrow transplant. Unenhanced images suggest thickening of multiple loops of small bowel. Immediately after intravenous contrast, intense mucosal enhancement of multiple loops of small bowel (arrows, *b*) is appreciated. On the interstitial-phase image (*c*), enhancement has spread to involve the majority of the wall (arrows). This enhancement pattern reflects hyperemia and capillary leakage, respectively. The decreased signal intensity of the liver (arrow, *a*) is consistent with iron overload secondary to multiple blood transfusions. (Reprinted with permission from Ascher SM, Semelka RC: MRI of the gastrointestinal tract. In Higgins CB, Hricak H, Helms CA (eds.), *Magnetic Resonance Imaging of the Body*. New York: Raven Press, 1997, p. 677–700.) Sagittal (*d*) and transverse (*e*) T2-weighted SS-ETSE and transverse interstitial-phase gadolinium-enhanced fat-suppressed SGE (*f*) images in a second

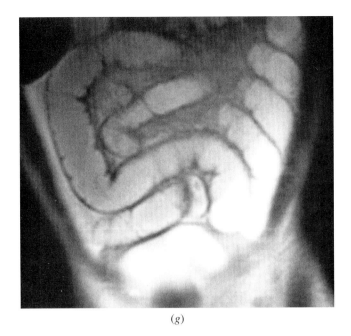

(g)

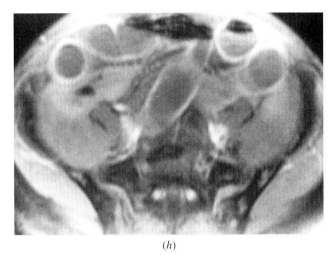

(h)

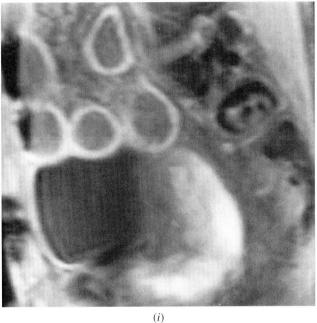

(i)

F I G . 6.87 (*Continued*) patient after bone marrow transplant. There is marked and diffuse wall thickening and increased mural enhancement of multiple bowel loops. Coronal T2-weighted SS-ETSE (g) and transverse (*h*) and sagittal (*i*) interstitial-phase gadolinium-enhanced fat-suppressed SGE images in a third patient after bone marrow transplant for ALL. There are dilated, fluid-filled small bowel loops associated with diffuse enhancement of the bowel wall.

multiple planes. This permits exact determination of the location and developmental status of the sphincter muscles as well as identification of associated anomalies of the kidneys and spine. MRI is also valuable for postoperative assessment of the neorectum and sphincteric muscles (figs. 6.91 and 6.92) [93].

Mass Lesions

Benign Masses

Polyps and Polyposis Syndromes. Adenomas are the most common form of colorectal polyp. Colonic adenomatous polyps are the most common large bowel neoplasm. All adenomatous polyps arise as the result

of epithelial proliferative dysplasia or deranged development (fig. 6.93). In this regard, adenomas are precursor lesions for colorectal adenocarcinoma. Three basic patterns of adenomatous polyps are discerned pathologically: tubular, tubulovillous, and villous. Villous adenomas are characterized by a neoplastic growth composed of fine fingerlets or villi that project from the muscularis mucosae to the outer tip of the adenoma and show a propensity for the rectum and rectosigmoid area. Villous architecture tends to be found more frequently in larger adenomas and is associated with a higher risk of malignancy (fig. 6.94) [94]. Multiple colonic adenomas are seen in association with familial adenomatous polyposis or Gardner syndrome, whereas

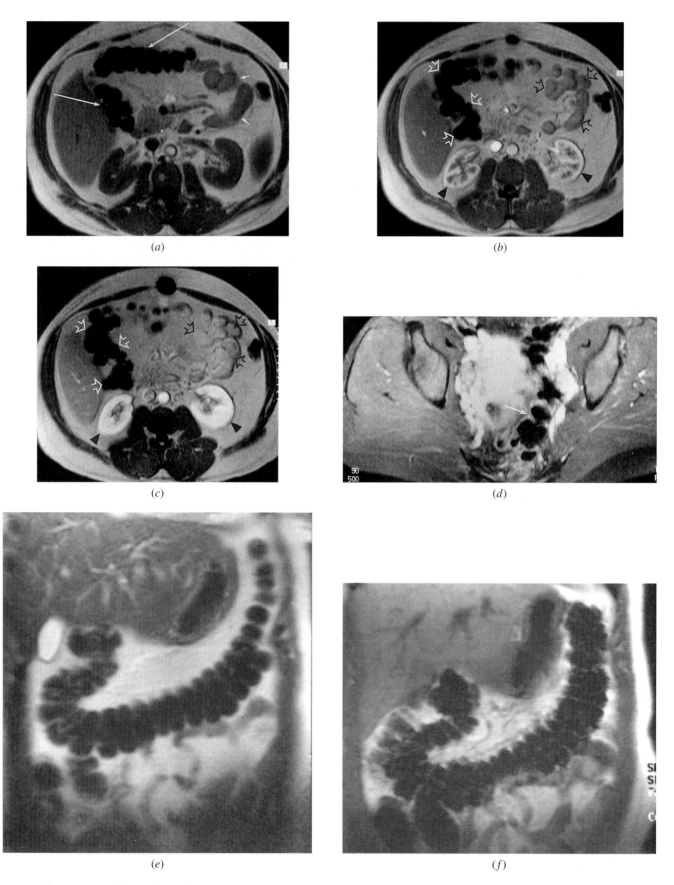

F I G . 6.88 Normal large bowel. SGE (*a*) and immediate (*b*) and 90-s (*c*) postgadolinium SGE images. Air-filled colon (long arrows) and normal small bowel (short arrows) are seen on the precontrast T1-weighted image (*a*). After intravenous gadolinium administration the walls of the large and small bowel (open arrows, *b*, *c*) enhance less than adjacent renal parenchyma (arrowheads, *b*, *c*) on capillary-phase (*b*) and interstitial-phase (*c*) images. Gadolinium-enhanced T1-weighted fat-suppressed spin-echo image (*d*) in another subject demonstrates a normal-appearing sigmoid colon that shows minimal mural enhancement, thin wall, and haustrations (arrow). Coronal T2-weighted SS-ETSE (*e*) and coronal SGE (*f*) images in a third patient demonstrate normal transverse colon with multiple haustrations.

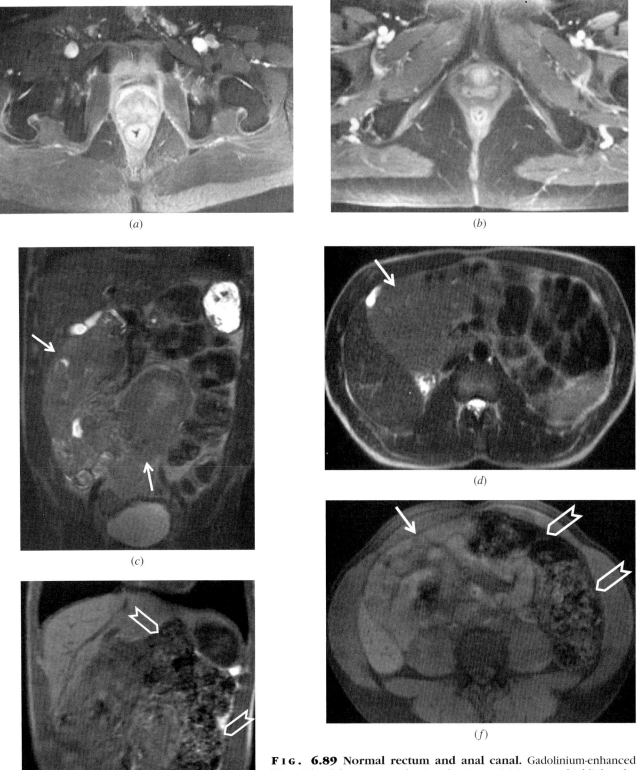

(a)

(b)

(c)

(d)

(e)

(f)

F I G . 6.89 Normal rectum and anal canal. Gadolinium-enhanced
T1-weighted fat-suppressed spin-echo image (*a*) in a man highlights the
different layers of the rectum (from inner layer to outer layer): high-signal-
intensity mucosa, low-signal-intensity muscularis mucosa and lamina
propria, high-signal-intensity submucosa, and low-signal-intensity muscularis propria. The rectum contains air within the lumen. Gadolinium-
enhanced T1-weighted fat-suppressed spin-echo image (*b*) in a woman
demonstrates the same enhancement features of the anal canal. Note that
the anal canal is collapsed and does not contain air. **Malrotation.** Coronal
(*c*) and transverse (*d*) T2-weighted single-shot echo-train spin-echo and
coronal (*e*) and transverse (*f*) T1-weighted SGE images demonstrate malrotation of the small and large bowel. While the small bowel (arrows, *c*,
d, *f*) is located at the midline and right side of the abdomen, the large
bowel (including the cecum) (open arrows, *e, f*) is located at the midline
and the left side of the abdomen.

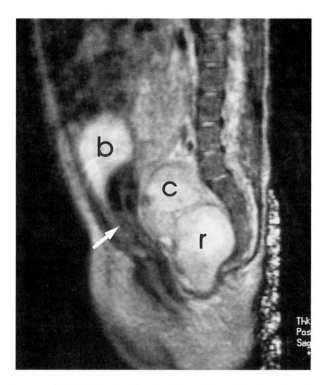

FIG. 6.90 Colonic duplication. T2-weighted spin-echo image in a patient with colonic duplication. The uterus (arrow) and bladder (b) are anteriorly displaced by two fluid-filled viscous structures that represent the rectum (r) and the duplication cyst (c).

multiple colonic hamartomas may be seen in Peutz–Jeghers syndrome or juvenile polyposis syndromes.

A number of polyposis syndromes have been described. The most common are familial adenomatous polyposis, Gardner and Peutz–Jeghers syndromes, and the juvenile polyposis syndromes. Familial adenomatous polyposis syndrome is an autosomal dominant disorder characterized by numerous adenomas affecting primarily the colon and the rectum. Familial adenomatous polyposis represents a prototype of a hereditary precancerous syndrome because the risk of malignant transformation to colorectal carcinoma approaches 100%. Patients with familial adenomatous polyposis syndrome have an increased risk of developing periampullary duodenal carcinoma. Gardner syndrome is an autosomal dominant condition with diffuse adenomatous polyps, bony abnormalities (osteomas), and soft tissue tumors. Presently regarded as a variation of familial adenomatous polyposis syndrome, Gardner syndrome confers the same risk of progression to colon adenocarcinoma. Peutz–Jeghers syndrome is an autosomal dominant disorder characterized clinically by skin and mucosal pigmented macules and gastrointestinal hamartomas. The hamartomas favor the small bowel in 95% of cases, with colonic and stomach involvement in up to 25%. Although the hamartomatous polyps themselves do not have malignant potential, patients with this syndrome have an increased

incidence of both benign and malignant tumors arising in many organs. Up to 3% of patients with Peutz–Jeghers syndrome will develop adenocarcinoma of the stomach or duodenum, and 5% of women will have ovarian cysts or tumors. There are three distinct syndromes associated with juvenile polyps of the alimentary tract: juvenile polyposis, gastrointestinal juvenile polyposis, and the Cronkhite–Canada syndromes. Hamartomas are common to all three syndromes [95, 96].

Gadolinium-enhanced fat-suppressed SGE or 3D-GE images can demonstrate polyps, whether they occur in isolation or in association with a polyposis syndrome. Semelka and Marcos reported on the MR appearance of polyposis syndromes [65]. In that series, polyps were well seen with a combination of gadolinium-enhanced fat-suppressed SGE images and T2-weighted single-shot echo-train spin-echo images. The importance of demonstrating polyp enhancement by comparing precontrast and postcontrast fat-suppressed SGE images was emphasized, because this observation permitted distinction between polyps and colon contents. Polyps smaller than 1 cm in familial polyposis syndrome were not commonly observed. The most common appearance is an enhancing sessile or pedunculated mass arising from the bowel wall and protruding into the lumen (figs. 6.95 and 6.96). If frondlike polyp morphology or enhancement is observed, the possibility of a villous adenoma should be raised. Similarly, extension beyond the bowel wall signifies malignant degeneration.

Lipomas. Lipomas are the second most common benign neoplasm of the large bowel. They usually originate in the submucosa. Most are asymptomatic, although changes in bowel habits, bleeding, or both have been reported in patients with large lesions. The most common locations for colonic lipomas are the cecum, ascending colon, and sigmoid colon. The MRI appearance of lipomas with T1-weighted and fat-suppressed T1-weighted sequences are pathognomonic: high in signal intensity on T1-weighted images and diminished in signal intensity on fat-suppressed T1-weighted images (fig. 6.97) [97]. Additional use of out-of-phase SGE may demonstrate fat-water black ring phase cancellation surrounding the polyp (fig. 6.98). Lipomas may also act as lead point for intussusceptions (fig. 6.99).

Other Mesenchymal Neoplasms. Leiomyomas, hemangiomas (fig. 6.100), and neurofibromas are all rare.

Mucocele. A mucocele is defined as a dilatation of the appendiceal lumen resulting from mucus accumulation associated with luminal obstruction. Mucoceles are frequently asymptomatic unless they become secondarily infected or rupture. Pathologically, it is important to distinguish between nonneoplastic lesions (retention) and neoplastic mucoceles. Nonneoplastic

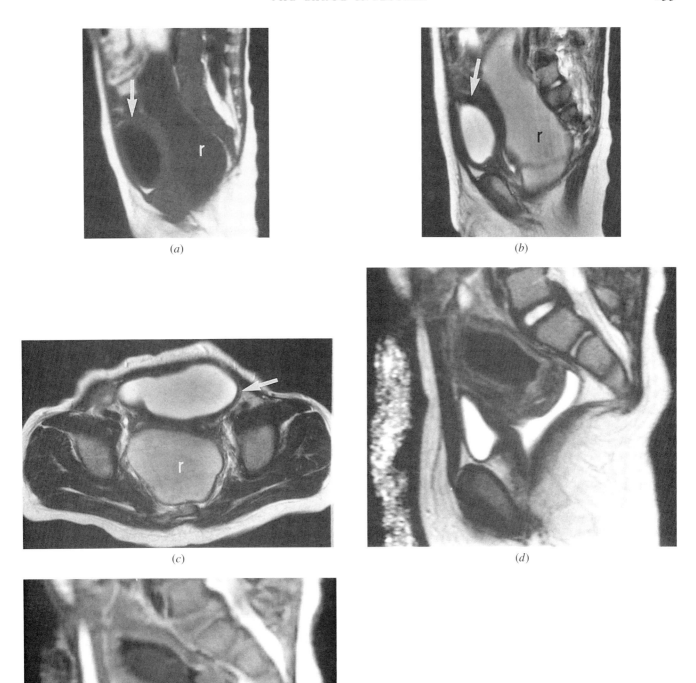

FIG. 6.91 Surgical repair of persistent cloaca. Sagittal T1-weighted spin-echo (*a*), sagittal T2-weighted echo-train spin-echo (*b*), and transverse T2-weighted echo-train spin-echo (*c*) images. A capacious neorectum (r, *a–c*) is present. The bladder (large arrow, *a–c*) is thick-walled and anteriorly displaced. Absence of the vagina is noted. Sagittal T2-weighted SS-ETSE (*d*) and T1-weighted SGE (*e*) images in a second patient with cloacal anomaly who had undergone multiple surgeries. The levator ani complex is diminutive in size, and distal sacral segments are absent. There is a fluid-filled structure situated posterior to the uterus that represents the anal canal and rectum.

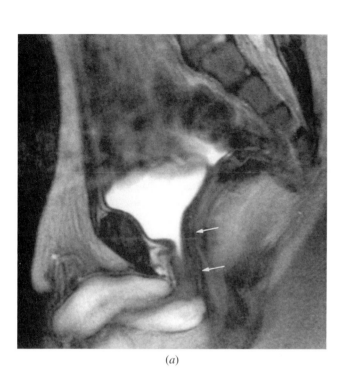

(a)

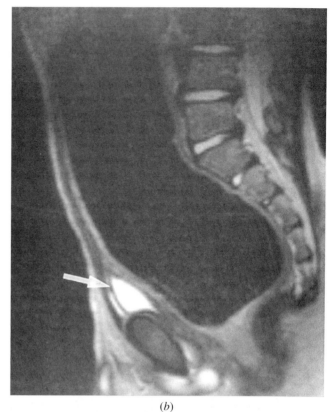

(b)

FIG. 6.92 Reconstructed imperforate anus. Sagittal T2-weighted SS-ETSE (*a*) image in a 1-year old boy shows that the anal canal is situated in an anterior location, just posterior to the prostate. The levator ani muscle is intact. Sagittal T2-weighted echo-train spin-echo images in a second (*b*) and a third (*c*) patient demonstrate a markedly dilated air-filled rectum, compressing and displacing the bladder anterosuperiorly (arrow, *b*).

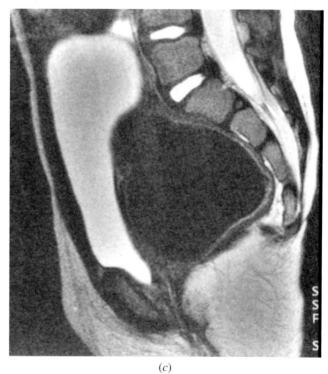

(c)

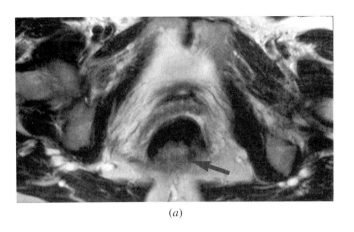

(a)

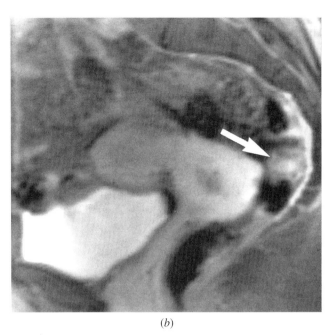

(b)

FIG. 6.93 Adenomatous polyp of rectum. Transverse T2-weighted echo-train spin-echo (*a*) and sagittal interstitial-phase gadolinium-enhanced fat-suppressed SGE (*b*) images. There is a 1.6-cm polypoid mass (arrows, *a, b*) arising from the posterior wall of the rectum, without evidence of extension beyond the rectal wall.

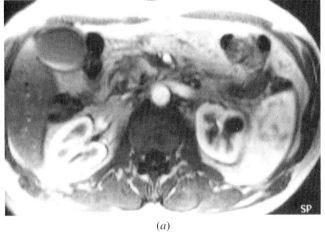

(a)

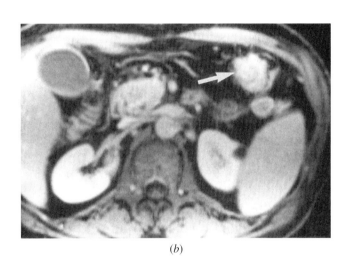

(b)

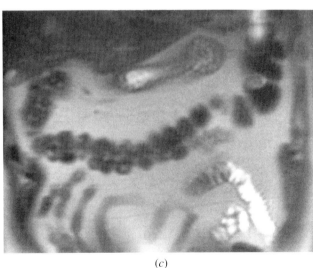

(c)

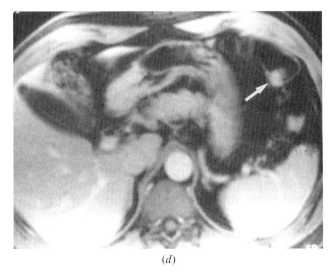

(d)

FIG. 6.94 Villous adenoma. Immediate postgadolinium SGE (*a*) and interstitial-phase gadolinium-enhanced fat-suppressed SGE (*b*) images. A polypoid mass is seen within the distal transverse colon. The mass enhances minimally on immediate postgadolinium images (*a*) and in a moderately intense fashion with mild heterogeneity on 2-min postgadolinium image (arrow, *b*). Coronal T2-weighted SS-ETSE (*c*) and transverse interstitial-phase gadolinium-enhanced fat-suppressed SGE (*d*) images in a second patient with villous adenoma of transverse colon (arrow, *d*) demonstrate an appearance similar to the previous patient. Most tumors show moderately intense enhancement with mild heterogeneity on 2-min postgadolinium interstitial-phase images, reflecting a larger and more irregular interstitial space than adjacent normal bowel. Sagittal (*e*) and coronal (*f*) single shot echo train spin echo and transverse (*g*) high resolution fast spin echo T2-weighted images and transverse (*h, i*) and sagittal (*j*) T1-weighted fat-suppressed postgadolinium interstitial phase 3D-GE images at 3.0 T demonstrate a villous adenoma (white thick arrows; *e-g*) located in

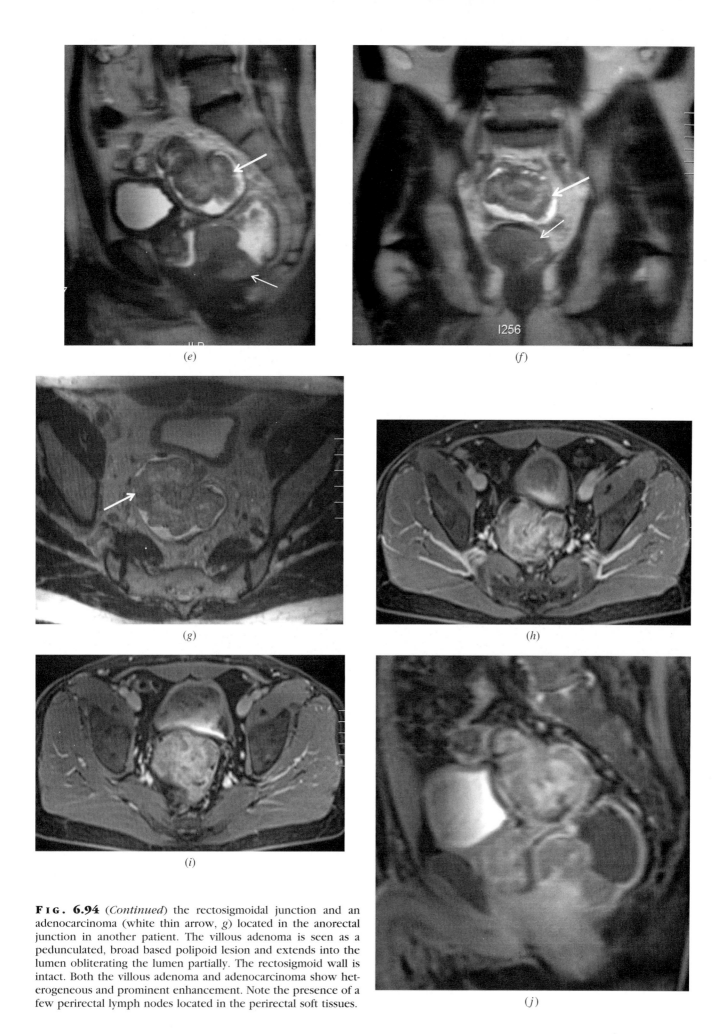

(e)

(f)

(g)

(h)

(i)

(j)

FIG. 6.94 (*Continued*) the rectosigmoidal junction and an adenocarcinoma (white thin arrow, *g*) located in the anorectal junction in another patient. The villous adenoma is seen as a pedunculated, broad based polipoid lesion and extends into the lumen obliterating the lumen partially. The rectosigmoid wall is intact. Both the villous adenoma and adenocarcinoma show heterogeneous and prominent enhancement. Note the presence of a few perirectal lymph nodes located in the perirectal soft tissues.

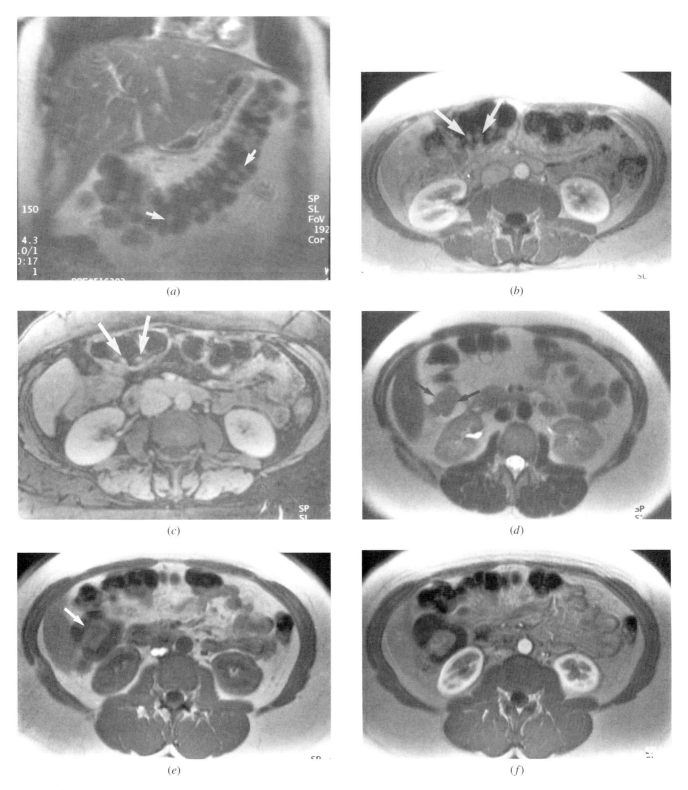

(a)

(b)

(c)

(d)

(e)

(f)

FIG. 6.95 Familial adenomatous polyposis syndrome. Coronal T2-weighted SS-ETSE (*a*), immediate postgadolinium SGE (*b*), and interstitial-phase gadolinium-enhanced fat-suppressed SGE (*c*) images. Numerous polyps are seen measuring less than 1 cm in diameter in the transverse colon (arrows, *a*). The signal void of the air in the colon provides good contrast from the soft tissue polyps on the T2-weighted image (*a*). The polyps are mildly enhanced (arrows) on the immediate postgadolinium image (*b*). Polyps demonstrate persistent enhancement on interstitial-phase images (arrows, *c*). This patient underwent total colectomy, which demonstrated numerous adenomatous polyps. Transverse T2-weighted SS-ETSE (*d*), SGE (*e*), and immediate postgadolinium SGE (*f*) images in another patient with familial polyposis syndrome. A 2.5-cm polyp is present that arises in the ascending colon. The high signal intensity of the fluid contents of the colon permits good delineation of the low signal intensity of the polyp on the SS-ETSE image (arrows, *d*).The polyp is isointense to the bowel wall on the precontrast T1-weighted image (arrow, *e*). On the early postgadolinium image, the polyp shows mild heterogeneous enhancement comparable to the bowel wall. Note the intense enhancement of the normal renal cortex, which is greater than the enhancement of the bowel wall or the polyp. This patient underwent sigmoidoscopy with biopsy followed by total colectomy (Reprinted with permission from Semelka RC, Marcos HB: Polyposis syndromes of the gastrointestinal tract. *J Magn Reson Imaging* 11: 51–55, 2000.). Coronal SS-ETSE (*g*, *h*) images in a third patient with

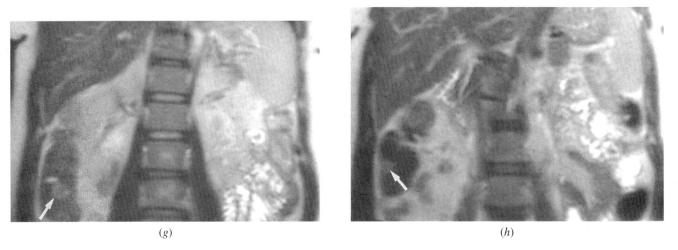

(g)   (h)

F i g . 6.95 (*Continued*) familial adenomatous polyposis demonstrate polypoid lesions in the ascending colon (arrows, *g, h*).

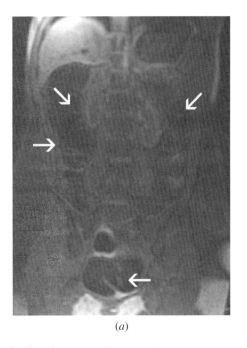

(a)

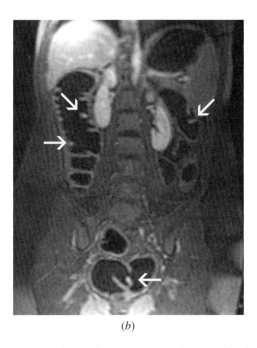

(b)

F i g . 6.96 Polyposis coli. With dark-lumen water enema contrast MR colonography, multiple colonic polyps can be detected in this 12-year-old female patient with polyposis coli. These lesions show an avid contrast enhancement comparing precontrast (arrows, *a*) and postcontrast (arrows, *b*) T1-weighted sequences.

lesions show an inflamed mucosa or hyperplastic epithelium. Neoplastic mucoceles are best classified as mucinous cystoadenoma or mucinous cystadenocarcinoma. In mucinous cystoadenocarcinoma, spread of malignant cells beyond the appendix in the form of peritoneal implants is frequently present. Pseudomyxoma peritonei, with the findings of adenocarcinomatous cells, distinguishes this malignant process from simple mucinous spillage, which may occur with rupture of a retention mucocele or cystadenoma. Because of the possibility of an underlying malignancy and the risk of rupture, mucoceles should be prophylactically removed.

T2-weighted single-shot echo-train spin-echo images show a high-signal-intensity tubular structure in the region of the appendix. Mucoceles have a higher signal intensity than simple fluid on T1-weighted sequences owing to their protein content. In uncomplicated cases, the wall of the mucocele is thin and enhances minimally after intravenous gadolinium administration (fig. 6.101).

Varices. Rectal varices develop in patients with portal hypertension. The incidence of hemorrhoids is not increased in these patients [98].

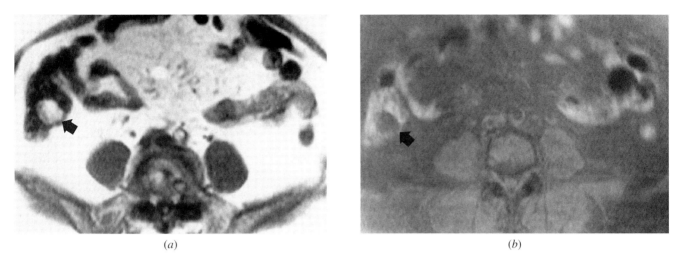

(a)   (b)

F IG . 6.97 Cecal lipoma. SGE (*a*) and T1-weighted fat-suppressed spin-echo (*b*) images. A mass in the cecum is high in signal intensity on the T1-weighted image (arrow, *a*) and diminishes in signal intensity on the fat-suppressed image (arrow, *b*). These imaging characteristics are pathognomonic for a fat-containing tumor. The cecum is a common location for large bowel lipomas. (Reprinted with permission from Shoenut JP, Semelka RC, Silverman R,Yaffe CS, Mickflikier AB: Magnetic resonance imaging evaluation of the local extent of colorectal mass lesions. *J Clin Gastroenterol* 17: 248–253, 1993.)

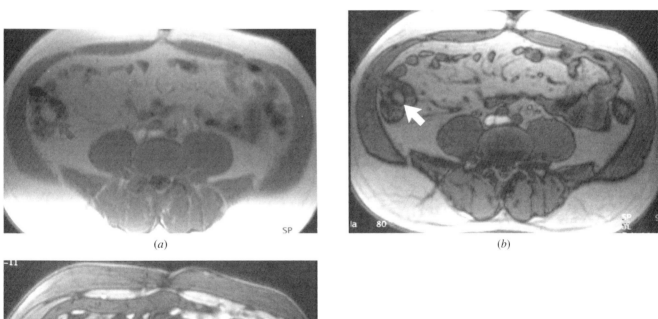

(a)   (b)

(c)

F IG . 6.98 Cecal lipoma. Precontrast SGE (*a*), precontrast out-of-phase SGE (*b*), and 90-s postgadolinium fat-suppressed SGE (*c*) images. A 2-cm mass in the cecum is high in signal intensity in the precontrast SGE image (arrow, *a*) and demonstrates a phase cancellation artifact in the out-of-phase SGE image (arrow, *b*). Markedly diminished signal intensity of the mass is noted on post-contrast fat-suppressed SGE image (arrow, *c*). (Reprinted with permission from Chung JJ, Semelka RC, Martin DR, Marcos HB: Colon diseases: MR evaluation using combined T2-weighted single-shot echo train spin-echo and gadolinium-enhanced spoiled gradient-echo sequences. *J Magn Reson Imaging* 12: 297–305, 2000.)

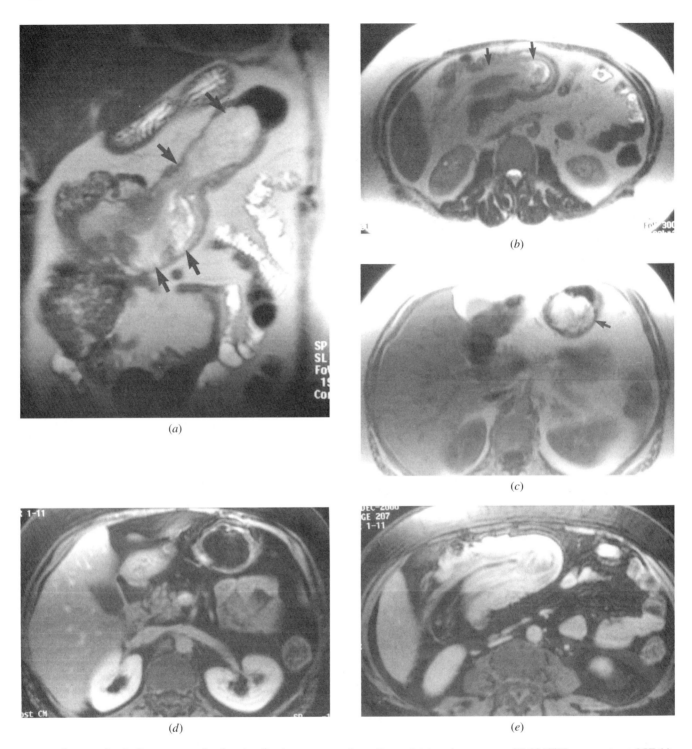

F i g . 6.99 Colonic lipoma as a lead point for intussusception. Coronal (*a*) and transverse (*b*) SS-ETSE, precontrast SGE (*c*), and 90-s postgadolinium fat-suppressed SGE (*d*, *e*) images. There is a lipoma situated within the lumen of the mid-transverse colon (arrow, *c*) at the end of a colo-colonic intussusception (arrows, *a*, *b*), which arose from the mid-ascending colon.

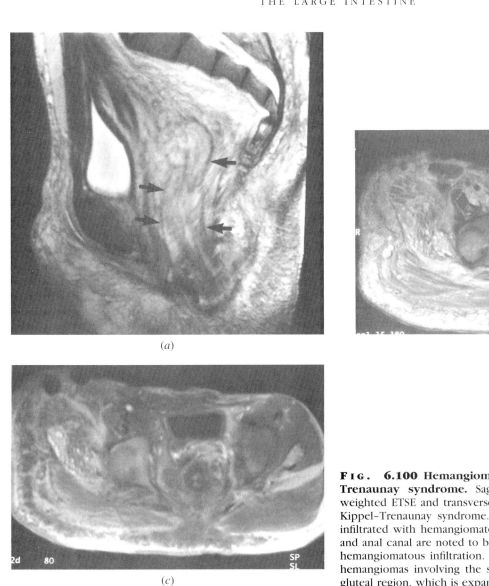

(a)

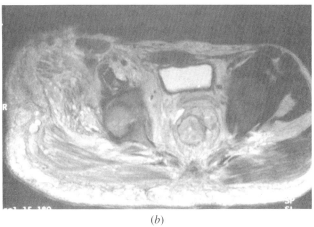

(b)

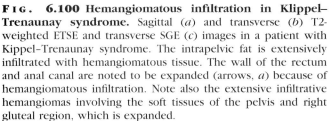

(c)

FIG. 6.100 Hemangiomatous infiltration in Klippel–Trenaunay syndrome. Sagittal (a) and transverse (b) T2-weighted ETSE and transverse SGE (c) images in a patient with Kippel–Trenaunay syndrome. The intrapelvic fat is extensively infiltrated with hemangiomatous tissue. The wall of the rectum and anal canal are noted to be expanded (arrows, a) because of hemangiomatous infiltration. Note also the extensive infiltrative hemangiomas involving the soft tissues of the pelvis and right gluteal region, which is expanded.

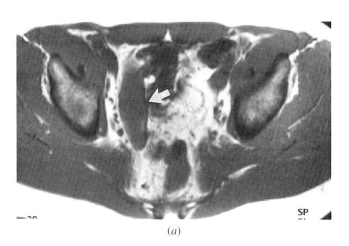

(a)

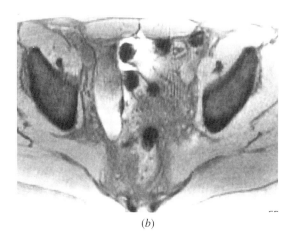

(b)

FIG. 6.101 Mucocele of the appendix. SGE (a), fat-suppressed SGE (b), SS-ETSE (c), sagittal SS-ETSE (d), and immediate postgadolinium fat-suppressed SGE (e) images. An oblong-shaped mucocele of the appendix is present (arrow, a) that contains high-signal-intensity material in the dependent portion of the cyst on the T1-weighted image (a), which is accentuated with the application of fat suppression (b). The mucocele is high in signal intensity on the T2-weighted image, with slight heterogeneity in

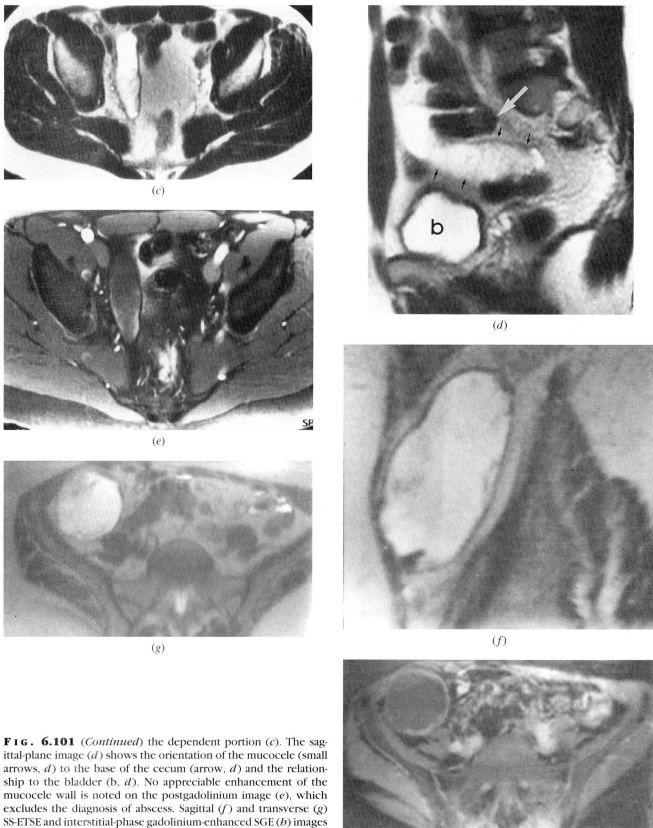

FIG. 6.101 (*Continued*) the dependent portion (*c*). The sagittal-plane image (*d*) shows the orientation of the mucocele (small arrows, *d*) to the base of the cecum (arrow, *d*) and the relationship to the bladder (b, *d*). No appreciable enhancement of the mucocele wall is noted on the postgadolinium image (*e*), which excludes the diagnosis of abscess. Sagittal (*f*) and transverse (*g*) SS-ETSE and interstitial-phase gadolinium-enhanced SGE (*h*) images in a second patient show a large cystic mass in the lower right quadrant of the abdomen extending into the pelvic inlet. Note the presence of septations and a thin rim of enhancement.

Malignant Masses

Adenocarcinoma. Adenocarcinoma of the colon is the most common gastrointestinal tract malignancy and the second most common visceral cancer in North America. The estimated incidence in the United States is 138,000 new cases per year, and the 5-year survival is 50–60% [39]. The incidence of adenocarcinoma of the colon increases with advancing age. Sporadic cancers are increased in first-degree family relatives of patients with known colorectal carcinoma. Other conditions that predispose to the development of colon cancer include familial adenomatous polyposis, Gardner syndrome, Lynch syndrome, ulcerative colitis, Crohn colitis, and previous ureterosigmoidostomies. Cancers occur most often in the rectosigmoid colon, but right-sided cancers are reported to occur in increasing frequency [99]. Tumors may be polypoid, circumferential ("apple core"), or plaquelike. Symptoms reflect tumor location and morphology, with most patients reporting a combination of change in bowel habits, bleeding, pain, and weight loss. A TNM system is used for staging (Table 6.3).

Good correlation is observed between gadolinium-enhanced fat-suppressed MRI techniques and surgical specimens for tumor size, bowel wall involvement, peritumoral extension, and lymph node detection [5].

Table 6.3 TNM Staging for Cancer of the Colon

T—Primary Tumor

Tx Primary tumor cannot be assessed

T0 No evidence of primary tumor

Tis Pre-invasive carcinoma (carcinoma in situ)

T1 Tumor limited to the mucosa or mucosa and submucosa

T2 Tumor with extension to muscle or muscle and serosa

T3 Tumor with extension beyond the colon to immediately contiguous structures

T3a Tumor without fistula formation

T3b Tumor with fistula formation

T4 Tumor with deep infiltration occupying more than one-half but not more than one region or extending to neighboring structures

N—Regional lymph nodes

Nx Regional lymph nodes cannot be assessed

N0 No evidence of regional lymph node metastasis

N1 Evidence of regional lymph node involvement

N2, N3 Not applicable

N4 Evidence of involvement of juxta-regional lymph nodes

M—Metastases

Mx Distant metastases cannot be assessed

M0 No distant metastases

M1 Distant metastases

Malignant lymph nodes are usually not enlarged in gastrointestinal adenocarcinoma. However, the presence of more than five lymph nodes that measure smaller than 1 cm in a regional distribution related to the tumor correlates well with tumor involvement. All segments of the colon and the appendix are well shown on MR images. The combination of T2-weighted single-shot echo-train spin-echo and gadolinium-enhanced fat-suppressed SGE or 3D-GE images results in the most reproducible image quality for the colon above the rectum (figs. 6.102–6.109). Rectal and colon cancers

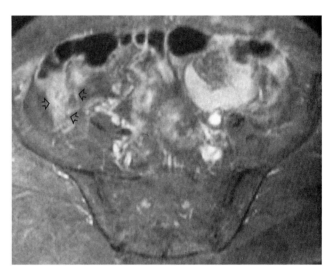

F I G . 6.102 Appendiceal adenocarcinoma. Gadolinium-enhanced T1-weighted fat-suppressed spin-echo image demonstrates heterogeneous enhancing infiltrative tumor arising from the appendix (open arrows).

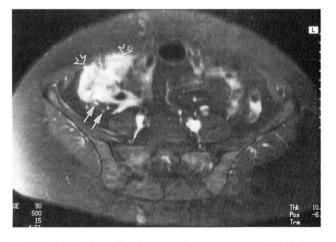

F I G . 6.103 Colonic adenocarcinoma, cecum. Gadolinium-enhanced T1-weighted fat-suppressed spin-echo image demonstrates a large heterogeneous intensely enhancing cecal carcinoma (open arrows) that extends to the anterior peritoneal wall. Multiple enhancing lymph nodes smaller than 5 mm are identified (arrows), which are malignant.

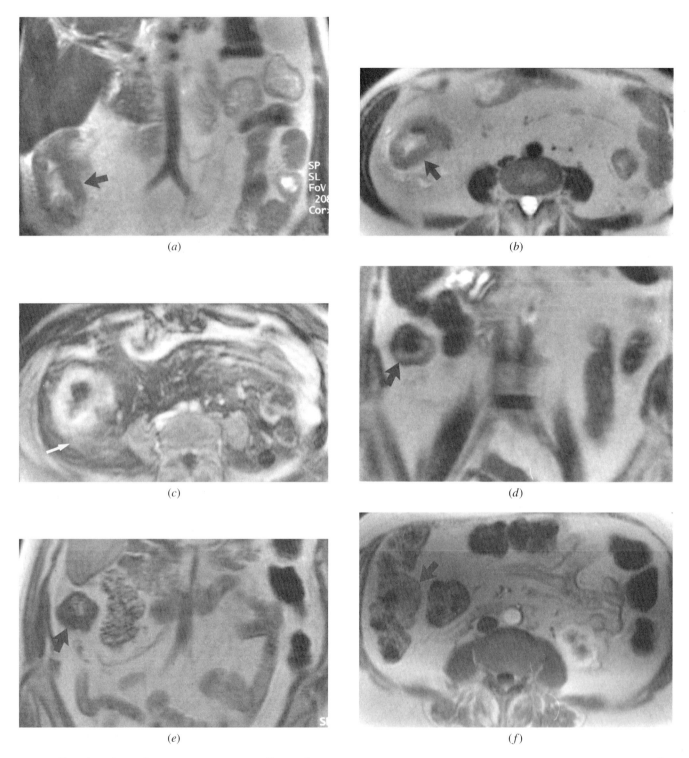

F I G . 6.104 Colon adenocarcinoma, ascending colon. Coronal (*a*) and transverse (*b*) SS-ETSE and 90-s postgadolinium fat-suppressed SGE (*c*) images. Irregularly thickened bowel wall with intermediate signal intensity representing cancer is noted in the ascending colon (arrows, *a*, *b*). The cancer enhances in a moderate and slightly heterogeneous fashion. Pericolonic fat infiltration is demonstrated in the ascending colon on postcontrast fat-suppressed SGE image as enhancing strands of tissue (arrow, *c*). Coronal SS-ETSE (*d*), coronal precontrast SGE (*e*), and transverse immediate postcontrast SGE (*f*) images in a second patient also demonstrate an irregular thickening of the ascending colon wall (arrow, *d-f*). There is no evidence of pericolonic fat infiltration with sharp external margins to the tumor.

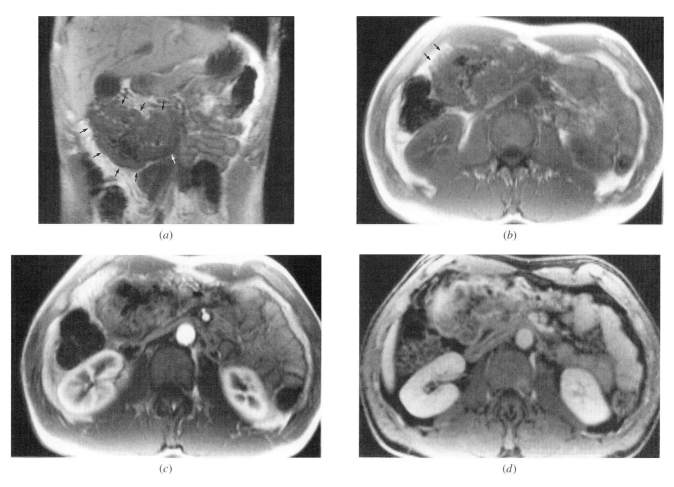

(a) (b)

(c) (d)

F I G. 6.105 Colon adenocarcinoma, transverse colon. Coronal SGE (*a*), SGE (*b*), immediate postgadolinium SGE (*c*), and 90-s postgadolinium fat-suppressed SGE (*d*) images. A large cancer arises from the transverse colon (small arrows, *a*). The outer margin of the tumor is indistinct (small arrows, *b*), a finding consistent with lymphovascular extension. The tumor is heterogeneous and moderate in signal intensity on capillary-phase (*c*) and interstitial-phase (*d*) images.

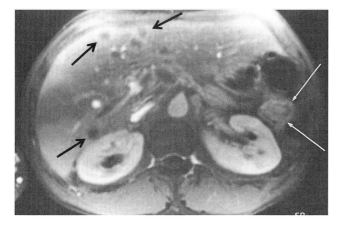

F I G. 6.106 Colon adenocarcinoma, proximal descending colon. Transverse 90-s postgadolinium SGE image demonstrates a heterogeneously enhancing tumor (white arrows) in the proximal descending colon with prominent enhancing strands in the surrounding mesentery consistent with lymphovascular extension. Multiple ring-enhancing liver metastases are apparent (black arrows).

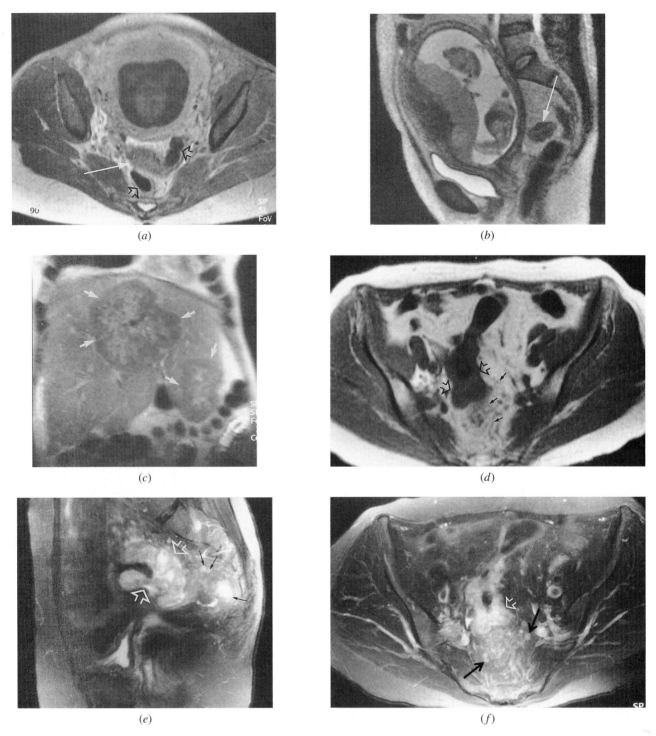

F I G . 6.107 Sigmoid adenocarcinoma. SGE (*a*) and sagittal (*b*) and coronal (*c*) SS-ETSE images in a pregnant patient with colon cancer. The SGE image shows air-filled colon (open arrows, *a*) proximal and distal to the 4-cm sigmoid cancer (arrow, *a*). The SS-ETSE images show the primary tumor (arrow, *b*) and the liver metastases (arrows, *c*). The gravid uterus is well imaged with the single-shot T2-weighted breathing-independent technique (*b*). SGE (*d*), sagittal T2-weighted fat-suppressed spin-echo (*e*), and gadolinium-enhanced T1-weighted fat-suppressed spin-echo (*f*) images in a second patient with advanced sigmoid adenocarcinoma. The precontrast image demonstrates abnormal thickening of the sigmoid colon (open arrows, *d*) with low-signal-intensity strands infiltrating the pericolonic fat (small arrows, *d*). The primary tumor (open arrows, *e, f*) and pericolonic extension are well shown as high-signal-intensity structures in a low-signal-intensity background on both fat-suppressed T2-weighted (*e*) and gadolinium-enhanced T1-weighted fat-suppressed (*f*) images. Multiple small regional malignant lymph nodes are identified (black arrows, *e, f*).

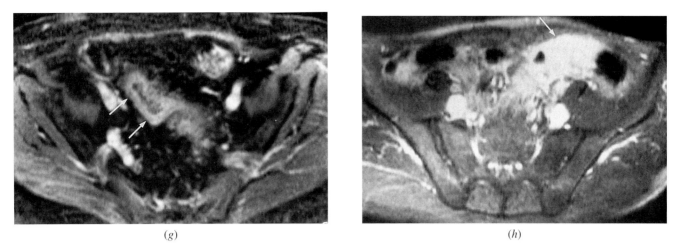

(g)   (h)

F I G . 6.107 (*Continued*) Transverse 90-s postgadolinium SGE image (*g*) in a third patient demonstrates a circumferential 4-cm sigmoid colon cancer (arrows, *g*) that does not show lymphovascular extension. Gadolinium-enhanced T1-weighted fat-suppressed spin-echo image (*b*) in a fourth patient demonstrates an intensely enhancing sigmoid colon cancer (arrow) involving the anterior peritoneum.

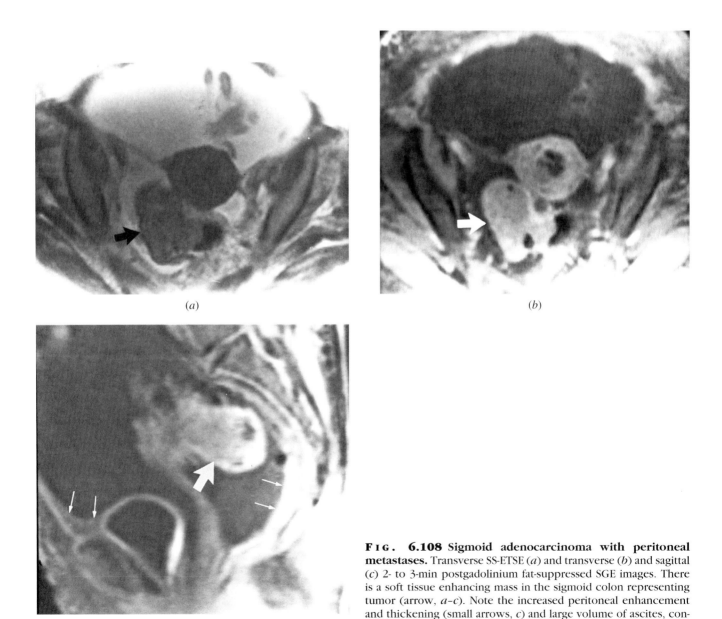

(a)   (b)

(c)

F I G . 6.108 Sigmoid adenocarcinoma with peritoneal metastases. Transverse SS-ETSE (*a*) and transverse (*b*) and sagittal (*c*) 2- to 3-min postgadolinium fat-suppressed SGE images. There is a soft tissue enhancing mass in the sigmoid colon representing tumor (arrow, *a–c*). Note the increased peritoneal enhancement and thickening (small arrows, *c*) and large volume of ascites, consistent with peritoneal disease.

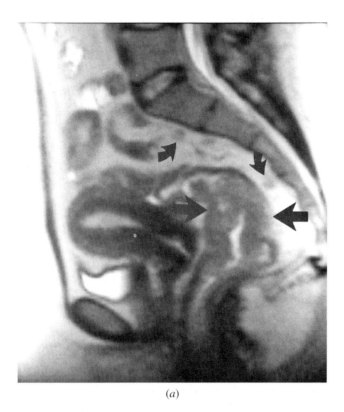

(a)

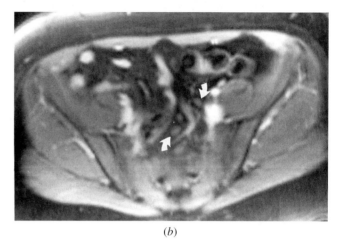

(b)

F I G . 6.109 Rectosigmoid colon adenocarcinoma. Sagittal SS-ETSE (*a*) and 90-s postgadolinium fat-suppressed SGE (*b*) images. Markedly thickened tumor mass (large arrows, *a*) is noted in the rectosigmoid region on the SS-ETSE image. Multiple regional lymph nodes less than 1 cm in diameter are well demonstrated in the pelvis (curved arrows, *a*, *b*). Small nodes are best shown on gadolinium-enhanced fat-suppressed SGE images. (Reprinted with permission from Chung JJ, Semelka RC, Martin DR, Marcos HB: Colon diseases: MR evaluation using combined T2-weighted single-shot echo train spin-echo and gadolinium-enhanced spoiled gradient-echo sequences. *J Magn Reson Imaging* 12: 297–305, 2000.)

benefit from the combined use of gadolinium-enhanced fat-suppressed SGE or 3D-GE and high-resolution T2-weighted echo-train spin-echo images (fig. 6.110). MR colonography employing a bowel cleansing preparation and administration of rectal water enema has been shown effective in demonstrating small polyps (figs. 6.96 and 6.111) and tumors (figs. 6.112, 6.113) [90–92].

Gadolinium-enhanced fat-suppressed GE imaging is valuable in demonstrating perirectal tumor extension, regional lymph nodes, and seeding of peritoneum by tumor. This reflects the high-contrast resolution of this technique for detecting enhancing diseased tissue (figs. 6.114, 6.115). Thin-section 3D-GE may be of particular value to assess tumor extension to the perirectal fascia, the presence of which will affect surgical technique and patient prognosis. Image acquisition of T2-weighted echo-train spin echo or single-shot echo-train spin echo after the administration of gadolinium is commonly done when abdomen and pelvis studies are combined in one examination. As an additional benefit to a shortened MR examination, dependent, concentrated gadolinium in the bladder, which is low in signal intensity, may increase the conspicuity of high-signal-intensity rectal tumor invasion of the bladder wall (see fig. 6.114).

MRI has established an important role in the evaluation of rectal cancer based on the combination of overall topographic display and appreciation of soft tissue contrast resolution [100–102]. One of the strengths of MRI is to evaluate the integrity of the mesorectum, which may be observed as a thin linear structure that envelops the immediate perirectal fat [101, 102]. The ability to routinely visualize this thin structure, which is low signal on T2-weighted images and exhibits enhancement on postgadolinium fat-suppressed images, allows for improved staging of rectal cancer and guidance of appropriate therapy. A large multicentric European prospective observational study showed a MRI specificity of 92% (327/354, 90% to 95%) in predicting curative resection of rectal cancer [103].

When feasible, surface torso coils (e.g., phased-array torso coil) should be employed to ensure better definition of perirectal tumor extension [104]. Phased-array torso coils also provide good overall topographic display that improves detection of features such as regional lymph nodes.

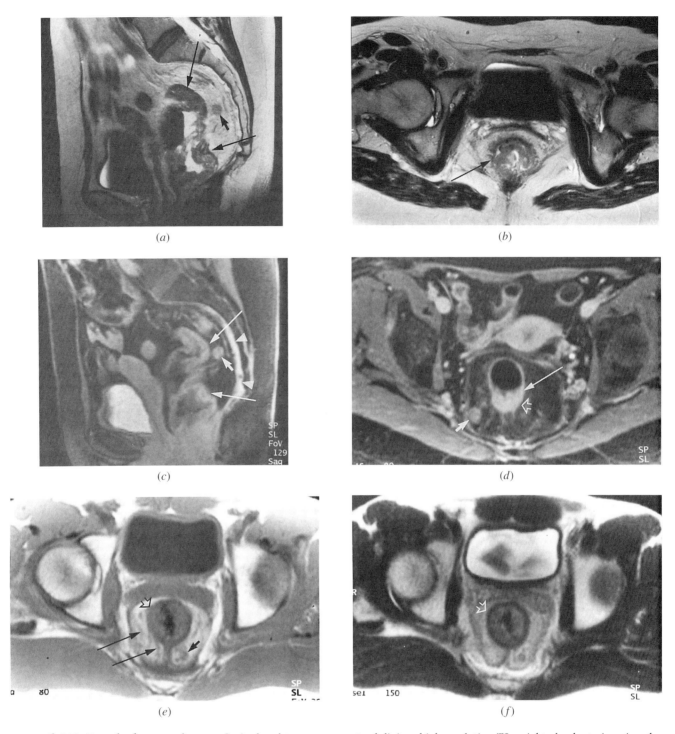

F I G . 6.110 Rectal adenocarcinoma. Sagittal and transverse postgadolinium high-resolution T2-weighted echo-train spin-echo (*a, b*) and sagittal and transverse postgadolinium fat-suppressed SGE (*c, d*) images in a patient with advanced colon cancer. A large rectal cancer is present (long arrows, *a, c*). The craniocaudal extent of tumor is well shown on sagittal images (*a, c*). The tumor extends inferiorly in the rectum (arrow, *b*) to the anal verge. Lymphovascular extension with involved lymph nodes (small arrows, *a, c, d*) is present. At the superior margin, the tumor is mainly posterior in location (open arrow, *d*). The transition from normal colon to tumor (long arrow, *d*) is clearly shown. Presacral spread of tumor is shown as enhancing tissue on the sagittal gadolinium-enhanced fat-suppressed image (arrowheads, *c*). SGE (*e*), SS-ETSE (*f*), and postgadolinium fat-suppressed SGE (*g*) images in a second patient with rectal adenocarcinoma and similar imaging findings. The rectal tumor (open arrows, *e, f, g*), lymphovascular extension (long arrows, *e, g*), and perirectal lymph nodes (short arrows, *e, g*) are well shown. Sagittal and transverse postgadolinium

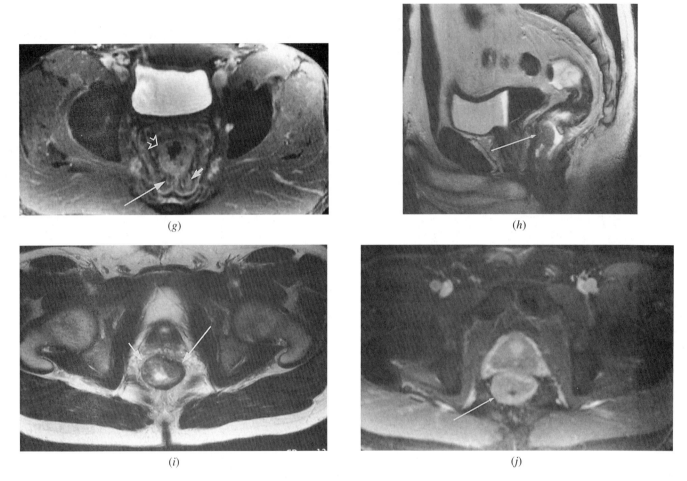

FIG. 6.110 (*Continued*) 512-resolution T2-weighted echo-train spin-echo (*h, i*) and interstitial-phase gadolinium-enhanced fat-suppressed SGE (*j*) images in a third patient. Asymmetric tumor involvement of the rectal wall is apparent on the 512-resolution T2-weighted images (long arrows, *h, i*). Tumor penetrates the full thickness of the right aspect of the rectum (short arrow, *i*). This is shown by interruption of the muscular wall that appears low signal intensity on the T2-weighted image (long arrow, *i*). On the gadolinium-enhanced fat-suppressed SGE image, lower-signal-intensity tumor (arrow, *j*) penetrates the full thickness of the higher-signal-intensity wall. Postgadolinium T2-weighted imaging is a novel technique for assessing possible bladder invasion. Enhancing tumor is conspicuous against the low signal intensity produced by concentrated gadolinium excreted into the bladder. In this case, the bladder is spared.

Endorectal coil imaging permits differentiation of the anatomic layers of the rectal wall on T2-weighted fat-suppressed images [10]. Local staging of rectal carcinoma also benefits from endorectal coil imaging (fig. 6.116) [9, 10].

Recurrence rates for rectosigmoid carcinoma, which are reported to range from 8% to 50%, are a function of the stage of the primary tumor at initial presentation [12]. Tumors tend to recur locally, and curative surgery is feasible. The sagittal imaging plane facilitates MRI detection of recurrent rectal carcinoma. Using T1-weighted, T2-weighted, and gadolinium-enhanced T1-weighted sequences, one study reported a 93.3% accuracy in detecting recurrent disease [12]. Others have shown that MRI is superior to conventional CT imaging and is more specific than transrectal ultrasound for identifying recurrent tumor [11, 13–15]. Specifically, MRI correctly diagnosed recurrent rectal carcinoma in 83.2% of patients versus transrectal ultrasound, which diagnosed recurrence in only 41.6% [16].

Recurrent tumor tends to be low in signal intensity on T1-weighted images and enhances moderately after intravenous gadolinium (figs. 6.117–6.119) [6, 11, 105]. On T2-weighted images, recurrent tumor usually is moderately high in signal intensity. This may be difficult to appreciate on echo-train spin-echo sequences because the surrounding fat is also moderately high in signal intensity on these sequences (see fig. 6.118). Caution must be exercised in interpreting images in patients with possible recurrent disease on echo-train spin-echo sequences: Tumor appears lower in signal intensity compared to its appearance on conventional

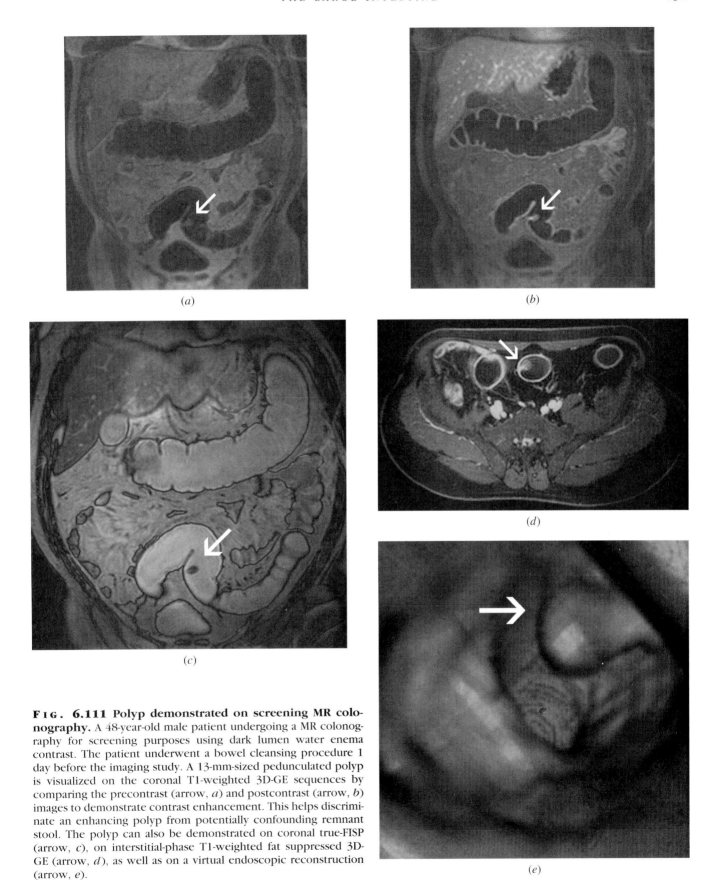

(a)

(b)

(c)

(d)

(e)

F I G . 6.111 Polyp demonstrated on screening MR colonography. A 48-year-old male patient undergoing a MR colonography for screening purposes using dark lumen water enema contrast. The patient underwent a bowel cleansing procedure 1 day before the imaging study. A 13-mm-sized pedunculated polyp is visualized on the coronal T1-weighted 3D-GE sequences by comparing the precontrast (arrow, *a*) and postcontrast (arrow, *b*) images to demonstrate contrast enhancement. This helps discriminate an enhancing polyp from potentially confounding remnant stool. The polyp can also be demonstrated on coronal true-FISP (arrow, *c*), on interstitial-phase T1-weighted fat suppressed 3D-GE (arrow, *d*), as well as on a virtual endoscopic reconstruction (arrow, *e*).

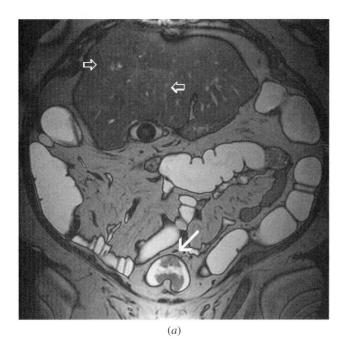

(a)

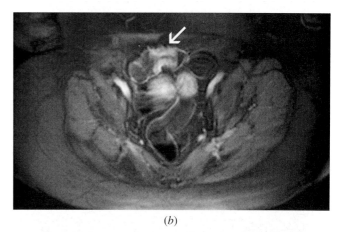

(b)

FIG. 6.112 Adenocarcinoma of the sigmoid colon. A 58-year-old male patient with colon adenocarcinoma arising from the sigmoid colon showing an apple core lesion growth pattern. The adenocarcinoma can be easily depicted on the coronal true-FISP image (arrow, *a*) as well as on the transverse gadolinium-enhanced T1-weighted fat-suppressed 3D-GE image (arrow, *b*). Simultaneous display of the parenchymal abdominal organs show multiple hepatic metastases, which can be accurately detected and characterized on gadolinium-enhanced T1-weighted fat-suppressed 3D-GE image (arrows, *c*), whereas the diagnosis is difficult to make on true-FISP images (open arrows, *a*).

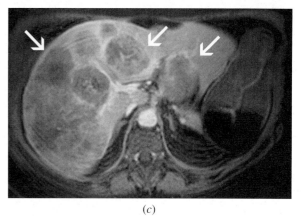

(c)

spin-echo sequences. This reflects the relatively high signal intensity of fat on echo-train spin-echo sequences.

Demonstration of sacral invasion is well shown on T2-weighted fat-suppressed echo-train spin-echo and gadolinium-enhanced T1-weighted fat-suppressed images. Marrow is low in signal intensity on both of these sequences, particularly in the setting of postradiation fatty replacement, which is often present in these patients, and tumor extension is conspicuous because of its high signal intensity (figs. 6.120, 6.121). In the assessment of sacral involvement, imaging in the sagittal plane is essential for visualizing invasion of the cortex of the sacrum. In selected cases, oblique coronal images (following the angulation of the sacrum) are helpful (see fig. 6.120). Recurrent tumor often has a nodular configuration. Recurrent rectosigmoid cancer and post-treatment (surgical and/or radiation) fibrosis frequently coexist (figs. 6.121, 6.122).

Postradiation fibrosis in patients more than 1 year after therapy often demonstrates low signal intensity in the surgical bed on T1- and T2-weighted images and may show negligible enhancement after intravenous gadolinium administration (fig. 6.123) [6, 11, 106]. Enhancement of fibrosis with gadolinium, particularly on fat-suppressed images, often persists for 1.5–2 years after therapy, which is longer than the period of time that fibrosis is high in signal intensity on T2-weighted images. Morphologically, fibrosis often has a plaquelike appearance. Unfortunately, the imaging features of postradiation changes, especially in patients receiving doses in excess of 45 Gy, may not always follow a predictable time course, and overlap in signal behavior between recurrent tumor and posttreatment fibrosis exists [105]. On echo-train spin-echo images, the high signal intensity of fat admixed with fibrous tissue may simulate recurrence (fig. 6.124). Although the T2-weighted signal intensity of fibrosis usually decreases 1

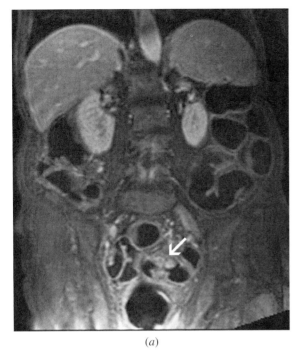

(a)

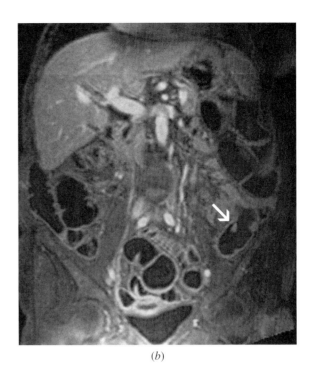

(b)

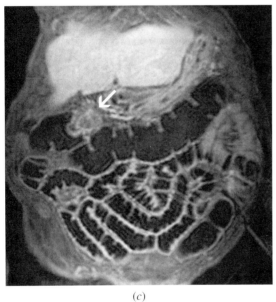

(c)

F I G . 6.113 Multifocal adenocarcinoma and polyp. A 61-year-old female patient is examined with dark-lumen water enema contrast MR colonography in conjunction with contrast-enhanced T1-weighted imaging after a bowel cleansing preparation. A stenotic tumor in the sigmoid colon is conspicuous and demonstrated as an enhancing mass (arrow, *a*). In addition, a pedunculated polyp is noted in the descending colon (arrow, *b*) and a metachronous second focus of adenocarcinoma is identified near the hepatic flexure (arrow, *c*). In this patient, a conventional colonoscopy only demonstrated the distal sigmoid lesion, but because of the stenotic nature of this mass, the scope could not be passed and the more proximal lesions were not observed.

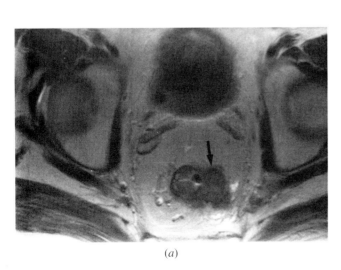

(a)

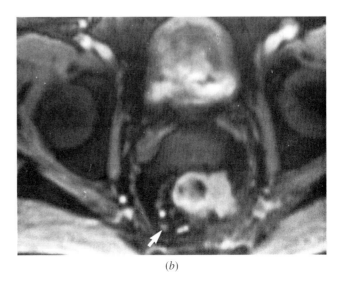

(b)

F I G . 6.114 Rectal cancer. Transverse T2-weighted ETSE (*a*) and interstitial-phase gadolinium-enhanced SGE (*b*) images. There is a soft tissue mass involving the wall of the rectosigmoid with gross tumor extension through the left aspect of the wall (arrow, *a*). Small regional lymph nodes are also identified (arrow, *b*). Sagittal postgadolinium SS-ETSE (*c*) and interstitial-phase

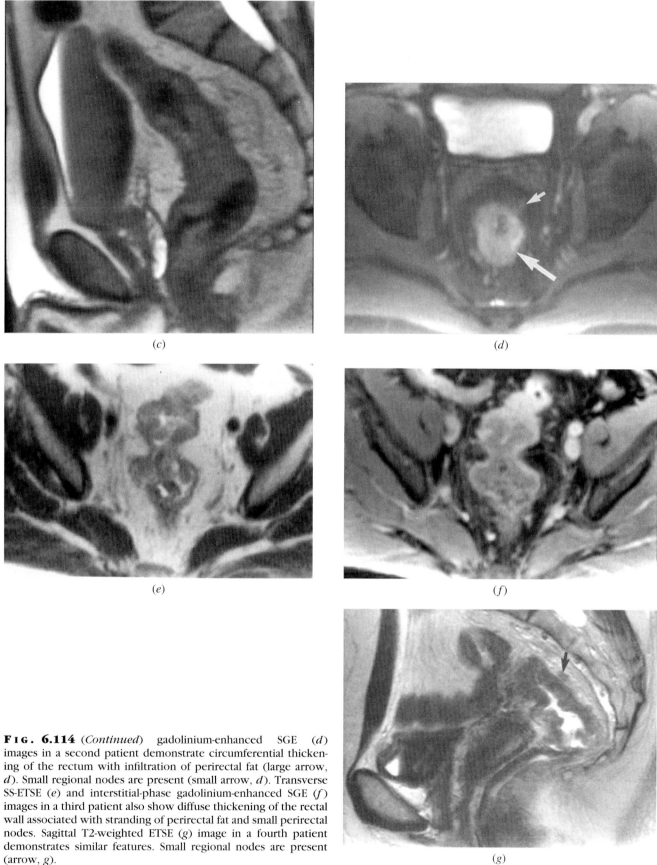

(c)

(d)

(e)

(f)

Fig. 6.114 (*Continued*) gadolinium-enhanced SGE (*d*) images in a second patient demonstrate circumferential thickening of the rectum with infiltration of perirectal fat (large arrow, *d*). Small regional nodes are present (small arrow, *d*). Transverse SS-ETSE (*e*) and interstitial-phase gadolinium-enhanced SGE (*f*) images in a third patient also show diffuse thickening of the rectal wall associated with stranding of perirectal fat and small perirectal nodes. Sagittal T2-weighted ETSE (*g*) image in a fourth patient demonstrates similar features. Small regional nodes are present (arrow, *g*).

(g)

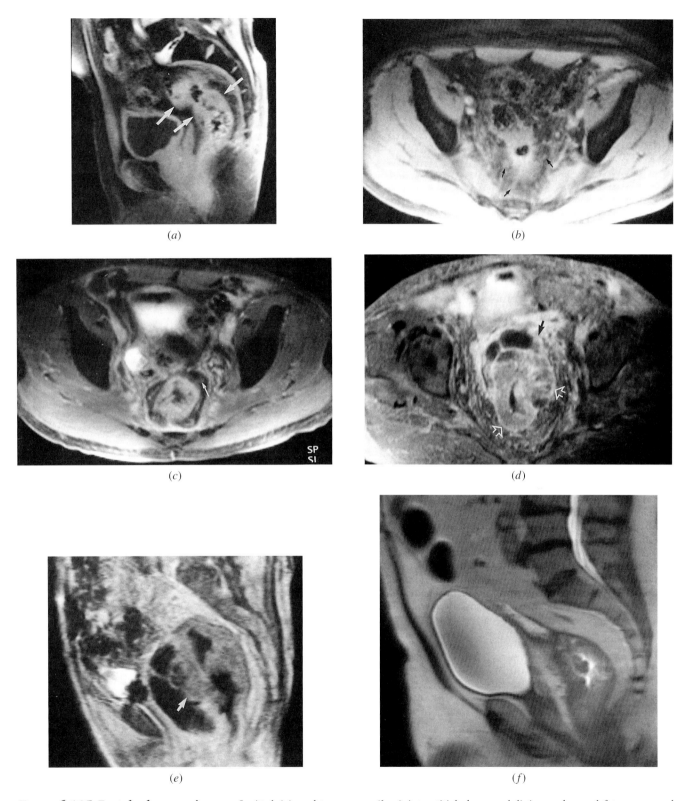

(a) (b) (c) (d) (e) (f)

F I G . 6.115 Rectal adenocarcinoma. Sagittal (*a*) and transverse (*b*, *c*) interstitial-phase gadolinium-enhanced fat-suppressed SGE images demonstrate a large rectal adenocarcinoma (arrows, *a*) with prominent lymphovascular extension and multiple small malignant lymph nodes (arrows, *b*, *c*). The sagittal imaging plane (*a*) highlights the inferior and superior extent of the tumor. Transverse gadolinium-enhanced fat-suppressed SGE (*d*) and sagittal postgadolinium SGE (*e*) images in a second patient demonstrate a large rectal cancer (open arrows, *d*) that has prominent lymphovascular invasion. Invasion of adjacent small bowel (arrow, *d*, *e*) is shown. Sagittal T2-weighted single-shot echo-train spin-echo (*f*), transverse T2-weighted high-resolution fast spin-echo (*g*), and transverse T1-weighted postgadolinium interstitial-phase fat-suppressed 3D-GE (*h*, *i*) images at 3.0 T demonstrate rectal adenocarcinoma in another patient. The rectal wall is diffusely thickened (arrow, *h*) and shows intense enhancement (arrow, *h*) due to

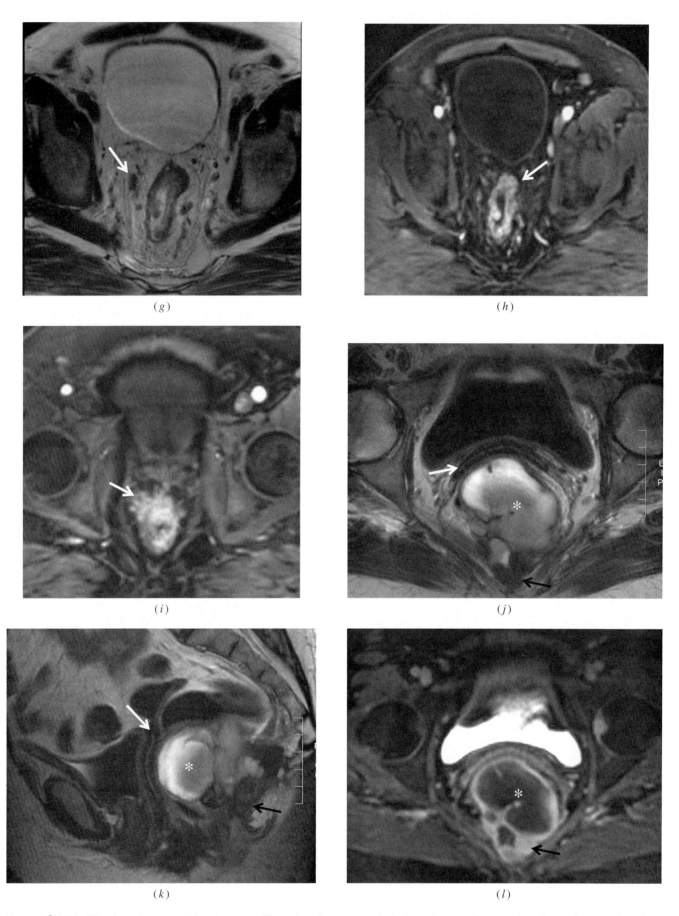

FIG. 6.115 (*Continued*) tumoral involvement. Note that there are spiculations (arrow, *i*) extending from the rectal wall to surrounding perirectal soft tissue, suggesting the presence of serosal invasion. Perirectal lymph nodes (arrow, *g*) are also detected. Transverse (*j*) and sagittal (*k*) T2-weighted high-resolution fast spin-echo and transverse T1-weighted postgadolinium interstitial-phase fat-suppressed 3D-GE (*l*) images at 3.0 T demonstrate a complex structure containing cystic (*, *j-l*) and solid (black arrows, *j-l*) components in another patient with rectal adenocarcinoma. High-resolution imaging is helpful for the staging. The vagina (arrows, *j*, *k*) is displaced anteriorly without any invasion. The wall and the solid component of the tumor show intense enhancement.

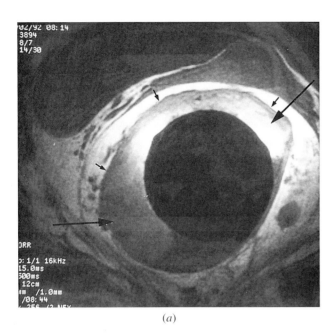

(a)

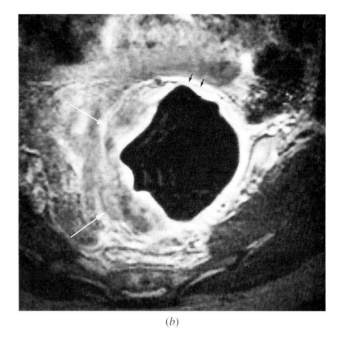

(b)

F i g . 6.116 Endorectal coil imaging of rectal cancer. Gadolinium-enhanced T1-weighted image (*a*) demonstrates a T2 rectal cancer (long arrows). Preservation of low-signal-intensity muscular wall (short arrows, *a*) along the outer margin of the tumor confirms lack of full-thickness involvement. Gadolinium-enhanced T1-weighted fat-suppressed spin-echo image (*b*) in a second patient with T3 rectal cancer. Heterogeneous moderate enhancing tumor (long arrows, *b*) is noted to extend beyond the confines of muscularis propria (short arrows, *b*). [Courtesy of Rahel A. Kubik Huch.]

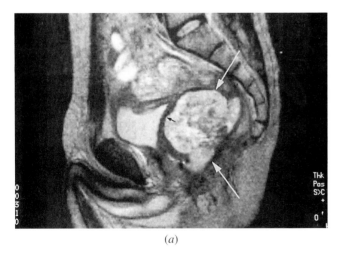

(a)

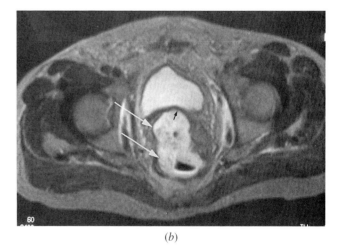

(b)

F i g . 6.117 Recurrent rectal adenocarcinoma. Sagittal and transverse T2-weighted echo-train spin-echo (*a, b*) and interstitial-phase gadolinium-enhanced T1-weighted fat-suppressed spin-echo (*c*) images. A large heterogeneous mass occupies the rectal fossa, a finding consistent with recurrence. Recurrent tumors are usually moderately high in signal intensity on T2-weighted images (long arrows, *a, b*) and enhance moderately after intravenous contrast (long arrows, *c*). Central necrosis is well shown on the gadolinium-enhanced T1-weighted fat-suppressed image. The tumor is contiguous with the bladder wall (short arrow, *a–c*), but the low signal intensity of the bladder wall on the T2-weighted images shows that the bladder wall is not invaded. Sagittal and

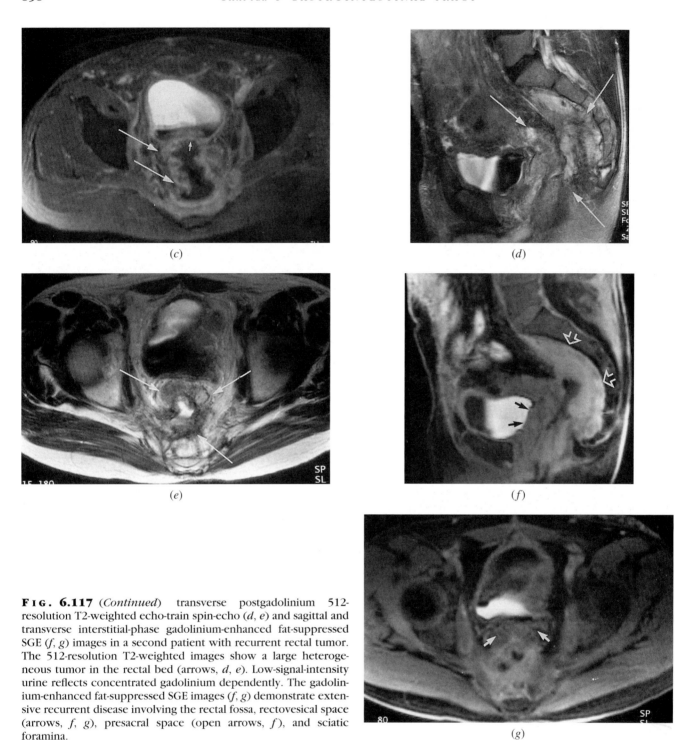

FIG. 6.117 (*Continued*) transverse postgadolinium 512-resolution T2-weighted echo-train spin-echo (*d, e*) and sagittal and transverse interstitial-phase gadolinium-enhanced fat-suppressed SGE (*f, g*) images in a second patient with recurrent rectal tumor. The 512-resolution T2-weighted images show a large heterogeneous tumor in the rectal bed (arrows, *d, e*). Low-signal-intensity urine reflects concentrated gadolinium dependently. The gadolinium-enhanced fat-suppressed SGE images (*f, g*) demonstrate extensive recurrent disease involving the rectal fossa, rectovesical space (arrows, *f, g*), presacral space (open arrows, *f*), and sciatic foramina.

year after radiation, granulation tissue may show persistent high signal intensity up to 3 years after therapy, particularly if intervening inflammation or infection has developed. Persistent increased signal intensity is most pronounced on gadolinium-enhanced T1-weighted fat-suppressed images. Finally, recurrent tumor may mimic radiation fibrosis when desmoplastic features predominate [6, 11]. Clinical history will often aid radiologic

diagnosis: elevation of CEA levels, onset of presacral pain, or both, are harbingers of tumor recurrence irrespective of imaging features.

Evidence of distant metastases in the setting of recurrent disease is also well shown with MRI. Liver metastases are optimally shown on MRI, and peritoneal disease and lymphadenopathy are also revealed (see fig. 6.119).

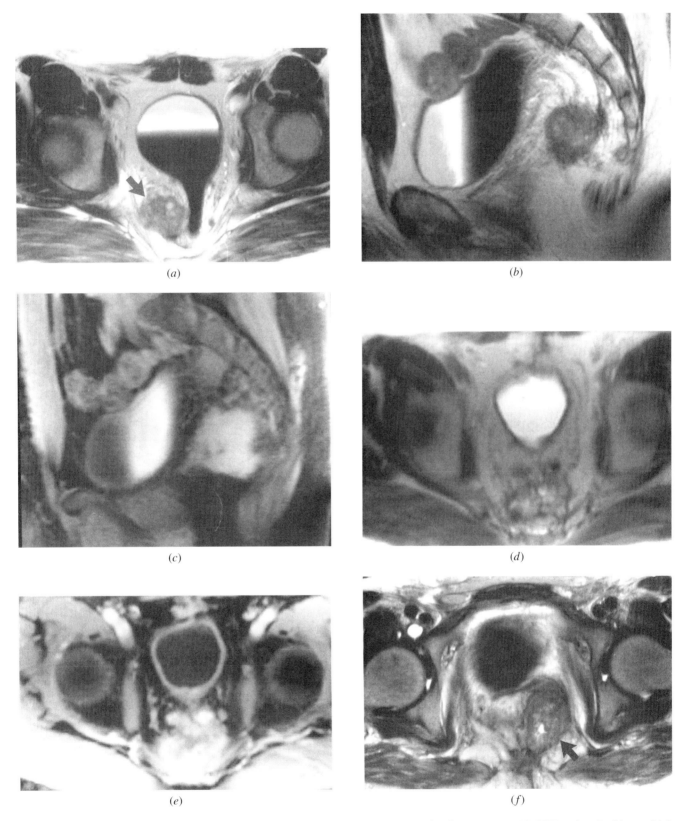

FIG. 6.118 Recurrent rectal cancer. Transverse (*a*) and sagittal (*b*) T2-weighted postcontrast SS-ETSE and sagittal interstitial-phase gadolinium-enhanced SGE (*c*) images in a patient after abdominoperineal resection (APR) for rectal cancer. There is a 4-cm mass in the right presacral space that is mildly heterogeneous on T2 (arrow, *a*) and heterogeneously enhancing consistent with tumor recurrence. Note the abnormal posterior position of the bladder after APR surgery. T2-weighted SS-ETSE (*d*) and interstitial-phase gadolinium-enhanced SGE (*e*) images in a second patient demonstrate an irregular presacral mass, which enhances heterogeneously after gadolinium administration. T2-weighted ETSE (*f*) image in a third patient with tumor recurrence also shows a mass (arrow, *f*) in the presacral space.

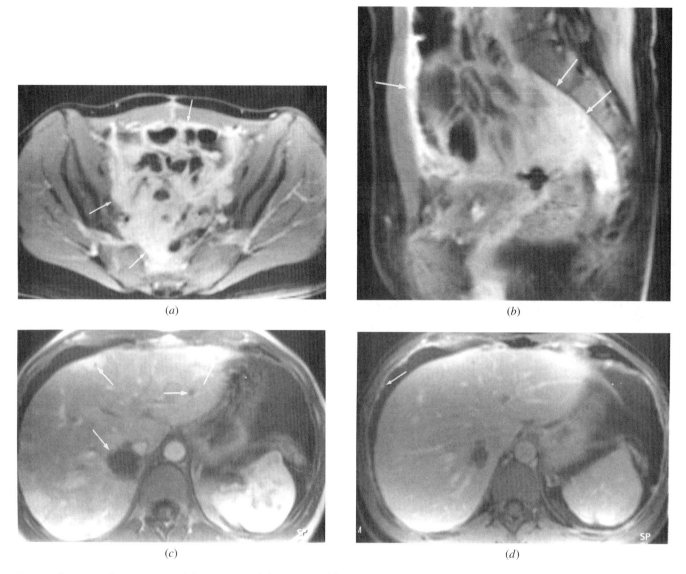

(a)

(b)

(c)

(d)

F I G . 6.119 Colon cancer with peritoneal disease and hepatic metastases. Transverse (*a*) and sagittal (*b*) T2-weighted SSETSE, transverse immediate postgadolinium SGE (*c*), and 90-s postgadolinium fat-suppressed SGE (*d*) images demonstrate a large recurrent rectal carcinoma in the presacral space, with extensive local infiltration in the pelvis (arrows, *a*, *b*). Immediate postgadolinium image demonstrates the presence of hepatic metastases (arrows, *c*). The peritoneal involvement in the upper abdomen is well shown on interstitial-phase postcontrast image (arrow, *d*).

Squamous Cell Carcinoma. Squamous cell cancer occurs in the anal canal, and its imaging characteristics resemble those of adenocarcinoma. Evaluation of local and distant spread is aided by gadolinium-enhanced fat-suppressed SGE or 3D-GE images (fig. 6.125).

GIST. Less than 10% of GISTs are seen in the colon and rectum (fig. 6.125). MR imaging findings are similar to the findings of gastric or small bowel GISTs.

Lymphoma. Primary non-Hodgkin lymphoma accounts for approximately 0.5% of all colorectal malig- nancies. Primary lymphoma is most often seen in patients with human immunodeficiency virus (HIV) infection or chronic ulcerative colitis [107, 108]. The cecum is the most common site of involvement, followed by the rectosigmoid colon. Secondary involvement of the colon by lymphoma occurs in the setting of widespread disease, especially in the elderly population. The MRI appearance includes isolated or multiple enhancing masses. Alternatively, diffuse nodularity with wall thickening may be seen after intravenous gadolinium administration (fig. 6.126) [48, 49]. Coexistent lymphadenopathy and splenic lesions may aid in the diagnosis.

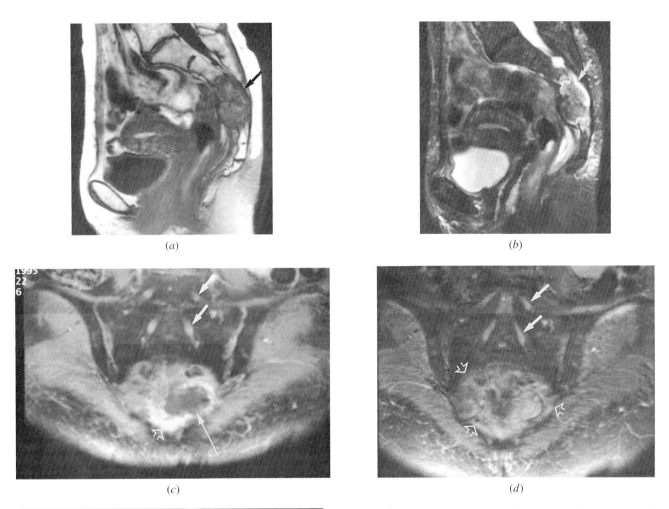

(a)

(b)

(c)

(d)

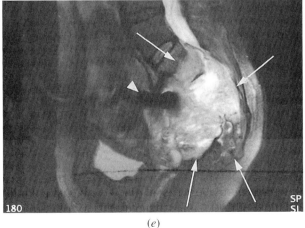

(e)

FIG. 6.120 Recurrent rectal adenocarcinoma invading sacrum. Sagittal T1-weighted SGE (*a*), sagittal 512-resolution T2-weighted fat-suppressed echo-train spin-echo (*b*), and oblique coronal postgadolinium fat-suppressed SGE (*c*, *d*) images. A large recurrent tumor mass invades the sacrum and is intermediate in signal intensity on the T1-weighted image (arrow, *a*) and heterogeneously high in signal intensity on the T2-weighted image (arrow, *b*). After contrast the tumor enhances heterogeneously (open arrows, *c*, *d*) and contains an area of central necrosis (long arrow, *c*). S1 and S2 sacral segments are not involved, and uninvolved S1 and S2 nerve roots are shown (short arrows, *c*, *d*). Sparing of the upper two sacral segments is a finding on which surgeons used to base surgical resection. At surgery, the upper margin of the tumor involved S3, sparing the S2 sacral segment. Sagittal 512-resolution T2-weighted echo-train spin-echo image (*e*) in a second patient demonstrates sacral invasion by a large recurrent rectal adenocarcinoma (arrows). This tumor involves the entire sacrum and precludes a surgical resection attempt. Surgical clip from prior resection produces a signal-void susceptibility artifact (arrowhead, *e*).

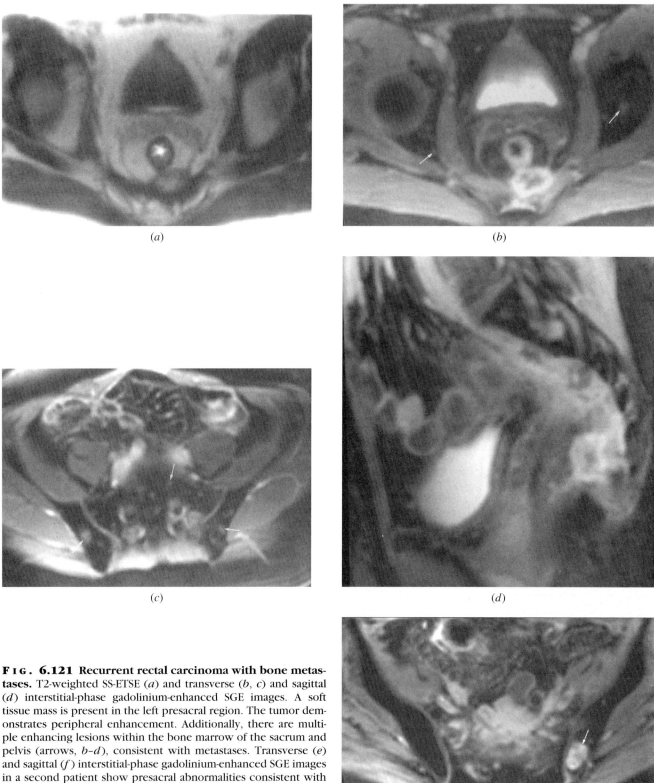

(a)

(b)

(c)

(d)

FIG. 6.121 Recurrent rectal carcinoma with bone metastases. T2-weighted SS-ETSE (*a*) and transverse (*b*, *c*) and sagittal (*d*) interstitial-phase gadolinium-enhanced SGE images. A soft tissue mass is present in the left presacral region. The tumor demonstrates peripheral enhancement. Additionally, there are multiple enhancing lesions within the bone marrow of the sacrum and pelvis (arrows, *b–d*), consistent with metastases. Transverse (*e*) and sagittal (*f*) interstitial-phase gadolinium-enhanced SGE images in a second patient show presacral abnormalities consistent with tumor recurrence associated with radiation changes. Note the presence of metastatic lesions (arrows, *e*, *f*) within the sacrum and left iliacus.

(e)

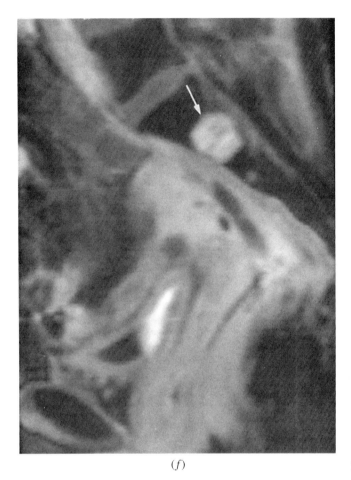

(f)

FIG. 6.121 (*Continued*)

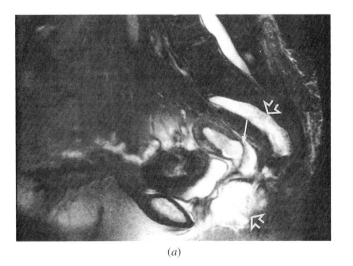

(a)

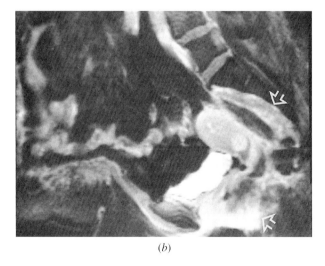

(b)

FIG. 6.122 Recurrent rectal adenocarcinoma and postradiation therapy changes. Sagittal postgadolinium 512-resolution T2-weighted fat-suppressed echo-train spin-echo (*a*) and sagittal interstitial-phase gadolinium-enhanced fat-suppressed SGE (*b*) images in a woman status post radiotherapy for rectal adenocarcinoma. Recurrent tumor is high in signal intensity on the T2-weighted fat-suppressed image and enhances after gadolinium administration (open arrows, *a*, *b*). Cervical stenosis (arrow, *a*) secondary to radiation therapy causes widening of the proximal endocervical and endometrial canal.

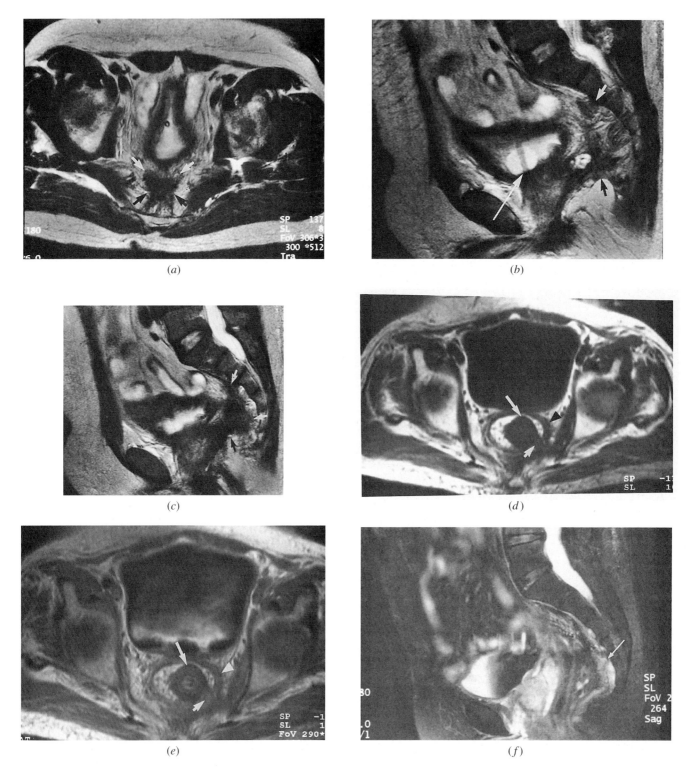

F I G . 6.123 Posttreatment fibrosis. Transverse (*a*) and sagittal (*b*, *c*) 512-resolution T2-weighted echo-train spin-echo images demonstrate low signal intensity in the surgical bed (arrows, *a–c*) consistent with fibrosis. Fibrosis has a plaquelike morphology, whereas recurrence tends to be more nodular. A Foley catheter is in place (long arrow, *b*). SGE (*d*) and 4-min postgadolinium SGE (*e*) images in a second patient show thickening of the rectal wall (long arrows, *d*, *e*) and perirectal tissue (arrowheads, *d*, *e*). Prominent perirectal strands are also present (short arrows, *d*, *e*). Negligible enhancement is consistent with perirectal fibrosis. The perirectal halo of fibrotic tissue is a common finding after radiation therapy for rectal cancer. Sagittal (*f*) and transverse (*g*) 512-resolution T2-weighted fat-suppressed echo-train spin-echo images and interstitial-phase gadolinium-enhanced fat-suppressed SGE image (*h*) in a third patient demonstrate platelike tissue in the presacral space that is low in signal intensity on T2-weighted images (arrows, *f*, *g*) and does not enhance substantially after gadolinium administration (arrow, *h*). Normal seminal vesicles have a cluster-of-grapes appearance (large arrow, *g*) on T2-weighted images, which permits distinction from recurrent tumor.

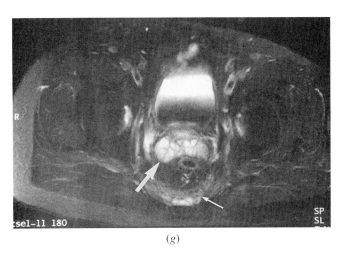

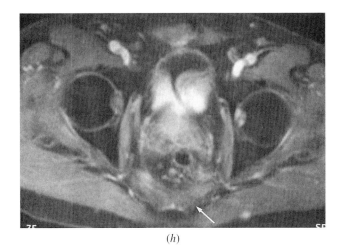

(g) (h)

FIG. 6.123 (*Continued*)

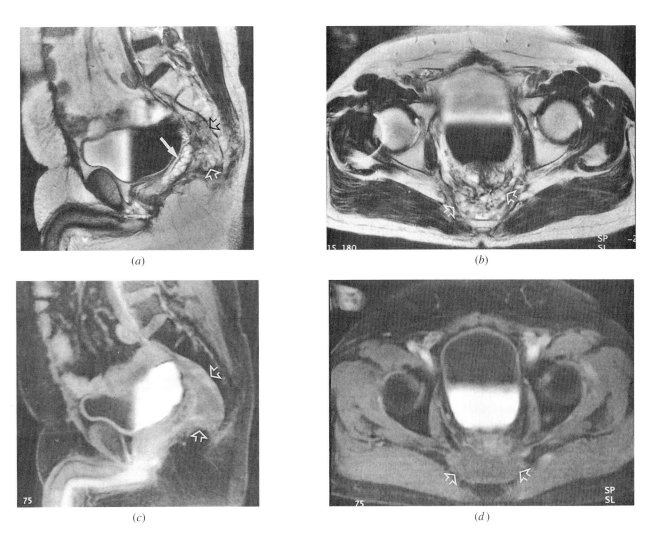

(a) (b)

(c) (d)

FIG. 6.124 Radiation fibrosis simulating recurrence. Sagittal (*a*) and transverse (*b*) postgadolinium 512-resolution T2-weighted echo-train spin-echo and sagittal (*c*) and transverse (*d*) interstitial-phase gadolinium-enhanced fat-suppressed SGE images in a patient 1.5 years after treatment for rectal cancer. Heterogeneous, bulky high-signal-intensity tissue occupies the rectal fossa (open arrows, *a*, *b*), on the T2-weighted echo-train spin-echo images, worrisome for recurrent disease. Other diagnostic possibilities include granulation tissue associated with radiation, inflammation, or infection. The heterogeneity is misleading because it reflects low-signal-intensity fibrotic tissue interspersed with high-signal-intensity fat. The high signal of fat is a consequence of the echo-train spin-echo technique. Minimal enhancement on the gadolinium-enhanced fat-suppressed SGE is consistent with fibrosis (open arrows, *c*, *d*). The seminal vesicles are distinguished from tissue in the rectal bed by the normal high signal intensity and grapelike morphology on the T2-weighted image (arrow, *a*).

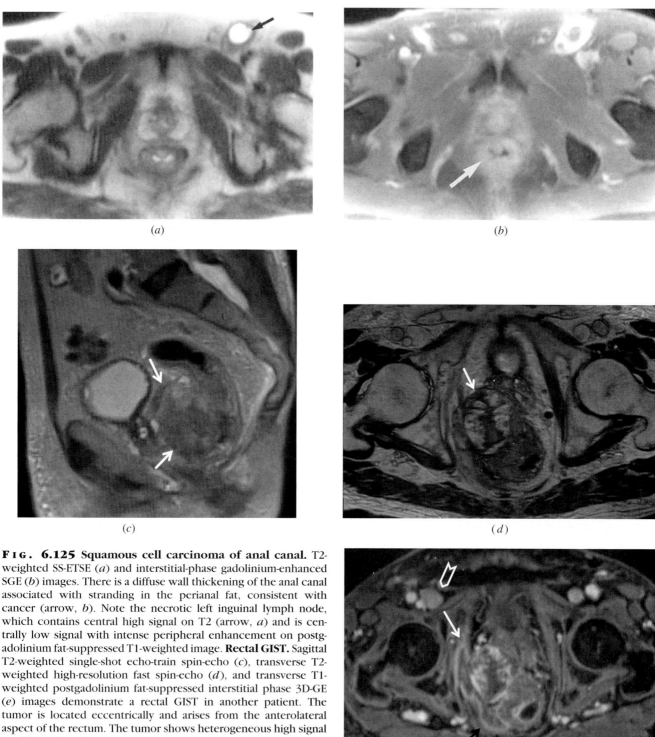

(a)

(b)

(c)

(d)

(e)

FIG. 6.125 Squamous cell carcinoma of anal canal. T2-weighted SS-ETSE (*a*) and interstitial-phase gadolinium-enhanced SGE (*b*) images. There is a diffuse wall thickening of the anal canal associated with stranding in the perianal fat, consistent with cancer (arrow, *b*). Note the necrotic left inguinal lymph node, which contains central high signal on T2 (arrow, *a*) and is centrally low signal with intense peripheral enhancement on postgadolinium fat-suppressed T1-weighted image. **Rectal GIST.** Sagittal T2-weighted single-shot echo-train spin-echo (*c*), transverse T2-weighted high-resolution fast spin-echo (*d*), and transverse T1-weighted postgadolinium fat-suppressed interstitial phase 3D-GE (*e*) images demonstrate a rectal GIST in another patient. The tumor is located eccentrically and arises from the anterolateral aspect of the rectum. The tumor shows heterogeneous high signal on T2-weighted image and contains central necrosis. It invades the right internal obturator muscle (white arrow, *e*) laterally and perirectal soft tissue (black arrow, *e*) posteriorly. The rectal wall is also thickened, suggesting the tumoral involvement posteriorly. Note that an enlarged right inguinal lymph node (open arrow, *e*) is present.

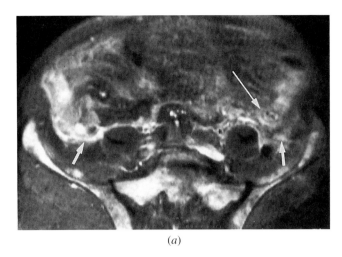

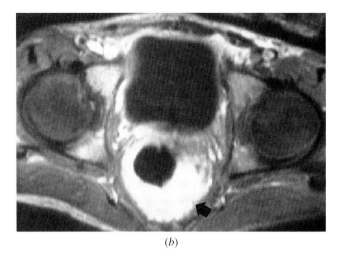

(*a*)   (*b*)

F I G. 6.126 Colonic lymphoma. Gadolinium-enhanced T1-weighted fat-suppressed spin-echo images (*a*, *b*) in two patients with lymphoma. In the first patient with Burkitt lymphoma (*a*), there is enhancing soft tissue in both paracolic gutters (arrows), thickening of the descending colon (long arrow), and ill-defined stranding in the mesentery. Note the diffuse enhancing bone marrow involvement. The second patient (*b*) has HIV infection and a primary rectal lymphoma (arrow). HIV patients are at risk for developing primary large bowel lymphoma. (Reprinted with permission from Shoenut JP, Semelka RC, Silverman R, Yaffe CS, Mickflikier AB: The gastrointestinal tract. In Semelka RC, Shoenut JP (eds.), *MRI of the Abdomen with CT Correlation*. New York: Raven Press, 1993, pp. 119–143.)

Carcinoid Tumors. The rectum is a common location for carcinoid tumor (fig. 6.127). A retrospective report of 170 carcinoid tumors found that 94 (55%) were primary rectal lesions. Larger tumors were associated with metastatic disease and poor survival [109]. The imaging features of carcinoid tumors have been discussed elsewhere. As with other rectal diseases, direct sagittal-plane imaging is useful. Liver metastases are best studied with dynamic gadolinium-enhanced SGE or 3D-GE technique.

Melanoma. Primary colonic melanoma is rare and carries a poor prognosis [110]. Owing to the paramagnetic effects of melanin, the lesion can have characteristic high signal intensity on T1-weighted images (fig. 6.128). Tumors may demonstrate ring enhancement after gadolinium administration.

Metastases. The large intestine may be the site of metastasis from a number of tumors including lung and breast carcinoma. The most common mode of secondary colonic involvement is peritoneal seeding [111]. Ovarian carcinoma commonly extends along peritoneal surfaces to involve the large bowel. Prostate or cervical carcinoma may affect the rectum by direct extension. Colorectal involvement is well shown on gadolinium-enhanced fat-suppressed T1-weighted images [71] (fig. 6.129).

Inflammatory and Infectious Disorders

Ulcerative Colitis

Ulcerative colitis is a chronic ulcero-inflammatory disease limited to the large bowel. It has a predictable distribution: disease begins in the rectum and extends proximally in a continuous fashion to involve part or all of the colon. "Skip" lesions, such as occur in Crohn disease, are absent. The incidence of ulcerative colitis is greatest in the second through fourth decades of life. There is a Caucasian, Jewish, and female predominance, and a positive family history is reported in up to 25% of cases [112]. The cause is unknown, but, similar to Crohn disease, a multifactorial etiology has been postulated. Ulcerative colitis is variable in presentation, but symptoms tend to be indolent with intermittent diarrhea and rectal bleeding. Patients with ulcerative colitis are at risk for developing toxic megacolon, which may be the presenting feature. Chronic ulcerative colitis is associated with an increased risk of colon cancer.

In contrast to Crohn disease, which affects full-thickness bowel wall, ulcerative colitis is a mucosal disease. In active ulcerative colitis, there are multifocal full-thickness ulcerations of the mucosa. Adjacent to these sites, edematous, inflammatory tags of mucosa may bulge upward toward the lumen as "pseudopolyps." In longstanding ulcerative colitis, intestinal shortening with loss of haustral folds may occur. This abnormality is ascribed to muscular abnormalities and is most marked in the distal colon and rectum.

The MRI appearance of ulcerative colitis reflects the underlying physiology: 1) rectal involvement progressing in a retrograde fashion to involve a variable amount of colon and 2) submucosal sparing (fig. 6.130). The latter is especially well seen on gadolinium-enhanced fat-suppressed SGE or 3D-GE images showing marked mucosal enhancement and negligible submucosal

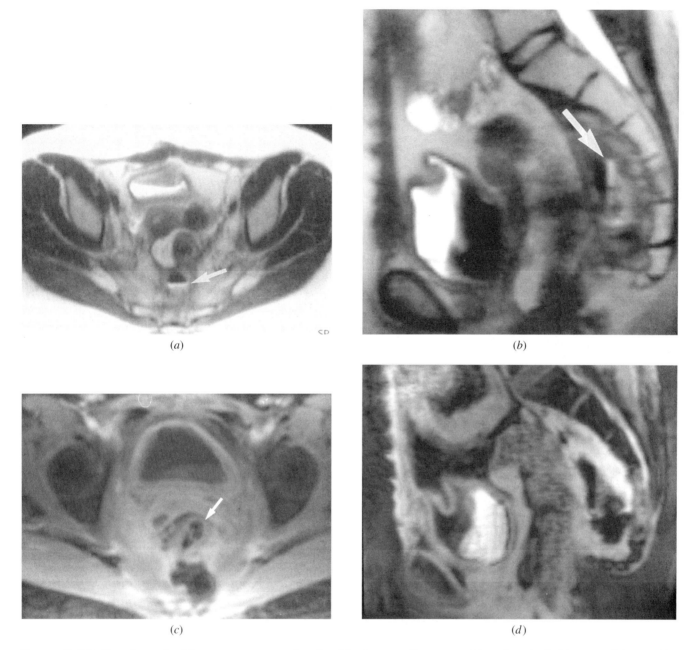

(a)

(b)

(c)

(d)

F I G . 6.127 Rectal carcinoid recurrence associated with abscess. Transverse (*a*) and sagittal (*b*) postgadolinium T2-weighted SS-ETSE and transverse (*c*) and sagittal (*d*) interstitial-phase gadolinium-enhanced T1-weighted SGE fat-suppressed images. There is thickening and enhancement of the rectal wall (arrow, *c*) associated with soft tissue stranding within the pelvis. An air-fluid level is present in the presacral space (arrow, *a*, *b*), consistent with a small abscess.

enhancement. Comparable to other inflammatory processes, the vasa rectae are prominent. The appearance of submucosal sparing is particularly pronounced in longstanding disease because of the combination of submucosal edema and lymphangiectasia [1–3, 6].

Toxic megacolon is characterized by total or segmental colonic dilatation with loss of its contractile ability. Toxic megacolon usually affects patients with universal colonic involvement ("pancolitis") and, unlike

acute exacerbation and chronic indolent ulcerative colitis, is a transmural process. The entire bowel wall enhances after intravenous contrast administration (fig. 6.131). Patients are prostrate with debilitating bloody diarrhea, fever, leukocytosis, and abdominal pain.

Inflammatory bowel disease may be exacerbated during pregnancy. These patients are particularly well suited for MR examination because of the relative safety of the procedure (fig. 6.132).

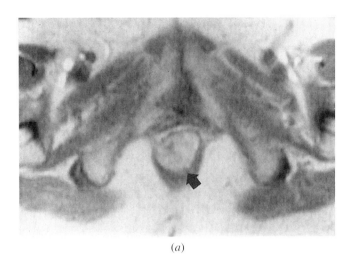

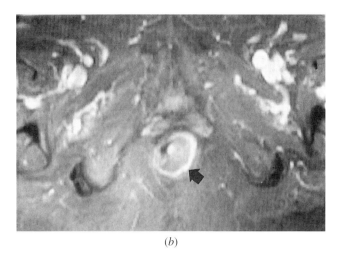

(a)   (b)

F I G . 6.128 Anorectal malignant melanoma. SGE (*a*) and gadolinium-enhanced T1-weighted fat-suppressed spin-echo (*b*) images in a patient with melanoma. Melanoma may be bright on T1-weighted sequences (arrow, *a*) owing to the paramagnetic properties of melanin. Rim enhancement is apparent after contrast and allows accurate determination of mural extent (arrow, *b*) (Reprinted with permission from Shoenut JP, Semelka RC, Silverman R, Yaffe CS, Mickflikier AB: The gastrointestinal tract. In Semelka RC, Shoenut JP (eds.), *MRI of the Abdomen with CT Correlation.* New York: Raven Press, 1993, pp. 119–143.)

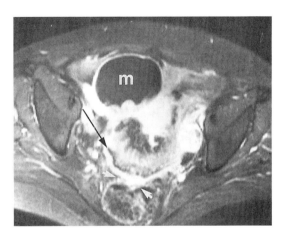

F I G . 6.129 Ovarian carcinoma metastatic to colon. Gadolinium-enhanced T1-weighted fat-suppressed spin-echo image in a patient with metastatic ovarian carcinoma. A complex cystic mass (m) encases the sigmoid colon (long arrow) and invades the rectum (short arrows). Tumor extension is clearly defined as enhancing tissue in a background of suppressed fat. (Reprinted with permission from Shoenut JP, Semelka RC, Silverman R, Yaffe CS, Mickflikier AB: The gastrointestinal tract. In Semelka RC, Shoenut JP (eds.), *MRI of the Abdomen with CT Correlation.* New York: Raven Press, 1993, p. 119–143.)

Crohn Colitis

Isolated colon involvement is noted in approximately one-fourth of cases. When Crohn colitis is limited to the anorectal region, differentiation from ulcerative colitis may be difficult [74]. In rare instances, Crohn colitis also may present with toxic megacolon (fig. 6.133). Crohn colitis is distinguished from ulcerative colitis by the following features: 1) persistence of colonic redundancy and haustrations in pancolonic disease and 2) transmural enhancement, which at times may show the most intense enhancement in the submucosal layer, a layer that is spared in ulcerative colitis (fig. 6.134). As with ulcerative colitis, submucosal edema may also be present (fig. 6.135).

Diverticulitis

Diverticula occur throughout the colon and tend to be most numerous in the sigmoid colon (fig. 6.136). Inflamed diverticula favor the left colon, whereas hemorrhagic diverticula tend to occur in the right colon. Several studies have shown cross-sectional imaging to be equivalent to, and in some cases superior to, barium enema in the evaluation of diverticulitis (fig. 6.137) [113, 114]. Bowel wall thickening and diverticular abscesses are well seen with a combination of gadolinium-enhanced fat-suppressed T1-weighted SGE or 3D-GE images and T2-weighted single-shot echo-train spin echo images (figs. 6.138 and 6.139) [115]. Similarly, sinus tracts and fistulas can be identified with this technique. On unenhanced T1-weighted SGE images, inflammatory changes appear as low-signal-intensity curvilinear strands located within the high signal intensity of the pericolonic fat. Sinus tracts, fistulas, and abscess walls enhance and are well shown in a background of suppressed fat on gadolinium-enhanced fat-suppressed SGE or 3D-GE images. It may be difficult to distinguish a perforated colon cancer from diverticulitis, and the two may coexist (fig. 6.140).

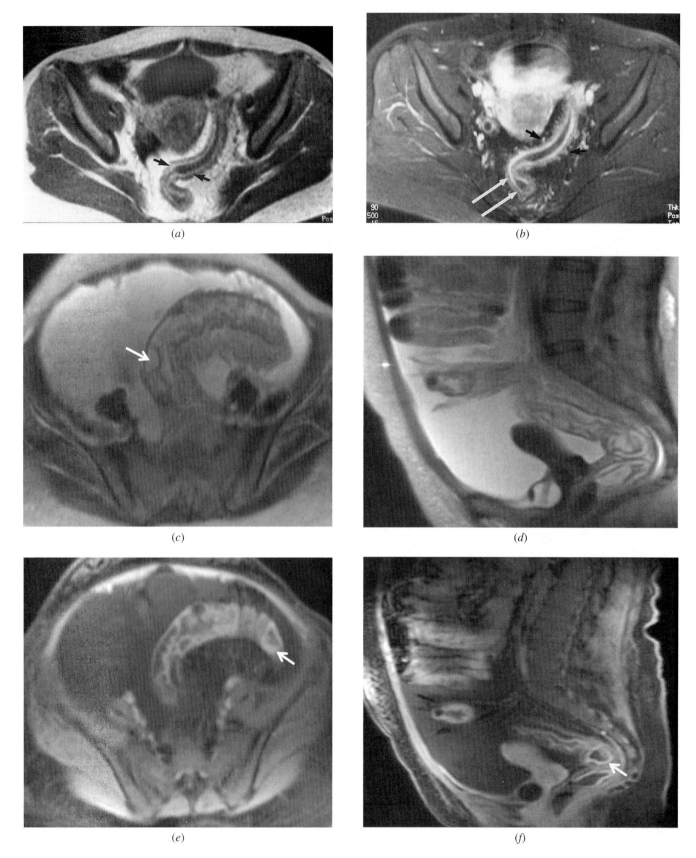

FIG. 6.130 Ulcerative colitis. Immediate postgadolinium SGE (*a*) and gadolinium-enhanced T1-weighted fat-suppressed spin-echo (*b*) images in a patient with ulcerative colitis. Increased enhancement on the immediate postgadolinium image (*a*) reflects increased capillary blood flow observed in severe disease. On the interstitial-phase image (*b*), there is marked mucosal enhancement with prominent vasa rectae (short arrows) and submucosal sparing (long arrows). Transverse (*c*) and sagittal (*d*) T2-weighted single-shot echo-train spin-echo, and transverse (*e*) and sagittal (*f*) postgadolinium fat-suppressed T1-weighted SGE images demonstrate ulcerative colitis and ascites in another patient. Submucosal edema (arrow, *c*) is detected in the sigmoid colon on T2-weighted images (*c*, *d*). Prominent mucosal enhancement (arrows, *e*, *f*) is detected on postgadolinium images (*e*, *f*). Note that no haustra is detected in the sigmoid colon.

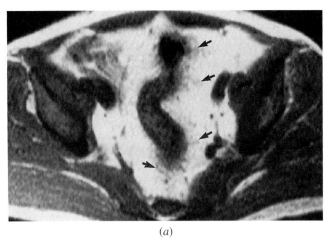

(a)

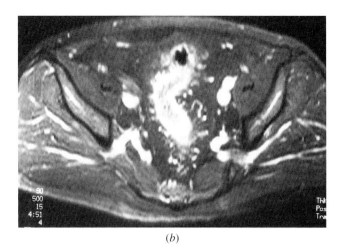

(b)

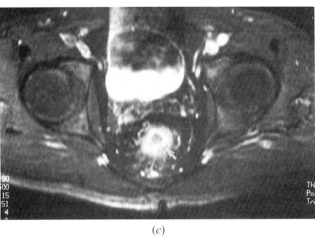

(c)

FIG. 6.131 Ulcerative colitis, toxic colon. SGE (*a*) and gadolinium-enhanced T1-weighted fat-suppressed spin-echo (*b, c*) images. The precontrast image shows irregular low-signal-intensity strands (arrows, *a*) related to a thick-walled sigmoid colon. After contrast there is marked mural enhancement. Enhancement of the pericolonic strands reflects prominent vasa rectae. Submucosal sparing is apparent (arrow, *c*), which is a feature of ulcerative colitis. Note the very intense enhancement of the colon wall, which appears to involve full thickness in the sigmoid colon. This is consistent with the patient's presentation of toxic colon.

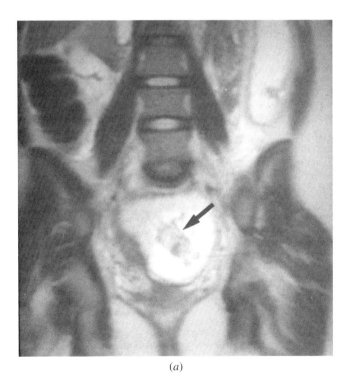

(a)

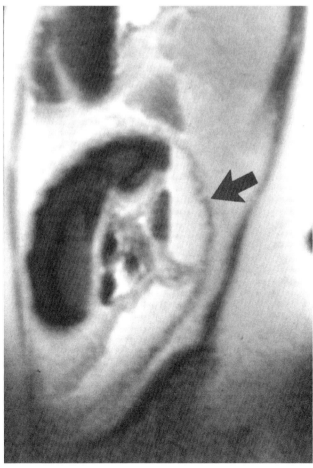

(b)

FIG. 6.132 Ulcerative colitis with acute exacerbation in pregnancy. Coronal (*a*) and sagittal (*b*) T2-weighted SS-ETSE images in a pregnant patient with history of ulcerative colitis. Diffuse irregular circumferential wall thickening of the descending (arrow, *b*) and sigmoid colon is present. Note the fetus (arrow, *a*) in the gestational sac.

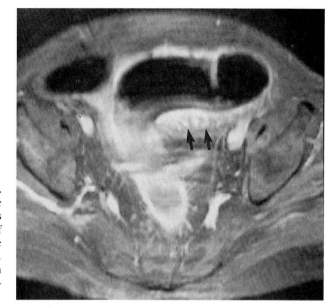

FIG. 6.133 Crohn disease presenting as toxic megacolon.
Gadolinium-enhanced T1-weighted fat-suppressed spin-echo image
in a patient with toxic megacolon. Dilatation and full-thickness
involvement characterize toxic megacolon, a complication of
inflammatory bowel disease (IBD). Note the prominent vasa rectae
(arrows), a common finding in the setting of bowel inflammation.
(Reprinted with permission from Shoenut JP, Semelka RC, Silverman
R, Yaffe CS, Mickflikier AB: Magnetic resonance imaging in inflammatory bowel disease. *J Clin Gastroenterol* 17: 73–78, 1993.)

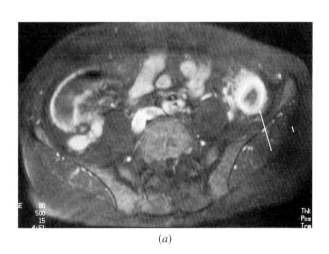

(a)

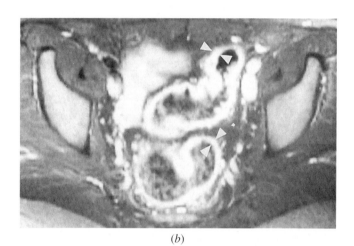

(b)

FIG. 6.134 Crohn colitis. Gadolinium-enhanced T1-weighted
fat-suppressed spin-echo image (*a*) demonstrates transmural
enhancement with greater enhancement of the submucosa
(arrow) than the other bowel wall layers, which is diagnostic of
Crohn disease and excludes the diagnosis of ulcerative colitis. In
a second patient with Crohn colitis, gadolinium-enhanced T1-
weighted fat-suppressed spin-echo image (*b*) shows full-thickness
enhancement of the sigmoid colon (arrowheads). The distribution
of colon involvement is compatible with ulcerative colitis.
However, the colon has remained redundant with persistence of
haustrations despite severe disease. These findings combined with
transmural enhancement are consistent with Crohn colitis. Note
the enhancing pericolonic inflammation in both patients.
(Reprinted with permission from Shoenut JP, Semelka RC, Magro
CM, Silverman R, Yaffe CS, Mickflikier AB: Comparison of magnetic resonance imaging and endoscopy in distinguishing the type
and severity of inflammatory bowel diseases. *J Clin Gastroenterol*
19: 31–35, 1994) Interstitial-phase gadolinium-enhanced T1-
weighted SGE (*c*) image in a third patient with Crohn colitis shows
thickening and enhancement of the ascending and descending
colon (arrows).

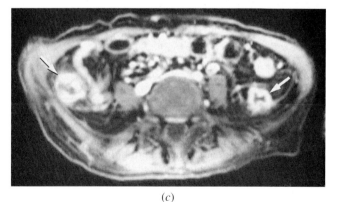

(c)

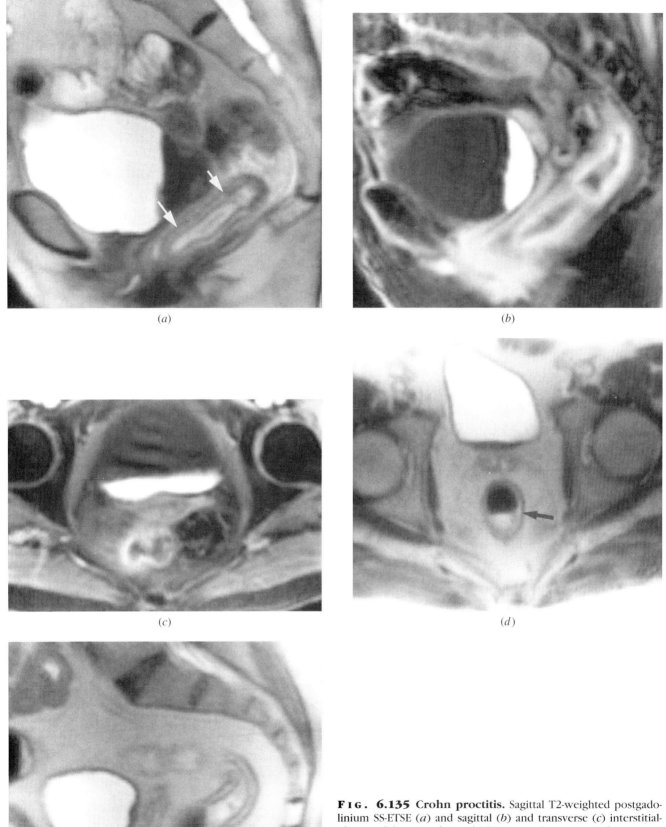

FIG. 6.135 Crohn proctitis. Sagittal T2-weighted postgadolinium SS-ETSE (*a*) and sagittal (*b*) and transverse (*c*) interstitial-phase gadolinium-enhanced SGE images. Prominent enhancement and thickening of the rectal wall are observed. Submucosal edema is appreciated as a high-signal stripe on the T2-weighted image (arrows, *a*). There is also diffuse perirectal soft tissue enhancement consistent with perirectal inflammatory changes. Transverse (*d*) and sagittal (*e*) T2-weighted SS-ETSE images in a second patient demonstrate thickening of the rectum associated with submucosal edema (arrow, *d*). Sagittal T2-weighted high-resolution

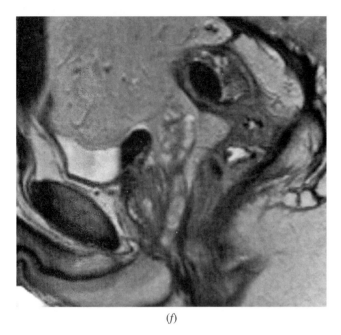

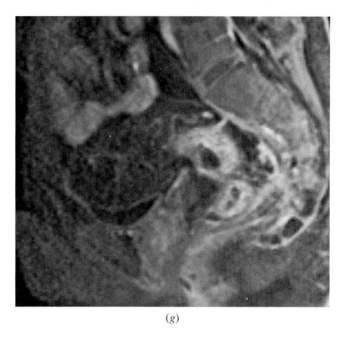

(f)   (g)

FIG. 6.135 (*Continued*) fast spin-echo (*f*) and sagittal T1-weighted postgadolinium fat-suppressed interstitial phase 3D-GE (*g*) images demonstrate rectal wall thickening and prominent rectal wall enhancement in another patient with Crohn proctitis. Note that perirectal tissue shows increased enhancement due to inflammation.

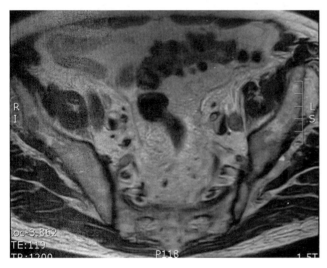

FIG. 6.136 Diverticulosis. Transverse T2-weighted 3D SPACE image demonstrates multiple signal void sacculations arising from the sigmoid colon consistent with diverticulosis. Diverticula are common and often incidental findings. Complications of diverticula include diverticulitis and frank abscess.

Appendicitis

Diagnostic imaging in cases of appendicitis is typically reserved for unusual presentations. Although CT imaging and ultrasound have surpassed barium enema in the workup of appendicitis [116, 117], MRI has several features that make it an attractive alternative. Specifically,

MRI has high contrast resolution for inflammatory processes and does not involve ionizing radiation. The latter feature is not inconsequential, because appendicitis is most common in children and young adults of reproductive age. MRI is especially useful to accurately show abdominal and pelvic disease in pregnant patients, including appendicitis and appendiceal abscess [118]. On gadolinium-enhanced T1-weighted fat-suppressed images, the inflamed appendix and surrounding tissues show marked enhancement (fig. 6.141). Inflammatory stranding in the surrounding fat is well visualized on unenhanced T1-weighted SGE images. In cases complicated by a periappendiceal abscess, the abscess wall shows enhancement with intravenous contrast administration, whereas the cavity remains signal void (fig. 6.142). Acute appendicitis can be diagnosed based on the findings of noncontrast sequences, particularly T2-weighted sequences in pregnant patients (see fig. 6.141).

Abscess

Abscess formation may be a complication of gastrointestinal or biliary surgery, diverticulitis, appendicitis, or inflammatory bowel disease (IBD). CT imaging and ultrasound are the mainstays of diagnosis and have the added advantage of ease of percutaneous drainage capabilities. For MRI to compete effectively with these modalities, automatic table motion, MRI-compatible needle and drainage equipment, and ultrafast imaging techniques must be in common usage.

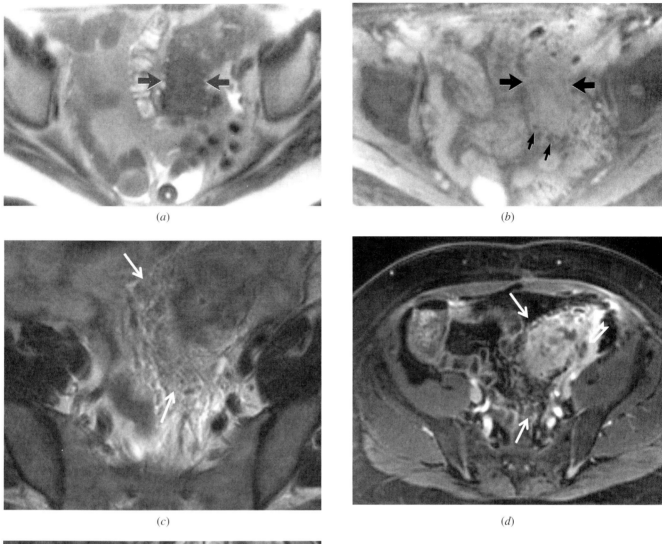

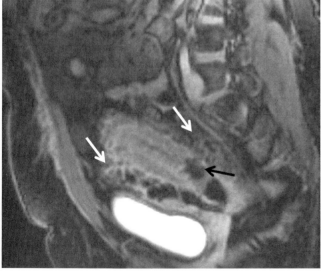

F I G . 6.137 Diverticulitis. T2-weighted SS-ETSE (*a*) and 90-s postgadolinium fat-suppressed SGE (*b*) images. Marked concentric wall thickening of an 8-cm segment of sigmoid colon is noted on the T2-weighted SS-ETSE image (arrows, *a*). The thickness of the colon wall measures up to 1 cm. Moderate contrast enhancement and marked wall thickening in the sigmoid colon (large arrows, *b*) are shown, with small diverticula (small arrows, *b*) on the postcontrast fat-suppressed SGE image. (Reprinted with permission from Chung JJ, Semelka RC, Martin DR, Marcos HB: Colon diseases: MR evaluation using combined T2-weighted single-shot echo train spin-echo and gadolinium-enhanced spoiled gradient-echo sequences. *J Magn Reson Imaging* 12: 297–305, 2000.) Transverse T2-weighted high-resolution fast spin-echo (*c*) and transverse (*d*) and sagittal (*e*) T1-weighted postgadolinium interstitial-phase fat-suppressed 3D-GE images demonstrate diverticulitis in another patient. The wall of the sigmoid colon is thickened and shows intense enhancement. Multiple diverticula (open arrow, *d*) are detected in the sigmoid colon. Associated inflammatory stranding (white arrows, *c–e*) in the mesocolon is detected. Note that small abscesses (black arrow, *e*) are also present.

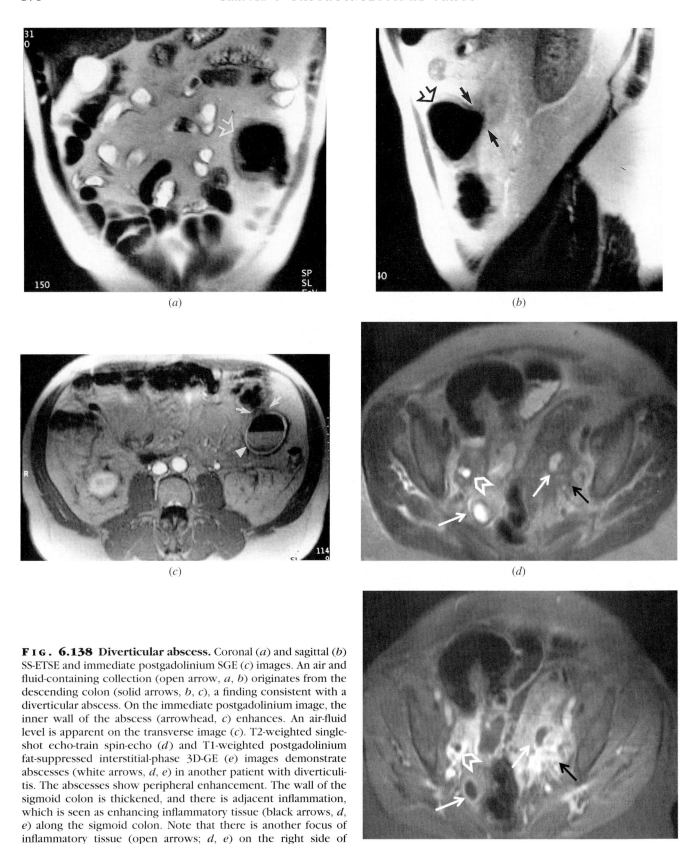

FIG. 6.138 Diverticular abscess. Coronal (*a*) and sagittal (*b*) SS-ETSE and immediate postgadolinium SGE (*c*) images. An air and fluid-containing collection (open arrow, *a*, *b*) originates from the descending colon (solid arrows, *b*, *c*), a finding consistent with a diverticular abscess. On the immediate postgadolinium image, the inner wall of the abscess (arrowhead, *c*) enhances. An air-fluid level is apparent on the transverse image (*c*). T2-weighted single-shot echo-train spin-echo (*d*) and T1-weighted postgadolinium fat-suppressed interstitial-phase 3D-GE (*e*) images demonstrate abscesses (white arrows, *d*, *e*) in another patient with diverticulitis. The abscesses show peripheral enhancement. The wall of the sigmoid colon is thickened, and there is adjacent inflammation, which is seen as enhancing inflammatory tissue (black arrows, *d*, *e*) along the sigmoid colon. Note that there is another focus of inflammatory tissue (open arrows; *d*, *e*) on the right side of the pelvis. T2-weighted single-shot echo-train spin-echo (*f*) and

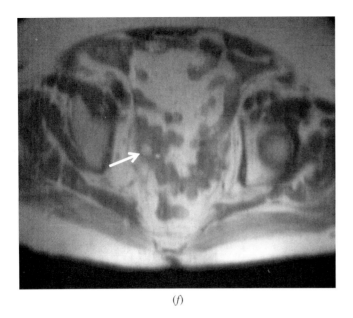

(f)

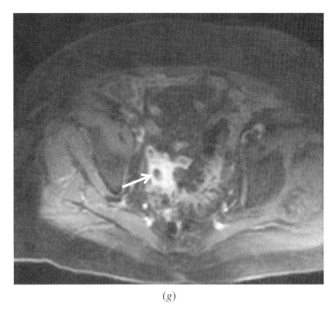

(g)

FIG. 6.138 (*Continued*) T1-weighted postgadolinium fat-suppressed interstitial phase 3D-GE (*g*) images demonstrate an abscess (white arrows, *f*, *g*) in another patient with diverticulitis. The abscess shows intense peripheral enhancement. Multiple sigmoid diverticula and associated mesenteric inflammation are present.

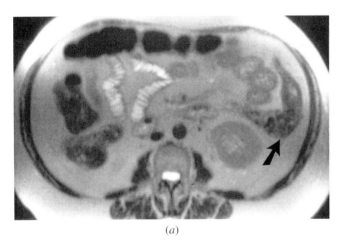

(a)

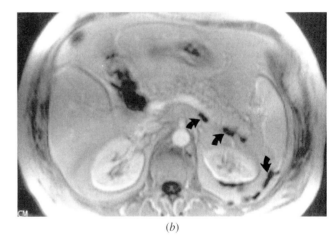

(b)

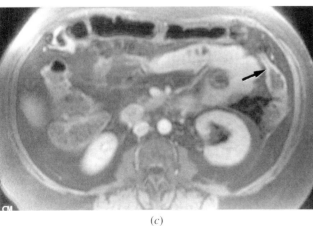

(c)

FIG. 6.139 Diverticulitis with pericolonic abscess. T2-weighted SS-ETSE (*a*), immediate postgadolinium SGE (*b*), and 90-s postgadolinium fat-suppressed SGE (*c*) images. An irregularly shaped gas collection is noted in the left anterior pararenal space, posterior to the descending colon, on the T2-weighted image (arrow, *a*). This appears to be in direct communication with a thickened segment of descending colon with an irregular focus of mural discontinuity. Multiple small gas pockets in the left retroperitoneal space are also apparent on the immediate postcontrast SGE image (curved arrows, *b*). The involved descending colon shows marked contrast enhancement (arrow, *c*) with an adjacent gas-containing abscess in the pericolonic fat on the 90-s postgadolinium fat-suppressed SGE image. (Reprinted with permission from Chung JJ, Semelka RC, Martin DR, Marcos HB: Colon diseases: MR evaluation using combined T2-weighted single-shot echo train spin-echo and gadolinium-enhanced spoiled gradient-echo sequences. *J Magn Reson Imaging* 12: 297–305, 2000.)

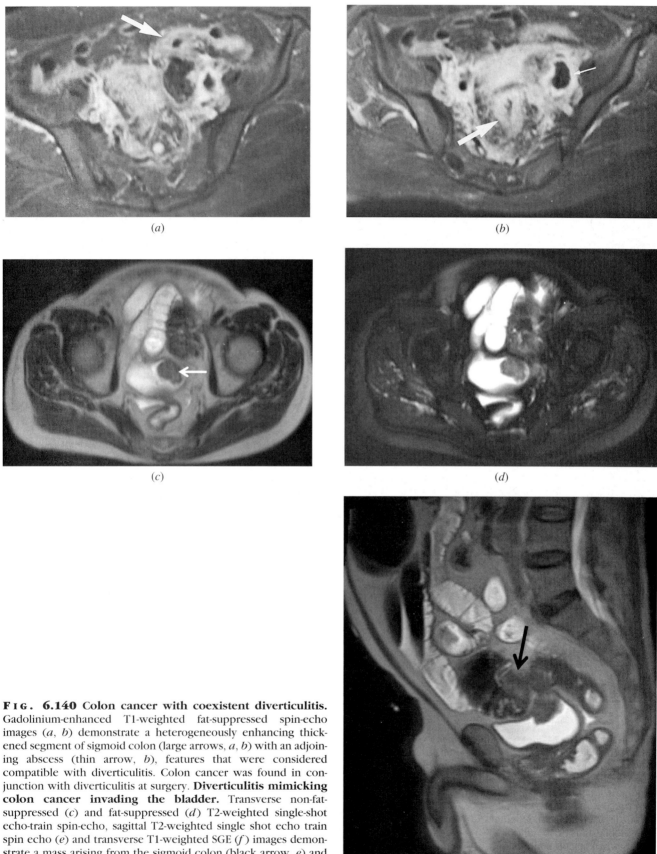

FIG. 6.140 Colon cancer with coexistent diverticulitis.
Gadolinium-enhanced T1-weighted fat-suppressed spin-echo
images (*a, b*) demonstrate a heterogeneously enhancing thickened segment of sigmoid colon (large arrows, *a, b*) with an adjoin-
ing abscess (thin arrow, *b*), features that were considered
compatible with diverticulitis. Colon cancer was found in conjunction with diverticulitis at surgery. **Diverticulitis mimicking
colon cancer invading the bladder.** Transverse non-fat-
suppressed (*c*) and fat-suppressed (*d*) T2-weighted single-shot
echo-train spin-echo, sagittal T2-weighted single shot echo train
spin echo (*e*) and transverse T1-weighted SGE (*f*) images demonstrate a mass arising from the sigmoid colon (black arrow, *e*) and
invading the bladder (white arrow, *c*) in another patient with
diverticulitis. The wall of the sigmoid colon (black arrow, *f*) is

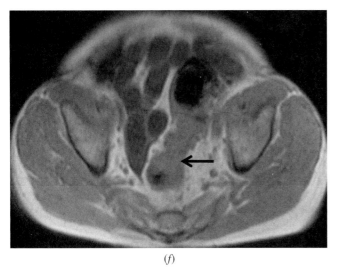

(f)

FIG. 6.140 (*Continued*) thickened on noncontrast T1-weighted image. The mass was diagnosed as colon cancer invading the bladder based on MR findings, and also on the basis of colonoscopy. Colectomy was performed, and the diagnosis was inflammatory tissue secondary to diverticulitis histopathologically. The inability to perform postgadolinium imaging in this patient because of end-stage renal disease hindered demonstrating post-contrast findings of diverticulitis and may have masked the correct diagnosis. It should be emphasized that diverticulitis can both mask and mimic colon cancer.

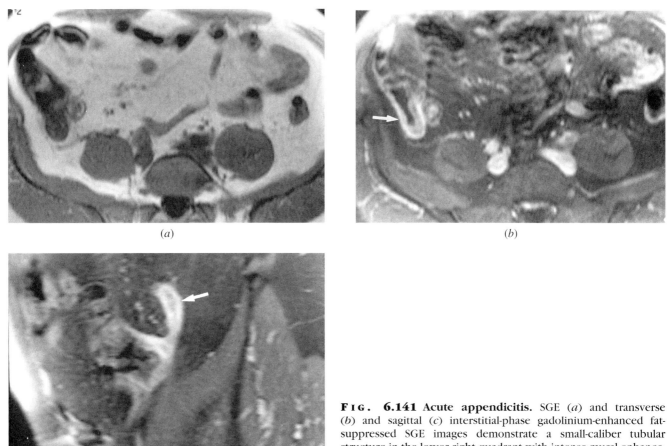

(a)

(b)

(c)

FIG. 6.141 Acute appendicitis. SGE (*a*) and transverse (*b*) and sagittal (*c*) interstitial-phase gadolinium-enhanced fat-suppressed SGE images demonstrate a small-caliber tubular structure in the lower right quadrant with intense mural enhancement. The findings are consistent with acute appendicitis. The direct multiplanar imaging permits display of a low segment of the inflamed retrocecal abscess on the sagittal projection (*c*).

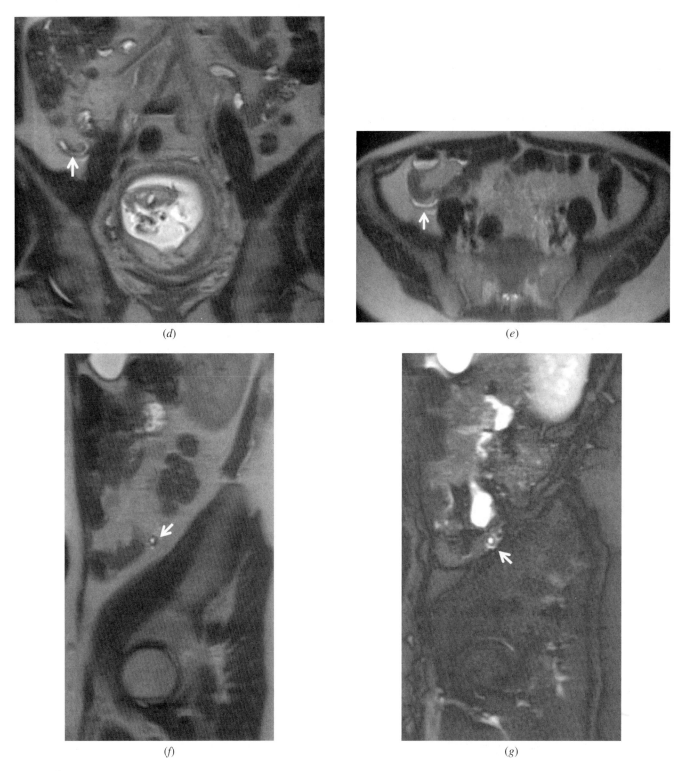

(d)

(e)

(f)

(g)

F i g . 6.141 *(Continued)* **Acute appendicitis in pregnant patients.** T2-weighted single-shot echo-train spin-echo non-fat-suppressed coronal (*d*), transverse (*e*), and sagittal (*f*) and fat-suppressed sagittal (*g*) images demonstrate mild acute appendicitis in a pregnant patient. The appendix is mildly dilated, and its wall is mildly thickened. Note that there is minimal free fluid around the appendix. Acute appendicitis can be diagnosed based on the findings of noncontrast sequences, particularly T2-weighted sequences. Postgadolinium imaging should not be performed routinely and should be avoided unless maternal and/or fetal survival depends on it. For further descriptions, see Chapter 16.

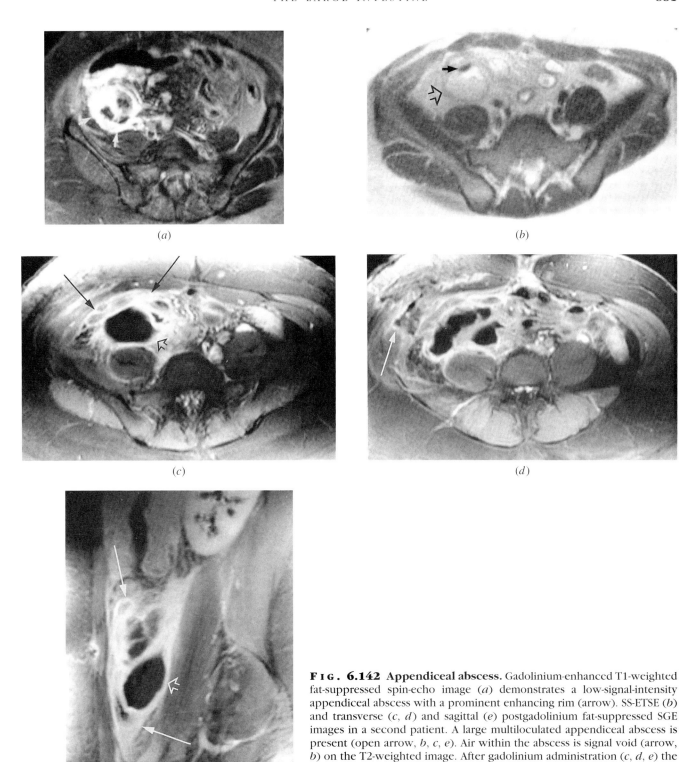

(a)

(b)

(c)

(d)

(e)

FIG. 6.142 Appendiceal abscess. Gadolinium-enhanced T1-weighted fat-suppressed spin-echo image (a) demonstrates a low-signal-intensity appendiceal abscess with a prominent enhancing rim (arrow). SS-ETSE (b) and transverse (c, d) and sagittal (e) postgadolinium fat-suppressed SGE images in a second patient. A large multiloculated appendiceal abscess is present (open arrow, b, c, e). Air within the abscess is signal void (arrow, b) on the T2-weighted image. After gadolinium administration (c, d, e) the abscess rim enhances (open arrow, c, e), and extensive enhancement of periabscess tissue is present (long arrows, c, d, e).

Noone et al. [119] reported a high diagnostic accuracy of MRI in evaluating suspected acute intraperitoneal abscess. In that series, abscesses were visualized as well-defined fluid collections with peripheral rim enhancement on gadolinium-enhanced T1-weighted fat-suppressed images.

The presence of signal-void air within the collection confirms the diagnosis (fig. 6.143) [120]. The role of oral or rectal contrast in distinguishing bowel from abscess is not firmly established. Most abscesses can be confidently differentiated from bowel with gadolinium-enhanced T1-weighted fat-suppressed SGE or 3D-GE

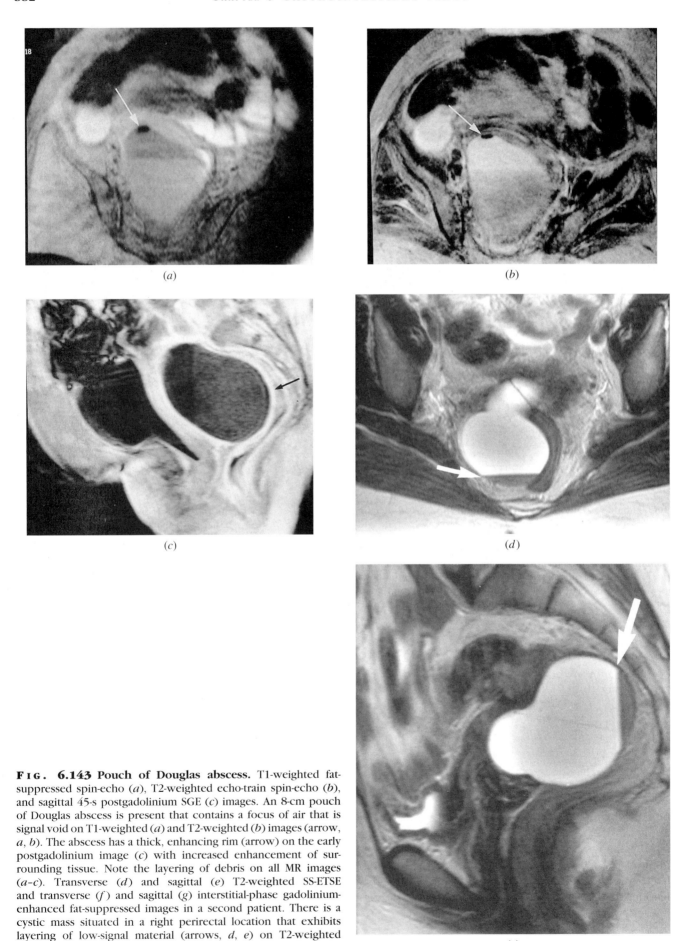

FIG. 6.143 Pouch of Douglas abscess. T1-weighted fat-suppressed spin-echo (*a*), T2-weighted echo-train spin-echo (*b*), and sagittal 45-s postgadolinium SGE (*c*) images. An 8-cm pouch of Douglas abscess is present that contains a focus of air that is signal void on T1-weighted (*a*) and T2-weighted (*b*) images (arrow, *a, b*). The abscess has a thick, enhancing rim (arrow) on the early postgadolinium image (*c*) with increased enhancement of surrounding tissue. Note the layering of debris on all MR images (*a–c*). Transverse (*d*) and sagittal (*e*) T2-weighted SS-ETSE and transverse (*f*) and sagittal (*g*) interstitial-phase gadolinium-enhanced fat-suppressed images in a second patient. There is a cystic mass situated in a right perirectal location that exhibits layering of low-signal material (arrows, *d, e*) on T2-weighted images. Moderately intense enhancement is observed of the

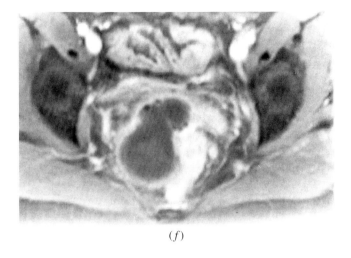

(f)

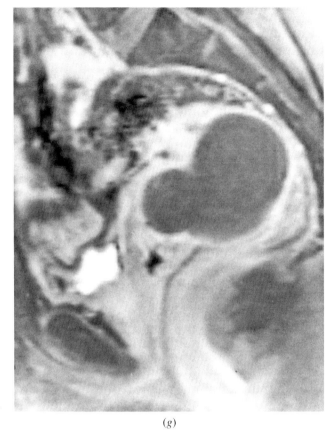

FIG. 6.143 (*Continued*) abscess wall (*f*). The abscess displaces the rectal-sigmoid region to the left. Layering of low-signal material on T2-weighted images is a relatively specific feature of abscesses.

(g)

and T2-weighted single-shot echo-train spin-echo images acquired in two planes. This approach demonstrates the oval shape of abscesses and permits their distinction from adjacent tubular bowel. Enhancement of periabscess tissues on gadolinium-enhanced T1-weighted fat-suppressed SGE or 3D-GE images confirms the inflammatory nature of the fluid collections (fig. 6.144). The layering effect of low-signal-intensity material in the dependent portion of the abscess on T2-weighted images is an important ancillary feature observed in the majority of abscesses [120]. The absence of motion artifact on T2-weighted single-shot echo-train spin echo facilitates identification of the dependent low-signal material in abscesses. The low signal reflects the high protein content of products of infection.

In patients with a contraindication to iodinated intravenous contrast secondary to allergy, MRI should be considered for the evaluation of abscess. MRI is particularly advantageous over CT in patients in whom high-density barium is present in bowel, because the barium creates severe artifacts on CT and may, if anything, improve the image quality in MRI. MRI also may be effective as a method to follow therapeutic interventions (fig. 6.145).

Colonic Fistulas

MRI is an effective imaging modality for evaluating colonic fistulas [7, 8, 121–123]. In particular, the multiplanar imaging capability of MRI has been shown to be useful for surgical planning for perirectal/perianal fistulas. The relationship of fistulas to the levator ani muscle is well shown on a combination of transverse, coronal, and sagittal plane images. T1-weighted images, T2-weighted images, and gadolinium-enhanced T1-weighted fat-suppressed images all provide good contrast between fistulas and surrounding tissues (fig. 6.146).

Infectious Colitis

Pseudomembranous colitis is defined as an acute colitis characterized pathologically by the formation of an adherent inflammatory "membrane" (pseudomembrane) overlying areas of mucosal damage. This disease occurs in the setting of broad-spectrum antibiotic use. The infectious organism most frequently implicated is *Clostridium difficile* [124]. The severity of the disease varies from mild to life-threatening. MRI shows thickening of the affected large bowel with marked enhancement (figs. 6.147 and 6.148).

In the past, neutropenic enterocolitis (typhlitis) was a disease affecting predominantly children treated for leukemia. The disorder also affects healthier neutropenic patients with solid tumors and other conditions. The cecum and ascending colon are the segments most commonly affected (fig. 6.149). MRI findings are nonspecific in patients with infectious colitis and generally demonstrate increased wall thickness and enhancement. Other infectious agents and infections that target the colon include *Shigella*, *Salmonella*, *Escherichia coli*, amebiasis, and cholera.

Patients with AIDS are prone to *Mycobacterium avium-intracellulare* colitis. *Mycobacterium avium-intracellulare* also affects the large bowel and produces

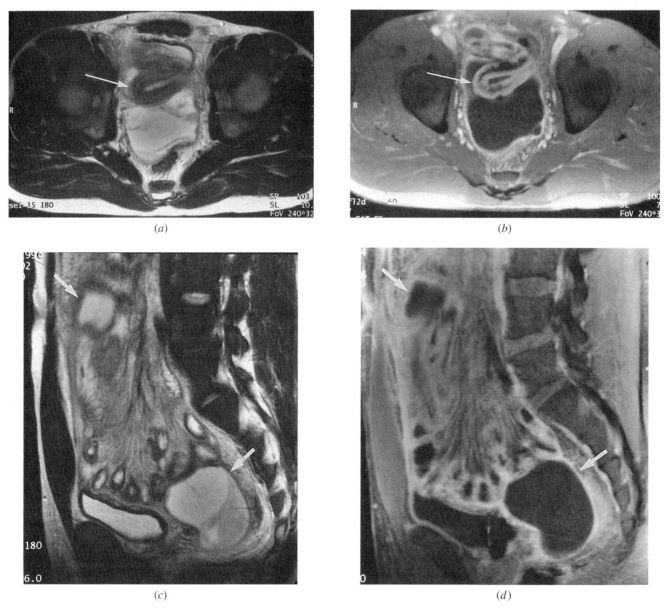

(a)

(b)

(c)

(d)

F I G . 6.144 Midabdominal and pelvic abscesses. Transverse 512-resolution echo-train spin-echo (*a*) and gadolinium-enhanced fat-suppressed SGE (*b*) images through the pelvis and sagittal 512-resolution echo-train spin-echo (*c*) and sagittal gadolinium-enhanced fat-suppressed SGE (*d*) images through the pelvis and midabdomen. An 8-cm, irregular, oval-shaped abscess is present in the recto-vesicle space that demonstrates dependent layering of low-signal-intensity debris on the T2-weighted image (*a*) and substantial enhancement of the abscess wall (*b*). Inflammatory thickening of a loop of ileum (arrow, *a*) abutting the abscess is identified. Enhancement of the serosal surface of the bowel is appreciated (arrow, *b*). The sagittal plane images demonstrate the pelvic and midabdominal abscesses (arrows, *c*, *d*). Layering of low-signal-intensity material in the dependent portion of the pelvic abscess is shown on the T2-weighted image (*c*). Enhancement of the abscess wall and increased enhancement of multiple loops of small bowel are noted on the gadolinium-enhanced fat-suppressed SGE image (*d*). Transverse 512-resolution T2-weighted echo-train

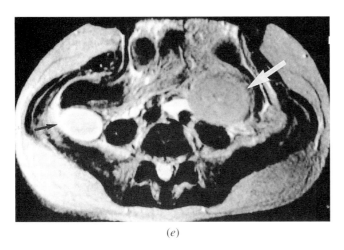

(e)

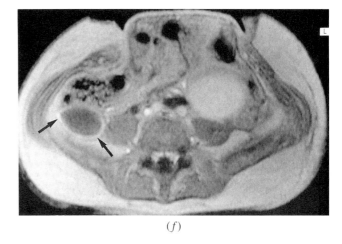

(f)

FIG. 6.144 (*Continued*) spin-echo (*e*) and immediate postgadolinium SGE (*f*) images in a second patient. This patient with chronic renal failure had undergone multiple abdominal surgical procedures for bowel ischemia and has a large anterior abdominal wall dehiscence with exposed peritoneal lining. A retrocecal abscess collection is present (black arrows, *e, f*) that is high in signal intensity on the T2-weighted image and demonstrates ring enhancement on the immediate postgadolinium image. A chronically failed renal transplant is also identifiable (large arrow, *e*).

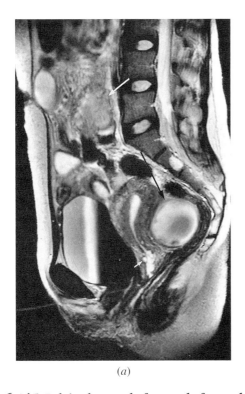

(a)

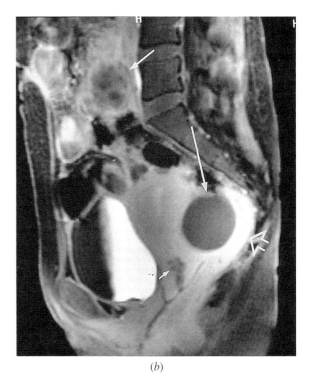

(b)

FIG. 6.145 Pelvic abscess, before and after catheter drainage. Sagittal 512-resolution T2-weighted echo-train spin-echo (*a*) and sagittal (*b*) and transverse (*c*) interstitial-phase gadolinium-enhanced fat-suppressed SGE images. The sagittal images demonstrate a 5-cm abscess in the pouch of Douglas (long arrow, *a, b*) and a smaller midabdominal abscess (short arrow, *a, b*). On the T2-weighted image, heterogeneous low signal is present in the dependent portion, which is a common finding in abscesses. On the postgadolinium images, substantial enhancement of the abscess wall and the adjacent rectum (open arrow, *b*) is present. Multiple Nabothian cysts are present in the cervix (small arrow, *a, b*). The transverse gadolinium-enhanced fat-suppressed image through

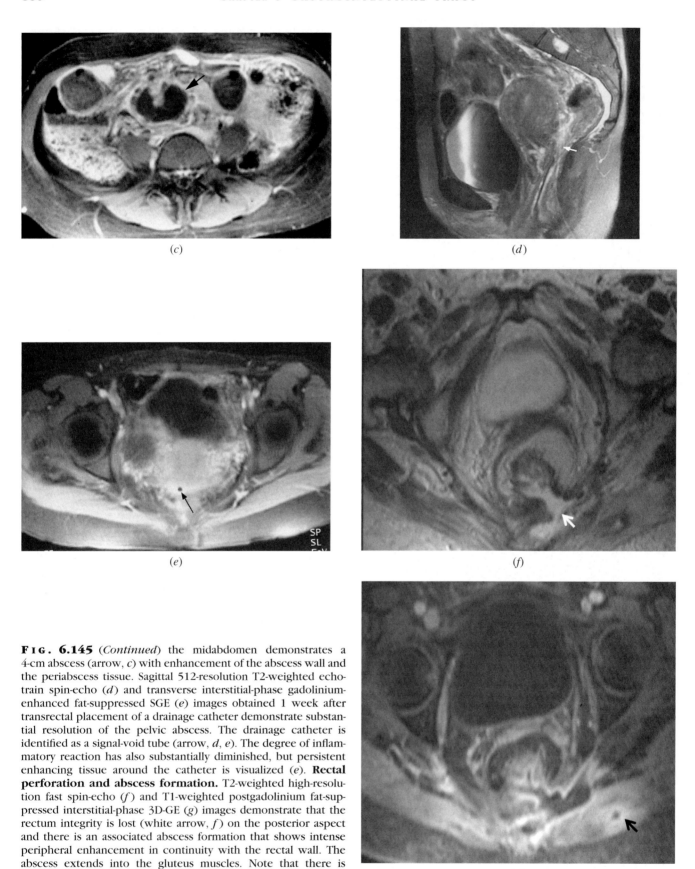

(c)

(d)

(e)

(f)

(g)

FIG. 6.145 (*Continued*) the midabdomen demonstrates a 4-cm abscess (arrow, *c*) with enhancement of the abscess wall and the periabscess tissue. Sagittal 512-resolution T2-weighted echotrain spin-echo (*d*) and transverse interstitial-phase gadolinium-enhanced fat-suppressed SGE (*e*) images obtained 1 week after transrectal placement of a drainage catheter demonstrate substantial resolution of the pelvic abscess. The drainage catheter is identified as a signal-void tube (arrow, *d*, *e*). The degree of inflammatory reaction has also substantially diminished, but persistent enhancing tissue around the catheter is visualized (*e*). **Rectal perforation and abscess formation.** T2-weighted high-resolution fast spin-echo (*f*) and T1-weighted postgadolinium fat-suppressed interstitial-phase 3D-GE (*g*) images demonstrate that the rectum integrity is lost (white arrow, *f*) on the posterior aspect and there is an associated abscess formation that shows intense peripheral enhancement in continuity with the rectal wall. The abscess extends into the gluteus muscles. Note that there is another small abscess (black arrow, *g*) in the left gluteus muscle.

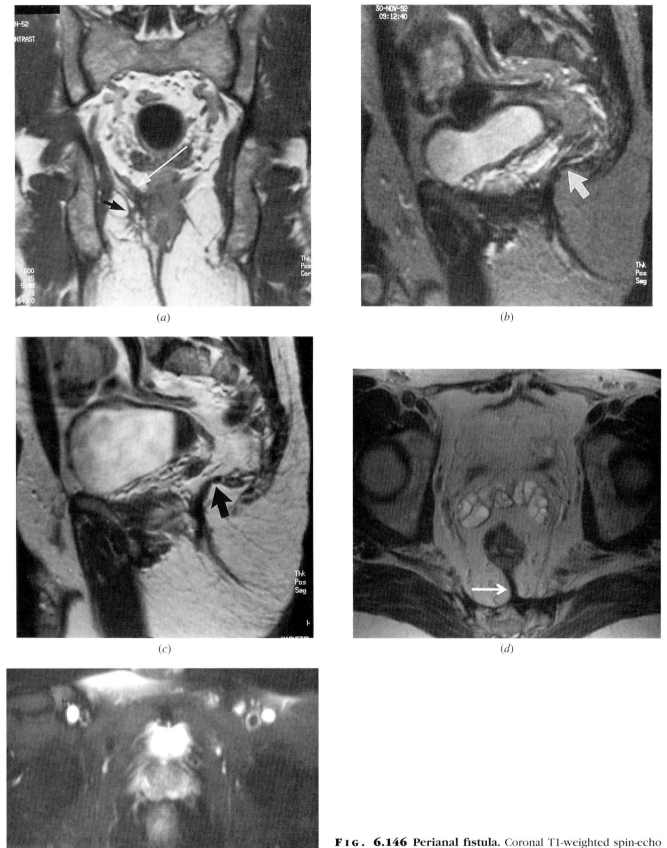

(a)

(b)

(c)

(d)

(e)

FIG. 6.146 Perianal fistula. Coronal T1-weighted spin-echo (*a*), sagittal T2-weighted spin-echo (*b*), and gadolinium-enhanced T1-weighted spin-echo (*c*) images. A complex fistula (arrow, *a*) is present in a right perianal location that extends to the levator ani muscle (long arrow, *a*). The fistula is low in signal on T1-weighted (arrow, *a*), T2-weighted (arrow, *b*), and postgadolinium (arrow, *c*) images, reflecting its the chronic fibrotic nature. T2-weighted high-resolution fast spin-echo (*d*), T2-weighted fat-suppressed single-shot echo-train spin-echo (*e*), and T1-weighted postgadolinium

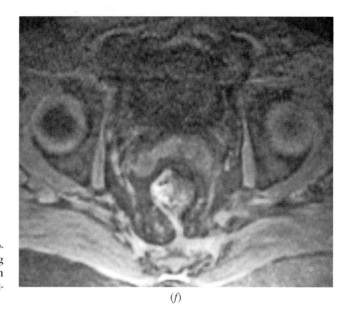

(f)

FIG. 6.146 (*Continued*) interstitial-phase fat-suppressed 3D-GE (*f*) images demonstrate a pelvic fistula (arrow, *d*) extending from the rectum to the presacral soft tissue in another patient with Crohn proctitis. The fistulous tract shows enhancement on post-gadolinium image (*f*).

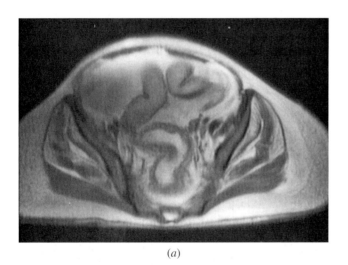

(a)

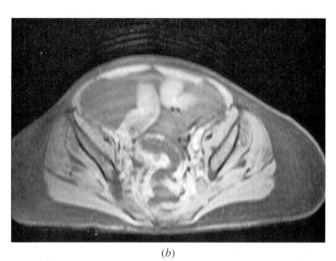

(b)

FIG. 6.147 *Clostridium difficile* colitis. T2-weighted single-shot ETSE (*a*) and T1-weighted fat-suppressed gadolinium-enhanced interstitial-phase T1 (*b*) images through the pelvis show marked diffuse wall thickening and edema of the sigmoid colon and proximal rectum. A moderate amount of free fluid is noted within the peritoneum.

wall thickening (fig. 6.150) [46]. Cytomegalovirus colitis (fig. 6.150) may also be seen in these patients. Bowel wall thickening secondary to submucosal hemorrhage is the most characteristic finding. Patients with AIDS frequently develop proctitis. Opportunistic infection leads to rectal wall thickening and stranding in the perirectal space. Occasionally, frank perirectal abscesses occur. Gadolinium-enhanced T1-weighted fat-suppressed SGE and 3D-GE images demonstrate bowel wall thickening with increased enhancement and abscess formation. Unenhanced SGE imaging is effective for showing perirectal stranding, which appears low in signal intensity in a background of high-signal-intensity fat.

Radiation Enteritis

The rectum is the segment of large bowel most susceptible to radiation enteritis. This finding may be attributed to the large radiation doses used to treat tumors arising in the pelvic area and the relatively fixed position of the rectosigmoid colon. Pathologic changes of acute radiation injury include prominent submucosal edema, ulceration, inflammatory polyps, and ischemic changes. Chronic radiation injury may show the histologic features of mucosal atrophy, vascular occlusion, and fibrosis. Late effects of radiation damage are evidenced pathologically by mucosal, submucosal, and muscular fibrosis with stricture formation [125]. In one study, the T1- and T2-weighted MRI features of the rectum in 42

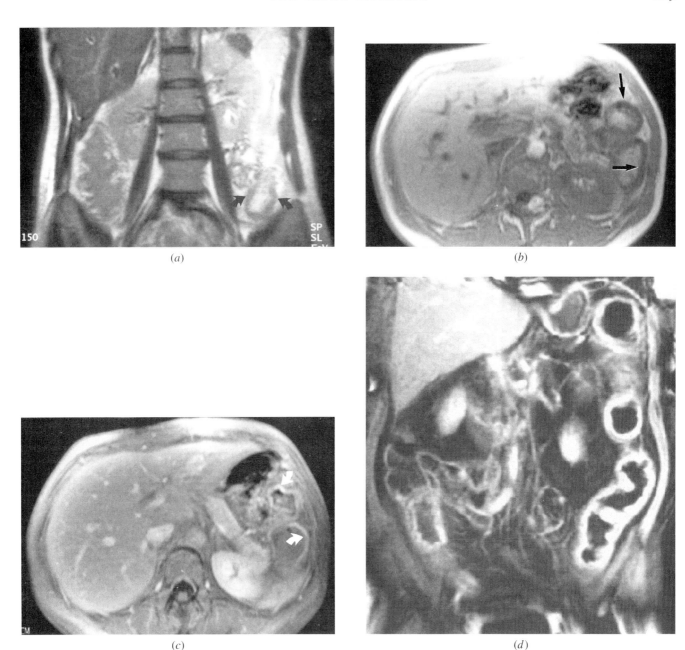

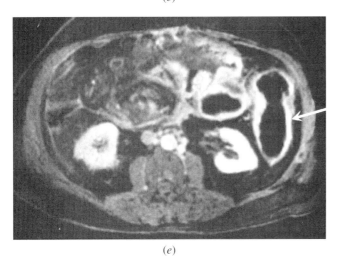

F I G . 6.148 Pseudomembranous colitis. T2-weighted SS-ETSE (*a*), precontrast SGE (*b*), and 90-s postgadolinium fat-suppressed SGE (*c*) images. Diffuse bowel wall thickening is noted in the descending colon on the coronal T2-weighted image (curved arrows, *a*). Circumferential bowel wall thickening is seen in the splenic flexure of the large bowel on the precontrast SGE image (arrows, *b*). Moderately increased enhancement and wall thickening of the splenic flexure is noted on the postcontrast fat-suppressed SGE image (curved arrows, *c*). (Reprinted with permission from Chung JJ, Semelka RC, Martin DR, Marcos HB: Colon diseases: MR evaluation using combined T2-weighted single-shot echo train spin-echo and gadolinium-enhanced spoiled gradient-echo sequences. *J Magn Reson Imaging* 12: 297–305, 2000.) Coronal (*d*) and transverse (*e*) interstitial-phase gadolinium-enhanced fat-suppressed SGE images in a second patient demonstrate diffuse thickening of the descending colon (arrow, *e*) with intense mural enhancement. (Courtesy of Russel Low, M.D., Sharp Clinic, San Diego.)

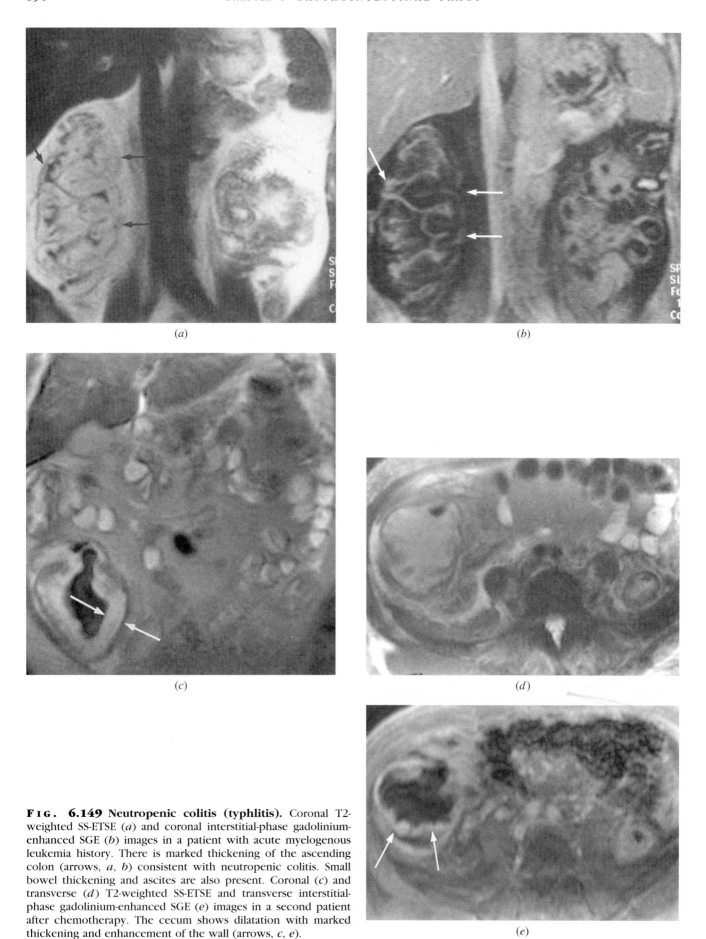

FIG. 6.149 Neutropenic colitis (typhlitis). Coronal T2-weighted SS-ETSE (*a*) and coronal interstitial-phase gadolinium-enhanced SGE (*b*) images in a patient with acute myelogenous leukemia history. There is marked thickening of the ascending colon (arrows, *a*, *b*) consistent with neutropenic colitis. Small bowel thickening and ascites are also present. Coronal (*c*) and transverse (*d*) T2-weighted SS-ETSE and transverse interstitial-phase gadolinium-enhanced SGE (*e*) images in a second patient after chemotherapy. The cecum shows dilatation with marked thickening and enhancement of the wall (arrows, *c*, *e*).

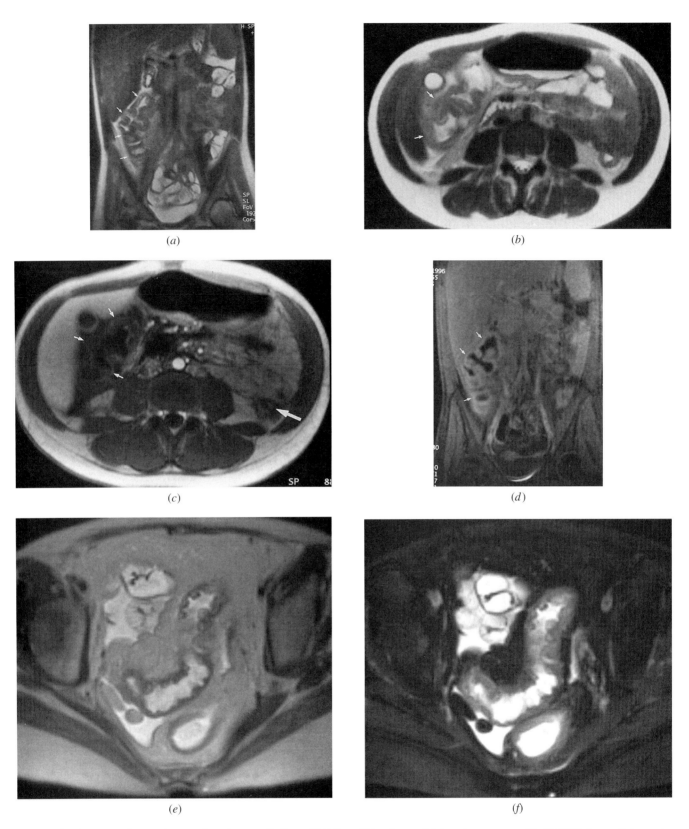

FIG. 6.150 *Mycobacterium avium-intracellulare (MAI) colitis.* Coronal (*a*) and transverse (*b*) SS-ETSE, immediate postgadolinium SGE (*c*), and coronal 90-s postgadolinium fat-suppressed SGE (*d*) images in a patient with *Mycobacterium avium-intracellulare* colitis. SS-ETSE images (*a, b*) demonstrate marked wall thickening of the ascending colon (small arrows, *a, b*) with relative sparing of the descending colon. The mucosal surface enhances on the immediate postgadolinium image (small arrows, *c*), with negligible enhancement of the thickened outer wall. Less severe involvement of the descending colon is also seen (arrow, *c*). Enhancement of the wall increases and becomes more uniform (small arrows, *d*) on interstitial-phase images, reflecting capillary leakage. ***Cytomegalovirus colitis.*** Transverse T2-weighted non-fat-suppressed (*e*) and fat-suppressed (*f*) single-shot echo-train spin-echo, T1-weighted SGE (*g*), and T1-weighted postgadolinium fat-suppressed interstitial-phase 3D-GE (*h*) images demonstrate cytomegalovirus colitis in another patient. The sigmoid colon and rectum walls are edematous and thickened, and show intense enhancement. Note that mesenteric inflammation and free fluid are also present.

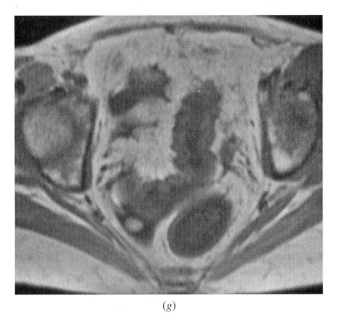

(g)   (h)

F I G . 6.150 (*Continued*)

patients status post radiation therapy were graded with respect to wall thickness and signal intensity of the muscular layers and submucosa. A spectrum of tissue changes were seen in the rectum regardless of the time from initiation of therapy. MRI had excellent sensitivity for depicting abnormalities, but specificity was limited [106]. The results of this study emphasize the need for detailed clinical history to ensure optimal MRI. The routine use of gadolinium-enhanced T1-weighted fat-suppressed imaging is effective for evaluating postradiation changes because of the high sensitivity of this technique for inflammatory changes. High-resolution T2-weighted images demonstrate the findings of submucosal edema in acute radiation proctocolitis well (figs. 6.151 and 6.152).

Rectal Surgery

A number of surgical procedures are performed for rectal cancer and other disease processes. Abdominoperineal resection (APR) is performed for tumors that are distal in the rectum, in which a tumor-free distal margin may not be achievable. After APR, more anteriorly positioned pelvic structures reposition more posteriorly, including the bladder, the prostate and seminal vesicles, and the uterus. The pelvis is often packed with omental fat to prevent small bowel from filling the potential space when postoperative radiation therapy is contemplated (fig. 6.153).

Intraluminal Contrast Agents

The goals of intraluminal contrast agent use are twofold: 1) reliable differentiation of bowel from adjacent struc-

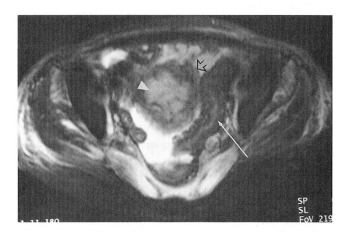

F I G . 6.151 Radiation enteritis. Transverse 512-resolution T2-weighted echo-train spin-echo image in a patient after radiation therapy. The sigmoid colon is thick-walled with marked submucosal edema (long arrow). The circumferential and symmetric nature of the bowel wall changes are suggestive of radiation enteritis. Note the thick-walled bladder (open arrow) and its heterogeneous contents (arrowhead), findings consistent with hemorrhagic cystitis, another sequela of radiation therapy. Free pelvic fluid is also present.

tures and 2) better delineation of pathologic processes involving the bowel wall. Oral contrast agents fall into two major categories, positive (signal intensity increasing) and negative (signal intensity decreasing) agents. Positive agents shorten T1-relaxation time, whereas negative agents either shorten T2-relaxation time or rely on immobile protons to decrease intraluminal signal intensity. Biphasic intraluminal agents are formulated to produce high signal intensity on T1-weighted images and low signal intensity on T2-weighted images [126].

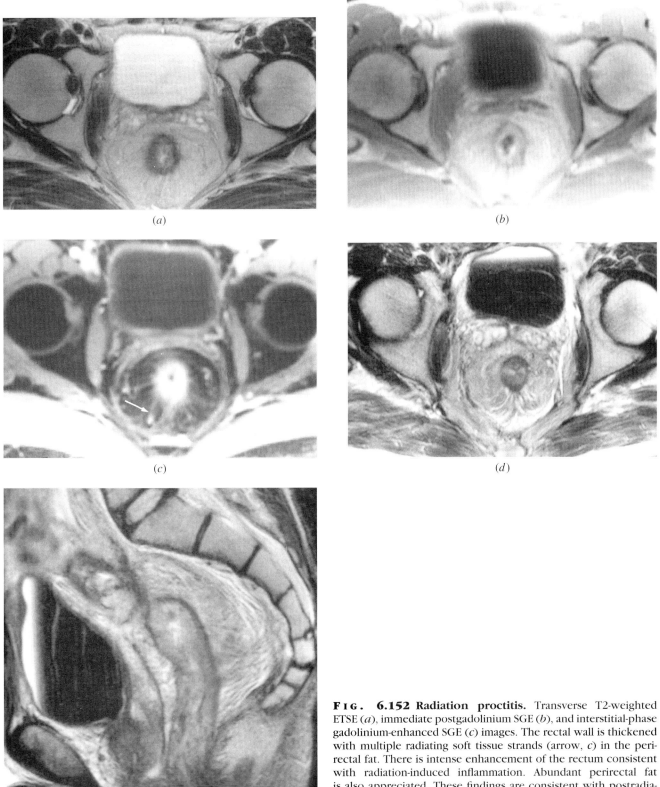

(a)

(b)

(c)

(d)

(e)

F I G . 6.152 Radiation proctitis. Transverse T2-weighted ETSE (*a*), immediate postgadolinium SGE (*b*), and interstitial-phase gadolinium-enhanced SGE (*c*) images. The rectal wall is thickened with multiple radiating soft tissue strands (arrow, *c*) in the perirectal fat. There is intense enhancement of the rectum consistent with radiation-induced inflammation. Abundant perirectal fat is also appreciated. These findings are consistent with postradiation changes. Transverse (*d*) and sagittal (*e*) T2-weighted ETSE and transverse (*f*) and sagittal (*g*) interstitial-phase gadolinium-enhanced SGE images in a second patient after radiation therapy show substantial thickening of the rectal wall with extensive linear strands in the enlarged perirectal fat.

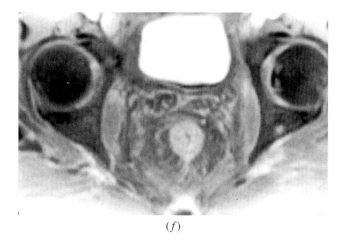

(f)

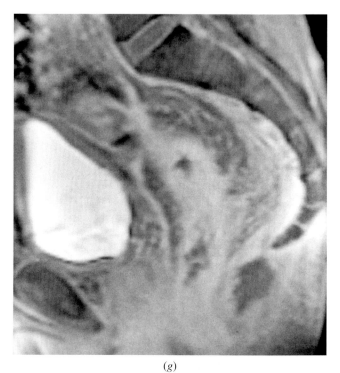

FIG. 6.152 (Continued)   (g)

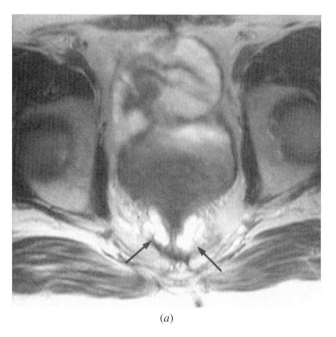

(a)

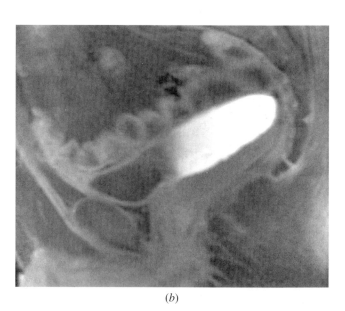

(b)

FIG. 6.153 Abdominoperineal resection (APR). Axial T2-weighted ETSE (a) and sagittal interstitial-phase gadolinium-enhanced fat-suppressed SGE (b) images. The bladder and the seminal vesicles (arrows, a) are located posteriorly in the pelvis.

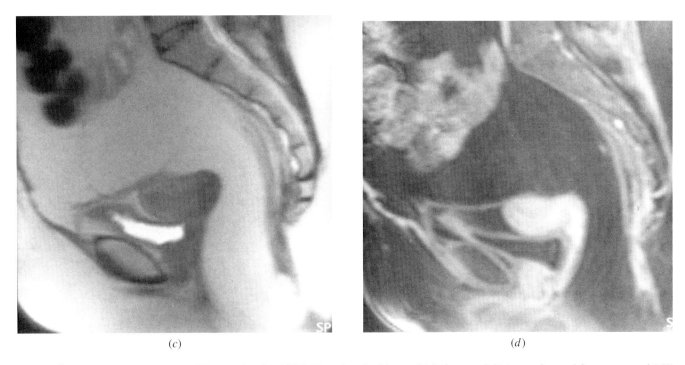

(c)   (d)

FIG. 6.153 (*Continued*) Sagittal T2-weighted SS-ETSE (*c*) and sagittal interstitial-phase gadolinium-enhanced fat-suppressed SGE (*d*) images in a second patient show increase of pelvic fat consistent with omental packing.

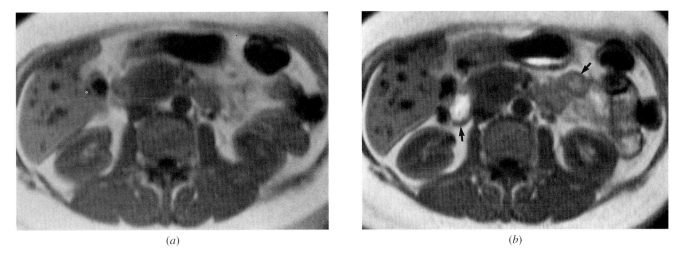

(a)   (b)

FIG. 6.154 Positive oral contrast agent. SGE images before (*a*) and after (*b*) ingestion of ferric ammonium citrate (FAC). Oral contrast causes high signal intensity within the bowel (arrows, *b*). The bowel loops are readily distinguished from the adjacent pancreas after oral contrast administration. Note that FAC not only results in signal intensity change of the bowel lumen but distends it as well.

Positive Intraluminal Contrast Agents

Manganese-containing agents, ferric ammonium citrate, and gadolinium-containing agents have been employed as positive intraluminal agents (fig. 6.154). They are all paramagnetic [127–129]. To date, none of these agents is in routine use. Positive intraluminal agents may be useful to distinguish bowel (which would be rendered as high signal) from encapsulated fluid collections such as abscesses (which would remain low signal). Opacification of fistulous tract could also be demonstrated with these agents. On the other hand, positive intraluminal agents may mask the enhancement of inflammatory bowel wall or bowel masses.

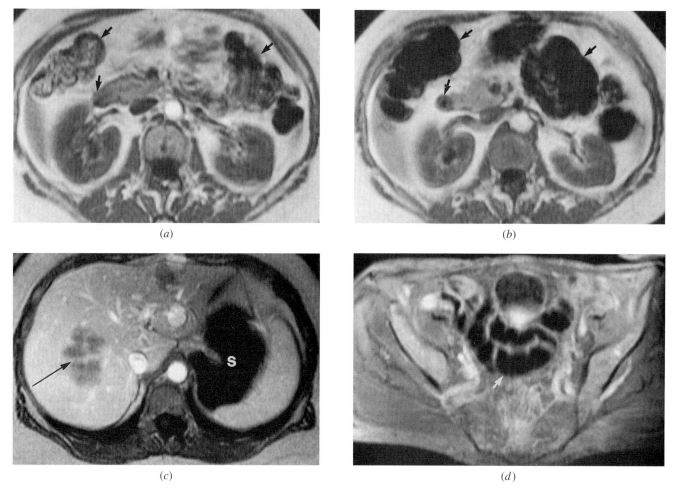

F I G . 6.155 Negative oral contrast agent. SGE images before (*a*) and after (*b*) perfluorooctylbromide (PFOB) ingestion, intravenous gadolinium-enhanced SGE image after PFOB ingestion (*c*), and gadolinium-enhanced T1-weighted fat-suppressed spin-echo image after PFOB ingestion (*d*) in three patients. In the first patient (*a*, *b*), bowel contents are heterogeneous before PFOB intake (arrows, *a*), but after ingestion of PFOB they become nearly signal void (arrows, *b*). PFOB is signal void in the stomach (s, *c*) of a woman with hepatic metastases (arrow, *c*) from cervical carcinoma. In a third patient (*d*), distal small bowel is signal void (arrow, *d*) after PFOB administration. Oral agents distend the bowel, which may aid detection of mucosal abnormalities.

Negative Intraluminal Contrast Agents

Intraluminal contrast agents may result in darkening of the bowel lumen because of lack of mobile protons (perfluorooctylbromide) (fig. 6.155) [130] or superparamagnetic susceptibility effects (oral magnetic particles) (fig. 6.156) [131]. Because of high cost, perfluorooctylbromide is not available at present. A drawback of oral magnetic particles is occasional disturbing susceptibility artifact on T1-weighted SGE images, particularly in the region of the pancreas. Dilute barium results in a high fluid content of bowel and therefore low signal intensity on T1-weighted images and has achieved routine clinical use by some investigators [126]. Water functions well as a low-signal agent on T1-weighted images in the stomach (by oral administration) and colon (by rectal administration) (figs. 6.111–6.113) and has been proposed for screening examinations [90].

FUTURE DIRECTIONS

Future directions include the use of oral contrast agents described above, new intravenous agents, and new imaging techniques. Regarding intravenous agents, iron oxide particle agents have been used for MR lymphography in pilot studies [132]. These agents are taken up by normal lymphoid tissue and hyperplastic lymph nodes, which decrease uniformly in signal intensity on T2-weighted images, whereas nodes involved with malignant disease retain signal intensity. This agent may increase the specificity of detecting malignancy involvement in normal-sized (<1 cm) lymph nodes. Normal-sized malignant lymph nodes are a common occurrence with gastrointestinal malignancies; therefore, improved specificity is of particular value for these tumors. Future imaging directions include real-time,

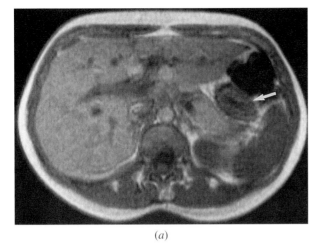

(a)

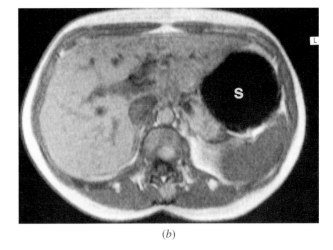

(b)

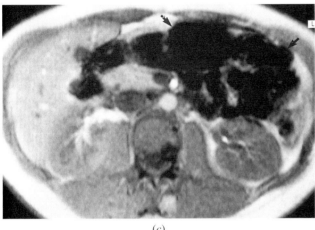

(c)

FIG. 6.156 Negative oral contrast agent. SGE before (*a*) and after (*b*, *c*) oral magnetic particle (OMP) ingestion. Before OMP ingestion, the stomach is collapsed, with apparent wall thickening. Once distended with oral contrast, the stomach wall is barely perceptible. Similarly, the small and large bowel are distended and marked by OMP (arrows, *c*). Susceptibility artifact is visualized in many of the loops of bowel (*c*).

dynamic alimentary track imaging (MRI upper GI), 3D intraluminal display (MRI endoscopy, colonography), and therapeutic interventions (e.g., abscess drainage).

REFERENCES

1. Semelka RC, Shoenut JP, Silverman R et al. Bowel disease: prospective comparison of CT and 1.5-T pre- and postcontrast MR imaging with T1-weighted fat-suppressed and breath-hold FLASH sequences. *J Magn Reson Imaging* 1(6): 625–632, 1991.

2. Shoenut JP, Semelka RC, Silverman R et al. Magnetic resonance imaging in inflammatory bowel disease. *J Clin Gastroenterol* 17(1): 73–78, 1993.

3. Shoenut JP, Semelka RC, Magro CM et al. Comparison of magnetic resonance imaging and endoscopy in distinguishing the type and severity of inflammatory bowel disease. *J Clin Gastroenterol* 19(1): 31–35, 1994.

4. Kettritz U, Isaacs K, Warshauer DM et al. Crohn's disease. Pilot study comparing MRI of the abdomen with clinical evaluation. *J Clin Gastroenterol* 21(3): 249–253, 1995.

5. Shoenut JP, Semelka RC, Silverman R et al. Magnetic resonance imaging evaluation of the local extent of colorectal mass lesions. *J Clin Gastroenterol* 17(3): 248–253, 1993.

6. Shoenut JP, Semelka RC, Silverman R et al. The gastrointestinal tract. In: Semelka RC, Shoenut JP, editors. *MRI of the Abdomen with CT Correlation.* New York: Raven Press; 1993. p. 119–143.

7. Outwater E, Schiebler ML. Pelvic fistulas: findings on MR images. *AJR Am J Roentgenol* 160(2): 327–330, 1993.

8. Semelka RC, Hricak H, Kim B et al. Pelvic fistulas: appearances on MR images. *Abdom Imaging* 22(1): 91–95, 1997.

9. Chan TW, Kressel HY, Milestone B et al. Rectal carcinoma: staging at MR imaging with endorectal surface coil. Work in progress. *Radiology* 181(2): 461–467, 1991.

10. Schnall MD, Furth EE, Rosato EF et al. Rectal tumor stage: correlation of endorectal MR imaging and pathologic findings. *Radiology* 190(3): 709–714, 1994.

11. de Lange EE, Fechner RE, Wanebo HJ. Suspected recurrent rectosigmoid carcinoma after abdominoperineal resection: MR imaging and histopathologic findings. *Radiology* 170(2): 323–328, 1989.

12. Balzarini L, Ceglia E, D'Ippolito G et al. Local recurrence of rectosigmoid cancer: what about the choice of MRI for diagnosis? *Gastrointest Radiol* 15(4): 338–342, 1990.

13. Gomberg JS, Friedman AC, Radecki PD et al. MRI differentiation of recurrent colorectal carcinoma from postoperative fibrosis. *Gastrointest Radiol* 11(4): 361–363, 1986.

14. Krestin GP, Steinbrich W, Friedmann G. [Diagnosis of recurrent rectal cancer: Comparison of CT and MR]. *Rofo* 148(1): 28–33, 1988.

15. Pema PJ, Bennett WF, Bova JG et al. CT vs MRI in diagnosis of recurrent rectosigmoid carcinoma. *J Comput Assist Tomogr* 18(2): 256–261, 1994.

16. Waizer A, Powsner E, Russo I et al. Prospective comparative study of magnetic resonance imaging versus transrectal ultrasound for preoperative staging and follow-up of rectal cancer. Preliminary report. *Dis Colon Rectum* 34(12): 1068–1072, 1991.

17. Martin DR, Danrad R, Herrmann K et al. Magnetic resonance imaging of the gastrointestinal tract. *Top Magn Reson Imaging* 16(1): 77–98, 2005.

18. Macpherson RI. Gastrointestinal tract duplications: clinical, pathologic, etiologic, and radiologic considerations. *Radiographics* 13(5): 1063–1080, 1993.

19. Rafal RB, Markisz JA. Magnetic resonance imaging of an esophageal duplication cyst. *Am J Gastroenterol* 86(12): 1809–1811, 1991.

20. Mutrie CJ, Donahue DM, Wain JC et al. Esophageal leiomyoma: a 40-year experience. *Ann Thorac Surg* 79(4): 1122–1125, 2005.

21. Taylor FH, Christenson W, Zollinger RW 2nd et al. Multiple leiomyomas of the esophagus. *Ann Thorac Surg* 60(1): 182–183, 1995.

22. Blot WJ, Devesa SS, Fraumeni JF Jr. Continuing climb in rates of esophageal adenocarcinoma: an update. *JAMA* 270(11): 1320, 1993.

23. Bujanda L. The effects of alcohol consumption upon the gastrointestinal tract. *Am J Gastroenterol* 95(12): 3374–3382, 2000.

24. Maram ES, Kurland LT, Ludwig J et al. Esophageal carcinoma in Olmsted County, Minnesota, 1935–1971. *Mayo Clin Proc* 52(1): 24–27, 1977.

25. Adler DG, Romero Y. Primary esophageal motility disorders. *Mayo Clin Proc* 76(2): 195–200, 2001.

26. Takashima S, Takeuchi N, Shiozaki H et al. Carcinoma of the esophagus: CT vs MR imaging in determining resectability. *AJR Am J Roentgenol* 156(2): 297–302, 1991.

27. Trenkner SW, Halvorsen RA Jr., Thompson WM. Neoplasms of the upper gastrointestinal tract. *Radiol Clin North Am* 32(1): 15–24, 1994.

28. Halvorsen RA Jr., Thompson WM. Primary neoplasms of the hollow organs of the gastrointestinal tract. Staging and follow-up. *Cancer* 67(4 Suppl): 1181–1188, 1991.

29. Marcos HB, Semelka RC. Stomach diseases: MR evaluation using combined T2-weighted single-shot echo train spin-echo and gadolinium-enhanced spoiled gradient-echo sequences. *J Magn Reson Imaging* 10(6): 950–960, 1999.

30. Hamed MM, Hamm B, Ibrahim ME et al. Dynamic MR imaging of the abdomen with gadopentetate dimeglumine: normal enhancement patterns of the liver, spleen, stomach, and pancreas. *AJR Am J Roentgenol* 158(2): 303–307, 1992.

31. Scholz FJ, Vincent ME. The stomach. In: Putnam CE, Ravin CE (eds.), *Textbook of Diagnostic Imaging*. Philadelphia: Saunders, 1988. p. 778–807.

32. Hsia CY, Wu CW, Lui WY. Heterotopic pancreas: a difficult diagnosis. *J Clin Gastroenterol* 28(2): 144–147, 1999.

33. Ciftci AO, Tanyel FC, Hicsonmez A. Gastric diverticulum: an uncommon cause of abdominal pain in a 12 year old. *J Pediatr Surg* 33(3): 529–531, 1998.

34. Velanovich V. Gastric diverticulum. Endoscopic and radiologic appearance. *Surg Endosc* 8(11): 1338–1339, 1994.

35. Nakamura T, Nakano G. Histopathological classification and malignant change in gastric polyps. *J Clin Pathol* 38(7): 754–764, 1985.

36. Eisenberg RL. Single filling defects in the colon. In: Eisenberg RL, editor. *Gastrointestinal Radiology*. Philadelphia: Lippincott; 1983. p. 681–710.

37. Fenoglio-Preiser CM, Noffsinger AE, Stemmermann GN et al. Gastrointestinal Pathology. *Gastrointestinal Pathology*. Philadelphia: Lippincott; 1999, p. 232.

38. Ming SC, Goldman H. *Pathology of the Gastrointestinal Tract*. Philadelphia: Lippincott, 1998.

39. Wingo PA, Tong T, Bolden S. Cancer statistics, 1995. *CA Cancer J Clin* 45(1): 8–30, 1995.

40. Lambert R, Guilloux A, Oshima A et al. Incidence and mortality from stomach cancer in Japan, Slovenia and the USA. *Int J Cancer* 97(6): 811–818, 2002.

41. Parkin DM. International variation. *Oncogene* 23(38): 6329–6340, 2004.

42. Auh YH, Lim TH, Lee DH et al. In vitro MR imaging of the resected stomach with a 4.7-T superconducting magnet. *Radiology* 191(1): 129–134, 1994.

43. Semelka RC, Shoenut JP, Kroeker MA et al. Focal liver disease: comparison of dynamic contrast-enhanced CT and T2-weighted fat-suppressed, FLASH, and dynamic gadolinium-enhanced MR imaging at 1.5 T. *Radiology* 184(3): 687–694, 1992.

44. Hasegawa S, Semelka RC, Noone TC et al. Gastric stromal sarcomas: correlation of MR imaging and histopathologic findings in nine patients. *Radiology* 208(3): 591–595, 1998.

45. Chadrasoma P. *Gastrointestinal Pathology*. Stamford: Appleton & Lange, 1999, p. 371.

46. Jeffrey RB Jr. Abdominal imaging in the immunocompromised patient. *Radiol Clin North Am* 30(3): 579–596, 1992.

47. Liang R, Todd D, Chan TK et al. Prognostic factors for primary gastrointestinal lymphoma. *Hematol Oncol* 13(3): 153–163, 1995.

48. Chou CK, Chen LT, Sheu RS et al. MRI manifestations of gastrointestinal lymphoma. *Abdom Imaging* 19(6): 495–500, 1994.

49. Chou CK, Chen LT, Sheu RS et al. MRI manifestations of gastrointestinal wall thickening. *Abdom Imaging* 19(5): 389–394, 1994.

50. Modlin IM, Lye KD, Kidd M. Carcinoid tumors of the stomach. *Surg Oncol* 12(2): 153–172, 2003.

51. Chadrasoma P. *Gastrointestinal Pathology*. Stamford: Appleton & Lange, 1999, p. 110.

52. Ming SC, Goldman H. *Pathology of the Gastrointestinal tract*. Philadelphia: Lippincott, 1998, p. 563.

53. Yamada T, Alpers DH. *Textbook of Gastroenterology*. Philadelphia: Lippincott, 1991, p. 1302–1305.

54. Ming SC, Goldman H. *Pathology of the Gastrointestinal tract*. Philadelphia: Lippincott, 1998, p. 583.

55. Lee JK, Marcos HB, Semelka RC. MR imaging of the small bowel using the HASTE sequence. *AJR Am J Roentgenol* 170(6): 1457–1463, 1998.

56. Torres AM, Ziegler MM. Malrotation of the intestine. *World J Surg* 17(3): 326–331, 1993.

57. Marcos HB, Semelka RC, Noone TC et al. MRI of normal and abnormal duodenum using half-Fourier single-shot RARE and gadolinium-enhanced spoiled gradient echo sequences. *Magn Reson Imaging* 17(6): 869–880, 1999.

58. Levy AD, Hobbs CM. From the archives of the AFIP. Meckel diverticulum: radiologic features with pathologic correlation. *Radiographics* 24(2): 565–587, 2004.

59. Chew FS, Zambuto DA. Meckel's diverticulum. *AJR Am J Roentgenol* 159(5): 982, 1992.

60. Gill SS, Heuman DM, Mihas AA. Small intestinal neoplasms. *J Clin Gastroenterol* 33(4): 267–282, 2001.

61. Perzin KH, Bridge MF. Adenomas of the small intestine: a clinicopathologic review of 51 cases and a study of their relationship to carcinoma. *Cancer* 48(3): 799–819, 1981.

62. Chappuis CW, Divincenti FC, Cohn I, Jr. Villous tumors of the duodenum. *Ann Surg* 209(5): 593–598; discussion 598–599, 1989.

63. Shekitka KM, Sobin LH. Ganglioneuromas of the gastrointestinal tract. Relation to Von Recklinghausen disease and other multiple tumor syndromes. *Am J Surg Pathol* 18(3): 250–257, 1994.

64. Losty P, Hu C, Quinn F et al. Gastrointestinal manifestations of neurofibromatosis in childhood. *Eur J Pediatr Surg* 3(1): 57–58, 1993.

65. Semelka RC, Marcos HB. Polyposis syndromes of the gastrointestinal tract: MR findings. *J Magn Reson Imaging* 11(1): 51–55, 2000.

66. Teplick SK. The duodenum. In: Putnam CE, Ravin CE, editors. *Textbook of Diagnostic Imaging.* Philadelphia: Saunders, 1988, p. 808.

67. Semelka RC, John G, Kelekis NL et al. Small bowel neoplastic disease: demonstration by MRI. *J Magn Reson Imaging* 6(6): 855–860, 1996.

68. Al-Mondhiry H. Primary lymphomas of the small intestine: east-west contrast. *Am J Hematol* 22(1): 89–105, 1986.

69. Rubesin SE, Gilchrist AM, Bronner M et al. Non-Hodgkin lymphoma of the small intestine. *Radiographics* 10(6): 985–998, 1990.

70. Bader TR, Semelka RC, Chiu VC et al. MRI of carcinoid tumors: spectrum of appearances in the gastrointestinal tract and liver. *J Magn Reson Imaging* 14(3): 261–269, 2001.

71. Semelka RC, Lawrence PH, Shoenut JP et al. Primary ovarian cancer: prospective comparison of contrast-enhanced CT and pre-and postcontrast, fat-suppressed MR imaging, with histologic correlation. *J Magn Reson Imaging* 3(1): 99–106, 1993.

72. Low RN, Barone RM, Lacey C et al. Peritoneal tumor: MR imaging with dilute oral barium and intravenous gadolinium-containing contrast agents compared with unenhanced MR imaging and CT. *Radiology* 204(2): 513–520, 1997.

73. Brahme F, Lindstrom C, Wenckert A. Crohn's disease in a defined population. An epidemiological study of incidence, prevalence, mortality, and secular trends in the city of Malmo, Sweden. *Gastroenterology* 69(2): 342–351, 1975.

74. Goldberg HI, Caruthers SB Jr., Nelson JA et al. Radiographic findings of the National Cooperative Crohn's Disease Study. *Gastroenterology* 77(4 Pt 2): 925–937, 1979.

75. Marcos HB, Semelka RC. Evaluation of Crohn's disease using half-Fourier RARE and gadolinium-enhanced SGE sequences: initial results. *Magn Reson Imaging* 18(3): 263–268, 2000.

76. Tomei E, Semelka RC, Braga L et al. Adult celiac disease: what is the role of MRI? *J Magn Reson Imaging* 24(3): 625–629, 2006.

77. Feeny PC, Stevenson GW. *Margulis.* 5th ed. St Louis: Mosby, 1994, pp. 678–679.

78. Deutsch AA, McLeod RS, Cullen J et al. Results of the pelvic-pouch procedure in patients with Crohn's disease. *Dis Colon Rectum* 34(6): 475–477, 1991.

79. Gutmann LT. *Yersinia enterocolitica* and *Yersinia pseudotuberculosis.* In: Gorbach SI, editor. *Infectious Diarrheia.* Boston: Blackwell Scientific, 1986, p. 65.

80. Lambert ME, Schofield PF, Ironside AG et al. Campylobacter colitis. *Br Med J* 1(6167): 857–859, 1979.

81. Leonardou P, Kierans AS, Elazazzi M, et al. MR imaging findings of small bowel hemorrhage: two cases of mural involvement and one of perimural. *J Magn Reson Imaging* 29(5):1185–1189, 2009.

82. Guingrich JA, Kuhlman JE. Colonic wall thickening in patients with cirrhosis: CT findings and clinical implications. *AJR Am J Roentgenol* 172(4): 919–924, 1999.

83. Warshauer DM, Lee JK. Adult intussusception detected at CT or MR imaging: clinical-imaging correlation. *Radiology* 212(3): 853–860, 1999.

84. Ajaj W, Goehde SC, Schneemann H et al. Dose optimization of mannitol solution for small bowel distension in MRI. *J Magn Reson Imaging* 20(4): 648–653, 2004.

85. Prassopoulos P, Papanikolaou N, Grammatikakis J et al. MR enteroclysis imaging of Crohn disease. *Radiographics* 21 Spec No: S161–172, 2001.

86. Laghi A, Carbone I, Catalano C et al. Polyethylene glycol solution as an oral contrast agent for MR imaging of the small bowel. *AJR Am J Roentgenol* 177(6): 1333–1334, 2001.

87. Hussain SM, Stoker J, Lameris JS. Anal sphincter complex: endoanal MR imaging of normal anatomy. *Radiology* 197(3): 671–677, 1995.

88. Hussain SM, Stoker J, Zwamborn AW et al. Endoanal MRI of the anal sphincter complex: correlation with cross-sectional anatomy and histology. *J Anat* 189 (Pt 3): 677–682, 1996.

89. Okizuka H, Sugimura K, Ishida T. Preoperative local staging of rectal carcinoma with MR imaging and a rectal balloon. *J Magn Reson Imaging* 3(2): 329–335, 1993.

90. Ajaj W, Pelster G, Treichel U et al. Dark lumen magnetic resonance colonography: comparison with conventional colonoscopy for the detection of colorectal pathology. *Gut* 52(12): 1738–1743, 2003.

91. Ajaj W, Lauenstein TC, Pelster G et al. MR colonography: how does air compare to water for colonic distention? *J Magn Reson Imaging* 19(2): 216–221, 2004.

92. Martin DR, Yang M, Thomasson D et al. MR colonography: development of optimized method with ex vivo and in vivo systems. *Radiology* 225(2): 597–602, 2002.

93. Sato Y, Pringle KC, Bergman RA et al. Congenital anorectal anomalies: MR imaging. *Radiology* 168(1): 157–162, 1988.

94. Chadrasoma P. *Gastrointestinal Pathology.* Stamford: Appleton & Lange, 1999, p.319.

95. Chadrasoma P. *Gastrointestinal Pathology.* Stamford: Appleton & Lange, 1999, p. 333.

96. Eisenberg RL. Multiple filling defects in the colon. In: Eisenberg RL, (ed). *Gastrointestinal Radiology.* Philadelphia: Lippincott, 1983. p. 711–739.

97. Younathan CM, Ros PR, Burton SS. MR imaging of colonic lipoma. *J Comput Assist Tomogr* 15(3): 492–494, 1991.

98. Bernstein WC. What are hemorrhoids and what is their relationship to the portal venous system? *Dis Colon Rectum* 26(12): 829–834, 1983.

99. Kee F, Wilson RH, Gilliland R et al. Changing site distribution of colorectal cancer. *Bmj* 305(6846): 158, 1992.

100. Shihab OC, Moran BJ, Heald RJ et al. MRI staging of low rectal cancer. *Eur Radiol* 19(3): 643–650, 2009.

101. Brown G, Radcliffe AG, Newcombe RG et al. Preoperative assessment of prognostic factors in rectal cancer using high-resolution magnetic resonance imaging. *Br J Surg* 90(3): 355–364, 2003.

102. Videhult P, Smedh K, Lundin P et al. Magnetic resonance imaging for preoperative staging of rectal cancer in clinical practice: high accuracy in predicting circumferential margin with clinical benefit. *Colorectal Dis* 9(5): 412–419, 2007.

103. MERCURY Study Group. Diagnostic accuracy of preoperative magnetic resonance imaging in predicting curative resection of rectal cancer: prospective observational study. *BMJ* 333(7572): 779, 2006.

104. de Lange EE, Fechner RE, Edge SB et al. Preoperative staging of rectal carcinoma with MR imaging: surgical and histopathologic correlation. *Radiology* 176(3): 623–628, 1990.

105. Ito K, Kato T, Tadokoro M et al. Recurrent rectal cancer and scar: differentiation with PET and MR imaging. *Radiology* 182(2): 549–552, 1992.

106. Sugimura K, Carrington BM, Quivey JM et al. Postirradiation changes in the pelvis: assessment with MR imaging. *Radiology* 175(3): 805–813, 1990.

107. Bartolo D, Goepel JR, Parsons MA. Rectal malignant lymphoma in chronic ulcerative colitis. *Gut* 23(2): 164–168, 1982.

108. Dragosics B, Bauer P, Radaszkiewicz T. Primary gastrointestinal non-Hodgkin"s lymphomas. A retrospective clinicopathologic study of 150 cases. *Cancer* 55(5): 1060–1073, 1985.

109. Jetmore AB, Ray JE, Gathright JB, Jr. et al. Rectal carcinoids: the most frequent carcinoid tumor. *Dis Colon Rectum* 35(8): 717–725, 1992.

110. Pack GT, Oropeza R. A comparative study of melanoma and epidermoid carcinoma of the anal canal: a review of 20

melanomas and 29 epidermoid carcinomas (1930 to 1965). *Dis Colon Rectum* 10(3): 161–176, 1967.

111. Fenoglio-Preiser CM, Noffsinger AE, Stemmermann GN et al. *Gastrointestinal Pathology.* Philadelphia: Lippincott, 1999, p. 1050.

112. Acheson ED. The distribution of ulcerative colitis and regional enteritis in United States veterans with particular reference to the Jewish religion. *Gut* 1: 291–293, 1960.

113. Hulnick DH, Megibow AJ, Balthazar EJ et al. Computed tomography in the evaluation of diverticulitis. *Radiology* 152(2): 491–495, 1984.

114. Cho KC, Morehouse HT, Alterman DD et al. Sigmoid diverticulitis: diagnostic role of CT—comparison with barium enema studies. *Radiology* 176(1): 111–115, 1990.

115. Chung JJ, Semelka RC, Martin DR et al. Colon diseases: MR evaluation using combined T2-weighted single-shot echo train spin-echo and gadolinium-enhanced spoiled gradient-echo sequences. *J Magn Reson Imaging* 12(2): 297–305, 2000.

116. Balthazar EJ, Megibow AJ, Siegel SE et al. Appendicitis: prospective evaluation with high-resolution CT. *Radiology* 180(1): 21–24, 1991.

117. Keyzer C, Zalcman M, De Maertelaer V et al. Comparison of US and unenhanced multi-detector row CT in patients suspected of having acute appendicitis. *Radiology* 236(2): 527–534, 2005.

118. Birchard KR, Brown MA, Hyslop WB et al. MRI of acute abdominal and pelvic pain in pregnant patients. *AJR Am J Roentgenol* 184(2): 452–458, 2005.

119. Noone TC, Semelka RC, Worawattanakul S et al. Intraperitoneal abscesses: diagnostic accuracy of and appearances at MR imaging. *Radiology* 208(2): 525–528, 1998.

120. Semelka RC, John G, Kelekis NL et al. Bowel-related abscesses: MR demonstration preliminary results. *Magn Reson Imaging* 16(8): 855–861, 1998.

121. Lunniss PJ, Armstrong P, Barker PG et al. Magnetic resonance imaging of anal fistulae. *Lancet* 340(8816): 394–396, 1992.

122. Barker PG, Lunniss PJ, Armstrong P et al. Magnetic resonance imaging of fistula-in-ano: technique, interpretation and accuracy. *Clin Radiol* 49(1): 7–13, 1994.

123. Myhr GE, Myrvold HE, Nilsen G et al. Perianal fistulas: use of MR imaging for diagnosis. *Radiology* 191(2): 545–549, 1994.

124. Larson HE, Price AB, Honour P et al. Clostridium difficile and the aetiology of pseudomembranous colitis. *Lancet* 1(8073): 1063–1066, 1978.

125. Fenoglio-Preiser CM, Noffsinger AE, Stemmermann GN et al. *Gastrointestinal Pathology.* Philadelphia: Lippincott; 1999. p. 819.

126. Pels Rijcken TH, Davis MA, Ros PR. Intraluminal contrast agents for MR imaging of the abdomen and pelvis. *J Magn Reson Imaging* 4(3): 291–300, 1994.

127. Bernardino ME, Weinreb JC, Mitchell DG et al. Safety and optimum concentration of a manganese chloride-based oral MR contrast agent. *J Magn Reson Imaging* 4(6): 872–876, 1994.

128. Wesbey GE, Brasch RC, Goldberg HI et al. Dilute oral iron solutions as gastrointestinal contrast agents for magnetic resonance imaging; initial clinical experience. *Magn Reson Imaging* 3(1): 57–64, 1985.

129. Kaminsky S, Laniado M, Gogoll M et al. Gadopentetate dimeglumine as a bowel contrast agent: safety and efficacy. *Radiology* 178(2): 503–508, 1991.

130. Brown JJ, Duncan JR, Heiken JP et al. Perfluoroctylbromide as a gastrointestinal contrast agent for MR imaging: use with and without glucagon. *Radiology* 181(2): 455–460, 1991.

131. Rubin DL, Muller HH, Sidhu MK et al. Liquid oral magnetic particles as a gastrointestinal contrast agent for MR imaging: efficacy in vivo. *J Magn Reson Imaging* 3(1): 113–118, 1993.

132. Hovels AM, Heesakkers RA, Adang EM et al. Cost-analysis of staging methods for lymph nodes in patients with prostate cancer: MRI with a lymph node-specific contrast agent compared to pelvic lymph node dissection or CT. *Eur Radiol* 14(9): 1707–1712, 2004.

INDEX

For each index term, the volume number(s) for the page entries is given (*V1*, *V2*).

Pseudotumor:
hepatic inflammatory disease, *V1*: 415, 418–422
retroperitoneal inflammatory, *V2*: 1247
testes, scrotum and epididymis, *V2*: 1388, 1390
Psoas muscle:
abscess, *V2*: 1273–1274, 1276–1279
MR imaging, *V2*: 1271, 1273–1280
neurogenic tumor, *V2*: 1271, 1273
Pulmonary emboli, magnetic resonance angiography, *V2*: 1673, 1675–1677
Pulmonary hyperplasia, fetal assessment, *V2*: 1605
Pulmonary infiltrates, *V2*: 1666, 1668–1671
Pulmonary nodules, MR imaging, *V2*: 1654, 1657, 1662–1665
"Pure gonadal dysgenesis," *V2*: 1415
Pyelonephritis:
acute, *V2*: 1142, 1147–1149
renal transplants, *V2*: 1177, 1179–1180
chronic, *V2*: 1126, 1128, 1130
in pregnancy, maternal imaging, *V2*: 1564, 1566
xanthogranulomatous, *V2*: 1152
Pyeloureteral anastomosis, renal transplants, *V2*: 1184
Pyogenic abscesses, hepatic, *V1*: 418, 422–432
Pyonephrosis, *V2*: 1155–1156
Pyosalpinx. *See* Tubo-ovarian abscess (TOA)

Radial scarring, breast lesions, *V2*: 1714–1715, 1717
Radiation therapy:
bladder changes, *V2*: 1331, 1337
breast cancer, post-therapy imaging, *V2*: 1744, 1747
breast carcinoma from, *V2*: 1743
cervical cancer metastases:
bladder fistulae, *V2*: 1486, 1489
recurrence and posttreatment change, *V2*: 1493–1495
Crohn disease, *V1*: 791
esophagitis, *V1*: 730–731
gastric ulceration and gastritis, *V1*: 761, 763
hepatitis, *V1*: 321, 331
large intestine:
enteritis, *V1*: 888, 892
proctitis, *V1*: 888, 893–894
liver metastases following, *V1*: 257, 262–264
pancreatic cancer and, *V1*: 589–590
peritoneal metastases, differential diagnosis, *V2*: 923–924
prostate cancer, *V2*: 1368–1373
rectosigmoid colon adenocarcinoma, *V1*: 852, 858, 861–865
small intestine, metastases *vs.*, *V1*: 815–816, 818
vaginal effects, *V2*: 1421, 1428

Radiofrequency ablation:
hepatocellular carcinoma, *V1*: 278, 280–286
liver metastases, *V1*: 278–280
renal cell carcinoma, *V2*: 1088–1089, 1095–1096
Radiofrequency power deposition, 3T MR imaging, *V1*: 31
Radiological Diagnostic Oncology Group (RDOG), ovarian cancer, epithelial tumors, *V2*: 1533
Rapid acquisition with relaxation enhancement (RARE) sequences, *V1*: 6
magnetic resonance cholangiopancreatography, *V1*: 456, 460
Rapidly involuting congenital hemangioma (RICH), fetal assessment, *V2*: 1604, 1607
Real-time ("on-the-fly") bolus-tracking method, liver imaging protocol, *V1*: 20
Receiver coil, pediatric MRI, *V2*: 1644–1645
Recipient assessment, hepatic transplantation protocol, *V1*: 287, 291–292
Reconstructive surgery:
bladder, *V2*: 1331, 1335–1336
imperforate anus, *V1*: 827, 834
Rectal cancer:
adenocarcinoma, *V1*: 843, 848–850, 852, 855–857
bone metastases, *V1*: 858, 861–863
bone metastases and sacral invasion, *V1*: 852, 861–863
endorectal coil imaging, *V1*: 850, 857
recurrent, *V1*: 850, 857–866
bladder metastases from, *V2*: 1320, 1323–1324
carcinoid tumors, *V1*: 867–868
MR imaging techniques, *V1*: 843, 848, 850, 852–865
penis and urethra metastases, *V2*: 1376–1377
vaginal metastases, *V2*: 1426–1427
Rectoceles, female urethra, *V2*: 1408–1410
Rectosigmoid colon:
adenocarcinoma, *V1*: 843, 848
fibrosis and, *V1*: 852, 861–863
recurrence rates, *V1*: 850, 857–860
bladder metastases from, *V2*: 1320, 1323–1324
lymphoma, *V1*: 860, 867
Rectourethral fistulas, *V2*: 1408
Rectovaginal fistula, *V2*: 1421, 1426, 1429–1430
Rectum:
anorectal anomalies, *V1*: 827, 831, 833–834
cloacal repair, *V1*: 827, 833
metastases to:
cervical cancer, *V2*: 1492–1495
gastrointestinal stromal tumors, *V1*: 860, 866
vaginal carcinoma, *V2*: 1416, 1423

MR imaging techniques, *V1*: 824, 827
normal anatomy, *V1*: 824, 827, 831
perforation and abscess, *V1*: 874, 886
postsurgical infection, *V1*: 892, 894–895
varices, *V1*: 838
Recurrent malignant disease imaging, echo-train spin-echo sequences, *V1*: 6–7
Recurrent pyogenic cholangitis, MR imaging, *V1*: 502, 507
Redundant sequences, MR imaging strategies and, *V1*: 16–24
Reflux nephropathy, *V2*: 1126, 1128, 1130
Regenerative nodules (RNs), cirrhosis, *V1*: 333–334, 339–345
iron-containing, *V1*: 334, 340, 344–346
Reidel lobe, MR imaging, *V1*: 58–60
Relaxation times, 3T MR imaging, *V1*: 32–36
Reliability issues, parallel MR imaging, *V1*: 29, 31
Remote table motion, MR imaging strategies, *V1*: 20
Renal adenomas, *V2*: 1068
Renal agenesis, fetal assessment, *V2*: 1613
Renal arterial disease, *V2*: 1128–1129, 1131–1133
abdominal aortic aneurysm, *V2*: 1201–1207
renal transplants, *V2*: 1177, 1182–1183
Renal blood flow evaluation, *V2*: 1173
Renal calculi, *V2*: 1159, 1166–1167
Renal cell carcinoma (RCC):
adrenal gland metastases, *V2*: 998–1002
autosomal dominant polycystic kidney disease and, *V2*: 1098, 1101
bilateral cancer, *V2*: 1088, 1093
chronic renal failure, *V2*: 1098–1101
cystic changes with, *V2*: 1088, 1090–1092
cystic disease, differential diagnosis, *V2*: 1052, 1061–1062
granulocytic sarcoma (chloroma), differential diagnosis, *V2*: 1109, 1111
hemorrhage, *V2*: 1088–1094
chronic renal failure, *V2*: 1098–1101
hypervascular tumors, *V2*: 1084, 1086
imaging protocol for, *V1*: 16, 19–20
infiltrative, *V2*: 1088, 1095
metastases, pancreas, *V1*: 619, 625
MR imaging, *V2*: 1098, 1102
radiofrequency ablation, *V2*: 1088–1089, 1095–1096
recurrence, *V2*: 1089, 1096–1097
renal cysts, differential diagnosis, *V2*: 1053, 1098
renal transplants, *V2*: 1177, 1181, 1184
staging, *V2*: 1073–1095
stage 1, *V2*: 1073–1077
stage 2, *V2*: 1076, 1078, 1087–1089
stage 3a, *V2*: 1076–1077, 1079–1081
stage 3b, *V2*: 1077, 1081
stage 3c, *V2*: 1082–1083
stage 4, *V2*: 1082, 1084–1085
subtraction image, *V2*: 1037, 1040
von Hippel-Lindau syndrome, *V1*: 549–550